Endodontics

Endodontics

SECOND EDITION

John Ide Ingle, D.D.S., M.S.D.

Senior Professional Associate, Institute of Medicine
National Academy of Sciences
Washington, D.C.
Formerly Dean and Professor of Endodontics and Periodontics
University of Southern California School of Dentistry
Los Angeles, California
Formerly Chairman and Professor of Endodontics and Periodontics
University of Washington School of Dentistry
Seattle, Washington

Edward Edgerton Beveridge, D.D.S., M.S.D.

Late Associate Dean and Professor of Endodontics
University of Southern California School of Dentistry
Los Angeles, California

Plates by Virginia E. Brooks, B.A.

23 Contributors

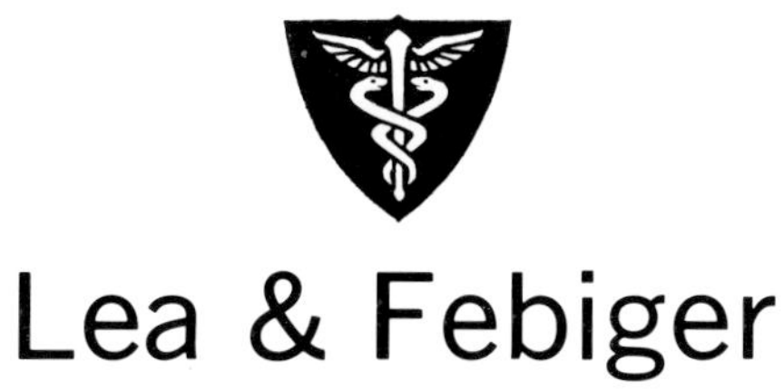

Lea & Febiger

Philadelphia

Library of Congress Cataloging in Publication Data

Ingle, John Ide.
Endodontics.

Includes bibliographies and indexes.
1. Endodontics. I. Beveridge, Edward Edgerton, 1931–1972.
RK351.I5 1976 617.6'34 76–25018
ISBN 0–8121–0542–7

Published in Great Britain by Henry Kimpton Publishers, London

PRINTED IN THE UNITED STATES OF AMERICA

Print number: 6 5 4 3 2

Dedicated to the late

Edward Edgerton Beveridge

July 1931–May 1972

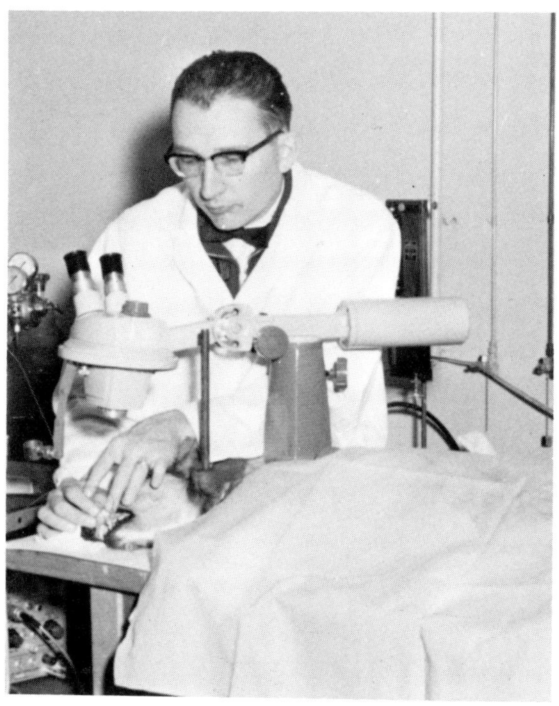

Have you ever seen a book dedicated to one of its authors? The memory of Ed Beveridge deserves such dedication. It matches in only small measure his personal dedication to life.

Knowing he was faced with death, Ed devoted the last six months of his life to the revision of this text. More than anyone I have ever known, Ed Beveridge had the monumental integrity and the "gift of giving" John Steinbeck must have had in mind when he wrote Doc's soliloquy in *Sweet Thursday:*

> What has my life meant so far, and what can it mean in the time left? What have I contributed in the great ledger? What am I worth? And this isn't vanity or ambition. Men seem to be born with a debt they can never repay no matter how hard they try. It piles up ahead of them. Man owes something to man. If he ignores the debt, it poisons him, and if he tries to make payments, the debt only increases; the quality of his *gift* is the measure of the man. Yes, man owes something to man, and the quality of his gift is the measure of the man.

Preface

If PULL AND BE DAMNED ROAD was the symbol of the first edition of this text, then surely the WASHINGTON MONUMENT will symbolize the second. And this for two reasons:

First, the revision has been done virtually in the shadow of the Monument. And second, the WASHINGTON MONUMENT, more than any other symbol, epitomizes the discipline of endodontics.

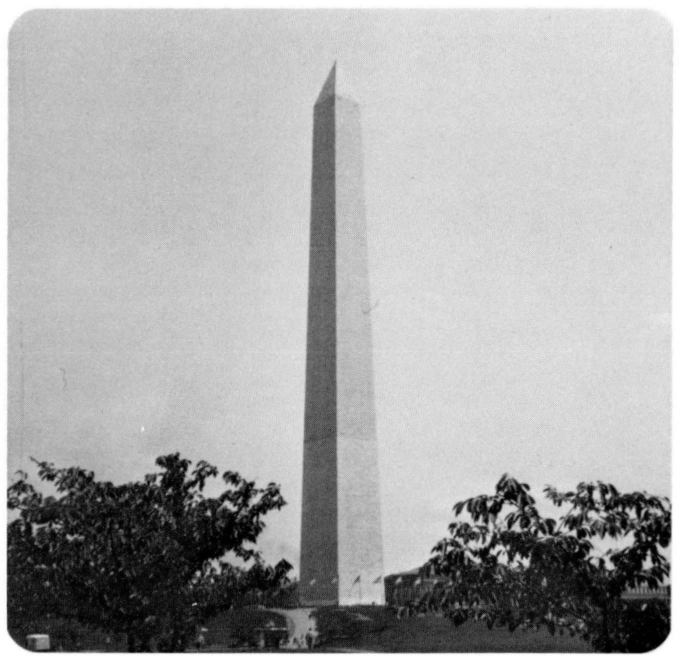

At first blush this analogy seems somewhat ridiculous. But is it? Proper preparation of the root canal has often been likened to the shape of the Washington Monument. But even more than that, the Washington Monument stands for solidity, for integrity—the integrity expected of every member of the profession.

Today, integrity is being scoffed at. Time and profits are held out as first priority. Quality is shunted aside. The American dentist is being told that root canal therapy, as advocated in this text, is too time-consuming to practice profitably. The answer, they say, is the "quick fix"—an admittedly casual cavity preparation immediately followed by a "magic paste" of questionable stability and toxicity.

The fakirs have a new rope trick; the "medicine men" are peddling a new brand of snake oil. Led by a Pied Piper, the *children* of the profession are seeking the panacea. Rather than nirvana, they will end in a debacle. The entire movement is a shoddy approach to man's laze and greed.

Root canal therapy *can* be done properly in a modest amount of time—not fifteen minutes, mind you, but during a reasonable appointment. Knowing exactly what needs to be done and being skillful and organized in performance is the secret to success, not some shabby shortcut learned on a weekend.

The endodontic specialist has been made the whipping boy by this movement. Is the American dentist so naive as to believe that only 500 specialists could hoard the endodontic care of nearly 200 million people? The answer, of course, lies with the general practitioners of America—the backbone of the profession. The answer also lies with the dental schools—to prepare their students so thoroughly there is only occasional need for the specialist, and this should include meaningful continuing education for the practicing dentist as well as the predoctoral student.

It is in the dental schools that a *monumental* integrity and skill will be built, not by some slick huckster in a hotel ballroom. It is in the general practices of the nation this skill and integrity will be put to the test.

Washington, D.C. John I. Ingle, D.D.S.

Acknowledgments

Revising this text has been like perusing a menu in a French restaurant. There are so many items to choose from, and they all sound so good. How does one make a choice? The menu of endodontic literature from the past ten years is enormous and exciting—a veritable explosion of investigation and reevaluation. Much of it good, some not so good. But how to choose? This is the question. I hope we have chosen wisely. We have avoided being verbose, while including all relevant material.

I have tried to keep this a how-to-do-it text. In this I have been encouraged by practicing dentists who have taught themselves to do root canal therapy by reading the book. At the same time, this revision broadly expands on the background material that makes endodontics a separate discipline in dentistry. The chapters on diagnosis have been broadly expanded, for this is the truly challenging area of dental practice that can be performed only by the full professional. If I have erred, it is on the side of inclusion not exclusion. This is particularly true of photographs. My friends and colleagues around the world have plied me with an avalanche of outstanding material. I could not use it all; I hope I have not included too much. Only an indulgent publisher would allow the inclusion of so many germane examples. If the book weighs too much, blame endodontics for its decade of growth, and blame the publisher for using such excellent paper.

Some of this text will be controversial. I have deliberately chosen contributing authors who are controversial because I believe them to be at the forefront of the profession. I predict our material will stand the test of time because it is based on a sound knowledge of the field. It is also based on integrity.

I acknowledge to my contributing author colleagues the great debt I owe them for being so patient and productive. The profession and the public will owe them a debt as well. I only wish Ed Beveridge had lived to see the outcome of our efforts.

I am also pleased to acknowledge once again the magnificent photomicrographic contributions by Dr. Seiichi Matsumiya of Tokyo and the late Dr. Balint Orban as well as the outstanding contributions by Clifford Freehe, photographer, and Virginia Brooks, illustrator, of the University of Washington. To them I must add James Butler, illustrator at the National Academy of Sciences, and Carol Oswald at the University of Washington as well as Claude E. (Pete) Petrone, photographer at the National Geographic Society.

I would have liked to acknowledge here every person who has contributed, in even a small way, to this text. They are far too numerous to list. I hope I have properly credited the contributor under each photograph. With each credit goes my gratitude. Special thanks go to Thomas Mullaney at the University of Kentucky as well as Henry Van Hassel, Gerald Harrington and Robert Oswald at the University of Washington for editorial review and comment.

I am grateful to my colleagues at the Institute of Medicine and the National Academy of Sciences for their forbearance while this revision was under way.

To my publishers, the four partners of Lea & Febiger; to Martin Dallago and Mary Mansor, my editors; and Thomas J. Colaiezzi, production manager at L & F; I acknowledge the great patience they have exhibited and the confidence they have shown that this revision would be forthcoming. *Nonpareil.*

And finally to my wife, Joyce, my undying gratitude for not only being so loving and tolerant over the years, but for typing this entire manuscript as well. Could one ask more?

J. I. I.

Preface to the First Edition

This book was begun at Snee-oosh Beach, a quiet retreat overlooking Puget Sound and the San Juan Islands. At Snee-oosh it is possible to escape from complex civilization, and to concentrate upon the job at hand—writing a text.

Hard by Snee-oosh is an old Indian trail called PULL AND BE DAMNED ROAD. One can hardly imagine a more fitting location while writing a text on the *pulpless tooth* than nearby PULL AND BE DAMNED ROAD, for "Pull and be damned" could well be the motto of the dental profession from its inception.

PULL AND BE DAMNED ROAD goes down to the shores of Skagit Bay, an inside passage of the gentle Pacific leading ominously to DECEPTION PASS. This delusive inlet which so easily deceived the early explorers, reminds us how our profession has practiced *self-deception* over the years. Unfortunately, many pass into the "pull and be damned," deceptive phase of dental practice, never to return.

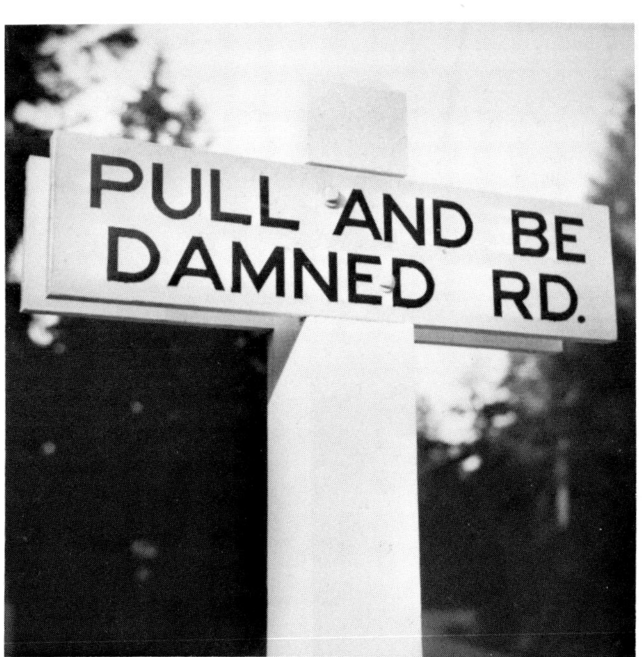

Inside DECEPTION PASS, however, lies HOPE ISLAND, a symbol of the future. HOPE we must have, coupled with resolve. HOPE that the future of dentistry will noticeably improve. HOPE that an enlightened profession will be guided by the concept of *retention* and *rehabilitation* of the dental apparatus. HOPE for the rejection of "oral amputation."

To say that the ideas contained within this text are ours or are original is ridiculous. Nothing really is new under the dental sun. We have liberally borrowed from our contemporaries as well as the past. We only hope we give credit where credit is due.

The student who chooses this text for an encyclopedia will be disappointed. In this age of "do it yourself" this is a "how to do it" book. We have attempted to discuss and illustrate in great detail the operative aspects of endodontic therapy, for we estimate that in treating a pulpless tooth the dentist will spend at least 75 per cent of treatment time in endodontic cavity preparation, canal debridement and filling. Operative endodontics is therefore presented first in the text, and a correspondingly significant section deals with these matters.

We leave to other authors the *detailed* discussion of anti-infectives, local anesthesia, or oral microbiology. Although these subjects are dealt with in this text, we have tried to keep the material in proper context; brief, and to the point. We have spent, however, an unusual amount of space and time in developing the chapter on DIFFERENTIAL DIAGNOSIS OF ORAL AND PERIORAL PAIN.

Diagnosis of pain is an area of dental practice which more frequently is falling into the province of

Endodontics. It has often been said that any well-trained person can practice the mechanics of dentistry, but that proper diagnosis is the discipline that separates the really competent dentist from the merely mechanical; hence the extensive coverage of the subject.

A great deal of thought and talent was put into developing the four chapters on the normal and pathologic pulp and periapical tissues. This discussion builds the background for diagnosis of endodontic problems and sets the stage for a better understanding of oral and perioral pain.

Snee-oosh Beach is no Walden Pond, nor we Thoreau for that matter. But we may learn a lesson from Walden. "Simplify, simplify!" was Thoreau's text, and simplification is one text we may well take to heart. There has been far too much complicated mumbo-jumbo in endodontic treatment, a significant factor in discouraging the profession from including endodontic therapy in their practices.

We will attempt to present the subject not only in a simplified form but in a systematic manner; for the simplified systematic practice of endodontics will lead to successful results achieved with pleasure and profit. We have attempted to remove the mystery and retain the basic core of the subject. We only hope we succeed in bringing some order out of the present chaos.

Finally, we would like to eulogize Dr. Balint J. Orban to whom the first edition was dedicated. Dr. Orban's death was a great loss to the profession and an even greater loss to those of us fortunate enough to have known him well. His ability to clarify and delineate a problem is apparent in the Classification of Pulpal and Periapical Pain which we discussed just prior to his death. The profession is forever in the debt of Balint Orban; not the least for his matchless decriptions of pulpal histopathology. We are proud to be the recipients of this priceless collection of microscopic material. We are more proud to have been his friends and disciples.

Seattle, Washington JOHN I. INGLE

Contributors

Edward Edgerton Beveridge, D.D.S., M.S.D.*
Associate Dean for Academic Affairs
Professor and Chairman
Department of Endodontics
School of Dentistry
University of Southern California

Raleigh Reed Cummings, D.D.S., M.S.
Associate Professor and Chairman
Section of Endodontics
School of Dentistry
Loma Linda University

Alfred L. Frank, D.D.S.
Clinical Professor
Graduate and Undergraduate Endodontics
School of Dentistry
University of Southern California
Consultant, Endodontic Graduate Program
Long Beach Veterans Administration Hospital

Cyril Gaum, D.D.S.
Clinical Professor
School of Dental Medicine
Tufts University
Lecturer in Endodontics
School of Dental Medicine
Harvard University

Dudley H. Glick, B.S., D.D.S.
Clinical Professor
Graduate and Undergraduate Endodontics
School of Dentistry
University of Southern California
Consultant
Endodontic Graduate Program,
Long Beach Veterans Adminstration Hospital

*Deceased.

John Ide Ingle, D.D.S., M.S.D.
Senior Professional Associate
Institute of Medicine
National Academy of Sciences
Formerly Dean and Professor of Endodontics and Periodontics
School of Dentistry
University of Southern California
Formerly Professor and Chairman
Department of Periodontics and Endodontics
School of Dentistry
University of Washington

Hugh M. Kopel, D.D.S., M.S.
Professor and Chairman
Department of Pedodontics
School of Dentistry
University of Southern California

Kaare Langeland, D.D.S., Ph.D.
Professor and Chairman
Department of Endodontics
Formerly Professor Department of General Dentistry
School of Dental Medicine
University of Connecticut Health Center

Raymond G. Luebke, D.D.S., M.S.D.
Professor and Chairman
Department of Endodontics
School of Dentistry
Louisiana State University

Eugene Natkin, D.D.S., M.S.D.
Professor and Chairman
Department of Endodontics
School of Dentistry
University of Washington

Edwin B. Nutting, D.D.S.
Professor of Oral Medicine (Endodontics)
School of Dentistry
Loma Linda University
Formerly Chief of Endodontic Service
U.S. Naval Dental School
Bethesda, Maryland

Alfred L. Ogilvie, D.D.S., M.S.
Professor of Oral Medicine
Faculty of Dentistry
University of British Columbia
Formerly Professor of Periodontics
School of Dentistry
University of Washington

Thomas J. Pallasch, D.D.S., M.S.
Associate Professor of Pharmacology and Periodontics
Chairman
Department of Pharmacology
School of Dentistry
University of Southern California

Leonard Parris, D.D.S.
Formerly Chairman and Professor of Endodontics
School of Dentistry
Temple University

L. Daniel Schaeffer, B.S., M.S., Ph.D.
Associate Professor and Chairman
Department of Physiology
School of Dentistry
University of Southern California

Ronald R. Slowey, D.D.S., M.S.D.
Endodontist
San Carlos, California

Stephen Teel, B.S., D.D.S.
Associate Professor of Restorative Dentistry
School of Dentistry
University of Washington

Richard E. Walton, B.S., D.M.D., M.S.
Associate Professor of Endodontics and Oral Biology
Chairman
Department of Endodontics
School of Dentistry
Medical College of Georgia

David H. Wands, D.D.S., M.S.D.
Assistant Professor
Department of Prosthodontics
School of Dentistry
University of Washington

Jack A. Weichman, B.A., D.D.S.
Clinical Professor
Department of Endodontics
School of Dentistry
University of Southern California
Chief of Endodontics
St. Johns Hospital
Santa Monica, California

Edward White, D.D.S., M.S., Ph.D.
Professor and Chairman
Department of Endodontics
College of Dental Medicine
Medical University of South Carolina
Formerly Assistant Professor and Chairman
Department of Microbiology and Immunology
School of Dentistry
University of Southern California

Bertram L. Wolfsohn, D.D.S.
Clinical Professor of Endodontics
College of Dentistry
University of the Pacific

James D. Zidell, D.D.S., M.S.C.D.
Guest Lecturer
Formerly Director of Graduate Endodontics
School of Dentistry
University of Southern California

Contents

Chapter 3
ENDODONTIC CAVITY PREPARATION

John I. Ingle, Edward E. Beveridge, Raymond G. Luebke, Richard E. Walton, and James D. Zidell

Chapter 4

OBTURATION OF THE RADICULAR SPACE

John I. Ingle, Raymond G. Luebke, Richard E. Walton, and James D. Zidell

Chapter 5
PLAN OF TREATMENT
John I. Ingle

Chapter 6
HISTOLOGY AND PHYSIOLOGY OF THE DENTAL PULP
Alfred L. Ogilvie and L. Daniel Schaeffer

Chapter 7
ETIOLOGY AND PREVENTION OF PULP INFLAMMATION, NECROSIS, AND DYSTROPHY
John I. Ingle and Kaare Langeland

Chapter 8
PULP PATHOSIS
Alfred L. Ogilvie

Chapter 9
PERIAPICAL PATHOSIS
Alfred L. Ogilvie

Chapter 10
DIAGNOSTIC PROCEDURES
John I. Ingle, Edward E. Beveridge, Cyril Gaum, and Ronald R. Slowey

Chapter 11

DIFFERENTIAL DIAGNOSIS AND TREATMENT OF ORAL AND PERIORAL PAIN

John I. Ingle, Dudley H. Glick, and L. Daniel Schaeffer

Chapter 12

MICROBIOLOGIC CONSIDERATIONS IN ENDODONTICS

Edward White

Chapter 13
INTRACANAL MEDICATION AND SYSTEMIC ANTIBIOTIC THERAPY
Edward White and Thomas J. Pallasch

Chapter 14
ENDODONTIC INSTRUMENT STERILIZATION AND OPERATIVE FIELD DISINFECTION
Edward White

Chapter 15
ENDODONTIC SURGERY
John I. Ingle, Edward E. Beveridge, Raleigh R. Cummings, Alfred L. Frank, Dudley H. Glick, and Bertram L. Wolfsohn

Chapter 16

DIAGNOSIS AND TREATMENT OF TRAUMATIC INJURIES AND THEIR SEQUELAE

John I. Ingle, Alfred L. Frank, Eugene Natkin, and Edwin E. Nutting

Chapter 17

PEDIATRIC ENDODONTICS

Hugh M. Kopel

Chapter 18

RESTORATION OF THE PULPLESS TOOTH. PREPARATION FOR THE OVERDENTURE

Alfred L. Frank, Stephen Teel, and David H. Wands

Chapter 1

Modern Endodontic Therapy

JOHN I. INGLE, EDWARD E. BEVERIDGE, DUDLEY H. GLICK, and JACK A. WEICHMAN

The year 1959 marked the one-hundredth anniversary of the founding of the American Dental Association. For world dentistry, and particularly for North American dentistry, the year was spent evaluating the present status of the profession, heralding our advances in the past century, and forecasting the future.

The year was climaxed by a gigantic Centennial Meeting, held in New York City, at which a good share of the program was devoted to the historical analysis of a century of progress. In the field of endodontics, the signal honor of recapitulation was given to the late Dr. Edgar D. Coolidge of Chicago. Doctor Coolidge had lived through much of the century past and had undoubtedly contributed more to dentistry than any man present.

Doctor Coolidge's historical paper was concise, literate, accurate, and discouraging.[1] The conclusion may be drawn from his paper that basically endodontics had not advanced as far as other disciplines in dentistry, and for good reason.

For generations, progress in endodontic therapy was postponed for want of the x-ray. As a "blind" discipline, root canal therapy remained far too inexact. Unfortunately there was born with the roentgen ray the ***theory of focal infection.*** This theory, accepted as fact, reigned supreme for generations, condemning the pulpless tooth to extraction, and retarding root canal therapy some 25 years. Fortunately, during this "age of the one hundred percenters," when all pulpless teeth were condemned to extraction, a small band of nonconformists continued to practice and preach root canal therapy. Doctor Coolidge was joined in Chicago by Doctors Roy Blayney and G. R. Lundquist and later by Doctor Orban. Doctors Jasper in St. Louis, Weaver in Cleveland, Johnston in Atlanta, Rhein in New York, Sommer and Richert in Ann Arbor, Grossman in Philadelphia, Krueger in Toronto, Garvin in Winnipeg, Sharp in Pasadena, and Davis in Lincoln, as well as a number of distinguished foreign colleagues, disavowed the general attitude toward the treated pulpless tooth during the reign of "death and dentistry."

Today we have nearly discarded the shackles of the ***theory of focal infection;*** although a small core of our colleagues in both medicine and dentistry chooses to look upon the pulpless tooth as a convenient "whipping boy" for desperate diagnosis.

It was not until the period following World War II that endodontic treatment began to enjoy some confidence by the profession. Probably the introduction of the antibiotics once again turned the profession to saving the pulpless tooth. To Dr. Louis I. Grossman, of the University of Pennsylvania, goes most of the credit for the endodontic revival based on the intelligent use of antibiotics. Gradually, physicians and the lay public alike were aroused to an interest in endodontic results.

In his centennial paper, Doctor Coolidge pointed to the improvements in endodontics as, "largely a matter of trial and error."[1] "It is true," he said, "that we have discarded arsenic to devitalize the pulps of teeth, but this only recently in the century when local anesthetics were improved. Moreover, the preservation of the vital pulp has not progressed greatly since 1929 when Orban first discussed the reparative powers of the pulp."[2]

In the meantime, damage of the dental pulp goes forward relentlessly. Accidents and contact sports have increased the incidence of pulp death from impact, and in reality, little ***preventive*** headway has been made against dental caries. Even the communal fluoride program seems to have reached a plateau. The individual dentist, working the best he can against the disease, is often an unwelcome contributor to pulp death through the use of heat-generating cutting tools and the placement of toxic filling materials.

Although lip service has been paid to the preservation of healthy dental pulp, little has actually been done toward this end. Instead, too much time and literature have been spent arguing the merits of various magic formulas to mummify or sterilize this remarkable tissue and the space it occupies. Little ***true*** progress has been made since Walkhoff recommended chlorophenol in 1891.[3]

In the highly important area of ***operative endodontics,*** Pucci, almost alone, emphasized the importance of less colorful but highly important endodontic cavity preparations.[4] Unfortunately, his monumental encyclopedic contribution to the field is relatively unknown outside Latin America, never having been translated from the Spanish.

As was the case with cavity preparations, endodontic instruments had received little attention in the endodontic literature. Until 1955 the basic instruments for preparation, reamers and files, remained unnoticed, unstandardized, and unimproved.[5,6] In the past twenty years, however, there have been some remarkable improvements. Even power-driven endodontic instruments have been developed, only to be abused by a profit hungry segment of the profession masquerading as "do-gooders."

Root canal filling or obturation, on the other hand, has been extensively covered in the dental writing of the past century. Starting with the introduction of gutta percha by G. A. Bowman in 1867,[7] we have slowly moved through a gamut of filling materials into modern petrochemical plastics. Only at this time does it appear that a simplified filling procedure is enticingly close. One can foresee on the horizon cementification closure of the apical foramen stimulated by such biologically active materials as calcium hydroxide or a gel of colloidal collagen and mineral salts.[8] Canal obturation by injection of new petrochemicals seems excitingly near.[9]

Over the years, improvement has been made in dental education in the field of root canal therapy. Today, every dental school in the nation teaches endodontics—and this could not be said in 1950. On the other hand, a study by Beveridge in 1972 proved most embarrassing to endodontic education.[10] Beveridge learned by questionnaire of the paucity of qualified teachers of endodontics. In some schools, however, root canal therapy involves a considerable amount of curricular and clinical time, and along with periodontics and restorative dentistry has become the keystone to present concepts of retentive dentistry, gradually replacing the old concept of extraction-replacement dentistry.

In continuing education, endodontic courses have proved most popular, as dentists return to school to learn a subject that was poorly taught or ignored when they studied dentistry. Graduate education in endodontics has also flourished. The future teacher or specialist continues his education for at least two years following graduation.

"Organized endodontics" began in 1943 when a group of 20 men met in Chicago to form the ***American Association of Endodontists,*** an organization grown to over 1400 domestic and foreign members by 1975. The culmination of progress by the association was reached in 1963 when Endodontics was recognized as a special area of dental practice by the American Dental Association, and the ***American Board of Endodontics*** was established. At that time, over 500 American dentists were limiting their practices exclusively to root canal therapy.

The three greatest improvements in the field of endodontics are associated with general improvements in the overall discipline of the health sciences: antibiotics for the control of severe infections, profound anesthetics for the control of pain, and the relegation of the theory of focal infection into proper perspective.

Direct improvements in the practice of endodontic therapy center around the application of time and motion practices to treatment; the standardization of instruments and filling materials; the standardization of cavity preparation and filling techniques; the improved techniques of apexification, endodontic implants, and overdentures; the use of accelerated speed cutting instruments; the optimal use of auxiliaries; prepackaged-presterilized equipment, and the rapid development of roentgenograms. With all of these improvements, many patients must still be convinced that root canal therapy is an intelligent, practical solution to an age-old problem—the loss of teeth. The "case for endodontic treatment" must be presented to the patient in a straightforward manner. The patient with the correct "oral image" will be anxious to proceed with therapy.

ENDODONTIC CASE PRESENTATION

"Is this tooth worth saving, doctor?" This sentiment is voiced more often than not by the patient who has been informed that his tooth will require endodontic therapy. Superficially, this appears to be a simple question that requires a direct, uncomplicated answer. It should not be interpreted as hostile or as a challenge to the diagnosis and decision you have offered for the retention of his tooth. However, psychologically, this initial question in effect is a prelude to a Pandora's Box of additional queries that disclose doubts, fears, apprehensions, and economic considerations. For example, "Is it painful?," "Will this tooth have to be extracted later?," "How long will this tooth last?," "Is it a dead tooth?," "Will it turn black?" and "How much will it cost?"

Following the first question, the dentist should anticipate a series of questions. By including the answers to anticipated questions in the presentation, the dentist will gain a decided psychologic advantage. By this apparent insight into his problems the patient is assured that the dentist is cognizant of the very questions he was about to raise or possibly was too reticent to raise. Most of the patient's fear and doubts can be allayed by giving a concise answer to each question. The dentist should be able to explain procedures intelligently as he exchanges ideas with the patient. To do this he must be endodontically oriented. That is, he must believe in the value of endodontic therapy himself, and in believing, he cannot help but influence the patient favorably. The dentist will soon gain the confidence of the patient who realizes that professional decisions emanate from an honest desire to preserve his mouth's functional efficiency. To answer patients' questions, the American Dental Association has available an inexpensive pamphlet entitled ***Your Teeth Can be Saved by Endodontic Treatment.***[11] In addition a clever pamphlet entitled ***Am I Losing My Nerve?*** written and illustrated by Dr. Richard Burns may be given to the patient to read while waiting.[12] Although this approach is a little impersonal, it gives the patient a tangible reference, particularly when he returns home and tries to explain to an interested spouse what endodontic therapy involves.

Based on his previous experiences in the office, the average patient has sufficient confidence in the dentist's ability to help him. He is ready to accept the professional knowledge and advice offered him, but he likes to have some part in evaluating the reasonableness of the treatment. The professional man must spend the time and thought necessary to understand the patient's initial resistance, a resistance possibly based on false assumptions and beliefs in matters dealing with pulpless teeth. Once the patient is secure in the thought that this is the correct treatment, however, most of the fears and apprehensions related to an unfamiliarity with endodontic therapy will be dissipated.

A dental appointment is still associated with fear in the minds of many people. The mere thought of treating the "nerve" of a tooth implies pain! These patients require reassurance, which is supported by all available psychologic and therapeutic methods of relaxation and pain control. The patient must be reassured that endodontic therapy will be pain-free, and requires no more than a local anesthetic.

It should be explained to the patient that root canal therapy is a specialized form of dental procedure designed to retain a tooth safely and comfortably. This tooth, when properly treated and restored, will be retained as long as a vital tooth. It is not a "dead tooth" as long as the root of the tooth is imbedded in healthy surrounding tissues that "bathe" the external surface and offer it nutrition. Seldom do teeth turn "black" in this day because precautions are taken to maintain the natural color, but if appearance becomes a prime concern and there is discoloration, the tooth may be bleached. In the event the bleaching is not successful, a jacket crown can be made. Most often, retention of the tooth and crowning are preferable to extraction and replacement with a prosthetic appliance.

There is little doubt that economic considerations play an important role (and for some a supreme role) in the final decision. Some patients "think financially," and even though able to afford treatment, they allow financial considerations to govern decisions that should logically be made on a physiologic basis only. It is necessary to point out to these people the ***financial*** advantage of retaining a tooth by endodontic therapy rather than by extraction and prosthetic replacement. The properly informed patient is quick to recognize that the fee for a bridge is more than that for root canal therapy and proper restoration. In addition, it should be mentioned in all honesty that any vital tooth prepared for a crown could become a possible condidate for future endodontic therapy. Also, the patient who states, "Pull it out," should be informed of the problems that arise if a space is left unfilled, *i.e.*, tilting, reduced masticatory efficiency, future periodontal problems, and cosmetic effects.

Another commonly heard statement by the patient is, "It's only a back tooth, anyway," or "If it were a front tooth I would save it, but no one sees it in back." This patient "thinks cosmetically." To him must be explained the disadvantages of the loss of any tooth, let alone a posterior one, which is so essential for mastication.

Fortunately, today's patient is becoming more sophisticated, too "tooth conscious" to permit indiscriminate extraction without asking whether there is an alternative. Extraction contributes to a crippling aberration from the normal dentition. There is no doubt that a normally functioning, endodontically treated, and well-restored tooth is vastly superior to the best prosthetic replacement.

INFORMED CONSENT

If today's patients are becoming more sophisticated about their dental wants, they are also becoming more sophisticated about their legal rights. As Milgrom and Ingle have noted,[13] the dentist can no longer consider himself immune to malpractice litigation by hiding behind a doctrine of "local community standards." The paucity in the dental literature of warning or discussion of patients' rights is now taking its toll in the increase in malpractice suits.

Only Serene has alerted the endodontic profession to litigation, pointing out a $390,000 award to a plaintiff who had suffered brain damage from anesthesia during root canal therapy.[14] Too frequently, a court case ensues when a reamer has been swallowed because a rubber dam was not used.

Weiner has observed that "a tooth severely traumatized will nearly always require eventual endodontic therapy," and that it is in the patient's best interest, when estimating future costs, to include the affected tooth in the estimate.[15] Surely this is true when an insurance settlement is being considered.

Weichman has pointed out the importance of the ***doctrine of informed consent*** as well as other steps that must be taken by the dentist to protect his patient as well as himself.[16]

According to the ***doctrine of informed consent,*** a dentist must: (1) describe the proposed treatment so that it is fully understood by the patient; (2) explain all the risks attendant to such treatment; and (3) discuss alternative procedures or treatments that might apply to the patient's particular problem.

The courts have decided that a patient can give a valid, or informed, consent for treatment only after he has been given all of this information. If a dentist does not obtain such an informed consent, he is guilty of professional negligence and is liable for any injury resulting from so-called unauthorized treatment. The options listed by the dentist should be noted in writing on the patient's chart and signed by the patient.

Weichman points out that at a minimum the dentist must tell the patient what he intends to accomplish and what any follow-up treatment, such as final restoration, might entail; he must list other ways of treating the condition a well as their advantages and disadvantages, such as extraction versus root canal therapy; and, above all, he must discuss possible complications—what might go wrong, or the fact that treatment could lose its effectiveness after a few months. It should be pointed out, however, that in some states "guaranteeing" the outcome of professional services is against the law.

Another type of informed consent is ***parental consent.*** Never should a minor be treated without the written consent of a parent. Again, "age of consent" varies by state.

Weichman goes on to list other aspects of practicing "defensive dentistry." He recommends showing concern for the patient's welfare by: (1) establishing good anesthesia; (2) anticipating problems such as unavoidable pain and forewarning the patient; (3) telephoning patients after treatment to inquire about their comfort; (4) placing high priority on emergencies; (5) consulting with other professionals to provide the best possible care for each patient; (6) providing competent "coverage" in the event the dentist himself is unavailable.

The importance of maintaining good office records, not just financial ones, is also emphasized by Weichman. These records should consist, at a minimum, of good, well-processed radiographs; a health history signed by the patient; the patient's complaints, from "chief complaint" to any variance at subsequent appointments; any objective findings made during treatment, such as the state of the pulp's vitality found upon opening the chamber, as well as the results of all testing before treatment; any possible complications foreseen or encountered, such as curved roots, obliterated canals, postoperative problems, and associated periodontal problems; a list of allergies and illnesses; any prescription written or medications given; and full disclosure of any accidents occurring during treatment, such as broken instruments or fractured roots. Milgrom and Ingle have suggested an informed consent form that will cover most situations (see Form 1–1).

Weichman has stated that the statute of limitations does not begin ***until the patient discovers*** such problems as a broken instrument or a poorly filled canal. He also points out the futility of adding to or changing records at a later date, noting the dishonesty of the procedure as well as the culpability when proved a fraud in court.

A serious problem in patient management that has

H. QUALITY, DDS 65 W. FIFTH ST. CAPITAL CITY 35420

Patient's Name ______ Record # ______ Date ______

1. Procedures to be followed ______

2. Purpose of procedures ______

3. Benefits of treatment ______

4. Risks/Discomfort ______

5. Alternatives ______

6. Fee for Treatment Specified ______

7. I am pleased to answer any inquiries concerning these procedures. You are free to withdraw your consent and discontinue treatment at any time.

______ Date ______ Signature of Dentist

8. CONSULTANTS RECORD

______ Date ______ Signature of Consultant

9. Patient's Acceptance

I have read and understand the information provided by my dentist above. I know I am free to ask any questions I may have about my treatment and to discontinue treatment at any time.

______ Date ______ Patient's Signature

______ Date ______ Spouse (Parent or Guardian)

Form 1–1. Informed consent form based on HEW guidelines. (From Milgrom, P., and Ingle, J. I.: J. Oral Surg., *33*:515, July, 1975.)

developed in this age of specialization revolves around responsibility. Who among the many professionals caring for the patient shall assume responsibility? "Who should be captain of the ship?" asked Beveridge. "Let it become a mutual objective that no patient shall move from one practitioner to another without someone in command. Every patient deserves to have a clearly understood, readily identified, 'captain of his dental ship'," he stated. Ideally the dentist most responsible should be the general practitioner who has referred the patient to the endodontist, periodontist, or oral surgeon. His office should be the "clearing house" for central records and coordination of treatment. Group practice, of course, would greatly simplify this responsibility.

All in all, dental practice in the future will be much more aware of the patient's rights and consent (Fig. 1–1)—a spin-off from the consumer movement which flowered in the early 1970's.

ATTITUDES TOWARD ENDODONTIC THERAPY

Before endodontic indications and contraindications can be discussed, a certain number of "givens" must be accepted to explain the upsurge in root canal therapy. Unfortunately, however, tooth extraction is still an important exercise in the United States, where it has been estimated that 56,000,000 teeth are extracted annually,[17] and the average 17-year-old student has lost 1.1 permanent teeth.[18] Compare that figure to the annual extraction rate for the children of New Zealand,[19] which is 0.0018 permanent tooth per child, and one would have to say that endodontics is a much needed discipline in the United States. Or consider the fact that half of all Americans are fully edentulous by age 65, and nearly two-thirds are edentulous by age 75.[20]

In spite of these figures, there have been some remarkable changes of attitude by the public and the

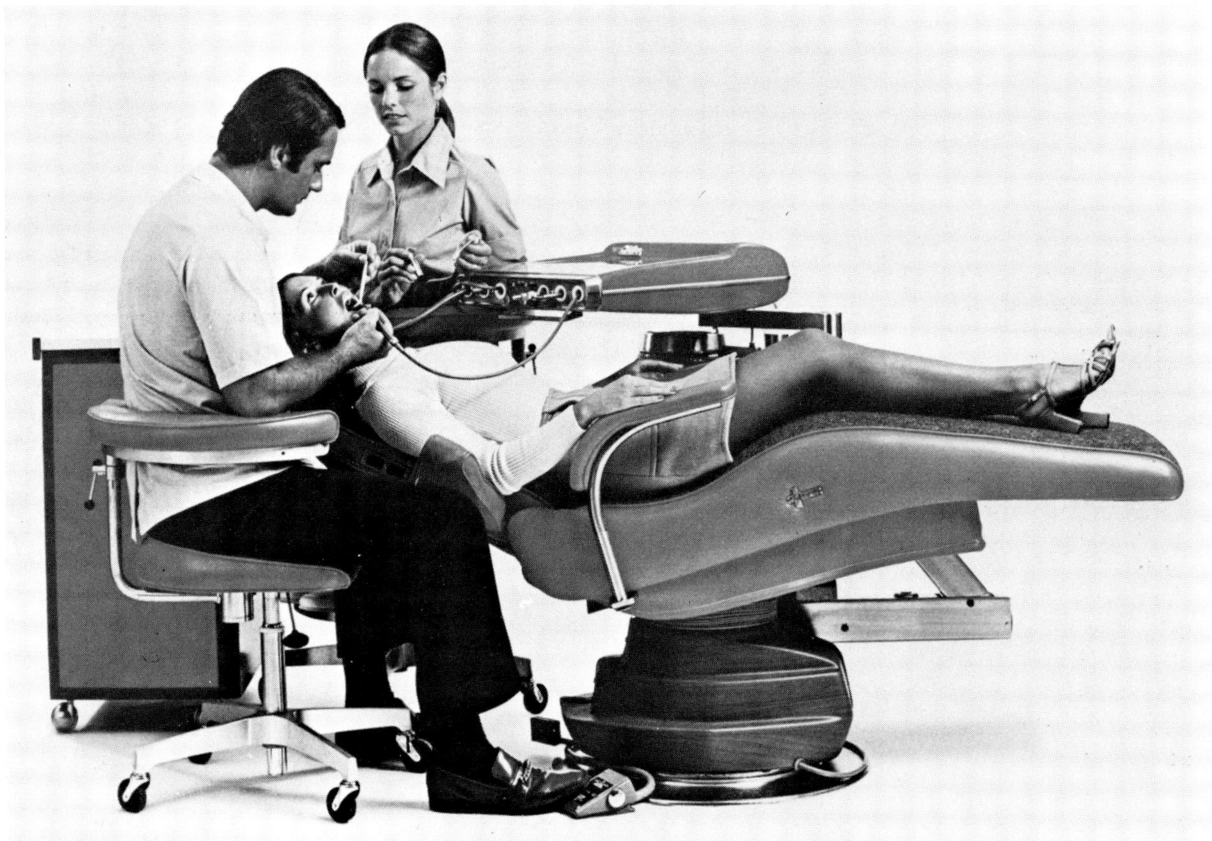

Fig. 1–1. Future dental practice is here today. Four-handed or six-handed dentistry involves coordination of dental team. Reclining patient and popular "over-the-patient" instrument delivery is ideal for endodontic therapy. (Courtesy Coastal Dynamics Corp.)

profession alike, and these are reflected in the following statements of fact:

1. A full complement of natural teeth with healthy support and esthetic in appearance is today's accepted ideal.

2. An attractive oral image, projected primarily through television, is being sought by an ever increasing segment of the public.

3. With improved life expectancy, more people need dental care to extend the "life" of their dentition.

4. There is every chance that a fully or partially edentulous person will sooner or later become a true dental "cripple."

5. Each lost tooth places an additional masticatory load on those remaining.

6. Well-treated pulpless teeth, properly restored, have a life expectancy equal to that of teeth with a healthy pulp.

7. Well-treated pulpless teeth are not foci of infection.

8. The age of the patient is not a limiting factor to endodontic practice or success.

9. With rare exceptions, general body health is not a limiting factor to endodontic practice or success.

10. There is no limit to the number of pulpless teeth that can be treated for any one patient.

11. Endodontic therapy does not require unusual or extraordinary skills.

12. Efficiently executed endodontic therapy is financially feasible for the patient and dentist alike.

13. Any dentist providing ***comprehensive*** dental care must include endodontic therapy in his practice.

These then are the "givens" of endodontics, so that the pulpless tooth can be safely and esthetically treated for more and more people. That most of this treatment will have to be done by the 100,000 general dentists of the nation seems obvious. All of the nation's endodontic needs cannot be satisfied by only 500 specialists, even though these specialists could be kept busy diagnosing and treating the baffling cases alone. Properly educating the future family-practice dentist in endodontic diagnosis and treatment is one of the important challenges facing dental education. This will undoubtedly include an increased use of expanded-duty auxiliaries in endodontic treatment.

Two congressional acts will have a decided impact on root canal therapy. The Health Maintenance Organization Act mandates "preventive dental care" for all children of families cared for by the HMO's. Slowly, but eventually, dental caries in these children will be controlled to a greater extent, and the number of pulpless teeth needing treatment should decline dramatically. Couple this with a reported drop in the caries rate in fluoridated areas and one could predict that by the year 2000 there will be fewer teeth needing endodontic treatment. That is not to say there will not be an immediate flurry of endodontic treatment demanded under federal legislation. This will merely be "catch up," however, and eventually this need will taper off.

On the other hand, if a strong dental component is retained in a National Health Insurance bill, the prevention and early treatment of dental caries will have a profound effect on future needs for root canal therapy. But again, this will be an initial flurry, as early needs are translated into demands.

The indications for endodontic therapy are legion. Every tooth from central incisor to third molar is a potential candidate for treatment. Far too often the expedient measure of extracting a pulpless tooth is a short-sighted attempt at solving a dental problem. Endodontic therapy, on the other hand, extends to the dentist and the patient the opportunity to save teeth.

The concept of retaining every possible tooth, and even the healthy roots of periodontally involved teeth, is based on the even distribution of the forces of mastication. The final success of any extensive restorative procedure depends on the root-surface area attached through the periodontal ligaments to the alveolar bone. Like the proverbial horseshoe nail, pulpless teeth may often be the salvation of an otherwise hopeless case.

To carry this concept one step further, recognized today is the importance of retaining even endodontically treated ***roots*** over which may be constructed a full denture, the so-called ***overdenture.***[21] On some occasions, attachments may be added to these roots to provide additional retention for the denture above. At other times the treated roots are merely left in place, on the assumption that the alveolar process will be retained around roots and there will not be the usual ridge resorption so commonly seen under full, or even partial, dentures.

The dentist who is honest with himself and his patient soon recognizes that the retained and restored individual tooth is better than a bridge replacement, and the bridge is better than the removable partial denture, which in turn is superior to the full denture. Treatment in every case should adhere to the standards set by the dentist for himself and his family.

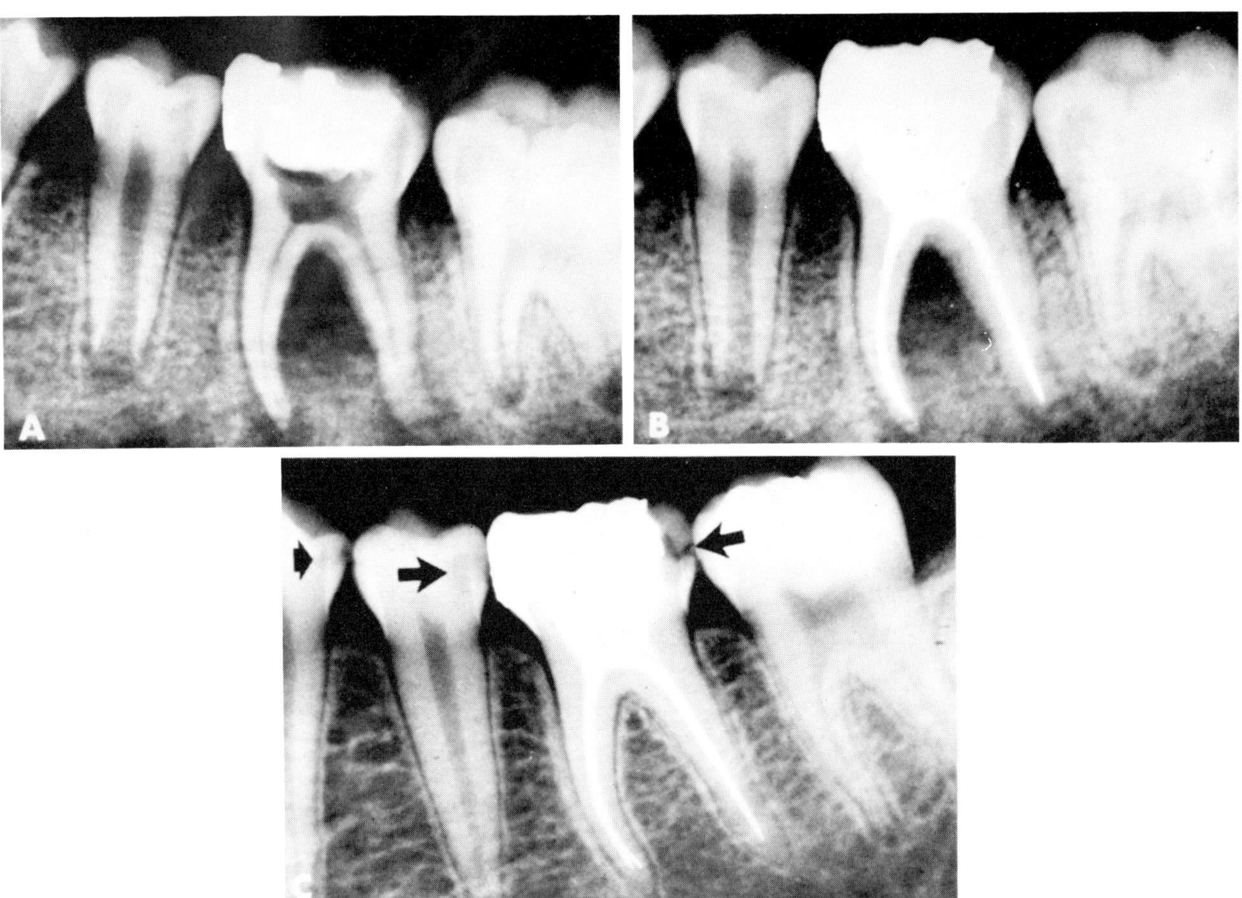

Fig. 1–2. *A,* Pulpless first molar following failure of pulpotomy. Note two periapical lesions and complete loss of intraradicular bone. Draining fistula opposite furca is also present. *B,* Completion of endodontic therapy without surgery. *C,* Two-year recall roentgenogram. Total healing was complete in six months. New carious lesions (arrows) now involve each interproximal surface.

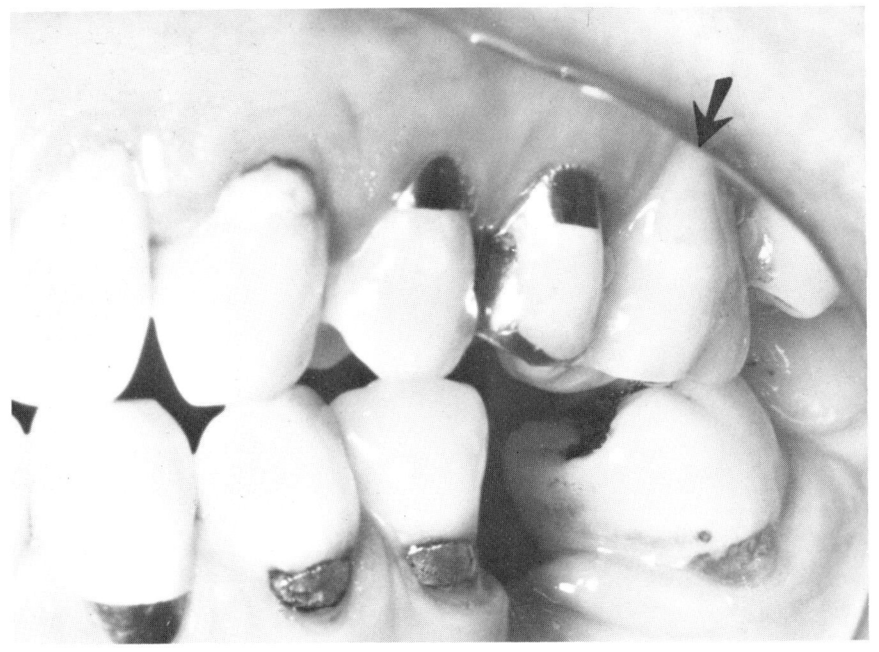

Fig. 1–3. Extrusion, recession (arrow), tipping, malocclusion, rotation, and gingival cemental caries are only a few of long-range consequences following early extraction of permanent first molar.

All too often a dentist treats his patients in one manner, and then seeks totally different treatment for the same condition in his own mouth.

One of the greatest services rendered by the profession is the retention of the first permanent molar (Fig. 1–2). The long-range consequences of breaking the continuity of either arch are well known (Fig. 1–3). Root canal therapy often provides the only rational method of saving first molars with pulp involvement.

In addition to saving molars for children, endodontic therapy for the posterior teeth for adults is also highly desirable. Frequently, saving a pulpless molar precludes the necessity of having to prepare two abutment teeth to place a fixed partial denture (Fig. 1–4). Moreover, root canal treatment may save an abutment tooth of an existing fixed prosthesis. The gain is doubled if the salvaged abutment is also the terminal posterior tooth in the arch, thus preventing its loss and the loss of its opponent in the opposite arch as well (Fig. 1–5).

Another candidate for endodontic therapy is the adolescent who arrives in the office with a grossly damaged dentition, and is faced with full mouth

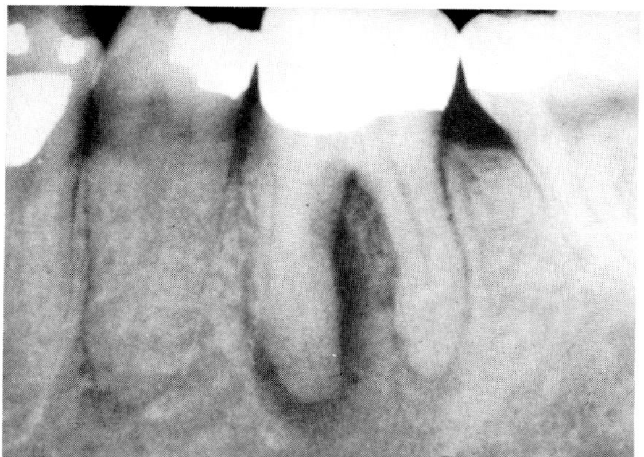

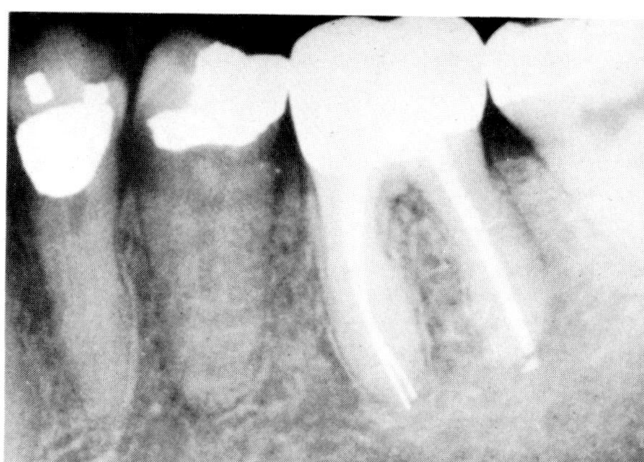

Fig. 1–4. Complete osseous repair following root canal therapy of permanent first molar in adult patient. Saving this well-restored, pulpless tooth precludes necessity for fixed prosthesis.

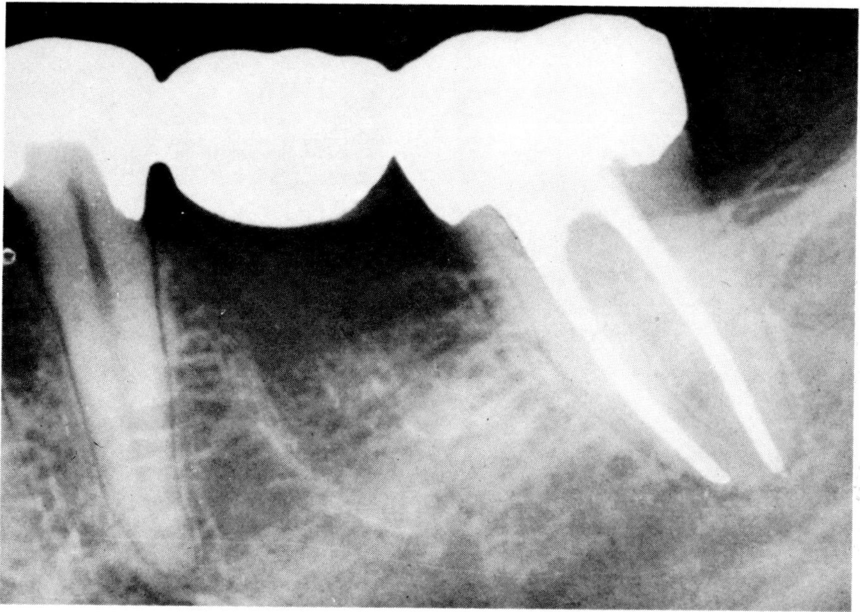

Fig. 1–5. Endodontic therapy of terminal, abutment tooth of recently placed fixed prosthesis. Endodontic preparation through full crown obviates necessity of removing bridge for treatment.

extraction and dentures (Fig. 1–6). Many of these children are mortified by their appearance. It is gratifying to see the blossoming personality when a cosmetic improvement has been achieved. The end result in these cases would not be possible without root canal therapy (Fig. 1–7).

Occasionally, intentional extirpation of a perfectly vital pulp may be necessary. More and more frequently dentists practicing periodontal prosthesis have learned to depend on intentional extirpation and root canal filling. This technique is used when hypererupted teeth or drifted teeth must be reduced so drastically that the pulp is certain to be involved.[22] In these cases the endodontic treatment may be completed before tooth reduction is started (Fig. 1–8).

Intentional extirpation and root canal filling are also

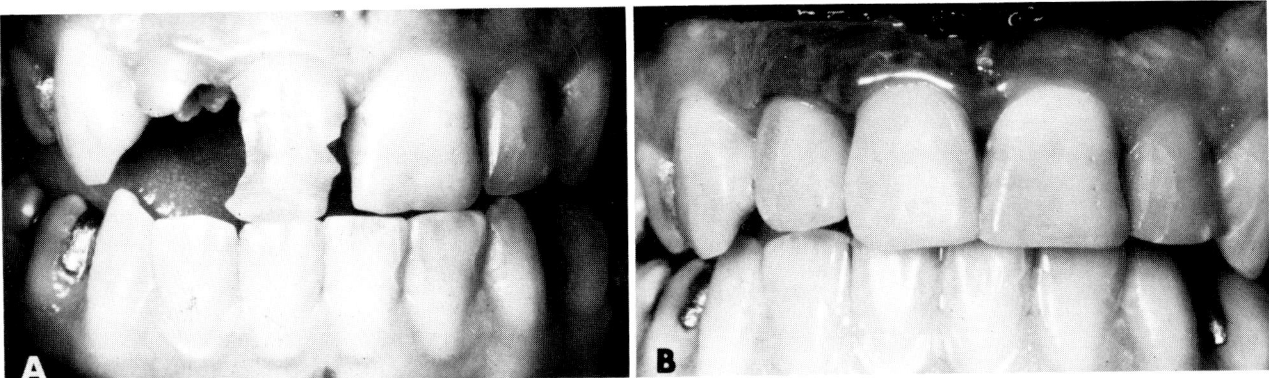

Fig. 1–6. *A*, Caries-decimated dentition in 14-year-old girl. Personality problems had developed in this youngster related to her embarrassing appearance. *B*, Provisional restoration following endodontic therapy has restored cosmetic appearance and confidence necessary for the adolescent.

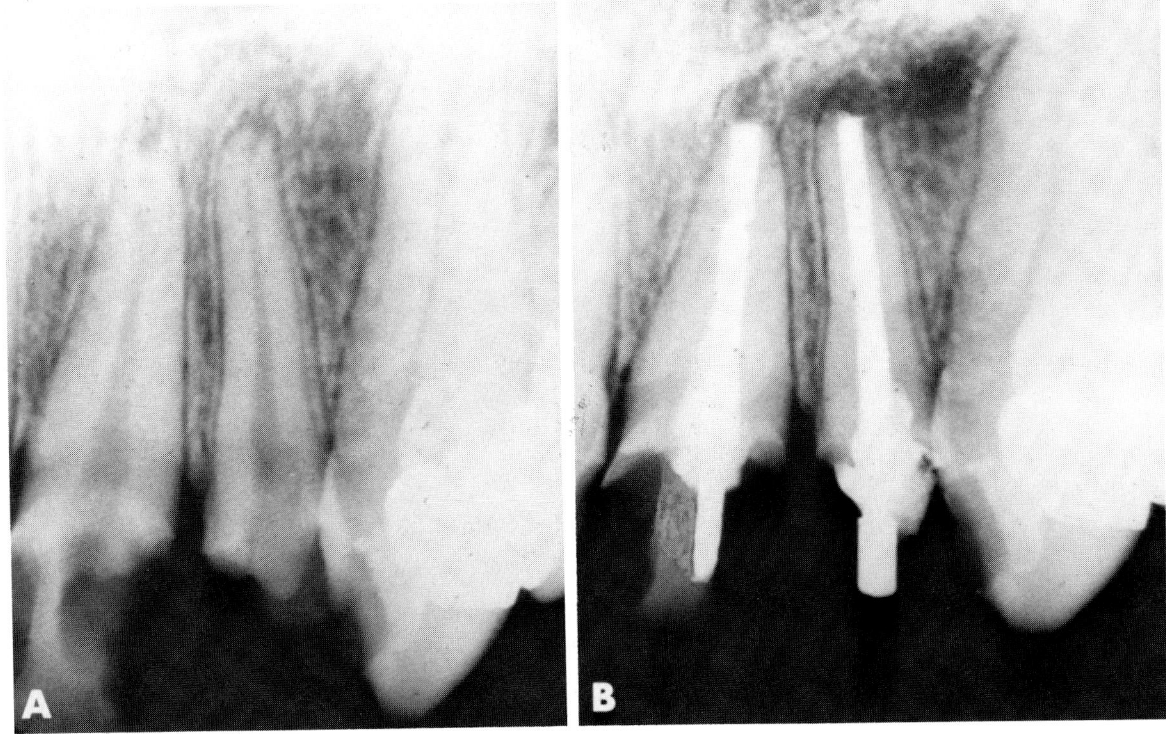

Fig. 1–7. *A*, Obvious pulp involvement of incisors shown in Figure 1–6. *B*, Root canal treatment of these incisors makes possible dowel restoration followed by cosmetic provisional plastic crowns.

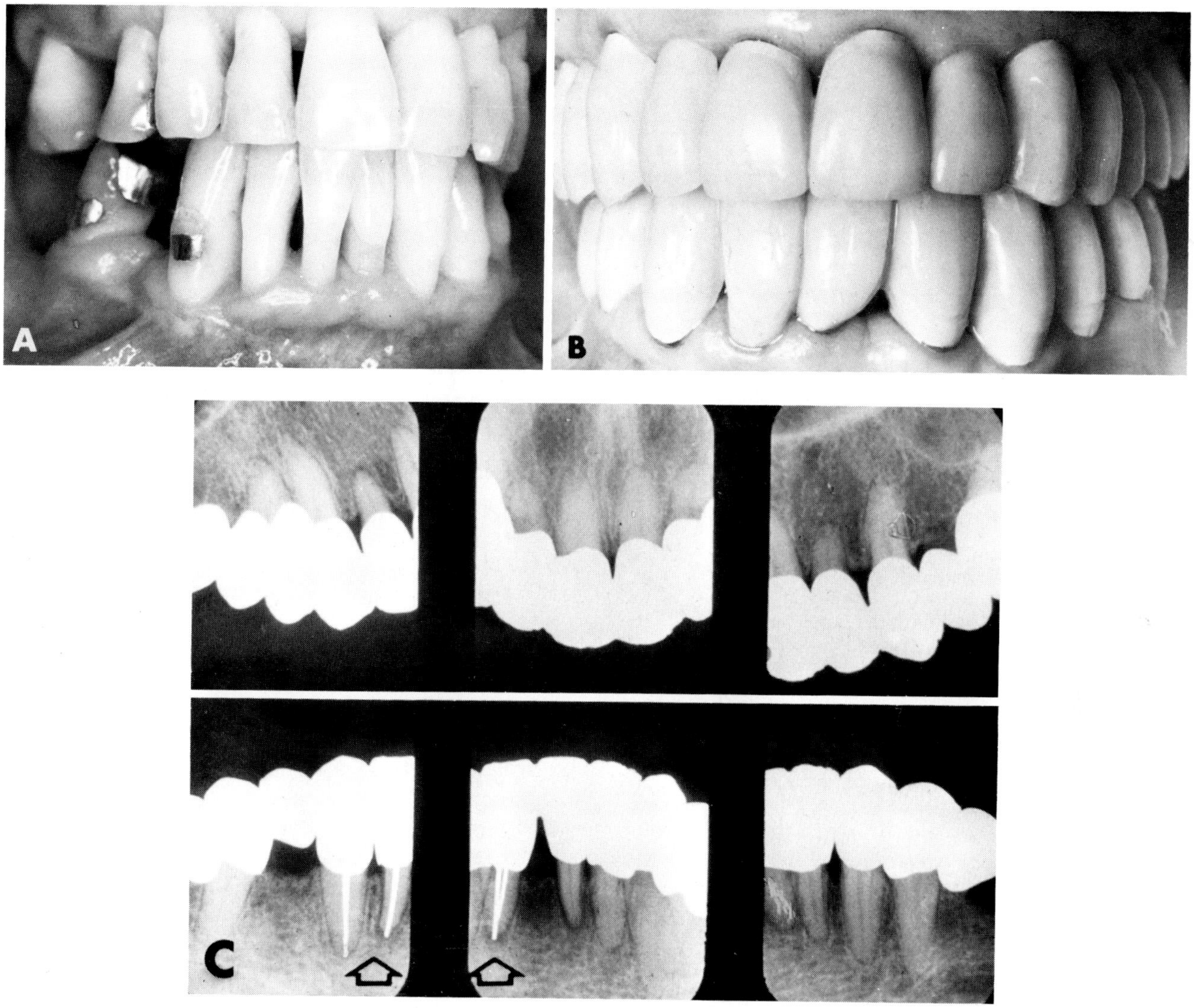

Fig. 1–8. *A*, Postoperative result following complete periodontal therapy. Over half the bony support has been lost around these remaining teeth. Advanced mobility forecasts necessity of full-arch splinting if dentition is to be saved. *B*, Final periodontal prosthesis at time of cementation. This satisfied female patient was horrified by possibility of having to wear full dentures. (Prosthesis by Dr. Harry Bohannan.) *C*, Importance of retaining every abutment tooth through root canal therapy is readily apparent.

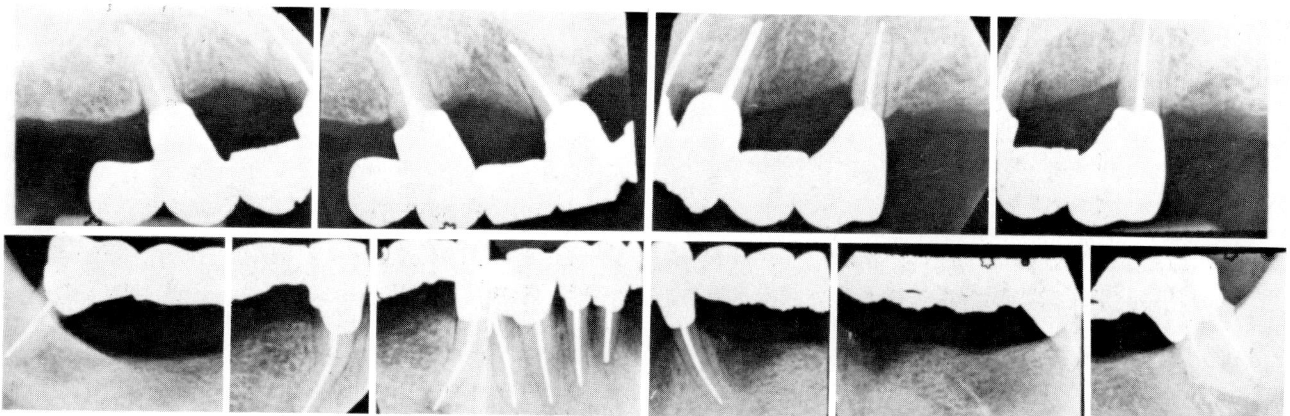

Fig. 1–9. Full periodontal prosthesis utilizing well-treated pulpless teeth. All thirteen remaining teeth required root canal therapy prior to rehabilitation. (Courtesy Dr. Morton Amsterdam.)

used when teeth have drifted labially, orthodontic treatment is impossible, and the tooth must be reduced drastically for jacket crown placement. On occasion a pulp is intentionally removed and the canal filled so that a dowel may be placed for increased crown retention.

In addition to intentional extirpation, successful periodontal prosthesis is frequently dependent on a number of well-treated pulpless teeth. Not only have some of the teeth been intentionally devitalized, but pulp death is a fairly common occurrence in these extensive cases. Five, six, or even eight pulpless teeth are not unusual in periodontal prosthesis (Fig. 1–9).

Indications for Endodontic Therapy

One may be quite dogmatic in listing the ***indications*** for endodontic therapy, possibly leaving the impression that every pulpless tooth, or every tooth in the arch may be treated endodontically. Such is not the case, for there are definite contraindications to endodontic treatment just as there are contraindications to all forms of therapy. ***On the other hand, there are a great number of so-called contraindications which, when examined, may be questioned.*** These charges will be dealt with later. For the moment, however, the true indications will be reviewed.

First of all, the pulpless tooth must be examined thoroughly and a decision to treat should be based on the following questions:

1. Is the tooth needed or important? Does it have an opponent? Will it some day serve as an abutment for prosthesis?
2. Is the tooth salvageable or is it so badly destroyed it cannot be restored?
3. Is the entire dentition so completely broken-down that it would be virtually impossible to restore?
4. Is the tooth serving esthetically, or would the patient be better served by its extraction and a more cosmetic replacement?
5. Is the tooth so severely involved periodontally that it would be lost soon for this reason?
6. Is the patient an appreciative dental patient who truly wants to save his teeth, or is he interested only in extraction?
7. Is the dentist capable of treating the case or are his abilities so limited in this area of practice that he, personally, should not undertake the treatment?

These are all necessary considerations before endodontic therapy can be undertaken. Of them all, the ability of the dentist to practice endodontic therapy is the least significant, because he can readily refer the patient. Unfortunately, many dentists stubbornly refuse to practice or to refer patients for endodontic therapy.

The philosophy some dentists develop toward root canal therapy is directly related to their abilities in the field. The practitioner not trained or not adept in endodontic treatment is often pessimistic about success. He makes excuses to his patient (and to himself) that "this work is generally not successful," or "this treatment is not indicated in molars, they have three canals, you know." What he really means is, he is not equipped by training or experience to handle the case, and rather than show his deficiency by referring the patient, he makes excuses such as, "This treatment is far too expensive and I know you could not afford it." To some extent, these same dentists have flocked to attend the "quick-fix" courses teaching "one-shot" root canal treatment. They would rather use these shoddy methods than learn proper therapy.

The modern, well-trained dentist has no fear of the pulpless tooth. If a large carious exposure develops during cavity preparation, he does not panic and begin procrastinating. On the contrary, he immediately informs the patient of the occurrence and receives permission to proceed with endodontic therapy while the tooth is anesthetized. He is properly equipped to begin pulpectomy within the minute, using completely sterile instruments, packaged and stored for just such an emergency.

The better a dentist is prepared for endodontic therapy, the more treatment he will undertake. Each dentist, on the other hand, must honestly assess his own abilities in endodontics. The decision to treat a case personally or to refer the patient to a colleague must be based on the clinician's evaluation of the difficulty of the case and his own degree of dexterity. The wise dentist will know his limitations and, for the patient's good, will refer the case to a colleague better qualified in the field.

Contraindications to Endodontic Therapy

The literature is replete with contraindications for root canal treatment. These objections are listed according to: (1) status of the patient, (2) dental reasons, and (3) local reasons.

Many of these contraindications, gleaned from the literature, may be questioned. For this reason they are under ***contention.***

Contended Contraindications by Status of the Patient

It is contended that endodontic therapy may be contraindicated by:

1. Age
2. Health of the patient
    a. Rheumatic fever and rheumatic heart disease
    b. Other heart disease
    c. Diabetes
    d. Leukemia and terminal cancer
    e. Radiation necrosis
    f. Tuberculosis and syphilis
    g. Pregnancy
3. Too many treated pulpless teeth
4. Financial position of the patient

CONTENTION: Endodontic Therapy is Contraindicated for Patients Past Middle Life. To consider age, either young or old, as a contraindication for root canal therapy is patently ridiculous. Root canal therapy has been successfully completed for patients as young as two and a half years of age and as old as ninety-six. The infant poses a problem in behavior; yet, if endodontic therapy is indicated, it may be successfully carried out under proper sedation.

The older patient is usually the easiest patient to care for. He has lived a long time, and if he has avoided dentures for sixty to eighty years, he is most appreciative of saving each tooth. The root canals in the "senior citizen" are very fine, having filled-in with secondary-reparative dentin. The major problem in treatment is finding the orifice to the canals, but once found, canal enlargement and obliteration are far simpler than for the youngsters. On the other hand, the elderly patient will be much slower to heal. Oftentimes, two years are required for a good-sized periapical lesion to heal, whereas in the adolescent the same lesion will heal in four to six months. The profession should also recognize that root canal therapy is far less traumatic for both extremes of age than is extraction.

CONTENTION: Endodontic Therapy is Contraindicated for the Very Ill, the Patient in Terminal Illness, or the Pregnant Patient. Many references are made to poor health as a contraindication for endodontic therapy. Actually, the reverse is true for the seriously ill patient. Root canal therapy is greatly preferred to extraction for these patients.

Rheumatic Fever and Rheumatic Heart Disease. For the rheumatic fever patient, elective extraction is contraindicated. Fish and MacLean[23] and Okell and Elliot[24] have shown the severe bacteremia that follows extraction, a shower of bacteria that might well turn mitral stenosis into subacute bacterial endocarditis. This leaves endodontic therapy as first choice of treatment for the pulpless tooth in these patients. For both extraction and endodontic therapy a "prophylactic umbrella" of antibiotics is recommended.[25]

If the acutely ill rheumatic fever patient develops a toothache, the dentist should temporize by removing the caries or restoration, and by placing a zinc oxide-eugenol sedative filling until the patient has recovered and may be treated as a regular office patient. The novice is warned, however, that some acutely ill rheumatic fever patients will have referred pain in their teeth.

Other Heart Disease. Again, root canal therapy is far less traumatic for the heart patient than is extraction. Moreover, a good deal of root canal therapy can be done painlessly and without anesthesia, which is not true of exodontia.

For the heart disease patient, as with any of these serious conditions, one must be careful to achieve a lasting endodontic result. A limited life expectancy is no excuse for shoddy treatment.

Diabetes. Diabetes, mellitus or insipidus, is certainly no contraindication for endodontic treatment. Here again, root canal therapy is far less traumatic and is preferred to extraction. Diabetes patients are frequently treated for advanced periodontal disease, and although healing is delayed, the diabetic usually responds well to therapy as long as his disease is reasonably well controlled.

Chronic Leukemia and Terminal Cancer. Endodontic therapy rather than extraction is by far preferable for the cancer or chronic leukemia victim. On a practical basis it is true: the patient will not live to "amortize his investment." He will, however, be able to live his last few months in oral comfort rather than risk the possibility of suffering an area of necrosis almost sure to follow extraction. Actually, most of the terminal patients suffering leukemia, Hodgkin's disease, or cancer are referred for endodontic therapy by oral surgeons, for many surgeons have had unfortunate experiences with neoplastic patients failing to heal. The patient with hemophilia or hemorrhagic purpura is in the same category as the leukemic victim. For these patients it is far better to practice conservative root canal therapy than to chance a fatal hemorrhage following extraction. For all of these patients periapical surgery is obviously contraindicated.

Some cancer victims, not aware of the terminal nature of their disease, have been referred for treatment. Graciously proceeding with treatment for these patients, in spite of the knowledge they are soon to die, frequently contributes to their optimism toward living. To refuse treatment, or to temporize, is often a crushing blow to their morale.

Radiation Necrosis. Endodontic therapy is indicated for patients who have had extensive radiation of the jaws just as it is for the chronic leukemic victim. Again, it is the oral surgeon who frequently refers these patients to the endodontist, knowing the dire results to follow extraction.[26]

Tuberculosis and Syphilis. These two diseases are grouped together, not because of common origin, but because of their present status of cure. Root canal therapy would certainly be indicated for these patients during a controlled state of their disease and it would be rare indeed to see a patient today in an uncontrolled state. Most luetics are treated as outpatients; the dentist is usually not even aware he is treating a syphilitic patient. Tuberculosis has been virtually wiped out. Most of the present victims are repeaters. Unfortunately, the majority (but by no means all) of the repeaters in today's sanatoria are derelicts from "skid row." They have usually let their oral cavity degenerate to the same level as the rest of their body and mind. Although deserving of dental attention, they are not necessarily appreciative of fine dental care such as root canal therapy.

It may be said that root canal therapy is not only indicated for patients with advanced health problems, but is almost always preferable to extraction.

Pregnancy. Endodontic treatment for the pregnant woman is greatly preferred by most obstetricians over extraction. On the other hand, elective endodontic treatment is best delayed until the second trimester of the pregnancy. The wisdom of waiting is quite apparent. If the patient is destined to miscarry, it will most likely happen during the first trimester. Even though the dental treatment is not responsible for the miscarriage, there is the chance the dentist and dental treatment will be blamed for the event. If a gravid patient develops a toothache during the first trimester of her pregnancy, it is recommended that the dentist temporize, if possible, with caries removal and a zinc oxide-eugenol dressing until the second trimester. Periapical surgery, ***if elective,*** should be avoided at any time during pregnancy.

There is no particular contraindication to endodontic treatment during the third trimester except for the comfort of the patient. Some women, on the other hand, have no complaints toward dental treatment during the final days of their pregnancy. One such patient had endodontic treatment completed while timing her labor contractions. She went directly to the hospital from the clinic and was delivered within two hours.

Many mothers prefer to have their dental treatment completed before delivery, knowing how difficult it will be to keep a dental appointment after the baby arrives.

CONTENTION: Endodontic Therapy is Contraindicated for the Patient Who Already Has Several Treated Pulpless Teeth. It is ridiculous to draw an arbitrary line by saying someone has too many treated pulpless teeth. The criterion for continuing root canal therapy in a certain mouth is the degree of success enjoyed by past endodontic therapy.

We have completed 11 anterior teeth for patients who have had all incisors devitalized in an automobile accident. Other patients, being prepared for extensive rehabilitation, have had 12 to 14 root canals filled. If one canal can be successfully treated, there is no reason why multiple successes cannot be enjoyed.

To fear numerous pulpless teeth as possible foci of infection is to admit pessimism toward success in endodontics and to bow to the adherents of the theory of focal infection. Careful attention to detail will assure almost total success.

Patients with multiple endodontic failures have been seen, having come from Europe where resorbable root canal pastes have long been used. Retreatment of these patients with proper endodontic therapy, enlarging and obturating the partially filled canals, has converted the multiple failures to multiple successes.

CONTENTION: Root Canal Therapy is Contraindicated for Those Patients Unable to Pay for the Therapy. In the past, many dentists, lacking confidence in endodontic therapy and in their ability to perform the treatment, either did not charge the patient for root canal therapy or charged him a pittance. This form of treatment was usually worth what the patient paid. A pessimistic attitude toward endodontics lowered the status of root canal therapy in the eyes of the profession and public alike.

Endodontic treatment, like any other dental treatment, deserves an adequate fee. The dentist's net income from endodontic therapy should be the same as it is from the other areas of dental practice. That some patients cannot afford root canal therapy is obvious. Many patients cannot afford orthodontic therapy, fine bridgework, or porcelain jacket crowns either. The dentist is not expected to give away these services, but he is obligated to seek possible alternative services for his patients. There may be a dental school clinic or a neighborhood health center for referral. Also there appears to be developing a turn-around in health care legislation as well as third-party payment, listing endodontic treatment as an alternative to extraction.

It is disappointing to hear a dentist explain that his patients cannot afford endodontic treatment. When this same dentist learns to perform good root canal therapy, however, he is suddenly surprised to find his patients can now afford endodontic treatment and, what's more, "are requesting treatment now rather than extraction."

In the long run, treating and thus retaining a pulpless tooth is far preferable to extracting the tooth (especially a first permanent molar) and allowing arch collapse. This is particularly true in youngsters. Moreover, root canal treatment and restoration are usually less expensive than extraction and a fixed replacement.

Contended Contraindications for Dental Reasons

Three particular dental situations are ***supposedly*** contraindications for endodontic therapy:

1. Pulpless teeth are not salvageable if there are associated periapical and periodontal lesions.
2. Pulpless teeth are not receptive to orthodontic therapy.
3. Pulpless teeth are not serviceable as abutment teeth.

CONTENTION: Endodontic Therapy is Contraindicated for Those Cases with an Associated Periapical and Periodontal Lesion. It is not always true that a pulpless tooth, also periodontally involved, is contraindicated for endodontic therapy. It is true, however, that the tooth literally has "two strikes against it," and the decision to save or sacrifice will depend, first, on the importance of saving the tooth and, second, on the treatability of the periodontal lesions.

Hiatt has shown that many associated periodontal defects will heal following successful endodontic treatment.[27] This has also been our experience (Fig. 1–10). The criterion for success is based on the origin of the periodontal pocket. If the ***periodontal*** lesion is a ***primary*** lesion that has advanced to meet the periapical lesion, the chance for successful therapy is slim. If, on the other hand, the ***periodontal lesion is secondary to the periapical lesion,*** the prognosis is greatly enhanced.

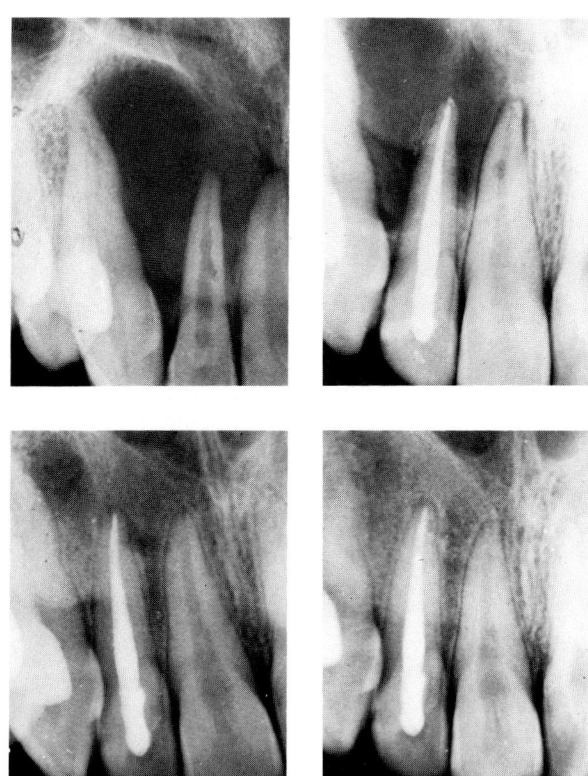

Fig. 1–10. Total osseous repair one year following root canal therapy of lateral incisor considered hopeless. Not only was bony support of this tooth almost totally destroyed, but periodontal ligament was completely detached on labial, and constant drainage through gingival sulcus was present. Primary lesion was periapical as sequela to necrotic pulp. Associated periodontal lesion was entirely secondary.

The dogmatic statement that treatment is contraindicated for "teeth with a fistulous tract connecting the periapical region with the gingival crevice" belies a knowledge of the anatomy of this region. The draining pus from a chronic periapical lesion may break out of the labial cortical plate, work under the periosteum, and evacuate through the gingival sulcus without ever involving the periodontal ligament. In other words, just because drainage comes from the

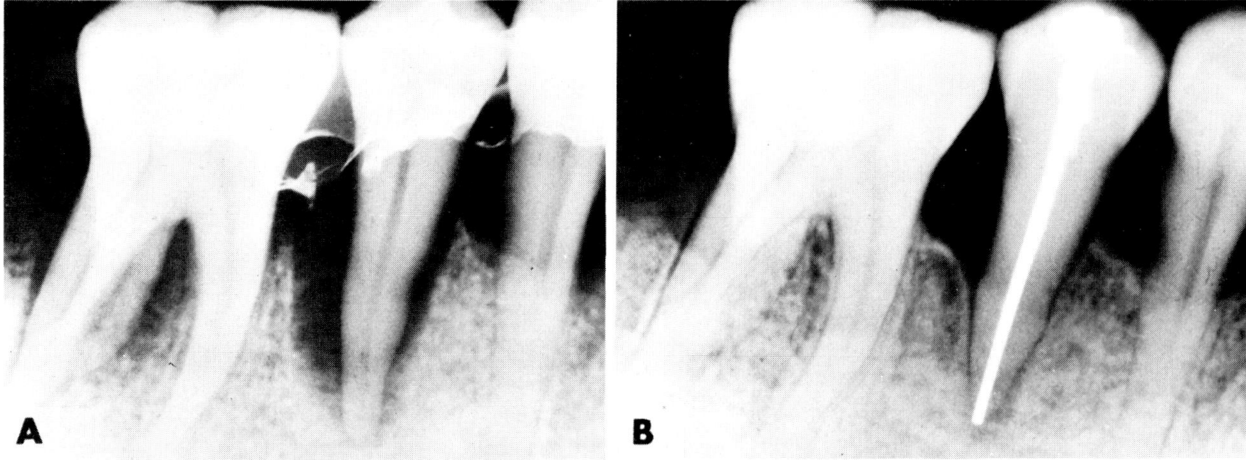

Fig. 1–11. *A,* Advanced periodontal lesions, intrabony in character. Retrogenic infection of pulp of second premolar has caused its death. *B,* Reattachment of periodontal ligaments and repair of alveolar process following curettage of three-wall intrabony lesions. Endodontic therapy of pulpless, second premolar was necessary to ensure this remarkable success. (From Prichard, J. E.: J. Perio., *28*:202, July, 1957.)

gingival sulcus does not necessarily mean it has arrived there via the periodontal ligament space.

If the periodontal and periapical lesions are treated concurrently, the chances for success are excellent (see p. 641). Even the case in which the involved periodontal lesion becomes distressingly apparent after treatment is often amenable to treatment if located in an accessible area. A favorite location for these draining sulci is the labial or lingual aspect of anterior teeth that have been involved in a traumatic accident. In these cases, not only has the pulp been devitalized, but the periodontal ligament and epithelial attachment have also been destroyed. The operation to repair this defect is shown on page 643.

Deep intrabony pockets in the molar region (Fig. 1–11) will respond to treatment in the manner early described by Prichard, if three bony walls exist.[28] If a pulpless tooth is also involved in the lesion, root canal therapy must be completed first to eliminate the toxic canal products that would act as a deterrent to healing.

Any time a ***periodontally involved pulpless*** tooth is treated, it is a risky undertaking. Therefore, this expensive and time-consuming procedure should be reserved for cases in which saving the tooth is highly important. The dentist must also be adept in performing the required periodontal procedures, for success depends so much on optimal treatment. Strategic abutment teeth for periodontal prosthesis (Fig. 1–12) and cases of single root involvement in the molars (Fig. 1–13) (amputation) are examples of advanced periodontal involvement often requiring endodontic intervention. All attempts should be made to save esthetic anterior teeth even though these teeth are involved pulpally and periodontally (Fig. 1–14).

CONTENTION: Pulpless Teeth Are Not Receptive to Orthodontic Movement. How this "old wives' tale" began is difficult to determine, but it is that, just that. Well-treated pulpless teeth will respond to orthodontic movement just as readily and successfully as vital teeth.[29] As a matter of fact, orthodontic movement might well stimulate periapical repair so that healing is accelerated (Fig. 1–15).

The pulpless tooth that cannot be moved orthodontically is the ankylosed tooth. Frequently, following partial avulsion or total avulsion and replantation, the root of the tooth and alveolar bone become inseparably attached, with no intervening periodontal ligament. This tooth is ankylosed. Orthodontic movement depends on the constant destruction, regrowth, and attachment of the periodontal ligament. Even a tiny area of ankylosis 2 mm. square will prevent orthodontic movement, or even eruption for that matter (Fig. 1–16).

CONTENTION: The Pulpless Tooth Is Not Serviceable as an Abutment Tooth for Fixed or Removable Partial Dentures. Here again we are dealing with a half-truth. If a pulpless tooth is well treated, even if

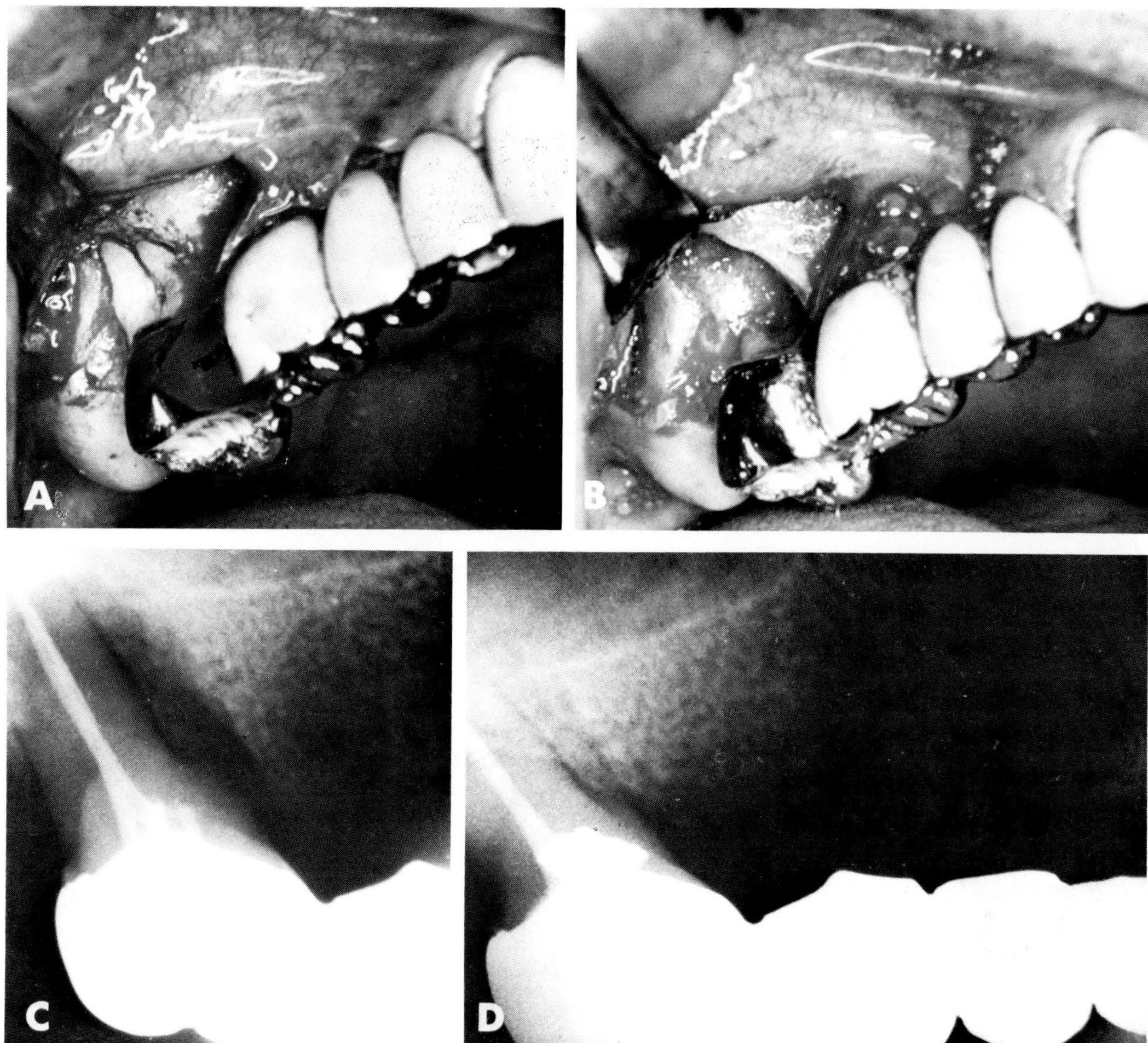

Fig. 1–12. *A,* Retraction of surgical flap reveals extent of periodontal lesion completely involving buccal roots of second molar abutment of full-arch periodontal prosthesis. Root canal therapy of healthy, palatal root is completed prior to surgery. *B,* Total amputation of buccal roots reveals extent of cavernous periodontal lesion. *C,* Extensive bone loss, seen above, is apparent in roentgenogram taken at time of treatment. (Root outline retouched for clarity.) *D,* Osseous repair, one year following buccal root amputation. Solidly supported palatal root serves as adequate terminal abutment for full-arch prosthesis. Endodontic therapy was completed in 1959 and has been successful since that time. (Courtesy Dr. Dudley H. Glick.)

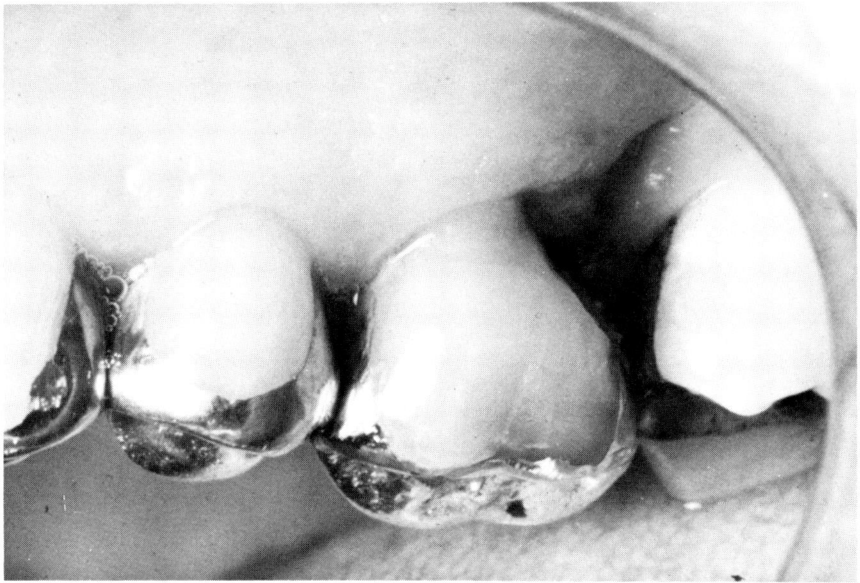

Fig. 1–13. Amputation of periodontally involved distobuccal root allows retention of well-restored maxillary first molar. Root canal therapy of two remaining roots is necessary. Buccal-lingual narrowing of occlusal table reduces forces of mastication on these roots. Vulva-like soft tissue defect should be corrected with gingivoplasty.

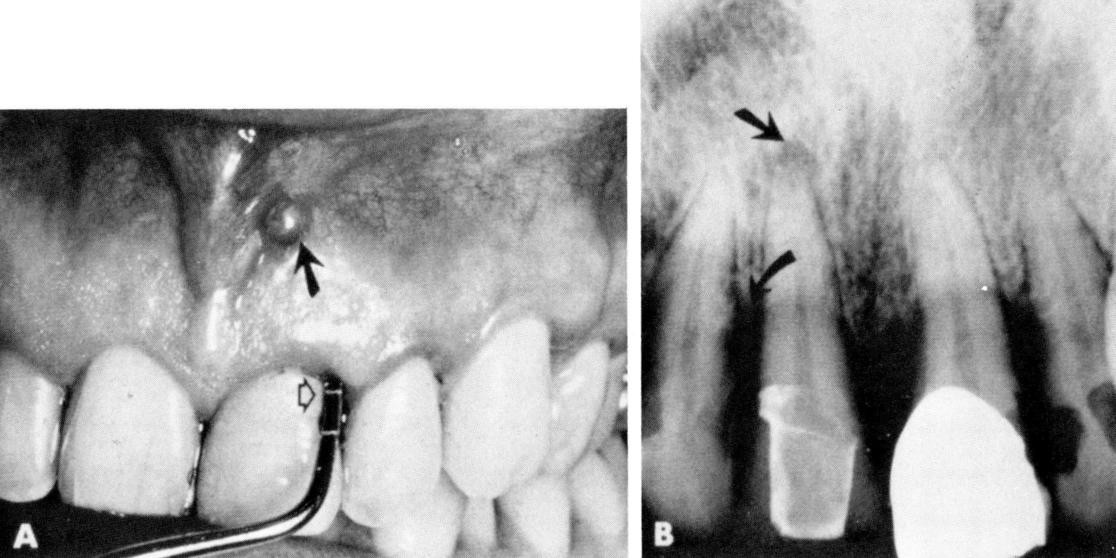

Fig. 1–14. Well-restored maxillary central incisor with periodontal and periapical involvement. Draining stoma (large arrow) associated with periapical lesion. Probing (white arrow) reveals total loss of labial periodontal attachment. Concomitant endodontic-periodontic therapy is indicated. *B,* Roentgenogram of case illustrated in *A*. Associated periodontal and periapical lesions (arrows) of periodontally involved tooth are also pulpless. Left central incisor is not pulpless, although stoma "points" above this tooth.

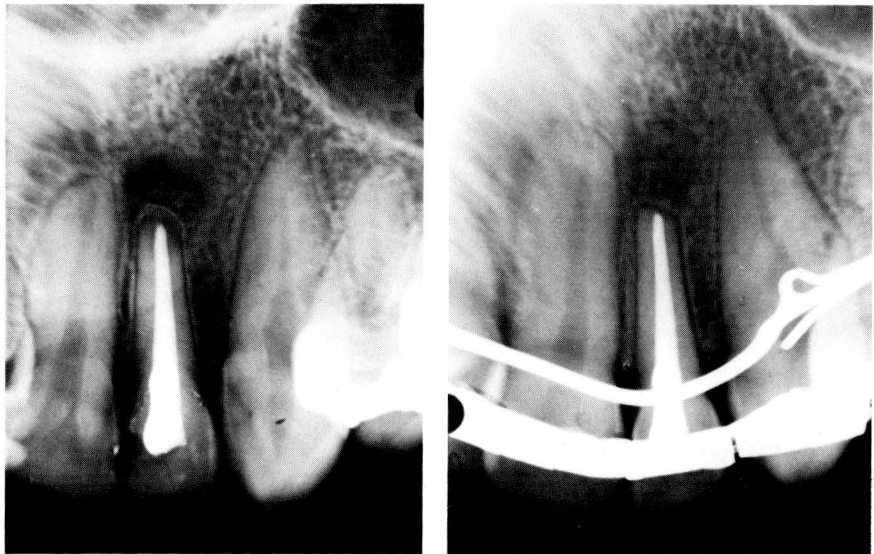

Fig. 1–15. Complete osseous repair *(right)* only four months following endodontic treatment, in spite of active orthodontic treatment apparent from width of periodontal ligament space.

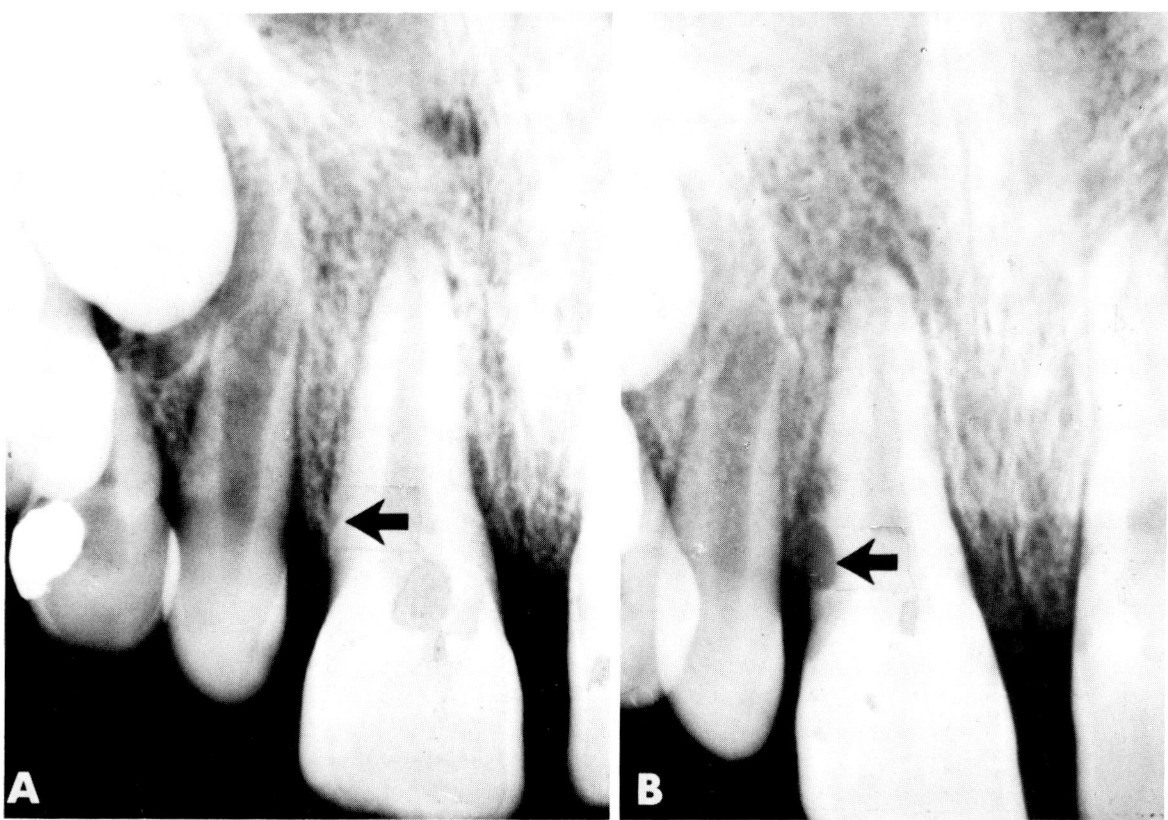

Fig. 1–16. *A,* Careful inspection (by hindsight) of roentgenogram taken one month following severe impact injury, reveals a point of ankylosis and beginning external root resorption (arrow). *B,* Roentgenogram taken six months after *A* reveals extensive resorption and ankylosis (arrow).

initially it had a periapical lesion present, it may well serve as an abutment. The key to success lies in the probable outcome of the endodontic therapy. If one is confident of success in the treated root canal, the tooth may be recommended for immediate crowning as an abutment tooth. Occasionally, the recommendation is made to wait six months to evaluate the result obtained from the root canal treatment.

If, on the other hand, a failure of endodontic treatment occurs, the abutment tooth may be retreated by entering back through the crown, removing the ineffective root canal filling, recleaning and reshaping the canal, medicating, and finally reobturating. In the event a large retention post blocks access to the canal, but the tooth is readily accessible to periapical surgical treatment, a retrofilling could be placed as a corrective measure.

Contended Contraindications for Local Oral Reasons

Endodontic local therapy is said to be contraindicated because of certain local conditions:

1. The periapical area associated with the pulpless tooth involves over one-third of the root length.
2. The periapical lesion is an apical cyst.
3. The involved tooth is badly broken down by caries.
4. The involved tooth is badly fractured.
5. The involved tooth has a tortuous canal.
6. The involved tooth has advanced pulpal recession.
7. The involved tooth has an open, flaring apex.
8. The involved tooth has a broken instrument in the canal.
9. The involved tooth has a mechanical root perforation.
10. The involved tooth has perforating internal root resorption.
11. The involved tooth has external root resorption.
12. The involved tooth is hopelessly discolored.
13. The involved tooth is wholly or partially luxated.
14. The involved tooth has had previous endodontic treatment which has failed.

The excuses listed above have all been given frequently for not treating a given pulpless tooth. Each of these reasons will be explored as to its verity.

CONTENTION: Endodontic Therapy Is Contraindicated if the Periapical Area Associated with a Pulpless Tooth Involves Over One-Third of the Root. The size of a periapical lesion apparently has no relation to the ability of the body to repair the lesion. As Figure 1–10 illustrates, enormous lesions will heal completely following endodontic therapy. By removing the source of the irritant, which lies within the canal, and thereafter completely filling the canal space, the periapical lesion should heal no matter what its size.

CONTENTION: Endodontic Therapy Is Contraindicated if the Periapical Lesion is an Apical Cyst. This contraindication to endodontic therapy is quite untrue. First of all, it is difficult, if not impossible, to diagnose accurately an apical cyst by roentgenogram.[30–32] For this reason, one would ***not*** be justified in rejecting endodontic treatment of a tooth involved with an apical cyst on the basis of roentgenographic evidence alone. Bhaskar has shown that over 42% of all periapical lesions are apical cysts.[33] It is quite obvious that when teeth involved with apical cysts are treated endodontically, whether or not the cyst is enucleated, the periapical osseous defect will repair as readily as any other intrabony lesion (Fig. 1–17).

CONTENTION: Endodontic Therapy is Contraindicated if the Pulp-Involved Tooth is Badly Broken Down by Caries. This is a charge of contraindication that may be true, but it is not entirely true. Each case must be decided on its own merits. First of all, is the tooth so badly destroyed that it cannot be restored even if treated endodontically? In some cases the carious destruction is so advanced (Fig. 1–18) it would be virtually impossible to restore the tooth to service.

If the tooth is this badly decayed, it must be evaluated on the basis of its usefulness. For example, a severely involved molar tooth that has no opponent or may be readily replaced by a bridge would not be a good candidate for endodontic therapy and restoration. On the other hand, a tooth needed as a bridge abutment must be saved at all costs. A strategic tooth can be saved by periodontic-endodontic therapy, restored with a dowel crown and serve as an excellent bridge abutment. One method of salvaging such a case is to resort to periodontal surgery. If the tooth is decayed to below the gingiva, and it is vital that the tooth be saved, a gingivoplasty or apically repositioned flap will be necessary to establish a gingival finish margin (Fig. 1–19). By performing this procedure before endodontic treatment, the clamp may be placed and the tooth treated under aseptic conditions.

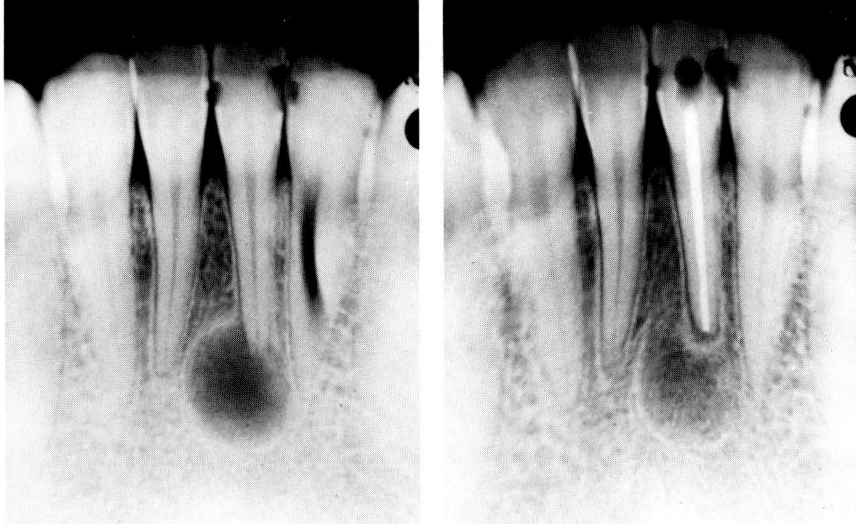

Fig. 1–17. Classic apical cyst *(left)* apparent in pretreatment roentgenogram. Total repair of cystic cavity in six-month recall film is signalled by complete lamina dura which has developed periapically. Biopsy confirmed initial diagnosis of apical cyst.

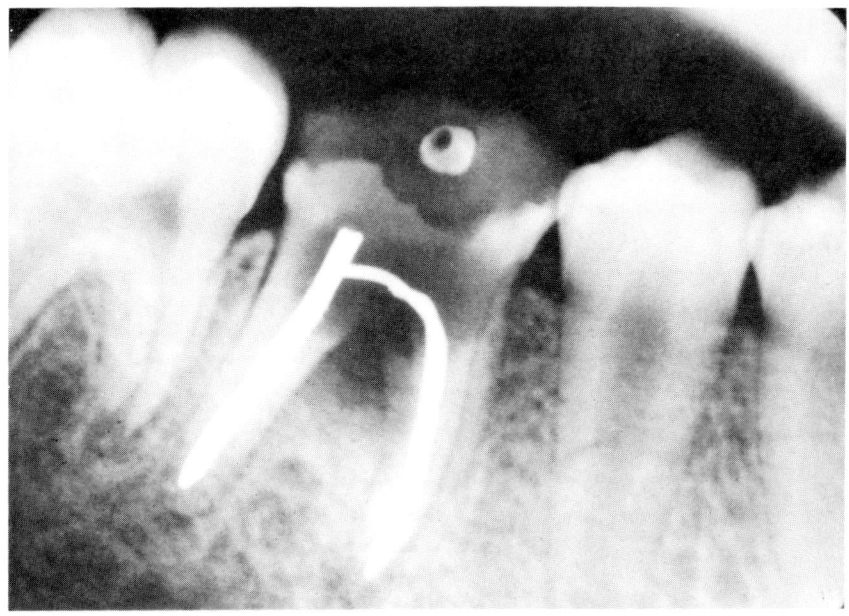

Fig. 1–18. Carious destruction of well-treated pulpless tooth demonstrates necessity for proper restoration immediately following endodontic therapy.

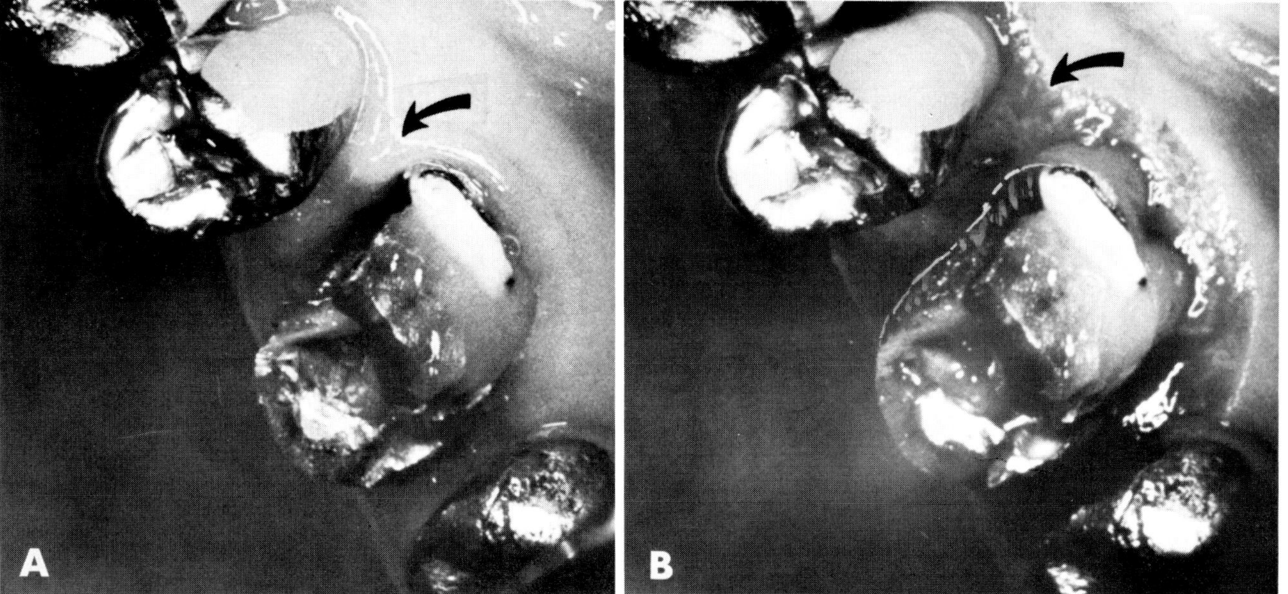

Fig. 1–19. *A,* Carious lesion beneath defective full crown has extended subgingivally as well as into pulp. *B,* Simple gingivoplasty has exposed apical extent of carious lesion. By this combined approach, rubber dam may be placed for endodontic therapy and finish line for new restoration is established. (Retouched to clarify margins.)

If it is ***absolutely necessary,*** virtually all teeth may be retained if caries or periodontal destruction has not advanced to an irreparable stage.

CONTENTION: Endodontic Therapy Is Contraindicated if the Tooth Is Badly Fractured. Here again, as with the problem of advanced caries, each case must be decided on its own evidence. Some teeth are hopelessly fractured (Fig. 1–20), but this fact may not be readily apparent unless the roentgenogram and the involved tooth are carefully examined (Fig. 1–21).

The dentist must be cautioned not to be too hasty about extraction in borderline cases. Just because a fracture of the crown in a youngster extends under the gingiva is no reason to consider the case hopeless. One must remember that the tooth has not yet reached full eruption and the cementoenamel junction may still be well below the margin of the gingiva, which in turn is probably swollen, and thus elongated, from the trauma.

Under these circumstances, the gingivectomy may again be used to uncover the margin and depth of fracture. If the fracture continues well down into the periodontal attachment of a single-rooted tooth, the prognosis is quite hopeless, for a periodontal defect will develop in spite of any attempt to restore the tooth following endodontic therapy.

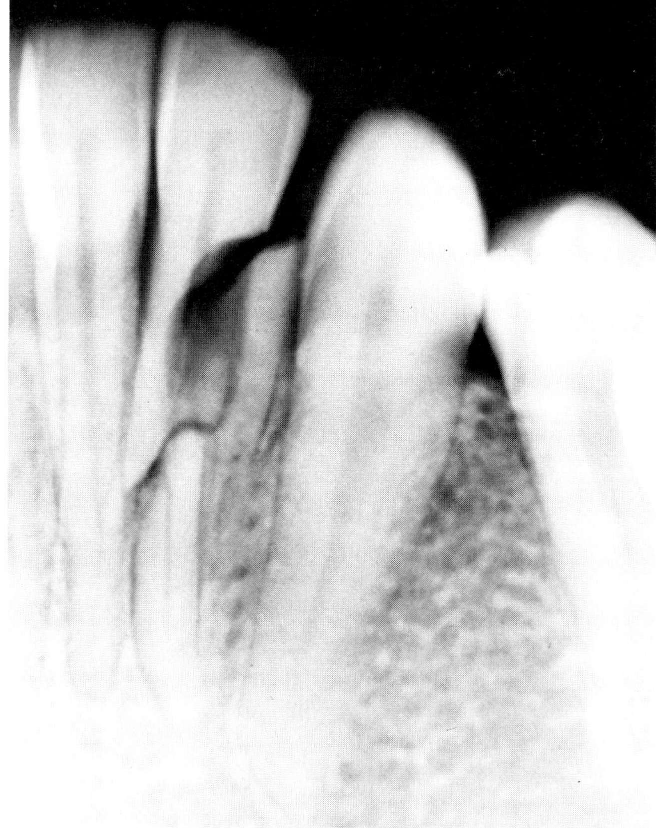

Fig. 1–20. Comminuted fracture of tooth requires no great diagnostic acumen to establish hopeless prognosis.

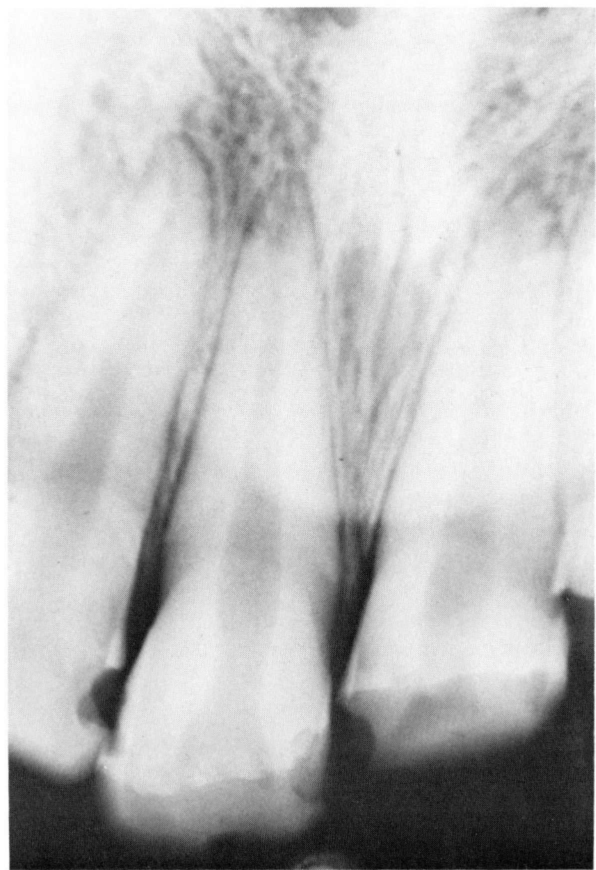

Fig. 1–21. Four maxillary incisors with coronal fractures into pulp. Roentgenogram is necessary to determine whether root fracture has occurred and stage of root development and apical closure. Immediate pulpectomy and root canal filling is indicated for all four incisors.

The multirooted teeth, on the other hand, may be saved if the fracture is along the lines of root design. Figure 16–26 shows just such a maxillary molar which split mesiodistally. The buccal roots have been retained by endodontic treatment and the tooth has been restored to service.

CONTENTION: Endodontic Therapy Is Contraindicated Because the Involved Tooth Has Tortuous Canal Anatomy or Very Fine Lumen. Although canal tortuosity contributes greatly to the problem of clinical endodontics, it does not render treatment impossible (Fig. 1–22). Canals with fine lumen, bayonet-shaped canals, or defalcation and bifurcation of root canals are other clinical situations that arise (Fig. 1–23).

Most of these problems may be solved with patience, perseverance, a lubricant, and fine sharp instruments. The standardized instruments, used in the presence of the chelating agent, ethylene diamine tetracetic acid (EDTA), or antiseptic lubricant such as R-C Prep, will, in the majority of cases, follow bizarre canal anatomy (pp. 202–205).

The extremely curved root canal may be handled with ingenuity. This situation may call for decuspation or amputation of the root if the canal cannot be enlarged (Fig. 1–24). If the canal has been instrumented but cannot be filled in a conventional manner, it has been found expedient to obliterate the canal with a new sterile instrument, broken off and cemented to place (Fig. 1–25) (see p. 252). In one manner or another, most cases may be completed in spite of the canal anatomy.

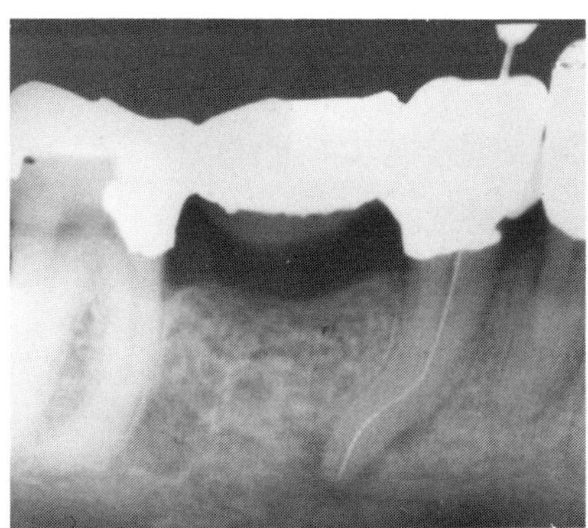

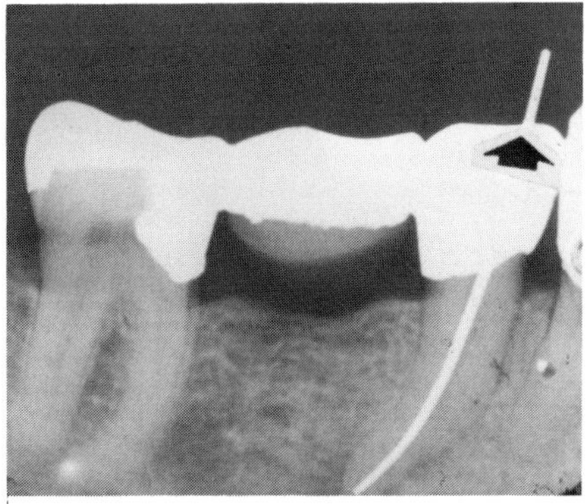

Fig. 1–22. Severe bayonet curve of this canal does not preclude its successful treatment. Roentgenogram on right reveals canal may be straightened into gradual curve and successfully obturated. Notice occlusal cavity has been skewed far to mesial (arrow) to accommodate instrumentation.

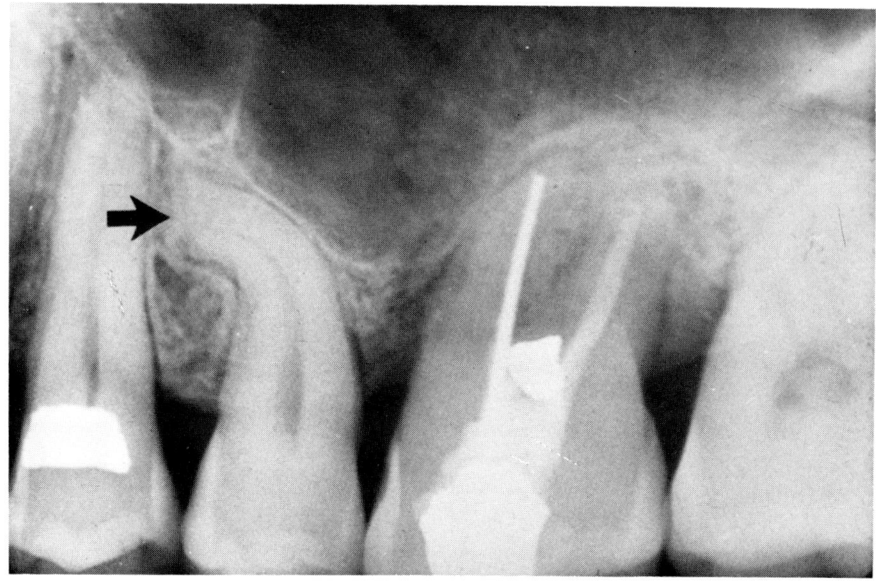

Fig. 1–23. Severe mesial defalcation (sickle shape) of maxillary second premolar. Careful instrumentation of this curve would be necessary to prevent shelf formation or perforation into maxillary sinus. (Courtesy Dr. Dudley H. Glick.)

CONTENTION: Endodontic Therapy Is Contraindicated Because the Involved Tooth Has Advanced Pulp Recession. There is no question that far-advanced pulp recession makes endodontic therapy much more difficult, but it certainly does not render treatment impossible.

The surgical-length contra-angle bur allows the operator to "reach" into the tooth 13 to 14 mm., which is 4 or 5 mm., further than one can advance with a standard-length contra-angle bur. By using the surgical-length bur in the miniature contra-angle, one may extend the cut another 2 or 3 mm. into the tooth (Fig. 1–26). This entire procedure must be handled with great care (see p. 181).

The retrosurgical approach may also be used, and the canal filled from the apex.

All in all, there are few cases that must be rejected for pulp recession.

CONTENTION: Endodontic Therapy Is Contraindicated Because the Involved Tooth Has an Open Flaring Apex. The pulpless tooth, devitalized at an early age before the root end has formed and closed, poses a special problem in obliteration. The tooth with the open flaring apex may be endodontically treated, however, and quite successfully. The first approach should be to encourage the continued growth of the root according to its genetic "blueprint"—the so-called ***apexification*** procedure (Fig. 1–27). Fortunately, this procedure leads to a reawakening of root formation which ceased with premature pulpal death. Following the new growth, root canal therapy must be completed, however, to obturate any tiny opening into the canal. Apexification has proved to be successful for youngsters. But in the event that this procedure fails, special techniques have been devised for filling through the apex; the so-called retrofilling (Fig. 1–28). If the methods used are designed specifically to overcome the problem of the "blunderbuss" canal, the great majority of these cases may be treated successfully (see pp. 689–699).

CONTENTION: Endodontic Therapy Is Contraindicated Because the Involved Tooth Has a Broken Instrument in the Canal. As the study of endodontic failures indicates (p. 34), the number of failures from broken instruments is negligible. As previously noted, the broken instrument itself may serve as an adequate root canal filling if it is locked into the dentin as it is twisted off. A broken instrument may also be bypassed and the canal obliterated beyond the instrument with softened or liquified gutta percha (p. 247). Broken instruments rarely can be removed. If the instrument cannot be removed or bypassed, it may be necessary to fill the apex by retrofilling.

All facts considered, the broken instrument need not be the formidable obstacle to success it once was.[34]

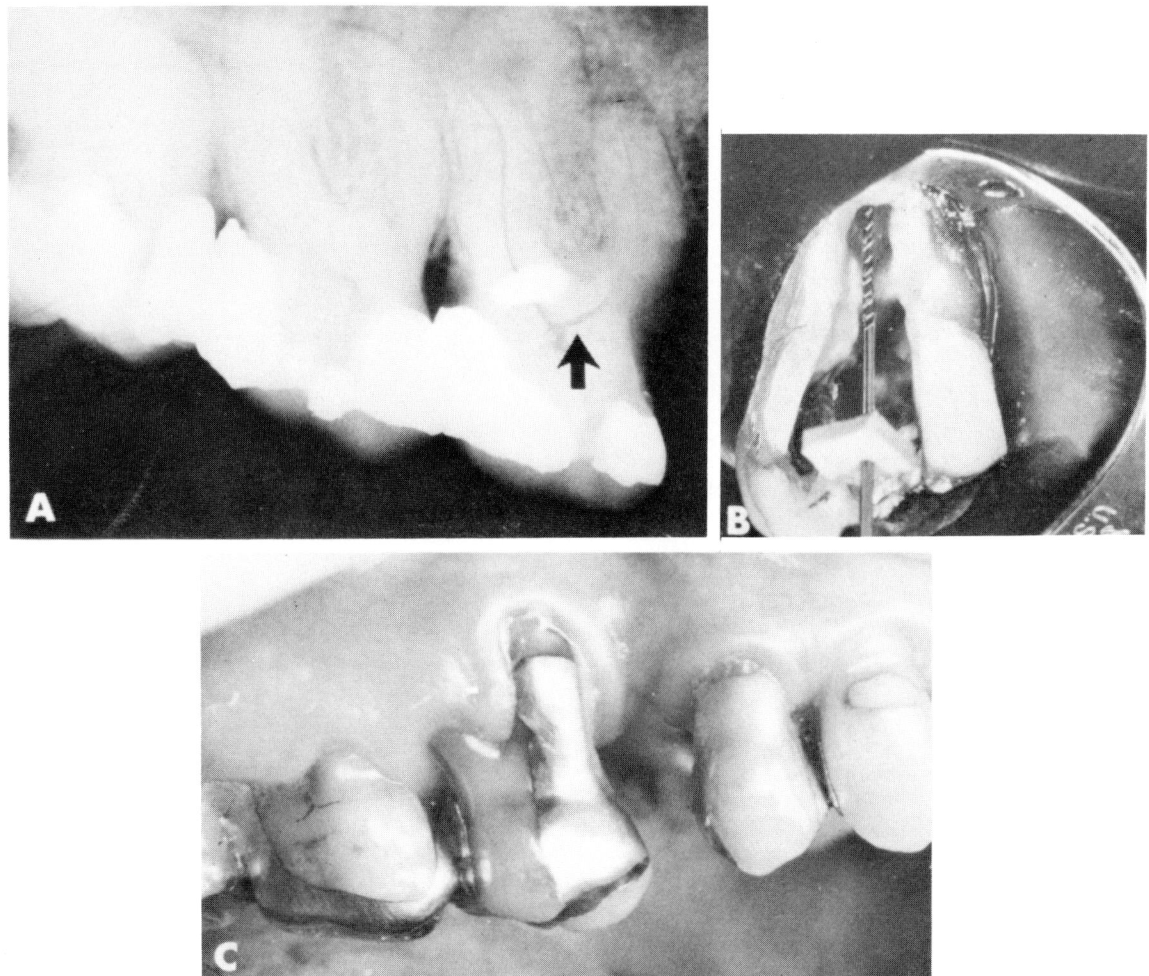

Fig. 1–24. *A*, Decuspation is necessary to establish adequate access into mesiobuccal canal of maxillary first molar which enters pulp chamber at acute angle (arrow). Without decuspation, instrument would be directed from distal and virtually impossible to use. *B*, Decuspation of entire mesiobuccal area grants perfect access into otherwise hopelessly curved canal. Notice verticality of operating instrument. *C*, Final restoration in amalgam of area of decuspation restores tooth to adequate function. Gingival recession was present prior to treatment.

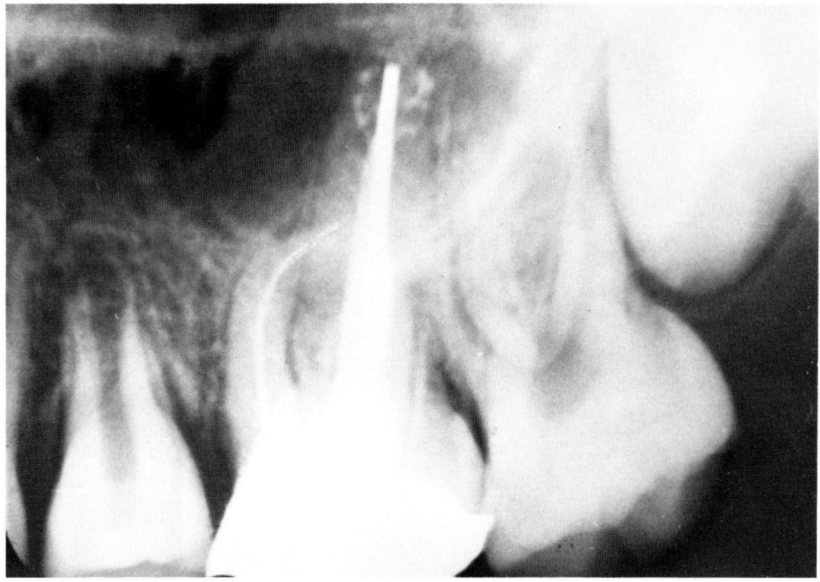

Fig. 1–25. Obturation of severely curved canal accomplished with sterile instrument purposely fractured and cemented in place to act as root canal filling. Silver or gutta percha points would be difficult to use in this canal.

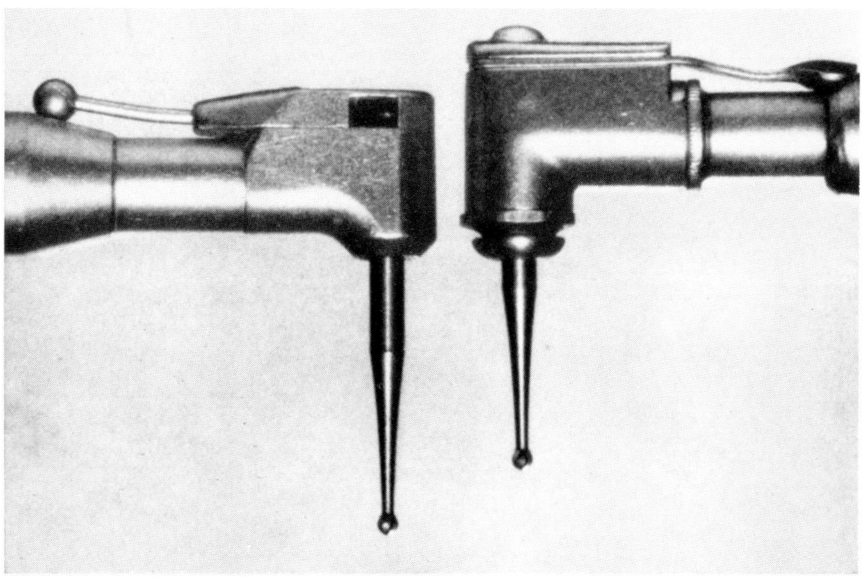

Fig. 1–26. Length of reach of surgical-length burs compared in two handpieces. When nose of miniature handpiece *(left)* rests against occlusal surface, "reach" of 17 mm. may be obtained with this bur. Surgical-length bur in regular contra-angle *(right)* reaches only 13 mm. In addition, "surgical" bur gives an "added" reach of 4 or 5 mm. over regular-length contra-angle bur.

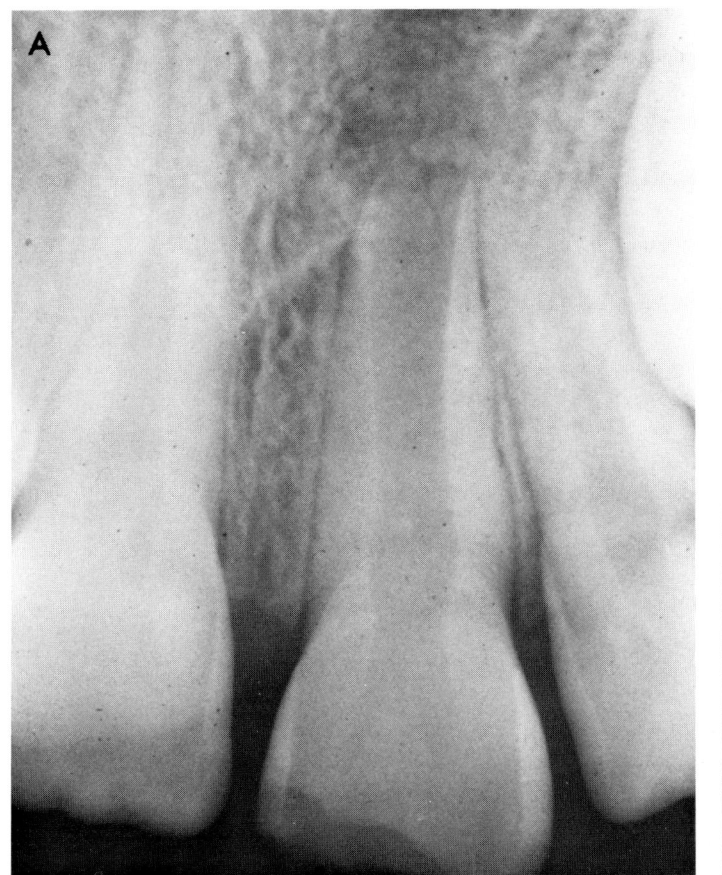

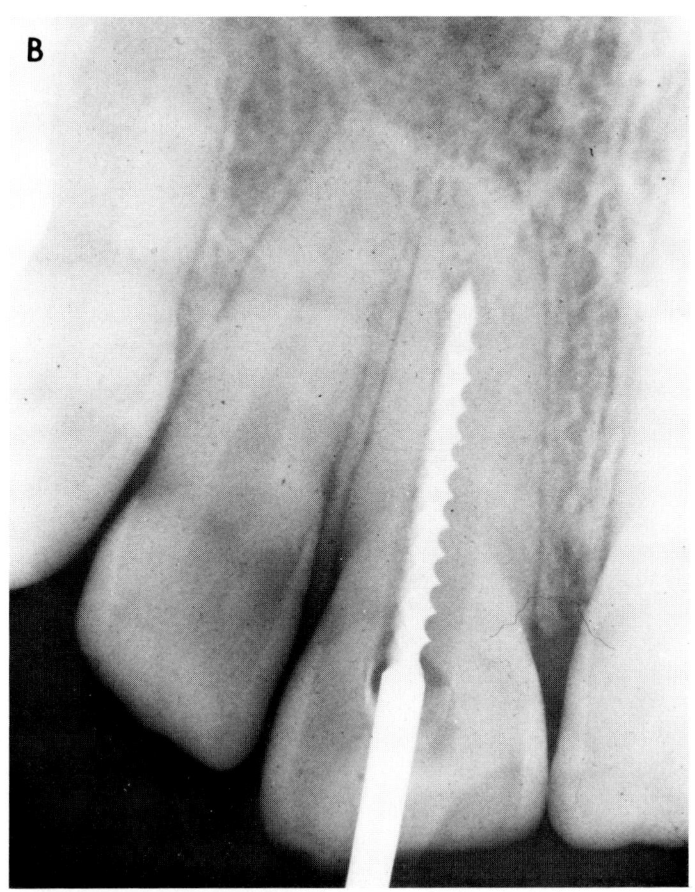

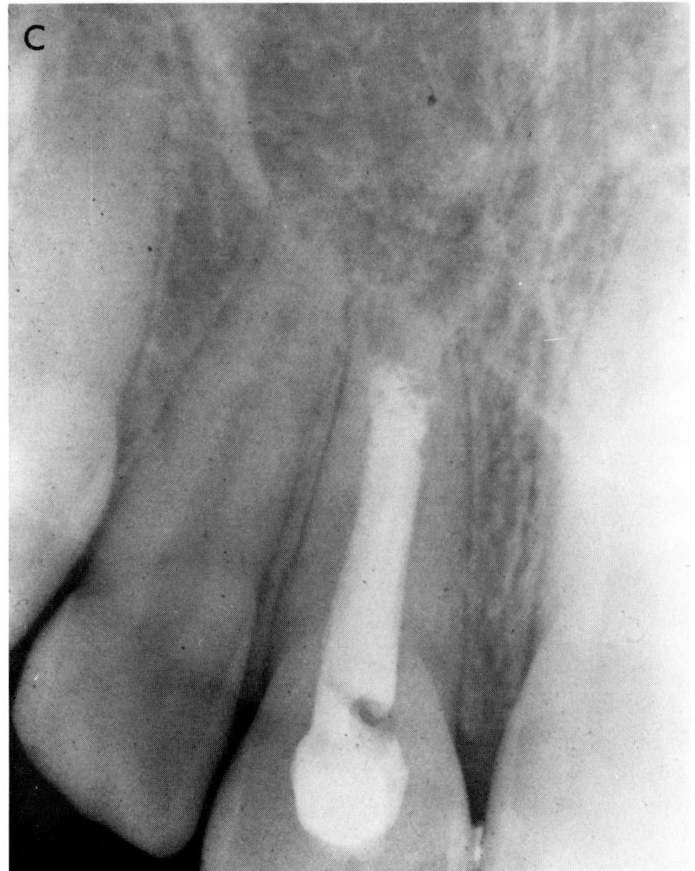

Fig. 1–27. Reawakened root growth termed "apexification." *A,* Pulp devitalized by trauma in 8-year-old child. Periapical inflammation develops and root growth ceases. *B,* Two-year recall. Probing with sharp instrument proves definite apical development. No improvement was apparent after one year of therapy. *C,* Permanent root canal filling placed after 24 months of treatment. No filling material could be expressed apically. (From Frank, A. L.: Dent. Clin. N. Amer., p. 675, Nov., 1967.)

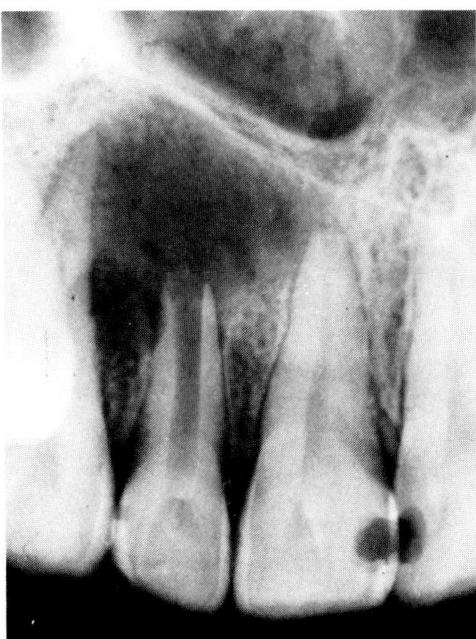
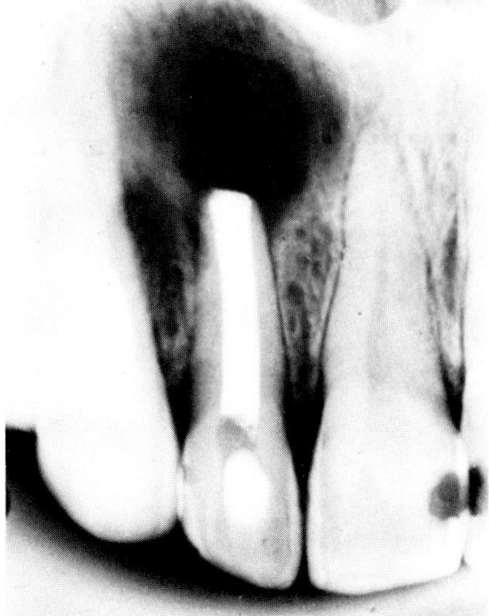

Fig. 1–28. *Left,* Flaring apex of incompletely formed root follows pulpal death caused by impact injury at early age. *Right,* Obturation of "blunderbuss" canal is accomplished by retrofilling from surgical approach. (Ingle, J. I., Dental Digest, *62*:410, Sept., 1956.)

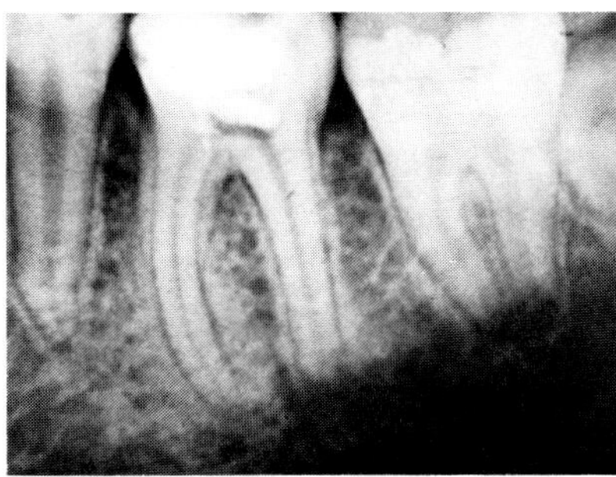
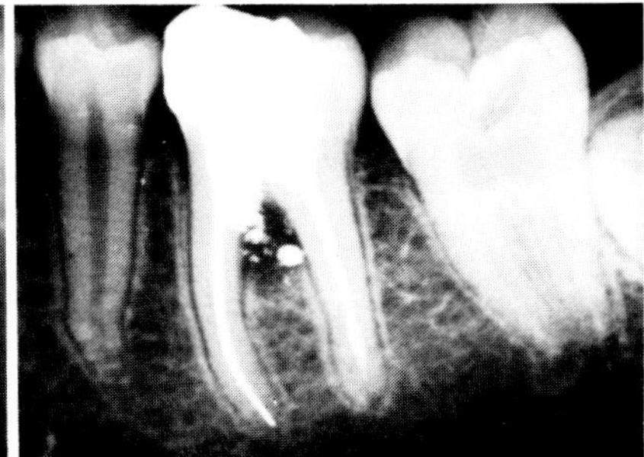

Fig. 1–29. Perforation through floor of pulp chamber during pulpotomy is not revealed until root canal therapy is completed *(right)* and filling material is forced into furca. Failure of pulpotomy could well have been related to initial perforation. Cavit should be used to repair such perforations before treatment.

CONTENTION: Endodontic Therapy is Contraindicated Because the Involved Tooth Has a Procedural Root Perforation. There is no question that procedural root perforation will condemn some teeth to extraction. Again, it is a matter of degree or position of the perforation that determines whether the tooth can be saved (Fig. 1–29).

Perforations through the pulp floor of a molar or premolar may frequently be repaired. Perforations through the labial aspect of an anterior tooth or premolar root canal may be repaired by using a surgical approach (p. 674). On the other hand, some perforations are too gross, or are perforated in a palatal or lingual position, factors that preclude an attempt to salvage the damaged tooth (Fig. 1–30).

CONTENTION: Endodontic Therapy Is Contraindicated Because the Involved Tooth Has Been Perforated by Internal Resorption. As is the case with procedural perforation, the degree and position of the perforation of the root by internal resorption is the determining factor in saving an involved tooth.

Occasionally the situation may be handled entirely as an internal problem; that is, the metaplastic pulp causing the internal resorption may be extirpated and the canal and defect obliterated through the coronal approach (pp. 244–245).

On the other hand, it may be necessary to approach the defect ***surgically*** and fill the defect with an extraradicular filling technique rather than the usual intraradicular approach. This would again call for the

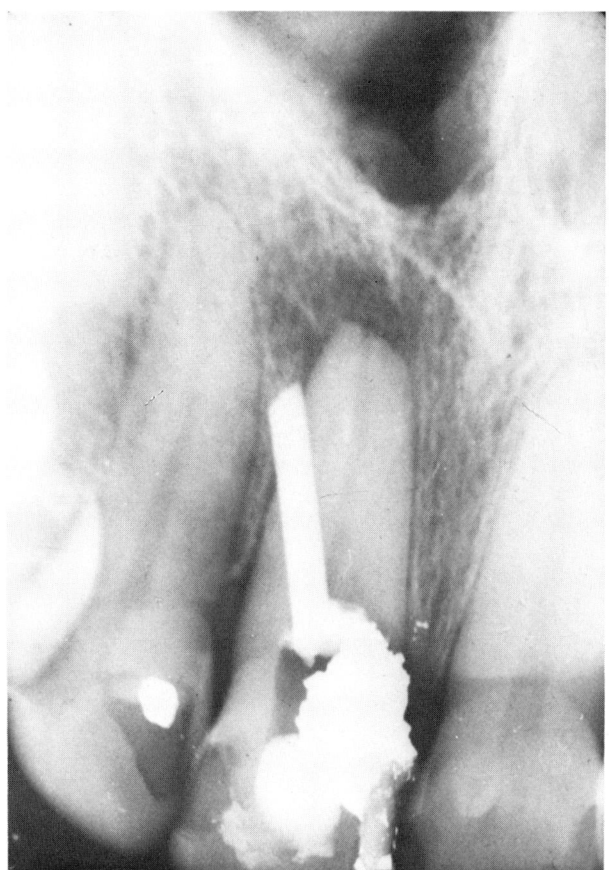

Fig. 1–30. Massive perforation probably caused by use of large bur for canal preparation. This error, combined with total destruction by gouging of mesial half of crown, condemned this tooth to extraction.

position of the defect to be toward the labial aspect of an anterior tooth or buccal in the maxillary posterior teeth. If the perforation from internal resorption involves one root of a multirooted tooth, it is altogether possible to totally amputate the involved root and treat the other canals by endodontic means (pp. 676–677).

All in all, decisions dealing with perforation by internal resorption must be made on an individual basis, each case to be reviewed on its own merits.

CONTENTION: Endodontic Therapy Is Contraindicated Because the Involved Tooth Has External Root Resorption Present. External root resorption is a controversial subject. Therefore, to make a categorical statement that teeth involved with external root resorption may or may not be saved is illogical. Again, each case must be reviewed on its own merits.

As shown in the evaluation of endodontic failures (p. 34), a number of failures (7.7%) were due to continuing external ***root end*** resorption. All of the cases that failed by resorption were maxillary lateral incisors (Fig. 1–31). On the other hand, external ***root end*** resorption of other teeth, particularly the mandibular molars, appears to be self-limiting when the root canals are filled and the inflammatory process is terminated by healing.

External root resorption of the lateral walls of the root is not comparable in healing capacity to external root end resorption. Lateral root resorption is frequently related to traumatic injury of the suspensory apparatus of the tooth. Once this process has begun, and ankylosis between bone and tooth develops, it is difficult to interrupt (p. 434).

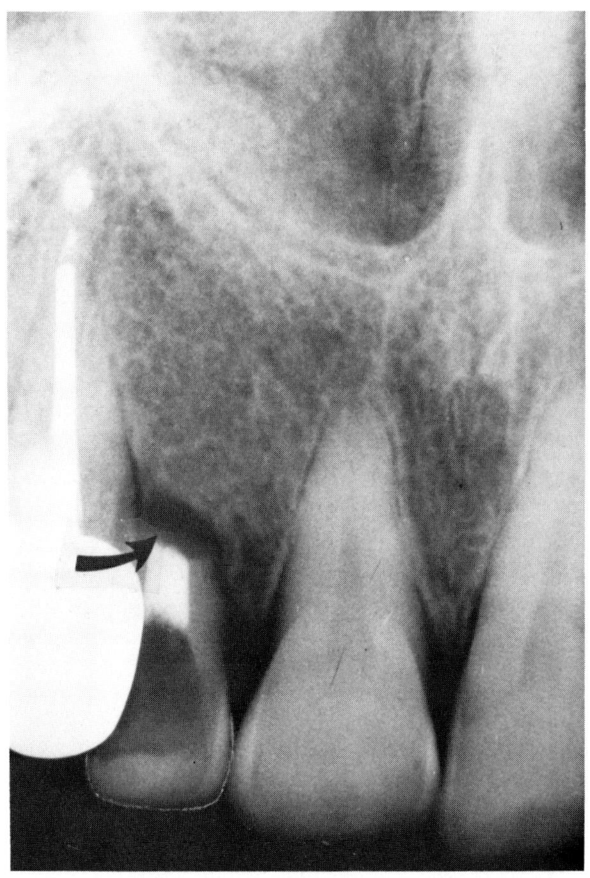

Fig. 1–31. Continued root resorption of maxillary lateral incisor following root canal therapy (arrow). Two attempts by surgical intervention to interrupt resorptive process have failed.

Occasionally, when the perforating defect is in an operable position, a successful result may be obtained. On the other hand, the resorbed defect may sometimes be restored only to have the resorption continue until the root is completely resorbed. There appears to be no rule of thumb for prognosticating the outcome of this type of resorption. This is especially true when internal root resorption perforates to the external surface of the root and concomitant external resorption also develops (Fig. 1–32).

CONTENTION: Endodontic Therapy Is Contraindicated Because the Involved Tooth Is Hopelessly Discolored. Discoloration of a pulpless tooth *per se* should never contraindicate endodontic therapy. First of all, many discolored pulpless teeth may be

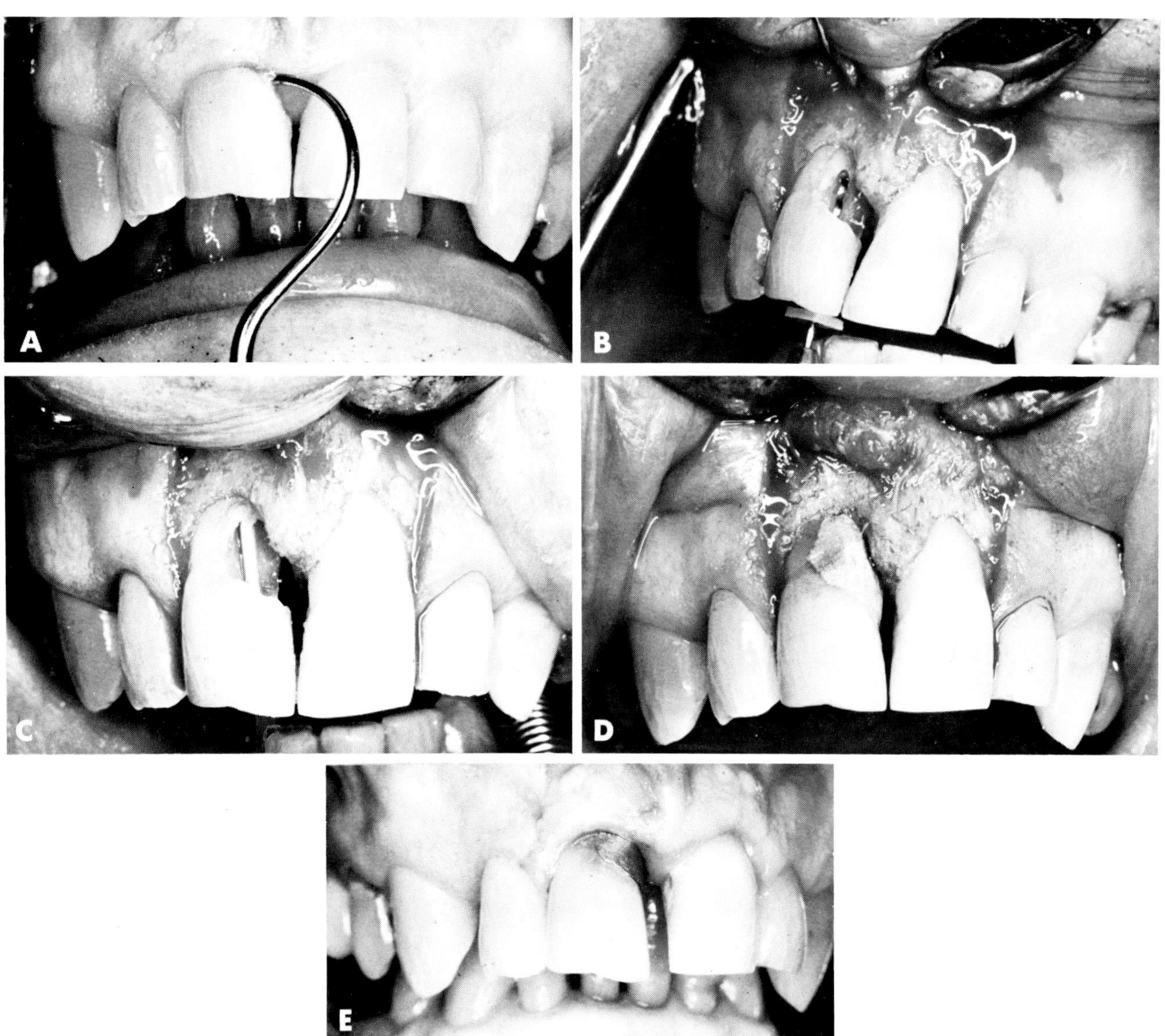

Fig. 1–32. *A,* Extensive defect by internal-external resorption is demonstrated by explorer in 67-year-old male. *B,* Retraction of rectangular flap reveals pathologic defect involving over half the tooth. Under no circumstances should root canal therapy be attempted from this lateral approach. *C,* Silver point root canal filling cemented to place prior to restoration of resorptive defect. *D,* Restoration of area of resorption with zinc-free amalgam. Case is completed by suturing flap into position. *E,* Five-year postoperative photograph (age 72) reveals gingival repair and toleration of sub-gingival amalgam filling.

successfully bleached and normal color restored (Fig. 1–33). Furthermore, a hopelessly discolored tooth, one that does not respond favorably to bleaching, may be successfully crowned with a jacket or a porcelain- or plastic-faced crown (p. 784).

CONTENTION: Endodontic Therapy Is Contraindicated if the Involved Tooth Is Wholly or Partially Luxated. Traumatic luxation *per se* is certainly not a singular contraindication for root canal therapy. If the root of the wholly or partially luxated tooth has not been fractured by the trauma, replantation of the tooth should be attempted (pp. 725–732).

The sooner the tooth is returned to the alveolus, the better the prognosis for retention. Most replanted teeth will ankylose and eventually be shed by external root resorption. On the other hand, one must consider the possible years of service gained by the simple expedient of replantation.

CONTENTION: Endodontic Therapy Is Contraindicated if the Involved Tooth Has Been Treated Previously and the Endodontic Treatment Has Failed. The previously treated pulpless tooth which has failed is far from a hopeless prognosis. Usually, an error in treatment or diagnosis has been made, which results in failure (Fig. 1–34). By careful examination the clinician must determine why the case has failed (p. 55). Then, if the cause of failure is correctible, he may correct the errors of omission or commission which led to failure, and thereby turn a failure into success (Fig. 1–35).

SUMMARY: As this review of the ***contended*** contraindications to endodontic therapy has revealed, there are ***few*** situations that present an absolute contraindication. If a tooth is vitally important, endodontic therapy may almost always be attempted, knowing full well in some cases that the prognosis is guarded. Nevertheless, the dentist and patient are frequently pleased by the outcome, especially if the final result of a full arch restoration is possible because of a successfully treated pulpless tooth.

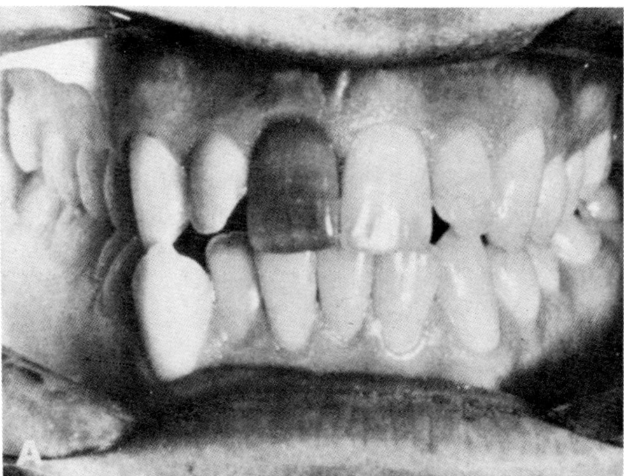

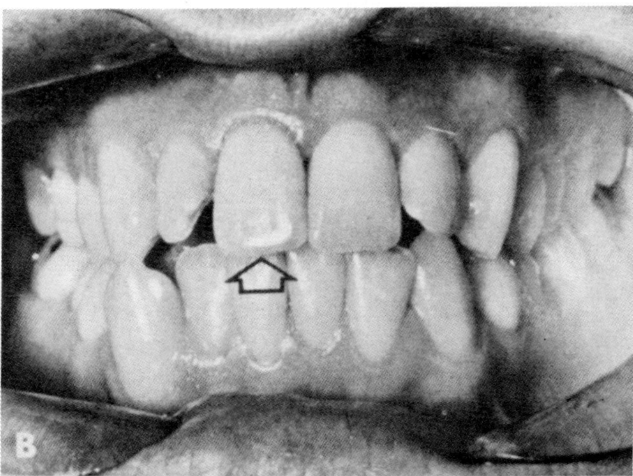

Fig. 1–33. *A*, Intense discoloration of pulpless maxillary central incisor. *B*, Successful bleaching with Superoxol. The incisor has been restored to its normal color.

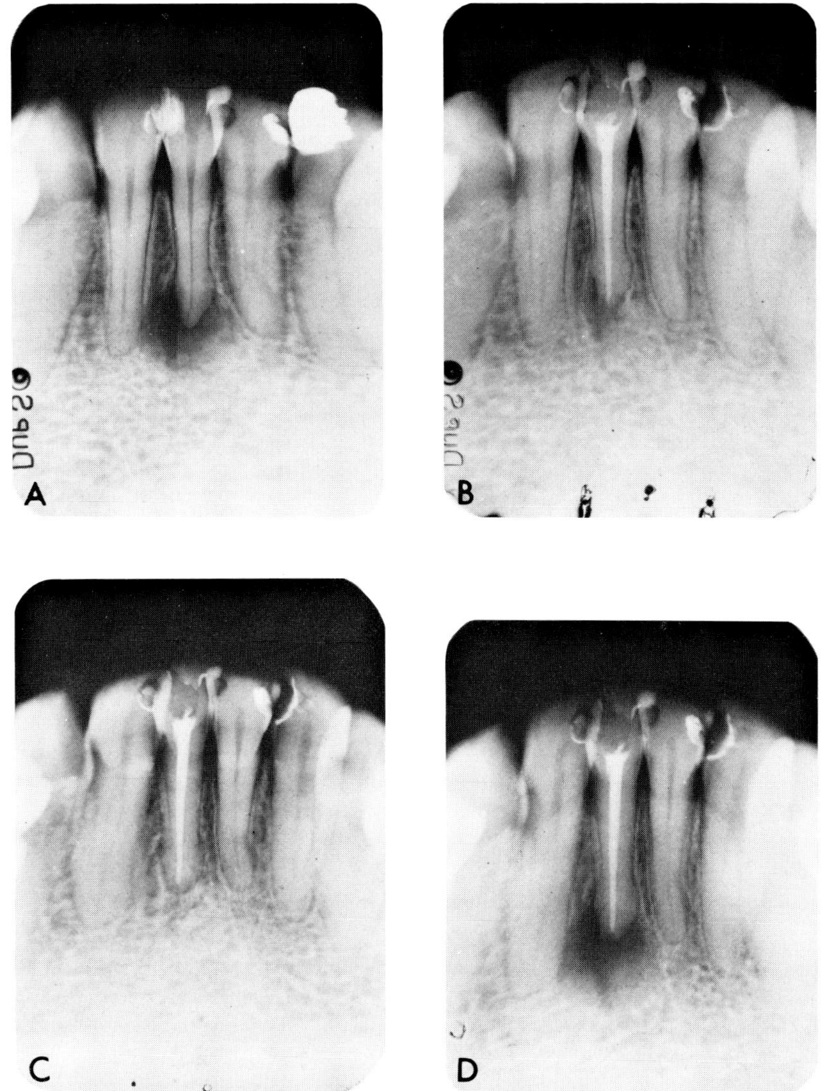

Fig. 1–34. Failure of "successfully" treated endodontic case. *A*, Pretreatment radiograph. *B*, Periapical healing well under way 20 months later. *C*, Apparently complete healing 9 years later. *D*, Complete breakdown 3 years later. Careful scrutiny of all films reveals multiple canals in other incisors. (Courtesy Dr. Juan H. Gutierrez, Concepcion, Chile.)

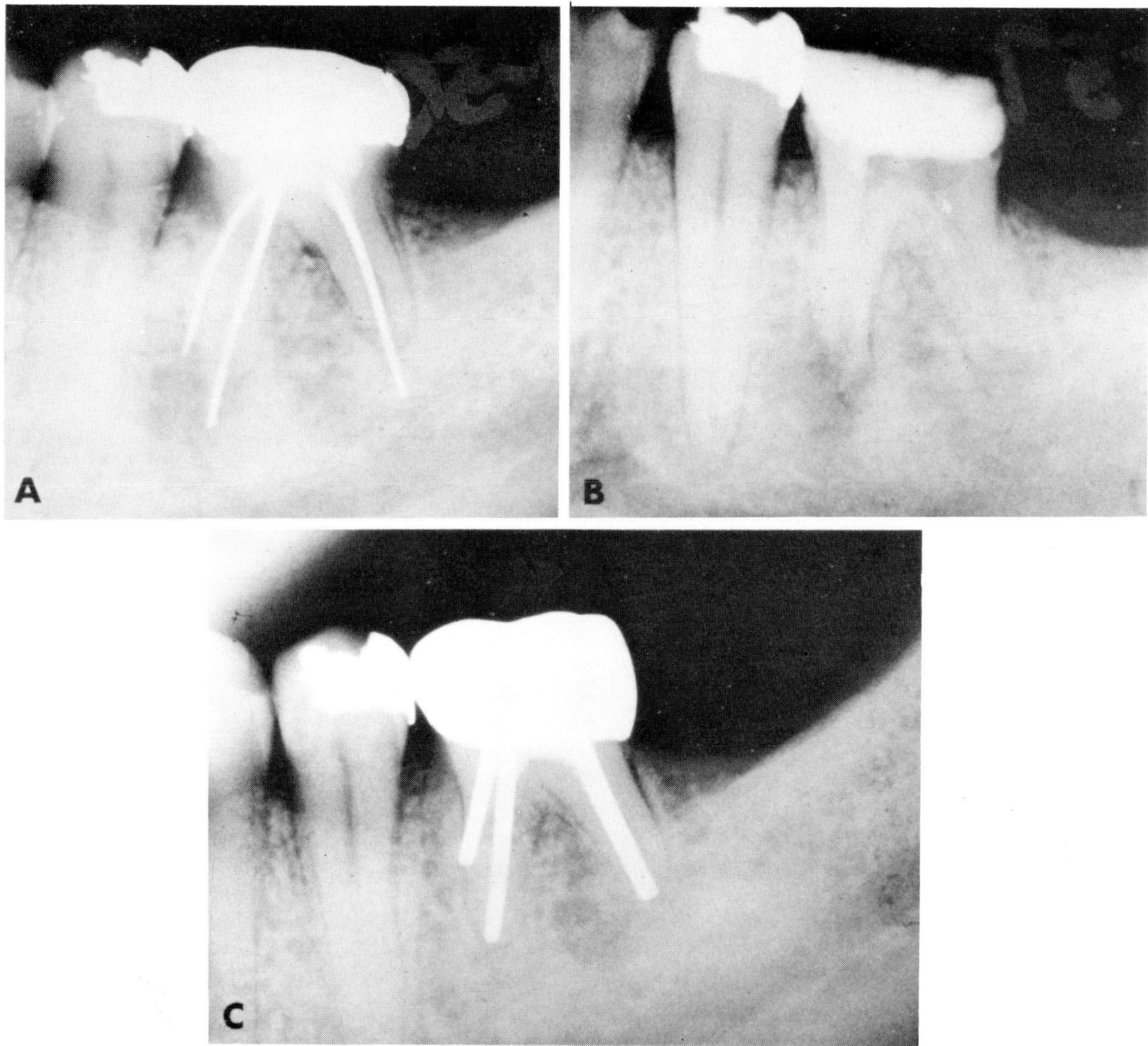

Fig. 1–35. *A,* Endodontic failure two years following treatment. Note severe root resorption associated with periapical lesion. *B,* Defective silver points are removed and canals are grossly enlarged and sterilized to be refilled with well-adapted silver points. Because of the open apical foramens, filling with gutta percha might have led to gross overfilling. *C,* Roentgenogram taken six months following treatment shows osseous repair. Successful therapy salvaged initial failure. (Courtesy Dr. Dudley H. Glick.)

ENDODONTIC SUCCESS AND FAILURE[35]

The first question to be asked of any discipline or technique in dentistry is, "What degree of success should be expected?" Success, in turn, should be measured in time—long-range success as opposed to short-term success. The beautiful resin restoration which has turned an ugly yellow in one year is not an unqualified success. By the same token, the denture "worn" in the bureau drawer is far from successful, nor is the well-fitting partial denture successful that has led to clasp caries in six months. Moreover, the treated pulpless tooth with a large periapical lesion remaining two years after treatment is not successfully treated.

In order to answer the question, "How successful is endodontic therapy?," a study was undertaken at the University of Washington School of Dentistry to evaluate treated endodontic cases and determine their rate of success. More important to the study, the rate of failure was also established and the causes of failure carefully examined. Examination of the failures led to modifications in technique and treatment. Finally, the entire discipline of endodontic therapy was re-examined, and decided improvements were made as a result. The improvements in treatment are reflected in the improvement in the degree of endodontic success, which had increased to 94.45% from a former success rate of 91.10%, an improvement of 3.35%. In other words, ***nearly 95% of all treated endodontic cases were successful.*** These figures compare favorably with other reports of success.[36–38]

The Washington Study

The foregoing figures are only a few from an exhaustive study encompassing many aspects of endodontic therapy. The modifications in treatment mentioned were instituted following the analysis of a pilot study of endodontic success and failure. Even with the limited number of cases in the pilot study, the causes of failure were apparent. Clinical techniques were then changed in an effort to overcome failure.

All endodontic cases at the University of Washington are recorded on a "Unisort Analysis Card," a 5" × 8" "punch card" which allows for rapid sorting and subsequent tabulation and analysis. In addition to the analysis card, each case has a corresponding x-ray mount in which are filed the applicable roentgenograms. Both the card and mount are filed chronologically. Patients are recalled for follow-up roentgenograms at six months, one year, two years, and five years. A recall postal card offering a "free x-ray" is sent to each patient just one week prior to each of the periods specified above.

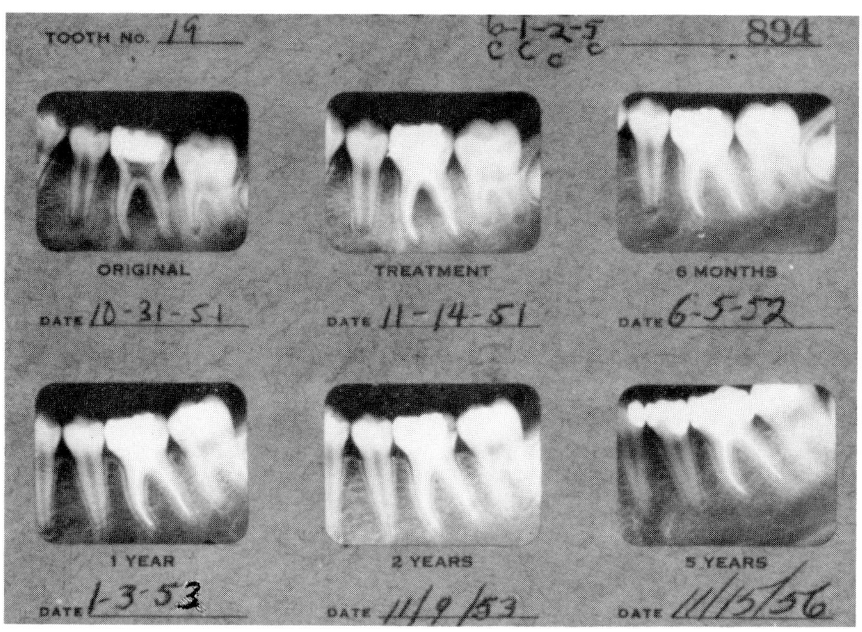

Fig. 1–36. Special mount for roentgenograms taken of each case. Note that recall films are exposed at six months, one year, two years, and five years following therapy. Figures at top of card indicate that ***complete*** healing had occurred at six months and was maintained for five years.

The recall roentgenograms are mounted in the appropriate "window" in the mount and are then carefully evaluated for improvement or lack of improvement. Included in the ***success*** group are those cases with decided periapical improvement (Figs. 1–36 and 1–37), and those cases with continuing periapical health (Fig. 1–38). The ***failure*** cases are made up of those cases which initially demonstrated

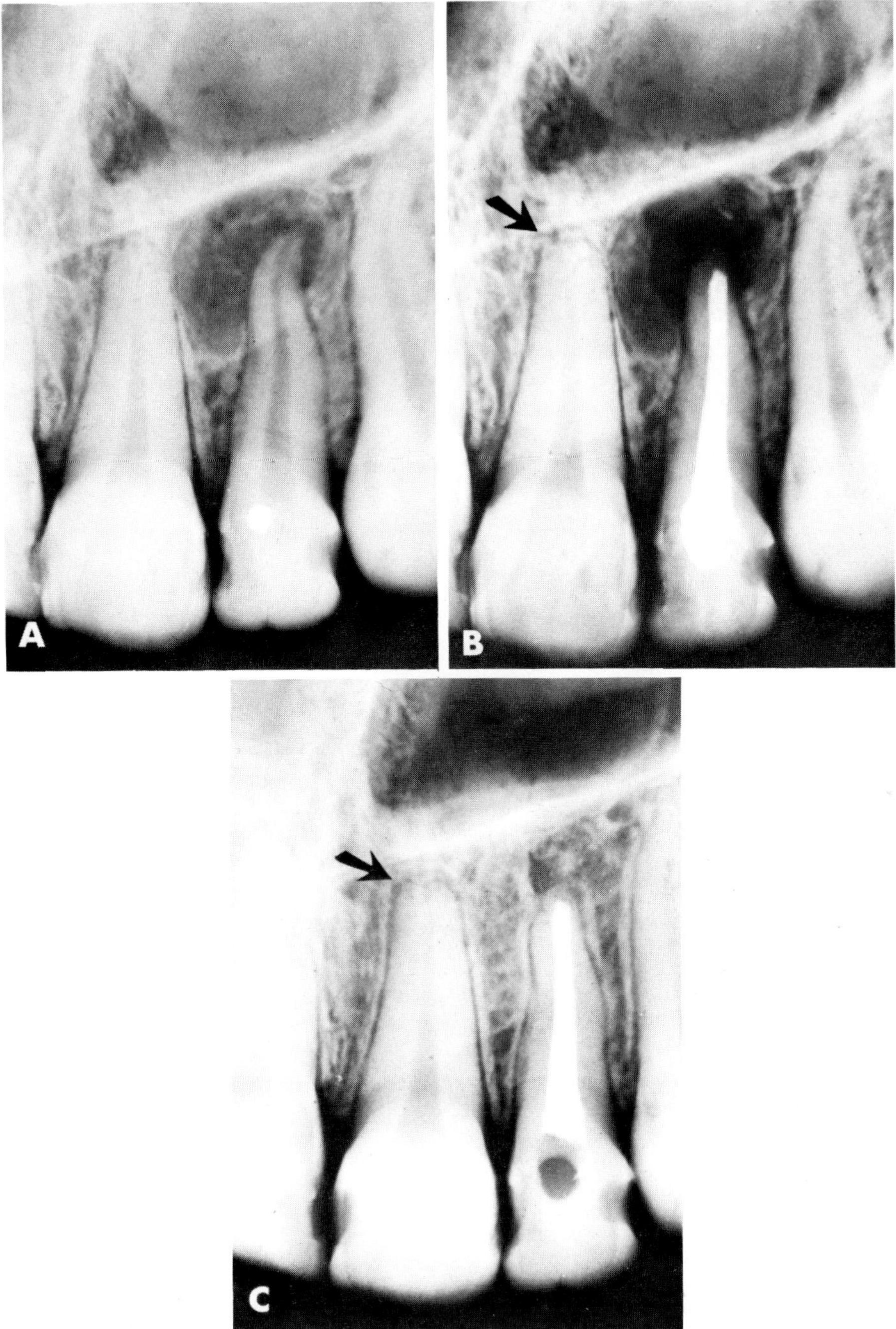

Fig. 1–37. *A,* "Before" roentgenogram with large periapical lesion. *B,* "Treatment" roentgenogram immediately following periapical surgery. Also note fractured root tip of central incisor (arrow) which tests vital. *C,* Two-year postoperative roentgenogram of successfully treated case. Lack of total periapical repair (moderate repair) is related to extensive surface of filling material over which cementum cannot grow. Also note fracture repair (arrow) of vital central incisor.

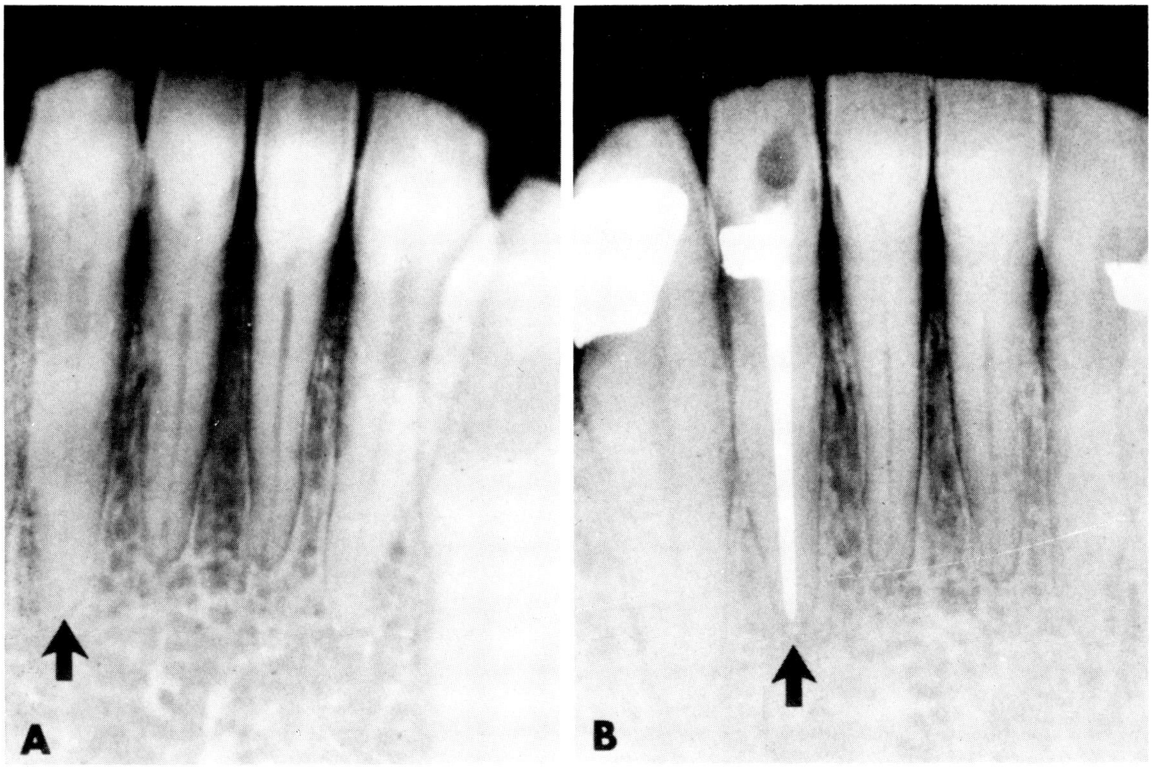

Fig. 1–38. *A,* Pulpless mandibular lateral incisor with no periapical lesion. *B,* Constant periapical health is revealed in two-year postoperative roentgenogram, a successful case.

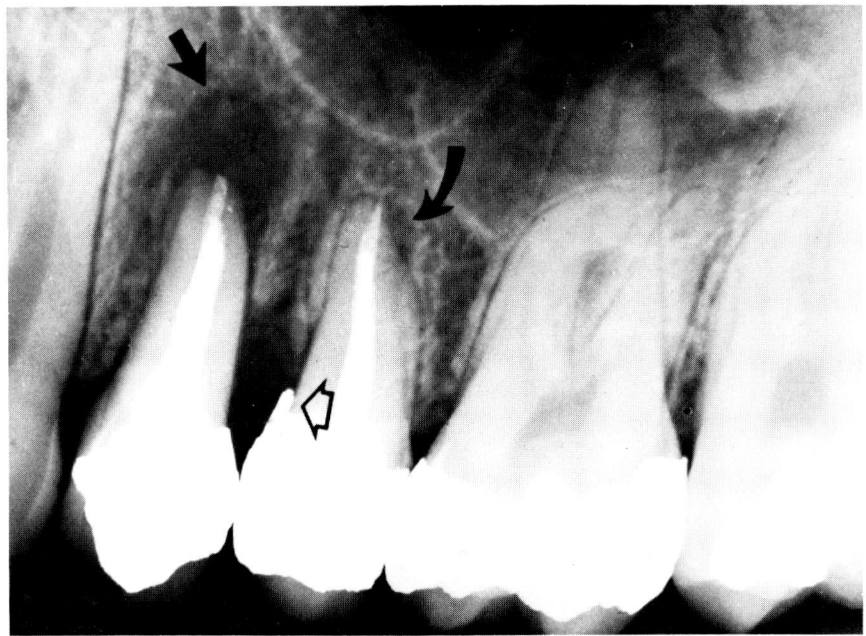

Fig. 1–39. Two failure cases demonstrated in single roentgenogram. Curved arrow *(right)* points to lesion which has failed to heal two years following endodontic treatment. Straight arrow *(left)* points to lesion which has grown worse two years following therapy. Lack of total obturation of canals is revealed by fuzzy appearance of root canal fillings. Defective amalgam restoration (open arrow) contributes to interproximal periodontal lesion.

Table 1–1. Distribution of Success and Failure in Treated Endodontic Cases—Two-Year Recalls

	Number of Cases	*Number of Successes*	*% Successes*	*Number of Failures*	*% Failures*
Cases treated after changes were instituted	162	153	94.45	9	5.55
Cases treated before changes were instituted	1,067	972	91.10	95	8.90
Total number of treated cases	1,229	1,125	91.54	104	8.46
IMPROVEMENT	—	—	3.35	—	3.35

Distribution of success and failure of endodontic cases two years following therapy. Technical changes were instituted in clinical program. Improvement which developed following these changes is reflected in 3.35% increase in success shown under "% Successes." Total failure rate is shown in final vertical column.

periapical damage and which ***have not*** improved (Fig. 1–39), as well as those cases which have deteriorated since treatment (Fig. 1–39). This information is recorded on the x-ray mount and is also transferred to the analysis cards. As soon as a statistically significant group of cases builds up in a file, the material is ready to be analyzed.

Early in the study it became apparent that the six-months and one-year films were valueless for analysis because periapical repair was frequently not complete for the middle-aged and elderly patients within one year. Most adolescents, however, had healed within six months. The two-year recall series was found to be ideal for study, for a statistically significant sample developed within this group. The five-year recall sample was also analyzed, but in understandably smaller, though significant, numbers.

The study did not take into consideration any illnesses or systemic differences between patients.

Two-Year Recall Analysis. A study of this type is no better than its returns. In other words, if only 5% of the total population returned on recall, the study might well be considered invalid. Moreover, a study of this type would tend toward the failure case, for the failure patient who is experiencing untoward symptoms would be more apt to return than would the healing patient who is symptom-free.

Out of a total population of 3,678 patients who could have returned for two years, 1,229 actually did return for a recall rate of 33.41%. In other words, one-third of the patients who could return did return, and statistically this is considered a significant group with which to work.

Out of the total of 1,229 returnees, 912 patients were treated in the University of Washington clinic, and 317 patients were from private practice. These figures will be separately analyzed later in the study. Of the 1,229 returnees there were 791 females and 438 males, figures which merely reflect the distribution of female to male patients in the University of Washington clinics and apparently in the average endodontic practice. There was no significant difference in endodontic success by sex.

Table 1–1 demonstrates the rate of success and failure, first in the cases treated ***after*** improvements in technique were instituted, followed by the cases treated ***before*** changes were instituted, and finally, the total two-year recall population of the entire sample.

As previously stated, an improvement of 3.35% was gained by improvements in technique. These improvements, which will be discussed later, raised the success rate from 91.10% to 94.45% and lowered the failure rate from 8.90% to 5.55%. Because of the preponderance of the reported cases treated before 1955, however (1,067 as against 162 treated after 1955), the overall failure rate for the entire study was 8.46%. Impressive as these gross figures might be, the differences are not statistically significant (X^2 = 2.038; $P > .10$).

Five-Year Recall Analysis. From the beginning of the study, enough five-year recalls had returned to

Table 1–2. Distribution of Success and Failure in Treated Endodontic Cases—Five-Year Recalls

Number of Cases	*Number of Successes*	*% Successes*	*Number of Failures*	*% Failures*
302	281	93.05	21	6.95

Distribution of success and failure of endodontic cases five years following therapy.

make a statistically valid analysis of these cases. Table 1–2 demonstrates the success and failure rate of this sample.

Of the 302 five-year recalls, 281 cases were successful for a success rate of 93.05%, and 21 cases were considered failures for a failure rate of 6.95%. These figures compare favorably with the two-year recall analysis and no significance would be attached to the slight improvement shown over the total two-year recalls.

Two-Year Recall Analysis—Private Practice Versus University Clinic. The value of comparing cases treated in the university clinic with cases treated in private practice was pointed out by Grossman in 1951.[39] In the Washington study little difference in the success rate was noted between the university clinic cases and private practice cases (Table 1–3). On the other hand, the ***reasons*** for failure were different between practice and clinic.

Most of the university clinic cases failed because of errors in treatment, whereas the majority of the private practice cases failed because of errors in case selection. As in most undergraduate clinics, the extremely difficult and unusual endodontic case were eliminated from the clinic load as too difficult for an undergraduate student. No graduate students were in residence at that time to treat the very difficult cases. The private practice case load, however, was replete with difficult and challenging cases, some of which should never have been undertaken (Fig. 1–40).

Table 1–3 demonstrates the relative success and failure rate between university clinic cases and private practice cases. The difference of only 1.63% is not statistically significant ($X^2 = .80$; $P > .30$).

Two-Year Recall Analysis by Age of Patient. Reference is frequently made to age as a criterion for endodontic treatment. The patient over 60 years of age has often been called a poor risk. The facts of this study do not bear out this contention. The youngest patient treated in the study was 2½ years of age; the oldest patient was 92.

Table 1–4 shows a fairly consistent rate of success and failure according to age. Three slight variances are noted, nevertheless; the higher failure rates for those patients in the first decade and sixth decade of life, and the lower failure rate for those patients age 60 and above. These differences appear significant, but when subjected to statistical analysis, they prove to be otherwise ($X^2 = 2.72$; $P > .09$).

Individual analysis of each of the failure cases arranged according to age leaves some impressions, however. First of all, a number of the failures in the young group are in incisor teeth and first permanent molars with enormous canals and large apical foramina, teeth with canals that are notoriously difficult to obturate. The second impression deals with molars. Over one-half of the failures in patients aged 50 to 59 years occurred in molar teeth. Undergraduate dental students often find molar endodontic cases difficult to prepare and fill, hence the increased failure rate.

For both of these problems (the large lumen canals in the very young and the molar problem in the middle-aged), changes in the technique were instituted in an effort to turn the tide of failure.

Table 1–3. Distribution of Success and Failure in Treated Endodontic Cases—Two-Year Recall Analysis by Private Practice and University Clinic Cases

	Number of Cases	*Number of Successes*	*% Successes*	*Number of Failures*	*% Failures*
Cases treated in private practice	317	294	92.75	23	7.25
Cases treated in university clinic	912	831	91.12	81	8.88
Total number of treated cases	1,229	1,125	91.54	104	8.46
IMPROVEMENT	—	—	1.63	—	1.63

Distribution of success and failure of endodontic cases two years following therapy. Analysis of private practice cases against university clinic cases. The 1.63% improvement held by private practice treatment is not statistically significant.

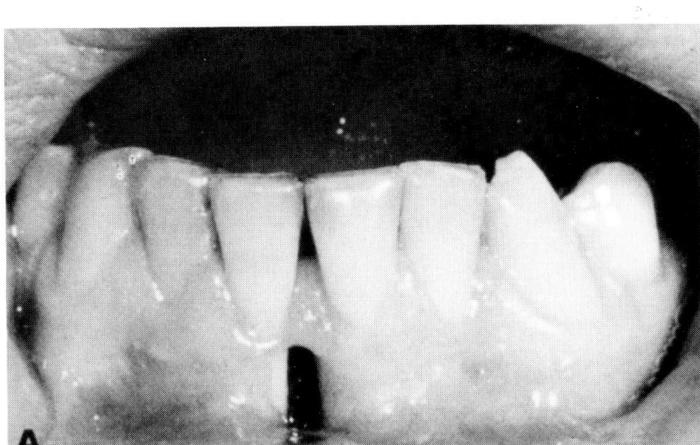

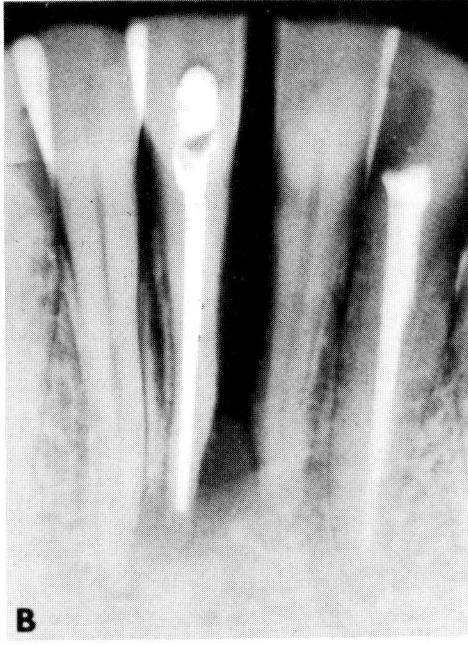

Fig. 1–40. *A,* Extended pathologic lesion as sequela of osteomyelitis. Exposed central incisor tested nonvital and treatment was undertaken. *B,* Total failure shown in two-year recall roentgenogram. Original prognosis was guarded and endodontic therapy was ill-advised.

Table 1–4. Distribution of Success and Failure in Treated Endodontic Cases—Two-Year Recall Analysis by Age of Patient

Age in Decades	*Number of Cases*	*Number of Successes*	*% Successes*	*Number of Failures*	*% Failures*
Under 10	112	99	88.40	13	11.60
10–19	327	304	93.97	23	7.03
20–29	251	226	90.04	25	9.96
30–39	265	243	91.70	22	8.30
40–49	145	136	93.80	9	6.20
50–59	79	69	87.34	10	12.66
60 and Over	50	48	96.00	2	4.0
Total number of treated cases	1,229	1,125	91.54	104	8.46

Distribution of success and failure of endodontic cases two years following therapy. No statistically significant difference exists between age groups.

Patients aged 60 and above, who enjoy the highest rate of success, have narrow root canals in all of their teeth due to the deposition of secondary and reparative dentin over the years. Although the canal orifices are difficult to find, once found these canals are relatively easy to prepare and obturate.

From the preceding discussion it is obvious that the size and shape of the lumen of the canal, and the direction of root curvature, play an important part in the successful completion of a root canal filling. Analysis of success, by individual tooth, will demonstrate these points.

Two-Year Recall Analysis by Individual Tooth. A glance at the column "% Failures" in Table 1–5, will confirm the fact that no significant difference in failure exists between any of the teeth ($X^2 = 2.43$; $P > .10$). Thus, no particular tooth can be considered a definite endodontic risk.

The wide discrepancy that exists between the mandibular second premolar with a failure rate of 4.54%, and the mandibular first premolar with a failure rate of 11.43%, requires an attempt at explanation. For the most part the mandibular first premolar can be the most difficult tooth in the mouth to treat and, at the same time, one of the easiest. Canal anatomy might account for the greater increase in failure in the first premolar. Pucci,[40] in his monumental work, ***Conductos Radiculares,*** points out the great anatomic differences between the two mandibular premolars. Whereas the mandibular second premolar has two canals and two foramina about 10% of the time, the mandibular first premolar has branching canals, apical bifurcation, and trifurcation 20% of the time.

Another factor affecting the failure rate in these teeth is the difference in perfectly straight, conical canals of the two premolars. In the mandibular first premolar the canal is straight 73.5% of the time, whereas the canal is straight in the second premolar 35% of the time. Paradoxically, the straight conical canal invites disaster. It is frequently the straight

Table 1–5. Distribution of Success and Failure in Treated Endodontic Cases—Two-Year Recall Analysis by Individual Tooth

Tooth	*Number of Cases*	*Number of Successes*	*% Successes*	*Number of Failures*	*% Failures*	*Frequency of Treatment*
Maxilla						
Central incisor	333	303	91.00	30	9.00	27.09
Lateral incisor	231	206	89.18	25	10.82	18.79
Canine	68	62	91.18	6	8.82	5.53
First premolar	65	59	90.77	6	9.23	5.29
Second premolar	51	48	94.12	3	5.88	4.15
First molar	67	61	91.05	6	8.95	5.45
Second molar	23	21	91.30	2	8.70	1.88
TOTAL	838	760	90.70	78	9.30	68.18
Mandible						
Central incisor	77	71	92.21	6	7.79	6.27
Lateral incisor	37	34	91.90	3	8.10	3.01
Canine	21	20	95.24	1	4.76	1.70
First premolar	35	31	88.57	4	11.43	2.85
Second premolar	44	42	95.46	2	4.54	3.59
First molar	127	118	92.92	9	7.08	10.33
Second molar	50	49	98.00	1	2.00	4.07
TOTAL	391	365	93.35	26	6.65	31.82
Total number of treated cases	1,229	1,125	91.54	104	8.46	100.00

Distribution of success and failure of endodontic cases two years following therapy. Lower failure rate for mandibular second molar and increased failure rates for maxillary lateral incisor and mandibular first premolar are of note. Success in mandible is not significantly greater than in maxilla.

Attention is also directed to frequency of treatment by arch and by individual tooth. Note maxillary incisors make up 45.88% of total sample. Mandibular first molar constitutes 10.33% of 1,229 total cases, and mandibular canine and maxillary second molar each account for less than 2% of total sample.

conical canal cases that have the apex perforated with instruments followed by gross overfilling. The frequent use of silver points in the obturation of mandibular premolars has also led to an increased failure rate in these teeth (Fig. 1–41). The widely tapering canals of these teeth should be filled with compressed gutta percha.

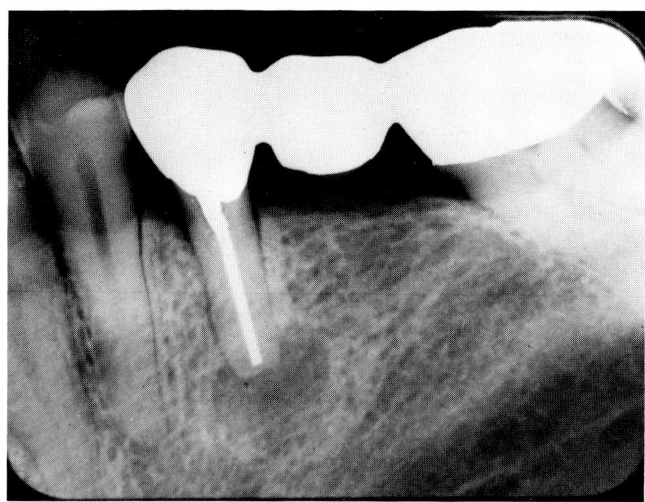

Fig. 1–41. Failure 20 years following treatment. Improper selection of silver point as filling material led to breakdown of cementing sealer and percolation into canal.

Anatomically, the ***mandibular*** first premolar more closely resembles the ***maxillary*** first premolar, and the same may be said for the second premolars. Again, Table 1–5 demonstrates this affinity with similar failure rates.

Failures in the maxillary lateral incisor may also be explained by anatomic differences. Pucci shows extensive distal curvature of the maxillary lateral incisor root 49.2% of the time.[41] Here again, poor judgment and preparation frequently prevent adequate instrumentation and obturation, with root perforation at the curvature a common occurrence (Fig. 1–42). Increased failure rate in the maxillary lateral incisor is also related to continuing root resorption, peculiar to these teeth, following treatment.

The overall failure rate, mandible to maxilla, is striking, but not statistically significant. Failure in the mandibular arch is encountered 6.65% of the time and 9.03% of the time in the maxilla.

Frequency of Occurrence of Treatment by Individual Tooth. Table 1–5, in the final column, shows numerically the frequency with which the individual teeth are treated by endodontic therapy. This column demonstrates over twice as much endodontic treatment in the maxillary arch as in the mandibular arch, 68.18 to 31.82% respectively. Furthermore, the

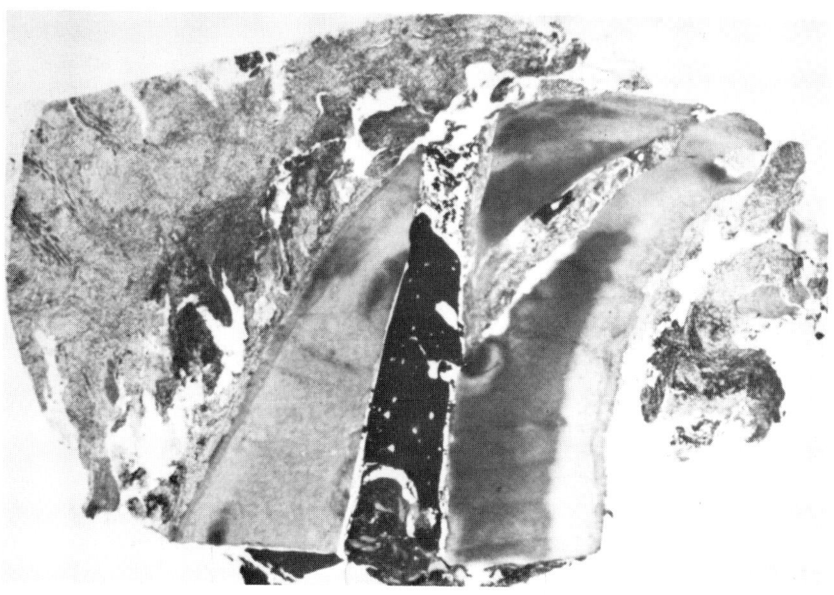

Fig. 1–42. Root tip biopsy from curved apex of maxillary lateral incisor. Severe inflammatory reaction surrounding root end is related to perforation as well as failure to debride and obturate curved portion of canal. (From Luebke, R. G., Glick, D. H., and Ingle, J. I.: Oral Surg., *18*:97, July, 1964.)

maxillary incisors alone account for 45.88%, or almost half, of the 1,229 cases in the study. The mandibular first molar is the third most frequently treated tooth, constituting 10.33% of all the cases. Other studies have shown this tooth to be the most frequently extracted as well.[42,43] Although these findings generally agree with the occurrence reported by Strindberg,[44] they are at variance with the findings of Sommer and Ostrander[45] of Michigan, who found the mandibular first molar the most frequently involved tooth and the maxillary central incisor to be next. The Michigan survey of 846 cases, however, was a "random sample ***picked*** from the clinic files."

The lowest frequency of treatment was for the mandibular canine, which made up only 1.70% of the total sample. That for the maxillary second molar was also low, occurring 1.88% of the time.

The frequency of occurrence in the maxillary incisors is easily explained. Of first importance: ***all*** incisors erupt early and so may decay early; on the other hand, caries rate for maxillary incisors is much higher than for the mandibular incisors. In addition to the caries rate is the desire on the part of patients to retain the maxillary incisors for esthetic and psychic reasons. This will account for a good deal of endodontic therapy in the premaxilla. Large pulpal horns, which lie in a mesiodistal direction, quickly become involved by interproximal caries; and the common use of silicate cement and autopolymerizing resins (materials shown to be pulpal irritants), account for another huge portion of the sample. Moreover, the maxillary incisors are more frequently traumatized by accident than any other teeth. All these factors go together to increase the incidence of pulpal involvement and endodontic therapy in the maxillary incisors.

Because of early eruption and early carious involvement, the four first molars constitute 15.78% of the total sample, this level in spite of the frequent early extraction of these teeth.[42,43]

Two-Year Recall Analysis by Nonsurgical or Surgical Intervention. The degree of success achieved by surgical intervention in the treated endodontic cases has long been a contentious point. There are those dentists who never resort to surgical intervention in an endodontic case, and then again, there are other dentists who use periapical surgery routinely. Both groups are wrong! As with any other surgical technique, periapical surgery may be positively indicated or elective. The "endodontic surgeons" who limit their practice to anterior teeth demonstrate their inferiority complex about endodontics as a total discipline.

Table 1–6 demonstrates that although the nonsurgical case appears to be slightly more successful than the surgical case, the differences are not statistically significant ($X^2 = 3.44$; $P > .05$).

It would be tempting to indict case selection as the basis for increased failure of the surgical case. One of the indications for surgical intervention has been the grossly involved periapical lesion where a lower rate of repair might be expected. Actually, this has not proved to be true. The 10- to 12-mm. periapical lesion appears to heal as readily, if not quite as rapidly, as the 2-mm. lesion (Fig. 1–43). This was recently confirmed by Selden, who stated, "healing rates were identical for periapical areas regardless of size."[46]

Careful analysis of the ***surgical*** failures reveals that incomplete filling of the canals occurs more frequently in the nonsurgical cases. Most of the surgical cases in the study were treated in one appointment; that is, the canal enlargement, sterilization, and obturation, as well as the periapical surgery, were completed in a single appointment. Here again,

Table 1–6. Distribution of Success and Failure of Treated Endodontic Cases—Two-Year Recall Analysis by Method of Therapy

Method of Therapy	*Number of Cases*	*Number of Successes*	*% Successes*	*Number of Failures*	*% Failures*	*Frequency of Treatment*
Nonsurgical treatment	870	808	92.88	62	7.12	65.74
Surgical treatment	359	317	88.30	42	11.70	34.26
Total number of treated cases	1,229	1,125	91.54	104	8.46	100.00

Distribution of success and failure of endodontic cases two years following therapy. Degree of success of nonsurgical therapy over surgical therapy is not significant. Note also that ***nonsurgical*** cases constitute 65.74% of total sample of 1,229 cases.

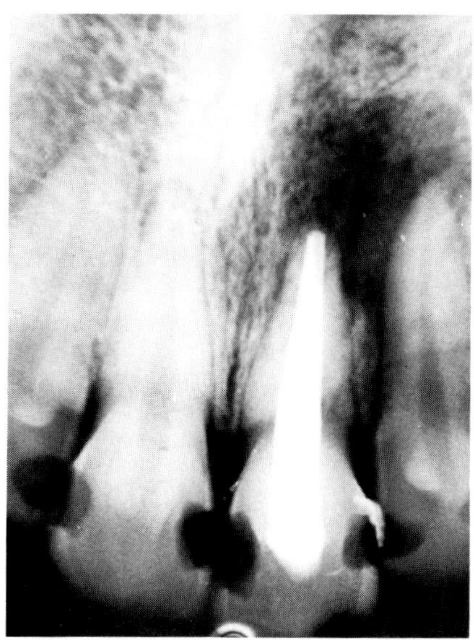
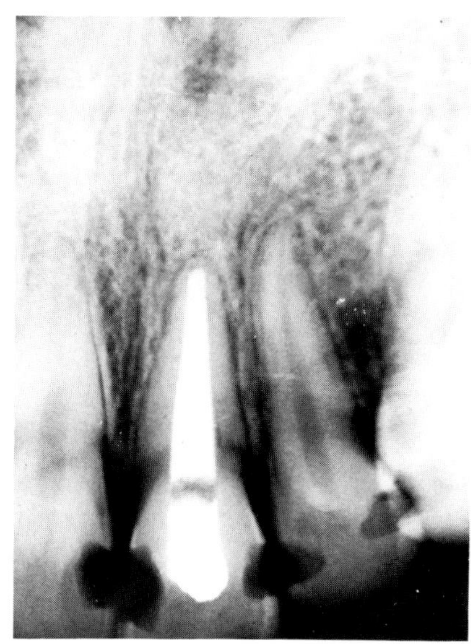

Fig. 1–43. Large periapical lesion *(left)* has healed completely *(right)* within six months in patient 20 years of age.

hurrying to complete the case could account for the lack of attention to detail, with incomplete obturation and increased failure the result. This should not be considered an indictment of surgery *per se*, but rather a fault of poor endodontic preparation and canal filling.

As far as frequency of treatment is concerned (65% nonsurgical versus 35 surgical) this figure has greatly changed in recent years. Far less surgical treatment is being performed today. Improved techniques and confidence in endodontic methods have led to this reduction.

Two-Year Recall Analysis of Endodontic Failures. The final and most important portion of the Washington Study dealt with the 104 failure cases as a group. Careful analysis of these particular cases is most revealing.

Arrangement of Failures by Frequency of Occurrence. As Table 1–7 will show, the most striking finding is the 58.66% of the failures caused by ***incomplete obturation*** of the canal (Fig. 1–44). This is a highly significant figure. This most common cause of failure is almost 50% ahead of the next greatest cause of failure, ***root perforation,*** which accounts for 9.61% of the failures. Thus, the two greatest causes of failure stand revealed, ***imperfect instrumentation*** and ***incomplete obturation.*** In other words, over two-thirds of all the endodontic failures in the study were related to imperfect performance of two points of the endodontic triad, "canal instrumentation and canal obtura-

Table 1–7. Distribution of Failures of Treated Endodontic Cases—Two-Year Recall

Arranged by Frequency of Occurrence

Causes of Failure	*Number of Failures*	*% Failures*
Incomplete obturation	61	58.66
Root perforation	10	9.61
External root resorption	8	7.70
Coexistent periodontal-periapical lesion	6	5.78
Canal grossly overfilled	4	3.85
Canal left unfilled	3	2.88
Developing apical cyst	3	2.88
Adjacent pulpless tooth	3	2.88
Silver point inadvertently removed	2	1.92
Broken instrument	1	0.96
Accessory canal unfilled	1	0.96
Constant trauma	1	0.96
Perforation, nasal floor	1	0.96
FAILURES, TOTAL	104	100.00

Distribution of 104 endodontic failures two years following therapy. When arranged by frequency of occurrence, note that ***Incomplete Obturation*** accounts for almost 60% of all failures, followed by ***Root Perforation,*** which accounts for nearly 10% of 104 failures. Cause of failure ranges down to infrequently encountered conditions which occur less than 1% of the time.

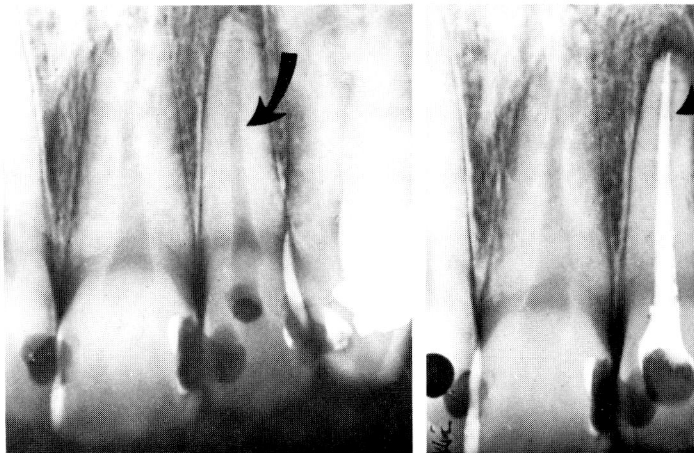

Fig. 1–44. *Left,* Careful examination of initial roentgenogram reveals internal resorption and widening of canal apical to the curved arrow. *Right,* In two-year recall roentgenogram periapical lesion persists due to failure to totally obliterate root canal space (arrow).

tion." This alone would call for improved technique and attention to detail.

Categorical Arrangement of Causes of Failure. The thirteen causes of endodontic failure may be arranged in three general categories of causes leading to failure: (1) apical percolation, (2) operative errors, and (3) errors in case selection (Table 1–8). Actually a clear-cut delineation of the agents of failure is difficult, for ultimately, percolation into the canal accounts for almost all failures as Table 1–8 shows.

Apical Percolation. Three of the causes of failure shown in Table 1–8 lead to apical percolation and subsequent diffusion stasis into the canal: (1) Incomplete obturation, 58.66% (Fig. 1–45); (2) canal left unfilled, 2.88% (Fig. 1–46); and (3) silver point removed inadvertently, 1.92%. These three causes together account for 63.47% of all endodontic failures, and demonstrate how vital to success is careful therapy. Apparently successful results following poorly executed root canal therapy attest to the inherent ability of the body occasionally to withstand noxious stimuli without great reaction.

Inadvertent removal of silver points during restorative procedures happens when the soft silver point is caught by a bur during cavity preparation and pulled from its seat in the canal. The dentist either fails to notice the error or is not aware of the consequence of its removal. Again, the empty canal invites percolation and failure.

Operative Errors. A category made up of errors in coronal cavity preparation and canal preparation

Table 1–8. Distribution of Failures of Treated Endodontic Cases—Two-Year Recall

Arranged by Category of Cause of Failure

Causes of Failure	*Number of Failures*	*% Failures*
Apical Percolation—Total	*66*	*63.46*
Incomplete obturation	61	58.66
Unfilled canal	3	2.88
Ag point inadvertently removed	2	1.92
Operative Error—Total	*15*	*14.42*
Root perforation	10	9.61
Canal grossly overfilled	4	3.85
Broken instrument	1	0.96
Errors in Case Selection—Total	*23*	*22.12*
External root resorption	8	7.70
Coexistent periodontal-periapical lesion	6	5.78
Developing aical cyst	3	2.88
Adjacent pulpless tooth	3	2.88
Accessory canal unfilled	1	0.96
Constant trauma	1	0.96
Perforation, nasal floor	1	0.96
FAILURES—TOTAL	104	100.00

Distribution of 104 endodontic failures two years following therapy. Causes of failure may be categorized into three general groupings: ***apical percolation,*** which accounts for 63.46% of failures, ***operative errors,*** which account for 14.42% of failures, and ***errors in case selection,*** which account for 22.12% of 104 failures.

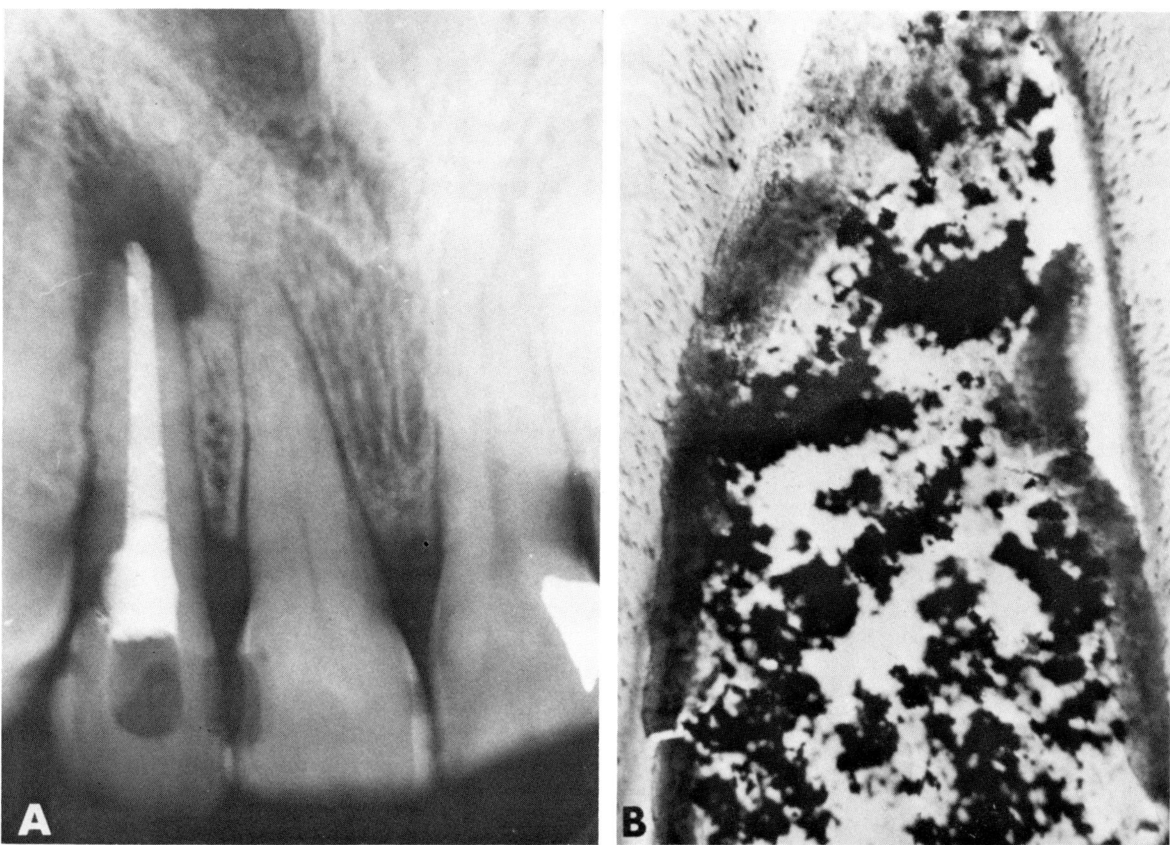

Fig. 1–45. *A,* Although root canal filling appears to be overextended, fuzzy appearance indicates lack of density necessary for total obturation. *B,* Root end biopsy of this failure case shows root canal cement and cellular debris rather than well-condensed gutta percha filling. Constant percolation into root canal space provides media for bacterial growth and breakdown of blood constituents.

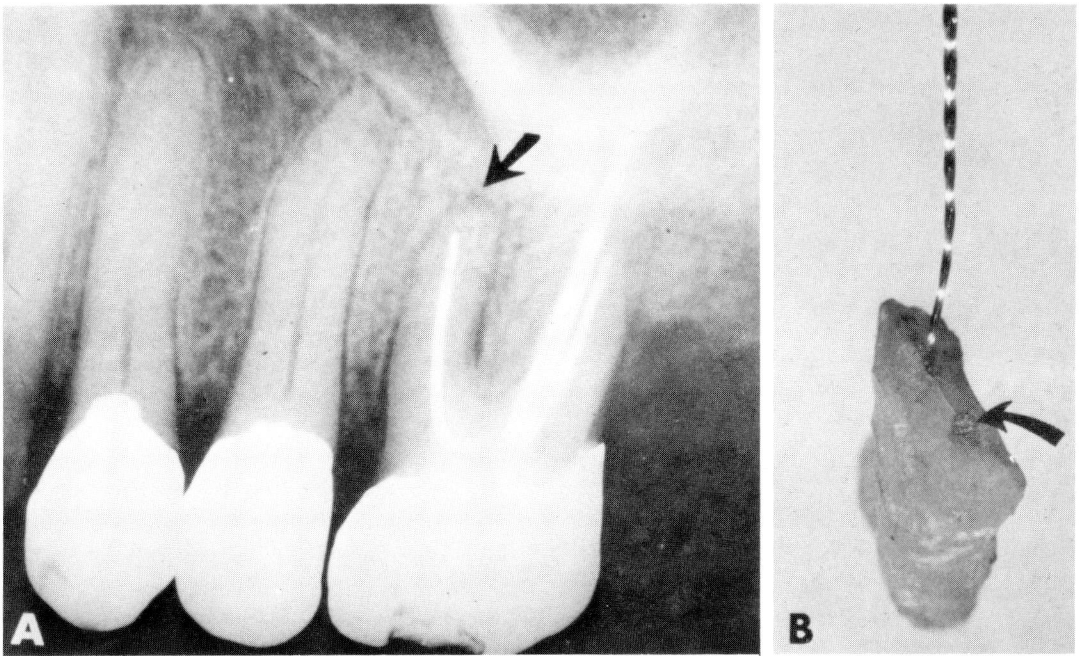

Fig. 1–46. *A,* Constantly draining fistula opposite mesiobuccal root of maxillary first molar (arrow) was thought to be related to advanced periodontal lesion. Total amputation of mesiobuccal root is indicated. *B,* Amputated root reveals error in diagnosis. Reamer is in undetected second canal, whereas the arrow points to obturated primary canal. Secondary canals in mesiobuccal roots of first permanent molars occur about one-third of the time.

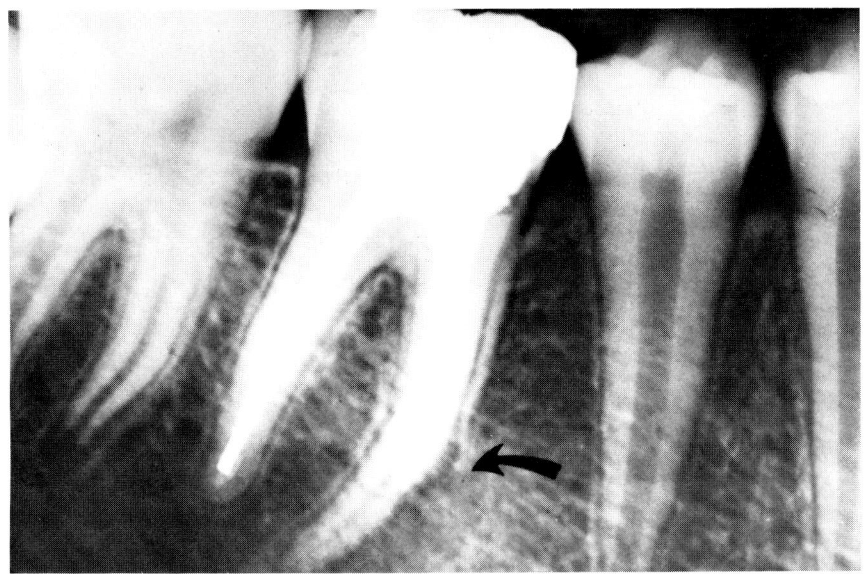

Fig. 1–47. Failure due to root perforation accompanied by incomplete debridement and imperfect obturation. Note break in lamina dura opposite perforation (arrow).

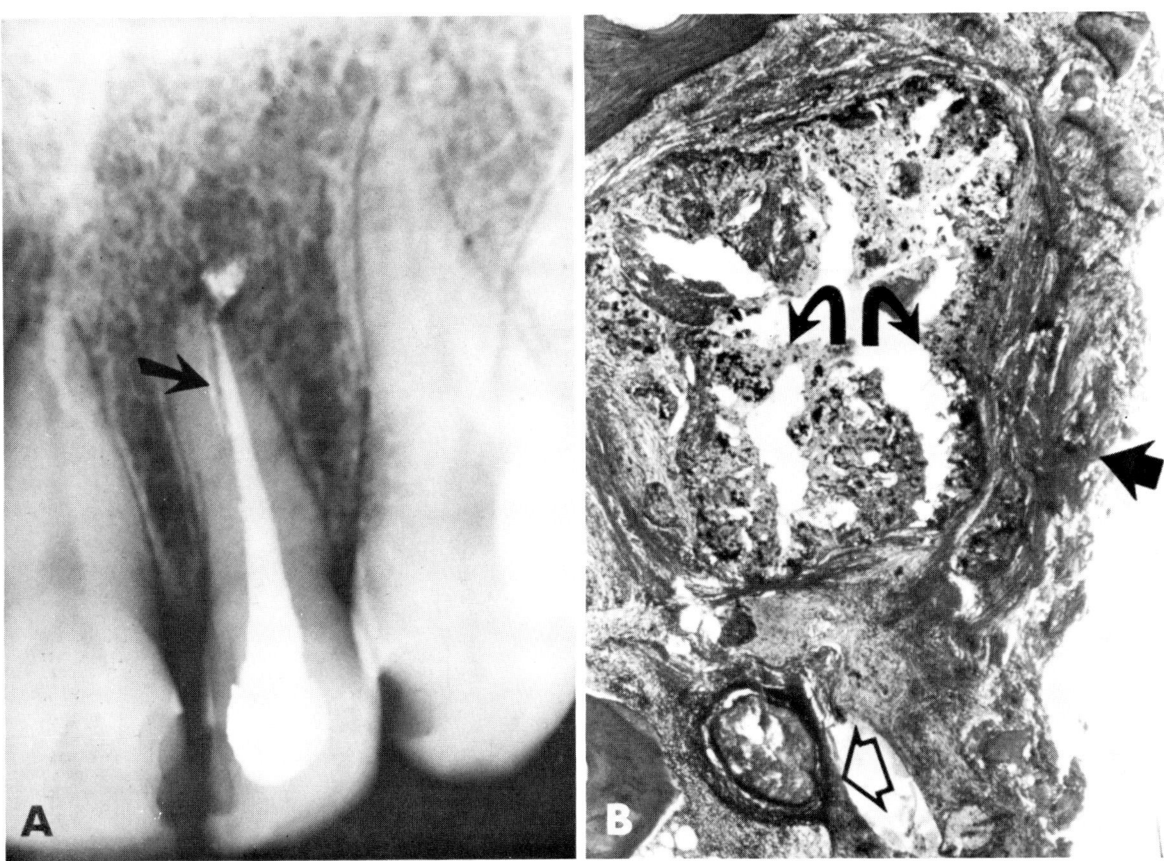

Fig. 1–48. *A,* Although this incisor appears to be grossly overfilled, careful examination (arrow) will reveal failure to totally obturate canal. *B,* Tissue reaction to overfilling and underfilling in single biopsy specimen from this failure case. Curved arrows direct attention to mass of cement forced into periapical tissue. Heavy black arrow *(right)* indicates noninflammatory tissue capsule which has developed as foreign body reaction. Open arrow *(bottom)* points to violent inflammatory reaction and abscess related to irritating products percolating from unfilled canal.

accounts for almost 15% of the failures. Root perforation, 9.61%; broken instrument, 0.96%; and canal grossly overfilled, 3.85%; total, 14.42% of all the failures. These operative errors are all related to improper use of endodontic instruments and filling materials as well as a lack of standardization of endodontic equipment and material as it arrives from the manufacturer. The latter problem has now been corrected.

On the one hand, delicate root canal instruments cannot be mistreated by the inexperienced, and one of the common complaints of the neophyte is "instrument breakage." On the other hand, improper use of the instruments causing root perforation and apex perforation accounted for 14 of the 104 failures in the study. Drilling out through the side of a curved root will ultimately lead to incomplete instrumentation and incomplete obturation (Fig. 1–47).

Opening wide the apical foramen during instrumentation is also a form of perforation and leads to gross overfilling. Healing is delayed and often incomplete around the grossly overfilled areas that may be due to foreign body reaction. Moreover, the open apical foramen does not allow for condensation during canal filling and, although the canal may appear overfilled, it is actually incompletely obturated, with resulting percolation and failure (Fig. 1–48).

A number of failures due to root perforation could be related to the total lack of standardization of endodontic instruments at that time. Sudden dimensional increase, from one size instrument to the next, will often result in the instrument binding in the canal. Inexperience in the tactile sensation and manipulation of the bound instrument may lead to breakage or perforation.

Actually, this study would indicate that the broken instrument is not the desperate situation it is often considered. During the eight years of the study, a great number of instruments were broken, yet the fact that failure involved a broken instrument in only one case out of the great number on record attests to the fact that a broken instrument will serve as an adequate root canal filling. Actually, it has been suggested as such (see p. 252). In analyzing the University of Washington case load, Crump and Natkin have found that failure following instrument fragmentation was the same as in other endodontic cases.[34]

Broken instruments are not favored any more than overfilling is favored, but occasionally both accidents may occur. Usually, periapical surgical treatment is the only corrective measure that can be used to reclaim either error. This procedure is recommended in operable teeth if the instrument is broken off in the apical one-third of the canal and ***is loose*** in the canal, or if the canal is grossly overfilled with irretrievable gutta percha and cement. Broken instruments, loose in the canal, have been seen to "rust out" (Fig. 1–49).

All these errors of operation may be prevented by careful cavity preparation and canal obturation. For example, if the operator is unsure of the instrument position in the canal, a roentgenogram should be taken. Also more accuracy in fitting the primary or initial filling point will lead to less overfilling. In the

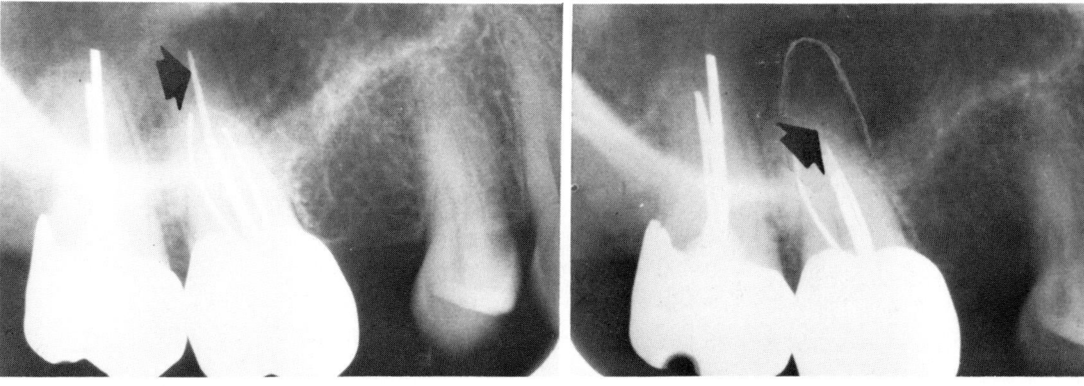

Fig. 1–49. Large broken, stainless file (arrow—*left*) in palatal root of maxillary first molar. In roentgenogram *(right),* broken instrument has disappeared (arrow) after one year. Apparently, even stainless instruments will dissolve or "rust out" if percolation into canal persists. (Root outline retouched—*right.)*

final analysis, operative error is the simplest cause of failure to control, and just requires more patience, care, and understanding to overcome.

Errors in Case Selection. Errors in case selection are not so easily overcome as operative errors, and may often be listed as the "bad breaks of the game" rather than errors in judgment. Who could predict, for example, that external root resorption would continue, or that an apical cyst would develop following treatment, or that an adjacent tooth would become pulpless? These are all factors that led to some of the failures in this study, factors added together to constitute 22.12% of the total failures. Some could well have been predicted at the time of therapy (such as Fig. 1–40), but others were entirely unpredictable. These are the cases that made up the bulk of the failure cases from private practice, merely because the endodontist, at the insistence of his colleagues, may extend himself into cases with a poor initial prognosis. The same fate awaits the experienced surgeon who attempts to save the hopeless and "inoperable" patient. His mortality rate often climbs with his skill and daring.

Each of the errors in selection will be dealt with separately.

External Root Resorption. The higher incidence of external root resorption at the apex of the pulpless tooth has been observed for some time and is dealt with in detail by Boyle.[47] Although every tooth in the mouth may be indicted for external resorption, the majority of the cases in this study are associated with pulpless maxillary lateral incisors and mandibular molars. Why these teeth in particular are affected to a greater degree than the other teeth is not known. The interesting fact is, however, that external resorption ***stops*** in most cases following successful endodontic therapy. The eight cases in this study in which apical resorption continued following therapy were all maxillary lateral incisors (see Fig. 1–31). Here again, why these particular teeth continue to resorb is a mystery. However, these eight cases were a contributing factor in raising the failure rate in the maxillary

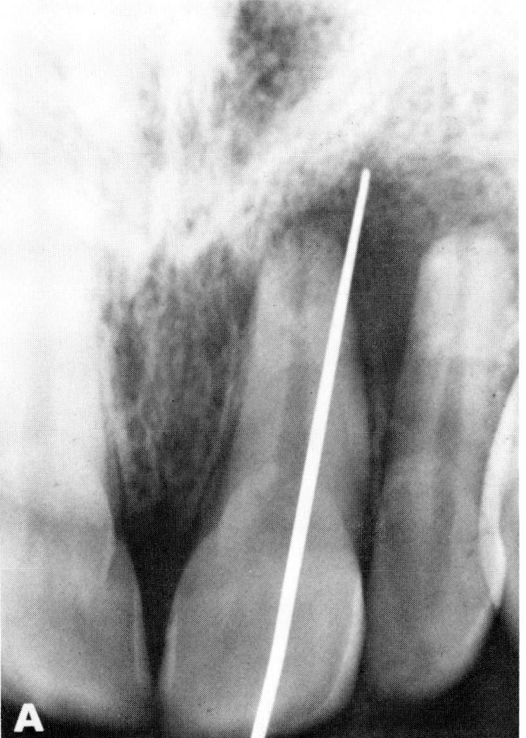

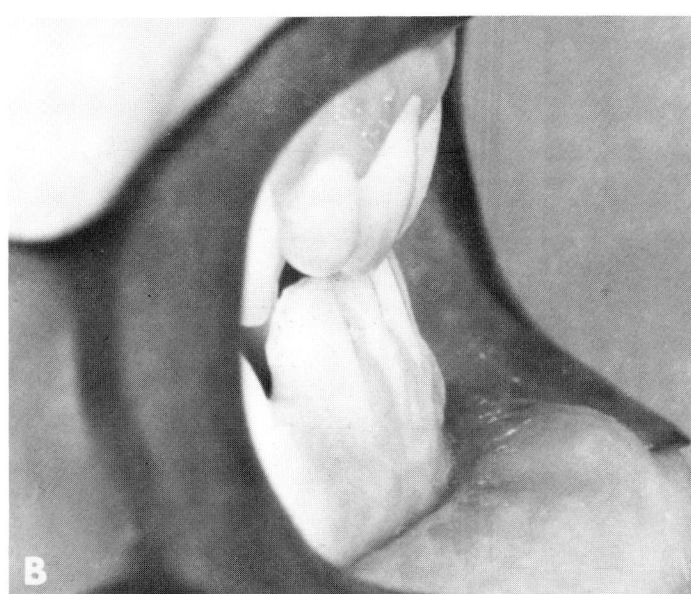

Fig. 1–50. *A,* Periapically positioned lesion associated with vital teeth is related to narrow, palatal, periodontal pocket in which probe has been placed to depth of 16 mm. Diagnosis by roentgenogram alone would undoubtedly lead to misdiagnosis as pulp-related lesion. *B,* Cause of periodontal lesions seen in *A* is tissue damage from deep overbite and incisal edges of mandibular incisors cutting into lingual gingiva of maxillary incisors.

lateral incisor. One should be wary in estimating the future of pulpless maxillary lateral incisors which exhibit extensive external root resorption. And this can be said for the surgical and nonsurgical approach alike, because half of the failure cases in these teeth had apicoectomies.

Concomitant Periodontal-Periapical Lesion. Of all the causes of failure which may be determined prior to treatment, the concomitant periodontal-periapical lesion may be discovered most frequently (Fig. 1–50). A careful periodontal examination using a fine explorer and a periodontal probe is an absolute necessity if these accompanying lesions are to be discovered prior to treatment. To find the narrow periodontal pocket which extends to the apex, it may be necessary to anesthetize the area before examining with the probe.* The necessity of this procedure is borne out by the fact that six cases in the study failed because of periodontal involvement, and in each of these cases the lesion existed prior to treatment.

*The area should never be anesthetized during examination until all tests for pulpal vitality are concluded.

The most common area where a coexistent periodontal pocket exists, but is missed at the time of examination, is in the maxillary incisor region. A number of these cases have a history of impact trauma which not only devitalized the pulp, but tore loose the attachment apparatus as well. Usually the periodontal ligament will reattach. However, in the presence of gingivitis, the inflamed area will not reattach and a narrow and sometimes tortuous pocket will develop in this region.[48] This pocket will then supply the periapical lesion with the irritants of bacteria and toxins from the infected sulcus, invalidating any treatment rendered by endodontic therapy.

The maxillary lateral incisor is frequently involved with anomalous defects coursing up the lingual surface to the apex. Dens en dente, invagination, lingual tubercles or even anomalous additional roots are the clues that a palatal pocket may be present in pulpless maxillary lateral incisors[49] (Fig. 1–51).

The concomitant lesion is also found with greater frequency in the mandibular molar area and often

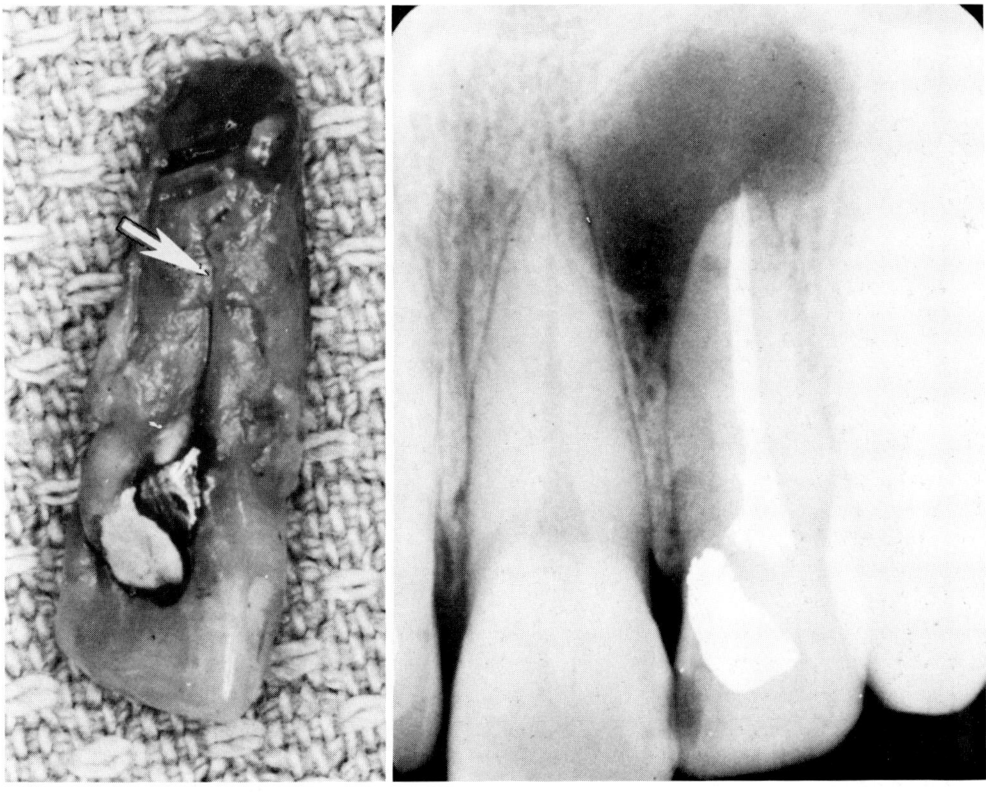

Fig. 1–51. Developmental defect, invagination, which results in unattached periodontal ligament tract to apex. Defect at cingulum probably communicated with pulp. Endodontic and periodontic therapy were to no avail. (From Simon, J. H. S., Glick, D. H., and Frank, A. L.: Oral Surg., 37:823, June, 1971.)

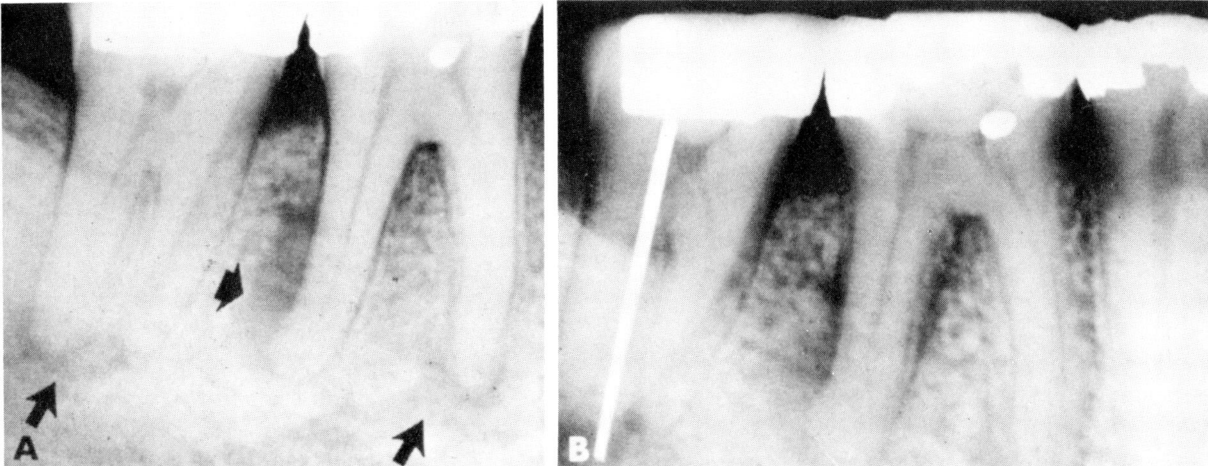

Fig. 1–52. *A,* Attention is directed (arrows) to three periapical lesions, all apparently related to necrotic pulps. Electric pulp testing proves pulp of first molar to be necrotic, but pulp of second molar to be vital. *B,* Careful periodontal probing, buccal to second molar, reveals periodontal lesion which extends to periapex. Second molar is being traumatized in nonfunctional excursion of mandible.

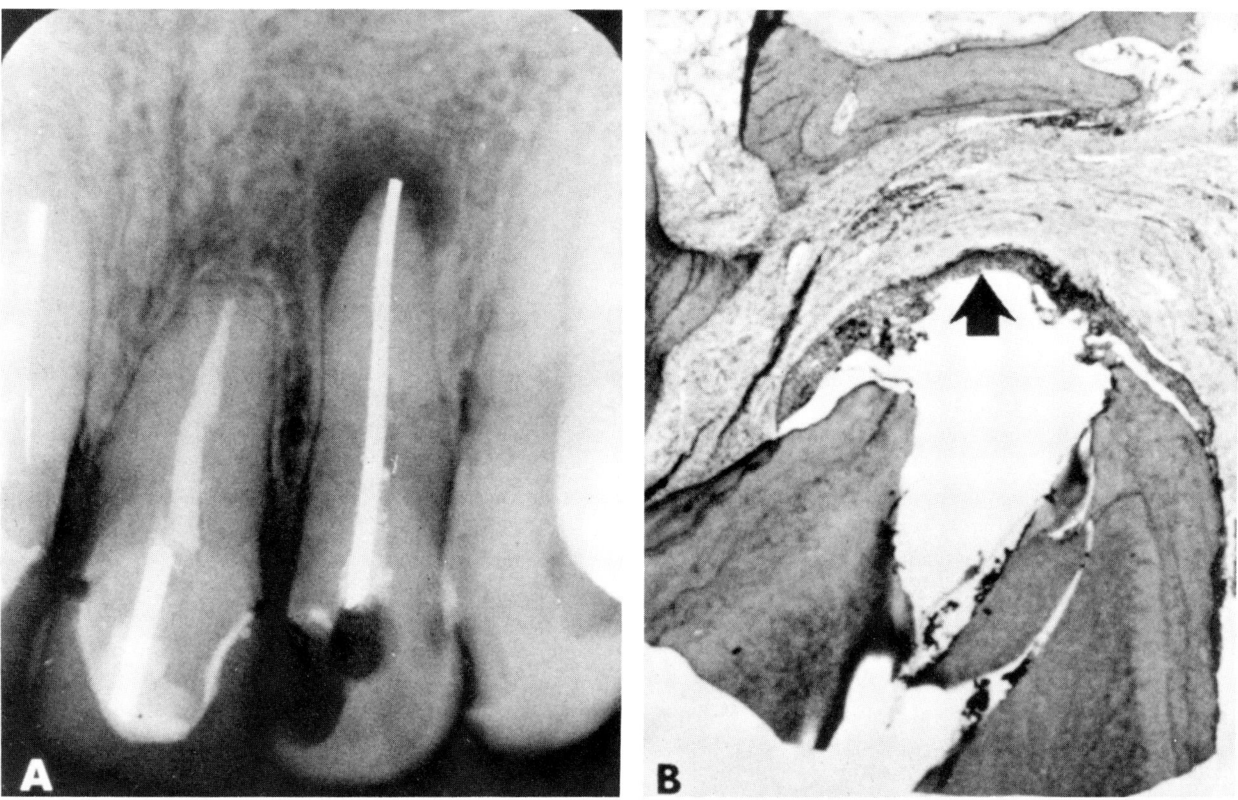

Fig. 1–53. *A,* Periapical lesion which persists two years following endodontic therapy appears to be either apical cyst or chronic apical periodontitis. *B,* Biopsy of periapex demonstrates epithelial lining of apical cyst (arrow). Persistence of development of apical cysts led to failure in three cases in study.

accompanies severe occlusal traumatism in ***nonfunction*** (balancing interferences). Quite commonly errors in diagnosis are made in this region, and what might appear roentgenographically to be a periapical lesion is in actuality a periodontal lesion (Fig. 1–52). How the pulp withstands the constant insult from the traumatism as well as the irritating products from the periodontal lesion remains a mystery. Few pulps succumb to this severe double irritant.

Fortunately, the concomitant periodontal lesion may often be corrected. Ideally, though, the two conditions should be treated concurrently, an approach which will materially improve the chances of success.[50]

Developing Apical Cyst. In three failure cases an apical cyst either developed or continued developing at the periapex following endodontic therapy. Diagnosis in each case was made by biopsy (Fig. 1–53). In one of the cases, no periapical lesion existed at the time endodontic therapy was completed. The apical cyst developed subsequently. In the other two cases, a small periapical lesion increased in size following therapy and, when examined by biopsy, proved to be cystic. This is not surprising when one considers that Bhaskar found 42% of all periapical lesions so examined to be cystic.[33] On the other hand, careful ***pretreatment*** diagnosis of the apical cyst is not an exacting procedure.

Adjacent Pulpless Tooth. An untreated pulpless tooth with a periapical area that communicates with a periapical lesion of a previously treated adjacent tooth is another condition that will cause ***apparent*** failure. This situation may well exist and frequently does in traumatic accident cases (Fig. 1–54). Again, the condition is seen more frequently in the anterior mouth because this area is more prone to injury by accident.

Undoubtedly, in many of these cases both teeth have nonvital pulps at the time of initial therapy. Faulty diagnosis, however, fails to reveal the fact. If a lesion exists at the periapex of only one tooth, the tendency might be to treat only this tooth without pulp testing the other teeth in the area. In time, a lesion may develop at the apex of the adjacent tooth and the two lesions coalesce. Then again, at the time of treatment the adjacent teeth may test vital, but later another pulp may die unbeknownst to the patient. The toxic products from this necrotic pulp may then act as an irritant to perpetuate the periapical lesion which the two teeth share in common.

These cases emphasize the necessity of complete examination and diagnosis prior to treatment as well as thorough diagnosis of the entire area for the patient who returns suspecting a failure.

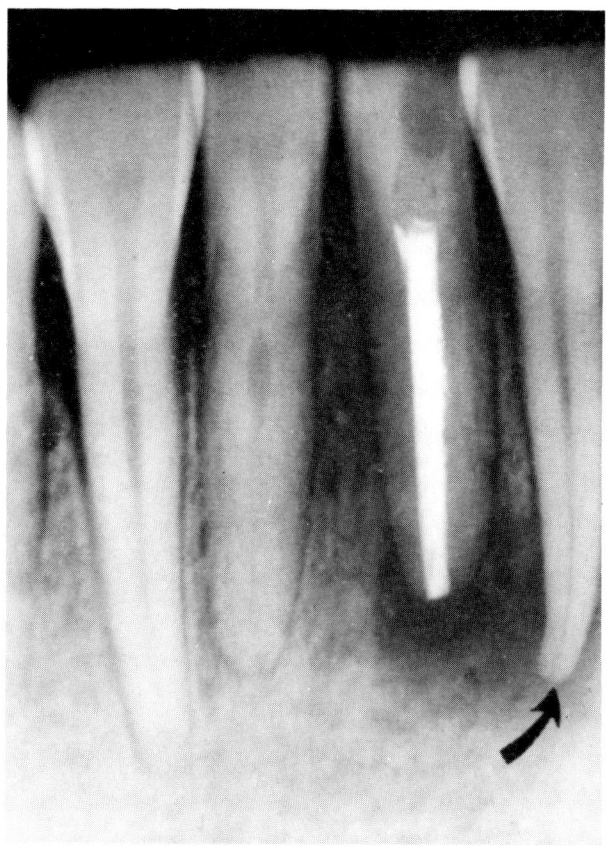

Fig. 1–54. Persistent periapical lesion, one year following endodontic therapy of mandibular central incisor, actually caused by pulpless, lateral incisor (arrow) whose periapical lesion joins lesion of previously treated central incisor. Pulpal necrosis in this case was caused by impact trauma. Note as well changes in canal shape in right central incisor indicating concomitant pulpal death and calcific activity. Misdiagnosis by roentgenogram alone points out importance of extended examination by electric pulp tester.

Accessory Canal Unfilled. Although a great "to-do" has been made over the accessory canal, in the Washington study only one failure could be associated with an unfilled accessory canal (Fig. 1–55). It is thought that in the majority of cases the tissue within the accessory canal remains vital even though the contents of the ***main canal*** become necrotic. Each accessory canal may have its own vascular supply from vessels in the periodontal space, and does not depend upon the major vessels of the pulp for blood supply.

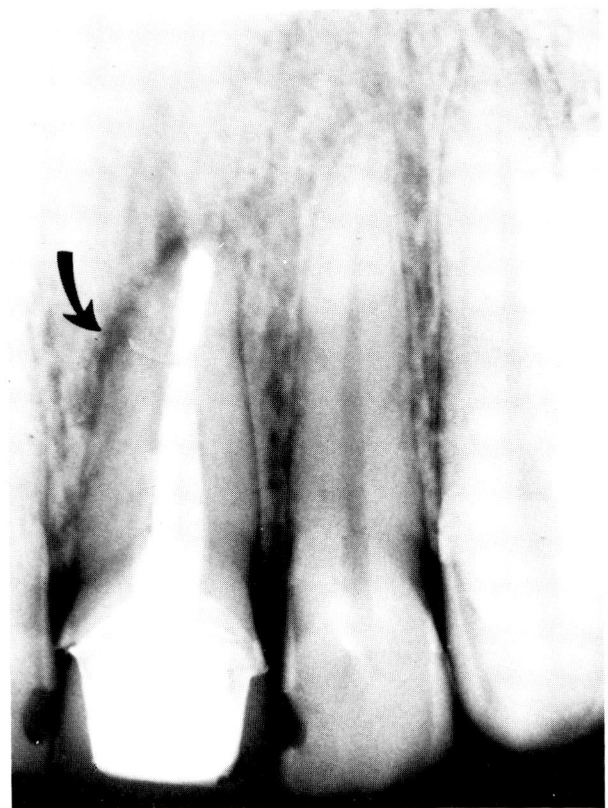

Fig. 1–55. Failure related to unfilled, lateral, accessory canal, although apical canal has been successfully obliterated with retrofilling. Accessory canal allows percolation into poorly filled portion of canal resulting in persisting, lateral lesion (arrow). (From Luebke, R. G., Glick, D. H., and Ingle, J. I.: Oral Surg., *18*:97, July, 1964.)

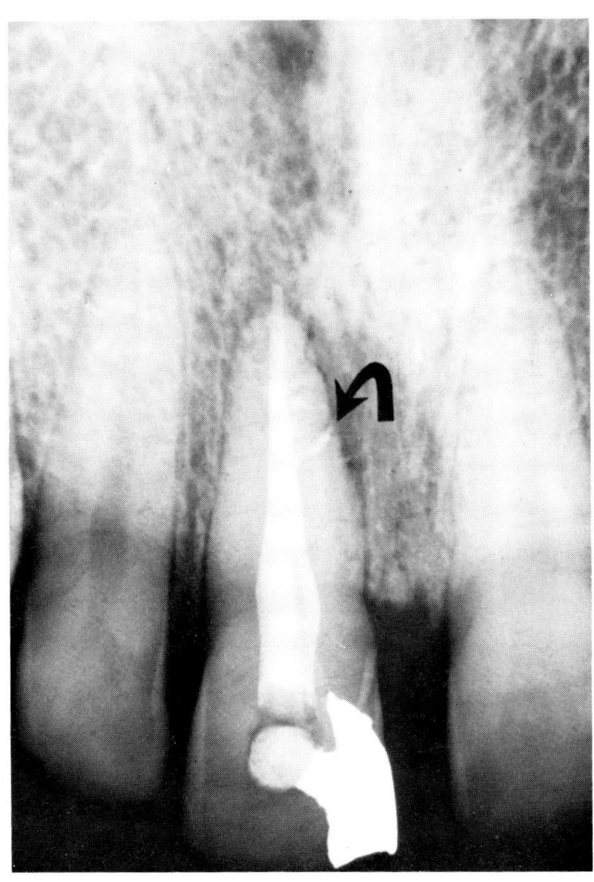

Fig. 1–56. Accessory canals filled by cement (arrow) in pulp devitalized in jackhammer accident. The root canal filling is gutta percha filled by lateral condensation.

Most of the cases with total devitalization of the tissue in the accessory canals as well as the body of the pulp are in teeth involved in severe traumatic accident (Fig. 1–56). In these cases not only are the pulpal vessels destroyed, but the periodontal ligament is ripped loose as well, and with it the vessels to the accessory canals. Here again, this problem usually arises in the premaxilla where the majority of traumatic damage occurs. Fortunately, when the canal filling is condensed, the accessory canals are frequently filled as well. Occasionally, however, the main canal is filled and the accessory canals remain patent and necrotic. The proponents of vertical obturation with softened gutta percha indicate the superiority of this technique for filling lateral or accessory canals (Fig. 1–57).

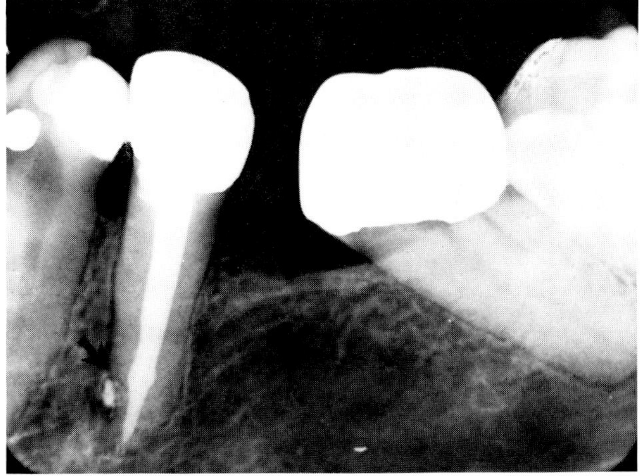

Fig. 1–57. Lateral canal obturated by softened gutta percha and vertical compression. Note lateral bony lesion and area of internal resorption opposite lateral canal. (Courtesy Dr. James D. Zidell.)

Constant Trauma. Constant trauma, usually from bruxism, is another factor to consider in failure of

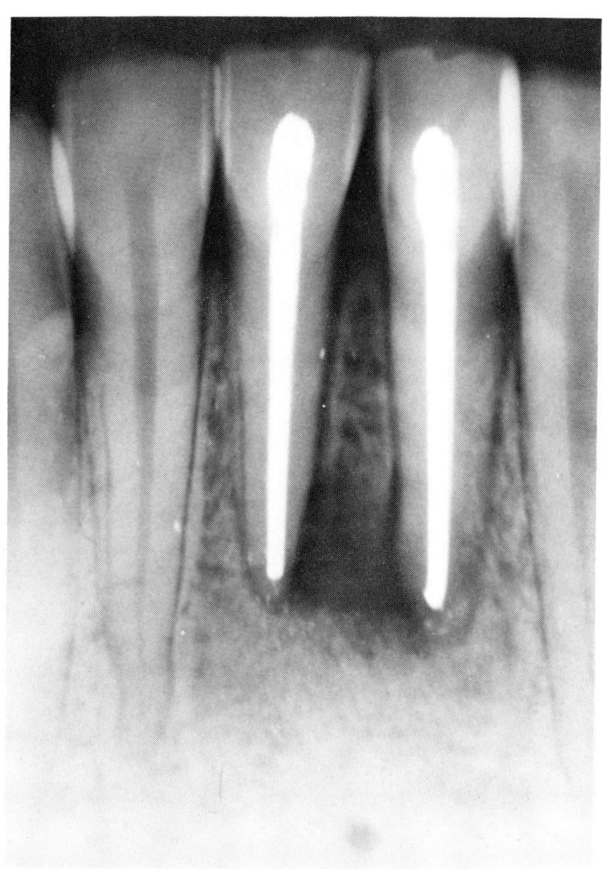

Fig. 1–58. Persistent periapical lesion one year following therapy. Pulps were devitalized in this adolescent female by constant protrusive bruxism. Continuation of traumatic habit prevents osseous repair. Plastic "night guard" was constructed to eliminate damaging effects of bruxism.

periapical repair. The one failure listed in Tables 1–7 and 1–8 in no way reflects the seriousness of this problem. Many treated patients had previously been seen with a complaint of periapical discomfort or swelling; however, relieving the occlusion and admonishing the patient not to grind traumatically on the affected tooth relieved the problem (Fig. 1–58).

Bruxism is not the only traumatic factor to consider. One patient constantly traumatized his chin following periapical surgery by practicing racing dives for hours each day. The constant slapping of the face into the water was enough to prevent complete healing. Another patient was a food faddist and used her anterior teeth to incise seven apples and three stalks (not sticks) of celery every day. As soon as she was convinced that she should cut the food into pieces and place them in her mouth with a fork, the necessary healing took place.

The most frequently encountered trauma, however, is related to the occlusally overcontoured restoration, upon which the patient cannot close without traumatizing the involved tooth. This phenomenon of healing failure related to traumatic occlusion should not be surprising when one considers the fact that pulps may be devitalized by bruxism.[51] It goes without saying that each restoration of a pulpless tooth should be thoroughly checked for overcontour and traumatism.

Perforation of the Nasal Floor. The single failure case involving perforation of the nasal floor was a retreatment case. The patient presented herself for retreatment of a failed endodontic case in which a

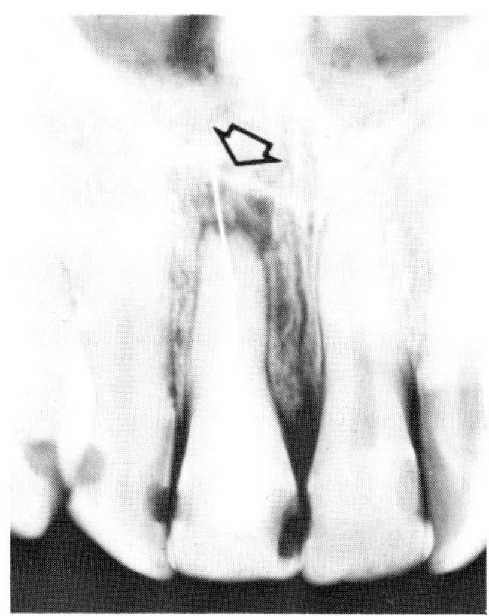

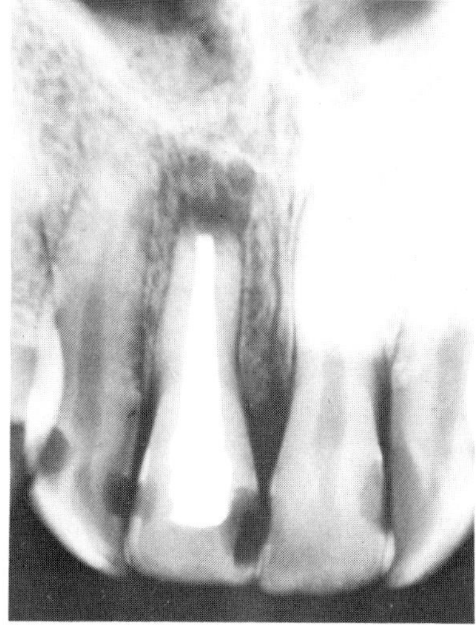

Fig. 1–59. Perforation of nasal floor (arrow) caused by extended "diagnostic wire" used as root canal filling. Persistent periapical lesion *(right)* is being maintained through fistulous tract into floor of nose.

diagnostic wire had been sealed in the canal and allowed to extend through the periapical lesion and past the nasal floor (Fig. 1–59). The patient commented when the wire was removed that, "the little loose bone (sic) in the floor of my nose is gone." When the recall roentgenogram demonstrated the continuing periapical lesion, an examination of the region revealed a small stoma in the floor of the right nostril and a fistulous tract leading to the periapex. The irritating bacteria, of course, were being supplied from the nose. Cautery by a rhinologist closed the tract and the lesion soon healed.

Causes of Failure Not Revealed by the Study. A number of causes of failure were not revealed by the study, mainly because the problem was encountered and corrected before the two-year recall roentgenogram was taken.

Three cases which involved the use of amalgam as a filling material in the retrofilling approach should be listed as failures. In an article by Omnell,[52] it was shown that failure in these cases was related to constant electrolysis between the zinc in the amalgam alloy and the other four constituents of the amalgam: silver, tin, copper, and mercury. The constant flow of electric current in this case will cause lysis of tissue in the affected area. The increased destruction of cells leads to an enlargement of the periapical lesion.

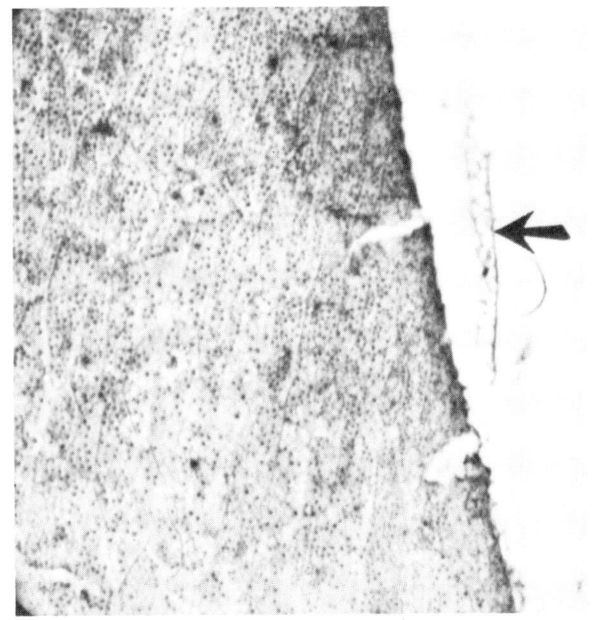

Fig. 1–60. Biopsy of what was thought to be root tip reveals columnar-like cells (arrow) of outer husk of popcorn kernel which was trapped in fresh surgical area and served as severe irritant.

Although not every case of retro-amalgam fillings of zinc-containing alloy has failed, use of a zinc-free alloy should improve success.

Another cause of failure involves a foreign body left in the periapical area following a surgical procedure. This particular patient complained of swelling and discharge from the periapical incision approximately two weeks following operation. A roentgenogram taken at this time failed to reveal any etiologic factor. Because the area was quiescent, reintervention into the surgical area was not undertaken.

About two weeks later the patient reported a swelling in the palate, lingual to the involved tooth, and the next day something fell out of this lingual area into a glass while she was drinking. The specimen looked like a root tip, but biopsy revealed the structure to be vegetable in nature, probably a seed (Fig. 1–60). The patient ultimately remembered stopping to see a motion picture on her way home after her previous appointment, and eating a bag of popcorn while watching the film. The foreign body was undoubtedly a popcorn kernel which worked into the surgical area through the still anesthetized incision.

Other cases that fail are treated internal root resorption cases which have perforated through to the cementum and then continue as external resorption cases. Also cases with root fenestration will fail if the dehiscence is so extensive that the periapical lesion is open to the irritants from the oral cavity, and healing is retarded if not arrested (Fig. 1–61). Occasionally the root of a pulpless tooth will split during or after treatment, causing failure. The persistent, fulminating periodontal-periapical lesion often is associated with the split root. In addition, dental caries may so involve the treated pulpless tooth as to destroy the value of the tooth (Fig. 1–62).

One of the most frequent causes of failure of the treated pulpless tooth is fracture of the crown. The tooth must be carefully protected by an adequate restoration.

It is interesting to note that in no case in this report has retained canal infection been listed as the primary cause of failure. Negative cultures were obtained prior to filling the nonsurgical cases in the study. The surgical cases were spot checked for sterility. Undoubtedly, in many of the failure cases, bacteria are ultimately the irritating force causing the failure. The infecting bacteria are not necessarily left in the canal, but have the freedom to invade from the apex and

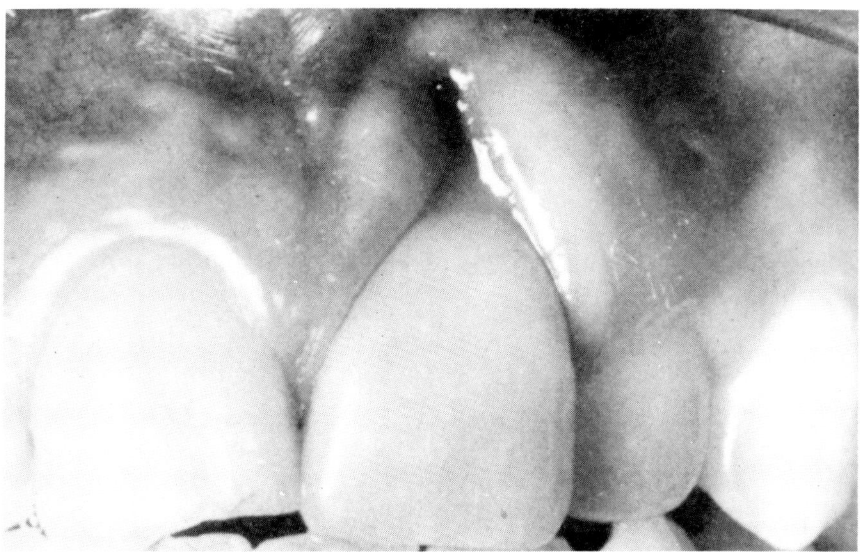

Fig. 1–61. Severe bony and soft tissue dehiscence which extends to periapex of traumatized incisor. Postoperative defects of this type may develop following surgery in area of osseous fenestration. (From Luebke, R. G., Glick, D. H., and Ingle, J. I.: Oral Surg., *18*:97, July, 1964.)

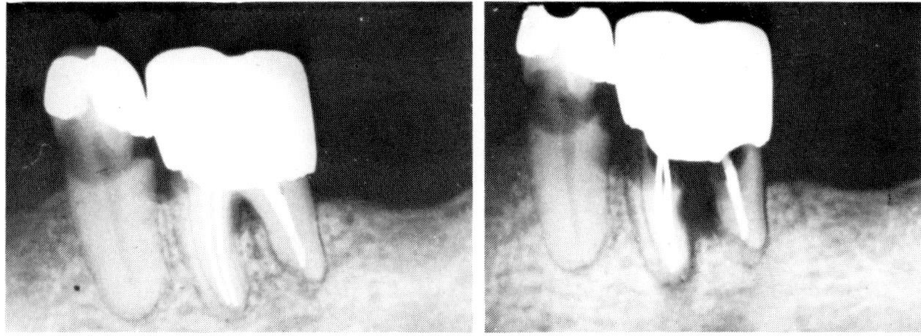

Fig. 1–62. Postoperative failure due to extension of dental caries rather than endodontic therapy *per se*. Loss of these abutment teeth led to full denture in this case.

multiply, because of some basic error in case selection or in operative or obturating technique. This emphasizes the point initially stressed; if the case is carefully selected before treatment, and if the canal is correctly instrumented and obturated, the ultimate outcome should be successful. The primary role of the anti-infectives is to prevent acute exacerbation of infection during therapy or after obturation.

Examination of the Failure Case. The examination of the failure case is important, for if the cause of failure can be determined and corrected, the failure may be turned into a success.

Before proceeding with a detailed examination, the most obvious causes of failure should be eliminated; is the canal incompletely obturated or, on the other hand, is there an obvious perforation of the root, or obvious overfilling? If all the obvious factors can be eliminated, then some more obscure cause of failure must be present.

The examiner should then begin a detailed examination following a four-stage procedure. One of these four steps in the examination should reveal the cause of failure.

1. Complete a thorough roentgenographic study of the involved tooth with exposures from three different horizontal projections—the standard buccal to lingual projection, 30 degrees from the mesial and 30 degrees from the distal. The central beam must pass directly through the apex. If this does not reveal incomplete obturation of the apical one-third of the canal, a canal obviously not filled, or an extra canal or root, then proceed to:

2. Examine the involved tooth for signs of occlusal traumatism. Test the mobility of the tooth and, using the forefinger, test for movement under the forces of centric closure and both lateral excursions. Be certain to check the tooth for trauma in the nonfunctional, lateral position or "balance." Look for telltale facets on occluding surfaces. If the tooth is not being traumatized by bruxism or an extra-oral habit, then proceed to:

3. Check the vitality of adjacent teeth to be sure the periapical lesion is not being maintained by an adjacent necrotic pulp. If all of these points of examination check out as normal, then:

4. Check the involved tooth and adjacent teeth for a coexistent periodontal lesion. This step should be left until last because the area may have to be anesthetized to complete the periodontal probing to depth.

If all of these causes are checked and eliminated by examination, one may assume that failure is due to an unusual factor such as a split root, or incomplete obturation which does not show roentgenographically. If the unusual can be eliminated by careful questioning, observation, and examination, the examiner should finally suspect incomplete obturation and steps should be taken to eliminate the cause.

Measures to be Employed to Improve Success. One may draw certain conclusions from this study, and finally list a number of procedures to improve the rate of success of treated endodontic cases. These are the Twelve Commandments of Endodontics:

1. *Use great care in case selection.* Be wary of the case that will be an obvious failure, but at the same time, be daring within the limits of capability.

2. *Use greater care in treatment,* not hurrying, maintaining an organized approach. Be certain of instrument position and procedure before progressing.

3. *Establish adequate cavity preparation,* both the access cavity, which can be improved by modifications of coronal preparation, and the radicular preparation, which can be improved by more thorough canal instrumentation.

4. *Determine the exact length of tooth to the foramen* and be certain to ***operate only*** to the cementodentinal junction which is about 0.5 mm. from the external orifice of the foramen.

5. *Utilize standardized instruments,* so that gross increases in size and taper of instrument sizes will not lead to shelf and ledge formation, broken instruments, and perforations. ***Always use sharp instruments.***

6. *Always use curved instruments in curved canals,* and especially remember to clean and reshape the curved instrument each time it is used. By adequate preparation, attempt to perfect a ***round tapered*** preparation at the apex, which will match the ***round tapered*** filling material to be used.

7. *Use standardized filling materials* to assure more perfect obturation in the apical one-third of the canal.

8. *Use great care in fitting the primary filling point.* One must be certain to obliterate the apical portion of the canal. Be more exacting in the total obturation of the entire root canal.

9. *Utilize periapical surgery only in those cases where surgery is definitely indicated.*

10. *Always check the apical density of the completed root canal filling* of the patient undergoing periapical surgical treatment, and this by using a sharp right-angle explorer. If found wanting, the apical foramen is retrofilled.

11. *Properly restore each treated pulpless tooth to prevent coronal fracture.*

12. *Practice endodontic techniques* until the procedures are as routine as the placement of an amalgam restoration or the extraction of a central incisor. Practice on extracted teeth mounted in acrylic blocks is especially recommended.

By careful attention to details in following the ***Twelve Commandments of Endodontics*** a degree of success approaching 100% will be assured.

REFERENCES

1. Coolidge, E. D.: Past and Present Concepts in Endodontics. J.A.D.A., *61*:676, Dec., 1960. (Presented before Centennial Meeting, American Dental Association, New York, 1959.)
2. Orban, B.: Contribution to the histology of the dental pulp and periodontal membrane with special reference to the cells of defense of these tissues. J.A.D.A., *16*:965, June, 1929.
3. Prinz, H.: A summary of Dr. Walkhoff's discussion of chlorophenol and treatment of diseases of the dental pulp. Ohio Dent. J., *19*:152, March, 1899.
4. Pucci, F. M.: *Conductos Radiculares*. Vol. II, Buenos Aires, Editorial Medico-Quirurgica, 1945, p. 625.
5. Ingle, J. I., and Levine, M.: The need for uniformity of endodontic instruments, equipment, and filling materials. In *Transactions of the Second International Congress on Endodontics*. Edited by L. I. Grossman, Philadelphia, 1958, p. 133-143.
6. Ingle, J. I.: A standardized endodontic technique utilizing newly designed instruments and filling materials. Oral Surg., *14*:83, Jan., 1961.
7. Bowman, G. A.: Quoted in *History of Dentistry in Missouri*. Fulton, Mo., The Ovid Bell Press Inc., 1938, p. 423.

8. Nevin, A.: The Stimulation of Calcified Tissue of the Nonvital Open Apex. Presented at meeting of Am. Assoc. of Endodont., April 24, 1975.
9. Goldman, L. B., Rosen, H., Goldman, M., and Kronman, J. H.: Further Report on Hydron as a Root Canal Filling Material. Presented at meeting of Am. Assoc. of Endodont., April 24, 1975.
10. Beveridge, E. E.: Endodontic teaching manpower report. Oral Surg., *34*:965, Dec., 1972.
11. Your Teeth Can be Saved . . . by Endodontic Treatment. Amer. Dental Association. Pamphlet No. G17.
12. Burns, R. C.: Am I Losing My Nerve? Long Island City, N.Y., Union Broach Co.
13. Milgrom, P., and Ingle, J. I.: Consent procedures as a quality control. J. Oral Surg., *33*:115, July, 1975.
14. Serene, T. P.: Endodontic litigation. Oral Surg., *36*:422, Sept., 1973.
15. Weiner, L.: Personal communication. Feb. 18, 1974.
16. Weichman, J. A.: Malpractice prevention and defense. Cal. Dent. Assoc. J., *3*:58, Aug., 1975
17. Survey of Dental Services Rendered-1969. J.A.D.A., *81*:35, July, 1970, Table 10.
18. Decayed, Missing and Filled Teeth Among Youths 12-17 Years. U.S. Dept. Health, Education & Welfare Publication #HRA 74-1626, Sept., 1974.
19. Dental Health and Care. Report of the New Zealand Public Health, 1974.
20. Loss of Teeth. U.S. Dept. of Health, Education & Welfare Publication #585-B22, 1967.
21. Lord, J., and Teel, S.: The overdenture: patient selection, use of copings. J. Prosth. Dent., *32*:41, July, 1974.
22. Bohannan, H. M., and Abrams, L.: Intentional vital extirpation in periodontal prosthesis. J. Prosth. Dent., *11*:781, July, 1961.
23. Fish, E. W., and MacLean, I.: The distribution of oral streptococci in the tissues. Brit. Dent. J., *61*:336, Sept., 1936.
24. Okell, C. C., and Elliot, S. D.: Bacteremia and oral sepsis. Lancet, *2*:869, 1935.
25. Bender, I. B., and Pressman, R. S.: Factors in dental bacteremia. J.A.D.A., *32*:836, July, 1945.
26. Hayward, J. R., Kerr, D. A., Jesse, R. H., and Ingle, J. I.: The management of teeth related to the treatment of oral cancer. CA, *19*:98, Mar.-Apr., 1969.
27. Hiatt, W. H.: Regeneration of the periodontium after endodontic therapy and flap operation. Oral Surg., *12*:1471, Dec., 1959.
28. Prichard, J.: The intrabony technique as a predictable procedure. J. Perio., *28*:202, July, 1957.
29. Moore, A. W.: Personal communication.
30. Sommer, R. F., Ostrander, F. D., and Crowley, M. C.: *Clinical Endodontics*. Philadelphia, W. B. Saunders Co., 2nd Ed., 1961, p. 446.
31. Grossman, L. I., and Rossman, S. R.: Correlation of clinical diagnosis and histopathologic findings in 101 pulpless teeth with areas of rarefaction. J. Dent. Res., *34*:692, Oct., 1955. (Abstract of paper read at 33rd meeting of Int. Assn. Dent. Res.)
32. Priebe, W. A., Lazansky, J. P., and Wuehrmann, A. H.: The value of roentgenographic film in the differential diagnosis of periapical lesions. Oral Surg., *7*:979, Sept., 1954.
33. Bhaskar, S. N.: Synopsis of Oral Pathology. St. Louis, C. V. Mosby Co., 4th Ed., 1973.
34. Crump, M. C., and Natkin, E.: Relationship of broken root canal instruments to endodontic case prognosis: a clinical investigation. J.A.D.A., *80*:1341, June, 1970.
35. Ingle, J. I.: Existos y Francasos en Endodoncia. Revista de la Asociacion Odontologica Argentina, Vol. 2, *50*:67, Feb., 1962.
36. Zeldow, B. J., and Ingle, J. I.: Correlation of the positive culture to prognosis of endodontically treated teeth: a clinical study. J.A.D.A., *66*:23, Jan., 1963.
37. Abramson, I. I.: A Frank Appraisal of the Present Status of the Bacterial Culture Test as a Routine Endodontic Procedure. Presented at the Annual Meeting of American Assn. of Endodontists, Feb., 1961, Chicago. (Personal Communication.)
38. Strindberg, L. L.: The dependence of the results of pulp therapy on certain factors. Acta Odontol. Scand., *14*:175, Supp. 21, 1956.
39. Grossman, L. I.: Polyantibiotic therapy of pulpless teeth. J.A.D.A., *43*:265, Sept., 1951.
40. Pucci, F. M., and Reig, R.: *Conductos Radiculares*, Vol. I, Buenos Aires, Editorial Medico-Quirurgica, 1944, pp. 219-225.
41. Ibid: pp. 185-188.
42. Miller, H. M.: Incidence of extraction at the University of Oregon Dental School. Oral Surg., *11*:1226, Nov., 1958.
43. Bossert, W. A., and Marks, H. H.: Prevalence and characteristics of periodontal disease in 12,800 persons under periodic dental observation. J.A.D.A., *52*:429, Apr., 1956.
44. Strindberg, L. I.: Op. cit., p. 61.
45. Sommer, R. F., Ostrander, F. D., and Crowley, M. C.: *Clinical Endodontics*. Philadelphia, W. B. Saunders Co., 1956, p. 514.
46. Selden, H. S.: Pulpoperiapical disease: diagnosis and healing. Oral Surg., *37*:271, Feb., 1974.
47. Boyle, P. E.: *Kronfield's Histopathology of the Teeth and Their Surrounding Structures*. Philadelphia, Lea & Febiger, 4th Ed., 1955, Chapter 11, pp. 273-296.
48. Ramfjord, S.: Experimental periodontal reattachment in Rhesus monkeys. J. Perio., *22*:73, Apr., 1951.
49. Slowey, R. R.: Radiographic aids in the detection of extra root canals. Oral Surg., *37*:271, Feb., 1974.
50. Simon, J. H., Glick, D. H., and Frank, A. L.: The relationship of endodontic-periodontic lesions. J. Perio., *43*:202, Apr., 1972.
51. Ingle, J. I.: Alveolar osteoporosis and pulpal death associated with compulsive bruxism. Oral Surg., *13*:1371, Nov., 1960.
52. Omnell, K. A.: Electrolytic precipitation of zinc carbonate in the jaw. Oral Surg., *12*:846, July, 1959.

Chapter 2

Preparation for Endodontic Therapy

JOHN I. INGLE, EDWARD E. BEVERIDGE, LEONARD PARRIS, RICHARD E. WALTON, and JAMES D. ZIDELL

Before the actual operative aspects of root canal therapy are begun, a number of preparatory procedures must first be completed.

1. Roentgenography is needed, first as an aid to diagnosis, then periodically during treatment.
2. Specialized endodontic instruments and equipment must be arranged for ready use.
3. Local anesthesia of the involved tooth or area may be necessary. Special problems of anesthesia also may arise, particularly in the case of an inflamed pulp.
4. Rubber dam placement sometimes requires special handling in endodontics.

ROENTGENOGRAPHY IN ENDODONTICS*

No single scientific development has contributed as greatly to improved dental health as the discovery of the amazing properties of cathode rays by Professor Wilhelm Konrad Roentgen in November, 1895. The significant possibilities of application to dentistry were seized upon fourteen days after Roentgen's announcement, when Doctor Otto Walkoff took the first dental roentgenogram in his own mouth.[1] In the United States, within five months, Dr. William James described Roentgen's apparatus and displayed several radiographs. Three months later, Dr. C. Edmund Kells gave the first clinic in this country on the use of the x-ray for dental purposes. Three years later (1899), Kells was using the x-ray to determine tooth length during root canal therapy.

*Abstracted in part from Walton, R. E.: Endodontic radiographic technics. Dental Radiography and Photography, *46*:51, 1973.

"I was attempting to fill the root canal of an upper central incisor," Kells later said. "It occurred to me to place a lead wire in this root canal and then take a radiogram to see whether it extended to the end of the root or not . . . The lead wire was shown very plainly in the root canal."

One year later (1900) Dr. Weston A. Price "called attention to incomplete root canal fillings as evidenced in radiographs." By 1901, Price was suggesting that radiographs be used to check the adequacy of root canal fillings.[2]

Though these early attempts were rarely of diagnostic quality, it was the beginning of a new era for all of dentistry. For the first time dentists could see the accumulation of past dental treatment—therapy done without knowledge of what lay beneath the gingiva. Needless to say, the calamitous findings must have disheartened the conscientious practitioner. Yet even today, with all the modern engineering refinements, the sleekness of operation, and the reduction of hazards, a discouraging segment of our profession continues to deprive the public by failure to utilize roentgenography to its full potential.

The total application of roentgen rays and the disciplined interpretation of the product are beyond the scope of this textbook. Only the utilization of roentgenography in endodontics will be discussed here. Suffice it to say that roentgenography is absolutely essential for root canal therapy.

Application of Roentgenography to Endodontics. The roentgen ray is used in endodontic therapy to (1) aid in the diagnosis of hard tissue alterations of the teeth and periradicular structures; (2) determine the

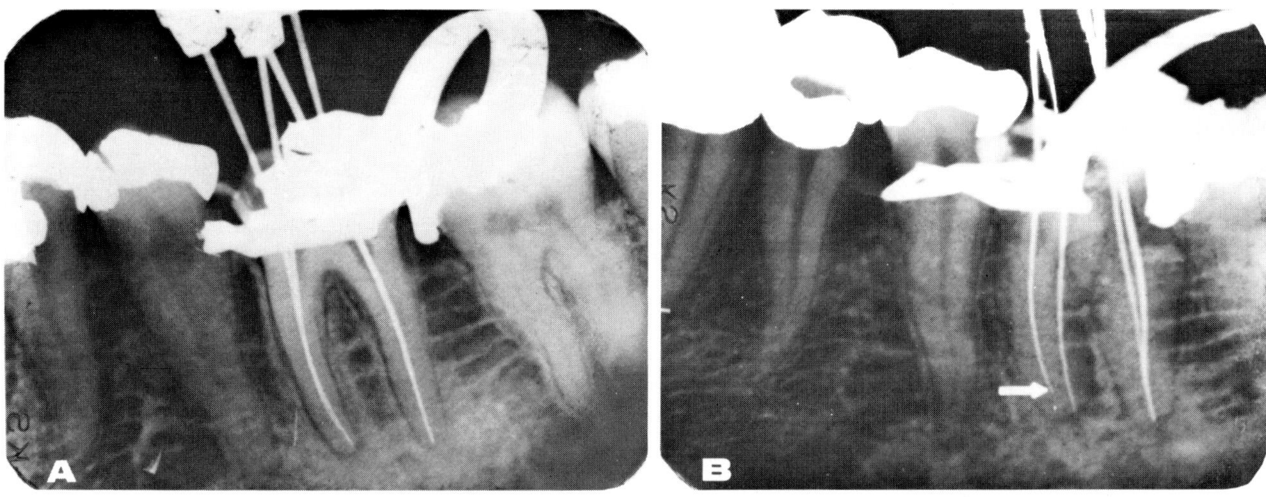

Fig. 2–1. Disclosing canals by radiograph. *A*, Right-angle horizontal projection reveals 4 files in separate canals superimposed. *B*, Horizontal angulation varied 30 degrees mesially reveals all 4 canals and file short of working length in mesiolingual canal (arrow). (From Walton, R. E.: Dental Radiog. Photog., *46*:51, Oct., 1973.)

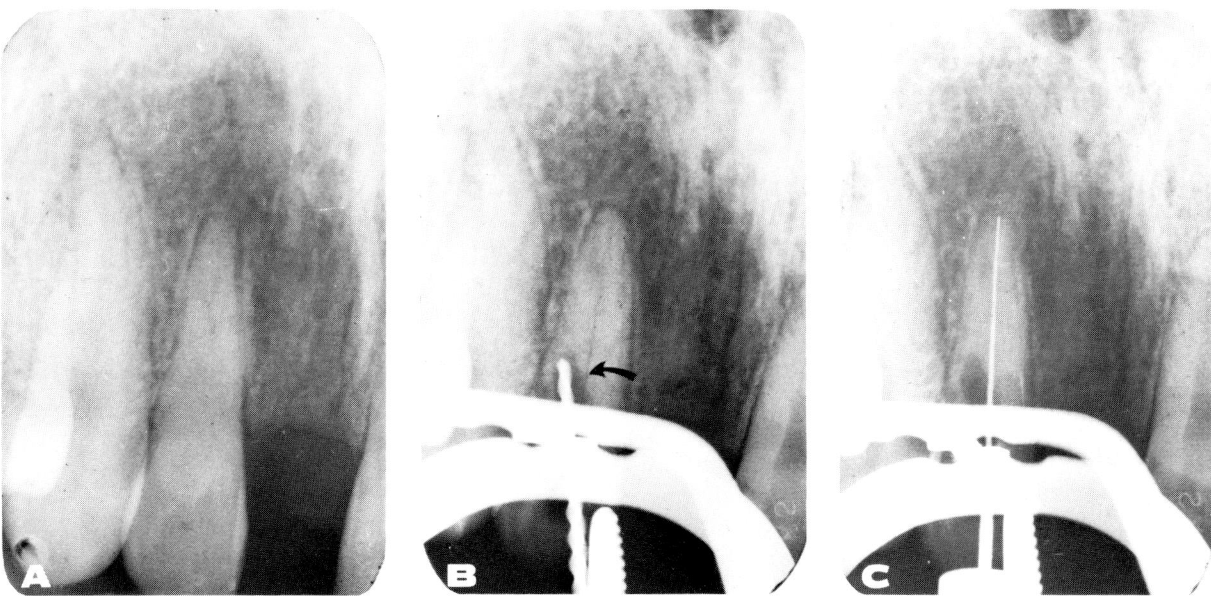

Fig. 2–2. Locating canal of receded pulp. *A*, Advanced calcification and receded pulp. *B*, Radiograph reveals angulation of preparation and canal (arrow) at mesial of cut. *C*, Canal, seen in radiograph, is discovered with fine file. (Courtesy Dr. Steven Koehler.)

numbers, location, shape, size, and direction of roots and root canals; (3) estimate and confirm the length of root canals prior to instrumentation; (4) localize hard-to-find or disclose unsuspected pulp canals by examining the position of an instrument within the root (Fig. 2–1); (5) aid in locating a pulp which is markedly calcified and/or receded (Fig. 2–2); (6) determine the relative position of structures in the facial-lingual dimension; (7) confirm the position and adaptation of the primary filling point; (8) aid in the evaluation of the final root canal filling; (9) aid in the examination of lips, cheeks, and tongue for fractured tooth fragments and other foreign bodies following traumatic injuries; (10) aid in localizing a hard-to-find apex during periapical surgery by relating an opaque object to the apex (Fig. 2–3); (11) confirm, prior to suturing, that all tooth fragments and excess filling material have been removed from the periapical region and the surgical flap, following periradicular surgery; and (12) evaluate, in recall films, success or failure of endodontic treatment.

Limitations of Roentgenograms. The roentgenogram has its limitations in endodontic treatment; roentgenograms are suggestive only and should not be considered the singular final evidence in judging any clinical problem. There must be correlation with other subjective and objective findings. The greatest fault with the roentgenogram relates to its physical state; it is a record of a shadow, and as such only two dimensions are shown on a single film. As with any shadow, these dimensions are easily distorted through improper technique and anatomic limitations. In addition, the buccal-to-lingual dimension is absent on a single film and is frequently forgotten, although techniques are available to define the third dimension. These techniques will be described later in detail.

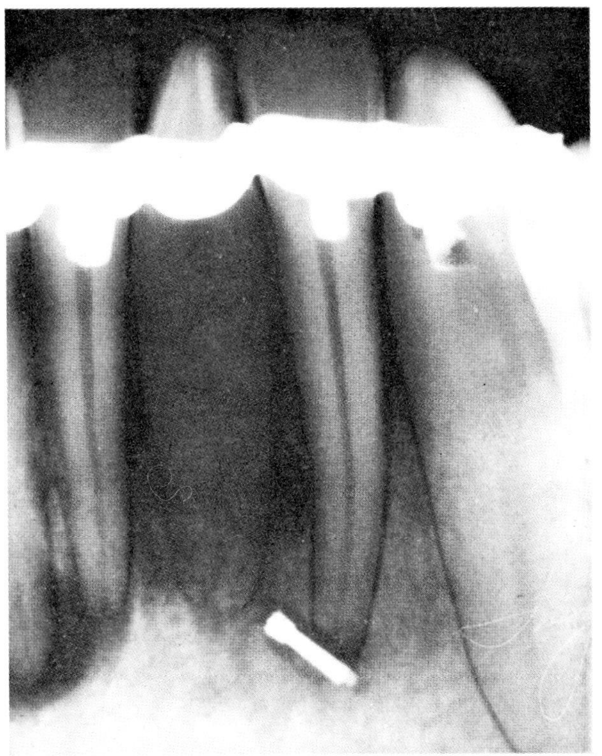

Fig. 2–3. Sterile, broken bur head positioned in surgical area and used to orient operator to periapical lesion.

Roentgenograms are not infallible. Various states of pulpal pathosis are indistinguishable in the roentgen-ray shadow. Neither healthy nor necrotic pulps cast an image. Correspondingly, the sterile or infected status of hard or soft tissue is not detectable other than by inference. Only bacteriologic evidence can determine this. Furthermore, periradicular soft tissue lesions cannot be accurately diagnosed by roentgenograms, but require histologic verification. Chronic inflammatory tissue cannot, for example, be differentiated from healed fibrous, "scar" tissue, nor can a differential diagnosis of periradicular radiolucencies usually be made on the basis of size, shape, and density of the adjacent bone.[3–7] A common misconception is that an inflammatory lesion is present only when there is at least a perceptible "thickening" of the periodontal ligament space. In fact, investigators have demonstrated that lesions of the medullary bone are likely to go undetected until the resorption has expanded into and eroded a portion of the cortical plate.[8–11]

The difficulties and inherent errors in roentgenographic interpretation were clearly demonstrated by Goldman, [12] who submitted recall radiographs of endodontic treatments, for clinical evaluation, to a group of radiologists and endodontists. They assessed success and failure by observation of radiodensities. There was ***more disagreement than agreement*** among the examiners.

Radiographs are an essential aid to diagnosis, but must be employed with discretion. However, roentgenograms are the only method whereby the endodontic operator can "visualize" that which he cannot see or feel during the process of diagnosis and treatment. He will discover that as his radiographic techniques and interpretation improve, so will the ease and success of his root canal treatment. The techniques outlined in the following sections have proved to be successful and predictable. If followed, they will greatly simplify difficulties in root canal treatment.

Instrumentation

Machines. Two basic types of x-ray machines are commonly employed in dental offices. One type has a range of kilovoltage and two milliamperage settings with which the long (16-inch) cone is frequently used. The other type offers only one kilovoltage and milliamperage setting and only the short (8-inch) cone. Either type provides adequate roentgenograms. However, each has advantages which, under different circumstances, will yield a more satisfactory result. The long-cone system is superior for diagnostic radiographs, whereas the flexible short-cone machine is more appropriate for treatment or "working" films. Any x-ray machine must be properly shielded and collimated by means of a lead diaphragm and filtered by aluminum discs to ensure proper radiation safeguards for the patient and the professional personnel. An additional protective measure is the draping of the patient with a lead apron to block scatter radiation.

Long cone. Because of the clarity of detail and minimum distortion inherent in the long-cone parallel technique,[13–16] it is preferred for exposing diagnostic, final, and recall roentgenograms.

Short cone. Because of the number of working roentgenograms taken in the course of endodontic therapy, the practitioner treating more than the occasional tooth will find that a short-cone machine, with a small, easily manipulated head, will save much time, energy, and frustration (Fig. 2–4). Although image sharpness is not so critical for working films as for diagnostic films, it must be emphasized that either machine will yield suitable films, provided other principles of roentgenography are applied.

Film. Industrial technologic advances have allowed film exposure time to be reduced to fractions of a second. Unfortunately, these high-speed, thick-emulsion films are not ideal for routine endodontic use, for they do not readily clear in the fixer, and a good deal of time may be lost waiting for the return of "wet films." Exposure of Kodak DF7 Radiatized film and a rapid processing method produce a highly acceptable ***working*** film.

A "slower" film, which is processed much more rapidly, can safely be recommended for all "working" films, such as the length-of-tooth and primary filling point roentgenograms, but "hi-speed" film should be used for all initial diagnostic and all final and recall roentgenograms.

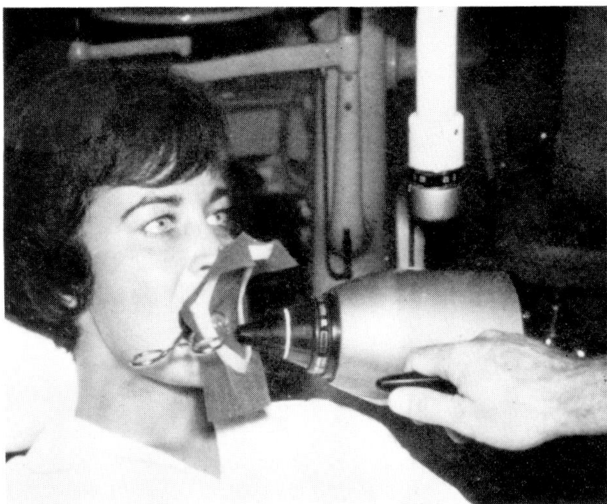

Fig. 2–4. Compact, short cone x-ray machine (Siemens) attached to dental unit is ideal for exposing endodontic "working" films.

For dentists with a referred endodontic practice, duplicate film packets are recommended for the diagnostic, final treatment, and recall roentgenograms—one set for his permanent office record, the other for the referring dentist.

The standard periapical size film is used for most situations. In addition, every office should have 2 × 3 inch ***occlusal*** film available to be used when: (1) periapical lesions are so extensive that they cannot be demonstrated in their entirety on one periapical film; (2) more than two adjacent anterior teeth are being examined or treated; (3) there is interest in or involvement of the nasal cavity, sinuses, or roof or floor of the mouth (Fig. 2–5); (4) trauma or inflammation prohibits the normal jaw opening required to place and hold a periapical film; (5) the location of a structure, lesion, or foreign body in the buccolingual dimension is necessry; (6) a handicapped person is unable to hold a periapical film by the usual means; and (7) detection of fractures of the anterior portion of the maxilla or mandible is needed.

Sheingorn has recommended the use of "occlusal" film as a lateral plate, to expose a mesiodistal view of the anterior teeth.[17] This is particularly valuable when questions arise about the number and placement of multiple canals in mandibular incisors. By placing instruments in the suspected canals and aiming the

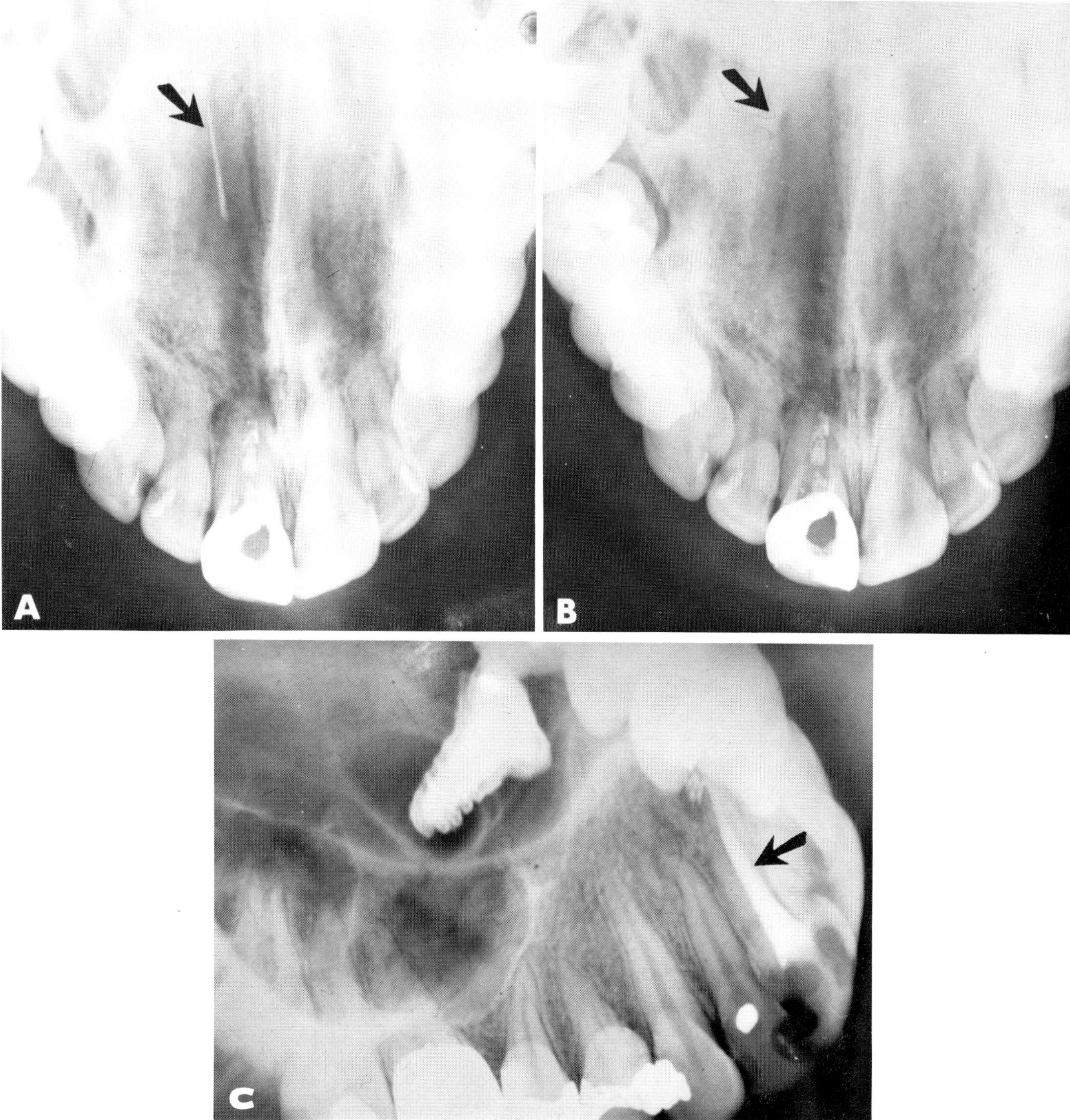

Fig. 2–5. *A,* Use of occlusal film to locate objects which extend beyond the limits of the standard periapical film. Piece of gutta percha (arrow) "lost" in a lesion extending beneath the floor of the nose is here revealed in an occlusal film. *B,* Check-up occlusal film reveals that "lost" filling material has been totally removed during surgical procedure (arrow). *C,* Treated central incisor (arrow) was suspected as origin of maxillary pain. Wider film, however, reveals wood screw buried in nose as source of inflammation. (Courtesy Dr. Thomas P. Serene.)

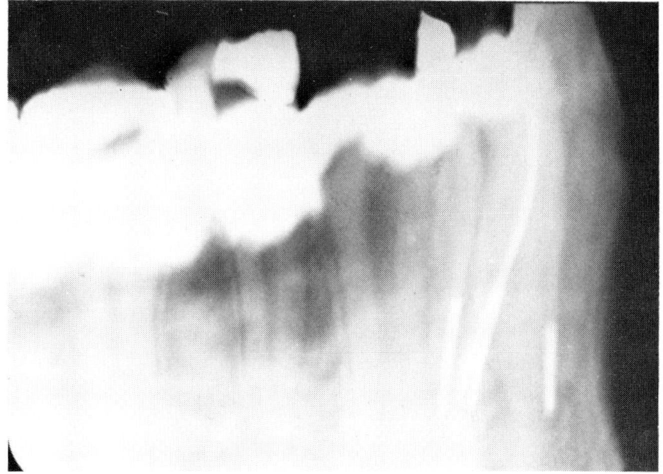

Fig. 2–6. Occlusal film used as lateral plate reveals multiple canals and position of incisors related to cortical plate. (Courtesy Dr. Abe Sheingorn.)

central beam across the mental region, from left to right rather than anterior to posterior, one may gain a somewhat distorted but valuable view of the incisor anatomy (Fig. 2–6).

Film Placement. Film placed parallel to the long axis of the teeth and exposed by cathode rays at a right angle to the surface of the film will yield accurate images, free of shortening or elongation.[18] If this principle is applied, it is unnecessary to memorize fixed cone angulations. In a modern, comfortable operating chair, moreover, with the patient in a semireclined position, he need not be returned to an upright position for each exposure.

Because of the complicating presence of the rubber dam, the methods for placement of ***working*** films differ somewhat from the methods for placement of diagnostic, final, and recall films.

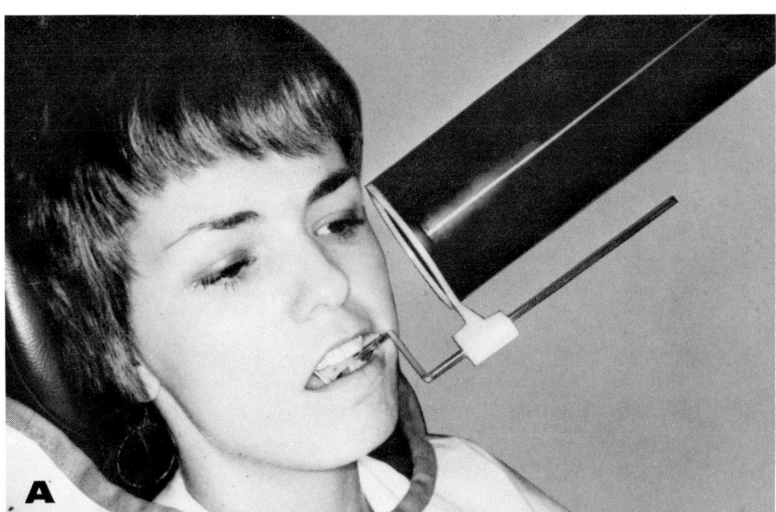

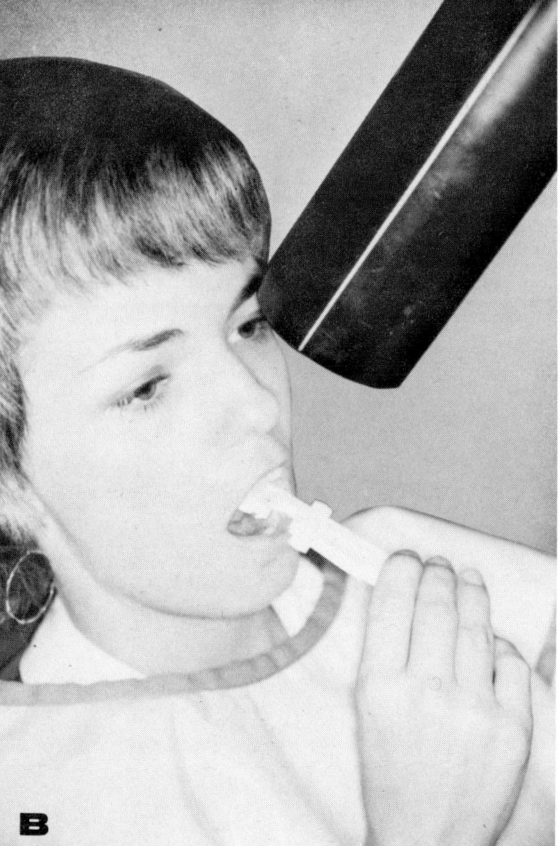

Fig. 2–7. Two film holders to improve parallelism. *A*, Rinn X-C-P holder properly places film as cone is aligned at right angles to handle. (Courtesy Dr. Richard E. Walton.)

Diagnostic roentgenograms. These must be the best roentgenograms possible. To achieve this goal there are advantages to parallelism, which permits more accurate visualization of structures as well as reproducibility. This facilitates comparison in recall roentgenograms. Examples are shown of two types of devices that simplify the procedure of parallelism. The Rinn X-C-P virtually guarantees distortion-free films, correct cone alignment, relative to the film, being assured. It is designed for use in any region (Fig. 2–7*A*). The Snap-A-Ray is a simpler holder, and is also suitable for all regions (Fig. 2–7*B*); however, it does not guarantee correct cone placement as does the X-C-P.

Film holders are preferred to finger retention of the film for several reasons: (1) there is less chance of film slippage and distortion; (2) because of the current emphasis on radiation hazards, many patients object to having their fingers repeatedly exposed; and (3) the necessarily wide opening of the mouth may be uncomfortable and cause inaccurate film placement. If it ***is*** necessary that the film be finger-held, cotton rolls will aid in obtaining parallelism of the film packet with the long axis of the tooth. Usually one large cotton roll placed horizontally, lingual to the crowns, will act as an adequate spacer to place the film in proper relationship to the tooth being examined (Fig. 2–8). Occasionally, because of restricting vault

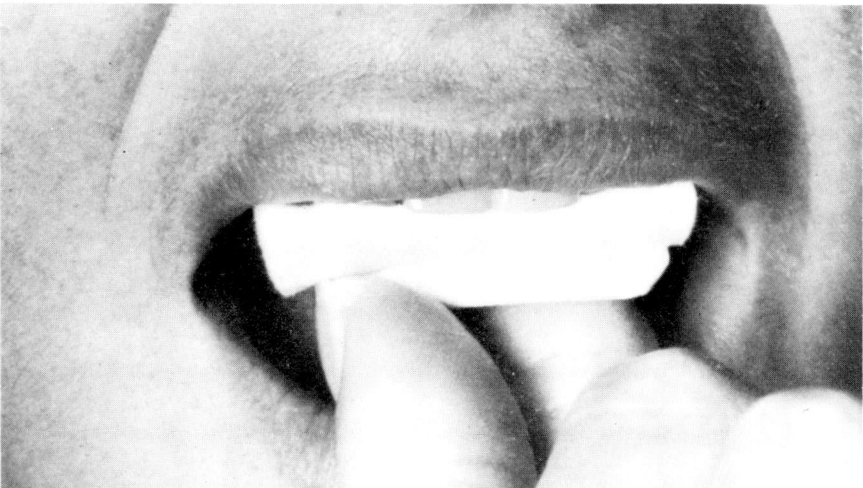

Fig. 2–8. Large cotton roll, placed horizontally, positions film packet parallel to long axis of anterior teeth. Index finger is placed at apical edge of film while thumb on incisal edge prevents it from slipping.

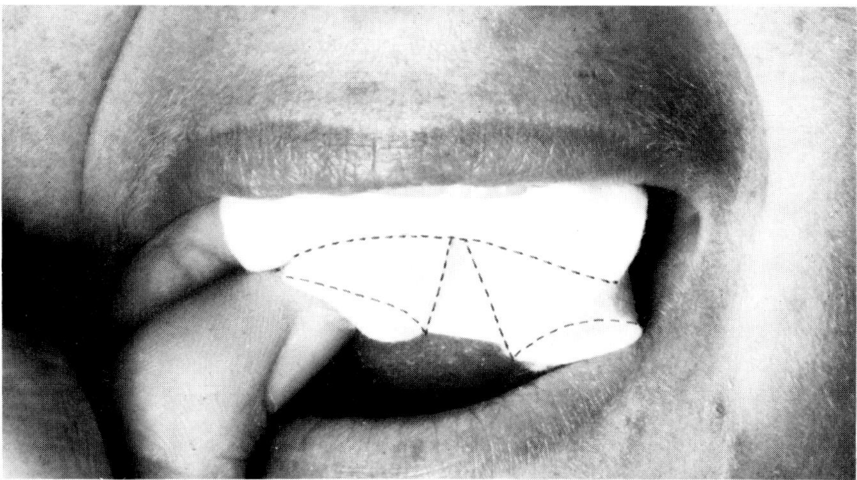

Fig. 2–9. Three cotton rolls may be required to parallel film with long axis of tooth. Two rolls are placed vertically and third roll in usual horizontal position. (Retouched)

form and/or tooth angulation, a wider "spacer" is required, and three cotton rolls may be used (Fig. 2–9). A cotton roll spacer is not required in the mandibular posterior regions.

Working roentgenograms. One great difficulty in the practice of root canal therapy is the clumsy, aggravating method of taking treatment roentgenograms with the rubber dam in place. Some dentists remove the rubber dam frame for access in film placement, and saliva enters to contaminate the operating field. It is therefore imperative that a film placement technique be utilized, so that the ***rubber dam frame need not be removed***. Use of a radiolucent N-O frame (Nygaard-Ostby) or the Starlite Visiframe type (see Figs. 2–51 and 2–52), will ensure that apices are not obscured.

With the rubber dam in place, the ***hemostat-held*** film has significant advantages over the finger-retained film: (1) the film placement is easier when the opening is restricted by the rubber dam and frame; (2) the patient may close with the film in place, a particular advantage in mandibular posterior areas where closing relaxes the mylohyoid muscle, permitting the film to be positioned further apically; (3) the handle of the hemostat is a guide to align the cone in the proper vertical and horizontal angulation (Fig. 2–10); (4) there is less risk of distortion of the roentgenogram caused by too much finger pressure bending the film (Fig. 2–11); and (5) patients can hold a hemostat handle more securely with less possibility of film displacement. In addition, any movement can be detected by the shift of the handles and corrected prior to exposure.

In all instances of film placement, the identifying ***dimple*** should be placed at the incisal or occlusal edge to prevent its obscuring an important structure.

Cone Placement. It is a mistake to rely on only one film. There is much to be learned from additional exposures taken from varied horizontal or vertical projections.

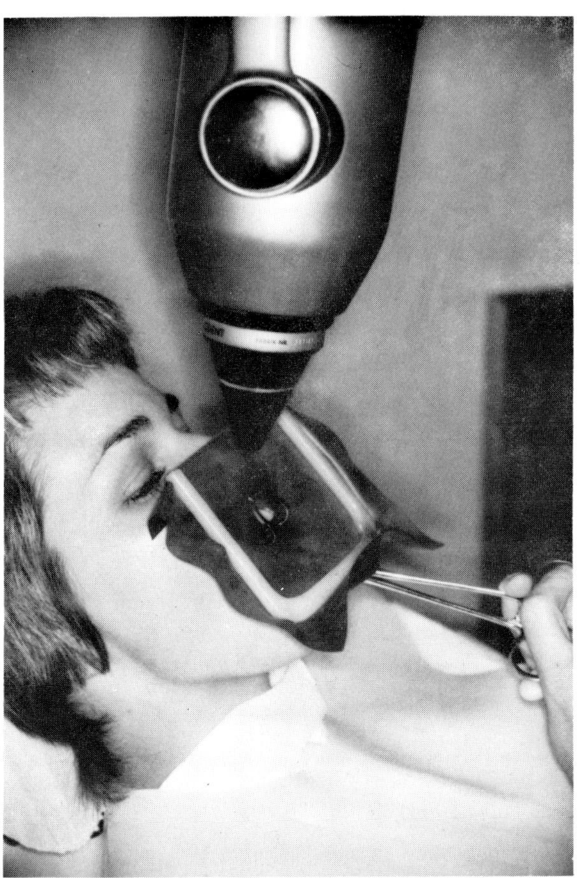

Fig. 2–10. "Working" film properly placed and held under rubber dam with hemostat. Cone is aligned at right angle to handle. (Courtesy Dr. Richard E. Walton.)

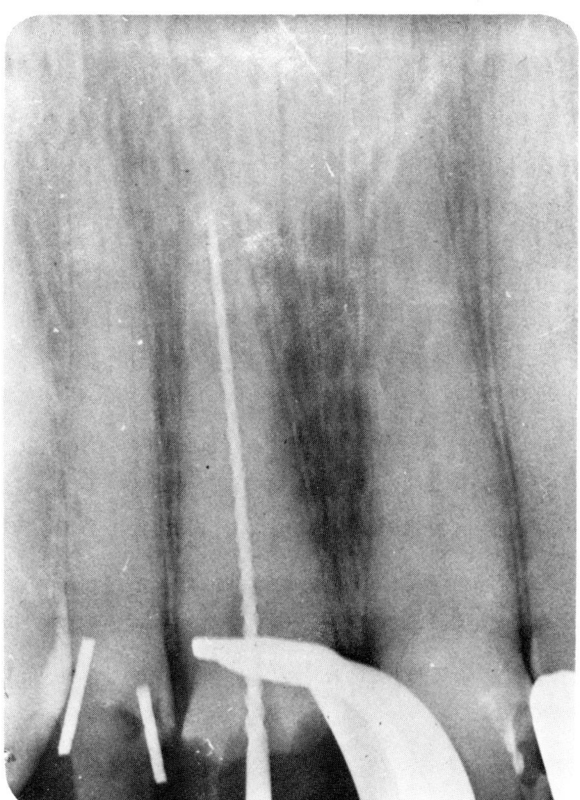

Fig. 2–11. Film bent by finger pressure to conform to narrow palate produces elongated distorted radiograph useless for diagnosis or treatment. (Courtesy Dr. Richard E. Walton.)

Vertical Angulation. Ordinarily, it is preferable to align the cone so that the beam strikes the film at a right angle. This alignment ensures a fairly accurate vertical image. Elongation of an image, however, may be corrected by ***increasing*** the vertical angle of the central ray. Conversely, foreshortening is corrected by decreasing the vertical angle of the central ray. To remember this, one should think of the sun, which casts a shortened shadow at noon when it is at its zenith, or increased vertical angle.

Frequently, an impinging palatal vault prevents parallel alignment of the film and the teeth. However, if the film angle is no greater than 20 degrees in relation to the long axis of the teeth, and the beam is directed at a right angle to the film, there is no distortion but a less effective orientation of structures.[18] The resulting roentgenogram is still adequate.

Horizontal Angulation. Walton has introduced an important refinement in dental roentgenography which will materially improve the endodontic interpretive film.[19] He has demonstrated a simple technique whereby the ***third dimension*** may be readily visualized. Specifically, the anatomy of superimposed structures, the roots and pulp canals, may be better defined.

The basic technique is to vary the ***horizontal*** angulation of the central ray of the x-ray beam. By this method overlying canals may be separated, and by applying Clark's rule,[20] the separate canals may then be identified. Clark's rule states that ***"the most distant object from the cone (lingual) moves toward the direction of the cone."*** Or, stated in another way, using the helpful mnemonic, MLM, aim the cone from the ***M***esial and the ***L***ingual root is always to the ***M***esial. Still another application of Clark's rule is: aim from the ***M***esial and the ***B***uccal root is always to the ***D***istal—MBD.

Horizontal Angulation Variations

Mandibular Molars. As previously emphasized, the film must be positioned parallel to the lower arch. The standard horizontal x-ray projection then is at a right angle to the film (perpendicular) as shown in Fig. 2–12. The two mesial canals are superimposed one upon the other and appear as a single line.

Through the ***Walton projection,*** however, the canals can be made to "open up." This is done by directing the central beam 20 or 30 degrees from the mesial (Fig. 2–13*A*). In Figure 2–13*B* (arrow), the two canals in ***each*** root can now be readily discerned. The contrast gained by varying the horizontal projection can best be seen in a clinical case with four canals. Figure 2–14*A*, taken at a right angle, clearly shows the four instruments superimposed upon one another. Figure 2–14*B*, on the other hand, taken from a 30-degree variance in horizontal projection, emphasizes the third dimension by the separation of the instruments in the canals. By applying Clark's rule (MLM), one also determines that the lingual canals are toward the mesial (the direction of the cone).

Another point should be made at this time concerning a frequent mistake in "reading" periapical

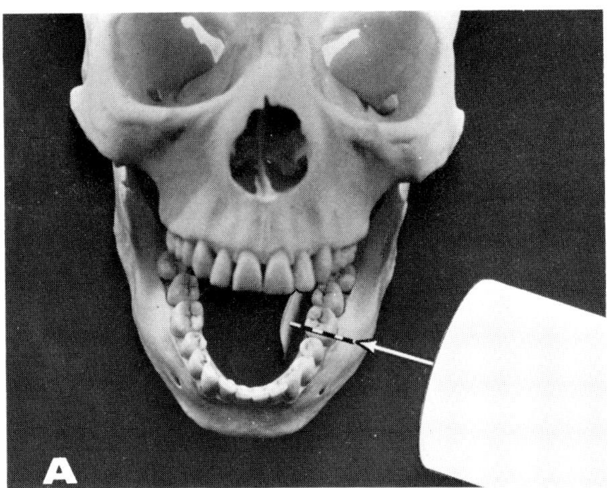

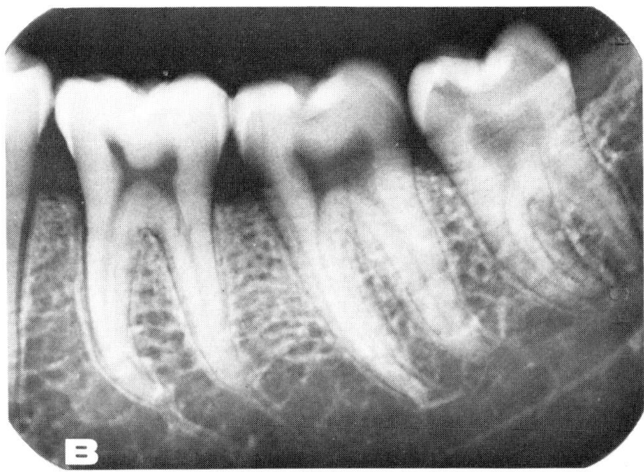

Fig. 2–12. Mandibular molars. *A*, Central ray directed at right angle to film positioned parallel to arch. *B*, Limited information is gleaned from radiograph because of superimposition of structures and canals. (From Walton, R. E.: Dental Radiog. Photog., *46*:51, Oct., 1973.)

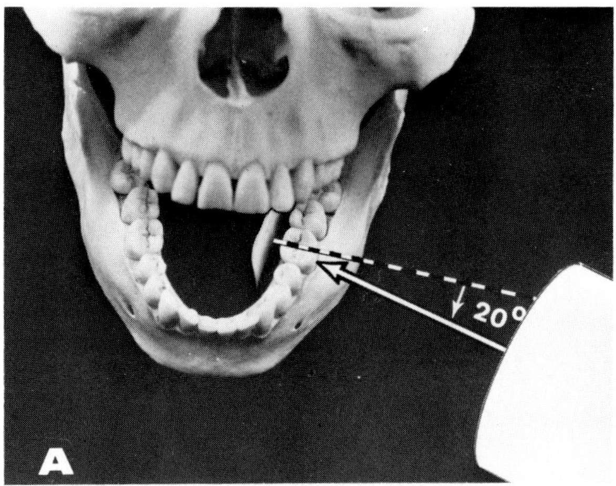

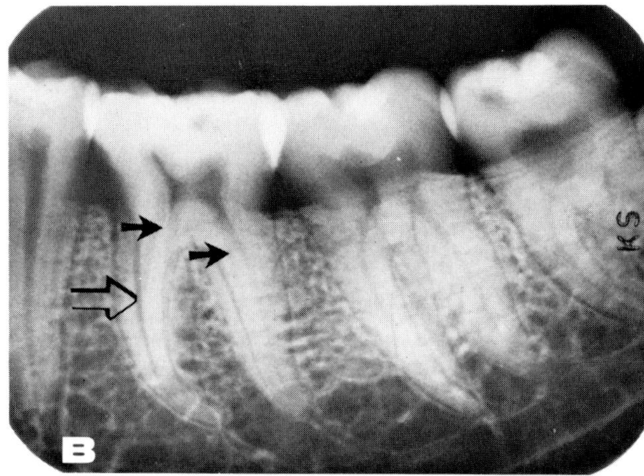

Fig. 2–13. Mandibular molars. *A,* Central ray directed at *20 degrees* mesially to film positioned parallel to arch. *B,* Two canals are now visible in *both* roots of the first molar (black arrows). Open arrow indicates confusing root outlines. (From Walton, R. E.: Dental Radiog. Photog., *46*:51, Oct., 1973.)

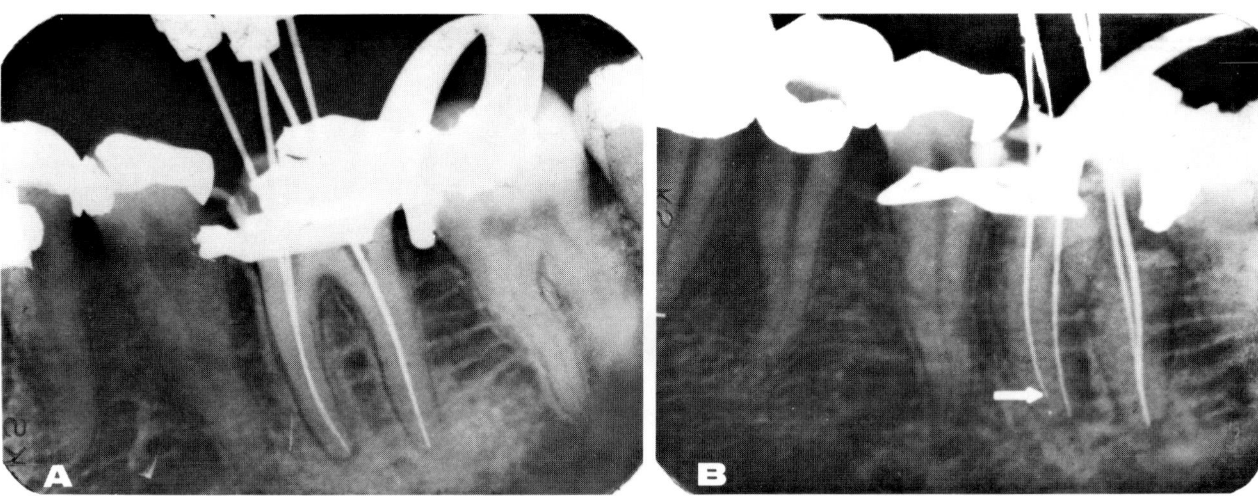

Fig. 2–14. Mandibular molars. *A,* Right-angle horizontal projection superimposes 4 files, one upon the other. *B,* Horizontal variance of 30 degrees separates 4 canals. Clark's rule (MLM) proves lingual canals are to mesial. (From Walton, R. E.: Dental Radiog. Photog., *46*:51, Oct., 1973.)

roentgenograms. It can best be illustrated by a cross-sectional drawing of molar root structure. Roots containing two canals are often hourglass-shaped, as Figure 2–15*A* indicates. When an x-ray beam passes directly through this structure, the buccal and the lingual portions of the root are in the same path (arrows). Because a double thickness of tooth structure is penetrated by the x-rays, it is seen in the film as a radiopaque root outline in close contact with the *lamina dura.* This is readily apparent on the radiograph (Fig. 2–15*B*).

By aiming the cone 20 degrees from the mesial, however, the central beam passes through the hourglass-shaped root at an angle (Fig. 2–16*A*). In this case the two thicknesses of the root are projected separately onto the film. Since less tooth structure was penetrated by the x-ray, the image on the film is less dense. A radiolucent line is clearly seen in Figure 2–16*B* (open arrow). This radiolucent line can be erroneously "read" as a root canal. One should take care to follow up the length of the line. Instead of entering the pulp chamber, it can be traced to emerge

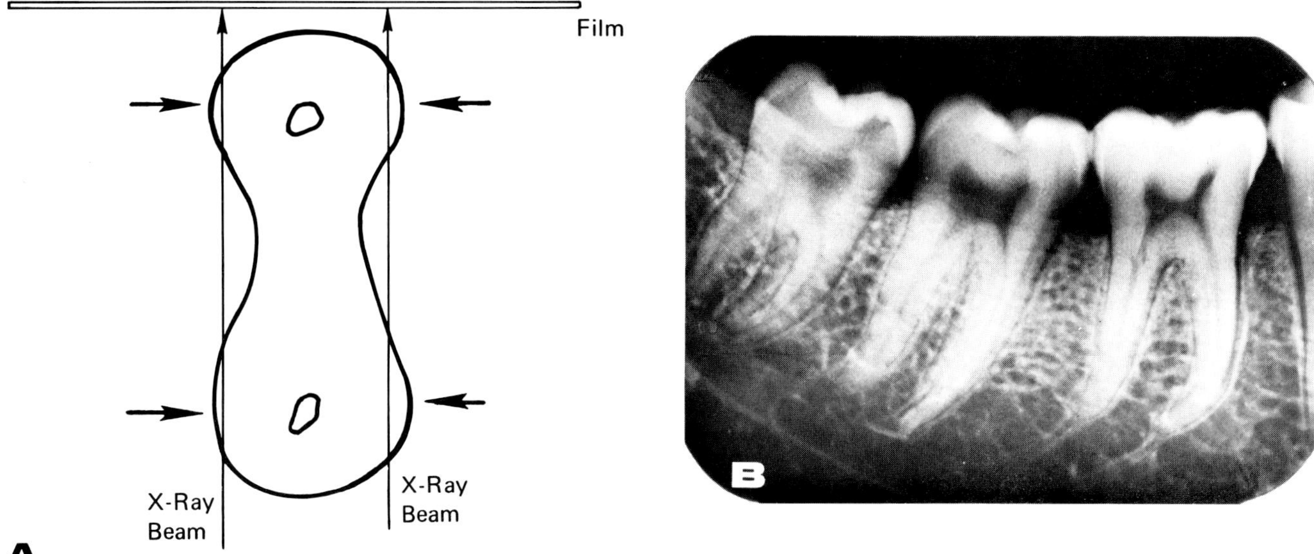

Fig. 2–15. *A,* X-ray beam passing directly through two thicknesses of root structure presents intensified image on film. *B,* Note radiopaque root outline inside *lamina dura.* (*B* part from Walton, R. E.: Dental Radiog. Photog., *46*:51, Oct., 1973.)

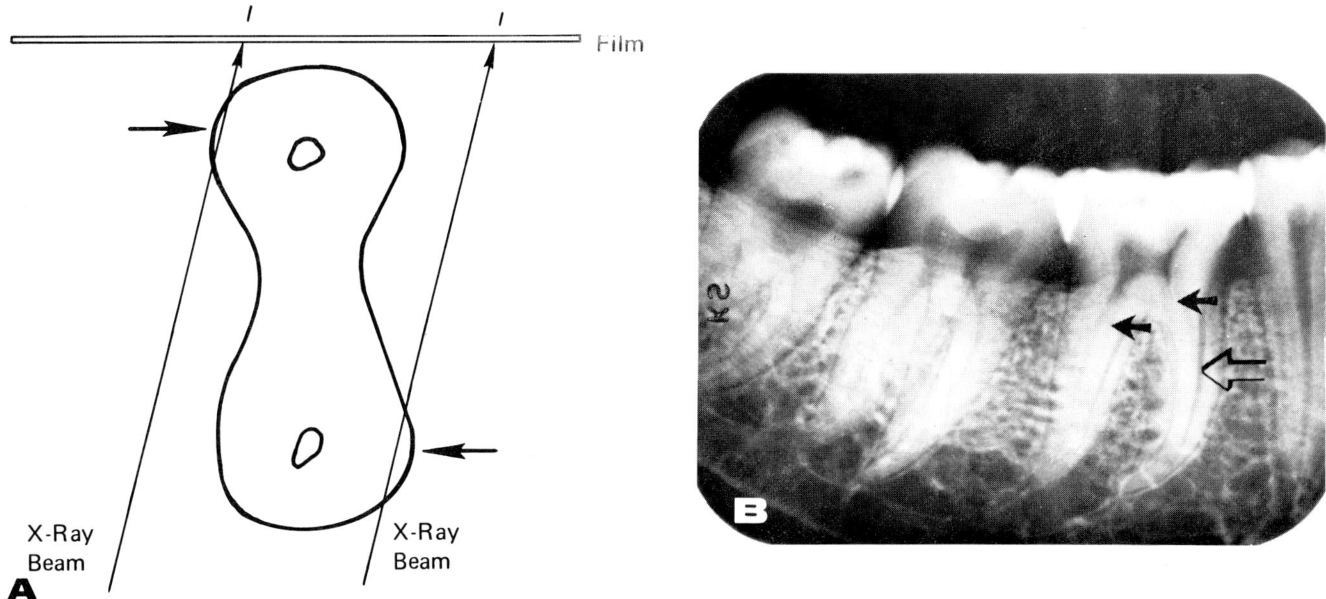

Fig. 2–16. *A,* X-ray beam aimed 20 degrees mesially passes through single thicknesses of hourglass root leaving less dense impression on film. *B,* Radiolucent line is apparent (open arrow) and may be confused with root canal. Note it emerges at gingival, not into pulp chamber. Black arrows indicate regular canals. (*B* part from Walton, R. E.: Dental Radiog. Photog., *46*:51, Oct., 1973.)

at the gingival surface of the root. This simple interpretive error can easily lead to gross mistakes in endodontic cavity preparation.

Mandibular Premolars. The importance of varying the horizontal angulation when radiographing mandibular premolars is demonstrated in Figure 2–17*A*, wherein the central ray is directed at a right angle to the film. What appears to be a single straight canal is discernible in each premolar (Fig. 2–17*B*). There is an indication, however, in the image of the first premolar, that the canal might bifurcate at the point of the abrupt change in density (arrow).

Directing the central ray 20 degrees from the mesial in the first premolar (Fig. 2–18A) causes the bifurcation into two separate canals to become readily apparent (Fig. 2–18*B*). The tapering outline of the tooth, seen in both projections, would indicate, on the other hand, that the two canals undoubtedly rejoin to form a common canal at the apex. In both

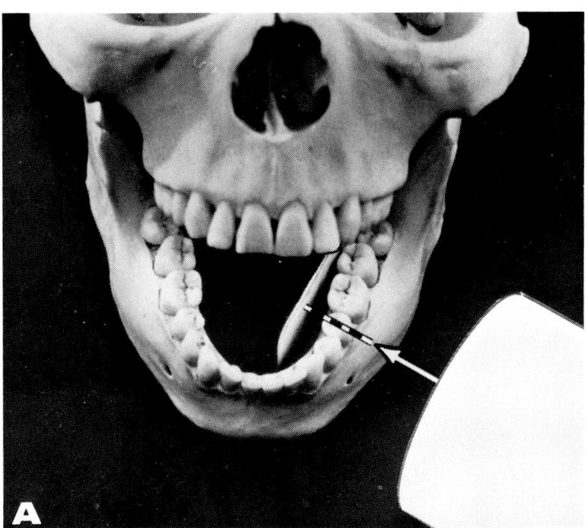

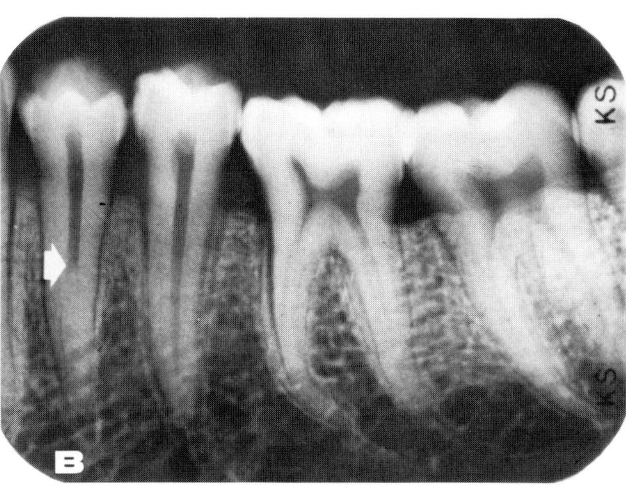

Fig. 2–17. Mandibular premolars. *A,* Central ray directed at right angle to film positioned parallel to arch. *B,* Radiograph reveals one canal in each premolar, although abrupt change in density (arrow) may indicate bifurcation. (From Walton, R. E.: Dental Radiog. Photog., *46*:51, Oct., 1973.)

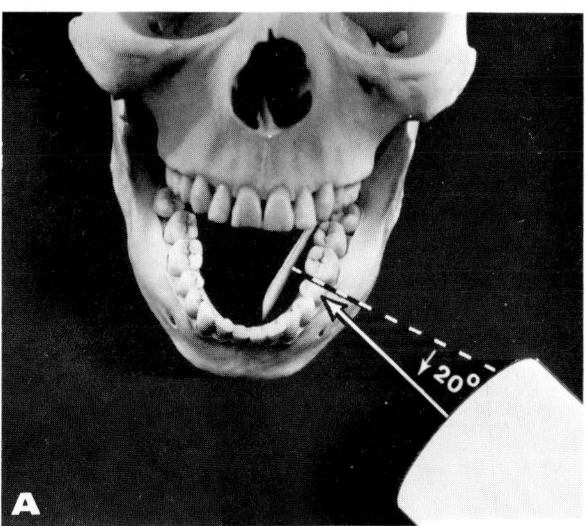

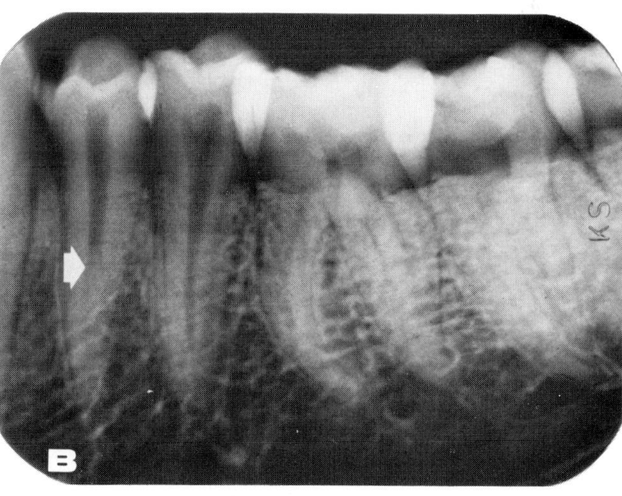

Fig. 2–18. Mandibular premolars. *A,* Central ray directed at 20 degrees mesially to film parallel to arch. *B,* In first premolar, two canals are clearly visible (arrow) which probably reunite, indicated by sharply tapered root. (From Walton, R. E.: Dental Radiog. Photog., *46*:51, Oct., 1973.)

the right-angle and 20-degree variance projections, the second premolar appears as a single canal.

Maxillary Molars. Maxillary molars are consistently the most difficult to radiograph because of (1) their more complicated root and pulp anatomy, (2) the frequent superimposition of portions of the roots upon each other, (3) the superimposition of bony structures (sinus floor, zygomatic process) upon root structures, and (4) the shape and depth of the palate, which is the major difficulty.

As is true of the mandible, the complex root anatomy and superimpositions may be dealt with by varying the horizontal angulations. Film placement must again be parallel to the posterior maxillary arch, not the palate.

The standard right-angle projection for a maxillary first molar illustrated in Figure 2–19*A* produces the

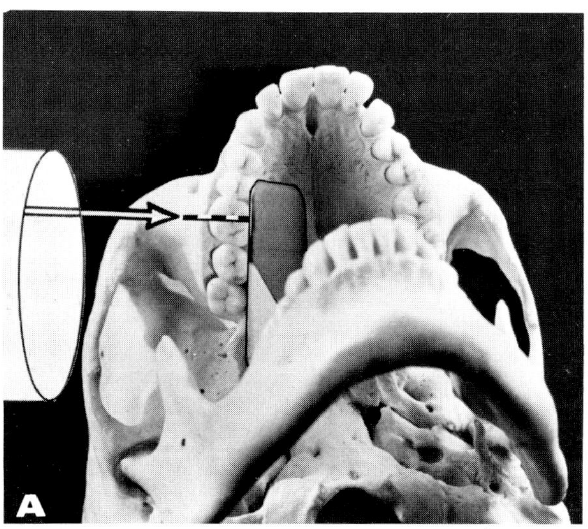

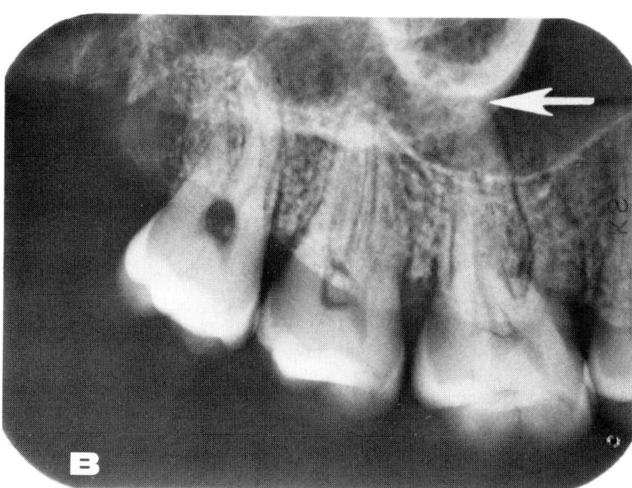

Fig. 2–19. Maxillary molars. *A,* Central ray is directed through maxillary molar at right angle to inferior border of film. Arrow and dotted line passing through malar process indicate it will superimpose over first molar. *B,* Superimposition of first molar roots, sinus floor, and malar process (white arrow) confuse diagnosis. (From Walton, R. E.: Dental Radiog. Photog., *46*:51, Oct., 1973.)

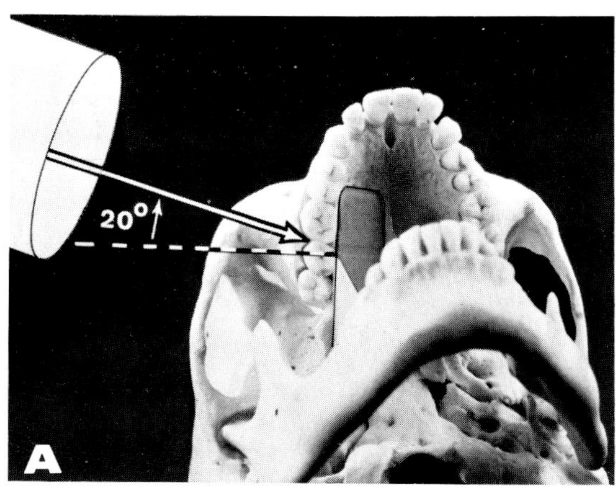

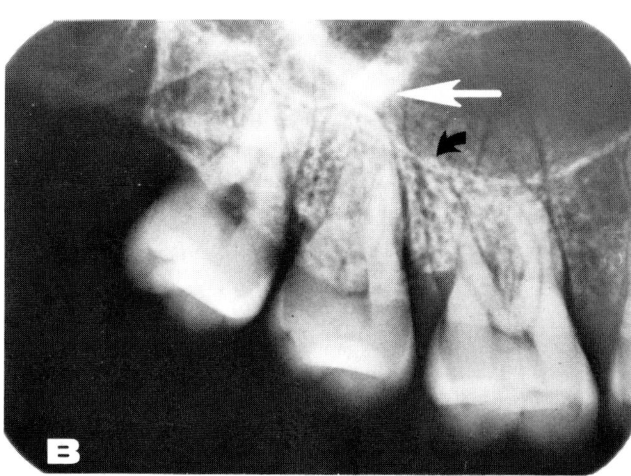

Fig. 2–20. Maxillary molars. *A,* Central ray directed at 20 degrees mesially skirts malar process projecting it distally. *B,* Distobuccal root is cleared of palatal root and malar process is projected far to distal (white arrow). Between right-angle and 20-degree projection, all three roots are clearly seen. (From Walton, R. E.: Dental Radiog. Photog., *46*:51, Oct., 1973.)

image seen in Figure 2–19*B*, wherein the zygomatic process is superimposed on the apex of the palatal root (arrow) and the distobuccal root appears to overlie the palatal root. The sinus floor is also superimposed on the apices of both the first and second molars.

When the horizontal angulation is varied by 20 degrees to the mesial (Fig. 2–20*A*), the zygomatic process is moved far to the distal of the first molar and the distobuccal root is cleared of the palatal root (Fig. 2–20*B*, arrows).

The opposite projection also can be used to isolate the mesiobuccal root of the first molar, that is, the central ray may be projected from 20 degrees ***distal*** to the right angle (Fig. 2–21*A*). Although this projection distorts the shape of the mesiobuccal root, it also isolates it (Fig. 2–21*B*), so that the canal is readily discernible (arrow). Also note that the zygomatic process is moved completely away from any root structure, including the second molar.

Clinical proof of the efficacy of this method is seen in Figure 2–22. In the standard right-angle projection in Figure 2–22*A*, one sees two instruments in the canals of the mesiobuccal root, but they are superim-

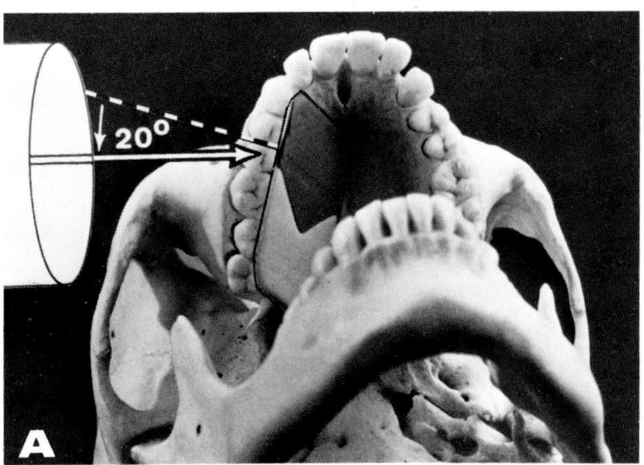

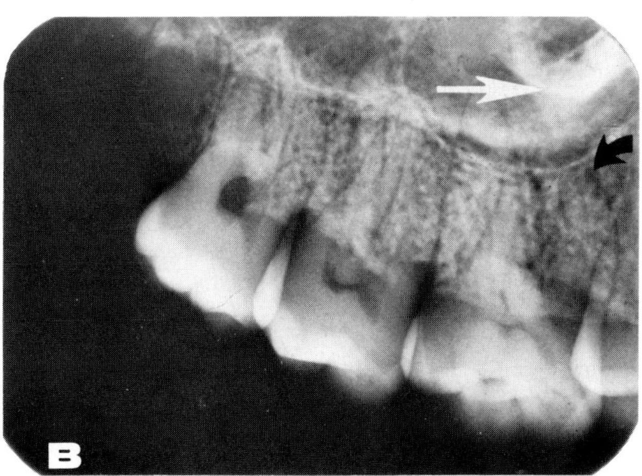

Fig. 2–21. Maxillary molars. *A,* Central beam projected 20 degrees from the *distal. B,* Mesiobuccal root of the *first* molar is isolated (black arrow) and second and third molars are cleared of malar process, which is projected forward (white arrow). Sinus floor may be "lowered" or "raised" by changing vertical angulation. (From Walton, R. E.: Dental Radiog. Photog., *46*:51, Oct., 1973.)

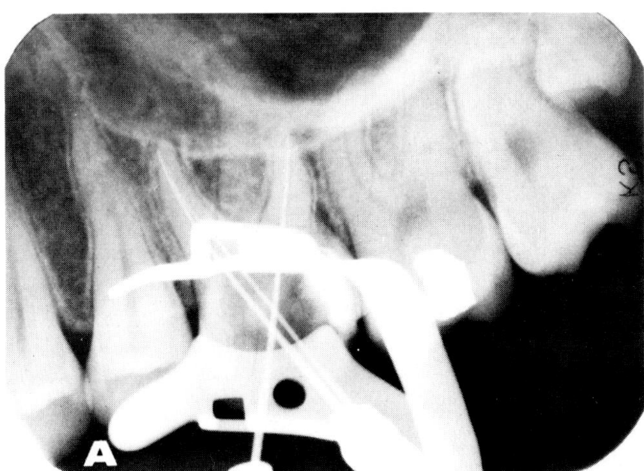

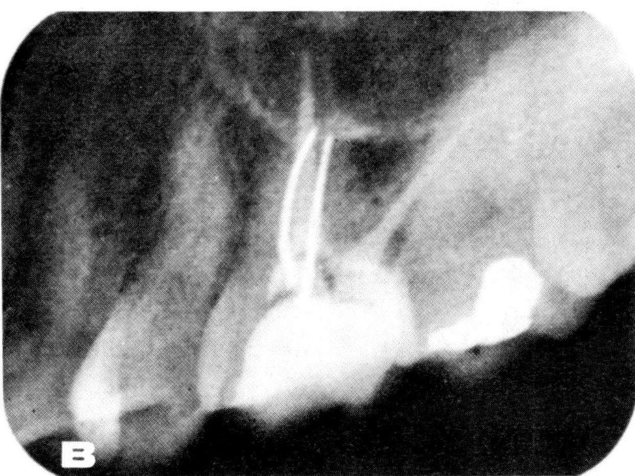

Fig. 2–22. Maxillary molars. *A,* Two files in separate canals of mesiobuccal root are superimposed in this horizontal right-angle projection. *B,* Two root canal fillings in mesiobuccal root are separated by projecting central beam 30 degrees from mesial. Distobuccal and palatal roots are separated as well. A 20-degree mesial projection would separate distobuccal root from second molar. (From Walton, R. E.: Dental Radiog. Photog., *46*:51, Oct., 1973.)

posed one upon the other. In the completion roentgenogram seen in Figure 2–22*B*, taken with a 30-degree variance from the mesial, the two separate canals in the mesiobuccal root are separated. All four canals can be seen. However, a 20-degree projection would have isolated the distobuccal root without superimposing it upon the second molar.

The same technique illustrated here for the maxillary first molar can be applied to the second or third molars by directing, at a horizontal variance, the central beam through those teeth.

Maxillary Premolars. Variance in the horizontal projection has great value in maxillary premolar radiography, particularly for the ***first*** premolar, which generally has two canals, but sometimes has three. The clinical efficacy of the Walton technique is well illustrated in Figure 2–23. The right-angle horizontal projection produces the single canal image seen in Figure 2–23*A*. By varying the angulation by 20 degrees, however, the two canals are separated (Fig. 2–23*B*), giving an unobstructed view of the quality of the fillings in both canals.

Again, the radiographic improvement by isolating structures is demonstrated in Figure 2–24. The bisecting angle projection seen in Figure 2–24*A* reveals the two maxillary premolars, apparently with a single canal in each tooth (Fig. 2–24*B*). In Figure

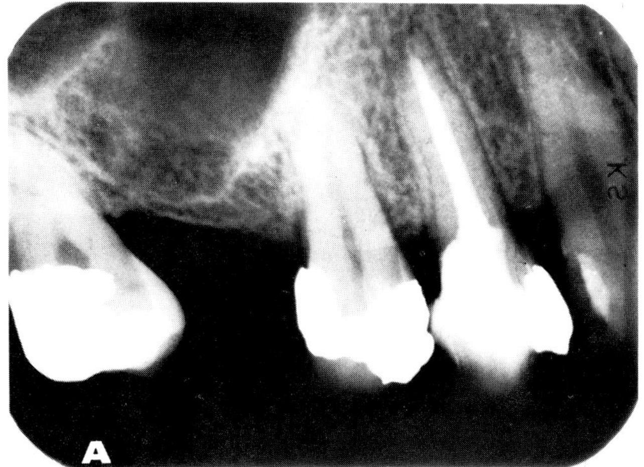

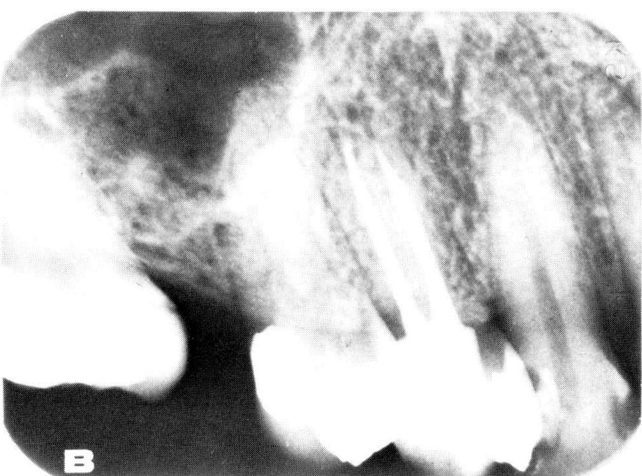

Fig. 2–23. Maxillary premolars. *A,* Horizontal right-angle projection produces illusion that maxillary first premolar has only one canal. *B,* Varying horizontal projection by 20 degrees mesially separates two canals. Buccal canal is toward distal (MBD). (From Walton, R. E.: Dental Radiog. Photog., *46*:51, Oct., 1973.)

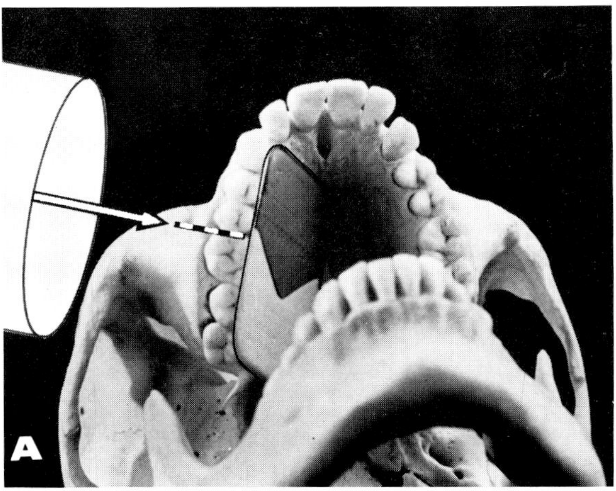

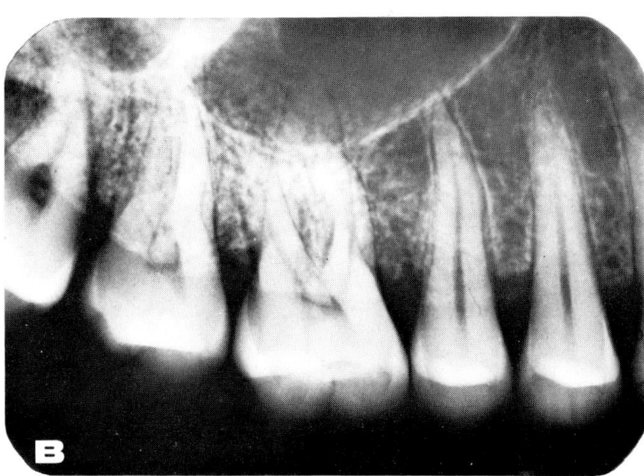

Fig. 2–24. Maxillary premolars. *A,* Central beam directed at right angle to film. *B,* Premolar canals and root shapes are superimposed. (From Walton, R. E.: Dental Radiog. Photog., *46*:51, Oct., 1973.)

2–25*B* (arrow), however, the two canals in the first premolar now become obvious. This separation of canals was achieved by varying the horizontal projection by 20 degrees (Fig. 2–25*A*). On the other hand, the single canal in the second premolar remains the same in both films.

Mandibular Anterior Teeth. Aberrations in canal anatomy in the ***mandibular*** anterior teeth are infamous. Variance of the horizontal x-ray projections in this region will bring out the differences. Figure 2–26*A* illustrates the standard x-ray projection bisecting the film held parallel to the arch. The incisor teeth

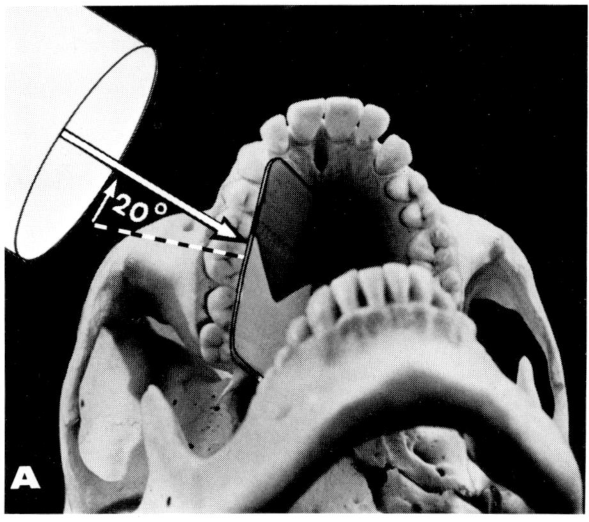

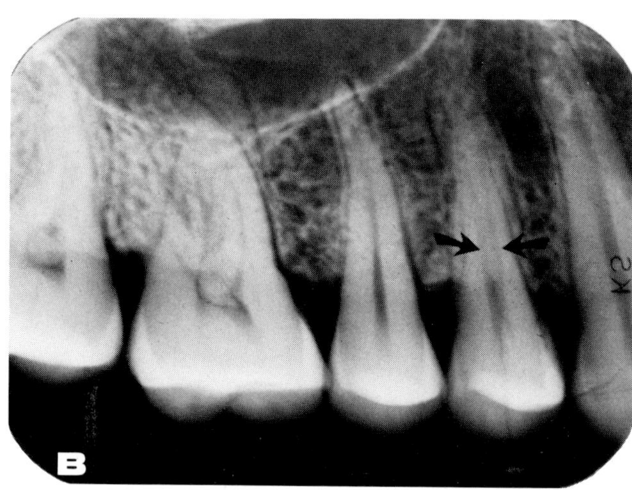

Fig. 2–25. Maxillary premolars. *A,* Central ray directed 20 degrees mesially from right-angle horizontal projection. *B,* Separation of two canals in first premolar becomes apparent (arrows). Single canal image remains in second premolar. (From Walton, R. E.: Dental Radiog. Photog., *46*:51, Oct., 1973.)

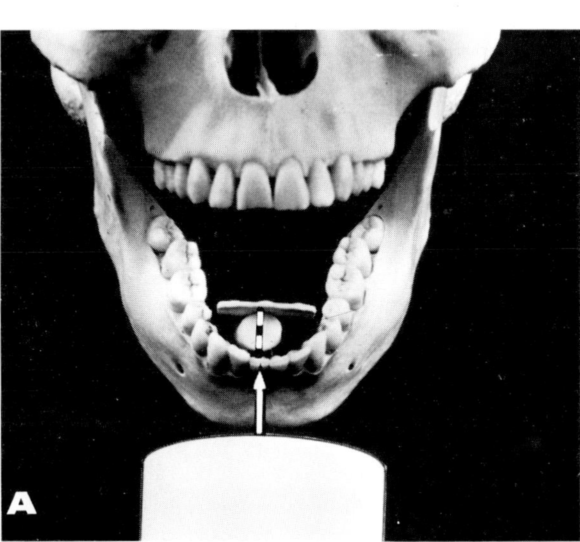

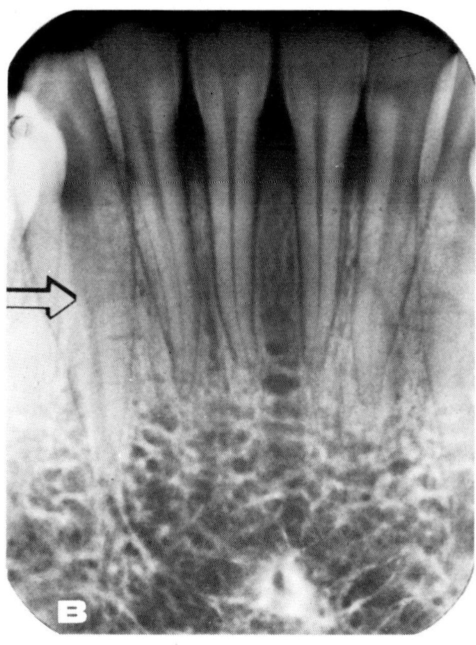

Fig. 2–26. Mandibular anterior teeth. *A,* Film placement for bisecting-angle technique. Horizontal central beam projection at right angle to film. *B,* Single canals seen in central incisors with only suggestion of two canals in lateral incisor. In distorted image of canine, note broad labiolingual canal dimension (arrow). (From Walton, R. E.: Dental Radiog. Photog., *46*:51, Oct., 1973.)

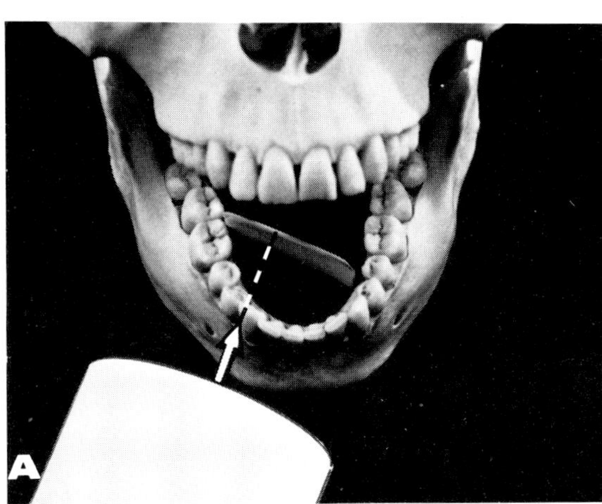

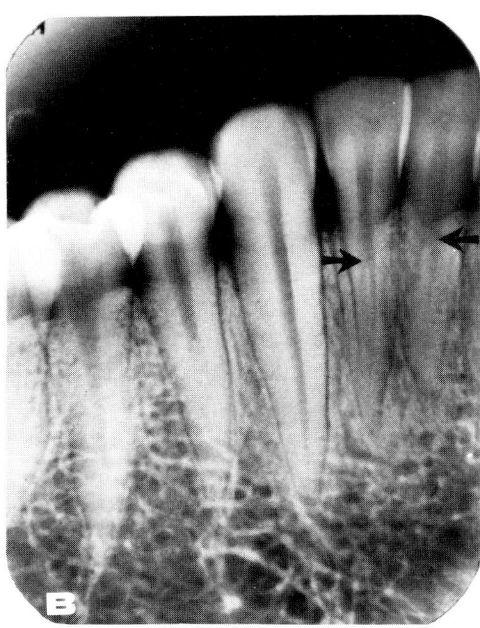

Fig. 2–27. Mandibular anterior teeth. *A,* Film is positioned for canine radiograph using bisecting-angle technique. Cotton rolls will prevent film curling. Horizontally, central beam is projected at right angle to film. *B,* Canine image is single straight canal, but incisor image reveals bifurcated canals that reunite in narrow tapered root (arrows). Note "bonus" image of bifurcated canals, first premolar. (From Walton, R. E.: Dental Radiog. Photog., *46*:51, Oct., 1973.)

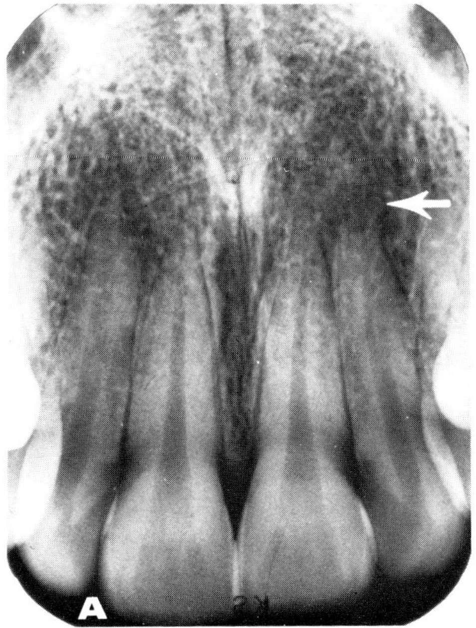

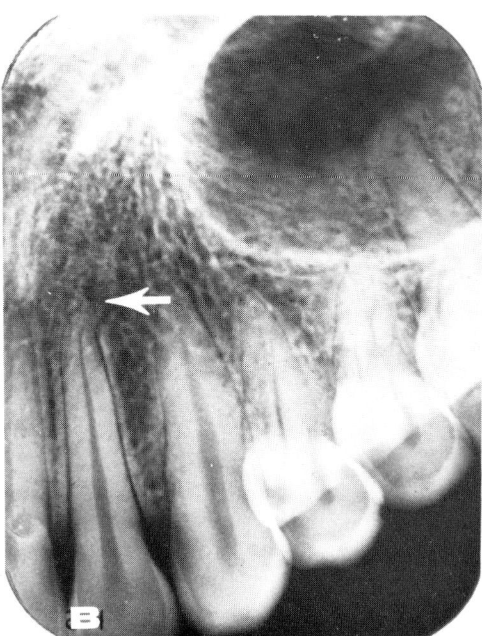

Fig. 2–28. Maxillary anterior teeth. Canal shape and root curvature can be demonstrated by varying horizontal angle. *A,* Distal curvature of lateral incisor is apparent in central incisor projection. *B,* Directing central ray more from distal increases distal curvature which leads one to believe root curve has lingual component. (From Walton, R. E.: Dental Radiog. Photog., *46*:51, Oct., 1973.)

appear to have single canals, and a broad single canal is seen in the distorted canine image (Fig. 2–26*B*).

By varying the film placement and projecting directly through the canine, as seen in Figure 2–27*A* (which is about 30 degrees variance for the incisors), separate canals appear in the incisors (Figure 2–27*B*, arrow) and are then seen to coalesce at the apex. This would be expected, however, when one views the tapered incisor roots seen in both horizontal projections; roots far too narrow to support two separate canals and foramina. Once again the abrupt change in canal radiodensity in the premolars (arrow) should make one suspicious of canal birfurcation, a fact that has already been confirmed in Figure 2–18*B*.

Maxillary Anterior Teeth. Although canal or root aberrations seldom appear in the maxillary anterior teeth, root curvature in the maxillary lateral incisors is a particularly vexing problem. In Figure 2–28, for example, the curvature of the apical third of the lateral incisor is revealed in the usual right-angle projection. But directed more from the distal, the distal curvature of the apex appears to have increased. Applying Clark's rule, that the image of the object most distant from the cone moves toward the cone, one would have to suspect that the distal curvature has a lingual component as well, a most valuable piece of information for optimum canal debridement and shaping.

Grady and Clausen have shown how difficult it is to determine when foramens exit to the labial or lingual.[21] Their radiographs of extracted teeth matched with photographs of instrument perforation short of the apex are a warning to all (Fig. 2–29).

Processing

Another deterrent to full endodontic utilization of roentgenography has been the length of time required in most offices to process films. Old, weakened

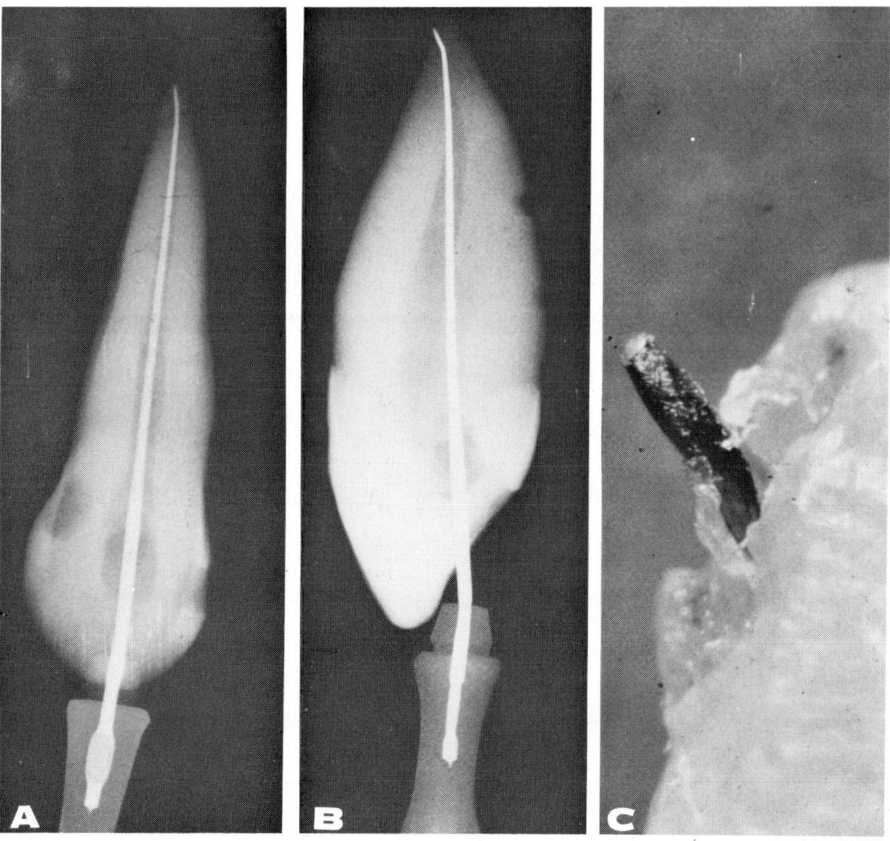

Fig. 2–29. *A*, Labiolingual projection through canine shows instrument apparently at apex with slight distal curvature. *B*, Mesiodistal projection reveals instrument actually emerging from labial short of apex. *C*, Instrument perforating foramen to labial well short of radiographic root end. (Courtesy Dr. John. R. Grady and Dr. Howard Clausen.)

solutions greatly increase the time required for processing. Moreover, adherence to the manufacturer's recommended temperature and time of 68° F for five to seven minutes for developing and clearing has retarded "on the spot" processing and viewing in most busy practices. Ingle, Beveridge and Olson demonstrated in a well-controlled blind study of the effects of varied processing temperatures, that a processing temperature of 92° F yielded, in less than one minute, the most acceptable roentgenograms.[22] A group of 37 physicians and dentists selected as "best" the films developed at 92° F from a coded selection of films processed at 4° intervals in the range of 68° to 100° F. At 92° F, using Kodak Developer and Fixer mixed to company specifications, development required only 30 seconds and fixation required 25 to 35 seconds, with no loss of quality. By comparison, the 68° F temperature recommended by the manufacturer required 4½ minutes for developing and clearing of 40 to 50 seconds.

In a practice limited to endodontic therapy, equipment designed for the processing of as many as 32 films at once is both unnecessary and uneconomical. The quart-sized rather than the standard gallon-sized processing tank permits the more rapid raising of solution temperature to 92° F. Films processed in solutions that have been maintained at 92° F for two weeks show only slight loss of contrast—more than adequate for endodontic working films. A weekly change of solutions in the quart-sized tank is recommended to maintain a constantly fresh solution without increased cost.

A compromise is suggested for the practitioner who wishes to retain the dark-room facilities to process full-mouth surveys at ordinary temperatures and still enjoy the convenience of rapid processing for endodontic treatment and emergencies. Three four-ounce jars or glasses are deep enough to suspend a periapical film on an individual film clip. They are adequate for developer, water, and fixer. If necessary, as many as three or four films can be processed at once. The temperature of the solutions can be easily and rapidly brought to the desired level in a compound heater converted to a processing tank. The volume of these "tanks" is small enough to allow even the most frugal practitioner to change solutions every other day, thus constantly maintaining fresh, active ingredients.

Also available are commercial rapid-processing solutions. They are more expensive, but require no heating bath since they may be kept at room temperature. Pestritto, in a blind study, evaluated the diagnostic quality of dental roentgenograms as processed by several rapid developing techniques.[23] Collits' Rapid X-ray Developer consistently produced the most diagnostic roentgenograms, requiring only 60 seconds for processing at room temperature. Examination of the films after one year disclosed little discoloration or deterioration of quality. Manson-Hing compared roentgenograms processed in conventional solutions with those rapidly processed.[24] He found the "rapid processing solutions produce radiographs with appreciably less image density than conventional solutions." He also recommended the obvious—not to use these solutions at 92° F. Concentrated Kodak replenisher and Kodak DX80R solutions proved to be good rapid processing solutions with small loss in image density.

When rapid developing solutions are used, the table top processing hood, into which the operator places his hands through light proof cuffs, has proved most effective in some offices. Hand movements inside the hood can be seen through the red plexiglass cover. Even the "trip down the hall to the darkroom" is eliminated if the hood is used right in the operatory.

Interpretation

Since a properly positioned, exposed and processed roentgenogram is only of value if it is properly interpreted, every advantage must be taken to obtain the most information from the film. For the student and seasoned practitioner alike, a good magnifying glass has often brought to light an extra root, root canal, or hard-to-find apex.

A superlative method for examining roentgenograms is the Brynolf magnifier-viewer.[25] This device enhances the viewing of individual films in two ways—the image is magnified several times and all peripheral light is effectively blocked out. Masking the light source around a roentgenogram ***greatly*** increases the ability of the viewer to distinguish grades of density.[26] A film that has been slightly overexposed, if magnified and inspected over a strong light, yields a remarkable amount of unsuspected information (Fig. 2–30). In a re-treated case, endodontic success had been denied for nine years until inspection under magnification of the original roentgenogram disclosed a previously overlooked third root on a maxillary first premolar.

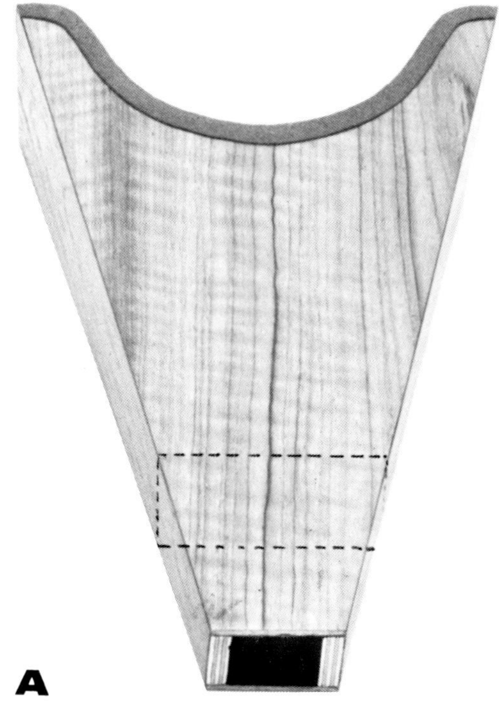

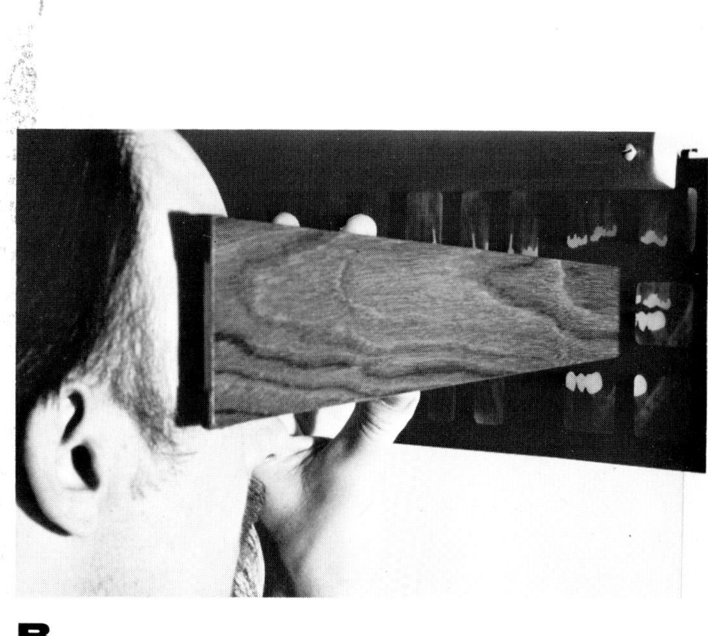

Fig. 2–30. The Swedish x-Producter, magnifier-viewer that greatly enhances radiographic interpretation. *A*, Opening is size of single film. A 4× magnifying glass is located at dotted lines. Inner walls are flat-black. *B*, Peripheral light is eliminated and image magnified. Markedly improved interpretation results. (Courtesy Dr. William Dowden.)

Many departures from classic roentgenographic procedures have been strongly advocated for endodontic therapy. This has been done with clear conscience and high motives. Many years of experience have proved these methods to be effective. Any variation that makes the exposure and processing of roentgenograms easier, faster, and better, and the interpretation more thorough, increases the value of these "eyes beneath the surface." It is when we don't see what we are doing that failures increase.

SPECIALIZED ENDODONTIC INSTRUMENTS AND EQUIPMENT

"The lack of proper equipment" is a reason often given by dentists who do not practice root canal therapy—and well it might be. Not only are special instruments imperative for endodontic treatment, but a special arrangement of these instruments is necessary.

The impractical, inefficient scurrying around the office to gather together a collection of unsterile, ill-adapted equipment completely discourages the average practitioner from endodontic therapy. These problems may be solved by ***procuring*** the correct equipment and supplies; by ***packaging*** the hand equipment into sterilized towel kits, or into canisters or on prearranged trays, and finally by storing the small endodontic instruments in an ***organized,*** compartmented instrument case.

Sterilized Towel Kit

Standard dental instruments, along with a few special instruments necessary for root canal therapy, are wrapped into a pack, in two layers of towel, which is fastened with a banker's pin or autoclave tape. This rolled kit can then be sterilized and stored, ready for use (Fig. 2–31). (See Chapter 14, Sterilizing Endodontic Equipment.)

When treatment is to begin the towel kit is unrolled on the working surface and the instruments arranged on the sterile towel according to their frequency of use (Fig. 2–32). A two- or three-well sterilizer containing tincture of Zephiran is then positioned at the rear of the tray. A sterile pair of cotton pliers is placed in the deep well. Fine gutta percha points and rubber instrument stops are in the shallow well.

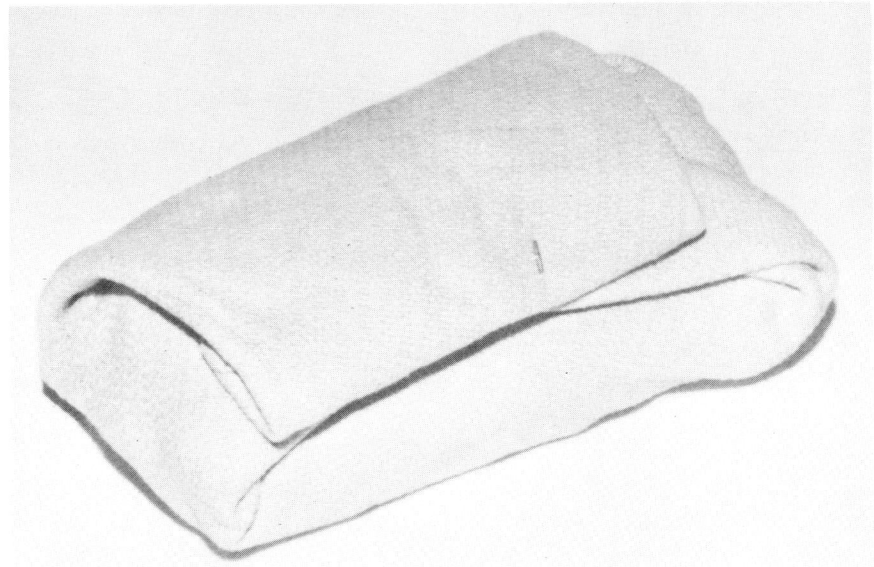

Fig. 2–31. Sterilized towel kit or pack which contains standard dental instruments necessary for endodontic treatment. Colored towels are used to identify special endodontic instrument pack which has been sterilized and conveniently stored for future use.

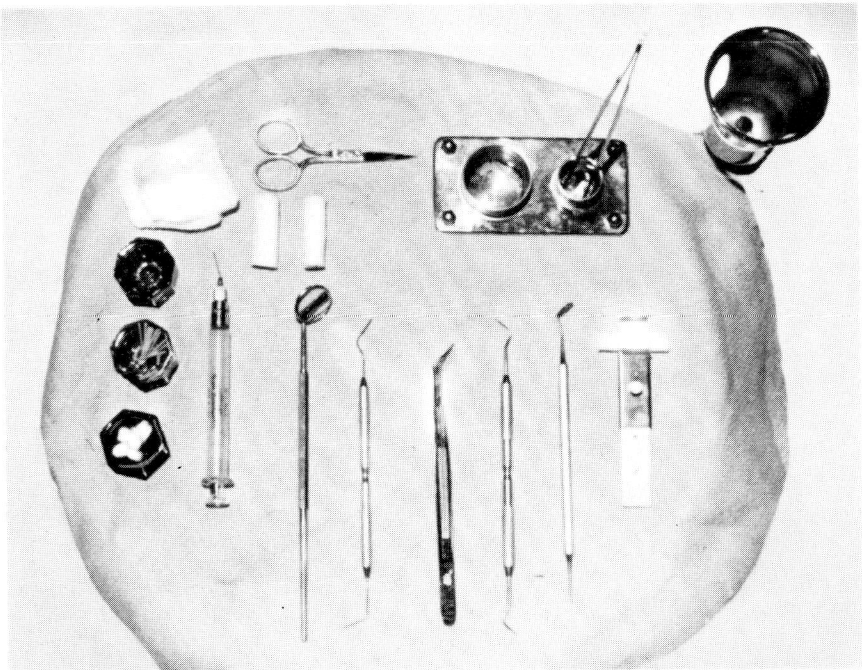

Fig. 2–32. Instruments in sterilized towel pack are laid out on dental tray or Mayo stand which is positioned in close proximity to field of operation. Three dappen dishes *(left)* are used to hold sterile cotton pellets, paper points, and irrigating solution. At right side of tray, resting on cotton roll, is endodontic measuring gauge. Two-well sterilizer (*top right*), which contains tincture of Zephiran, is repository for sterile pliers used to enter instrument case. Sterile gutta percha points and instrument stops are stored in large well. Cotton pliers on towel surface are used only to carry materials from tray to tooth.

The following instruments are contained in the towel kit:

Three dappen dishes
One Luer syringe, glass, 3 ml.
One Luer type 25-gauge needle, ¾-inch
One mouth mirror, "Front Surface" mirror—Kerr or Stardental
Two cotton pliers—Dixon Manufacturing Company
One DE spoon excavator, Starlite #31
One plastic instrument—Glick #1—Stardental
One measuring gauge—Stardental
One scissors, embroidery, 3¼ inch overall length
One D-G explorer—Stardental
Three gauze sponges, 2-inch
Three cotton rolls #3, 1 inch long

A banker's sponge, soaked with tincture of Zephiran, may also be placed on the tray. The banker's sponge serves as a handy receptacle for the endodontic instruments. Reamers and files are arranged by the assistant in numerical order (Fig. 2–33). It is impractical, if not impossible, for an assistant to pass the short-handled instruments to the operator—hence the practicality of arranging the instruments in order in the sponge. The sponge should be rinsed in soapy water after each use, and a fresh sponge, soaked in tincture of Zephiran, put out for the next patient.

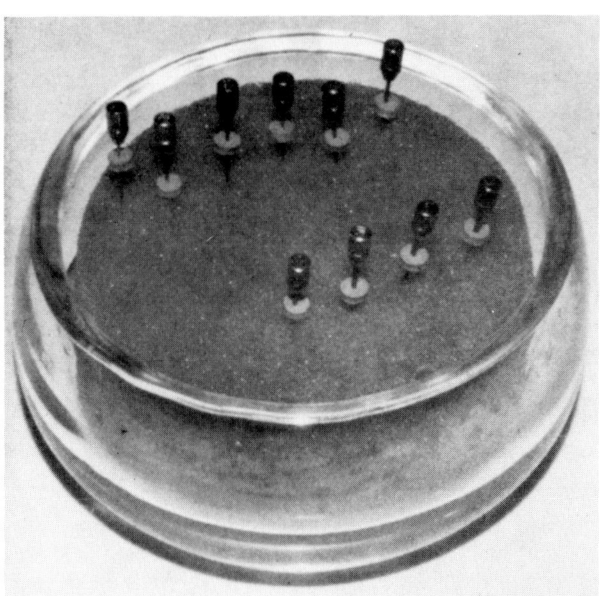

Fig. 2–33. Banker's sponge, soaked with tincture of Zephiran, serves as repository for endodontic instruments which are measured by assistant and arranged in numerical order. Plastic sponge should be washed after each use and fresh sponge, soaked in germicide, used for each patient.

Used instruments are not to be placed back in the sponge.

Handpieces

The only regular dental equipment needed, other than anesthetic syringes and rubber dam equipment, are the two contra-angle handpieces; one accelerated

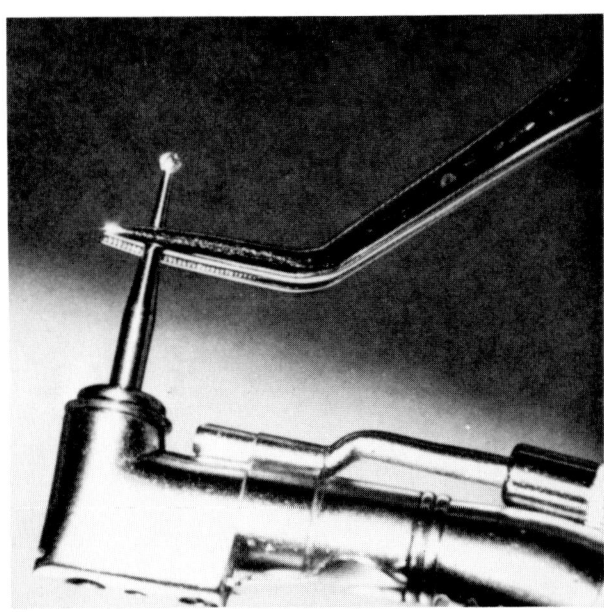

Fig. 2–34. Sterile burs are placed in contra-angle handpiece with sterile pliers. Bur is "dropped" into place by holding shaft of bur with pliers and spinning foot control.

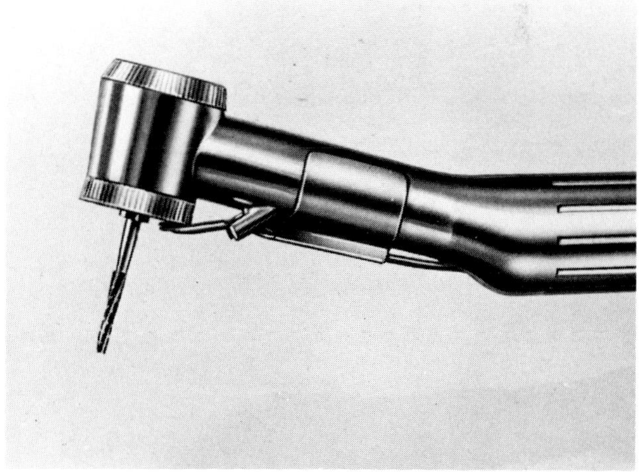

Fig. 2–35. Air rotor handpiece mounted with 702L carbide bur used in root amputation. True concentricity and accurate water spray are necessity. Fiber optic illumination is most helpful. (Courtesy Star Dental Manufacturing Co.)

speed, the other conventional speed. The heads of these contra-angles should be wiped down by the assistant with a sponge soaked in tincture of Zephiran. The assistant should then place the correct burs in the contra-angles, sized according to the case to be treated.

The burs, stored in the sterile instrument case, are removed from the case with the sterile cotton pliers, and placed in the contra-angle with the pliers (Fig. 2–34). While the shaft of the bur is held with the pliers, the foot control of the conventional handpiece is just tapped. As the bur spins it will drop down into place and the latch may be closed.

For the accelerated speed handpiece, the burs can be dropped down into the chuck, which is then tightened. The handpiece must be absolutely concentric. Whipping of the end of the bur, experienced with a worn chuck, will fracture teeth and is particularly dangerous when an extra long bur is being used to amputate an entire root (Fig. 2–35).

Endodontic Instrument Case

The collection of tiny endodontic instruments must be kept in an organized arrangement, yet lend itself readily to sterilization. The metal endodontic instru-

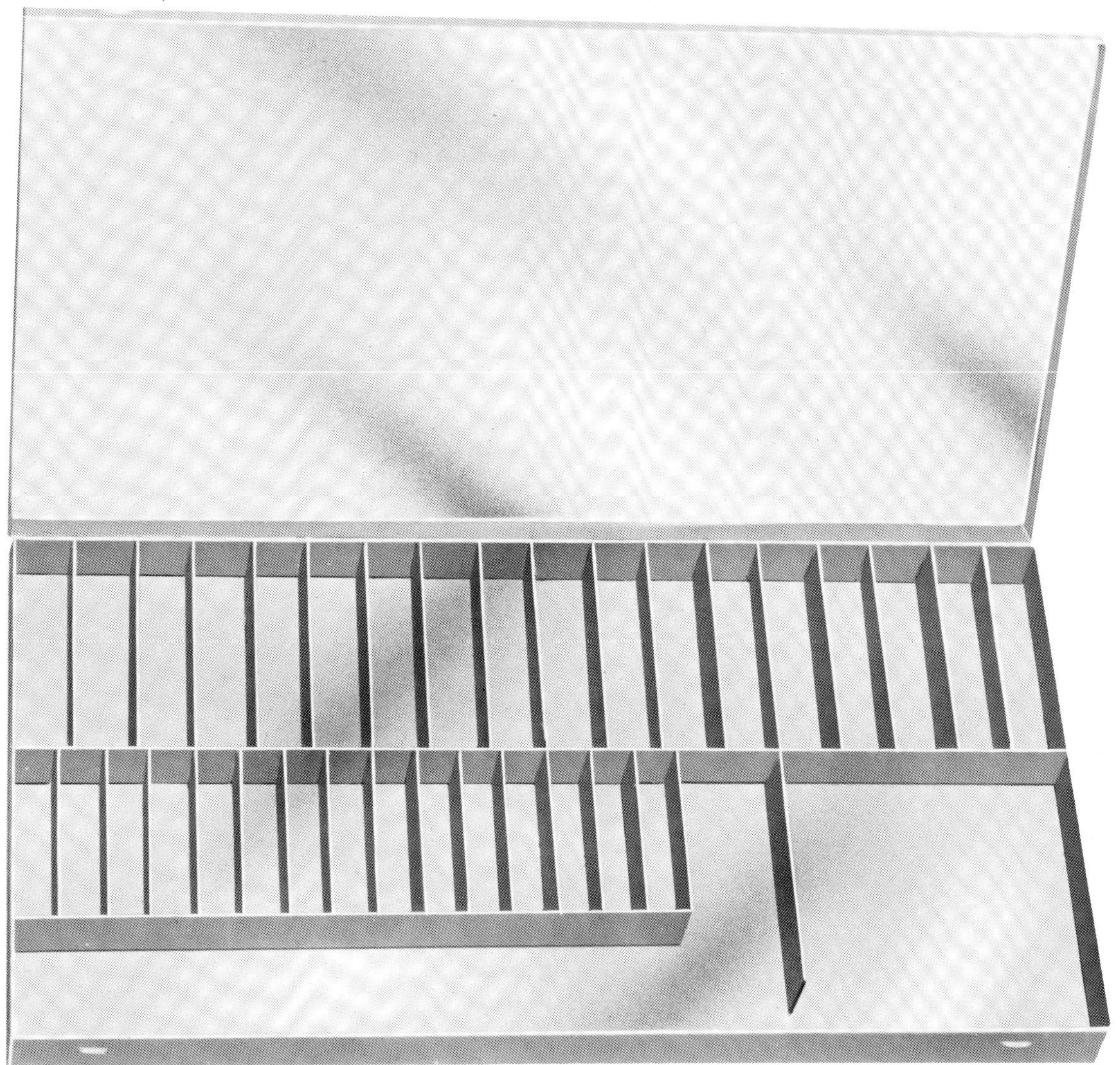

Fig. 2–36. USC design instrument case. Compartments at top hold full selection of files sizes 8 through 140 and compartment for special reamers or Hedstrom files. Small compartments are for broaches, burs, cotton pellets, and paper points. L-shaped compartment stores pluggers, spreaders, and spatulas; square compartment is for glass slabs. Loaded with *stainless* instruments, case is sterilized in autoclave. (Courtesy Union Broach Co.)

ment case meets these requirements. Storage cases have long been available, but never so refined as the modern case. All of the reamers, files, broaches, burs, and filling equipment, as well as paper points and cotton pellets, are stored and sterilized in the case. The dentist or assistant removes these with ***sterile pliers*** only as needed (Fig. 2–36).

The instrument case may be placed beside the dentist on a Mayo stand, or the assistant may obtain material from the case kept on the cabinet top. Supplies are transferred from the case to the open towel kit, which is the working surface. The case need only be resterilized when one of the instrument sizes is depleted. New instruments should replace the sizes 10 through 25, which should be used only once. The larger instruments may be thoroughly cleaned and reused when the case is replenished before sterilization.

A selection of instruments is available from the various distributors of endodontic supplies. These selections have been developed for the clinician treating all types of endodontic problems in a general practice of dentistry. The case and its contents are sterilized according to the directions given in Chapter 14, p. 591.

The surgical armamentarium is dealt with in the chapter on Endodontic Surgery, Chapter 15, pp. 625–626.

Contents of the Endodontic Instrument Case

Stainless Files—Color-Coded Handles

Style "B"—Short Handles

1 × 6 file, B, #10	1 × 6 file, B, #55
1 × 6 file, B, #15	1 × 6 file, B, #60
1 × 6 file, B, #20	1 × 6 file, B, #70
1 × 6 file, B, #25	1 × 6 file, B, #80
1 × 6 file, B, #30	1 × 6 file, B, #90
1 × 6 file, B, #35	1 × 6 file, B, #100
1 × 6 file, B, #40	1 × 6 file, B, #120
1 × 6 file, B, #45	1 × 6 file, B, #140
1 × 6 file, B, #50	

1 × 8 files Hedstrom, assorted #'s 50–110

Burs

1 × 3 bur, carbide #701U, RA
1 × 6 bur, #2 (3-surgical, 3-standard, RA)
1 × 6 bur, #4 (3-surgical, 3-standard, RA)
1 × 6 bur, #6 (3-surgical, 3-standard, RA)

Broaches

1 × 6 barbed broaches, fine
1 × 6 barbed broaches, medium
1 × 6 barbed broaches, coarse
1 × 6 barbed broaches, x coarse

Filling Instruments

2 only spreader, #3
2 only cement spatula, #3
2 only glass mixing slab, opal

Paper points—fine, medium, and coarse
Cotton pellets—large and small

Special Towel Kit

8 only—Pluggers, sizes 8, 9, 9½, 10, 10½, 11, 11½, 12

LOCAL ANESTHESIA FOR ENDODONTICS

Profound Pulp Anesthesia

Profound pulp anesthesia describes a state of local anesthesia of unusual "depth." It is necessary that ***profound*** pulp anesthesia be established if vital pulp tissue is to be removed without pain. Fortunately, today, profound local anesthetics are available. Lidocaine is a great improvement over procaine.

Complete anesthesia of pulp tissue is more difficult to obtain if the pulp is inflamed. That is to say, ***routine*** anesthesia injections which would anesthetize ***normal*** pulp tissue will not effectively anesthetize ***inflamed*** pulp tissue. Special ***supplementary injection techniques*** must be used, ***in addition*** to the routine anesthetic injections, to attain a depth of local anesthesia adequate for the removal of inflamed pulp tissue.

Importance of a Confident and Reassuring Manner

In addition to pulp inflammation, "patient inflammation" also may be present. The patient may be physically and mentally fatigued. He is usually apprehensive and fearful, although he may be able to mask his fears and hide his apprehensions. By training and experience, the dentist should be able to approach the endodontic patient and his problem with a confident and reassuring manner.

This may be the first meeting of the dentist and patient. The hour may be late, and the dentist has been called back to his office to treat an emergency. The patient is "keyed-up"—more than usually alert and responsive to all that goes on about him. Improperly managed, this visit is a traumatic experience. Properly managed, the visit should provide an efficient, painless solution to the problem. In any case, a sympathetic and reassuring manner will earn the patient's appreciation and respect.

Use of "Relaxing" or Superficial Anesthesia for Pulpless Teeth

When a tooth is found to have a ***nonvital pulp***, the dentist may choose to carry out endodontic procedures ***without*** using a local anesthetic. On the other hand, many dentists find patients more relaxed and cooperative if a ***minimum injection*** of local anesthetic solution is used routinely. Anesthesia of the gingival tissue will eliminate the discomfort from impingement of the rubber dam clamp. In addition, this superficial injection may anesthetize those surprisingly sensitive pulp fibers that have shown no sign of vitality; that is, until the canal is entered.

The various conduction injections—mandibular, mental, and long buccal in the mandible, and the "zygomatic" infraorbital, posterior palatine, and nasopalatine in the maxilla—are also used as initial injections. Although profound anesthesia is more apt to develop following conduction injections, they are not to be counted upon for total anesthesia and must often be backed up with ***supplementary*** injections.

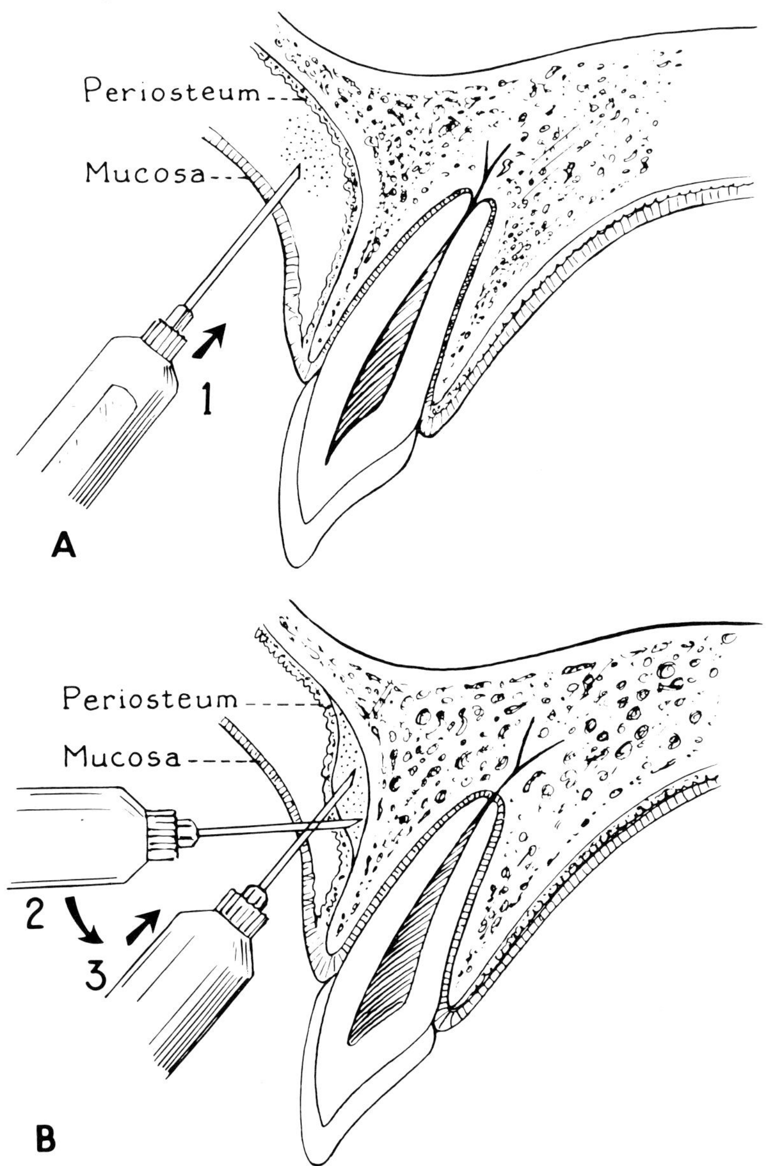

Fig. 2–37. Subperiosteal infiltration. *A,* Short needle enters soft tissue perpendicular to surface of bone (1). *B,* Tip of needle is carried just below periosteum and against bone (2). It is then advanced (3) beneath periosteum, and 0.5 ml. of solution is desposited *subperiosteally.*

If an acute abscess has developed apical to a pulpless tooth, ***superficial*** injection into the area of tissue involvement will accomplish nothing. The pulp chamber of such teeth can be opened to allow for drainage without the use of local anesthetic—without pain—if an ***ultraspeed handpiece*** is used and the tooth is supported against the light pressure of the handpiece. In fact, ultraspeed equipment is a godsend in these cases, for dentist and patient alike.

When to Use a Supplementary Injection

If ***vital*** pulp tissue is to be removed without pain, ***profound*** pulp anesthesia is necessary. This will require ***supplementary*** injections ***following*** the routine conductive or infiltrative injections. ***In every case involving the removal of vital pulp tissue, supplementary injections should be used*** before opening deeply into the pulp. There are three possible supplementary injections which may be made for any tooth. They are the ***subperiosteal*** injection, the ***intraseptal*** injection, or as a last resort, the ***intrapulpal*** injection.

Subperiosteal Infiltration. The needle is inserted into the ***previously anesthetized*** tissue slightly below the mucogingival junction. It approaches the bone surface at an angle slightly less than 90 degrees. The needle tip is pushed ***through*** the mucosa until the fibrous ***periosteal*** tissue overlying the bone is contacted in the area of the root apex. As pressure is maintained on the needle tip to keep it beneath the periosteum and against the bone, the angle of the needle is decreased and the tip is advanced one millimeter beneath the periosteum. Approximately 0.5 ml. of the anesthetic solution is deposited beneath the periosteal layer, against the cortical plate of bone. The fibers of the periosteum will force the anesthetic solution through the porous cortical plate and into the cancellous alveolar bone beneath, finally allowing it to contact those nerve fibers innervating the dental pulp (Fig. 2–37).

Palatal Infiltration (Anterior Palatine Nerve Injection). When a ***maxillary*** premolar or molar tooth is to be profoundly anesthetized, a supplementary injection of the palate is necessary. This injection anesthetizes the ***anterior palatine nerve***, which innervates the posterior half of the palate. It also ***reinforces*** the level of anesthesia obtained by the use of the ***supraperiosteal*** and ***subperiosteal*** injections on the buccal as well as the zygomatic sites.

Anesthesia of the anterior palatine nerve is accomplished by inserting the needle tip at a right angle into the palatal mucosa, halfway between the midline of the palate and the gingival margin of the tooth to be anesthetized (Fig. 2–38). The needle should penetrate deeply into the palatal mucosa. A small volume of the anesthetic solution (0.25 ml.) is deposited against the palatal periosteum. Blanching of the mucosa in the area of the injection is often evident.

Lingual Infiltration. When ***mandibular*** premolar and molar teeth are to be profoundly anesthetized, the ***lingual infiltration*** injection, together with the ***long buccal*** injection, are used to anesthetize possible anastomosing fibers from the cervical plexus.

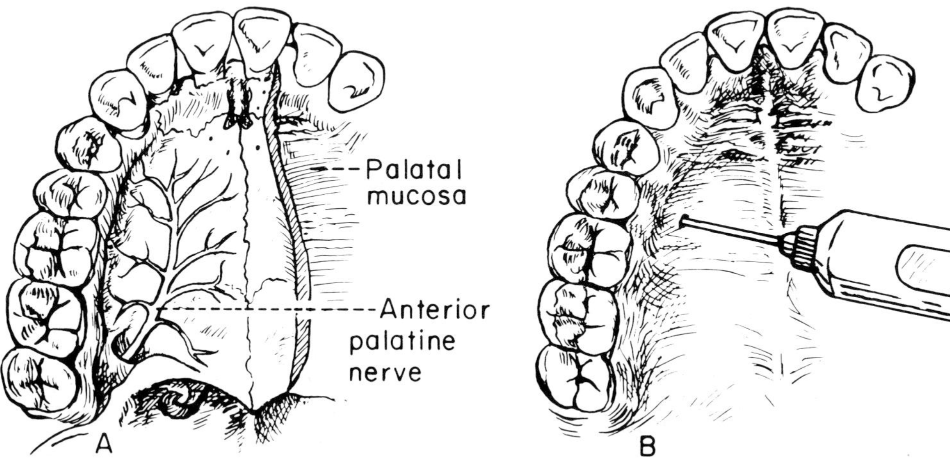

Fig. 2–38. Palatal infiltration. Infiltration of anterior palatine nerve will reinforce level of anesthesia obtained following injections of anterior and middle superior alveolar nerves.

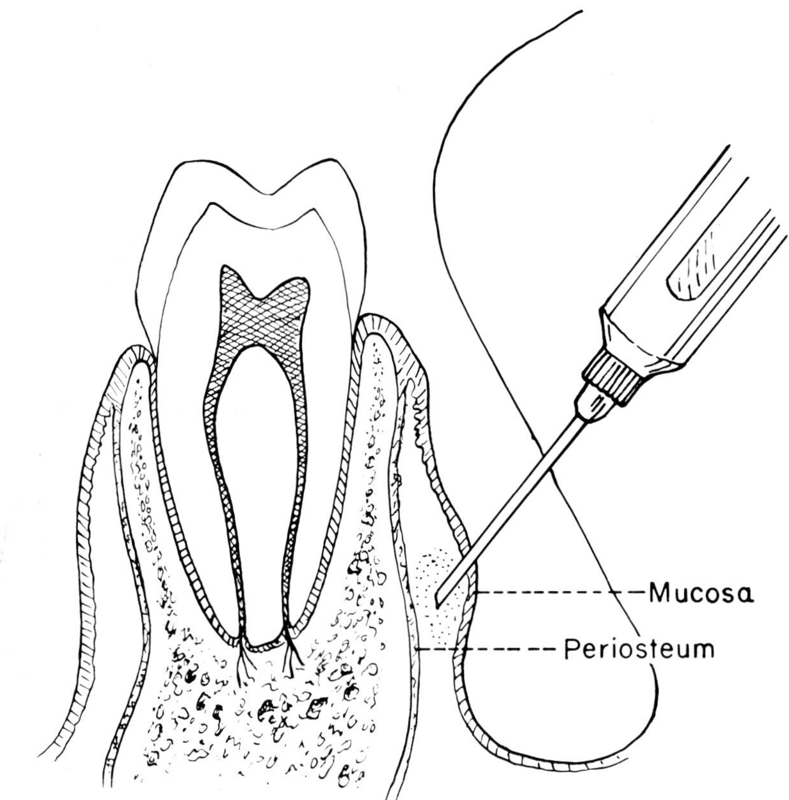

Fig. 2–39. Lingual infiltration. Infiltration to lingual of mandibular premolar and molar teeth will reinforce level of anesthesia obtained with long buccal and inferior alveolar injections. Needle tip should just penetrate thin lingual tissue and only 0.25 ml. of anesthetic is deposited.

Anatomists have long debated the existence of this "cross innervation," but the clinical fact is that without lingual and buccal infiltration injections, profound pulp anesthesia of mandibular premolar and molar teeth is frustratingly unpredictable.

The tissue on the lingual surface of the mandible adjacent to the involved premolar or molar is dried, and the tongue is retracted with a 2" × 2" gauze sponge. The needle tip should penetrate the thin tissue on the lingual surface of the mandible, rather than the tissue of the floor of the mouth. A small volume of anesthetic solution (0.25 ml.) is carefully injected beneath the surface of this delicate tissue adjacent to the tooth to be anesthetized (Fig. 2–39).

Intraseptal Infiltration. The ***intraseptal*** injection is really an intraosseous injection. It is accomplished by passing the needle tip through the ***previously anesthetized*** gingival papilla, as well as the thin cortical plate beneath, and finally penetrating ***into the cancellous*** bone of the interdental septum. At this point, a few drops of the anesthetic solution are deposited under pressure (Fig. 2–40).

Two separate intraseptal injections are usually used for each tooth—one into the interdental bony septum on the mesial, and a second on the distal. In making the ***intraseptal injection***, the angulation of the needle is 45 degrees to the long axis of the tooth. The needle should contact bone at the height of the interdental crest of bone, where the cortical layer is thinnest and most easily penetrated. A 1-inch 25-gauge needle is of correct length and "stiffness." Firm hand pressure is usually sufficient for osseous penetration, but ***penetration can be facilitated by rotation*** of the needle as it is pressed into the crestal bone. As the needle tip is felt to enter the bone, considerable pressure against the syringe plunger is applied. Blanching of the tissue in the area of the injection should be evident.

In the event the crestal bone cannot be penetrated by a needle, Pearce has recommended perforating the alveolar plate using a number three Busch power reamer (Fig. 2–41). Through this entrance a needle

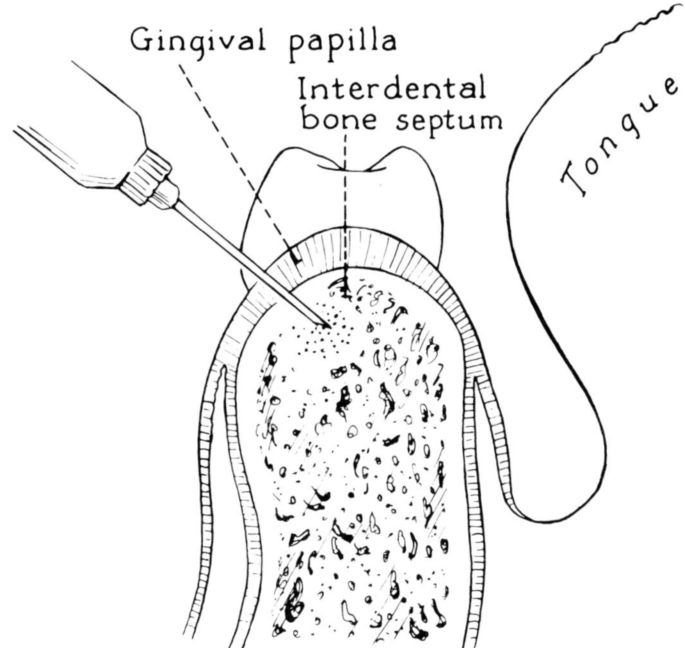

Fig. 2–40. Intraseptal infiltration. Intraseptal injection is made into cancellous bone of interdental septum from both buccal and lingual. Penetration into cancellous bone is facilitated by *rotating* needle through crestal bone. Injection is made until interdental papilla is blanched in appearance.

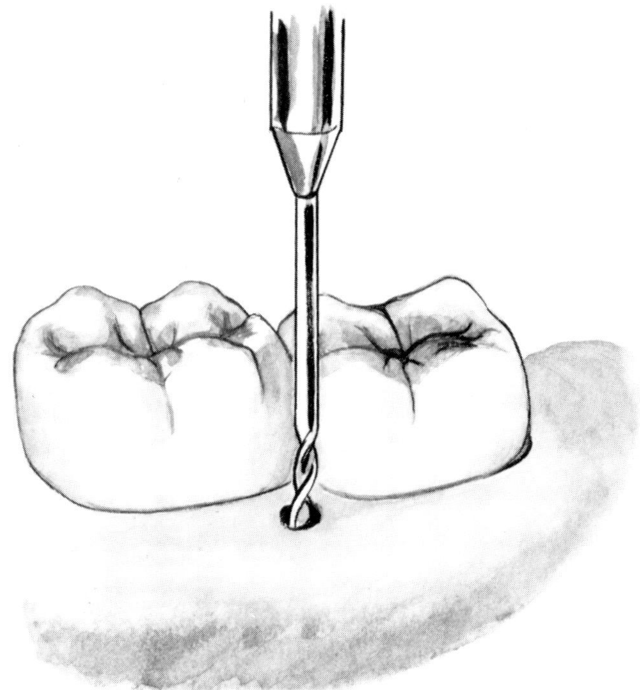

Fig. 2–41. Injection technique for case refractory to anesthesia. Power-driven reamer perforates alveolar plate and anesthetic is deposited under pressure in cancellous bone. (Courtesy Dr. James H. Pearce.)

can enter the cancellous bone and a solution deposited under pressure to anesthetize particularly refractory cases.

Intrapulp Injection. This injection into the pulp tissue itself is an "injection of last resort." It has been thought that the best anesthesia has been secured with lidocaine. However, a recent study concluded "there was no difference in the intrapulpal anesthesia that was produced whether sterile saline solution or lidocaine 2% with epinephrine 1:50,000 was used."[27] If the previously described injections are administered properly, the direct pulp injection is seldom necessary. In site of proper technique, however, the patient will sometimes experience pain as the pulp is exposed. It is at this critical moment that the intrapulp injection is useful.

Before proceeding with this injection, it is best to explain to the patient that despite your best efforts to anesthetize the "nerve" of his inflamed and "irritated" tooth, complete anesthesia has not been achieved. He is told that the injections he has received would certainly have produced complete and profound anesthesia if his tooth were normal. Because of the inflammation present in the pulp and surrounding tissues, however, profound anesthesia will only be attained if a drop of anesthetic is deposited directly into the partially anesthetized pulp. A momentary painful sensation will be felt as this is done, but this sensation is tolerable since the previous injections have partially anesthetized the pulp sensory nerves.

The tooth is isolated and any debris in the area of the pulp exposure is removed. The location of the opening in the dentin may be obvious; if it is not, a sharp explorer is used to pinpoint its exact position. Depending on the location of the pulp exposure, the needle is used straight, or it is bent at a 45-degree angle to facilitate insertion of the tip into the opening (usually necessary for posterior teeth). With a quick thrust, the needle tip penetrates the pulp tissue at the exposure site. ***The moment*** the needle tip touches the exposed pulp, a drop of the anesthetic solution is deposited into the tissue. This will immediately and profoundly anesthetize the tissue of the pulp chamber (Fig. 2–42).

If additional intrapulp injections are necessary to anesthetize completely the ***deeper tissue within the***

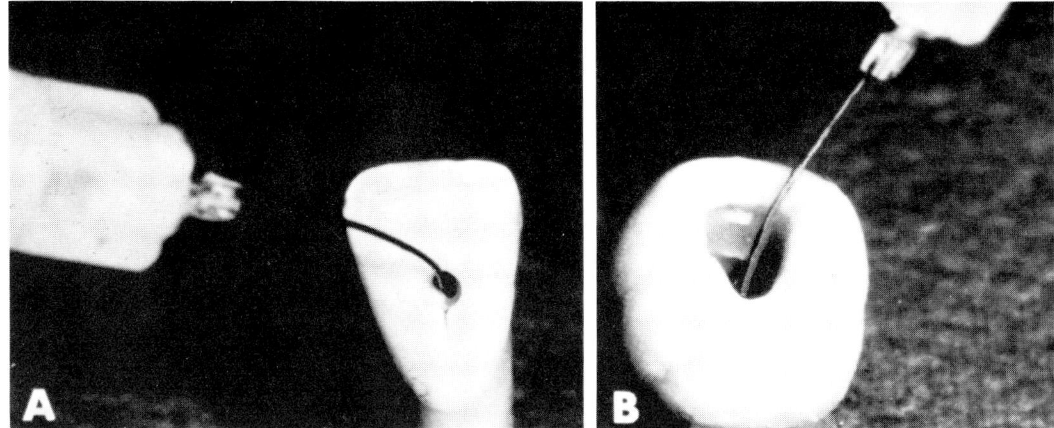

Fig. 2–42. *A,* Intrapulpal anesthesia is accomplished through tiny hole into pulp, allowing pressure to be exerted, which forces solution into tissue. Solution should be deposited at same instant needle touches exposed pulp. *B,* Intrapulpal anesthesia with lidocaine to develop complete anesthesia of pulpal shreds remaining in canals. Needle must fit tightly in canal with no backflow. Solution is deposited at instant needle locks in canal.

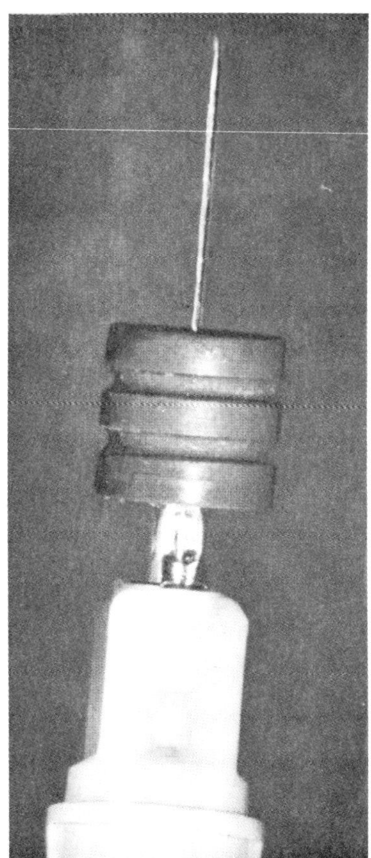

Fig. 2–43. Sterile rubber plunger from used carpule insures tight seal at cavity margin during intrapulpal anesthesia.

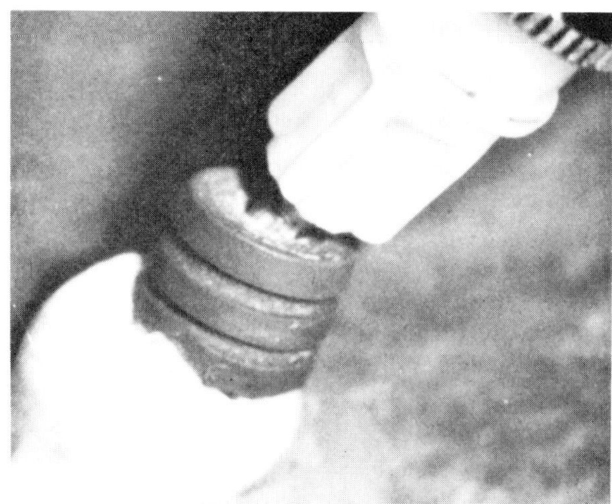

Fig. 2–44. Rubber plunger is jammed against occlusal cavity and acts to seal margins and thus improve pressure injection.

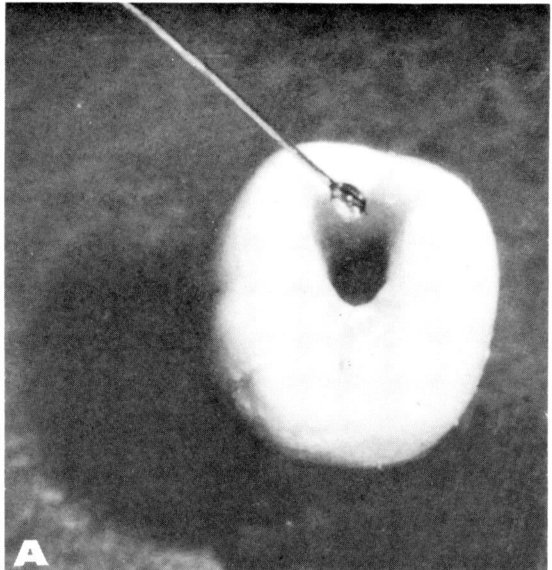

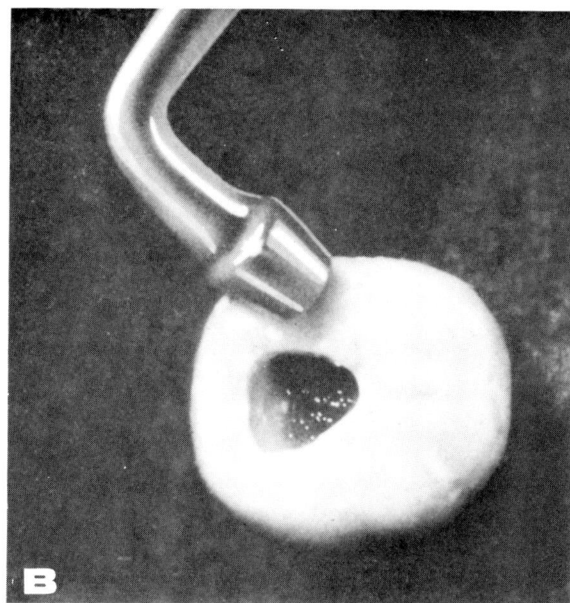

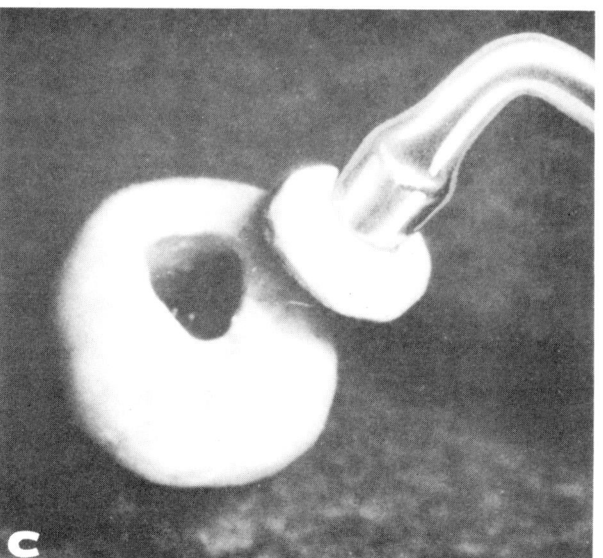

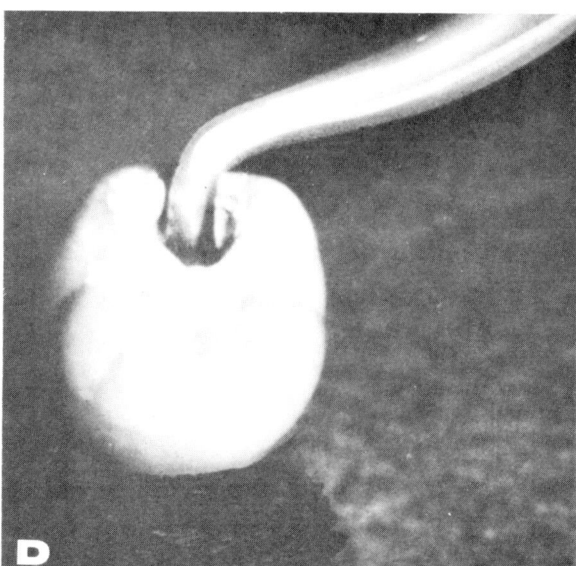

Fig. 2–45. Direct pressure anesthesia. *A,* Either lidocaine hydrochloride or cocaine solution is dripped onto cotton in cavity which opens into partially anesthetized pulp. Only*topical* anesthetics will give desired depth of pulpal anesthesia by pressure method. *B,* Plugger is selected which will just pass through cavity orifice. *C,* Warm (not hot) temporary stopping is added to plugger to act as plunger in driving topical anesthetic solution into pulpal fibers. *D,* Mass of temporary stopping is forced into closed cavity to apply pressure necessary to drive anesthetic solution to sensory nerves of pulp. Momentary pain will be experienced and patient should be warned of this possibility.

root canal, the needle must fit tightly in the canal. A return flow of the anesthetic solution signifies that anesthesia will not be gained. By adding on the needle a sterile rubber plunger from an anesthetic carpule (Fig. 2–43), and then tightly jamming the rubber against the cavity opening as the injection is made (Fig. 2–44), enough pressure may be developed to drive the solution into the pulp tissue and gain anesthesia.

Direct Pressure Anesthesia. "When all else fails, try direct pressure," the oldest form of pulp anesthesia. This is done by pressing a topical anesthetic solution directly into the pulp tissue.

Again, it must be explained to the patient that this is a last resort. Cotton is first placed loosely in the chamber and lidocaine is dripped from the needle into the cavity (Fig. 2–45*A*). (Originally, an aqueous solution of cocaine was used and is still recommended for refractory cases.) An amalgam plugger is then chosen which will just pass into the chamber. This will be used as a plunger (Fig. 2–45*B*). A mass of temporary stopping is then applied to the plugger. The stopping is rewarmed to the stage of firmness, not stickiness (Fig. 2–45*C*). The patient is warned that it will be momentarily painful, and the mass of stopping and the plugger are slowly but firmly forced into the cavity (Fig. 2–45*D*). The pressure is held for a few seconds, and the plugger and stopping are immediately removed before it hardens.

If the plugger fits too loosely, or if the solution can leak out of proximal cavities, the method will not be effective. Pulp vitality is checked by passing an instrument down the canals.

PREPARATION FOR ENDODONTIC THERAPY

Root canal therapy does not begin with the placement of the rubber dam, but rather with ***those restorative or periodontic procedures necessary to simplify its placement.*** These procedures determine the restorability of the tooth and establish a healthy periodontal relationship between tooth, gingiva, and bone. Pretreatment encompasses all procedures that ensure the ease of root canal treatment directed toward restoring and maintaining the involved tooth. The type of pretreatment varies with each case, but certain fundamental objectives must be considered.

1. Prevention of Postoperative Discomfort and the Inopportune Fracture of Teeth. Gross occlusal reduction should be performed on any decayed or filled posterior tooth undergoing root canal therapy. All such teeth will be required to have capped cusp restorations upon completion of treatment. This reduction should be done prior to rubber dam placement in order to check occlusal clearance in all excursive movements. It should also be done prior to the first endodontic treatment, rather than at the completion of that appointment, in order not to disturb cuspal reference points used to establish proper length of the tooth. Exempt from this pretreatment are posterior teeth adequately restored with capped cusp restorations, and anterior teeth from canine to canine.

2. Prevention of Bacterial Contamination from Salivary Leakage as well as the Prevention of Percolation of Intracanal Medication. All faulty restorations and carious defects must be removed and replaced with temporary filling material or alloy. Whenever possible Cavit is the filling material of choice because of its ease of manipulation and its excellent sealing properties.[28] For these same reasons it is used for the temporary closure of the access cavity.

To restore a minimal defect on the proximal that does not extend subgingivally, Cavit can be placed after the endodontic appointment is completed and prior to the removal of the rubber dam. On subsequent appointments, normal access can be made through the Cavit temporary, but if such access weakens the temporary filling, the entire Cavit temporary should be replaced at each visit. The use of Cavit is limited by its slow setting property, requiring one hour in a wet environment to reach a complete set.

Pretreatment often requires that a tooth be built up with temporary cement prior to the placement of the rubber dam. For example, a carious defect may extend subgingivally, permitting salivary leakage from beneath the rubber dam. In this situation a fast, hard-setting filling, such as zinc oxyphosphate cement or alloy, will permit the immediate placement of the rubber dam clamp, and will withstand repeated application of the clamp.

3. Provision of a Sound Margin of Tooth Structure for Rubber Dam Placement. The sound margin may be exposed by periodontal procedures or the crown may be restored with a temporary band.

Periodontal Therapy

Gingival hyperplasia or hypertrophy can be easily removed by gingivectomy or by the use of the

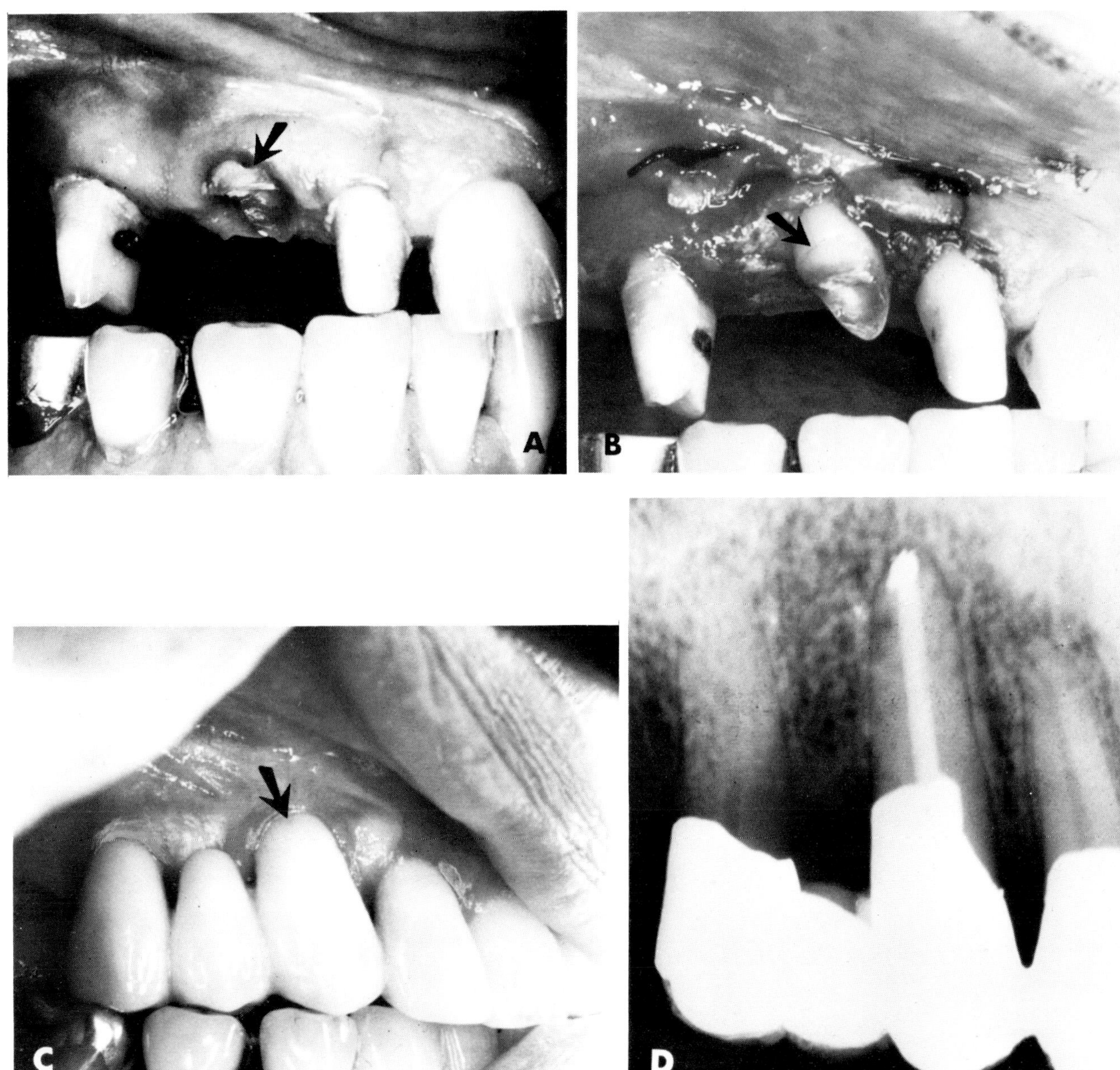

Fig. 2–46. *A,* Preoperative view of maxillary canine whose crown is totally destroyed by caries under defective bridge abutment. Level of gingival tissue (arrow) in relation to remaining root is apparent. *B,* View following root canal therapy and apical repositioning of attached gingiva. Elongation of clinical crown is seen *(arrow)* in comparison with prior photograph. *C,* View of final restoration. Important canine abutment *(arrow)* is salvaged by combined endodontic-periodontic procedures. (Restoration by Dr. James Haberman.) *D,* Retrofilling of pulpless canine abutment was done during mucogingival surgery. Previous endodontic filling was incomplete. (Endodontic-periodontic therapy by Dr. Edward E. Beveridge.)

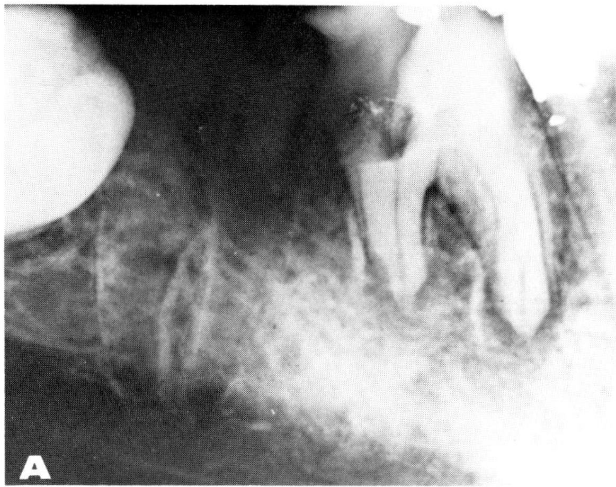

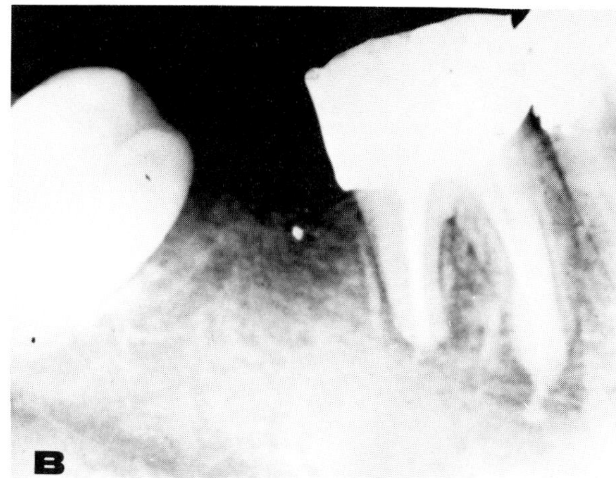

Fig. 2–47. *A,* Badly broken down pulpless molar with root resorption. Before endodontic treatment cavity must be sealed off. *B,* Custom fitted copper band allows for full treatment. (Courtesy Dr. James D. Zidell.)

electrosurgery. Both techniques are expedient, but have the disadvantage in some cases of producing large surface wounds, which may hemorrhage and must heal by secondary intention.

In such situations, and in cases in which the crown has been fractured or destroyed to the gingival level, a more refined mucogingival technique is indicated. The inflamed gingival margin is removed by means of an internally beveled horizontal incision. This measure eliminates an external wound and permits a rubber dam application immediately upon completion of the procedure without the problem of hemorrhage control. Two vertical relaxing incisions, extended from the gingival margin into the alveolar mucosa, create a mucogingival flap and permit the free movement of this flap to be repositioned apically and sutured to place. This technique permits the exposure of additional root surface for the placement of the rubber dam clamp and final restoration. In some cases, corrective osseous recontouring may be necessary (Fig. 2–46).

Copper Bands

The above periodontal procedures are expedient and can usually be limited to the endodontically involved tooth. However, there are some problems that cannot be easily corrected by periodontal therapy. Gross subgingival caries may be better treated by the cementation of a copper band custom fitted to the particular carious defect (Fig. 2–47). Or, the extraction of a partially erupted third molar may leave a bony defect and a deep carious lesion on the distal root of the second molar (Fig. 2–48). A copper band may be readily adapted to extend subgingivally in this area where anatomic considerations preclude definitive periodontal therapy. In severe cases the periodontal or carious defect may be beyond repair, requiring hemisection of the distal root of the lower second molar. Banding may then be helpful to seal off the bisected pulp chamber.

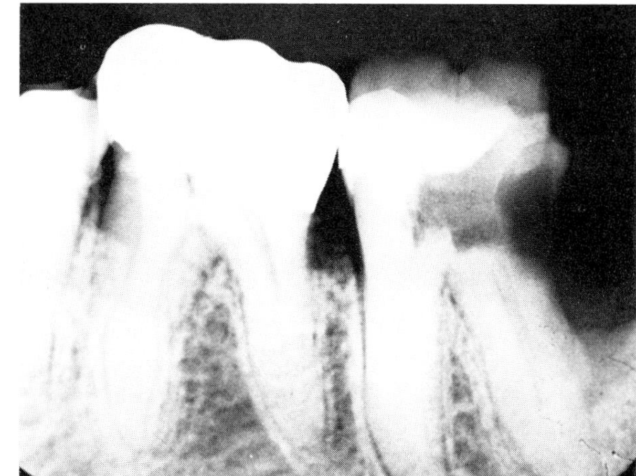

Fig. 2–48. Destruction caused by partially erupted third molar and caries. Extended copper band will isolate crown for endodontic treatment. (Courtesy Dr. James D. Zidell.)

Orthodontic Bands

Whereas the copper band is custom fitted to adapt to a carious defect extending ***well below*** the gingival margin, the orthodontic band is prefabricated to fit the tooth supragingivally. Thus, it is not used to replace the copper band, but to help retain a large temporary filling or support a tooth with undermined enamel walls. It is an essential step in the treatment of a tooth which is thought to be cracking or split (Fig. 2–49). It serves as an excellent temporary restoration to prevent splitting during extended treatment, or after treatment, when final restoration has to be postponed. All bands are cemented with zinc oxyphosphate cement.

Temporary Crowns and Restorations

Aluminum shell crowns and plastic crowns or bridges cemented with zinc oxide and eugenol cement are not acceptable as proper pretreatment temporization. The placement of the rubber dam clamp and the tension of the rubber dam displace these temporary crowns, as does repeated rubber dam application and endodontic manipulation. In addition, access attempted through the temporary crown and cement may easily be misdirected against one of the axial walls of the preparation, instead of directly into the pulp chamber.

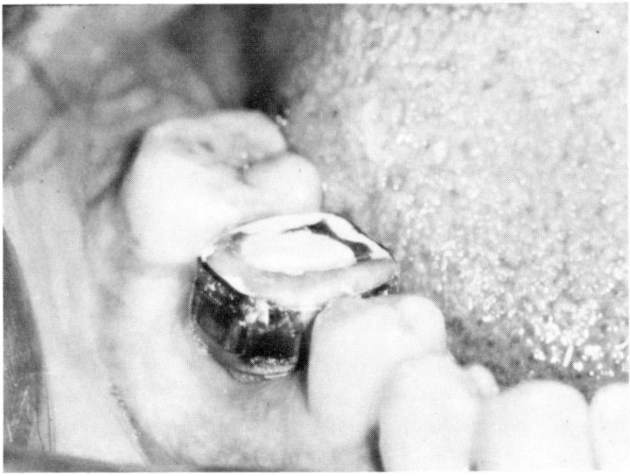

Fig. 2–49. Prefabricated orthodontic band for supragingival containment of large temporary proximal filling or to support weakened enamel walls. (Courtesy Dr. James D. Zidell.)

UTILIZATION OF THE RUBBER DAM

Many rubber dam techniques and concepts are time-consuming, frustrating, and discouraging when applied to endodontic therapy. For root canal treatment, a rapid, simple and effective method of dam application has developed. In all but the most unusual circumstances, the rubber dam can be placed in less than a minute.

Though the modern endodontic approach to the use of the dam has changed, the importance and purposes of the dam have remained the same:

1. It provides a dry, clean, and sterilizable field.
2. It protects the patient from the possible aspiration or swallowing of tooth and filling debris, bacteria, necrotic pulp remnants, and instruments or operating materials.
3. It protects the patient from rotary and hand instruments, drugs, and the trauma of repeated manual manipulation of the oral soft tissues.
4. It is faster, more convenient, and less frustrating than the repeated changing of cotton rolls or saliva evacuating devices.
5. It eliminates the interference, annoyance, and obscuring of vision by the tongue and cheeks.

Equipment

Time-and-motion studies have stressed the efficacy of kit or tray preparations which pool the instruments and materials to be utilized in a given procedure (Fig. 2–50). Applied to a rubber dam application, this system encourages the more routine use of the rubber dam in all phases of dentistry where it is indicated.

Dam Material. Rubber dam is available in a variety of thicknesses, colors, sizes, and methods of packaging. The medium-weight thickness is recommended for general all-around use. It has the advantage of cupping around the cervical of teeth, providing a hermetic seal without the use of floss ligatures tied around each tooth. Also, it does not tear or rip easily, and provides an unusual degree of protection from injury for the underlying soft tissues. It exerts a greater retracting force on the lips and cheeks than the thinner material, thus affording greater access and improved vision. There are advantages, however, in using the thin weight dam on mandibular anterior teeth and partially erupted posterior teeth. The problem of retaining a clamp on these tapering teeth, with little or no cervical undercut, is solved by applying the thinner dam, which exerts less dislodg-

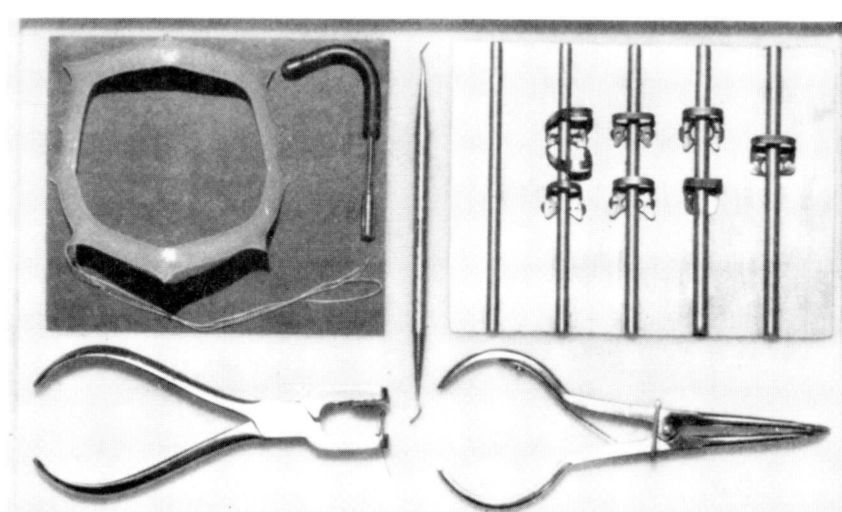

Fig. 2–50. Rubber dam tray, prearranged by dental assistant and ready for use. Tray contains pre-punched 6″ × 6″ rubber dam, rubber dam frame, saliva ejector, and ligature used in placement. Instrument for tucking dam into sulcus is beside rack which holds selection of clamps. Punch and forceps complete tray set-up.

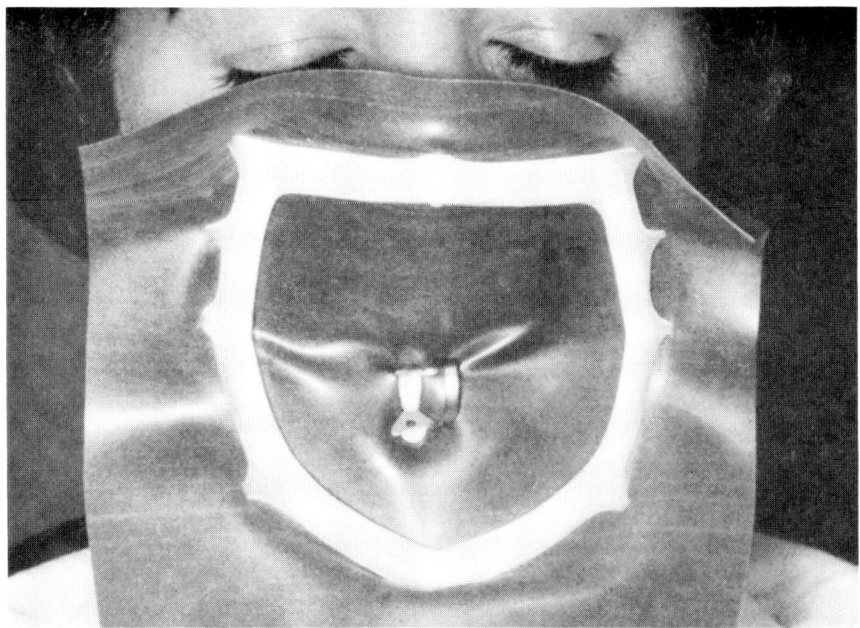

Fig. 2–51. Rubber dam frame, developed in nylon by Nygaard-Ostby, is radiolucent and will not impede x-rays. Frame is curved to fit patient's face and may be positioned so that patient breathes behind dam and not into operative field as he would with Wizard frame.

ing force on the clamp. The disadvantage is it is easily torn.

Dam material may be purchased in 5″ or 6″ wide rolls to be cut to size; precut sheets—either 5″ × 5″, 5″ × 6″ or 6″ × 6″ unsterilized and boxed; or precut and individually sterilized and packaged. A sheet 6″ × 6″ will fill all needs of various applications and is large enough to fit any size frame.

The choice of light- or dark-colored material is largely up to the individual. The dark material provides a contrasting color as a background for the light tooth.

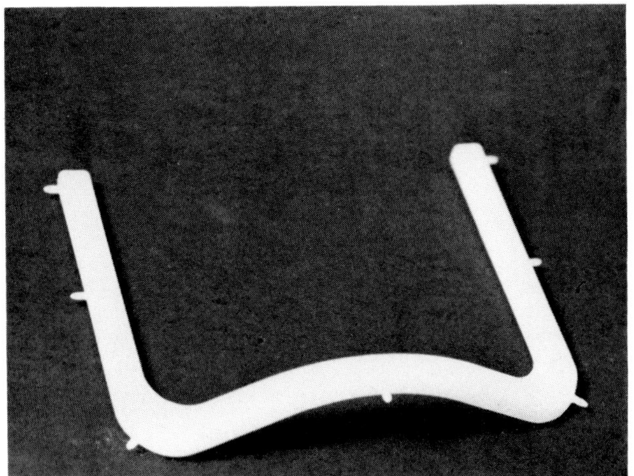

Fig. 2–52. Rigid glass-filled plastic rubber dam frame completely radiolucent. (Courtesy Star Dental Manufacturing Co.)

Frames. The Nygaard-Ostby (N-O) rubber dam frame is made of radiolucent nylon and may be left in place while a tooth is subjected to x-ray without interfering with the roentgenographic image (Fig. 2–51). It tends to hold the dam away from the patient's face and is thus cooler, drier, more comfortable, and requires no absorbent napkin. Because of its shape, it also directs the breath from the nostrils away from the operative field, thus minimizing the possible contamination by nasal staphylococci* (Fig. 2–51).

The metal Young's frame is easily manipulated, but is radiopaque and may cause obliteration of an important area on the radiograph. Another U-shaped frame, the Starlite Visuframe, is now made in radiolucent plastic, which is a great improvement (Fig. 2–52). Because of its shape, it exerts less tension on the dam and is easier to use than the Nygaard-Ostby frame when taking roentgenograms of molars. Like the N-O frame it requires no absorbent napkin, and stands away from the face.

The conventional "Wizard" or Hollenback frame, or any head-encompassing device, has no use in modern endodontic therapy. Placement requires

*This is a most important point and bears emphasis. All of the dental office personnel should have nose cultures, and if staphylococci are present, should apply Neosporin each day into their nostrils.

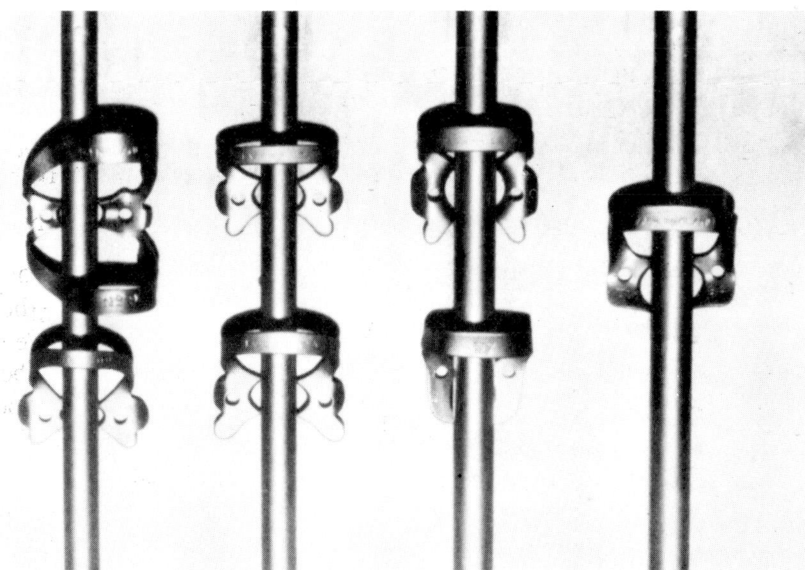

Fig. 2–53. Basic selection of rubber dam clamps, positioned on metal rack, developed by Dr. J. B. Freedland. These anterior, premolar and molar clamps will accommodate 90% of all endodontic cases. From left to right: first row, Ash #9, Ivory #00; second row, Ivory #2, Ivory #2A; third row, Ivory #14, S.S. White #18; fourth row, Ash #8A.

more time and manipulation and imposes a frustrating obstacle during roentgenography. It also requires the use of an absorbent napkin against the face. These frames exert considerable tension on the corners of the mouth and some patients, particularly mouth breathers, are frightened by the suffocating sensation.

Clamps. Although a basic selection of five to seven clamps (Fig. 2–53) will permit most dentists to place a clamp and dam on the majority of teeth encountered, the more experienced operator builds up a larger collection over the years. Teeth that are rotated, partially erupted, malaligned, malformed, fractured, hemisected, unusually large or small, or teeth with severe carious involvement, all present problems requiring special clamps or clamping techniques. A new rubber dam clamp holder, accompanied by a stainless sterilizing pan, has been developed by Dr. J. B. Freedland. Sixteen frequently used clamps, ranging from size 00 to molar clamps, may be stored in cold sterilizing solution. (See Fig. 14–4.)

Table 2–1 is a suggested minimum assortment of clamps for the various teeth. Incisor and premolar clamps that are losing their tension should be retained as they often make excellent clamps for unusual molar applications.

For endodontic therapy particularly, the use of clamps with wings allows a more rapid, efficient means of applying the rubber dam. A well-trained assistant is able to perform much of the usual technical procedure of application described later in this section. The wings allow the dentist to place the clamp dam and frame in one operation (Fig. 2–54). Also the wings cause a broader buccal-lingual deflection of the dam from the tooth involved, allowing increased access.

Table 2–1. Rubber Dam Clamp Selection

Maxillary Teeth	
Central Incisor	Ivory 0 or 2, S. S. White 27, Ash 8A Ash 9 (diagonally if partially erupted)
Lateral Incisor	Ivory 00, Ash 9
Canine	Ivory 2 or 2A
Premolars	Ivory 2 or 2A, S. S. White 20 or 27
Molars	Ivory 3 or 4, Ivory 14 or 14A, Ash 8A
Mandibular Teeth	
Incisors	Ivory 0 or 00, Ash 9
Canine	Ivory 2 or 2A
Premolars	Ivory 2 or 2A, S. S. White 20 or 27
Molars	S. S. White 18, Ivory 12 or 13, 14 or 14A, Ash 8A, Fatigued Ivory 2A.

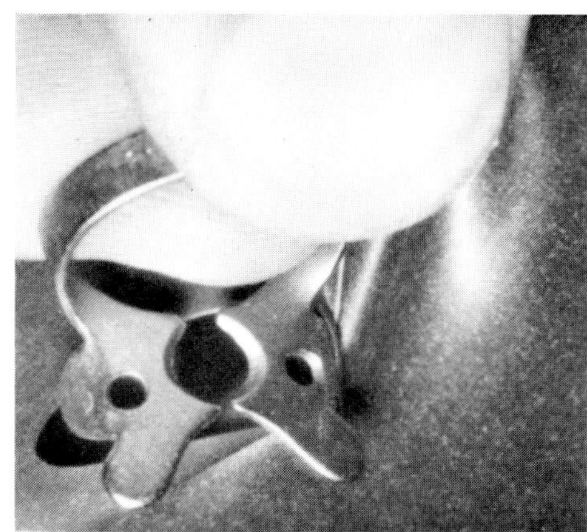

Fig. 2–54. Placement of wings of clamp by assistant prior to positioning dam on frame. Bow of clamp is oriented to distal.

Punch. Any rubber dam punch that is convenient for the operator and creates a sharp clean hole in the dam material is satisfactory. All too often the punch has not been correctly centered over a hole, and a "nick" on the cutting margin results, producing an incomplete or jagged cut in the dam material. This is easily corrected by "sharpening" the cutting edge of the hole with a carborundum stone. Failure to correct this punching error will result in the contamination of the field owing to salivary leakage at the site of the ragged hole in the dam.

Forceps. Either the Ash or Ivory style clamp forceps is satisfactory (Fig. 2–55). One advantage of the Ivory forceps, however, is the projections from the engaging beaks (Fig. 2–56). These allow the operator the opportunity to exert a gingivally directed force which often is necessary to force the clamp beyond the height of contour and into the proximal undercuts.

The projections on the beaks also allow positive control, so that the jaws of clamps may be tipped to depress either the "toe" or "heel" of the clamp. The Ash style forcep beaks, on the other hand, afford a fulcrum point for posterior or anterior rotation of the clamp.

Tucking Instrument. A plastic or cement instrument is used to shed the rubber dam off the wings of the clamp once the clamp has been positioned. It is also used, along with a stream of compressed air, to invert or "tuck" the edges of the dam into the gingival sulci, thus ensuring a moisture-proof seal. In

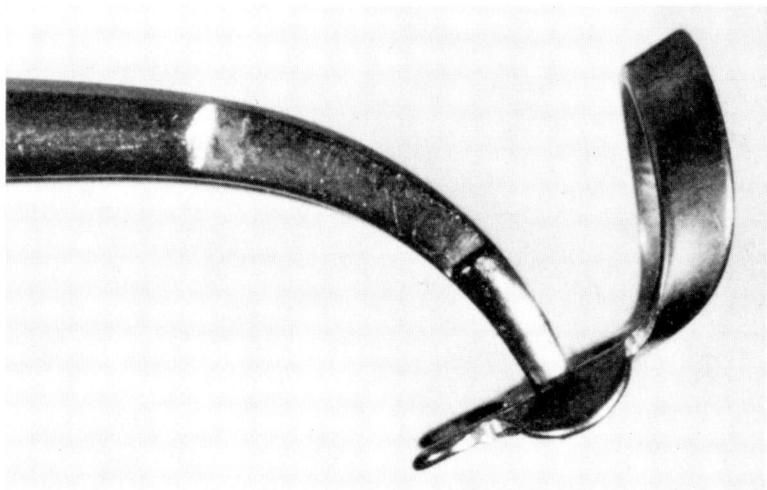

Fig. 2–55. Ash style rubber dam clamp forceps, valuable in clamp placement when bows of forceps must clear mandibular incisors.

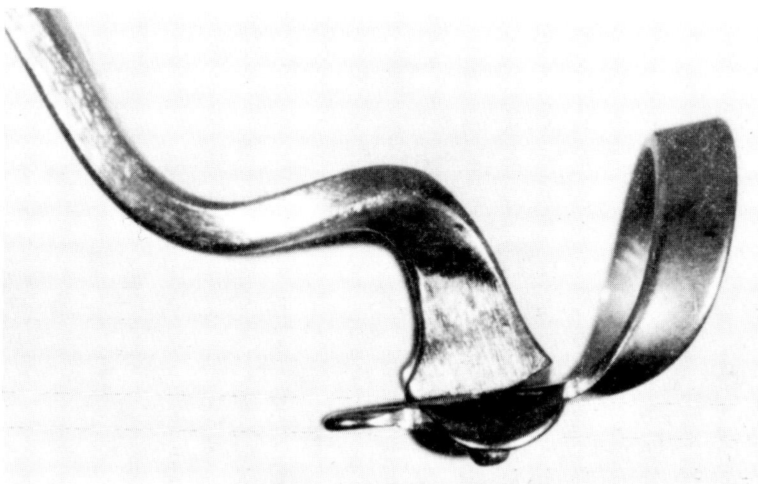

Fig. 2–56. Ivory style rubber dam clamp forceps. "Foot" on beaks affords more accurate placement of clamp, particularly when apical pressure must be applied to gain gingival undercut.

multiple-tooth applications this is particularly necessary.

The instrument is also occasionally needed to act as a lever in a gingival embrasure in order to open a tight contact and allow the rubber dam to pass through.

Dental Floss. At one time it was recommended that dental floss be routinely used as a ligature placed around the cervix of each tooth in order to invert or "tuck" the dam and provide a seal. Through the use of medium or heavy dam material, this is no longer necessary. Floss is still essential, however, for the testing of contacts prior to dam application, and for passing the dam material through the contacts. In both instances the operator should release his lingual grasp of the floss and pull it out to the buccal, rather than back through the contact point.

Saliva Ejector. Any sterilizable or disposable saliva ejector is acceptable. It should always be placed ***underneath*** the dam for endodontic use, in contrast to the procedure of cutting a hole through the dam. This will prevent possible salivary contamination of the field and be less of a hindrance while taking roentgenograms with the dam in place. Disposable plastic saliva ejectors have the advantage of being radiolucent.

Technique of Application

Preparation

Dentist:

1. Remove supra- and subgingival calculus and dental plaque.
2. Select clamp to be used.
3. Test contacts with floss to assure passability and to test for sharp edges which might tear the dam.

Assistant:

1. Punch one appropriate size hole ***just off center*** of a 6″ × 6″ piece of dam material. Ideally, only the teeth receiving therapy should be included in the dam application.
2. Stretch the dam over the frame.

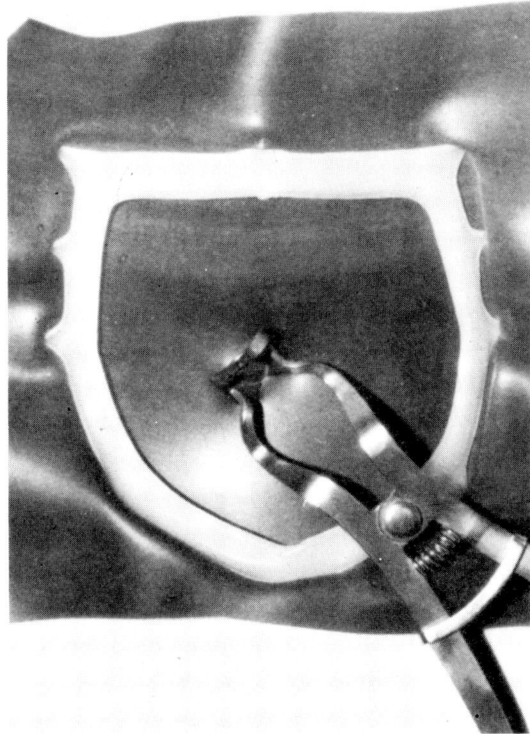

Fig. 2–57. Assistant has mounted rubber dam on frame and has positioned wings of clamp in dam. She presents assembled unit with forceps to dentist, ready for placement. Notice that hole is punched just off center of 6″ × 6″ rubber dam. Position of hole is identical for each tooth and dam is rotated for either right or left side, upper or lower.

3. Place the ***wings*** of the selected clamp in the punched hole with the bow of the clamp to the distal (see Fig. 2–54).
4. Place the forceps in the clamps with tension and hold in readiness for the dentist (Fig. 2–57).

Application by the Team

Dentist:

1. Place an index finger in the vestibule to retract the lip and cheek. The patient is instructed to place his tongue on the opposite side.
2. Sight the tooth to be clamped between the jaws of the clamp (Fig. 2–58*A*). Direct vision is essential.
3. Place the clamp into the cervical proximal undercuts on the tooth, as the index finger is removed from the vestibule (Fig. 2–58*B*). Finger pressure is sometimes used to ensure seating of the clamp.
4. Shed the dam off the clamp wings with the tucking instrument (Fig. 2–58*C*). Care is used not to rip the dam.
5. Use floss to aid in passing the dam through contacts—pull the floss through to the labial or buccal (Fig. 2–58*D*).
6. In multiple tooth applications, tuck the dam into the gingival sulci of the unclamped teeth, using the tucking instrument.

Assistant:

7. Use compressed air to dry the teeth; this aids in tucking.
8. Place the saliva ejector under the dam. Many patients will not need the saliva ejector on a maxillary dam application.

Completed dam application should take less than thirty seconds of the dentist's time, in all but the unusual cases (Fig. 2–59).

Advantages

There are many desirable features of this technique of application. First of all, there is an unobstructed view of the jaws of the clamp as it is placed on the tooth, thus preventing the impingement of the gingiva or inclusion of a fold of cheek or the tongue. Furthermore, it is a great time-saver for the dentist. The assistant is able to mount the clamp, frame, and forceps. Because of the efficiency, there is less manipulation in the mouth, there is no confusion about straightening out which corner of the dam goes where, the result is much neater in appearance, and there is less frustration for the dentist.

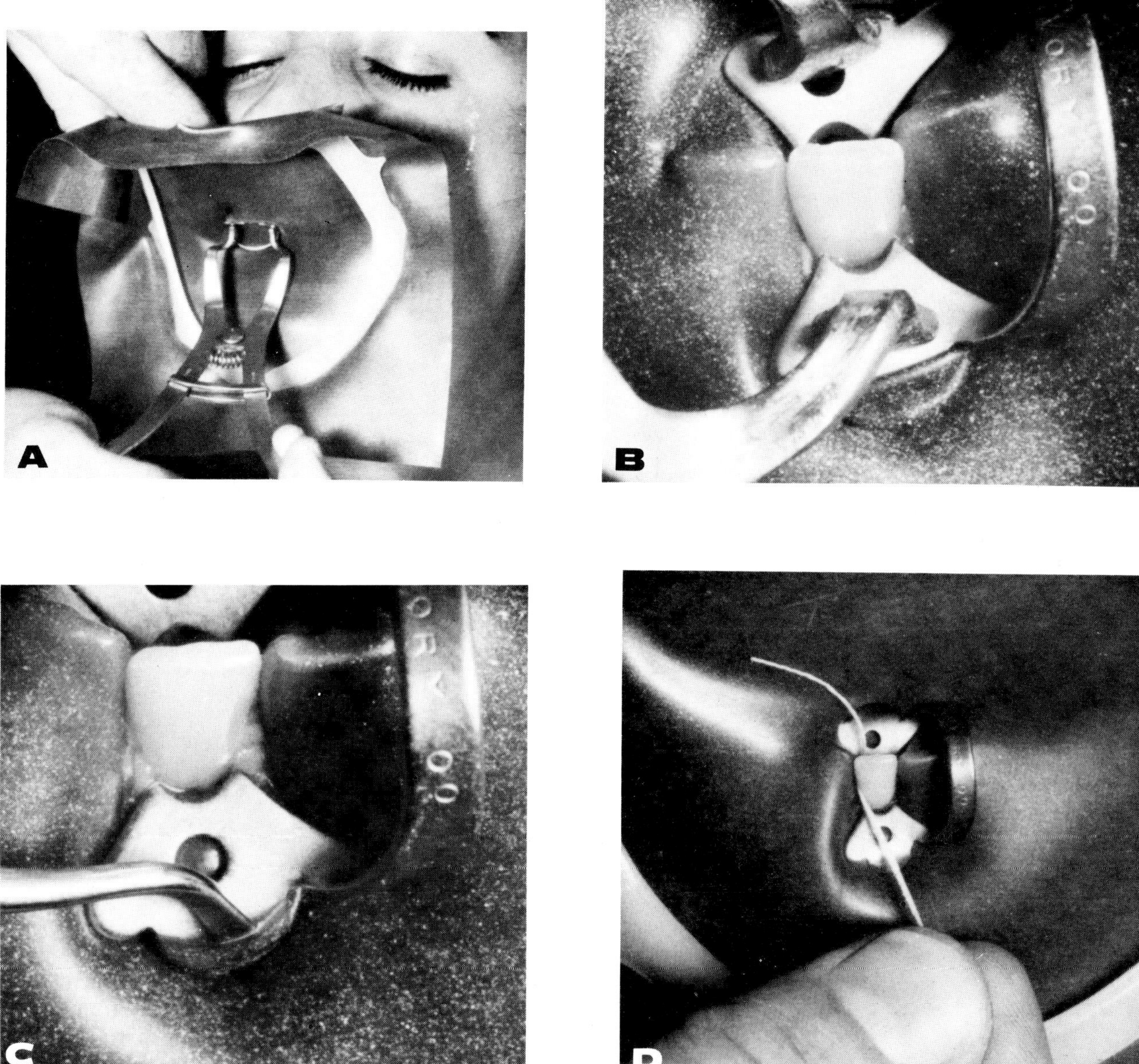

Fig. 2–58. *A,* Dentist retracts lip and cheek with thumb and index finger of left hand and sites tooth to be clamped (here a maxillary premolar) between bows of the clamp. Care must be taken not to clamp wrong tooth. *B,* Clamp is carried into gingival undercuts. If undercuts are slight, clamp may be rotated on tooth to take advantage of undercuts along labial and lingual-proximal long axis. *C,* Dam is shed from clamp wings with tucking instrument, which is also used to carry lip of dam under gingival sulcus after tooth is air-dried. *D,* Dental floss is used to carry dam past interproximal contacts. It should then be pulled to buccal rather than removed back past contact.

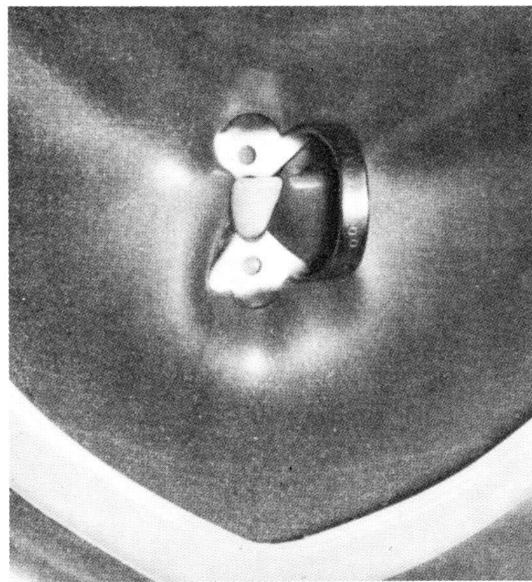

Fig. 2–59. Completed dam application, exposing only involved tooth. Team approach to placement of rubber dam materially speeds placement.

In applying the dam to a single tooth, however, the dentist must take great care that the correct tooth is clamped. After placement, the record is checked and the teeth are counted under the dam, first by the dentist and then independently by the assistant. If the team is hesitant about clamping the wrong tooth, the time-honored system of first placing the clamp, then the dam, then the frame should be used.

Removal of Dam

1. For single-tooth applications, simply remove the clamp with the forceps and remove the dam.
2. In the multiple-tooth applications first remove the clamp, then place a finger under the dam in the vestibule, and stretch the dam on the labial away from the teeth. Cut the stretched interproximal dam with scissors, and then remove the dam. It is essential that the dam be inspected to ensure that an interproximal dam septum has not been left between the teeth.

Circumstances Requiring Variations from the Usual Application

A number of circumstances require a variation from the standard dam application.

First Circumstance. A well-done gingival gold or porcelain baked-on gold veneer crown ***on the involved tooth,*** which could be fractured by clamps.

Variation. Clamp one or both ***adjacent*** teeth and tuck the dam around the involved tooth. Occasionally a floss ligature is needed on the involved tooth.

Second Circumstance. Multiple adjacent teeth requiring treatment.

Variation. The posterior tooth is clamped normally, while the clamp is reversed on the anterior tooth. By another approach, the most posterior tooth is clamped normally, while the anterior portion of the dam is retained and retracted without a clamp because of the retention of the several interproximal dam septa below their corresponding contact areas.

Third Circumstance. One or more teeth are being treated simultaneously in ***different*** quadrants. Include all involved teeth in the dam application.

Variation. Clamp each tooth separately as though it were the only one involved. Thought must be given in cross-arch and opposite-arch applications to avoid combinations that would make roentgenography difficult.

Fourth Circumstance. Bridge abutments, splints and orthodontic bands with wires.

Variation. Punch a larger than usual hole in the dam. Smear Orabase around the hole on the underside of the dam. This mucilaginous material prevents leakage. Clamp the tooth in the normal manner. In addition, place a toothpick through the gingival embrasure next to the pontic. If leakage is still a problem, softened modeling compound can then be applied to the toothpick and crown area, providing a good seal.

Fifth Circumstance. Partially erupted tooth.

Variation. An Ivory 14A or Ash 8A clamp forced subgingivally into the cervical undercut will often hold. On occasion, an Ash #9 clamp placed on the oblique will suffice.

Sixth Circumstance. Hemisected maxillary or mandibular molars.

Variation. The hemisected mandibular molars are treated as a premolar. Those that are wide buccolingually are best clamped with a fatigued SSW or Ivory 2 or 2A.

The hemisected maxillary molar with the lingual root remaining is also best treated as a large premolar. An SSW 27 clamp frequently adapts well.

When the two buccal roots of a maxillary molar are remaining, it is then best treated as a small molar, the Ash 8A frequently sufficing. Often the hemisected maxillary molar can be clamped only by placing the clamp obliquely.

Seventh Circumstance. Molar with root amputation but intact crown.

Variation. If the usual molar or fatigued premolar clamp will not hold, place the dam over the tooth, apply softened greenstick modeling compound into the undercut made by the amputation, harden it by cooling with air, and then seat the usual molar clamp onto both the tooth and the compound. If necessary, resoften the compound in the area where the clamp will rest; seat the clamp into the softened area and cool it while holding the clamp with the forceps. If the crown has been prepared and no undercut exists, an undercut may have to be cut into the preparation to hold the clamp beaks. The undercut must be eliminated before impressions for the crown are taken.

Eighth Circumstance. Full-crown preparation without cervical undercut to retain the clamp.

Variations. A proper full-crown preparation will shed toward the occlusal, and the clamp may not provide adequate resistance to the tension of the rubber dam. It may be necessary to place parallel horizontal grooves on the buccal and lingual axial walls of the preparation near the gingival margin to permit the clamp to grasp onto the preparation. The Ivory 2 or 2A clamp will fit into these grooves for retention.

Ninth Circumstance. Posterior teeth with minimal tooth structure for clamp retention.

Variation. The tension of the rubber dam as it is stretched taut over the frame exerts pressure, or a force of displacement, on the bow of the clamp. The clamp may be reversed on the working tooth; a second clamp is placed ***over*** the rubber dam on the next tooth posterior, to absorb the pressure of the rubber dam.

Periodontal preparation to "elongate" the crown of a fractured or badly decayed tooth was discussed under the section Preparation for Endodontic therapy, page 88.

SUMMARY

Students, recent graduates, and veteran practitioners alike will find restorative and endodontic practice more rewarding and less frustrating as their mastery of rubber dam applications increases. Utilization of the simplified techniques, improved materials and organized procedures, as well as patience, practice and perseverance, will hasten this mastery. The neophyte is urged to "give equal time" to this basic phase of his dental education. Should one find the routine use of the rubber dam impossible, he is best advised to forego the more demanding attention to detail required in endodontic therapy.

REFERENCES

1. Ennis, L. M., and Berry, H. M.: *Dental Roentgenology*, 5th Ed., Philadelphia, Lea & Febiger, 1959, p. 13.
2. Glenner, R. A.: Eighty years of dental radiography. J.A.D.A., *90*: 549, March, 1975.
3. Priebe, W. A., Lazansky, J. P., and Wuehrmann, A. H.: The value of the roentgenographic film in the differential diagnosis of periapical lesions. Oral Surg., *7*:979, Sept. 1954.
4. Baumann, L., and Rossman, S. R.: Clinical roentgenologic and histopathologic findings in teeth with apical radiolucent areas. Oral Surg., *9*:1330, Dec., 1956.
5. Wais, F. T.: Significance of findings following biopsy and histologic study of 100 periapical lesions. Oral Surg., *11*:650, June, 1958.
6. Linenberg, W. P., et al.: A clinical roentgenographic and histologic evaluation of periapical areas. Oral Surg., *17*:467, April, 1964.
7. LaLonde, E. R.: A new rationale for the management of periapical granulomas and cysts: an evaluation of histopathological and radiographic findings. J.A.D.A., *80*:1056, May, 1970.
8. Ardran, G. M.: Bone destruction not demonstrable by roentgenography. Brit. J. Radiol., *24*:107, Feb., 1951.
9. Bender, I. B., and Seltzer, S.: Roentgenographic and direct observation of experimental lesions of bone. J.A.D.A., *62*:153, Feb., 1961.
10. Ramadam, A. E., and Mitchell, D. F.: A roentgenographic study of experimental bone destruction. Oral Surg., *15*:934, Aug., 1962.
11. Schwartz, S. F., and Foster, J. K.: Roentgenographic interpretation of experimentally produced bony lesions. Part I. Oral Surg., *32*:606, Oct., 1971.
12. Goldman, M., Pearson, A., and Darzenta, N.: Endodontic success—who's reading the radiograph. Oral Surg. 23: 432–7, Mar., 1972.
13. Fitzgerald, G. M.: Dental roentgenography I: an investigation in adumbration, or the factors that control geometric unsharpness, J.A.D.A., *34*:1, Jan., 1947.
14. Fitzgerald, G. J.: Dental roentgenography II: vertical angulation, film placement and increased object-film distance. J.A.D.A., *34*:160, Feb., 1947.
15. Waggener, D. T.: The right-angle technique using the extension cone. Dent. Clin. No. Amer., Nov., 1968, p. 783.

16. Silha, R. E.: Paralleling long cone technique. Dent. Radiology Photog., *41*:3, 1968.
17. Sheingorn, A.: Personal Communication. 1972.
18. Barr, J. H., and Gron, P.: Palate contour as a limiting factor in intraoral x-ray technique. Oral Surg., *12*:459, April, 1959.
19. Walton, R. E.: Endodontic radiographic techniques. Dental Radiog. Photog., *46*:51, Oct., 1973.
20. Clark, C. A.: A method of ascertaining the relative position of unerupted teeth by means of film radiographs. Odont. Sec. Roy. Soc. Med. Trans., *3*:87, 1909–1910.
21. Grady, J. R., and Clausen, H.: Establishing Your Point. Clinic Am. Assoc. Endodont., April 25, 1975.
22. Ingle, J. I., Beveridge, E. E., and Olson, C.: Rapid processing of endodontic "working" films. Oral Surg., *19*:101, Jan., 1965.
23. Pestritto, S. T.: Comparison of diagnostic quality of dental radiographs produced by five rapid processing techniques. J.A.D.A., *89*:353, Aug., 1974.
24. Manson-Hing, L. R., and Monnier, P. Y.: Radiographic densitometric evaluation of seven processing solutions. Oral Surg., *39*:493, March, 1975.
25. Brynolf, I.: Improved viewing facilities for better roentgenodiagnosis. Oral Surg. *32*:808, Nov., 1971.
26. Spiegler, G.: Wiesollen Rontgenufrahmen Betrachtet Werden? Forstchr. Geb. Roentgenstr. *56*:662, 1937.
27. Birchfield, J. and Rosenberg, P. A.: Role of the anesthetic solution in intrapulpal anesthesia. J. Endodont., *1*:26, Jan., 1975.
28. Parris, L., and Kapsimalis, P.: Effect of temperature change on the sealing properties of temporary filling materials. Oral Surg., *13*:982, Aug., 1960.

Chapter 3

Endodontic Cavity Preparation*

JOHN I. INGLE, EDWARD E. BEVERIDGE, RAYMOND G. LUEBKE, RICHARD E. WALTON, and JAMES D. ZIDELL

The section on Success and Failure (Chapter 1) substantiates the endodontic dogma of ***careful cavity preparation and canal obturation*** as the keystones to successful root canal therapy. Apical moisture-proof seal, the first essential for success, is not possible unless the space to be filled is carefully prepared to receive the restoration. As in operative dentistry, the final restoration is rarely better than the initial cavity preparation.

Endodontic cavity preparation begins the instant the involved tooth is approached with a cutting tool, and the final obturation of the canal space will depend in great measure on the care and accuracy exercised in this initial preparation.

Divisions of Cavity Preparation. For descriptive convenience, endodontic cavity preparation may be separated into two anatomic divisions: ***(a) coronal preparation*** and ***(b) radicular preparation.*** Actually, coronal preparation is merely a means to an end, but to enlarge accurately and fill the radicular pulp space, intracoronal preparation must be correct in size, shape, and inclination.

CORONAL CAVITY PREPARATION

Basic Coronal Instruments

Preparations on and within the crown of the pulpless tooth are completed with power-driven rotary tools. For optimal operating efficiency, two separate handpieces are used to deliver widely divergent rates of speed. The correct burs are mounted by the dental assistant prior to their use. Rarely should a bur have to be placed or changed during the operation. For initial entrance through the enamel surface or through a restoration, the ideal cutting instrument is the round-end carbide fissure bur mounted in a contra-angle handpiece operating at accelerated speed (Fig. 3–1). With this instrument, enamel, plastic, or metal perforation is easily accomplished, and surface extensions may be rapidly

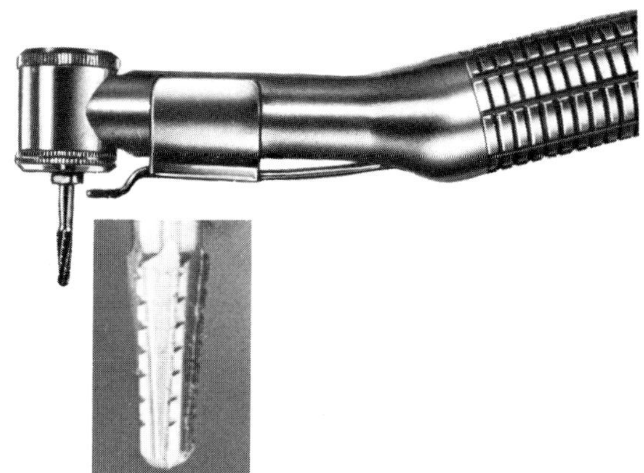

Fig. 3–1. Air rotor contra-angle handpiece mounted with No. 449 carbide bur (inset). Rounded end of bur is for initial opening and side blades for cavity wall extension. Small head of handpiece affords easier access to molars. (Courtesy Star Dental Manufacturing Co.)

*Originally published in part as: Endodontic Instruments and Instrumentation. Dental Clinics of North America, Philadelphia. W. B. Saunders Co., Nov., 1957, pp. 805-822.

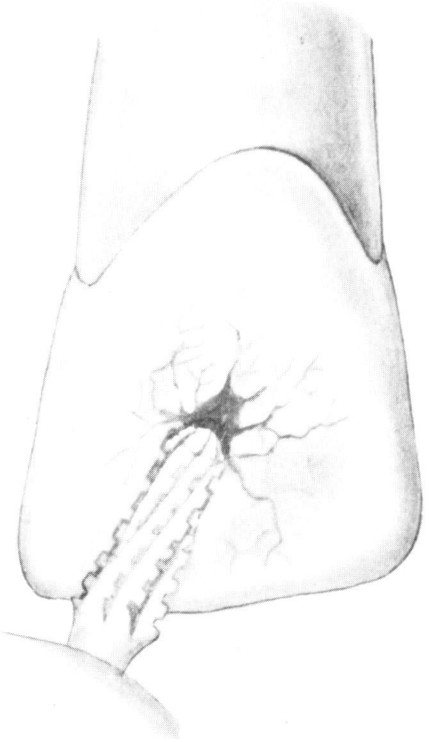

Fig. 3–2. Forcing accelerated tapered bur or stone will severely craze lingual enamel. Bur should be allowed to cut its own way.

completed. ***The tapered instrument should never be forced, but should be allowed to cut its own way with a light touch by the operator.*** Forcing a tapered instrument, it will act as a wedge. This causes the enamel to "check" or "craze" and will materially weaken the tooth (Fig. 3–2). If a porcelain jacket crown is to be entered, a small tapered diamond point should be used. Again, care must be exercised not to split the jacket by forcing the action of the tapered point.

As soon as the enamel or restorative penetration and minor surface extensions are complete, the accelerated handpiece is put aside, and the slow speed (3,000 to 8,000 rpm) contra-angle handpiece is used, mounted with a round bur, preferably carbide. Three sizes of round burs are routinely used, Nos. 2, 4, and 6, and two lengths, regular and surgical. The regular-length round bur in a conventional latch-type contra-angle will "reach" 9.0 mm. from the nose of the contra-angle. The surgical-length bur in a standard contra-angle will "reach" 14 or 15 mm. and is quite necessary in some deep preparations (Fig. 3–3). Numbers 8 and 11 round burs advocated for endodontic preparation by some authors are actually wider than most molar pulp chambers, and are far too large for ***optimal*** endodontic preparations.

The round burs are for dentin removal in both anterior and posterior teeth. These burs are first used to drill through the dentin and "drop" into the pulp chamber. The same bur is then employed in the

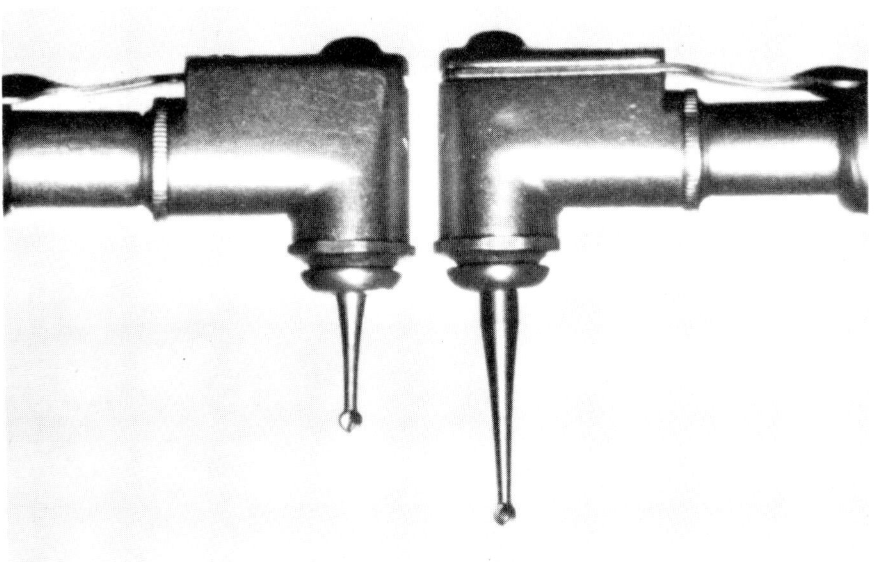

Fig. 3–3. Two identical contra-angle handpieces holding #4 round burs. Regular length bur on left will reach 9 mm. Surgical length bur on right will reach 14 mm.

removal of the roof and side walls of the pulp chamber. The choice of the size of the round bur is made by estimating the canal width and chamber size apparent in the initial roentgenogram.

The No. 2 round bur is generally used in preparing ***mandibular*** anterior teeth and most ***maxillary*** premolar teeth with narrow chambers and canals. It is also occasionally used in the incisal pulp horn area of ***maxillary*** anterior teeth.

The No. 4 round bur is generally used in the ***maxillary*** anterior teeth and the ***mandibular*** premolar teeth. It is also occasionally used in "young" ***maxillary*** premolars and "adult" molars in both arches, that is, molars with extensive secondary dentin.

The No. 6 round bur is used only in molars with large pulp chambers.

As soon as the bulk of the overhanging dentin is removed from the walls and roof of the chamber, the slower operating round burs are put aside, and once again the high-speed fissure bur is used to finish and slope the side walls in the visible portions of the preparation.

Rotary instruments operating at greatly accelerated speeds play a most important role in endodontic cavity preparation, especially for the patient with discomfort. At the same time, a good deal of damage may be rendered with these instruments because of the loss of tactile sense in their use. ***High-speed burs should not be used to penetrate into, or initially enlarge, the pulp chamber.*** In this operation the clinician depends almost entirely on the "feel" of the bur deep inside the tooth, against the roof and walls of the pulp chamber, in order to judge the extensions which are necessary. High-speed equipment is operated by sight alone and should never be employed in a blind area where reliance on tactile sensation is necessary.

Spade-shaped burs are advocated by a number of endodontists to "funnel-out" the coronal preparations in anterior teeth and to extend the walls of posterior preparations. Although efficient, the spade-shaped bur is uncomfortably vibratory. There are two other objections to its use. First, the spade-shaped bur can be a dangerous weapon in the hands of the neophyte. While the interest of the young operator is directed to the side-cutting action of the bur on the lingual side of the preparation, the point of the instrument may be ditching the dentin on the unseen labial wall deep within the cavity. The second objection deals with simplicity and speed of operation. If the two handpieces are set up prior to operation, with a fissure bur in the high-speed handpiece and the correct round bur in the low-speed handpiece, there should be no reason to change to a third bur which is both unnecessary and time consuming.

Pulp Anatomy in Relation to Cavity Preparation

The alliance between endodontic cavity preparation and pulp anatomy is inflexible and inseparable. In order to master the anatomic concept of cavity preparation, the operator must develop a mental, three-dimensional image of the inside of the tooth, from pulp horn to apical foramen. Unfortunately, the roentgenogram provides him only a two-dimensional "blueprint" of pulp anatomy. It is the third dimension that the clinician must visualize as a supplement to his two-dimensional thinking if he is to clean and enlarge accurately and fill the total pulp space (Plate I, A).

PRINCIPLES OF ENDODONTIC CAVITY PREPARATION

Any discussion of cavity preparation must ultimately revert to the basic ***Principles of Cavity Preparation*** established by G. V. Black.[1] By slightly modifying Black's principles, a list of ***Principles of Endodontic Cavity Preparation*** may be established. In laying down his principles, Black dealt completely with cavity preparations limited to the crowns of teeth. His principles can be applied, however, to radicular preparations as well. Endodontic preparations deal with both coronal and radicular cohorts—each prepared separately but ultimately flowing together into a single preparation. For convenience of description, ***Black's Principles*** are therefore divided into:

Endodontic Coronal Cavity Preparation

I. Outline form
II. Convenience form
III. Removal of the remaining carious dentin (and defective restorations)
IV. Toilet of the cavity

Endodontic Radicular Cavity Preparation

IV. Toilet of the cavity (continued)
V. Retention form
VI. Resistance form

In the first half of this chapter endodontic coronal cavity preparation will be discussed; the second half will be devoted to radicular preparation. A similar approach to coronal preparation was suggested by Pucci in 1944.[2]

Principle I—Outline Form (Plate I)

The outline form of the endodontic cavity must be correctly shaped and positioned to establish ***complete access for instrumentation,*** from cavity margin to apical foramen. Moreover, external outline form evolves from the ***internal anatomy*** of the tooth, the pulp. Because of this internal-external relationship, endodontic preparations must of necessity be done in a reverse manner, ***from the inside of the tooth to the outside.*** That is to say, ***external outline form is established*** during preparation by mechanically ***projecting the internal anatomy*** of the pulp onto the ***external surface.*** This may only be accomplished by drilling into the open space of the pulp chamber and then working with the bur from the inside of the tooth to the outside, cutting away the dentin of the pulpal roof and walls overhanging the floor of the chamber (Plate I, B).

This intracoronal preparation is contrasted to the extracoronal preparation of operative dentistry where outline form is always related to the ***external anatomy*** of the tooth. The tendency to establish endodontic outline form in the conventional operative manner and shape must be resisted (Plate I, C).

To achieve optimal preparation, three factors of internal anatomy must be considered: (1) the size of the pulp chamber, (2) the shape of the pulp chamber, and (3) the number of individual root canals and their curvature.

Size of Pulp Chamber. The outline form of endodontic access cavities is materially affected by the size of the pulp chamber. In the young patient these preparations must be more extensive than in the older patient where the pulp has receded and the pulp chamber is smaller in all three dimensions (Plate I, D). This becomes quite apparent in preparing the anterior teeth of youngsters, where larger root canals require larger instruments and filling materials; materials which in turn will not pass through a small orifice in the crown (Plate I, E).

Shape of Pulp Chamber. The finished outline form should accurately reflect the shape of the pulp chamber. For example, the floor of the pulp chamber in a molar tooth is triangular in shape owing to the triangular position of the orifices of the three canals. This triangular shape is extended up the walls of the cavity and out onto the occlusal surface, hence the final occlusal cavity outline form is triangular (Plate I, C). As another example, the coronal pulp of a maxillary premolar is flat mesiodistally, but is elongated buccolingually. The outline form of the endodontic cavity preparation in the maxillary premolars is, therefore, an elongated oval which extends buccolingually rather than mesiodistally, as does Black's operative cavity preparation (Plate I, F).

Number and Curvature of Root Canals. The third factor regulating outline form of endodontic coronal cavities is the number of and the curvature or direction of the root canals. In order to instrument each canal efficiently without interference, the cavity walls often have to be extended to allow an unstrained instrument approach to the apical foramen. When cavity walls are extended to improve instrumentation, the outline form is materially affected (Plate I, G). This change is for convenience in preparation, hence ***convenience form*** in part regulates the ultimate outline form.

Principle II—Convenience Form (Plate II).

Convenience form was conceived by Black as a modification of the cavity outline form, in order to establish greater convenience in the placement of intracoronal restorations. In the case of endodontic therapy, however, ***convenience form*** makes more convenient (and accurate) the ***preparation as well as filling of the root canal.*** Four important benefits are gained through convenience-form modifications: (1) unobstructed access to the canal orifice, (2) direct access to the apical foramen, (3) cavity expansion to accommodate filling techniques, and (4) complete authority over the enlarging instrument.

Unobstructed Access to the Canal Orifice. In endodontic cavity preparations of all teeth, enough tooth structure must be removed to allow instruments to be placed easily into the orifice of each canal without interference from overhanging walls. The clinician must be able to see each orifice and easily reach it with the instrument points. Failure to observe this principle not only endangers the successful outcome of the case, but also adds materially to the duration of treatment (Plate II, A–D).

In certain teeth, extra precautions must be taken to search for additional canals, the lower incisors being a case in point. Even more important is the high incidence of a second separate canal in the mesiobuccal root of maxillary first molars. A second canal sometimes is found in the distal root of mandibular molars as well. The premolars, both maxillary and mandibular, also can be counted on to have extra canals. During preparation, the operator is mindful of these variations from the norm, and searches conscientiously for additional canals. In many cases, the outline form has to be modified to facilitate this search and the ultimate cleaning, shaping, and filling of the extra canals.

Direct Access to the Apical Foramen. To provide direct access to the apical foramen, enough tooth structure must be removed to allow the endodontic instruments freedom within the coronal cavity so that they may extend down the canal in an unstrained position. This is especially true when the canal is severely curved or leaves the chamber at an obtuse angle (Plate II, E). Occasionally, total decuspation is necessary.

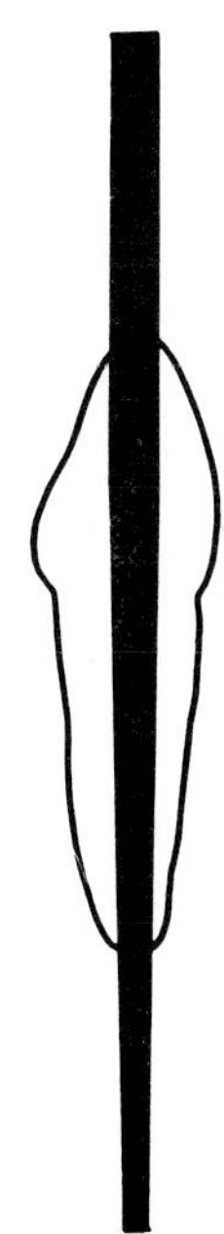

Fig. 3–4. Example of extension beyond normal outline form. In this case, incisal edge is invaded to provide access for rigid endodontic implant and instruments necessary for preparation. (From Frank, A. L.: Dent. Clin. No. Amer., Nov., 1967.)

Expansion to Accommodate Filling Techniques. It is often necessary to expand the outline form to make more ***convenient*** or practical certain filling techniques. If the softened gutta percha technique is used for filling, wherein rather rigid pluggers are used in a vertical thrust, then the outline form must be widely extended to accommodate these heavier instruments.

The same gross extensions of outline form are often necessary for successful ***endodontic implants.*** To accommodate the absolutely rigid (chrome cobalt) implant, the cavity preparation may have to invade the labial incisal edge of a lower incisor (Fig. 3–4).

Complete Authority over the Enlarging Instrument. It is imperative that the clinician maintain complete control over the root canal instrument. If the instrument is impinged at the canal orifice by tooth structure that should have been removed, the dentist will have lost control of the direction of the tip of the instrument and the intervening ***tooth structure*** will dictate the control of the instrument (Plate II, G).

If, on the other hand, the tooth structure is removed around the orifice so that the instrument stands free in this area of the canal (Plate II, H), the instrument will then be controlled by only two factors: (1) the clinician's fingers on the handle of the instrument, and (2) the walls of the canal at the tip of the instrument. Nothing is to intervene between these two points (Plate II, F).

Disturbances of controlling factors related to convenience form will ultimately lead to failure by either root perforation, "ledge" or "shelf" formation within the canal, instrument breakage, or the incorrect shape of the completed canal preparation.

Principle III—Removal of the Remaining Carious Dentin and Defective Restorations

The caries and defective restorations remaining in an endodontic cavity preparation must be removed for three reasons: (1) to eliminate mechanically as many bacteria as possible from the interior of the tooth, (2) to eliminate the discolored tooth structure, which may ultimately lead to staining the crown, and (3) to eliminate the possibility of any saliva leaking into the prepared cavity.

The last point is especially true of proximal or buccal caries that extend into the prepared cavity.

After the caries are removed, if a carious perforation of the wall is allowing salivary leakage, the area must be repaired with cement, ***preferably from inside***

PLATE I

Outline Form

A. Standard roentgenogram, in buccolingual projection, provides only two-dimensional view of what is ***actually three-dimensional problem*** (left). If ***mesiodistal*** x-ray projection could be made (right), one would find pulp of maxillary second premolar to be flat tapering "ribbon" rather than round "thread" visualized on initial roentgenogram. Final ovoid occlusal cavity preparation would mirror internal anatomy rather than buccolingual x-ray image.

B. Coronal preparation of maxillary first molar illustrating major principle of endodontic cavity outline form; ***internal anatomy of tooth (pulp) dictates external outline form.*** This is accomplished by extending preparation from inside of tooth to outside surface, that is, working from inside to outside.

C. Endodontic cavity preparation, mandibular first molar, superimposed upon inlay restoring proximal-occlusal surfaces. ***Black's outline form*** of ***inlay*** is related to external anatomy and environment of tooth, *i.e.* extent of carious lesions, grooves and fissures and position of approximating premolar. ***Triangular*** or ***rhomboidal outline form*** of ***endodontic preparation*** on the other hand, is related to internal anatomy of pulp. No relationship exists between the two outline forms.

D. Size and shape of endodontic coronal preparations in mandibular incisors related to ***size*** and ***shape*** of ***pulp*** and ***chamber.*** Contrast in outline form between "young" incisor (left) with large pulp and adult incisor (right) is apparent. Large triangular preparation in youngster reflects pulpal horn extension and size of pulp chamber, whereas ovoid preparation in adult relates to grossly receded pulp.

E. Large size and shape of coronal preparation in recently calcified incisor relates to huge pulp housing. To remove all pulp remnants and to accommodate large endodontic instruments and filling materials, coronal preparation must be extensive, triangular, funnel-shaped opening. Actually, no more than lingual wall of pulp chamber has been removed. When endodontic implant is to be used, outline form will have to be grossly extended to accommodate "enormous" instruments and rigid implant point. In lower incisors, outline form will frequently be extended into incisal edge, sometimes invading labial as well. This preparation allows absolutely ***direct*** access to apex.

F. Outline form of ***Endodontic*** coronal cavity in ***maxillary*** first premolar is narrow, elongated oval in buccolingual projection (bottom), which reflects size and shape of broad, flat pulp chamber of this particular tooth.

G. ***Buccal*** view of ***inadequate*** coronal preparation in maxillary molar with defalcated distal root. There has been no compensation in cavity preparation for severe curvature of distal canal or for obtuse direction by which canal leaves chamber. Operator can no longer maintain control of instrument, and ledge has been produced in distal canal (arrow). Extension of outline form and internal preparation to distal (dotted line) would have obviated this failure.

PLATE I

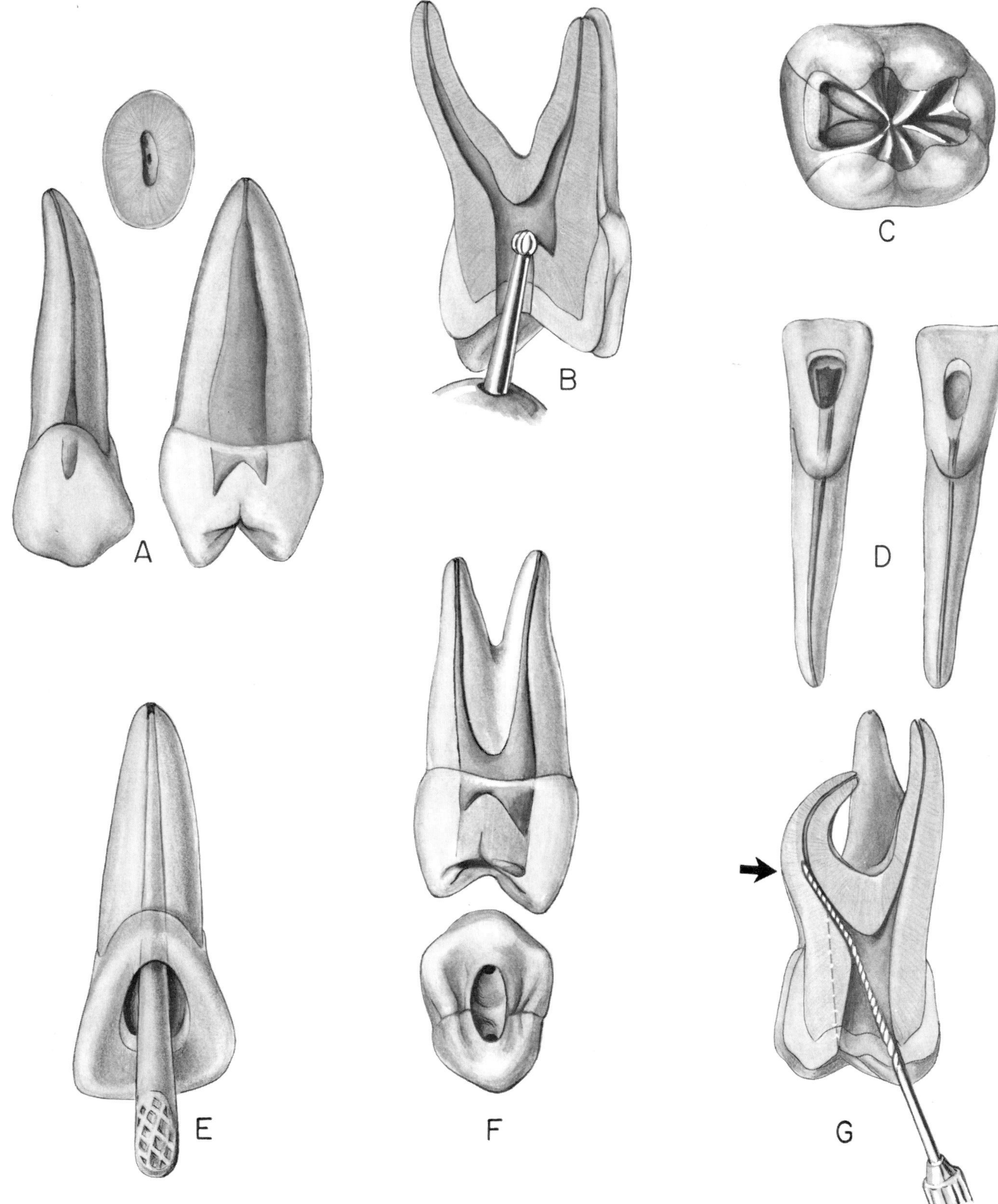

PLATE II

Convenience Form

A. ***Obstructed access*** to mesial canals in mandibular first molar. Overhanging roof of pulp chamber misdirects instrument mesially with resulting ledge formation in canal. It is virtually impossible to see, and difficult to locate, mesial canal orifices each time instrument is introduced.

B. ***Internal cavity preparation.*** Removing completely roof from pulp chamber will bring canal orifices into view and allow immediate access to each orifice. Using round bur and working from inside-out will accomplish this end.

C. ***Final finish of convenience form*** is completed with fissure bur. Entire cavity slopes toward mesial direction of approach, which greatly simplifies instrument placement.

D. ***Unobstructed access to canal orifices. Mesial*** wall has been ***sloped to mesial,*** for approach to mandibular molar is from mesial. Curved instrument, with curved tip pointed toward mesial, travels down mesial wall until tip engages orifice. ***Instrument*** is then given ***one-half turn*** so ***instrument curves*** in ***same directional*** curve as canal. After once determining position of each orifice, mouth mirror may be laid aside.

Distal wall of preparation also slopes to mesial and is easily entered from mesial approach.

E. ***Direct access to apical foramen.*** Extensive removal of coronal tooth structure is necessary to allow complete freedom of endodontic instruments in coronal cavity and ***direct access to apical canal.*** This is especially true when root is severely curved or leaves chamber at obtuse angle. Walls are generally reduced with burs (see B and C above) and with endodontic files at orifice. Burs are rarely used in floor or immediate orifice area. In the event a second canal is suspected in mesiobuccal root of maxillary molar, cavity outline would be extended in both these directions to broaden search.

Depending upon technique used to fill canal, outline form may also be expanded somewhat to accommodate pluggers used in obturation. Gross extension may also be necessary to accommodate huge instruments and rigid endodontic implants used in endodontic osseous implants. Extensions into incisal edge of lower incisor is case in point.

F. ***Complete authority of enlarging instrument is maintained*** when all intervening tooth structure is removed (arrow) and instrument is controlled by clinician's fingers on handle of instrument, and tip of instrument is free in lumen of canal.

G. ***Complete authority of enlarging instrument.*** If lateral wall of cavity has not been sufficiently extended and pulpal horn portion of orifice still remains in wall, orifice will have appearance of tiny "mouse hole." This ***lateral wall*** will then impinge upon enlarging instrument and dictate direction of instrument tip. Operator will have lost control of instrument and situation.

H. ***By extending lateral wall*** of cavity, thus removing all intervening dentin from orifice, "mouse hole" in wall will be eliminated and ***orifice*** will appear ***completely in floor.*** Now enlarging instrument will stand free of walls and ***operator will regain control of instrument*** (see F above).

PLATE II

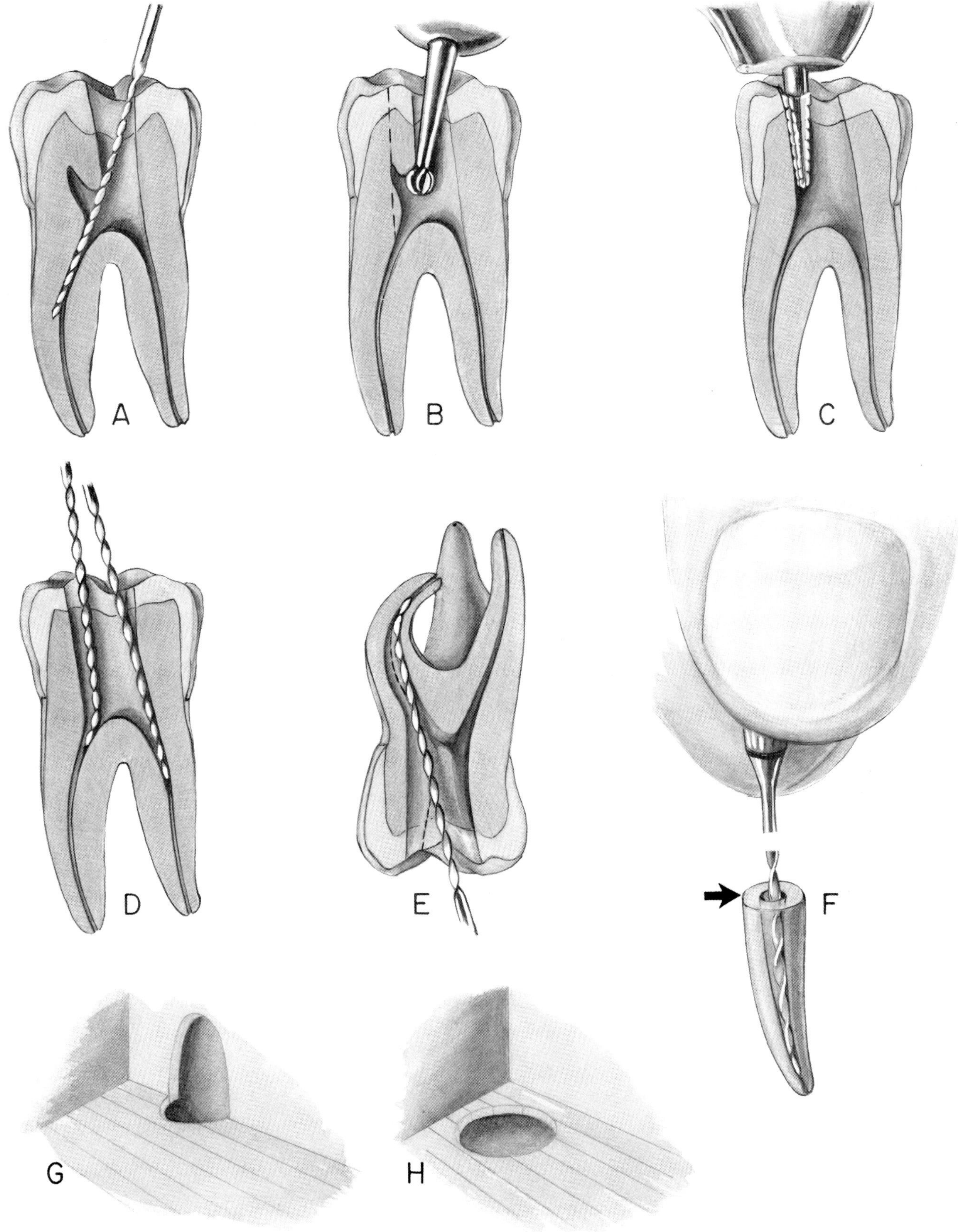

the cavity. A small piece of premixed temporary cement, Cavit or Cavit G, may be forced through the perforation and applied to the dry walls of the cavity, while care is taken to avoid forcing the cement into a canal orifice. A cotton pellet, moistened with any sterile aqueous solution such as saline or a local anesthetic, will cause the Cavit to set.

If the caries is so extensive that the lateral walls are destroyed, or if a defective restoration is in place which is loose and leaking, then the entire wall or restoration should be removed and later restored. It is important that restoration be postponed until the radicular preparation has been completed. It is much easier to complete the radicular preparation through an open cavity than through a restored crown. As a matter of fact, the more of the crown that is missing, the easier the radicular preparation becomes. The ultimate in ease of operation is the molar tooth broken off at the gingival (Fig. 3–5). As long as a rubber dam can be placed on the tooth, the tooth should not be built up with amalgam, cement, or a copper band; having to work through a hole only complicates the endodontic procedures. In addition, if the band comes off, the tooth measurements are invalidated and must be re-established. An adequate temporary filling can always be placed in the remaining pulp chamber (Fig. 3–6).

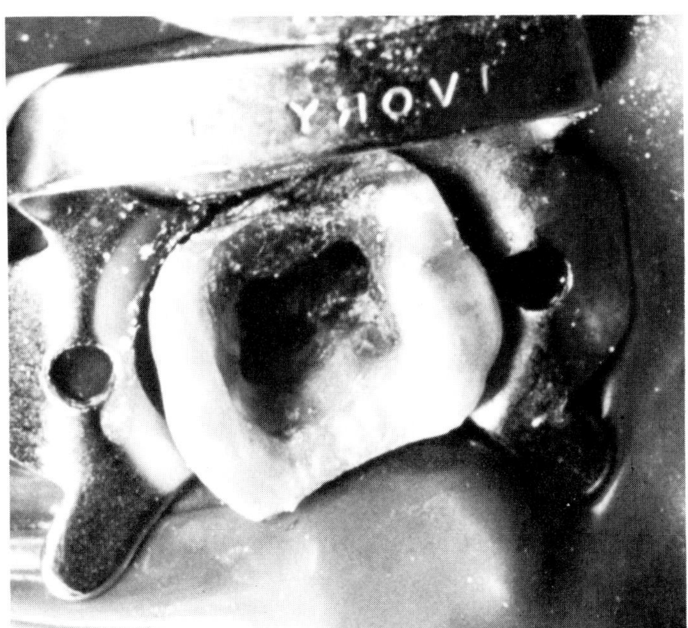

Fig. 3–5. Carious involvement of maxillary molar which has destroyed most of crown. Enough tooth structure remains to adapt rubber dam clamp. Wide open cavity allows greater ease of operation. If caries extends below gingival level, gingivectomy will expose solid tooth structure. Copper band placement is inadvisable.

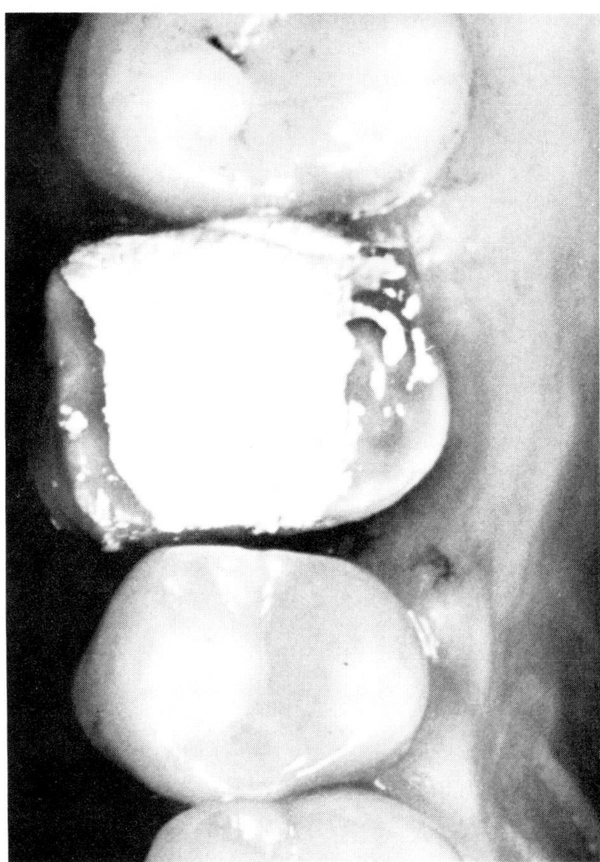

Fig. 3–6. Temporary filling may be placed as long as enough coronal cavity exists for retention.

If enough tooth does not remain above the gingiva to place a rubber dam clamp and seal against saliva, and if it is imperative that the tooth be retained, a simple gingivoplasty will establish the required "crown" length (see Fig. 18–15). In any case, this procedure is usually necessary before the tooth can be restored. In this case, the occlusal cavity may be sealed and the incised gingiva protected with the placement of a putty-like periodontal dressing over the entire stump and gingiva. Cotton, and then a thin layer of Cavit, should first cover the canal orifices.

Principle IV—Toilet of the Cavity

All of the caries, debris, and necrotic material must be removed from the chamber before the radicular preparation is begun. If the calcified or metallic debris is left in the chamber and carried into the canal, it may act as an obstruction during canal enlargement. Soft debris carried from the chamber might increase the bacterial population in the canal. Coronal debris may also stain the crown, particularly of anterior teeth.

Round burs, of course, are most helpful in cavity toilet. The long-blade, endodontic spoon excavator is ideal for debris removal (Fig. 3–7). Irrigation with sodium hypochlorite or hydrogen peroxide is also an excellent measure for cleansing the chamber and canals of persistent debris. If a bacterial culture is first required, the clinician must remember to culture the canal before irrigating with either of these drugs, for they will eliminate countless bacteria and make difficult the culture necessary for an antibiotic sensitivity test (p. 574). The chamber may finally be wiped out with cotton and a flush of air will eliminate the remaining debris. Air must never be aimed down the canals, however. Emphysema of the oral tissues has been produced by a blast of air escaping out the apex.

As previously stated, ***Toilet of the Cavity*** is important as a final step in coronal endodontic cavity preparation, but extends into the radicular preparation as well. As will be discussed later in the chapter, ***Toilet of the Cavity*** makes up a significant portion of the radicular preparation.

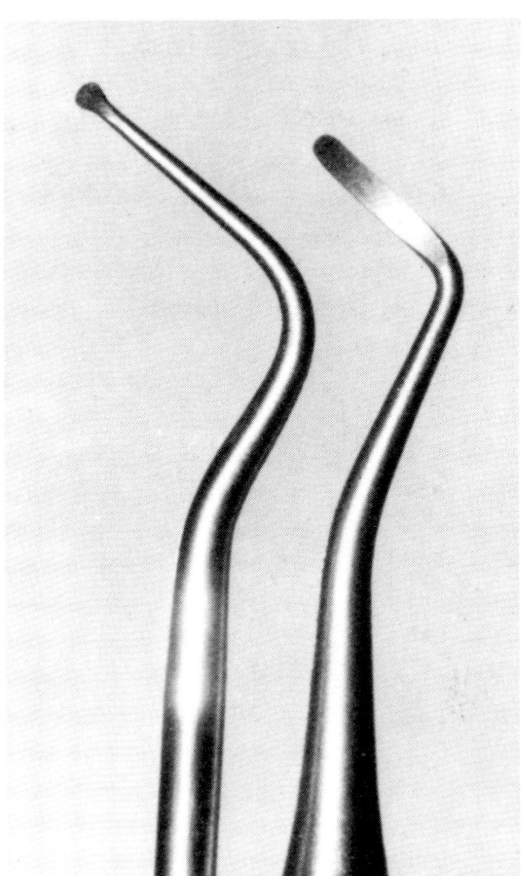

Fig. 3–7. Long blade endodontic spoon excavator compared to standard Black's spoon excavator. Long blade instrument *(left)* is needed to reach depths of molar preparations.

DETAILED CORONAL CAVITY PREPARATION

Descriptions and Caveats

With the basic principles of endodontic cavity preparation in mind, the student is urged to study the detailed plates that follow, each dealing with coronal preparation. Again, keep in mind the importance of the intracoronal preparation to the ultimate radicular preparation and filling.

For each group of teeth, e.g., maxillary anterior teeth, mandibular premolar teeth, there is a plate showing in detail the exact cavity preparation and operative technique applicable to that particular group of teeth. The technique plate is followed by plates of the individual teeth within the group. Four separate views of each tooth are presented: (1) the facial-lingual view as seen in the roentgenogram, (2) the mesiodistal view, impossible to obtain radiographically, but necessary to the three-dimensional mental image of the pulp anatomy, (3) a cross-sectional view at three levels, and (4) a view of the occlusal or lingual surface with cavity outline form.

Detailed variations in preparation related ***to each particular tooth,*** as well as information about tooth length, root curvature, and canal anatomy variations are presented. These plates are followed by a plate of ***errors*** commonly committed in the preparation of this group of teeth.

The ***mandibular*** incisors—centrals and laterals—are so anatomically similar they are confined to one plate.

The reader is reminded that the preparations illustrated here are ***minimal*** preparations, that the outline form is a direct reflection of the pulp anatomy, and if the pulp is expansive, the outline form will also be expansive. Furthermore, the outline form may have to be greatly enlarged to accept heavier instruments or rigid filling materials.

Finally, we are particularly indebted to Bjorndal et al. for the length of tooth measurements.[3] One must realize these measurements are only approximations, applying literally to Caucasian men between the ages of 17 and 21 years of age. Nonetheless, the measurements are helpful and should alert the dentist to what to expect as "normal." We have adapted liberally from the important work by Dempster and Adams on the angulation of the teeth in the alveolar process.[4] In addition, new information on multiple canals has been brought to light. The high incidence of additional canals in the maxillary molars and premolars, as well as multiple canal anatomy in the mandibular incisors and premolars, is a significant improvement in clinical knowledge. When there is lack of agreement between authors, we have chosen the larger figures, that is, the figures furthest from the normal.[5-13]

Plates III to XXVII

FOLIO OF CORONAL ENDODONTIC CAVITY PREPARATIONS

Illustrated by

VIRGINIA E. BROOKS

PLATE III

Endodontic Preparation of Maxillary Anterior Teeth

A. Entrance is ***always*** gained through lingual surface of ***all*** anterior teeth. Initial penetration is made in exact center of lingual surface at position marked "X." Common error is to begin cavity too far gingivally.

B. Initial entrance is prepared with tapering fissure bur in ***accelerated-speed*** contra-angle with air coolant, operated at ***right angle*** to long axis of tooth. ***Only enamel is penetrated at this time.*** Do not force bur; allow it to cut its own way.

C. ***Convenience extension*** toward incisal continues initial penetrating cavity. Maintain point of bur in central cavity and rotate handpiece toward incisal so bur ***parallels*** long axis of tooth. Enamel and dentin are beveled toward incisal. ***Entrance into pulp chamber should never be made with accelerated-speed instrument.*** Lack of tactile sensation with these instruments ***precludes their use inside*** tooth.

D. Preliminary cavity outline is funneled and fanned incisally with fissure bur. Enamel has ***short*** bevel toward incisal, and "nest" is prepared in dentin to receive round bur to be used for penetration.

E. ***Surgical length*** No. 4 round bur in ***slow-speed*** contra-angle is used to penetrate pulp chamber. If pulp has greatly receded, No. 2 round bur is used for initial penetration. Take advantage of ***convenience extension*** toward incisal to allow for shaft of penetrating bur, operated nearly parallel to long axis of tooth.

F. ***Working from inside chamber to outside,*** round bur is used to remove lingual and labial walls of pulp chamber. Resulting cavity is smooth, continuous, and flowing from cavity margin to canal orifice.

G. After outline form is completed, surgical length bur is carefully passed into canal. ***Working from inside to outside,*** lingual "shoulder" is removed to give continuous, smooth-flowing preparation.

H. Occasionally, No. 1 or 2 round bur must be used laterally and incisally to eliminate pulpal horn debris and bacteria. This also prevents future discoloration.

I. Final preparation relates to ***internal anatomy*** of chamber and canal. In "young" tooth with large pulp, outline form reflects large triangular internal anatomy—extensive cavity which allows thorough cleansing of chamber as well as passage of large instruments and filling materials needed to prepare and fill large canal.

J. Cavity preparations in "adult" teeth, with chamber obturated with secondary dentin, are ovoid in shape. Preparation ***funnels*** down to orifice of canal. The further pulp has receded, the more difficult to reach to this depth with round bur. Therefore, when roentgenogram reveals advanced pulpal recession, ***convenience extension must be advanced further incisally*** to allow bur shaft to operate in central axis.

K. Final preparation with reamer in place. Instrument shaft ***clears*** incisal ***cavity margin*** and ***reduced*** lingual "shoulder," allowing unstrained approach to apical third of canal. Instrument remains under complete control of clinician. Optimal, ***round, tapered cavity*** may be prepared in apical third, tailored to requirements of ***round, tapered filling*** materials to follow. Remaining ovoid part of canal is cleaned and shaped by extensive filing. Obturation by multiple points follows.

PLATE III

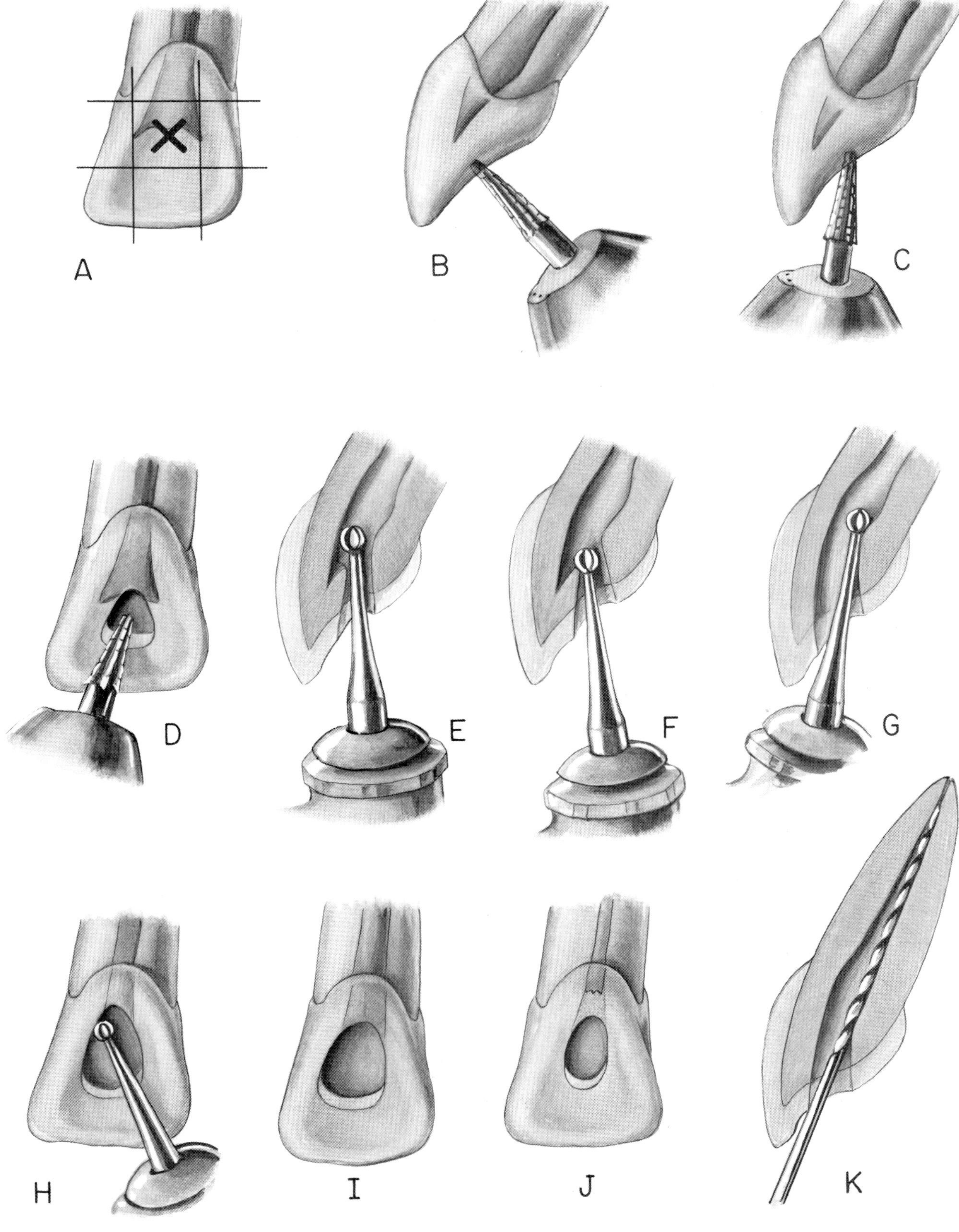

PLATE IV

Maxillary Central Incisor

Pulp Anatomy and Coronal Preparation

A. ***Lingual*** view of recently calcified incisor with large pulp. Roentgenogram will reveal:
   1. extent of pulp horns
   2. mesiodistal width of pulp
   3. apical-distal curvature (8% of time)
   4. 2-degree mesial-axial inclination of tooth

   These factors seen in roentgenogram are borne in mind when preparation is begun.

B. ***Distal*** view of same tooth demonstrating details ***not apparent in roentgenogram:***
   1. presence of ***lingual*** "shoulder" at point where chamber and canal join
   2. broad labiolingual extent of pulp
   3. 29-degree lingual-axial angulation of tooth.

   Operator must recognize that:
   a. lingual "shoulder" must be removed with surgical-length bur to allow better access to canal
   b. these "unseen" factors affect ***size, shape,*** and ***inclination*** of final preparation.

C. Cross sections at three levels: 1, cervical; 2, mid root; and 3, apical third:
   1. ***Cervical*** level: pulp is enormous in young tooth, wider in mesiodistal dimension. Debridement in this area is accomplished by ***extensive perimeter filing.***
   2. ***Mid root*** level: canal continues ovoid and requires perimeter filing and multiple point filling
   3. ***Apical third*** level: canal, generally round in shape, is enlarged by reaming cavity into ***round tapered*** preparation, which matches ***round tapered*** primary gutta percha filling point. Preparation terminates at cementodentinal junction, 0.5 mm. from apical foramen. Unusually large apical third canal is more ovoid in shape, must be prepared with ***perimeter filing*** rather than reaming, and obturated with multiple points.

D. Large, triangular, funnel-shaped ***coronal preparation*** is necessary to adequately debride chamber of all pulp remnants. (Pulp is "ghosted" in background.) Note beveled extension toward incisal which will carry the preparation labially and thus nearer central axis. Incisal extension allows better access for large instruments and filling materials used in apical third canal.

E. ***Lingual*** view of ***adult*** incisor with extensive secondary dentin formation.
   Roentgenogram will reveal:
   1. full pulpal recession
   2. apparently straight canal
   3. 2-degree mesial-axial inclination of tooth.

F. ***Distal*** view of same tooth demonstrating details ***not apparent in roentgenogram:***
   1. narrow labiolingual width of pulp
   2. reduced size of lingual shoulder
   3. apical-labial curvature (9% of time)
   4. 29-degree lingual-axial angulation of tooth.

   Operator must recognize that:
   a. small canal orifice is difficult to find
   b. ***apical***-labial curvature ***not usually seen roentgenographically,*** can be determined by exploration with fine curved file and mesially oriented x-rays
   c. axial inclination of root calls for careful orientation and alignment of bur to prevent "gouging."

G. Cross sections at three levels: 1, cervical; 2, mid root; and 3, apical third:
   1. ***Cervical*** level: canal, only slightly ovoid, becomes progressively more round
   2. ***Mid root*** level: canal varies from slightly ovoid to round
   3. ***Apical third*** level: canal is generally round in older patient.

H. Ovoid, funnel-shaped coronal preparation provides adequate access to root canal. Pulp chamber, obturated by secondary dentin, need not be extended for coronal debridement. "Adult" cavity preparation is narrow in mesiodistal width, but is almost as extensive in inciso-gingival direction as preparation in young tooth. This beveled incisal extension carries preparation nearer central axis, allowing better access to curved apical third.

PLATE IV

Length of Tooth[3]		*Canal*	*Curvature of Root*			
Average Length	23.7 mm.	1 canal	Straight	75%	*Labial Curve	9%
Maximum Length	27.3 mm.		Distal Curve	8%	*Lingual Curve	4%
Minimum Length	21.5 mm.	100%	Mesial Curve	4%		
Range	5.8 mm.					

*Not apparent on roentgenogram

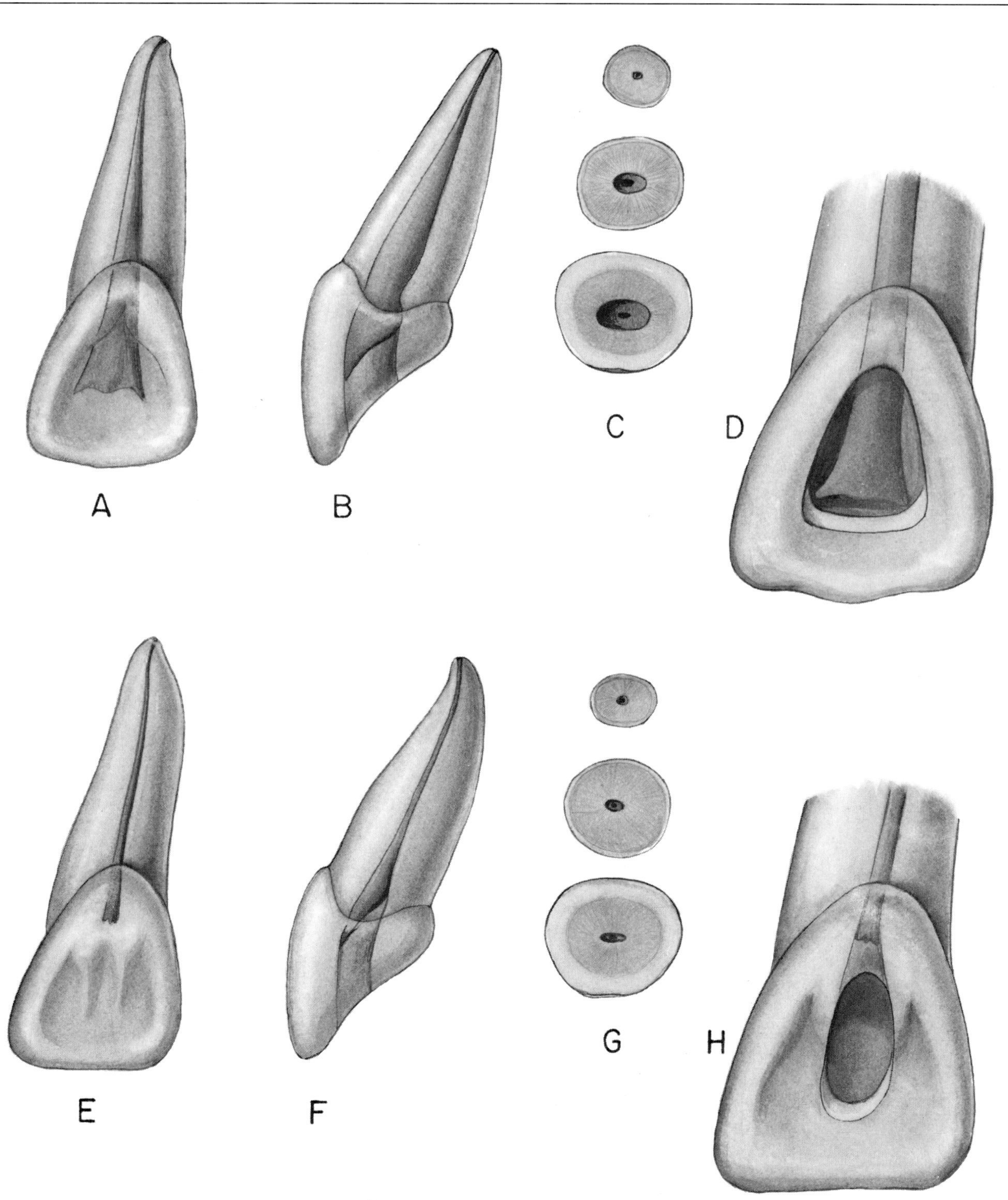

PLATE V

Maxillary Lateral Incisor

Pulp Anatomy and Coronal Preparation

A. Lingual view of recently calcified incisor with large pulp. Roentgenogram will reveal:
1. extent of pulp horns
2. mesiodistal width of pulp
3. apical-distal curvature (53% of time)
4. 16-degree mesial-axial inclination of tooth.

Factors seen in roentgenogram are borne in mind when preparation is begun.

B. ***Distal*** view of same tooth demonstrating details ***not apparent in roentgenogram:***
1. presence of ***lingual*** "shoulder" at point where chamber and canal join
2. broad labiolingual extent of pulp
3. 29-degree lingual-axial angulation of tooth.

Operator must recognize that:
a. lingual "shoulder" must be removed with surgical-length bur to allow better access to canal
b. these "unseen" factors will affect ***size, shape,*** and ***inclination*** of final preparation.

C. Cross sections at three levels: 1, cervical; 2, mid root; and 3, apical third:
1. ***Cervical*** level: pulp is large in young tooth, wider in labiolingual dimension. Debridement in this area is accomplished by extensive perimeter filing.
2. ***Mid root*** level: canal continues ovoid, and requires additional filing to straighten gradual curve. Multiple point filling is necessary.
3. ***Apical third*** level: canal, generally round and ***gradually curved,*** is enlarged by filing to straightened trajectory. Preparation is completed by reaming cavity into ***round, tapered*** preparation which matches ***round, tapered*** primary gutta percha filling point. Preparation terminates at cementodentinal junction, 0.5 mm. from apical foramen.

D. Large, triangular, funnel-shaped coronal preparation is necessary to adequately debride chamber of all pulpal remnants. (Pulp is "ghosted" in background.) Note beveled extension toward incisal, which will carry the preparation labially and thus nearer central axis. Incisal extension allows better access to apical third of canal.

E. ***Lingual*** view of ***adult*** incisor with extensive secondary dentin formation.
Roentgenogram will reveal:
1. full pulp recession
2. severe apical curve to distal
3. 16-degree mesial-axial inclination of tooth.

F. ***Distal*** view of same tooth demonstrating details ***not apparent in roentgenogram:***
1. narrow labiolingual width of pulp
2. reduced size of lingual shoulder
3. apical-***lingual*** curvature (4% of time)
4. 29-degree lingual-axial angulation of tooth.

Operator must recognize that:
a. small canal orifice is difficult to find
b. apical-lingual curvature ***not usually seen roentgenographically*** can be determined by exploration with fine curved file and mesially oriented roentgenograms
c. axial inclination of root calls for careful orientation and alignment of bur to prevent labial "gouging."

"Corkscrew" curve, to distal and lingual, complicates preparation of apical-third of canal.

G. Cross sections at three levels: 1, cervical; 2, mid root; and 3, apical third:
1. ***Cervical*** level: canal is only slightly ovoid and becomes progressively rounder.
2. ***Mid root*** level: canal varies from slightly ovoid to round.
3. ***Apical third*** level: canal is generally round in older patient.

Curved canal is enlarged by alternate reaming and filing. Ovoid preparation will require multiple point filling.

H. Ovoid, funnel-shaped coronal preparation should be ***skewed*** toward mesial to present better access to apical-distal. It is not necessary to extend preparation for coronal debridement, but bevel is necessary toward mesioincisal to carry preparation nearer central axis, allowing better access to apical third.

PLATE V

Length of Tooth[3]		*Canal*	*Curvature of Root*			
Average Length	23.1 mm.	1 canal	Straight	30%	*Labial Curve	4%
Maximum Length	26.0 mm.		Distal Curve	53%	*Lingual Curve	4%
Minimum Length	19.2 mm.	99.9%	Mesial Curve	3%	Bayonet & Gradual Curve	6%
Range	6.8 mm.					

*Not apparent on roentgenogram

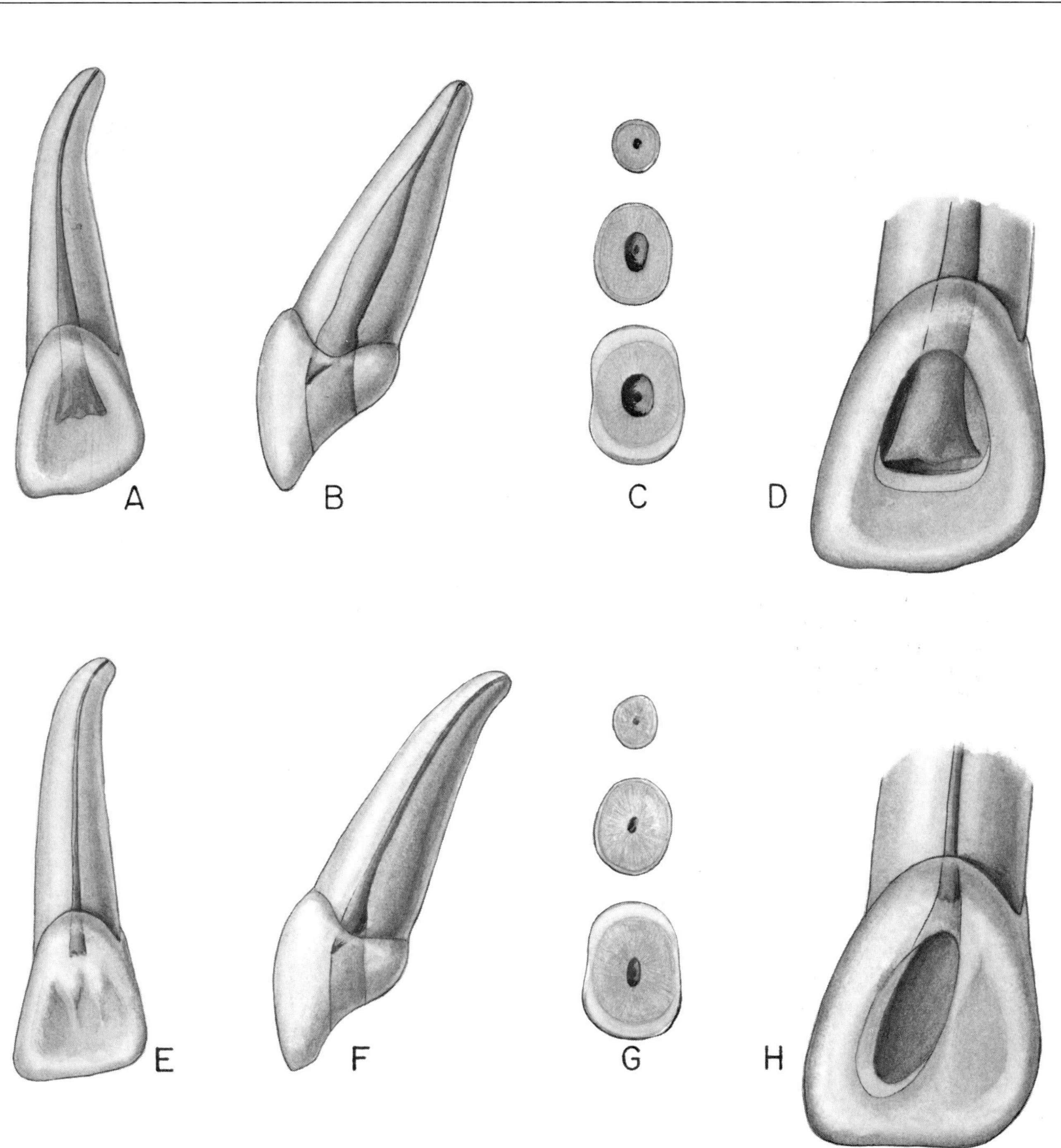

PLATE VI

Maxillary Canine

Pulp Anatomy and Coronal Preparation

A. ***Lingual*** view of recently calcified canine with large pulp. Roentgenogram will reveal:
   1. coronal extent of pulp
   2. ***narrow*** mesiodistal width of pulp
   3. apical-distal curvature (32% of time)
   4. 6-degree distal-axial inclination of tooth.

   These factors ***seen*** in roentgenogram are borne in mind when preparation is begun, particularly severe apical curve.

B. ***Distal*** view of same tooth demonstrating details ***not apparent in roentgenogram:***
   1. huge ovoid pulp, larger labiolingually than roentgenogram would indicate
   2. presence of ***labial*** "shoulder" just below cervical
   3. narrow canal in apical third of root
   4. 21-degree lingual-axial angulation of tooth.

   These "unseen" factors will affect ***size, shape,*** and ***inclination*** of final preparation.

C. Cross sections at three levels: 1, cervical; 2, mid root; and 3, apical third:
   1. ***Cervical*** level: pulp is enormous in young tooth, much wider in ***labiolingual*** direction. Debridement in this area is accomplished with surgical length bur and extensive perimeter filing.
   2. ***Mid root*** level: canal continues ovoid in shape and requires perimeter filing and multiple point filling.
   3. ***Apical third*** level: straight canal (39% of time), generally round in shape, is prepared by reaming cavity into ***round tapered*** preparation which matches round tapered ***primary*** gutta percha filling point. Preparation should terminate at cementodentinal junction, 0.5 mm. from apical foramen. If unusually large or curved, apical canal requires perimeter filing and multiple point filling.

D. Extensive, ***ovoid,*** funnel-shaped ***coronal preparation*** is necessary to adequately debride chamber of all pulpal remnants. (Pulp is "ghosted" in background.) Note long, beveled extension toward incisal which will carry preparation labially and thus nearer central axis. Incisal extension allows better access for large instruments and filling materials used in apical third canal.

E. ***Lingual*** view of ***adult*** canine with extensive secondary dentin formation. Roentgenogram will reveal:
   1. full pulp recession
   2. straight canal (39% of time)
   3. 6-degree distal-axial inclination of tooth.

F. ***Distal*** view of same tooth demonstrating details ***not apparent in roentgenogram:***
   1. narrow labiolingual width of pulp
   2. apical ***labial*** curvature (13% of time)
   3. 21-degree lingual-axial angulation of tooth.

   Operator should recognize that:
   a. small canal orifice is difficult to find
   b. apical ***labial*** curvature not seen roentgenographically can be determined only by exploration with fine curved file and mesially oriented roentgenograms
   c. distal-lingual axial inclination of root calls for careful orientation and alignment of bur to prevent "gouging"
   d. ***apical foramen*** toward labial is problem.

G. Cross sections at three levels: 1, cervical; 2, mid root; and 3, apical third:
   1. ***Cervical*** level: canal is slightly ovoid
   2. ***Mid root*** level: canal is smaller but remains ovoid
   3. ***Apical third*** level: canal becomes progressively rounder.

   Curved canal is enlarged by reaming and filing and filled with multiple points.

H. Extensive, ovoid, funnel-shaped preparation must be ***nearly as large*** as for young tooth. Beveled incisal extension carries preparation nearer central axis, allowing better access to curved apical third. Discovery by exploration of ***apical labial*** curve calls for even greater incisal extension.

PLATE VI

Length of Tooth[3]		*Canal*	*Curvature of Root*			
Average Length	27.3 mm.	1 canal	Straight	39%	*Lingual Curve	7%
Maximum Length	33.3 mm.		Distal Curve	32%	Bayonet & Gradual Curve	7%
Minimum Length	22.3 mm.	100%	Mesial Curve	0%	Dilaceration	2%
Range	11 mm.		*Labial Curve	13%		

*Not apparent on roentgenogram

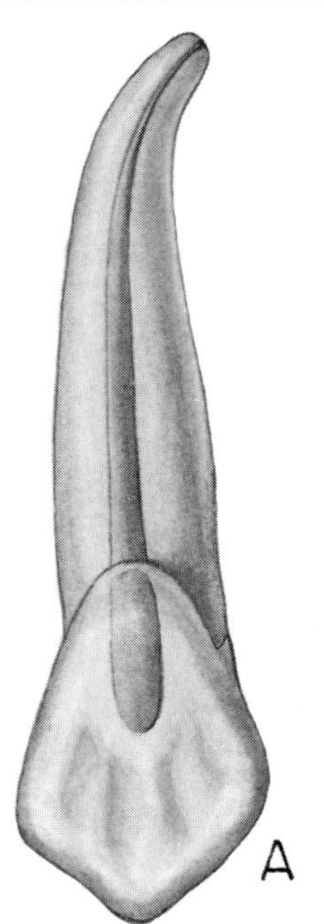

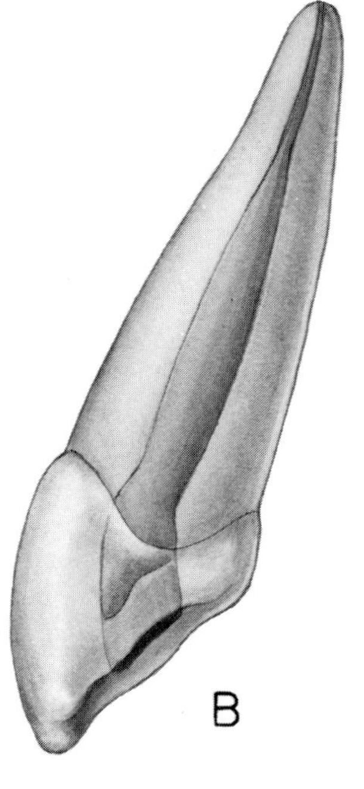

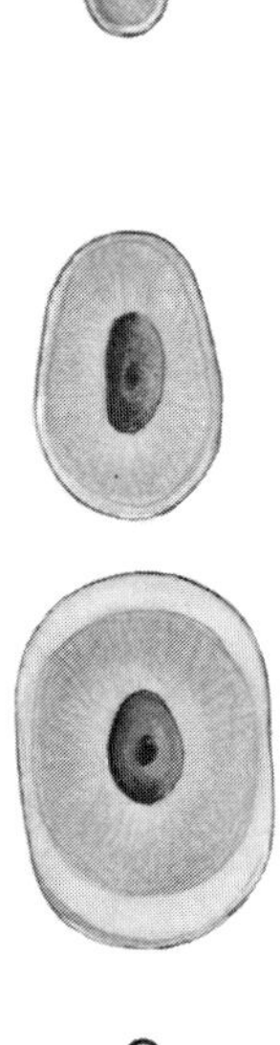

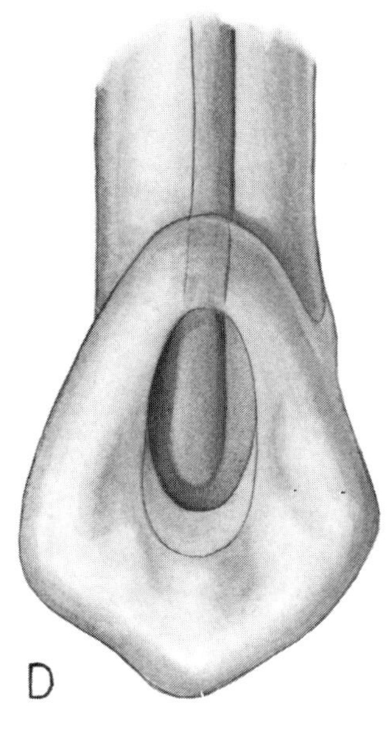

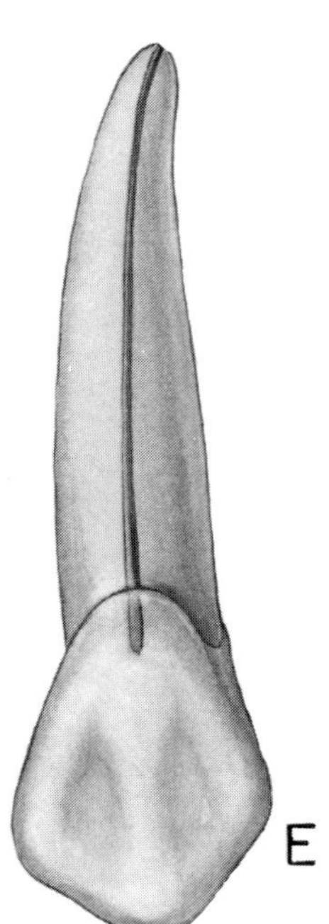

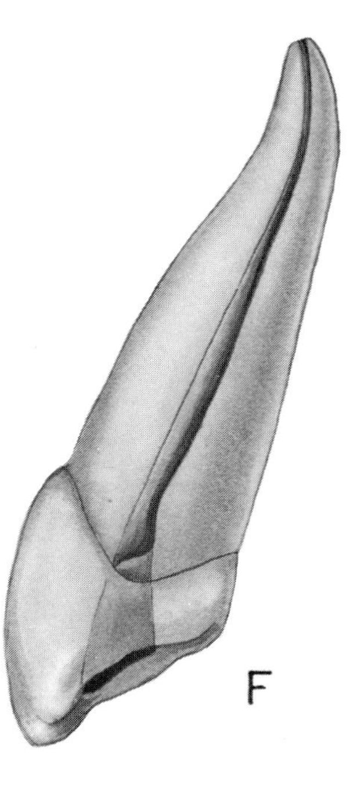

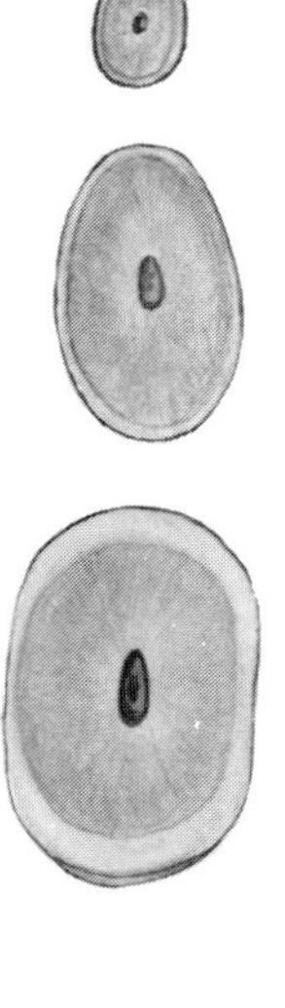

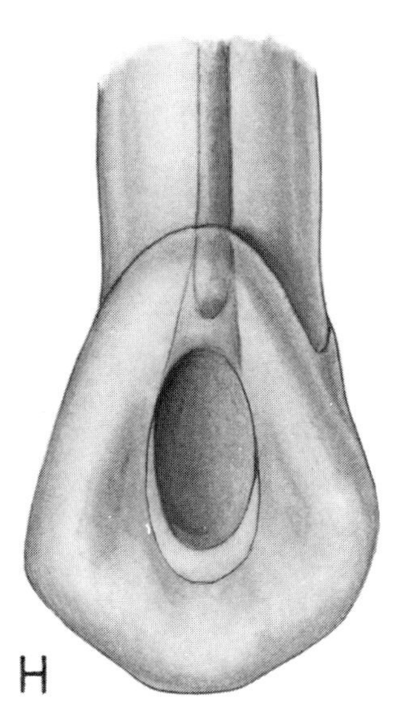

PLATE VII

Maxillary Anterior Teeth

ERRORS in Cavity Preparation

A. PERFORATION at labiocervical caused by ***failure to complete convenience extension*** toward incisal, prior to entrance of shaft of bur.

B. GOUGING of labial wall caused by ***failure to recognize*** 29-degree lingual axial angulation of tooth.

C. GOUGING of distal wall caused by ***failure to recognize*** 16-degree mesial axial inclination of tooth.

D. PEAR-SHAPED PREPARATION of apical canal caused by ***failure to complete convenience extensions.*** Shaft of instrument rides on cavity margin and lingual "shoulder." Inadequate debridement and obturation ensure failure.

E. DISCOLORATION of crown caused by failure to remove pulp debris. Access cavity is too far to gingival with no incisal extension.

F. LEDGE formation at apical-distal curve caused by using uncurved instrument too large for canal. Cavity is adequate.

G. PERFORATION at apical-distal curve caused by using too large an instrument through an ***inadequate*** preparation placed too far gingivally.

H. LEDGE formation at apical-labial curve caused by ***failure to complete convenience extension.*** Shaft of instrument rides on cavity margin and "shoulder."

PLATE VII

ERRORS

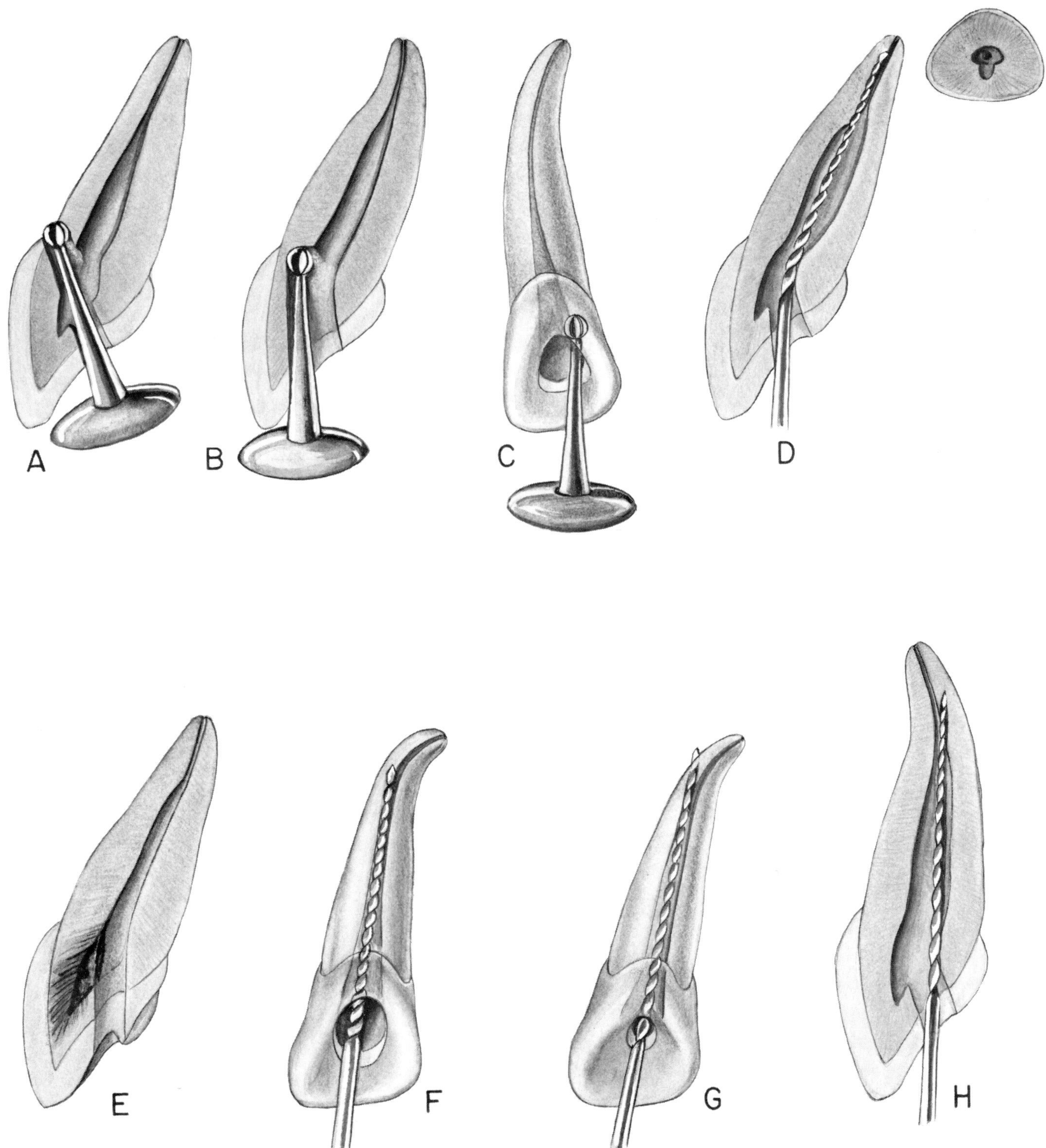

PLATE VII

ERRORS

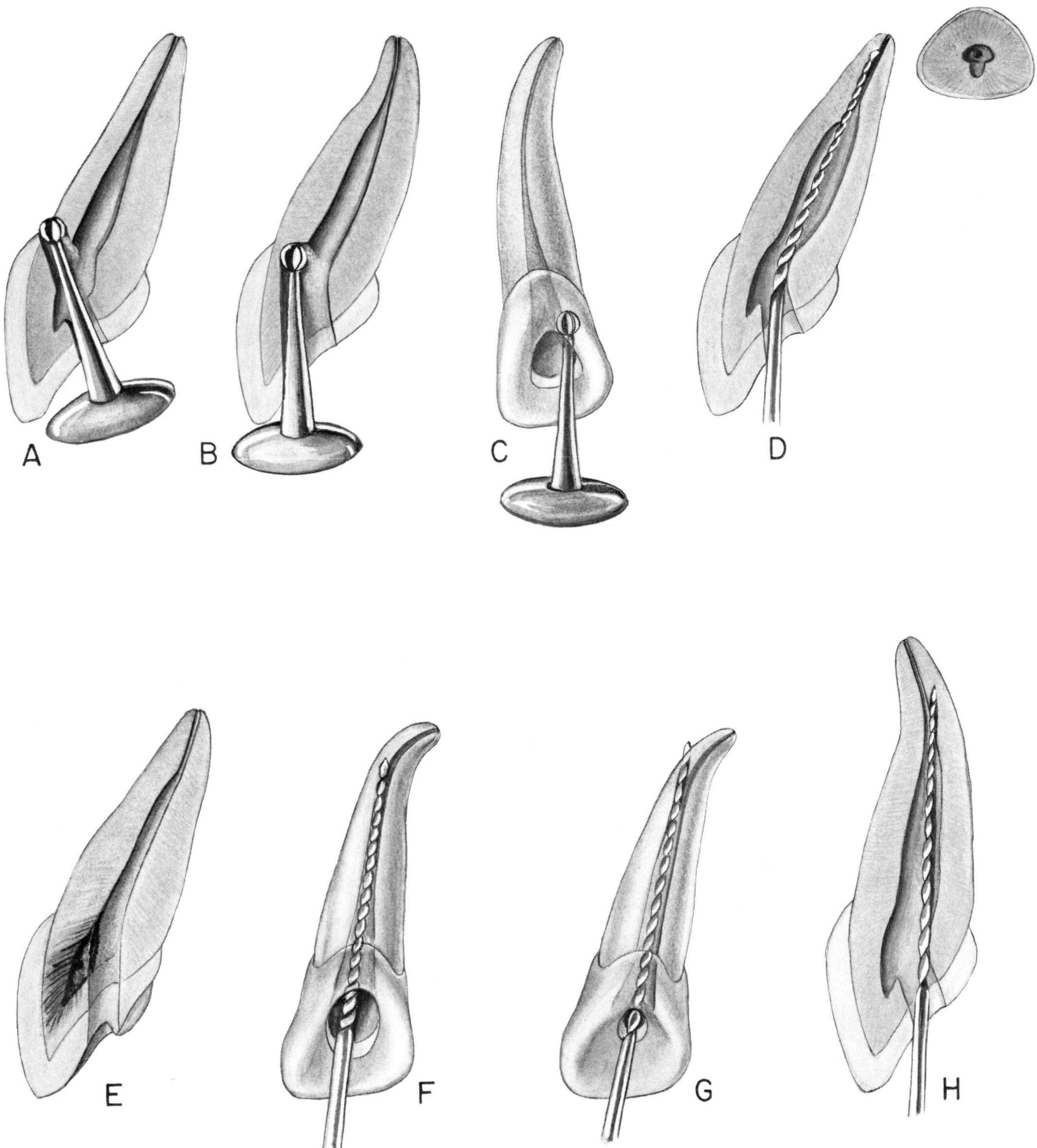

PLATE VIII

Endodontic Preparation of Mandibular Anterior Teeth

A. Entrance is ***always*** gained through lingual surface of all anterior teeth. Initial penetration is made in exact center of lingual surface at position marked "X." Common error is to begin too far gingivally.

B. Initial entrance cavity is prepared with 701U tapering fissure bur in ***accelerated-speed*** contra-angle with air coolant, operated at ***right angle*** to long axis of tooth. ***Only enamel is penetrated at this time.*** Do not force bur; allow it to cut its own way.

C. ***Convenience extension*** toward incisal continues initial penetrating cavity. Maintain point of bur in central cavity and rotate handpiece toward incisal so that bur ***parallels*** long axis of tooth. Enamel and dentin are beveled toward incisal. ***Entrance into pulp chamber should never be made with accelerated-speed instrument.*** Lack of tactile sensation with these instruments ***precludes their use inside*** tooth.

D. Preliminary cavity outline is funneled and fanned incisally with fissure bur. Enamel has short bevel toward incisal, and "nest" is prepared in dentin to receive round bur to be used for penetration.

E. ***Surgical-length*** No. 2 or 4 round bur in ***slow-speed*** contra-angle is used to penetrate into pulp chamber. If pulp has greatly receded, No. 2 round bur is used for initial penetration. Take advantage of ***convenience extension*** toward incisal to allow for shaft of penetrating bur, operated nearly parallel to long axis of tooth.

F. ***Working from inside chamber to outside,*** round bur is used to remove lingual and labial walls of pulp chamber. Resulting cavity is smooth, continuous, and flowing from cavity margin to canal orifice.

G. After outline form is completed surgical-length bur is carefully passed down into canal. ***Working from inside to outside,*** lingual "shoulder" is removed to give continuous, smooth-flowing preparation.

H. Occasionally No. 1 round bur must be used laterally and incisally in cavity to eliminate pulpal horn debris and bacteria. This also prevents future discoloration.

I. Final preparation related to ***internal anatomy*** of chamber and canal. In "young" tooth with large pulp, outline form reflects triangular internal anatomy—extensive cavity which allows thorough cleansing of chamber as well as passage of large instruments and filling materials needed to prepare and fill large canal.

J. Cavity preparations in "adult" tooth with chamber obliterated with secondary dentin are ovoid. Preparation ***funnels*** down to orifice of canal. The further pulp has receded, the more difficult to reach to this depth with round bur. Therefore, when roentgenogram reveals advanced pulpal recession, ***convenience extension*** must be advanced further incisally to allow bur shaft to operate in central axis.

K. Final preparation showing reamer in place. Instrument shaft ***clears*** incisal ***cavity margin*** and reduced lingual shoulder, allowing unstrained approach to apical third of canal. Instruments remain under complete control of clinician. ***Great care must be taken to explore for additional canals.*** Optimal ***round, tapered cavity*** may be prepared in the apical third, tailored to requirements of round, tapered filling materials to follow. Remaining ovoid part of canal is cleaned and shaped by extensive filing. Obturation by multiple points follows.

PLATE VIII

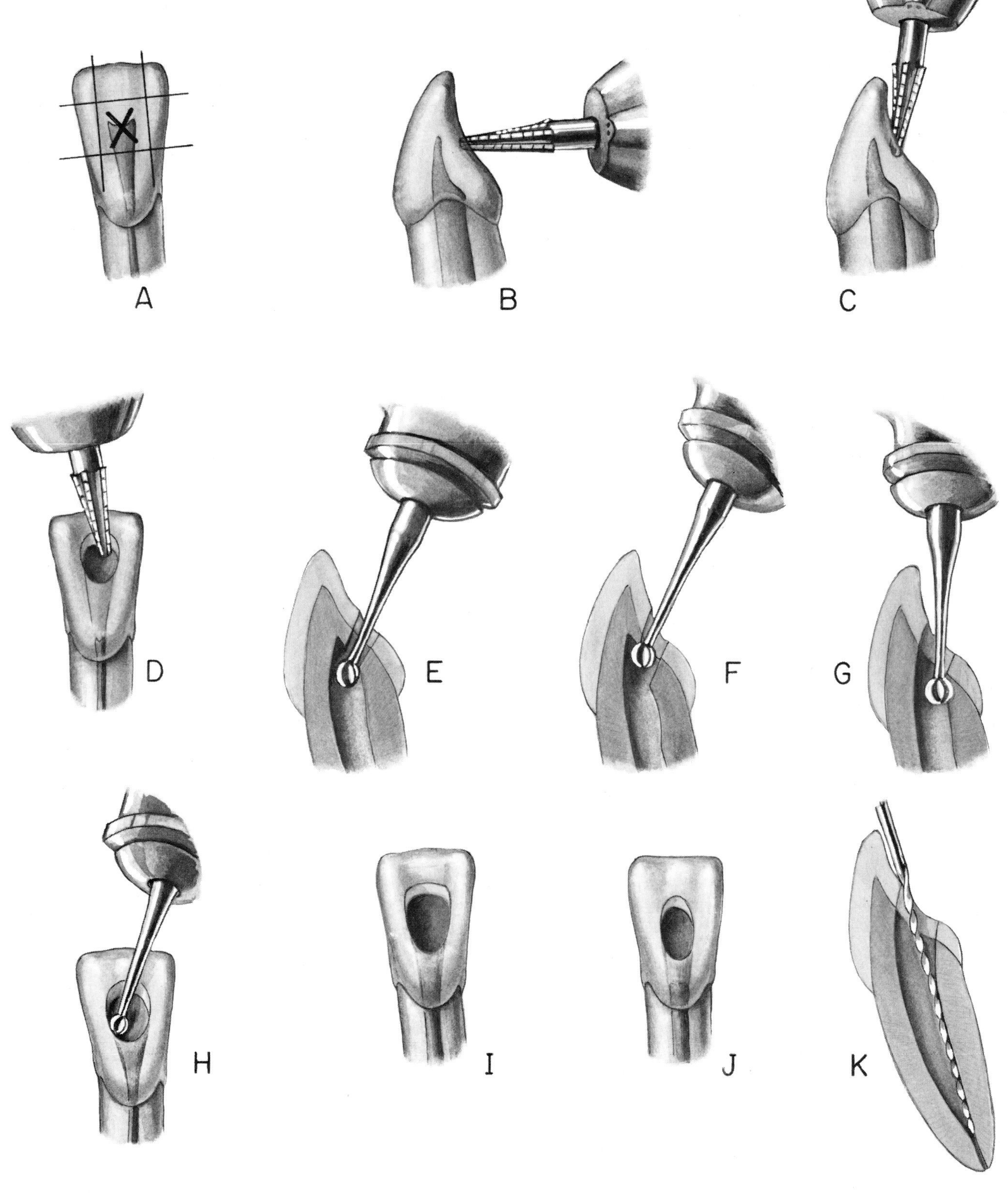

PLATE IX

Mandibular Central and Lateral Incisors

Pulp Anatomy and Coronal Preparation

A. ***Lingual*** view of recently calcified incisor with large pulp. Roentgenogram will reveal:
   1. extent of pulp horns
   2. mesiodistal width of pulp
   3. slight apical-distal curvature of canal (23% of time)
   4. mesial-axial inclination of tooth (central 2 degrees, lateral 17 degrees).

   These factors seen in roentgenogram are borne in mind when preparation is begun.

B. ***Distal*** view of same tooth demonstrating details ***not apparent in roentgenogram:***
   1. presence of lingual "shoulder" at point where chamber and canal join
   2. broad labiolingual extent of pulp
   3. 20-degree lingual-axial angulation of tooth.

   Operator must recognize that:
   a. lingual "shoulder" must be removed with surgical-length bur to allow better access to canal
   b. these "unseen" factors affect ***size, shape,*** and ***inclination*** of final preparation.

C. Cross sections at three levels: 1, cervical; 2, mid root; 3, apical third:
   1. ***Cervical*** level: pulp is enormous in young tooth, wider in labiolingual dimension. Debridement in this area is accomplished by ***extensive perimeter*** filing.
   2. ***Mid root*** level: canal continues ovoid and requires perimeter filing and multiple point filling.
   3. ***Apical third*** level: canal, generally round in shape, is enlarged by reaming cavity into ***round, tapered*** preparation, which matches ***round, tapered*** primary filling point. Preparation terminates at cementodentinal junction 0.5 mm. from apical foramen.

D. Large, triangular, funnel-shaped coronal preparation is necessary to adequately debride chamber of all pulp remnants. (Pulp is "ghosted" in background.) Note beveled extension toward incisal, which will carry preparation labially and thus nearer central axis. Incisal extension allows better access for instruments and filling materials used in apical third canal.

E. ***Lingual*** view of ***adult*** incisor with extensive secondary dentin formation.
   Roentgenogram will reveal:
   1. full pulp recession
   2. apparently straight canal
   3. mesial-axial inclination of tooth (central 2 degrees, lateral 17 degrees).

F. ***Distal*** view of same tooth demonstrating details ***not apparent in roentgenogram:***
   1. labiolingual width of pulp
   2. reduced size of lingual shoulder
   3. ***unsuspected presence of bifurcation of pulp into labial and lingual canal***
   4. 20-degree lingual-axial angulation of tooth.

   Operator must recognize that:
   a. smaller canal orifices are more difficult to find
   b. ***labial and lingual*** canals (4%) are discovered by exploration with fine curved file to ***both labial*** and ***lingual***
   c. axial inclination of root calls for careful orientation and alignment of bur to prevent "gouging."

G. Cross sections at three levels: 1, cervical; 2, mid root; and 3, apical third:
   1. ***Cervical*** level: canal is only slightly ovoid
   2. ***Mid root*** level: two canals are essentially round
   3. ***Apical third*** level: canals are round and curve toward labial.

   Both canals may be enlarged by reaming action and filled with single points. It is important that all mandibular anterior teeth be explored to both labial and lingual for possibility of two canals.

H. Ovoid, funnel-shaped coronal preparation provides adequate access to root canal. "Adult" cavity is narrow in mesiodistal width, but is as extensive in inciso-gingival direction as preparation in young tooth. This beveled incisal extension carries preparation nearer central axis allowing better access to ***both canals*** and ***curved apical third.*** Discovery of two canals calls for ***increased*** extension and better access.

PLATE IX

Central Incisor		Lateral Incisor					
Length of Tooth[3]				*Canals*[5,6]	*Curvature of Root*		
Average Length	21.8 mm.	***Average*** Length	23.3 mm.	1 canal	Straight 60%	*Labial Curve	13%
Maximum Length	25.1 mm.	Maximum Length	25.0 mm.	1 foramen 58%	Distal Curve 23%	*Lingual Curve	0%
Minimum Length	19.4 mm.	Minimum Length	21.0 mm.	2 canals	Mesial Curve 0%	Two Canals	4%
Range	5.7 mm.	Range	4.0 mm.	1 foramen 40%			
				2 canals			
				2 foramens 2–3%			

*Not apparent on roentgenogram

A B C D

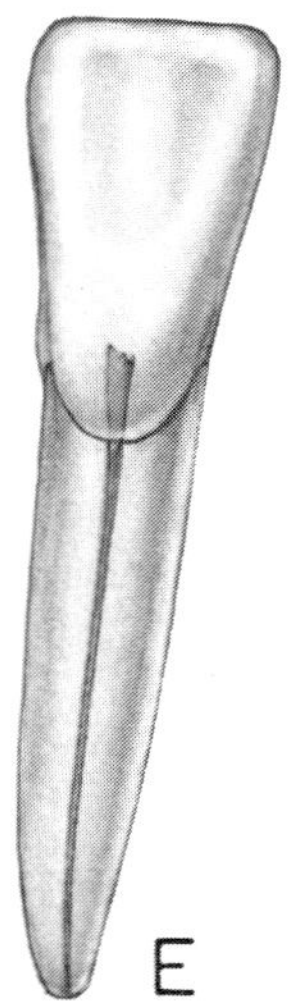

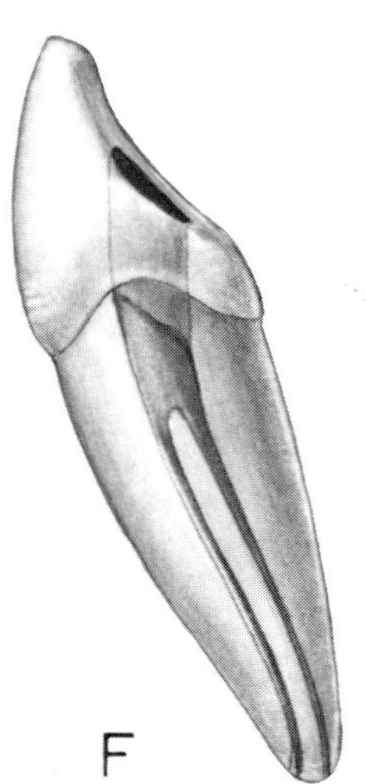

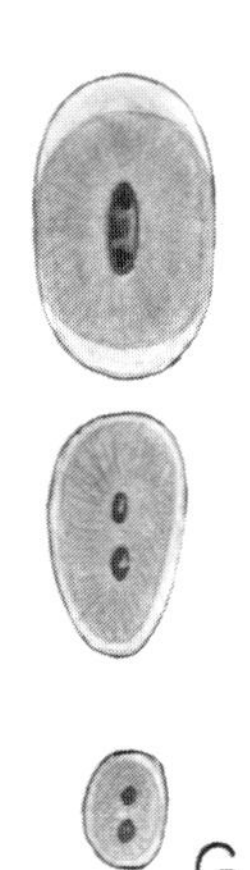

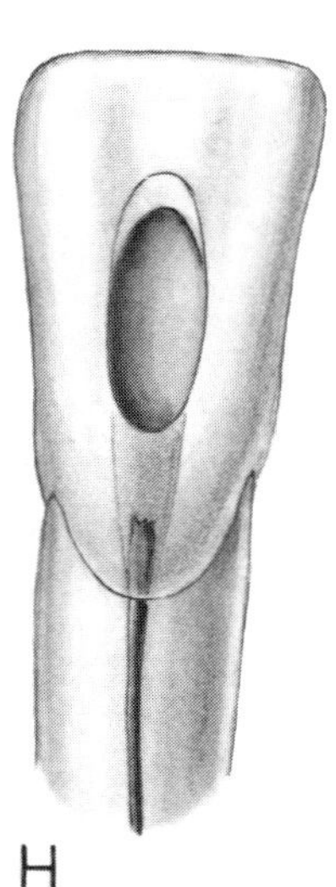

PLATE X

Mandibular Canine

Pulp Anatomy and Coronal Preparation

A. ***Lingual*** view of recently calcified canine with large pulp. Roentgenogram will reveal:
   1. coronal extent of pulp
   2. narrow mesiodistal width of pulp
   3. apical-distal curvature (20% of time)
   4. 13-degree mesial-axial inclination of tooth.

   These factors ***seen*** in roentgenogram are borne in mind when preparation is begun.

B. ***Distal*** view of same tooth demonstrating details ***not apparent in roentgenogram:***
   1. broad labiolingual extent of pulp
   2. narrow canal in apical third of root
   3. apical-labial curvature (7% of time)
   4. 15-degree lingual-axial angulation of tooth.

   These "unseen factors" affect ***size, shape,*** and ***inclination*** of final preparation.

C. Cross sections at three levels: 1, cervical; 2, mid root; and 3, apical third:
   1. ***Cervical*** level: pulp is enormous in young tooth, wider in labiolingual direction. Debridement in this area is accomplished with ***extensive perimeter filing.***
   2. ***Mid root*** level: canal continues ovoid and requires perimeter filing and multiple gutta percha point filling.
   3. ***Apical third*** level: canal, generally round, is enlarged by filing to reduce curve to relatively straight canal. This canal is then completed by reaming action into ***round, tapered*** preparation, which matches ***round, tapered*** primary gutta percha filling point. Total obturation is by multiple points. Preparation terminates at cementodentinal junction, 0.5 mm. from apical foramen. If unusually large or ovoid, apical canal requires perimeter filing and multiple point filling.

D. Extensive ovoid, funnel-shaped ***coronal preparation*** is necessary to adequately debride chamber of all pulp remnants. (Pulp is "ghosted" in background.) Note beveled extension toward incisal, which will carry preparation labially and thus nearer central axis. Incisal extension allows better access for large instruments and filling materials used in apical third canal.

E. ***Lingual*** view of ***adult*** canine with extensive secondary dentin formation. Roentgenogram will reveal:
   1. full pulp recession
   2. slight distal curve of canal (20% of time)
   3. 13-degree mesial-axial inclination of tooth.

F. Distal view of same tooth demonstrating details ***not apparent in roentgenogram:***
   1. narrow labiolingual width of pulp
   2. 15-degree lingual-axial angulation of tooth.

   Operator must recognize that:
   a. small canal orifice, positioned well to ***labial,*** is difficult to find
   b. lingual-axial angulation calls for careful orientation of bur to prevent "gouging"
   c. apical-labial curvature (7% of time).

G. Cross sections at three levels: 1, cervical; 2, mid root; and 3, apical third:
   1. ***Cervical*** level: canal is slightly ovoid
   2. ***Mid root*** level: canal is smaller but remains ovoid
   3. ***Apical third*** level: canal becomes progressively rounder.

   Canal is enlarged by filing, and is filled with multiple gutta percha points.

H. Extensive ovoid, funnel-shaped preparation must be as large as preparation for young tooth. Cavity should be extended inciso-gingivally for room to find orifice and enlarge apical third without interference. Apical-labial curve would call for increased extension incisally.

PLATE X

Length of Tooth[3]		*Canals*[6]		*Curvature of Root*			
Average Length	26.0 mm.	1 canal	94%	Straight	68%	*Lingual Curve	0%
Maximum Length	27.4 mm.	2 canals		Distal Curve	20%	Bayonet Curve	2%
Minimum Length	24.6 mm.	2 foramens	6%	Mesial Curve	1%	Two Canals	2%
Range	2.8 mm.			*Labial Curve	7%		

*Not apparent on roentgenogram

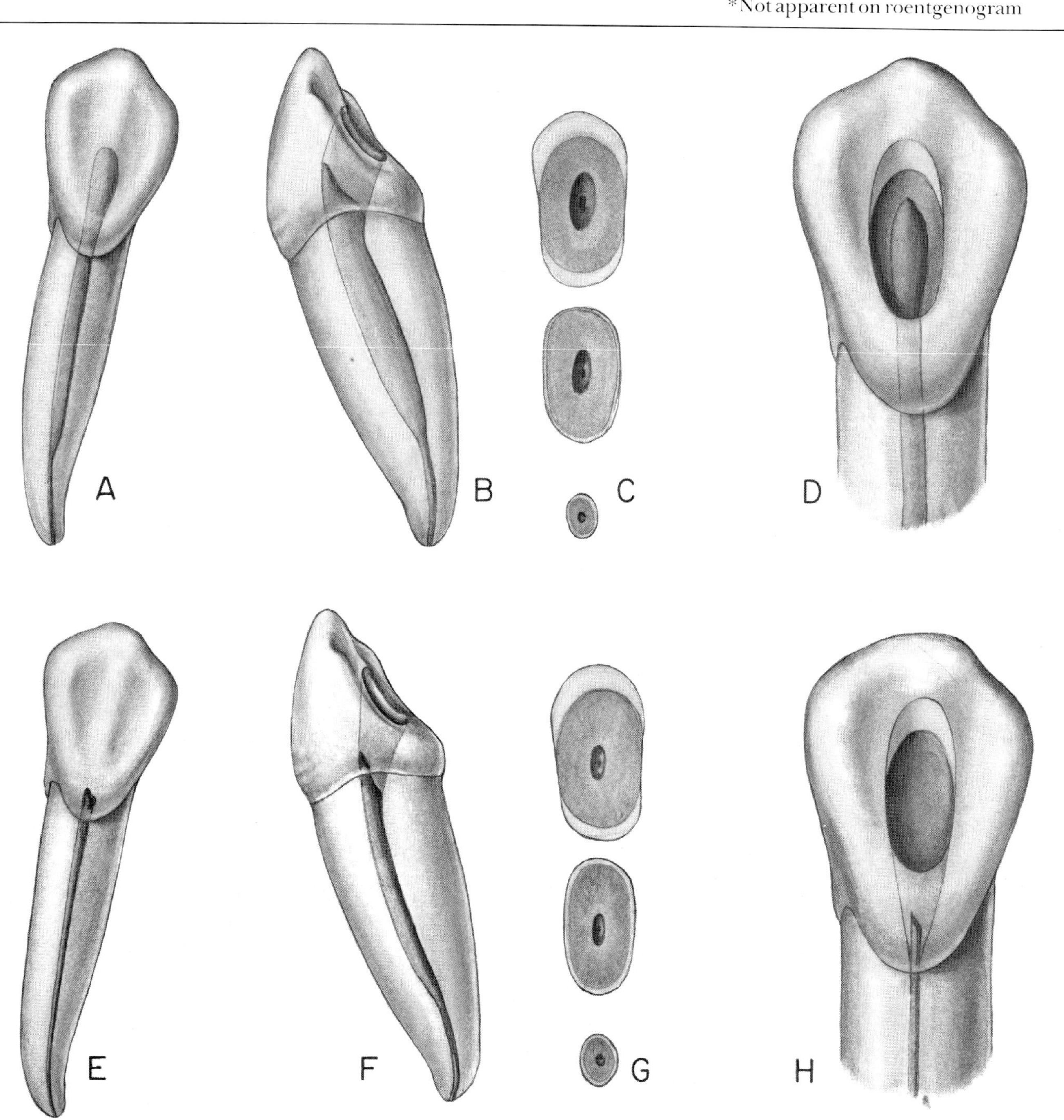

PLATE XI

Mandibular Anterior Teeth

ERRORS in Cavity Preparation

A. GOUGING at labiocervical caused by ***failure to complete convenience extension*** toward incisal prior to entrance of shaft of bur.

B. GOUGING of labial wall caused by failure to recognize 20-degree lingual-axial angulation of tooth.

C. GOUGING of distal wall caused by ***failure*** to ***recognize*** 17-degree mesial-axial angulation of tooth.

D. FAILURE to explore, debride, or fill second canal caused by ***inadequate access cavity.***

E. DISCOLORATION of crown caused by failure to remove pulp debris. Access cavity is too far to gingival with no incisal extension.

F. LEDGE formation caused by complete loss of control of instrument passing through access cavity prepared in proximal restoration.

PLATE XI

ERRORS

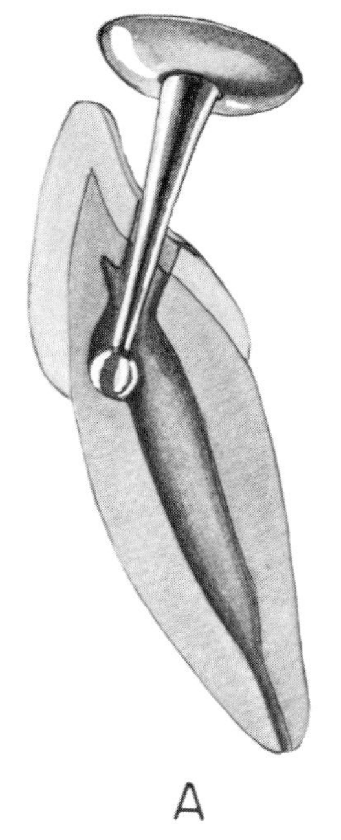
A

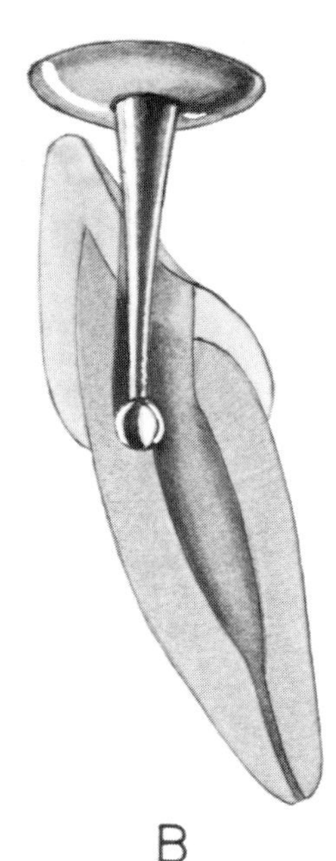
B

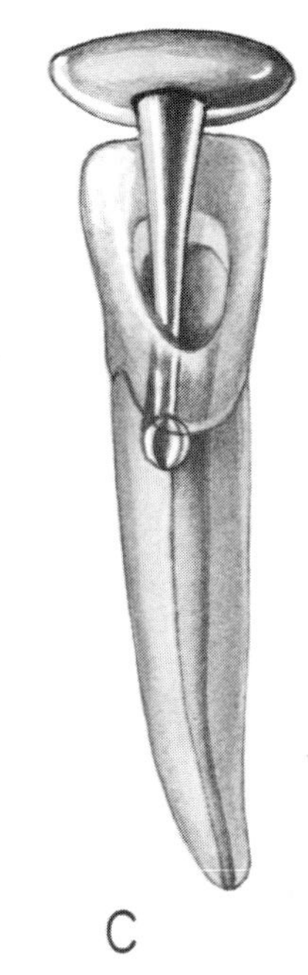
C

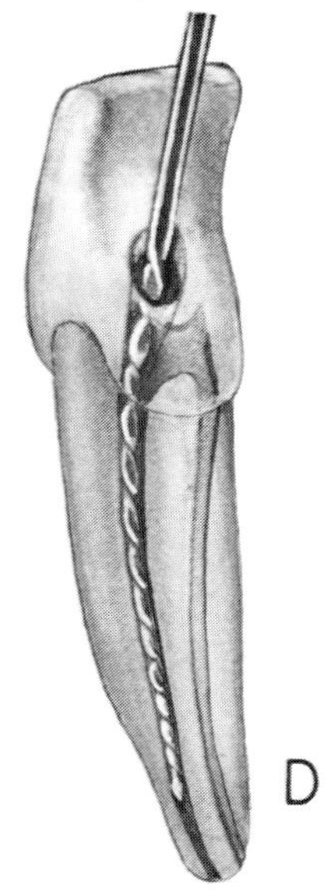
D

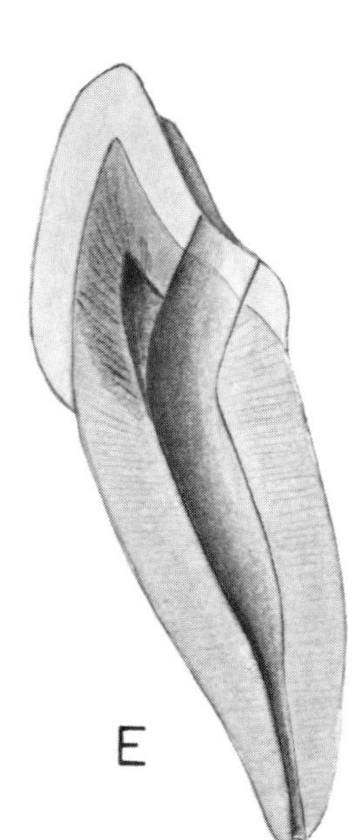
E

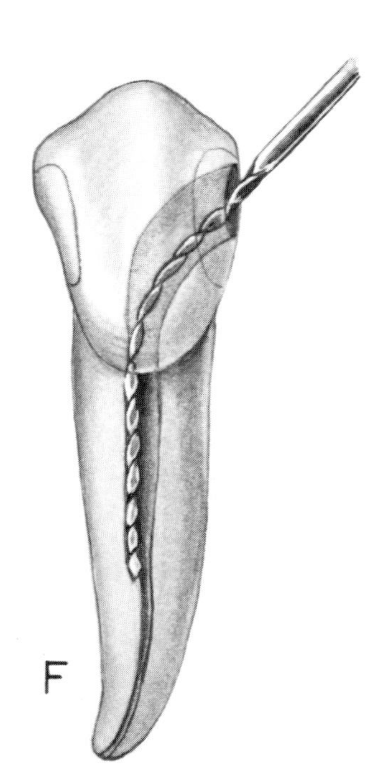
F

PLATE XII

Endodontic Preparation of Maxillary Premolar Teeth

A. Entrance is ***always*** gained through ***occlusal*** surface of all posterior teeth. Initial penetration is made parallel to long axis of tooth in exact center of central groove of maxillary premolars. The 701U tapering fissure bur in accelerated-speed contra-angle is ideal for penetrating gold casting or virgin enamel surface to depth of dentin. Amalgam fillings are opened with No. 4 round bur in slow-speed contra-angle.

B. ***Regular length,*** No. 2 or 4 round bur is used to open into pulp chamber. Bur will be felt to "drop" when pulp chamber is reached. If chamber is well calcified and "drop" is not felt, vertical penetration is made until contra-angle rests against occlusal surface. This depth is approximately 9 mm., the position of floor of pulp chamber which lies at cervical level. In removing bur, ***orifice is widened buccolingually*** to twice width of bur to allow room for exploration for canal orifices.

C. Endodontic explorer is used to locate orifices to ***buccal*** and ***lingual*** canals in ***first premolar*** or ***central canal*** in ***second premolar.*** Tension of explorer shaft against walls of preparation will indicate amount and direction of extension necessary.

D. Working from inside pulp chamber to outside, round bur is used at low speed to extend cavity buccolingually by removing roof of pulp chamber.

E. Buccolingual extension and finish of cavity walls is completed with 701U fissure bur at accelerated speed.

F. Final preparation should provide unobstructed access to canal orifices. Cavity walls should not impede complete authority over enlarging instruments.

G. ***Outline form*** of final preparation will be ***identical for*** both ***newly erupted*** and ***"adult" teeth.*** Buccolingual ovoid preparation reflects anatomy of pulp chamber and position of buccal and lingual canal orifices. Cavity must be extensive enough to allow for instruments and filling materials needed to enlarge and fill canals. ***Further exploration*** at this time is imperative. It may reveal orifice to additional canal; ***second canal*** in second premolar, or ***third canal*** in first premolar.

PLATE XII

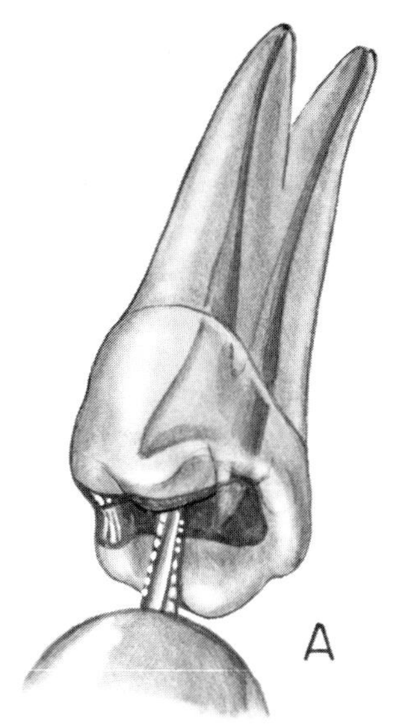
A

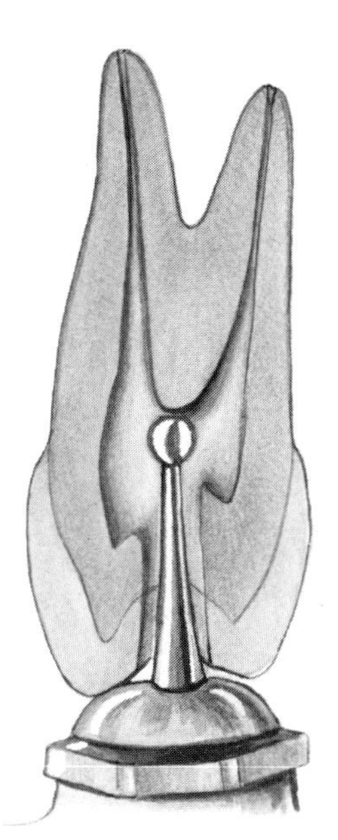
B

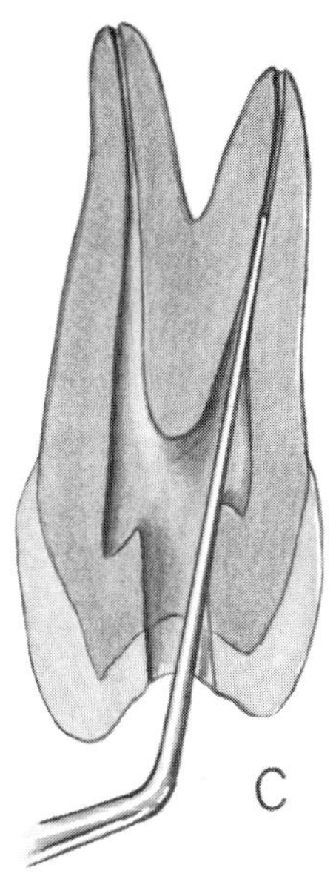
C

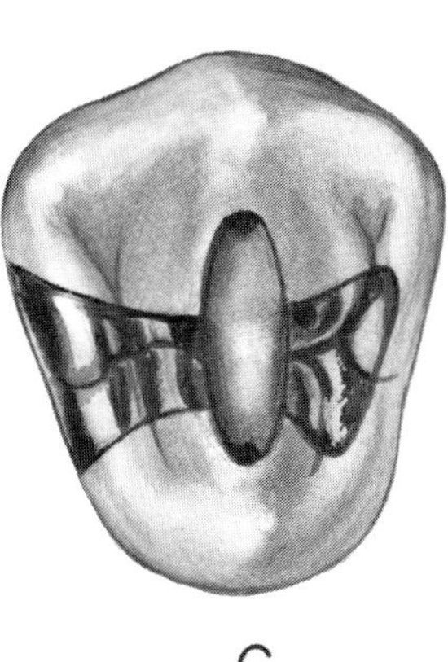
G

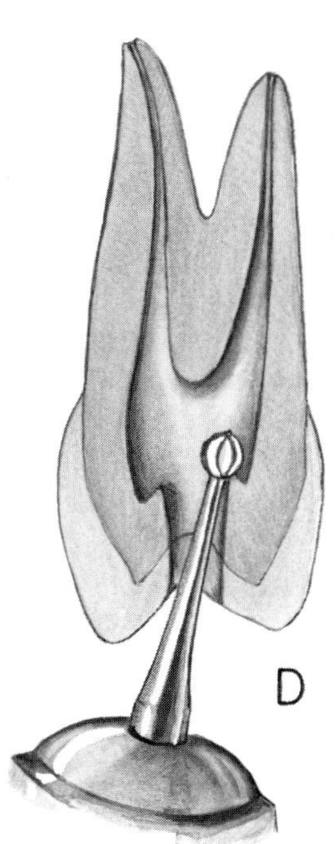
D

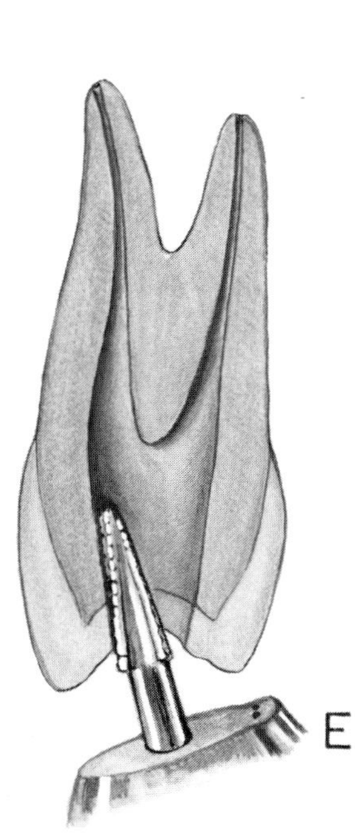
E

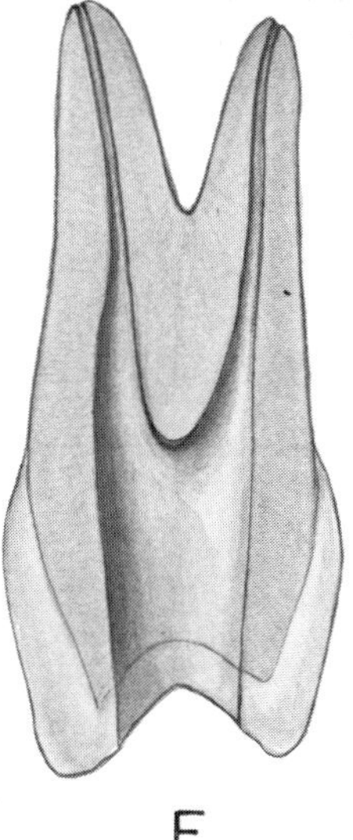
F

PLATE XIII

Maxillary First Premolar

Pulp Anatomy and Coronal Preparation

A. ***Buccal*** view of recently calcified first premolar with large pulp.
Roentgenogram, if exposed slightly from mesial, will reveal:
1. mesiodistal width of pulp
2. presence of two pulp canals
3. apparently straight canals
4. 10-degree distal-axial inclination of tooth.

These factors ***seen*** in roentgenogram are borne in mind when preparation is begun. One should always expect two canals and occasionally three canals.

B. ***Mesial*** view of same tooth demonstrating details ***not apparent in roentgenogram:***
1. height of pulp horns
2. broad buccolingual dimension of pulp
3. two widespread and separate roots, each with single straight canal
4. 6-degree buccal-axial angulation of tooth.

These "unseen" factors will affect size and shape of final preparation. Pulp horns in roof of pulp ***chamber*** are not to be confused with true canal orifices in cavity floor. Verticality of tooth simplifies orientation and bur alignment.

C. Cross sections at three levels: 1, cervical; 2, mid root; and 3, apical third:
1. ***Cervical*** level: pulp is enormous in young tooth, very wide in buccolingual direction. Debridement of chamber is completed in coronal cavity preparation with round bur. Canal orifices are found well to the buccal and lingual.
2. ***Mid root*** level: canals are only lightly ovoid and may be enlarged to round, tapered cavity.
3. ***Apical third*** level: canals are round and are reamed into ***round, tapered*** preparations which match ***round, tapered*** filling points. Preparations terminate at cementodentinal junction 0.5 mm. from apical foramen.

D. ***Ovoid*** coronal preparation need not be as long buccolingually as pulp chamber. However, ***outline form*** must be large enough to provide for two filling points at same time. Buccal and lingual walls smoothly flow to orifices.

E. ***Buccal*** view of ***adult*** first premolar with extensive secondary dentin formation. Roentgenogram will reveal:
1. full pulp recession and thread-like appearance of pulp
2. ***roentgen appearance*** of only one canal
3. 10-degree distal-axial inclination of tooth.

Due to misalignment of bur, ***perforation of mesiocervical, at point of mesial indentation, may occur.***

F. ***Mesial*** view of same tooth demonstrating details ***not apparent in roentgenogram:***
1. pulp recession and greatly flattened pulp chamber
2. buccolingual width revealing pulp to be "ribbon-shaped" rather than "thread-like"
3. single root with ***two parallel canals and single apical foramen***
4. 6-degree buccal-axial angulation of tooth.

Operator must recognize that:
a. small canal orifices are found well to the buccal and lingual and are difficult to locate
b. direction of each canal is determined only by exploration with fine curved instrument
c. single apical foramen cannot be determined, therefore two canals must be managed as two separate canals.
d. there will ***always*** be two canals, occasionally three, but never one canal.

G. Cross section at three levels: 1, cervical; 2, mid root; and 3, apical third:
1. ***Cervical*** level: chamber is very narrow ovoid and canal orifices are at buccal and lingual termination of floor
2. ***Mid root*** level: canals are round
3. ***Apical third*** level: canals are round.

Canals are enlarged by reaming and may sometimes be filled with silver points.

H. Ovoid coronal preparation must be more extensive in buccolingual direction because of parallel canals. More extensive preparation allows instrumentation without interference.

PLATE XIII

Length of Tooth[3]		*Canals*[7]		*Curvature of Roots*			
					Single	*Double Roots*	
				Direction	*Root*	*Buccal*	*Palatal*
Average Length	22.3 mm.	1 canal		Straight	38%	28%	45%
Maximum Length	25.8 mm.	1 foramen	9%	Distal	37%	14%	14%
Minimum Length	18.8 mm.	2 canals		Mesial	0	0	0
Range	7.0 mm.	1 foramen	13%	Buccal	15%	14%	28%
		2 canals		Lingual	3%	36%	9%
		2 foramens	72%	Bayonet	0	8%	0
		3 canals					
		3 foramens	6%				

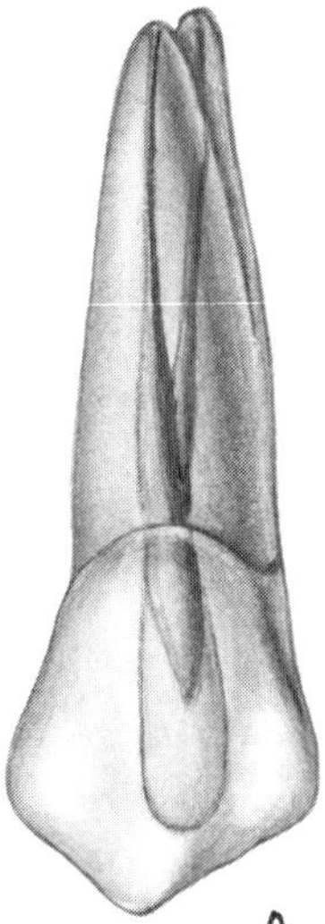

A 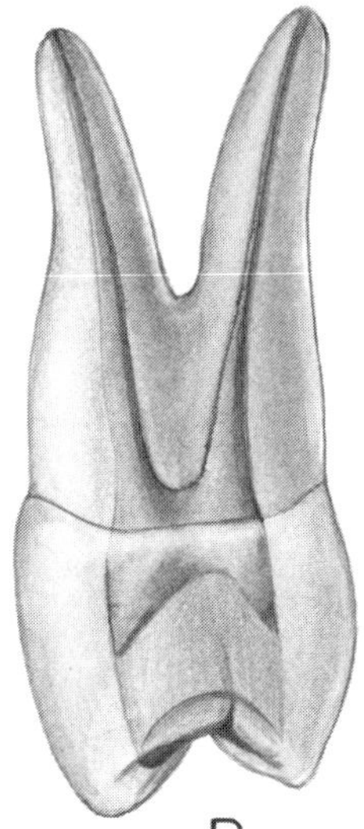 B 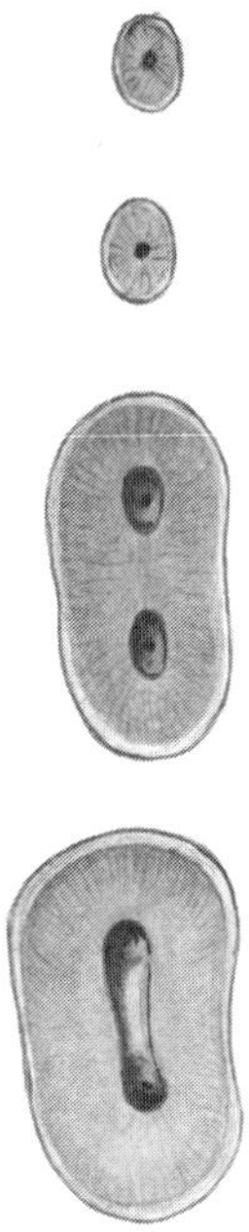 C 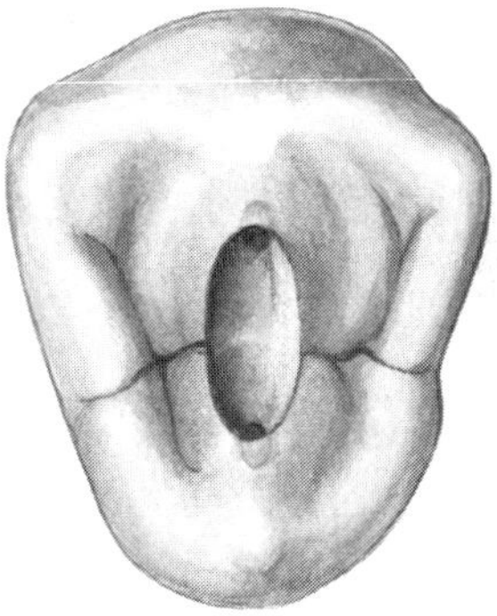 D

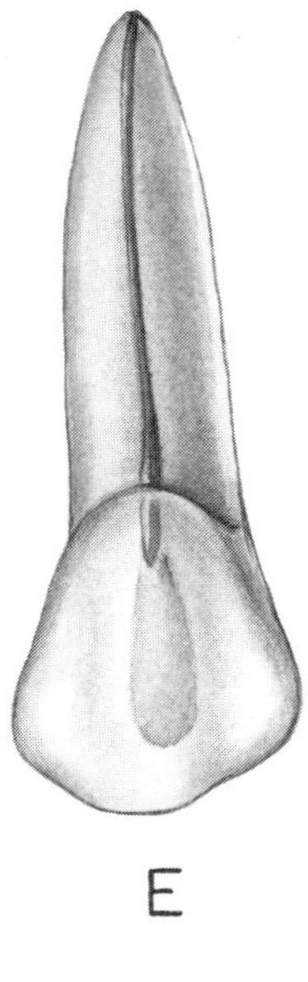

E 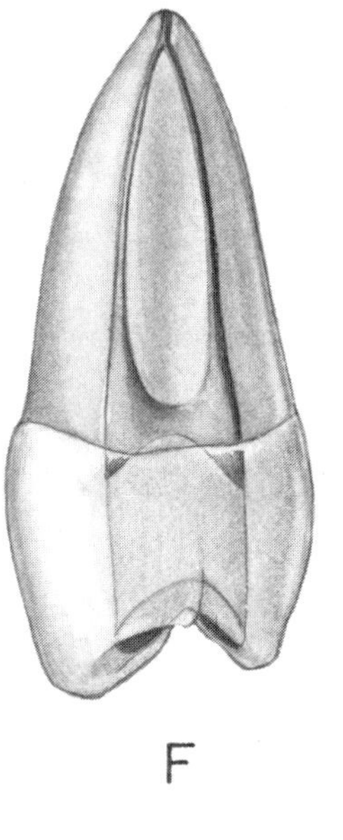 F 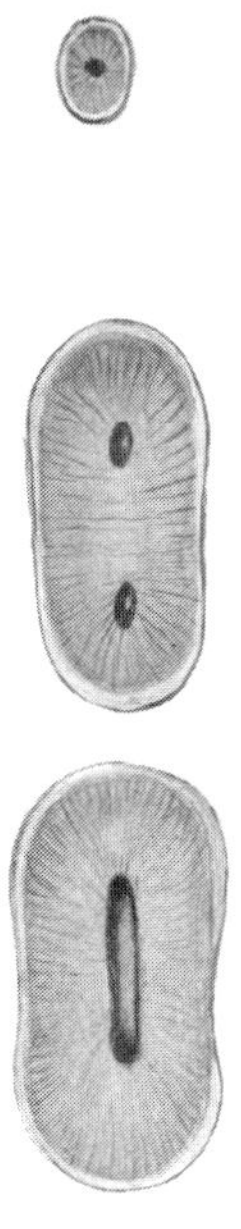 G 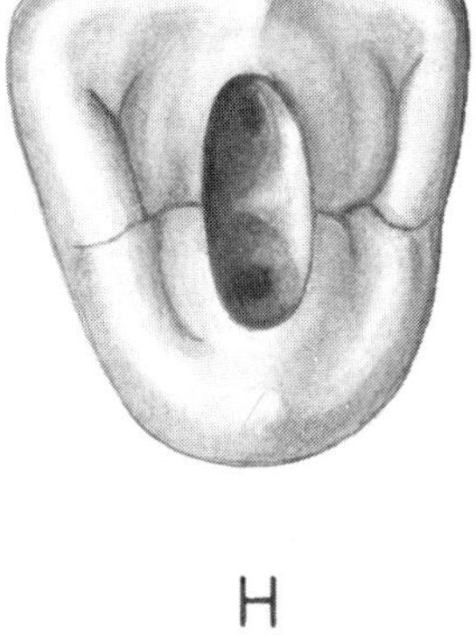 H

PLATE XIV

Maxillary Second Premolar

Pulp Anatomy and Coronal Preparation

A. ***Buccal*** view of recently calcified second premolar with large pulp. Roentgenogram will reveal:
   1. narrow mesiodistal width of pulp
   2. apical-distal curvature (34% of time)
   3. 19-degree distal-axial inclination of tooth

   These factors ***seen*** in roentgenogram are borne in mind when preparation is begun.

B. ***Mesial*** view of same tooth demonstrating details ***not apparent*** in ***roentgenogram:***
   1. broad buccolingual width revealing pulp to be "ribbon-shaped"
   2. single root with large single canal
   3. 9-degree lingual-axial angulation of tooth.

   Pulp is shown to be broad "ribbon" rather than "thread" it appears from roentgenogram. These "unseen" factors affect ***size, shape,*** and ***inclination*** of final preparation.

C. Cross sections at three levels: 1, cervical; 2, mid root; and 3, apical third:
   1. ***Cervical*** level: pulp is enormous in young tooth, very wide in buccolingual direction. Debridement of chamber is completed during coronal cavity preparation with round bur. Canal orifice is directly in center of tooth.
   2. ***Mid root*** level: canal remains ovoid in shape and requires perimeter filing and multiple point filling.
   3. ***Apical third*** level: canal, round in shape, is filed and then reamed into ***round, tapered*** preparation, which matches ***round, tapered*** primary filling point. Preparation terminates at cementodentinal junction, 0.5 mm. from apical foramen.

D. Ovoid preparation allows debridement of entire pulp chamber and funnels down to ovoid mid-canal.

E. ***Buccal*** view of ***adult*** second premolar with extensive secondary dentin formation. Roentgenogram, if exposed slightly from mesial, will reveal:
   1. pulp recession and "thread-like" appearance of pulp
   2. roentgen appearance of two roots (2% of time)
   3. bayonet curve of roots (20% of time)
   4. 19-degree distal-axial inclination of tooth.

F. ***Mesial*** view of same tooth demonstrating details ***not apparent in roentgenogram:***
   1. buccolingual width revealing coronal pulp to be "ribbon-shaped" rather than "thread-like"
   2. high bifurcation and two separate apical third roots
   3. 9-degree lingual-axial angulation of tooth.

   Operator must recognize that:

   a. small canal orifices are deeply placed in root and will be difficult to locate
   b. direction of each canal is determined by exploration with ***fine curved*** file carried down wall until orifice is engaged. Then, by half rotation, file is turned to match first curve of canal, followed by penetration until tip again catches on curved wall. Second half-turn and further penetration will carry tip of instrument to within 0.5 mm. of apical foramen. Retraction will remove dentin at both curves.

G. Cross sections at three levels: 1, cervical; 2, mid root; and 3, apical third:
   1. ***Cervical*** level: chamber, very narrow ovoid, extends deeply into root. This space will be finally filled with cement.
   2. ***Mid root*** level: bayonet curve and round canal orifices are apparent.
   3. ***Apical third*** level: canals are round. Severe curve at "bayonet" is reduced by filing action into gradual curve. Canals may then be completed by reaming action and filled with multiple points.

H. Ovoid coronal cavity is prepared ***well to mesial*** of occlusal surface, with depth of penetration ***skewed toward bayonet curvature. Skewing cavity*** allows unrestrained approach to first curve.

PLATE XIV

Length of Tooth[3]		*Canals*[8]		*Curvature of Roots*[8]			
Average Length	22.3 mm.	1 canal		Straight	9.5%	Buccal	12.7%
Maximum Length	26.4 mm.	1 foramen	75%	Distal	27.0%	Lingual	4.0%
Minimum Length	16.7 mm.	2 canals		Mesial	1.6%	Bayonet	20.6%
Range	9.7 mm.	2 foramens	24%				
		3 canals	1%				

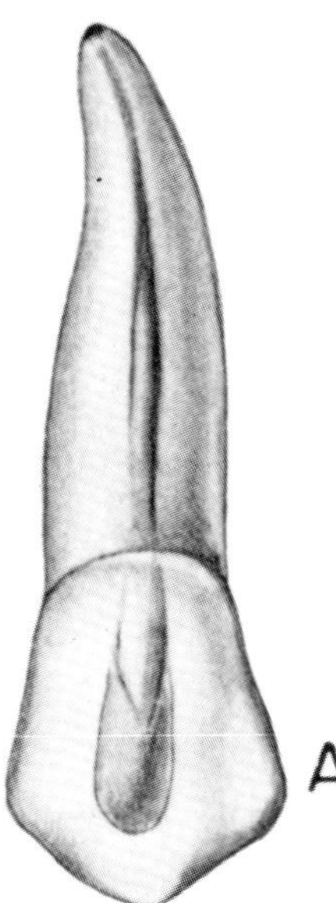

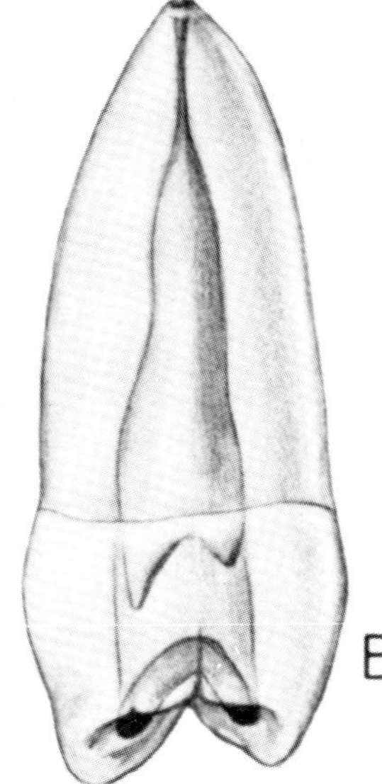

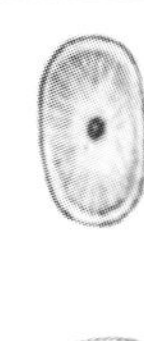

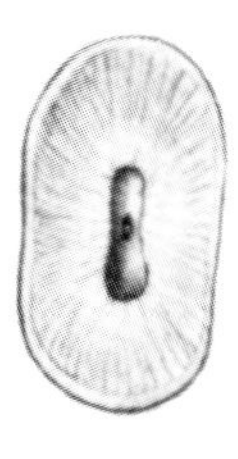

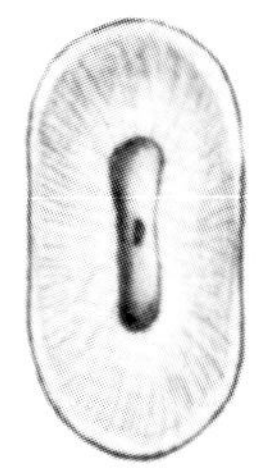

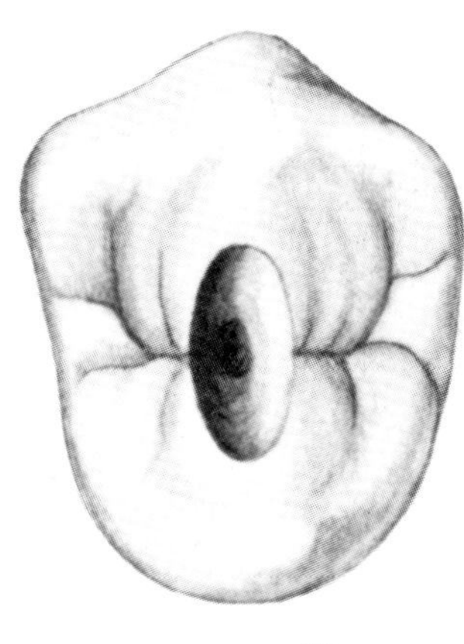

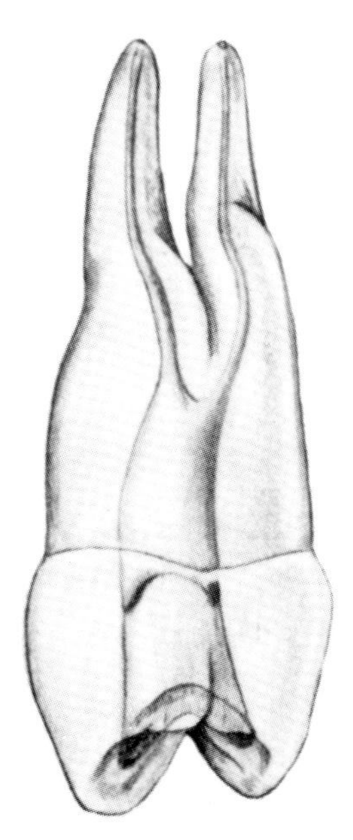

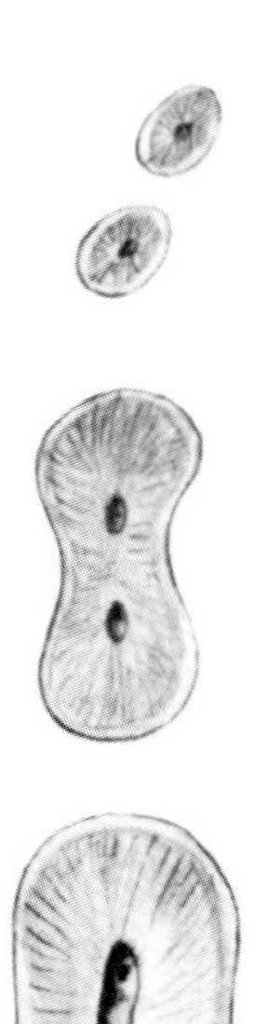

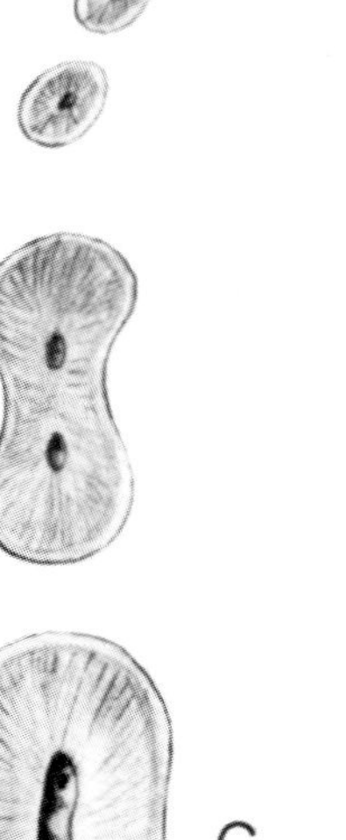

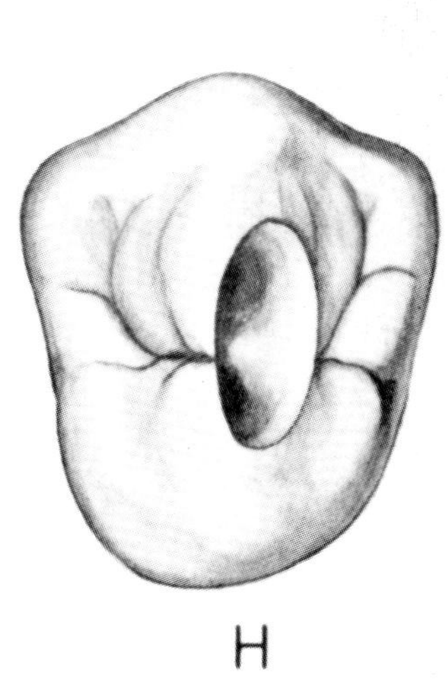

PLATE XV

Maxillary Premolar Teeth

ERRORS in Cavity Preparation

A. UNDEREXTENDED preparation exposing only pulp horns. Control of enlarging instruments is abdicated to cavity walls. ***White color*** of ***roof*** of ***chamber*** is clue to shallow cavity.

B. OVEREXTENDED preparation from fruitless search for receded pulp. Enamel walls have been completely undermined. Gouging relates to failure to refer to roentgenogram, which clearly indicates pulp recession.

C. PERFORATION at mesiocervical indentation. Failure to observe distal-axial inclination of tooth led to ***bypassing*** receded pulp and perforation.

D. FAULTY ALIGNMENT of access cavity through ***full veneer restoration*** placed to "straighten" crown of rotated tooth. Careful examination of roentgenogram would reveal rotated body of tooth.

E. BROKEN INSTRUMENT twisted-off in "cross-over" canal. This frequent occurrence may be obviated by filing internal preparation to straighten canals (dotted line).

F. FAILURE to explore, debride, and obturate third canal of maxillary ***first*** premolar (6% of time).

G. FAILURE to explore, debride, and obturate second canal of maxillary ***second*** premolar (24% of time).

PLATE XV

ERRORS

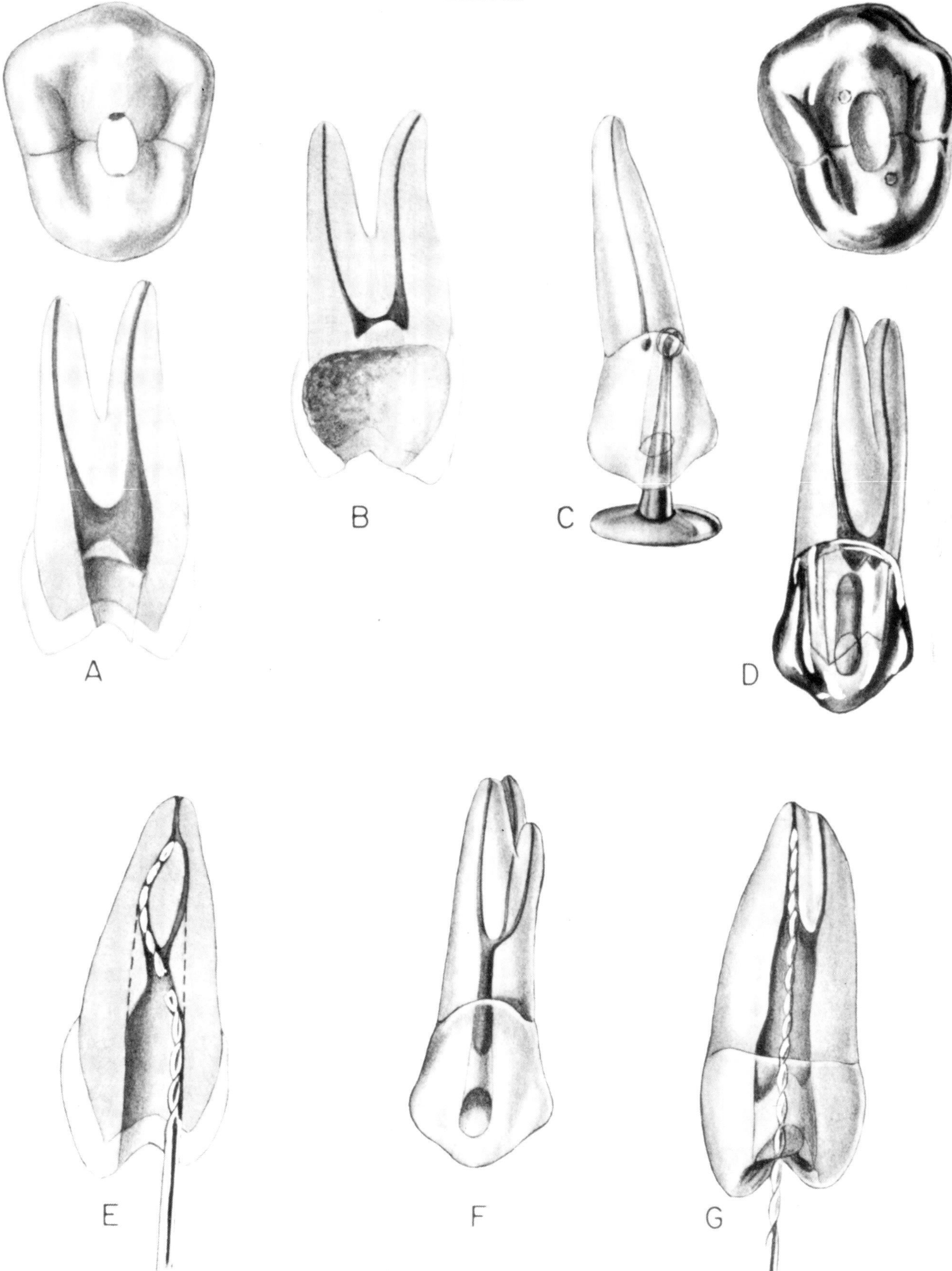

PLATE XVI

Endodontic Preparation of Mandibular Premolar Teeth

Pulp Anatomy and Coronal Preparation

A. Entrance is ***always*** gained through occlusal surface of ***all*** posterior teeth. Initial penetration is made in exact center of central groove of mandibular premolars. Bur is directed parallel to long axis of tooth. The 702 U taper fissure bur in ***accelerated-speed*** contra-angle is ideal for perforating gold casting or virgin enamel surface ***to depth of dentin.*** Amalgam fillings are penetrated with No. 4 round bur in slow-speed contra-angle.

B. Regular-length, No. 4 round bur is used to open vertically into pulp chamber. Bur will be felt to "drop" when pulp chamber is reached. If chamber is ***well-calcified,*** initial penetration is continued until contra-angle rests against occlusal surface. This depth of 9 mm. is usual position of canal orifice which lies at cervical level. In removing bur, occlusal opening is widened buccolingually to twice width of bur to allow room for exploration.

C. Endodontic explorer is used to locate central canal. Tension of explorer against walls of preparation will indicate amount and direction of extension necessary.

D. ***Working from inside pulp chamber to outside,*** regular-length No. 4 round bur is used to extend cavity buccolingually by removing roof of pulp chamber.

E. Buccolingual extension and finish of cavity walls is completed with 702 U fissure bur at accelerated speed.

F. Final ovoid preparation is tapered funnel from occlusal to canal, providing ***unobstructed access*** to canal. No overhanging tooth structure should impede complete authority over enlarging instruments.

G. Buccolingual ovoid ***outline form*** reflects anatomy of pulp chamber and position of centrally located canal. Cavity is extensive enough to allow for instruments and filling materials needed to enlarge and fill canals. ***Further exploration*** at this time ***may reveal*** orifice to ***additional canal,*** especially ***second canal*** in ***first premolar.*** Outline form of final preparation will be identical for both newly erupted and "adult" teeth.

PLATE XVI

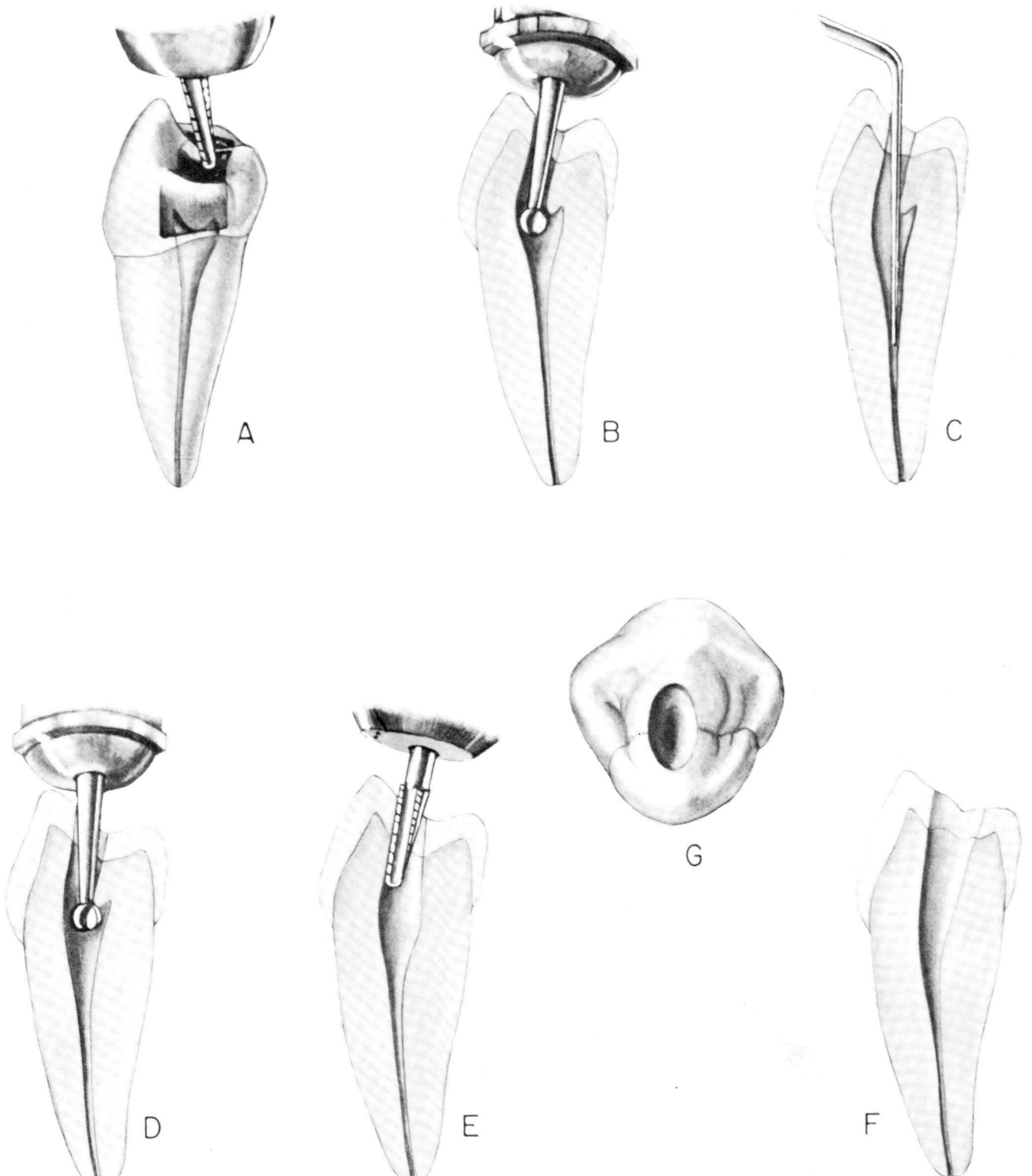

PLATE XVII

Mandibular First Premolar

Pulp Anatomy and Coronal Preparation

A. ***Buccal*** view of recently calcified first premolar with large pulp. Roentgenogram, if exposed slightly from mesial, will reveal:
   1. narrow mesiodistal width of pulp
   2. presence of one pulp canal
   3. relatively straight canal
   4. 14-degree distal-axial inclination of root.

   All of these factors ***seen*** in roentgenogram are borne in mind when preparation is begun.

B. ***Mesial*** view of same tooth demonstrating details not apparent from roentgenogram:
   1. height of pulp horn
   2. broad buccolingual extent of pulp
   3. apical-buccal curvature (2% of time)
   4. 10-degree lingual-axial angulation of root.

   These "unseen" factors will affect ***size, shape,*** and ***inclination*** of final preparation. Severe apical curvature can be detected only by exploration with fine curved file. Verticality of tooth simplifies orientation and bur alignment.

C. Cross sections at three levels: 1, cervical; 2, mid root; and 3, apical third:
   1. ***Cervical*** level: pulp is enormous in young tooth, very wide in buccolingual dimension. Debridement of ovoid chamber is completed during coronal cavity preparation with round bur.
   2. ***Mid root*** level: canal continues ovoid and requires perimeter filing and multiple point filling.
   3. ***Apical third*** level: canal, generally round in shape, is enlarged by reaming into ***round, tapered*** preparation, which matches ***round, tapered*** primary filling point. If primary point fits loosely in canal, it has been instrumented until ovoid and must be filled with multiple gutta percha points. Preparation terminates at cementodentinal junction, 0.5 mm from apical foramen.

D. ***Ovoid*** coronal preparation allows debridement of entire pulp chamber, funnels down to ovoid mid-canal, and is large enough buccolingually to allow passage of instruments used to enlarge and fill canal space.

E. ***Buccal*** view of ***adult*** first premolar with extensive secondary dentin formation. Roentgenogram will reveal:
   1. pulp recession and "thread-like" appearance of pulp
   2. roentgen appearance of only one canal
   3. 14-degree distal-axial inclination of root.

F. ***Mesial*** view of same tooth demonstrating details ***not apparent in roentgenogram:***
   1. buccolingual "ribbon-shaped" coronal pulp
   2. single root, bifurcated canal at mid-root level, and single apical foramen
   3. 10-degree lingual-axial angulation of root.

   Operator must recognize that:
   a. small orifices are difficult to locate
   b. presence of bifurcated canal is determined only by exploration with fine curved file
   c. single apical foramen can be determined by placing instruments in both canals at same time. Instruments will be heard and felt to grate against each other.

G. Cross sections at three levels: 1, cervical; 2, mid root; and 3, apical third:
   1. ***Cervical*** level: chamber is very narrow ovoid
   2. ***Mid root*** level: two branches of canal are round
   3. ***Apical third*** level: canal is round.

   Divisions of canal are enlarged by reaming. Buccal canal would be filled to apex and lingual canal to point where canals rejoin.

H. Ovoid funnel-shaped coronal preparation must be extensive enough buccolingually to allow for enlarging and filling both canals.

PLATE XVII

Length of Tooth[3]		*Canals*[9]		*Curvature of Root*			
Average Length	22.9 mm.	1 canal		Straight	48%	Buccal	2%
Maximum Length	24.2 mm.	1 foramen	73.5%	Distal	35%	Lingual	7%
Minimum Length	21.2 mm.	2 canals		Mesial	0%	Bayonet	7%
Range	3.0 mm.	1 foramen	6.5%				
		2 canals					
		2 foramens	19.5%				
		3 canals	0.5%				

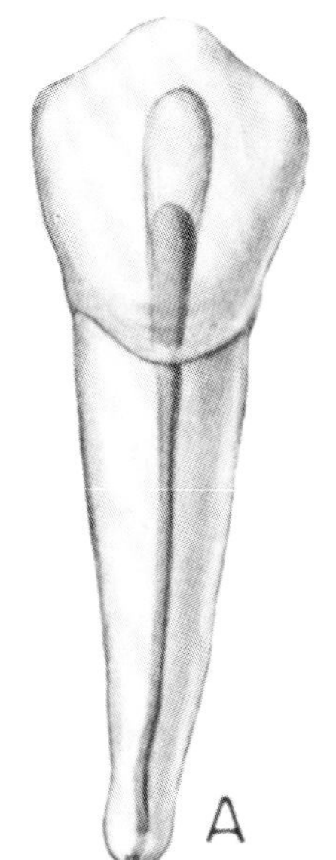
A

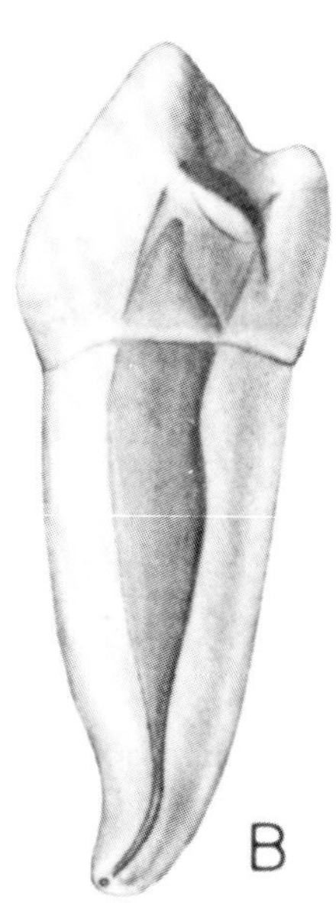
B

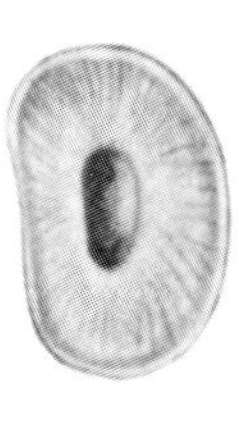
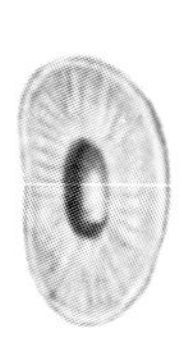
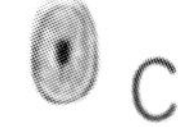
C

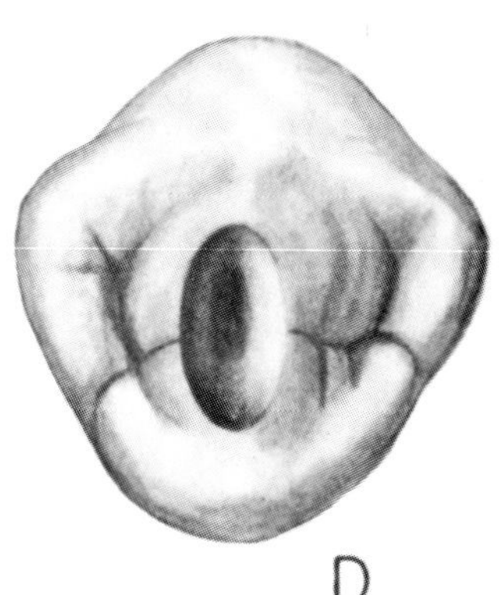
D

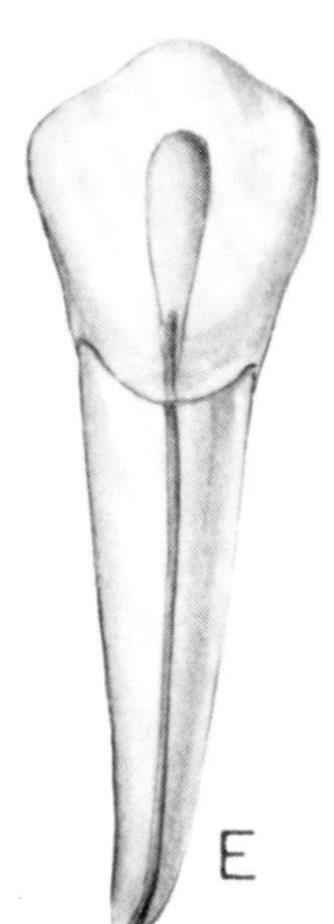
E

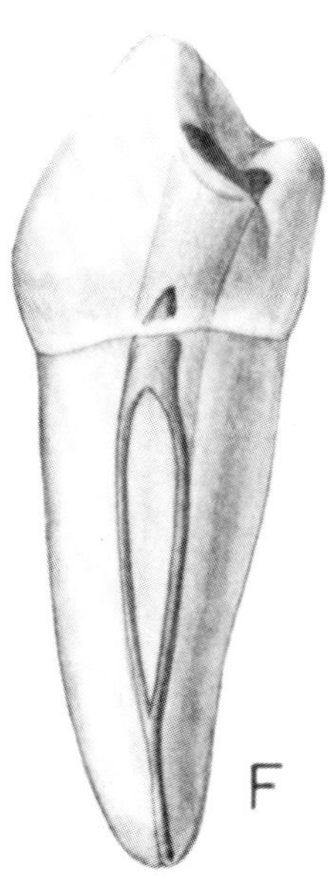
F

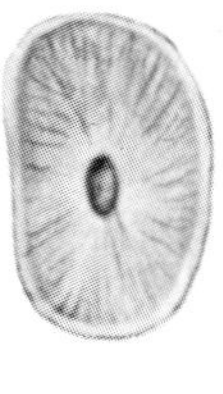
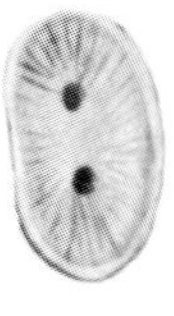
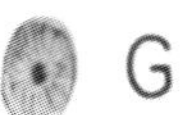
G

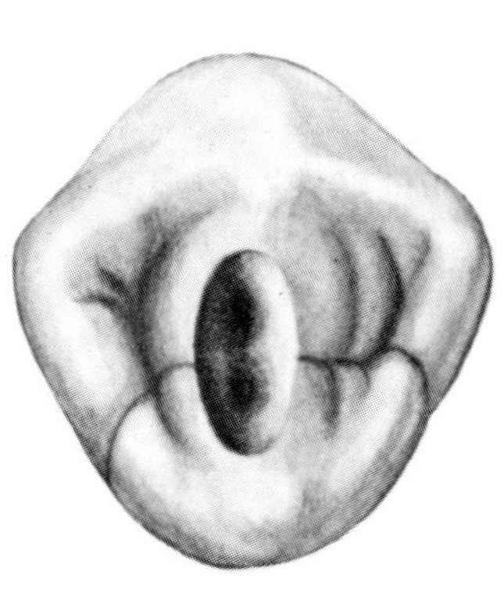
H

PLATE XVIII

Mandibular Second Premolar

Pulp Anatomy and Coronal Preparation

A. ***Buccal*** view of recently calcified second premolar with large pulp. Roentgenogram will reveal:
   1. mesiodistal width of pulp
   2. apical-distal curvature (40% of time)
   3. 10-degree distal-axial inclination of root.

   These factors ***seen*** in roentgenogram are borne in mind when preparation is begun.

B. ***Mesial*** view of same tooth demonstrating details ***not apparent in roentgenogram:***
   1. broad buccolingual "ribbon-shaped" coronal pulp
   2. single root with pulpal bifurcation in apical third
   3. −34-degree buccal-axial angulation of the root.

   These "unseen" factors affect ***size, shape,*** and ***inclination*** of final preparation. Apical third bifurcation, ***unseen in roentgenogram,*** emphasizes necessity of careful canal exploration.

C. Cross sections at three levels: 1, cervical; 2, mid root; and 3, apical third:
   1. ***Cervical*** level: pulp is large in young tooth, very wide in buccolingual dimension. Debridement of chamber is completed during coronal cavity preparation with round bur.
   2. ***Mid root*** level: canal continues to be long ovoid and requires perimeter filing and multiple point filling.
   3. ***Apical third*** level: canals generally round, are reamed into ***round, tapered*** preparations which match ***round, tapered*** primary filling points. Preparation terminates at the cementodentinal junction, 0.5 mm. from apical foramens.

D. ***Ovoid,*** coronal funnel-shaped preparation allows debridement of entire pulp chamber down to ovoid mid canal. Cavity is large enough buccolingually to allow enlarging and filling of both canals.

E. ***Buccal*** view of ***adult*** second premolar with extensive secondary dentin formation. Roentgenogram, if exposed slightly from mesial, will reveal:
   1. pulp recession and "thread-like" appearance of pulp
   2. sweeping distal curve of apical third of root of tooth (40% of time)
   3. 10-degree distal-axial angulation of root.

F. ***Mesial*** view of same tooth demonstrating details ***not apparent in roentgenogram:***
   1. buccolingual "ribbon-shaped" pulp.
   2. −34-degree buccal-axial angulation of root

   Operator should recognize that:
   a. small canal orifice will be difficult to locate
   b. direction of canal is best explored with fine curved file which is carried to within 0.5 mm. of apical foramen. Retraction will then remove dentin at curve.

G. Cross sections at three levels: 1, cervical; 2, mid root; and 3, apical third:
   1. ***Cervical*** level: chamber is very narrow ovoid
   2. ***Mid root*** level: canal is less ovoid
   3. ***Apical third*** level: canal is round.

   Sweeping curve at apical third is filed to gradual curve. Canal is then completed by reaming, and filled with multiple points.

H. ***Ovoid*** funnel-shaped coronal cavity is modest in size and skewed to mesial, allowing adequate room to instrument and fill curved apical third.

PLATE XVIII

Length of Tooth[3]		*Canals*[9]		*Curvature of Root*			
Average Length	22.3 mm.	1 canal		Straight	39%	Lingual	3%
Maximum Length	25.0 mm.	1 foramen	85.5%	Distal	40%	Bayonet	7%
Minimum Length	19.3 mm.	2 canals		Mesial	0%	Trifurcation	1%
Range	5.7 mm.	1 foramen	1.5%	Buccal	10%		
		2 canals					
		2 foramens	11.5%				
		3 canals	0.5%				

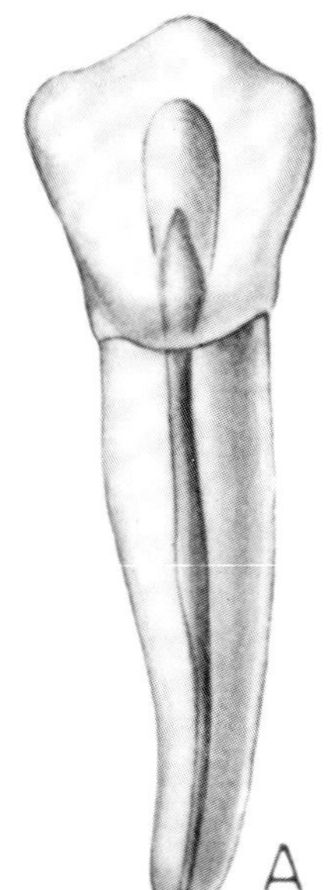
A

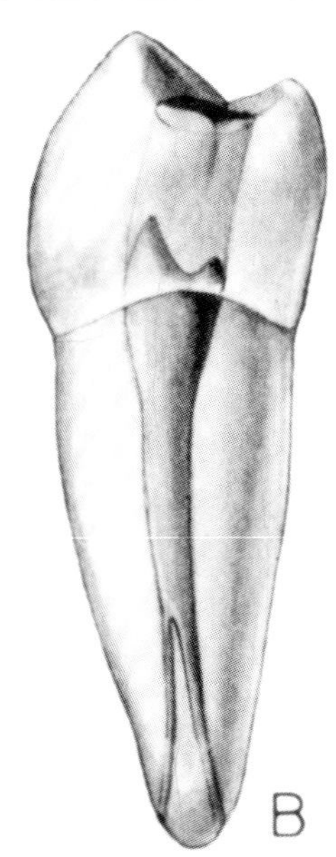
B

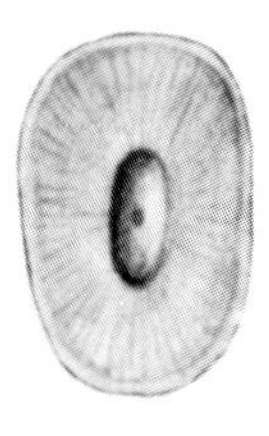
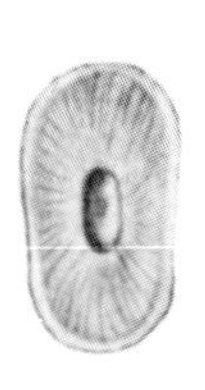
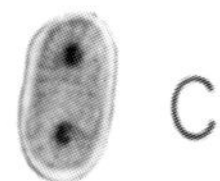
C

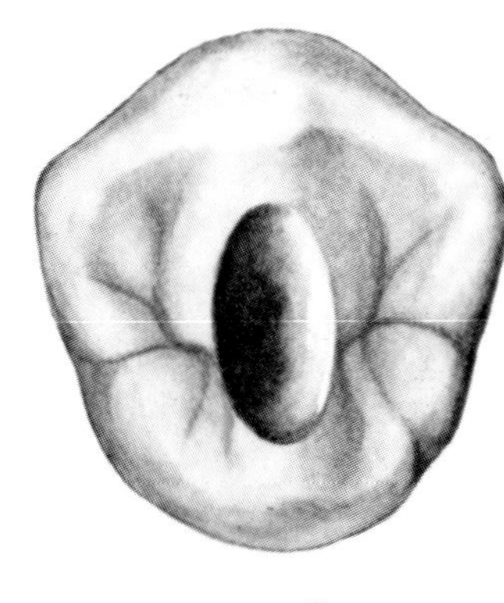
D

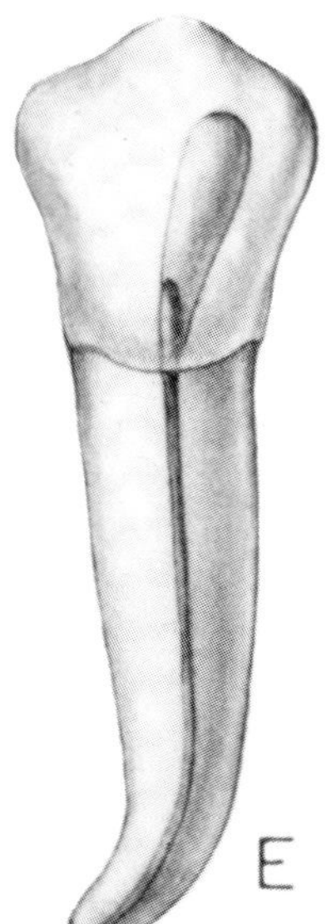
E

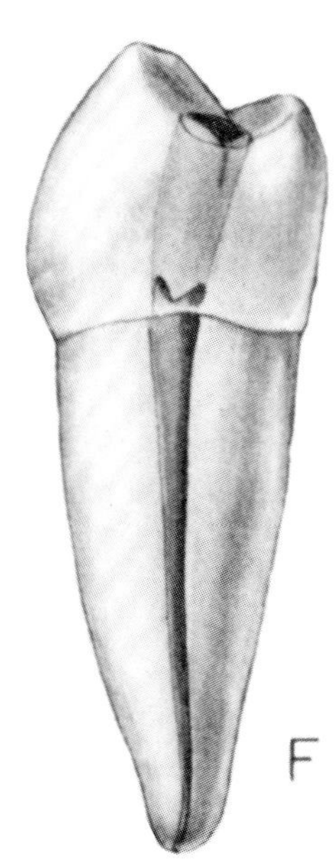
F

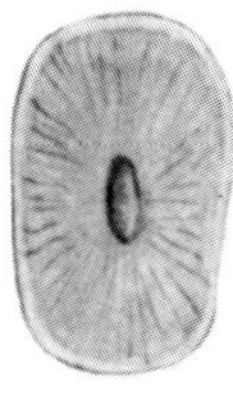
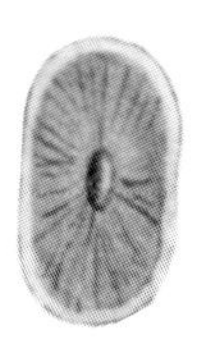
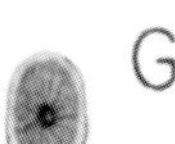
G

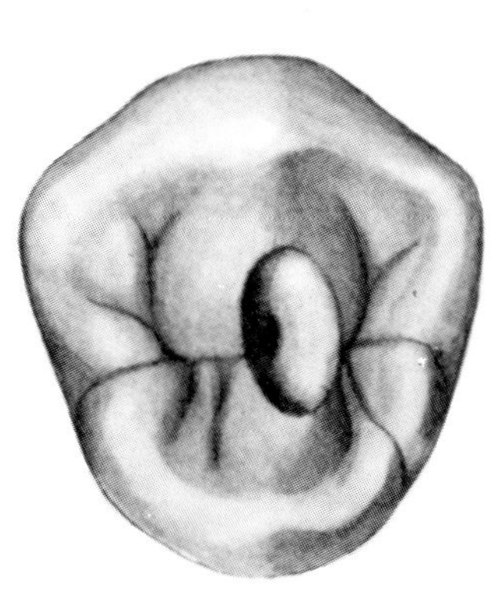
H

PLATE XIX

Mandibular Premolar Teeth

ERRORS in Cavity Preparation

A. PERFORATION at distogingival caused by failure to recognize that premolar has tilted to distal.

B. INCOMPLETE preparation and possible instrument breakage caused by total loss of instrument control. Use only occlusal access, never buccal or proximal access.

C. BIFURCATION of canal completely missed, caused by failure to adequately explore canal with curved instrument.

D. APICAL PERFORATION of invitingly straight conical canal. Failure to establish exact length of tooth leads to trephination of foramen.

E. PERFORATION at apical curvature caused by failure to recognize, by exploration, buccal curvature. Standard buccolingual roentgenogram will not show buccal or lingual curvature.

PLATE XIX

ERRORS

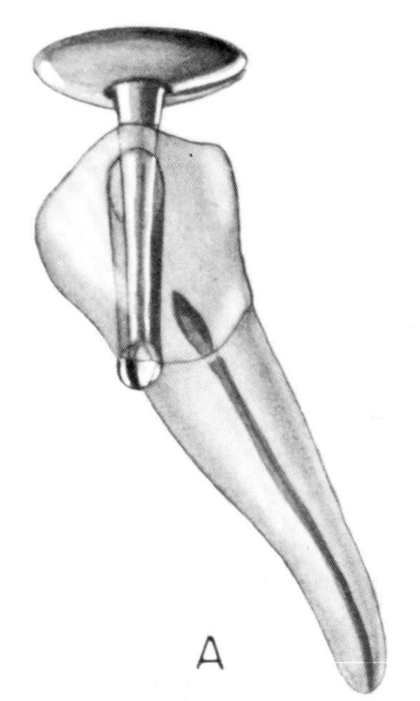

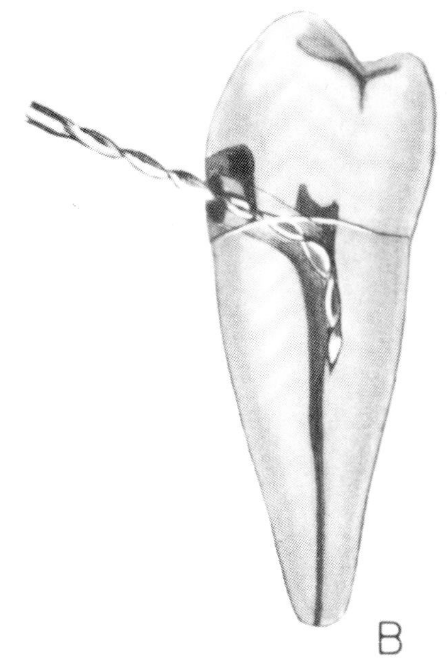

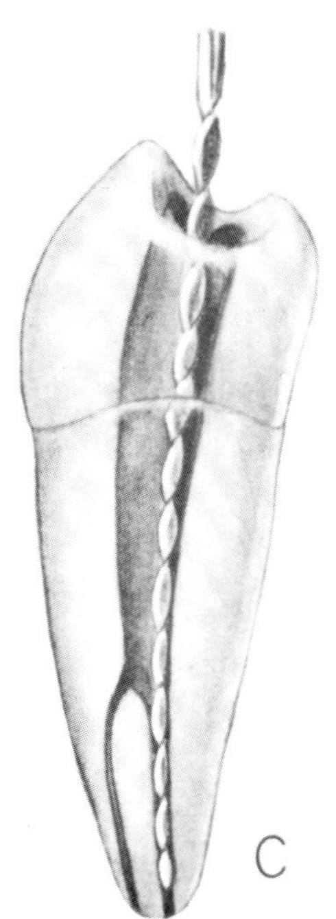

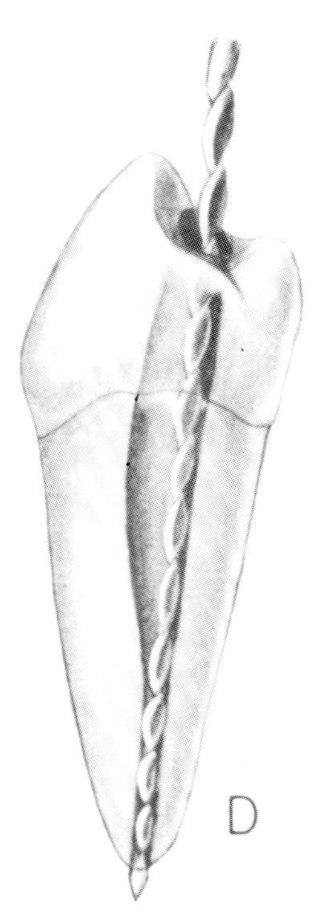

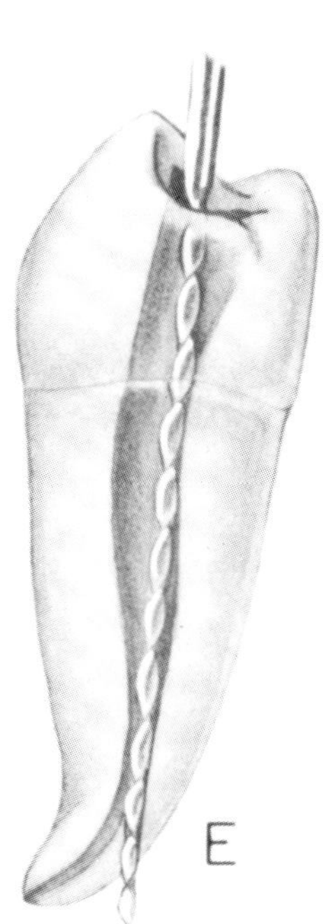

PLATE XX

Endodontic Preparation of Maxillary Molar Teeth

A. Entrance is ***always*** gained through occlusal surface of all posterior teeth. Initial penetration is made in the exact center of mesial pit, with bur directed toward lingual. The 702U tapering fissure bur in ***accelerated-speed*** contra-angle is ideal for perforating gold casting or virgin enamel surface ***to depth of dentin.*** Amalgam fillings are penetrated with No. 4 or 6 round bur operating in slow-speed contra-angle.

B. According to size of chamber, ***regular-length*** No. 4 or 6 round bur is used to open into pulp chamber. ***Bur*** should be ***directed toward orifice*** of ***palatal canal,*** where greatest space in chamber exists. It will be felt to "drop" when pulp chamber is reached. If chamber is ***well calcified,*** initial penetration is continued until contra-angle rests against occlusal surface. This depth of 9 mm. is usual position of floor of pulp chamber, which lies at the cervical level. Working from inside out, back toward buccal, bur removes enough roof of pulp chamber for exploration.

C. Endodontic explorer is used to locate orifices of ***palatal, mesiobuccal,*** and ***distobuccal*** canals. Tension of explorer against walls of preparation will indicate amount and direction of extension necessary. ***Orifices of canals form perimeter*** of preparation. ***Special care must be taken to explore for second canal in mesiobuccal root.***

D. Again, working at slow speed from inside to outside, round bur is used to remove roof of pulp chamber. Internal walls and floor of preparation should not be cut into unless difficulty is encountered in locating orifices. In that case, ***surgical-length*** No. 2 or 4 round burs are necessary to explore floor of chamber.

E. Final finish and funneling of cavity walls is completed with a 702U fissure bur at accelerated speed.

F. Final preparation provides unobstructed access to canal orifices and should not impede complete authority of enlarging instruments. Improve ease of access by ***"leaning" entire preparation toward buccal,*** for all instrumentation is introduced from buccal. Notice that preparation almost extends to height of buccal cusps. Walls are perfectly smooth and orifices located ***at exact pulpal-axial angles*** of cavity floor.

G. Triangular outline form reflects anatomy of pulp chamber. Base of triangle is toward buccal and apex is to lingual, with canal orifice positioned at each angle of triangle. Cavity is entirely within mesial half of tooth, need not invade transverse ridge, but is extensive enough, buccal to lingual, to allow positioning of instruments and filling materials. Outline form of final preparation is identical for both newly erupted and "adult" tooth. Note orifice to fourth canal.

PLATE XX

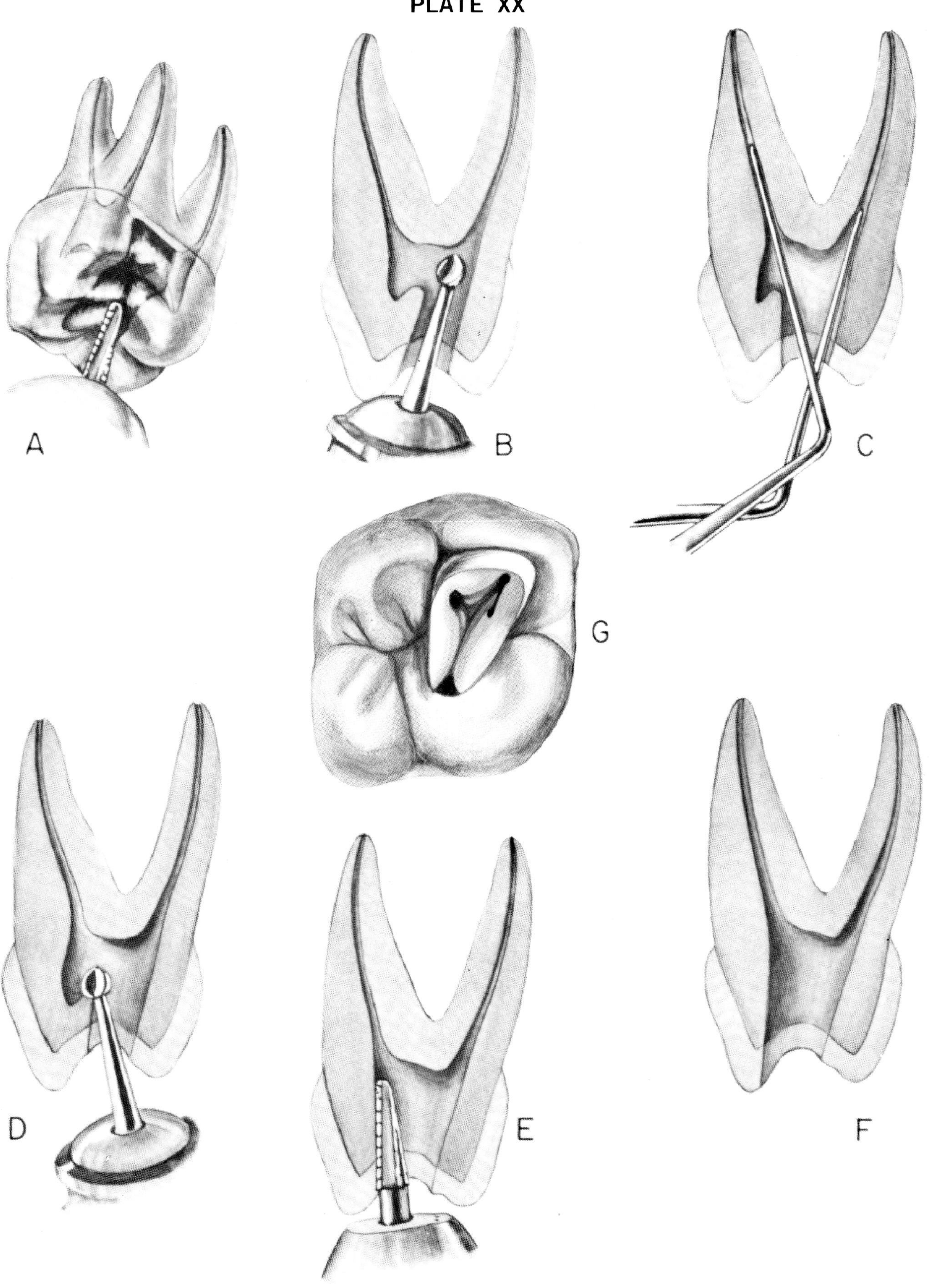

PLATE XXI

Maxillary First Molar

Pulp Anatomy and Coronal Preparation

A. ***Buccal*** view of recently calcified first molar with large pulp. Roentgenogram will reveal:
   1. large pulp chamber
   2. mesiobuccal, distobuccal, and palatal roots, each with one canal
   3. slightly curved buccal roots
   4. slightly curved palatal root
   5. vertical axial alignment of ***tooth.***

   These factors ***seen*** in roentgenogram are borne in mind when preparation is begun. Care must be taken to explore for additional mesiobuccal canal.

B. ***Mesial*** view of same tooth demonstrating details ***not apparent in roentgenogram:***
   1. buccolingual width of pulp chamber
   2. apical-buccal curvature of palatal root (55% of time)
   3. buccal inclination of buccal roots
   4. vertical axial alignment of ***tooth.***

   These "unseen" factors will affect ***size, shape,*** and ***inclination*** of final preparation. Sharp ***buccal curvature*** of ***palatal canal requires great care*** in exploration and instrumentation. Canals must be carefully explored with ***fine curved files.*** Enlargement of buccal canals is accomplished by reaming and filing, and palatal canal by filing with severely curved files.

C. Cross section at two levels: 1, cervical, and 2, apical third:
   1. ***Cervical*** level: pulp is enormous in young tooth. Debridement of ***triangular*** chamber is completed with round bur. ***Dark*** cavity floor with ***"lines"*** connecting orifices is in marked contrast to white walls. Palatal canal requires perimeter filing and filling with condensed primary gutta percha point and multiple points.
   2. ***Apical third*** level: canals are essentially round. Buccal canals are reamed into ***round, tapered*** preparations which match the ***round, tapered*** gutta percha filling points. Preparations terminate at cementodentinal junction, 0.5 mm. from apical foramens.

D. ***Triangular outline form,*** with base toward buccal and apex to lingual, reflects anatomy of pulp chamber, with orifice positioned at each angle of triangle. Both ***buccal*** and ***lingual walls slope buccally.*** Mesial and distal walls ***funnel*** slightly ***outward.*** Cavity is entirely within mesial half of tooth, and should be extensive enough to allow positioning of instruments and filling materials needed to enlarge and fill canals. Orifice to ***extra mesiobuccal canal*** will usually be found in groove connecting mesiobuccal and palatal canals.

E. ***Buccal*** view of ***adult*** first molar with extensive secondary dentin formation. Roentgenogram will reveal:
   1. pulp recession and "thread-like" pulp
   2. mesiobuccal, distobuccal, and palatal roots, each with one canal
   3. straight distal and palatal roots
   4. apical-distal curvature of mesial root (78% of time)
   5. vertical axial alignment of ***tooth.***

F. ***Mesial*** view of same tooth demonstrating details ***not apparent in roentgenogram:***
   1. pulp recession
   2. relatively straight palatal root
   3. buccal inclination of buccal roots
   4. vertical axial alignment of ***tooth.***

   Operator must recognize that:
   a. careful exploration for orifices and canals is imperative
   b. severe curvature of mesial root will require careful enlargement with curved instruments.

G. Cross section at two levels : 1, cervical, and 2, apical third:
   1. ***Cervical*** level: triangular chamber constricted from secondary dentin formation is debrided during coronal cavity preparation with round bur. Round palatal and distobuccal canals will be reamed to ***round, tapered*** preparation and might be filled with ***round, tapered*** silver point.
   2. ***Apical third*** level: canals are round. Curved mesiobuccal canal is enlarged by filing with curved files and filled by condensed gutta percha points. Preparations terminate at cementodentinal junction, 0.5 mm. from apical foramens.

H. ***Triangular outline*** form reflects anatomy of pulp chamber. Both ***buccal*** and ***lingual*** walls ***slope buccally. Mesial wall slopes mesially*** to allow for instrumentation of severely curved mesiobuccal canal. If ***additional canal*** is found in ***mesiobuccal*** root, its orifice will usually be in groove leading to palatal canal.

PLATE XXI

Length of Tooth[3]		*Canals in the Mesiobuccal Root*[10,11]	*Direction*	*Palatal*	*Mesial*	*Distal*	*Direction*	*Palatal*	*Mesial*	*Distal*
			Curvature of Roots							
Average Length	22.3 mm.	1 canal	Straight	40%	21%	54%	Buccal	*55%	0%	0%
Maximum Length	25.0 mm.	1 foramen 38%	Distal	1%	78%	17%	Lingual	0%	0%	0%
Minimum Length	19.6 mm.	2 canals	Mesial	4%	0%	19%	Bayonet	—	1%	10%
Range	5.4 mm.	1 foramen 37%								
		2 canals								
		2 foramens 25%								

*Not apparent in roentgenogram

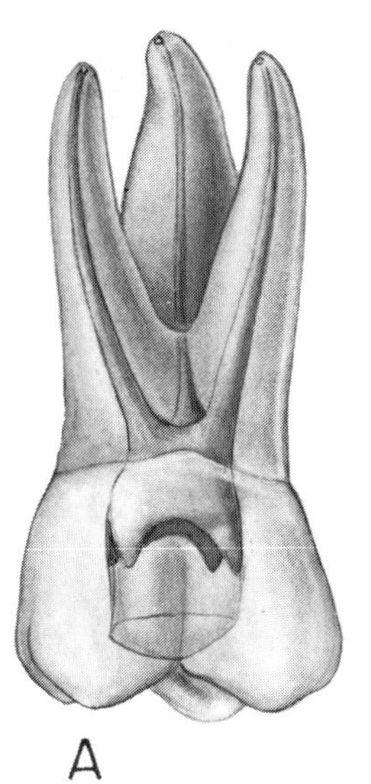
A

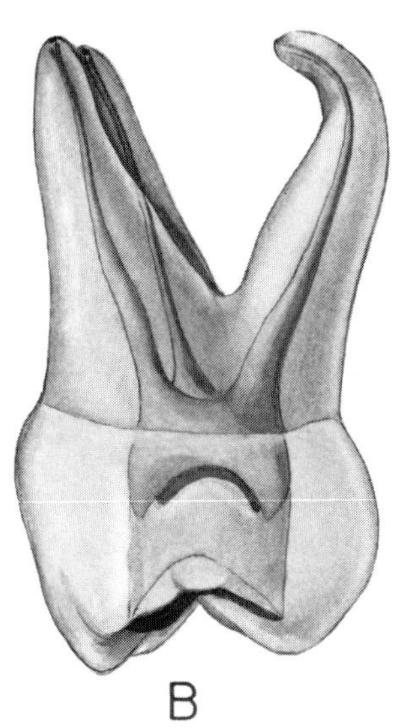
B

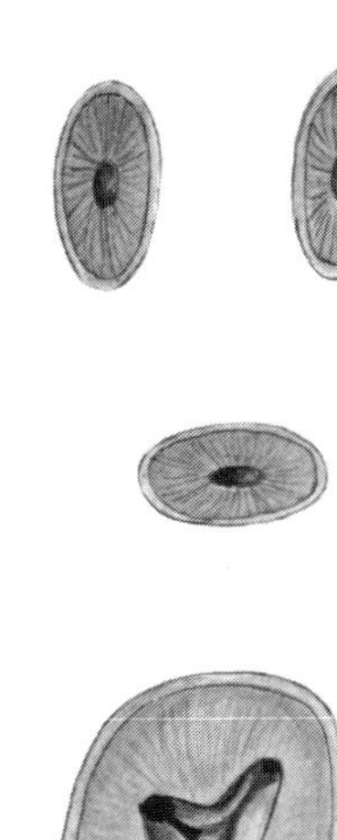
C

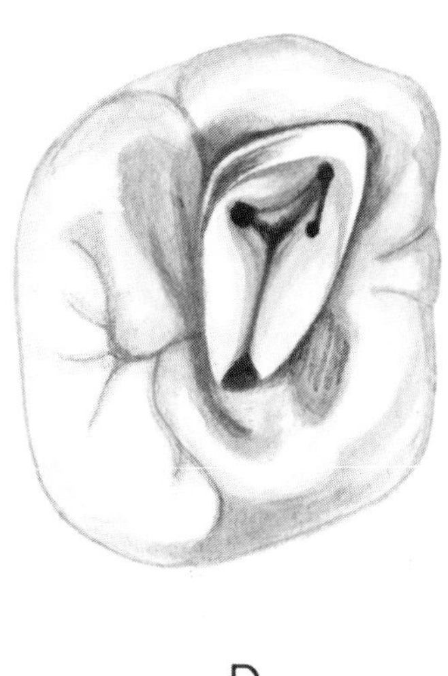
D

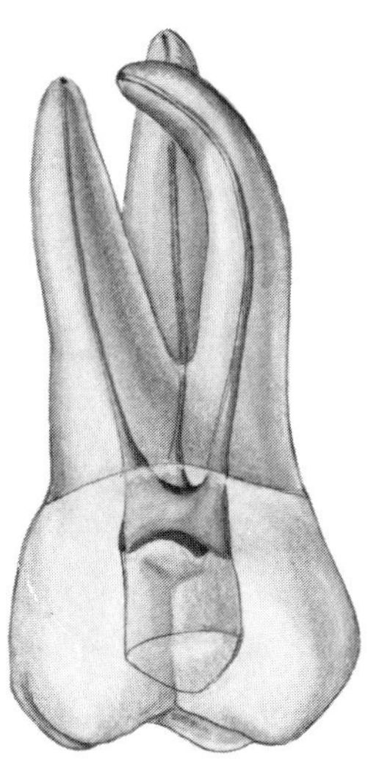
E

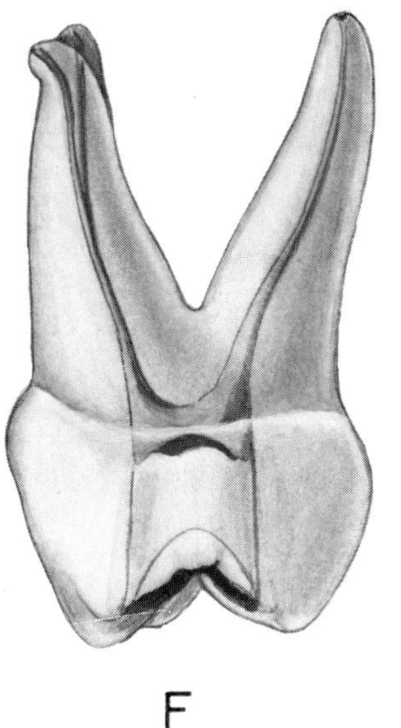
F

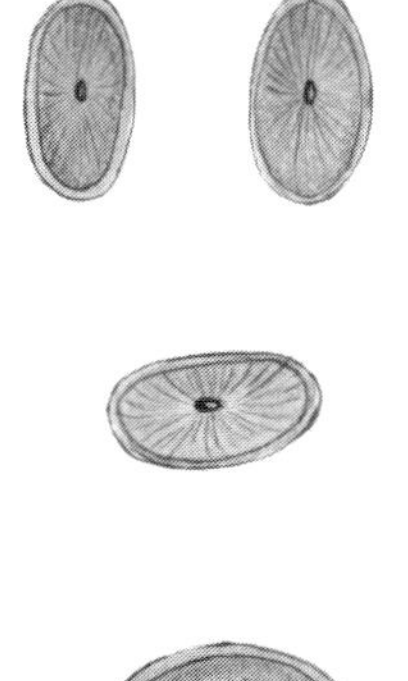

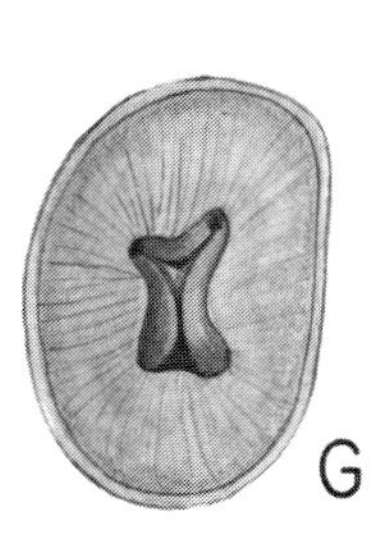
G

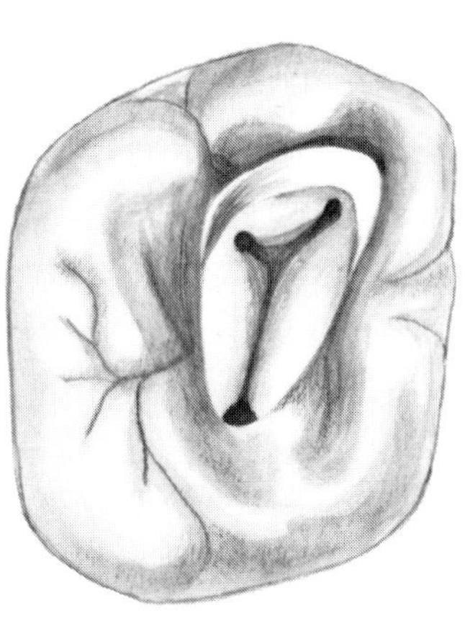
H

PLATE XXII

Maxillary Second Molar

Pulp Anatomy and Coronal Preparation

A. ***Buccal*** view of recently calcified second molar with large pulp. Roentgenogram will reveal:
1. large pulp chamber
2. mesiobuccal, distobuccal, and palatal roots each with one canal
3. gradual curvature of all three canals
4. vertical axial alignment of ***tooth.***

These factors ***seen*** in roentgenogram are borne in mind when preparation is begun.

B. ***Mesial*** view of same tooth demonstrating details ***not apparent in roentgenogram:***
1. buccolingual width of pulp chamber
2. gradual curvature of all three canals
3. buccal inclination of buccal roots
4. vertical axial alignment of ***tooth.***

These "unseen" factors will affect ***size, shape,*** and ***inclination*** of final preparation. Canals are all enlarged by ***alternate filing*** and ***reaming*** with curved instruments, and filled by multiple point fillings.

C. Cross section at two levels: 1, cervical, and 2, apical third:
1. ***Cervical*** level: pulp is enormous in young tooth. Debridement of ***triangular*** chamber is completed with round burs. ***Dark*** cavity floor with ***"lines"*** connecting orifices is in marked contrast to white walls.
2. ***Apical third*** level: canals are essentially round and are enlarged into ***round, tapered*** preparation which match ***round, tapered*** filling materials. Preparations terminate at cementodentinal junction, 0.5 mm. from the apical foramens.

D. ***Triangular outline form*** is "flattened" as it reflects internal anatomy of chamber. Note distobuccal canal orifice is nearer center of cavity floor. Entire preparation sharply slopes to buccal and is extensive enough to allow positioning of instruments and filling materials needed to enlarge and fill canals.

E. ***Buccal*** view of adult second molar with extensive secondary dentin formation.
Roentgenogram will reveal:
1. pulp recession and "thread-like" pulp
2. ***anomalous*** appearance of only ***one root*** and ***two canals***
3. vertical axial alignment of ***tooth.***

F. ***Mesial*** view of same tooth demonstrating details ***not apparent in roentgenogram:***
1. pulp recession
2. ***anomalous*** appearance of only ***one root*** and ***two canals***
3. sweeping curvature of lingual canal
4. vertical axial alignment of ***tooth.***

Operator must recognize that:
a. canal orifices are difficult to find by exploration
b. detailed search must be made for third canal
c. canals are reamed to ***round, tapered*** preparations which match ***round, tapered*** silver points.

G. Cross sections at two levels: 1, cervical, and 2, apical third:
1. ***Cervical*** level: ***ovoid*** pulp chamber is debrided during cavity preparation with round bur.
2. ***Apical third*** level: canals are round and may be filled with single silver points. Preparations terminate at cementodentinal junction, 0.5 mm. from the apical foramen.

H. ***Ovoid*** outline form reflects internal anatomy of pulp chamber and elongated parallelogram shape of occlusal surface. Entire preparation slopes sharply to buccal.

PLATE XXII

Length of Tooth[3]		*Roots*	*Canals in the Mesiobuccal Root*[12]		*Curvature of Roots* *Direction*	*Palatal*	*Mesial*	*Distal*	*Direction*	*Palatal*	*Mesial*	*Distal*
Average Length	22.2 mm.	Three 54%	1 canal		Straight	63%	22%	54%	Buccal	37%	?	?
Maximum Length	25.2 mm.	Fused 46%	1 foramen	63%	Distal	0%	54%	?	Lingual	0%	?	?
Minimum Length	20.1 mm.		2 canals		Mesial	0%	0%	17%	Bayonet	?	?	9%
Range	5.1 mm.		1 foramen	13%								
			2 canals									
			2 foramens	24%								

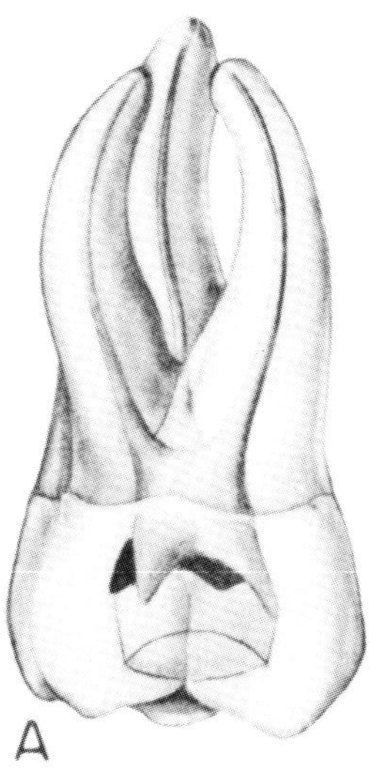
A

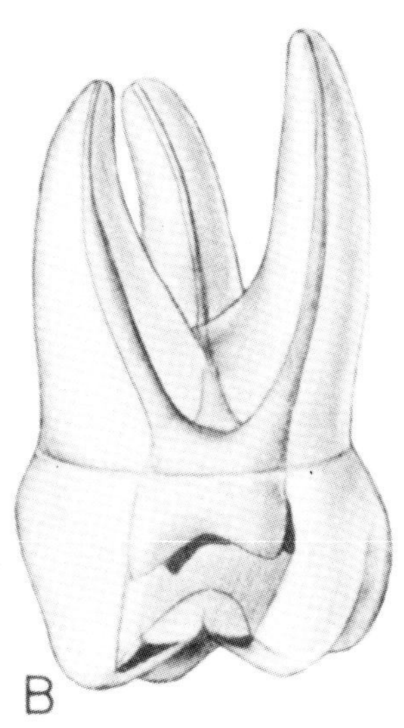
B

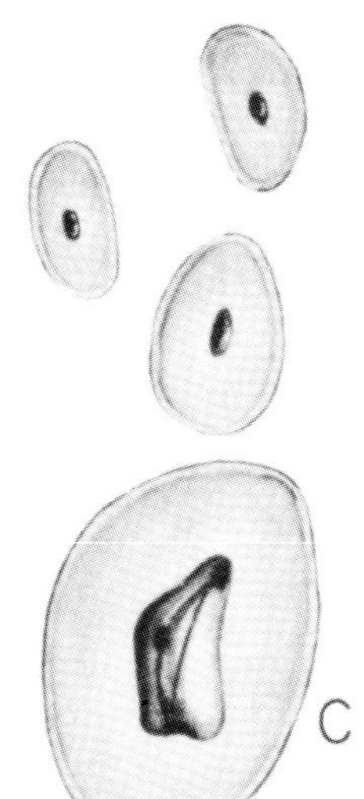
C

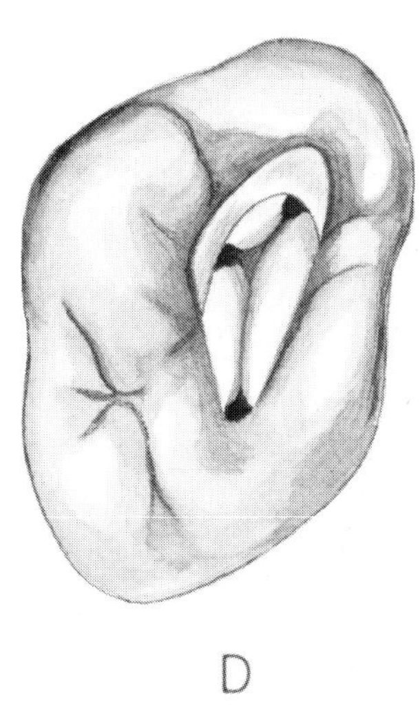
D

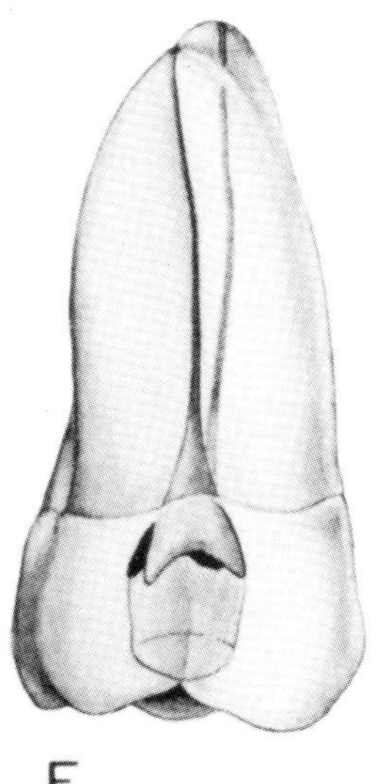
E

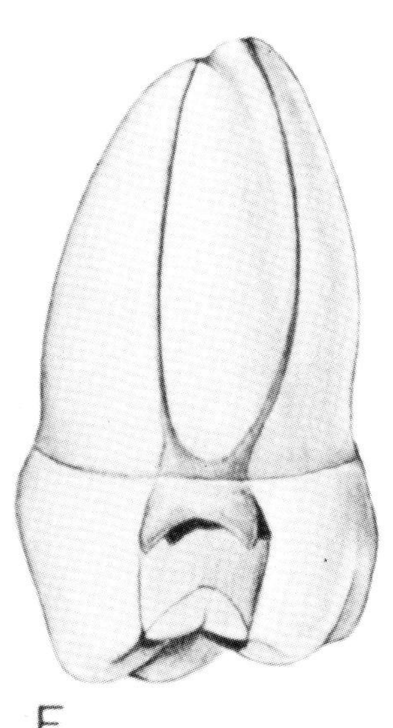
F

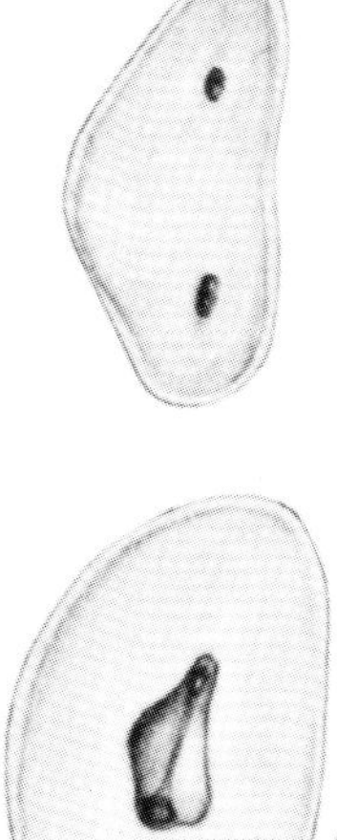
G

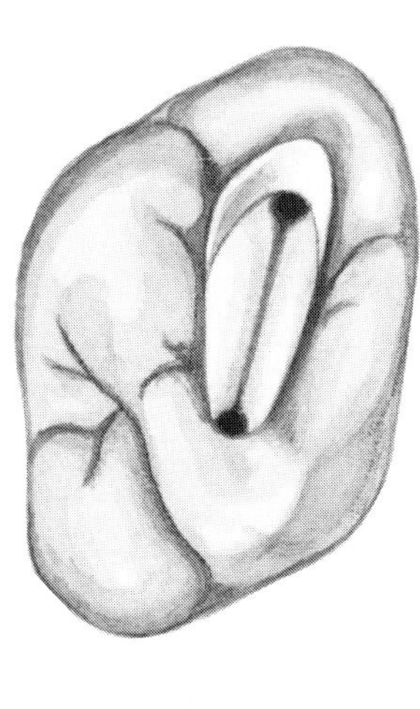
H

PLATE XXIII

Maxillary Molar Teeth

ERRORS in Cavity Preparation

A. UNDEREXTENDED preparation. Pulp horns have merely been "nicked" and entire roof of pulp chamber remains. "White" color dentin of roof is clue to underextension (A′). Instrument control is lost.

B. OVEREXTENDED preparation undermining enamel walls. Crown is badly gouged due to failure to observe pulp recession in roentgenogram.

C. PERFORATION into furca caused by using ***surgical-length*** bur and failing to realize narrow pulp chamber had been passed.

D. INADEQUATE vertical preparation related to failure to recognize severe buccal inclination of unopposed molar.

E. DISORIENTED occlusal outline form exposing only palatal canal. Faulty cavity has been prepared in full crown, which was placed to "straighten" ***rotated molar*** (E′).

F. LEDGE FORMATION caused by using large straight instrument in curved canal.

G. PERFORATION of palatal root commonly caused by assuming canal to be straight and failing to explore and enlarge canal with fine curved instrument.

PLATE XXIII

ERRORS

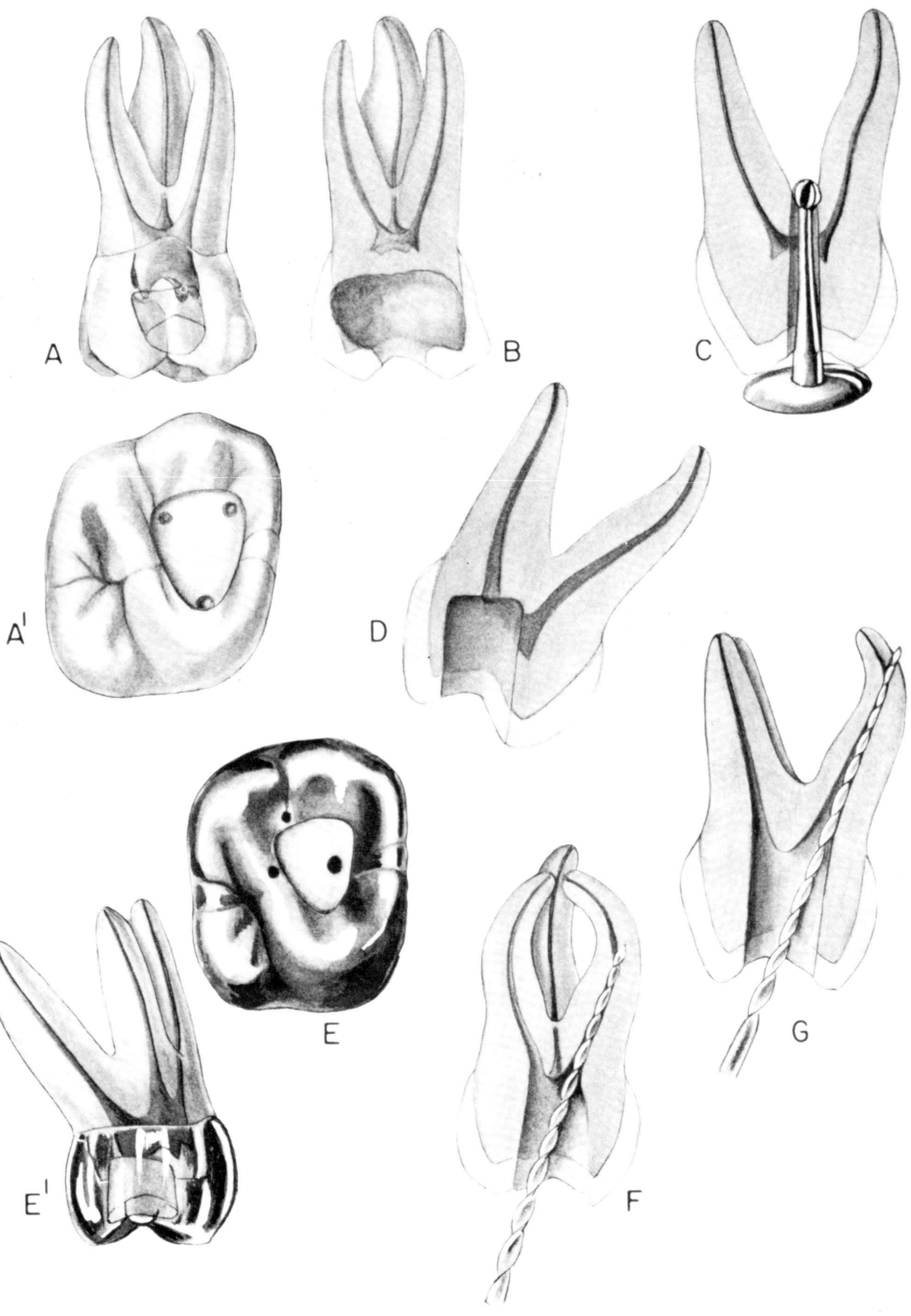

PLATE XXIV

Endodontic Preparation of Mandibular Molar Teeth

A. Entrance is ***always*** gained through occlusal surface of ***all*** posterior teeth. Initial penetration is made in exact center of mesial pit, with bur directed toward distal. The 702U tapering fissure bur in ***accelerated-speed*** contra-angle is ideal for perforating gold casting or virgin enamel surface to ***depth of dentin.*** Amalgam fillings are penetrated with No. 4 or 6 round bur operating in slow-speed contra-angle.

B. According to size of chamber, regular-length No. 4 or 6 round bur is used to open into pulp chamber. Bur should be ***directed toward orifice*** of ***distal canal*** where greatest space in chamber exists. It will be felt to "drop" when pulp chamber is reached. If chamber is well calcified, initial penetration is continued until contra-angle rests against occlusal surface. This depth of 9 mm. is usual position of floor of pulp chamber, which lies at cervical level. Working from inside out, back toward mesial, bur removes enough roof of pulp chamber for exploration.

C. Endodontic explorer is used to locate orifices of ***distal, mesiobuccal,*** and ***mesiolingual*** canals. Tension of explorer against walls of preparation indicates amount and direction of extension necessary. ***Orifices of canals form perimeter*** of preparation. ***Special care must be taken to explore for additional canal in distal root.*** It may be necessary to square-out outline form to distal to search for extra canal.

D. Again, working at slow speed from inside to outside, round bur is used to remove roof of pulp chamber. Internal walls and floor of preparation should not be cut into unless difficulty is encountered in locating orifices. In that case, ***surgical-length*** No. 2 or 4 round burs are necessary to explore floor of chamber.

E. Final finish and funneling of cavity walls is completed with 702U fissure bur at accelerated speed.

F. Final preparation provides unobstructed access to canal orifices and should not impede complete authority of enlarging instruments. Improve ease of access by ***"leaning" entire preparation toward mesial,*** for all instrumentation is introduced from mesial. Notice cavity outline extends almost to height of mesial cusps. Walls are perfectly smooth and orifices located ***at exact pulpal-axial angle*** of cavity floor.

G. "Rhomboidal" outline form reflects anatomy of pulp chamber. Both mesial and distal walls slope mesially. Cavity is primarily within mesial half of tooth, but is extensive enough to allow positioning of instrument and filling materials. Outline form of final preparation will be identical for both newly erupted and "adult" tooth. Further exploration should determine if fourth canal can be found in distal. If so, outline is extended in that direction. In that case an orifice will be positioned at each angle of rhomboid.

PLATE XXIV

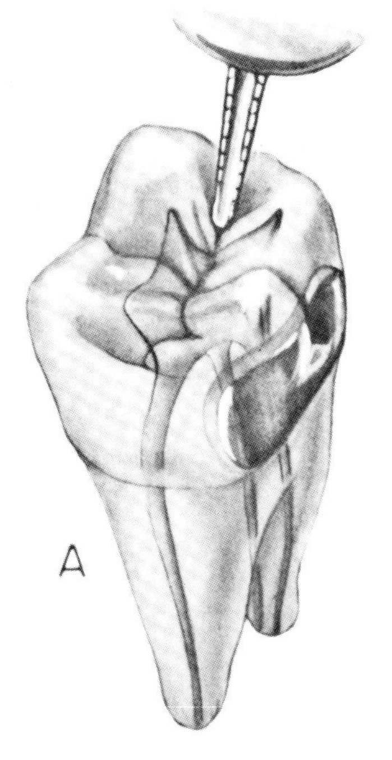

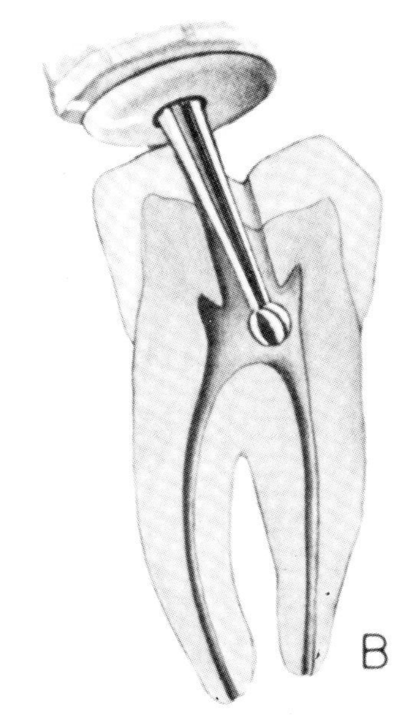

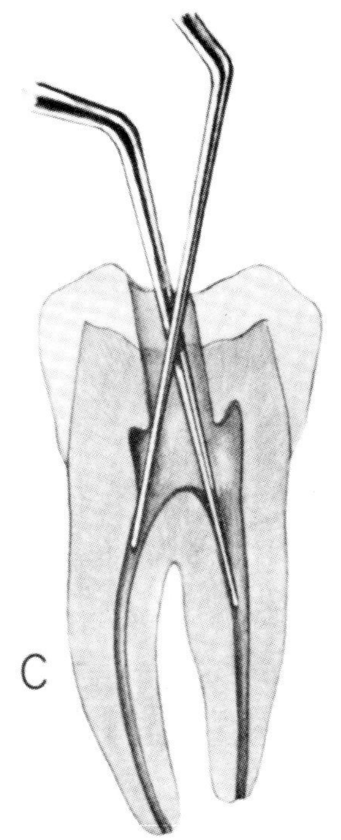

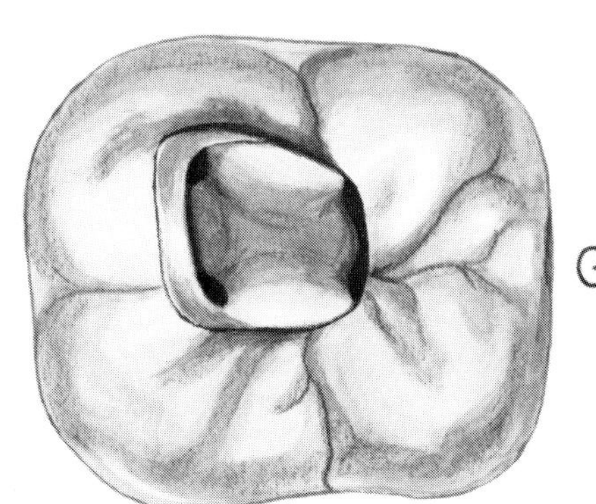

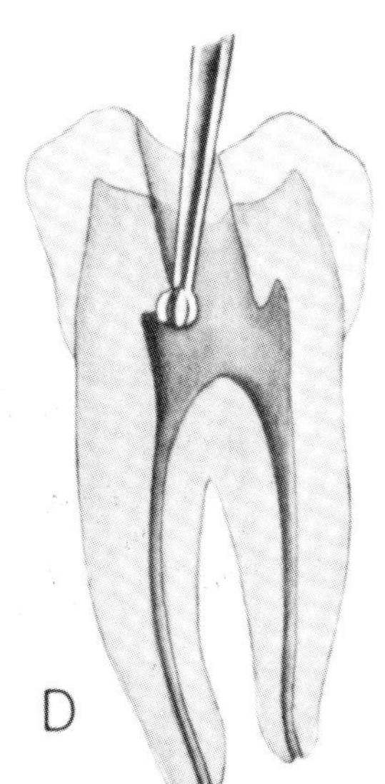

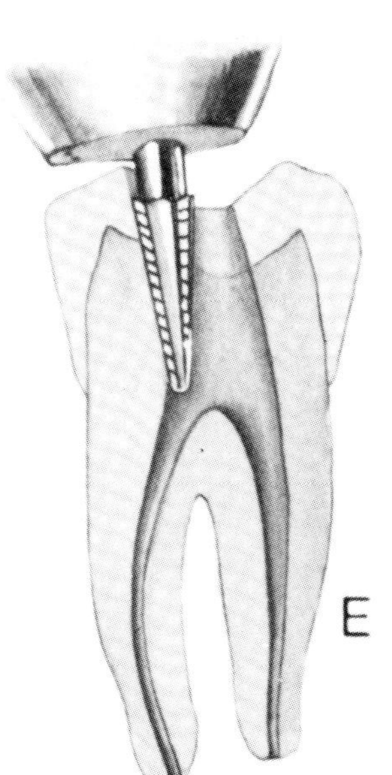

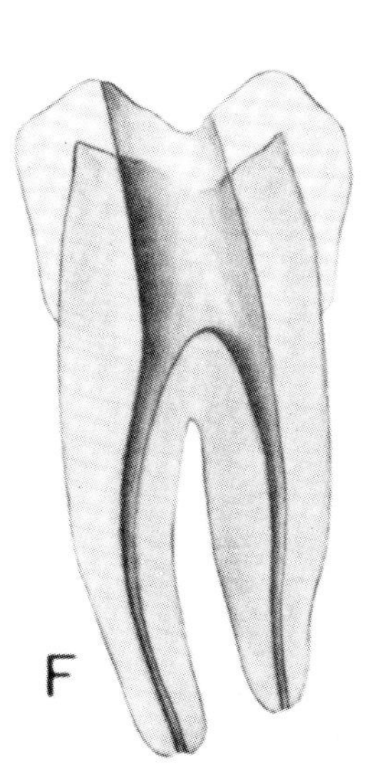

PLATE XXV

Mandibular First Molar

Pulp Anatomy and Coronal Preparation

A. ***Buccal*** view of recently calcified first molar with large pulp. Initial roentgenogram will reveal:
   1. large pulp chamber
   2. mesial and distal roots each ***apparently*** containing one canal
   3. vertical distal root (74%)
   4. curvature of mesial root (84%)
   5. distal-axial inclination of ***tooth.***

   These factors ***seen*** in roentgenogram are borne in mind when preparation is begun.

B. ***Mesial*** view of same tooth demonstrating details ***not apparent in roentgenogram:***
   1. single ***mesial root*** with ***two canals***
   2. −58-degree buccal-axial inclination of ***roots.***

   All of these ***unseen*** factors will affect ***size, shape,*** and ***inclination*** of final preparation.

C. Cross section at three levels: 1, cervical; 2, mid root; and 3, apical third:
   1. ***Cervical*** level: pulp, enormous in young tooth, is debrided during coronal cavity preparation with round bur.
   2. ***Mid root*** level: canals are ovoid. Distal canal requires perimeter filing and filling with multiple gutta percha points.
   3. ***Apical third*** level: canals are round and are reamed into ***round, tapered*** preparations which match ***round, tapered*** filling points. Preparations terminate at cementodentinal junction, 0.5 mm. from the apical foramens.

D. ***Distal*** view of same tooth demonstrating details ***not apparent in roentgenogram:***
   1. height of distal pulp horns
   2. "ribbon-shaped" distal canal.

E. ***Buccal*** view of ***adult*** first molar with extensive secondary dentin formation. Roentgenogram will reveal:
   1. pulp recession and "thread-like" pulp
   2. mesial and distal roots, each ***apparently*** containing one canal
   3. mesial curvature of distal root (5%) and distal curvature of mesial root (84%)
   4. distal-axial inclination of tooth.

F. ***Mesial*** view of same tooth demonstrating details ***not apparent in roentgenogram:***
   1. pulp recession
   2. ***mesial*** root, ***two canals*** and single foramen
   3. −58-degree buccal-axial inclination of ***roots.***

   Operator must recognize that:
   a. careful exploration with two instruments at same time reveals common apical foramen
   b. mesial canals curve in two directions.

G. Cross section at three levels: 1, cervical; 2, mid root; and 3, apical third:
   1. ***Cervical*** level: chamber is debrided during coronal cavity preparation with round bur
   2. ***Mid root*** level: canals are nearly round and are enlarged during reaming of apical third
   3. ***Apical third*** level: canals are round and are reamed into ***round, tapered*** preparation which matches ***round, tapered*** filling points. Preparations terminate at cementodentinal junction, 0.5 mm. from the apical foramens.

H. ***Distal*** view of same tooth demonstrating details ***not apparent in roentgenogram:***
   1. pulp recession
   2. ***distal*** root with ***two canals rather than usual single canal***
   3. buccal-axial inclination of roots.

   Operator should recognize that:

   Presence of fourth canal can only be determined by careful exploration.

I. ***"Rhomboidal" outline form*** reflects ***anatomy*** of pulp chamber. Both mesial and distal walls slope mesially. Cavity is primarily within mesial half of tooth, but is extensive enough to allow positioning of instruments and filling materials. Further exploration should determine whether fourth canal can be found in distal. In that case an orifice will be positioned at each angle of rhomboid.

PLATE XXV

Length of Tooth[3]		*Canals*[13] *Mesial Canals*		*Distal Canals*		*Curvature of Roots* *Direction*	*Mesial*	*Distal*	*Direction*	*Mesial*	*Distal*
Average Length	22.0 mm.	1 canal		1 canal		Straight	16%	74%	Buccal	0%	0%
Maximum Length	25.0 mm.	1 foramen	13%	1 foramen	92%	Distal	84%	21%	Lingual	0%	0%
Minimum Length	19.3 mm.	2 canals		2 canals		Mesial	0%	5%			
Range	5.7 mm.	1 foramen	49%	1 foramen	5%						
		2 canals		2 canals							
		2 foramens	38%	2 foramens	3%						

PLATE XXVI

Mandibular Second Molar

Pulp Anatomy and Coronal Preparation

A. ***Buccal*** view of recently calcified second molar with large pulp. Roentgenogram will reveal:
1. large pulp chamber
2. mesial and distal roots each ***apparently*** containing one canal
3. mesial curavature of distal root (18%)
4. bayonet curvature of mesial root (7%)
5. distal-axial inclination of ***tooth.***

These factors ***seen*** in roentgenogram are borne in mind when preparation is begun.

B. ***Mesial*** view of same tooth demonstrating details ***not apparent in roentgenogram:***
1. ***mesial*** root with ***two canals***
2. lingual curvature of mesiobuccal
3. "S" curvature of mesiolingual
4. −52-degree buccal-axial inclination of ***roots.***

These ***unseen*** factors will affect ***size, shape,*** and ***inclination*** of final preparation. Canals must be carefully explored with fine curved file. ***Double "S" curvature*** of ***mesiolingual*** canal is especially challenging. All three canals are enlarged by filing with curved files.

C. Cross section at three levels: 1, cervical; 2, mid root; and 3, apical third:
1. ***Cervical*** level: pulp, enormous in young tooth, is debrided during coronal cavity preparation with round bur.
2. ***Mid root*** level: canals are ovoid. Distal canal requires perimeter filing and filling with multiple gutta percha points.
3. ***Apical third*** level: canals are round and are filed into ***round, tapered*** preparations, which match ***round, tapered*** primary filing points. Preparations terminate at cementodentinal junction, 0.5 mm. from the apical foramens.

D. ***Distal*** view of same tooth demonstrating details ***not apparent in roentgenogram:***
1. height of the distal pulp horns
2. "ribbon-shaped" distal canal.

E. ***Buccal*** view of ***adult*** second molar with extensive secondary dentin formation. Roentgenogram will reveal:
1. pulp recession "thread-like" pulp
2. mesial and distal roots, each ***apparently*** containing one canal
3. straight distal root (58%) and distal curvature of mesial root (84%)
4. distal-axial inclination of ***tooth.***

F. ***Mesial*** view of same tooth demonstrating details ***not apparent in original roentgenogram:***
1. pulp recession
2. ***mesial*** root with ***two*** canals which join and "cross over"
3. −52-degree buccal-axial inclination of roots.

Operator should recognize that:

a. careful exploration with curved instruments is imperative
b. mesial canals curve in two directions.

G. Cross section at three levels: 1, cervical; 2, mid root; and 3, apical third:
1. ***Cervical*** level: chamber is debrided during coronal cavity preparation with round bur.
2. ***Mid root*** level: canals, only slightly ovoid in shape, will be enlarged by reaming of apical third of canals.
3. ***Apical third*** level: canals are round and are reamed into ***round, tapered*** preparation, which matches ***round, tapered*** filling points. Preparations terminate at the cementodentinal junction, 0.5 mm. from apical foramens.

H. ***Distal*** view of same tooth demonstrating details ***not apparent in roentgenogram:***
1. pulp recession
2. single distal root with usual single canal
3. buccal-axial inclination of tooth.

I. "Rhomboidal" outline form reflects anatomy of pulp chamber. Both mesial and distal walls slope mesially. Cavity is primarily within mesial half of tooth, but is extensive enough to allow positioning of instruments and filling materials. Further exploration should determine whether fourth canal can be found in distal. In that case an orifice will be found at each angle of rhomboid.

PLATE XXVI

Length of Tooth[3]		Canals[13] Mesial Canals	Canals[13] Distal Canals	Curvature of Roots Direction	Single Root	Double Root Mesial	Double Root Distal	Direction	Single Root	Double Root Mesial	Double Root Distal
Average Length	21.7 mm.	1 canal	1 canal	Straight	53%	27%	58%	Buccal	0%	4%	4%
Maximum Length	25.8 mm.	1 foramen 13%	1 foramen 92%	Distal	26%	61%	18%	Lingual	2%	0%	0%
Minimum Length	19.0 mm.	2 canals	2 canals	Mesial	0%	0%	10%	Bayonet	19%	7%	6%
Range	6.8 mm.	1 foramen 49%	1 foramen 5%								
		2 canals	2 canals								
		2 foramens 38%	2 foramens 3%								

A B C D

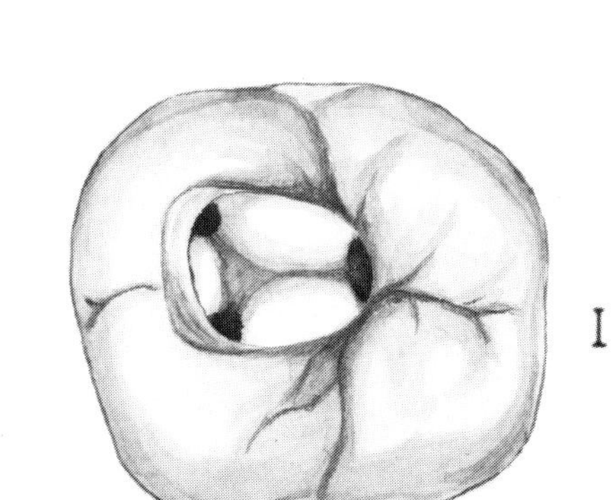

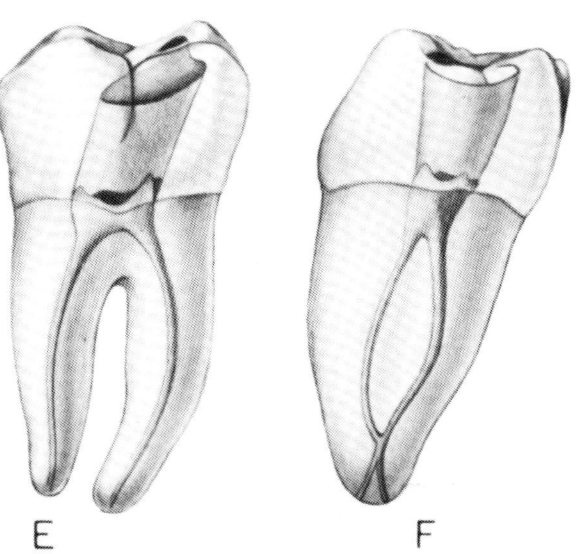

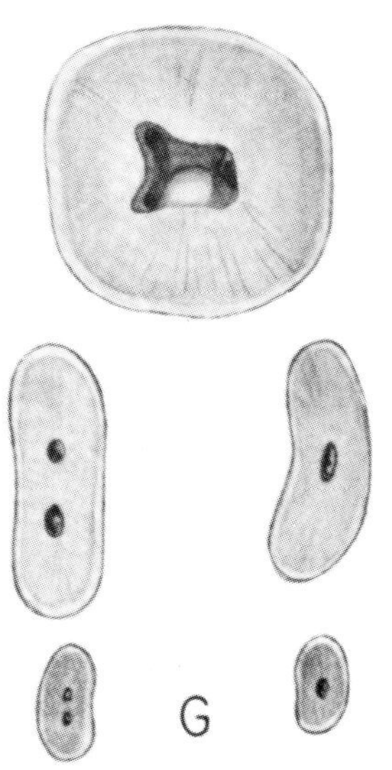

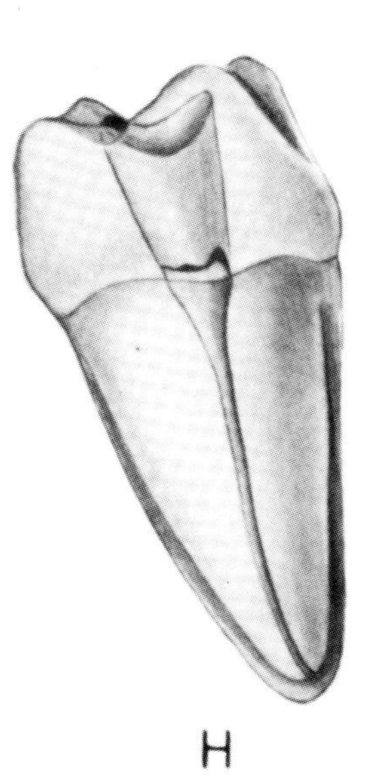

PLATE XXVII

Mandibular Molar Teeth

ERRORS in Cavity Preparation

A. OVEREXTENDED preparation undermining enamel walls. Crown is badly gouged due to failure to observe pulp recession in roentgenogram.

B. PERFORATION into furca caused by using ***surgical-length*** bur and failing to realize narrow pulp chamber had been passed.

C. PERFORATION at mesial cervical caused by failure to orient bur with long axis of molar severely ***tipped*** to mesial.

D. DISORIENTED occlusal outline form exposing only mesiobuccal canal. Faulty cavity has been prepared in full crown, which was placed to "straighten-up" lingually tipped molar (D′).

E. FAILURE to find ***second distal*** canal owing to lack of exploration for fourth canal.

F. LEDGE FORMATION caused by faulty exploration and using too large an instrument.

G. PERFORATION of curved distal root caused by using large straight instrument in severely curved canal.

PLATE XXVII

ERRORS

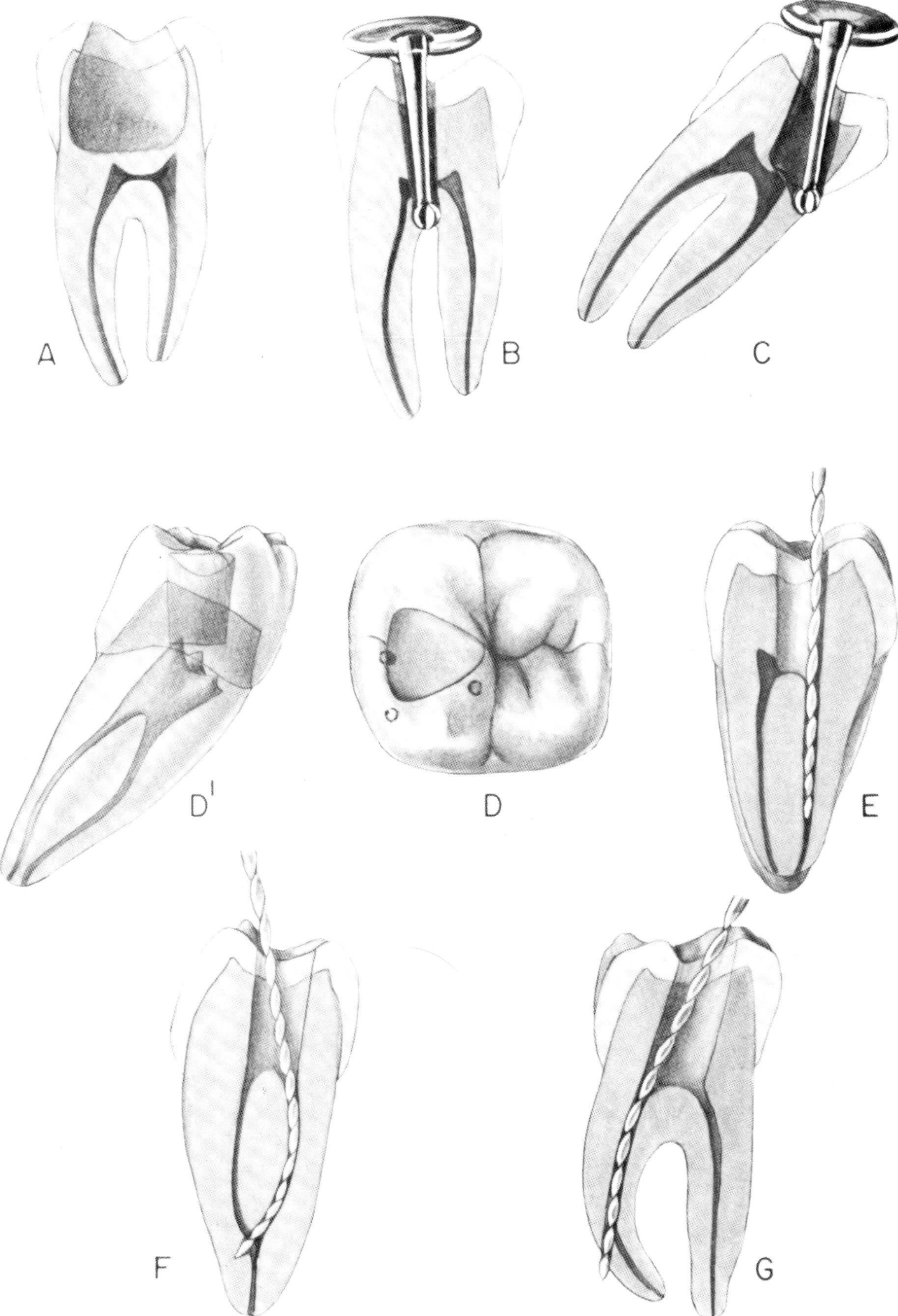

RADICULAR CAVITY PREPARATION

Objectives

With the completion of the coronal access cavity, preparation of the radicular cavity may be started. Root canal preparation has two objectives: (1) the cleaning and sanitation of the root canal system, and (2) the specific shaping of the root canal preparation to receive a specific type of filling. The ultimate objective of course is the total obturation of this designed space.

Cleaning and Sanitation of the Root Canal. This first objective is achieved by skillful instrumentation coupled with liberal irrigation. Ultimately, disinfection (hopefully sterilization) by intracanal medicaments completes the sanitation. Although mechanical debridement alone will only sterilize 4.6% of infected root canals,[14] it is still the principal method used to remove the majority of the debris and bacteria from the canal. This process is likened to the removal of the ***carious*** dentin in a restorative cavity preparation, i.e., enough of the dentinal wall of the canal must be removed to eliminate the attached necrotic debris, and insofar as possible, the bacteria and debris found in the dentinal tubuli (Fig. 3–8). Clean white dentin filings, in contrast to the earlier brown or "muddy" filings, must be seen to emerge when proper debridement is accomplished (Fig. 3–9). The debriding instruments, files and reamers, are to be constantly cleaned during use (Fig. 3–10). A sterile cotton roll, indented at one end and dipped in a germicide to prevent the loose fibers from clinging to the blades, is used to wipe the instruments. The color of the debris should finally match the white cotton.

Specific Shaping for a Specific Filling. The basis for this objective is the premise that the anatomic configuration of the canal (shape, size, and curvature) predetermines the enlarging technique and filling materials to be used. Again, this may be compared to restorative cavity preparations which vary according to the condition of the crown and the filling material (gold, silver, or plastic) to be used. The ultimate objective in either case, crown or root, is the total obturation of the prepared space.

Principles

Returning now to Black's Principles, the intraradicular cavity is prepared with the following principles in mind:

IV. Toilet of the cavity (continued)
V. Retention form
VI. Resistance form

In Figure 3–11 the entire endodontic cavity preparation is illustrated, from ***outline form*** at the enamel's edge to ***resistance form*** at the apical foramen (Fig. 3–11*A*). ***Retention form*** (Fig. 3–11*B*) is prepared in the apical 2 to 5 mm. of the cavity. The remainder of the preparation falls under the rubric, ***toilet of the cavity*** (Fig. 3–11*C*). At the margin of the cavity, the ***outline form*** must be continually evaluated as instrumentation or obturation proceeds. Access may have to be expanded by ***convenience form*** alteration (Fig. 3–11*D*) as larger, less flexible instruments are used.

The size and shape of the entire preparation is related to the internal anatomy of the pulp, but is modified throughout its length to accommodate the instruments and filling materials to be used in debridement and obturation. The total preparation, crown or apex, may be considered ***extension for prevention*** (Fig. 3–11*E*), that is, prevention of future periapical infection and inflammation.

Principle IV—Toilet of the Cavity (Continued)

Toilet of the cavity is continued from the same procedure in the crown, that is, the meticulous cleansing of the walls of the preparation until they are glassy smooth. Prior to completing the toilet of the cavity in the coronal two-thirds of the preparation, the apical one-third has been prepared into ***retention form,*** and it too is perfectly clean. Irrigation greatly assists toilet of the cavity, flushing out the necrotic and dentinal debris that results from filing.

Principle V—Retention Form

The apical one-third of the preparation must provide 2 to 5 mm. of nearly parallel walls to ensure the firm seating of the primary filling point. This modest taper provides retention of the point, the fit of which usually can be measured by the "tug back" or resistance felt when the point is withdrawn.

This final 2 to 3 mm. of the cavity is the most crucial and calls for meticulous care in its preparation. This is where the sealing against future leakage or percolation into the canal takes place. This is also the region where accessory or lateral canals are most apt to be present.

Coronally, from the area of retention, the cavity walls are deliberately flared, in a good many prepara-

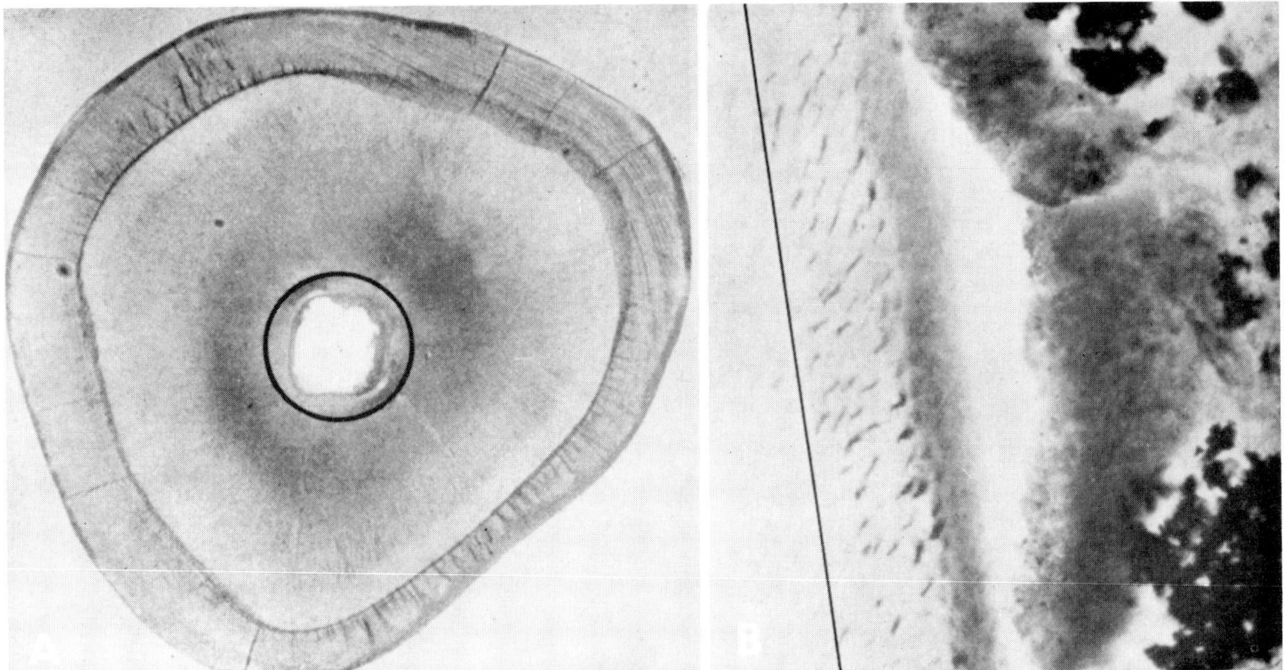

Fig. 3–8. *A,* Cross section through pulp canal showing round preparation which will remove canal debris and enough dentin to eliminate virtually all bacteria in tubuli. *B,* Cross section showing necrotic canal contents and debris-saturated dentin. Debridement of necrotic mass and instrumentation of the dentin to black line will remove necrotic and bacterial irritants from canal.

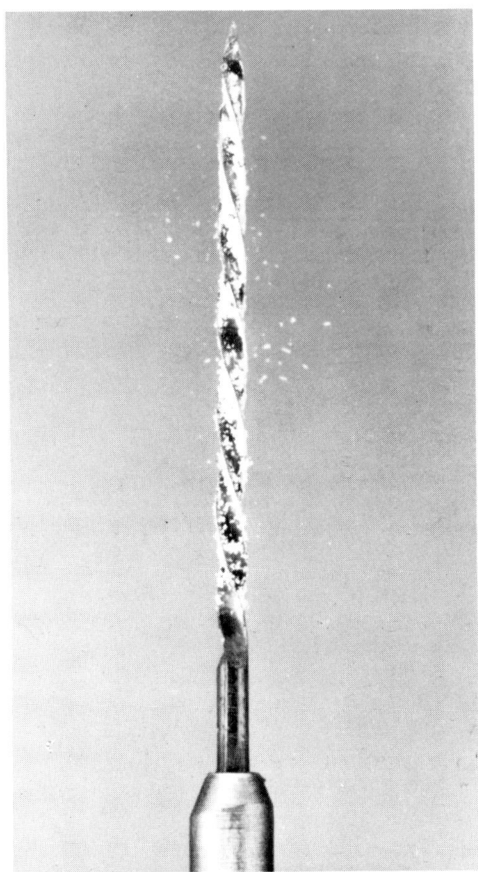

Fig. 3–9. Reamer with "clean white dentin" filings.

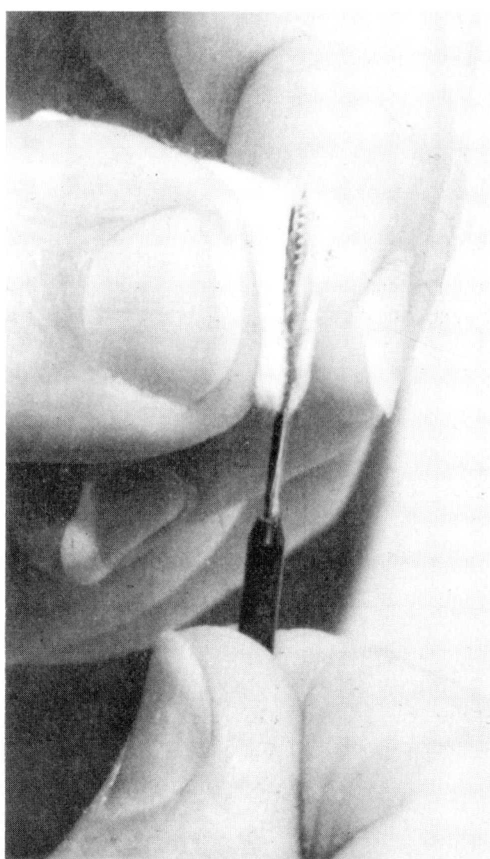

Fig. 3–10. Cleaning endodontic instrument by rotating through moistened, sterile cotton roll. Instrumentation is continued as long as cuttings on cotton roll appear dark or muddy.

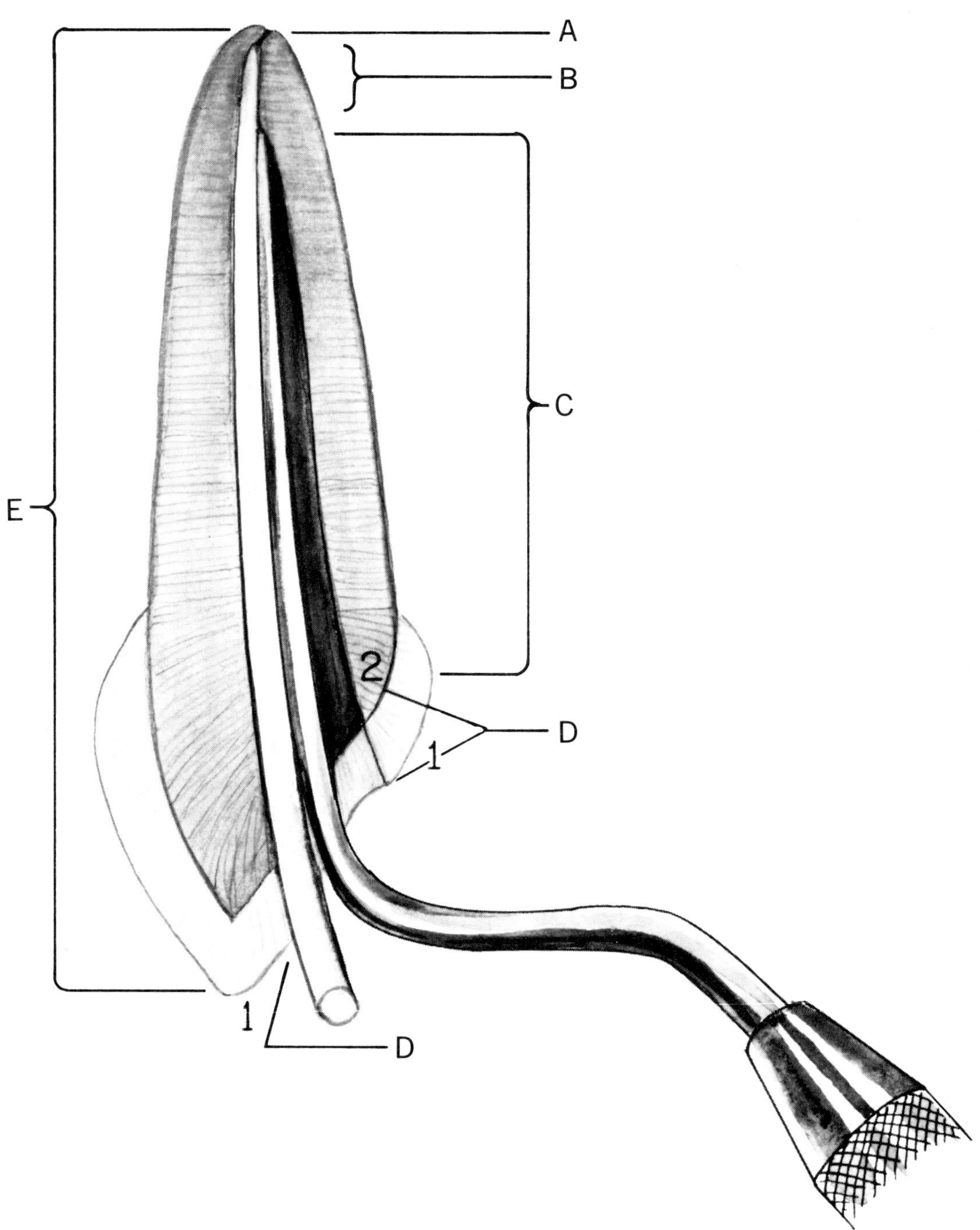

Fig. 3–11. Concept of total endodontic cavity preparation, coronal and radicular, based on Black's principles. Beginning at apex: *A, Resistance Form*—retaining or improving apical foramen to resist extrusion of filling material. *B, Retention Form*—to retain primary filling point in fully enlarged cavity from which all debris and necrotic dentin are removed in round preparation. The most critical 2 to 5 mm. of entire preparation. *C, Toilet of the Cavity*—extending from Resistance Form cavity through chamber. All debris and necrotic dentin are removed to "clean white dentin," walls filed glassy smooth. *D, Outline Form*—is subject to revision as needs present, such as larger less flexible instruments and filling materials. Internal modifications at D2. External modifications at D1 change Outline Form. *E, Extension for Prevention*—Basic preparation throughout its length is dictated by canal anatomy. Properly executed preparation is prevention against future breakdowns. (Courtesy Dr. James D. Zidell and USC Department of Endodontics, June, 1970.)

tions, during ***toilet of the cavity.*** The degree of flare will vary according to the filling technique to be used—lateral condensation of gutta percha, vertical condensation of softened gutta percha, custom-tailored gutta percha or cementation of a silver point.

Principle VI—Resistance Form

Resistance to overfilling is the primary objective of ***resistance form.*** Beyond that, however, maintaining the integrity of the natural constriction of the apical foramen is a key to successful therapy. Violating this integrity by overinstrumentation leads to complications: (1) acute inflammation of the periapical tissue from the injury inflicted by the instruments or canal debris forced into the tissue, (2) chronic inflammation of this tissue caused by the presence of a foreign body—the filling material forced there during obturation, and (3) the inability to compress the root canal filling because of the loss of the limiting apical termination of the cavity. This could be compared to an attempt to place a class II amalgam filling without the limiting presence of a proximal matrix band.

In some cases—youngsters, root fractures, apical root resorption—the apical foramen is open, and these cases always present difficulties in instrumentation and obturation. Special techniques, to be discussed later, have been devised to overcome the loss of ***resistance form.***

Kuttler has shown that the narrowest waist of the apical foramen lies at the dentinocemental junction (Fig. 3–12).[15] He established this point at approximately 0.5 mm. from the outer surface of the root in most cases. The older the patient, however, the greater this distance becomes, because continued cemental formation builds up the apex. One is also reminded that the dentinocemental junction, where ***resistance form*** is established, is the apical termination of the pulp. Beyond this point, one is dealing with the tissues of the periodontal ligament space, not the pulp.

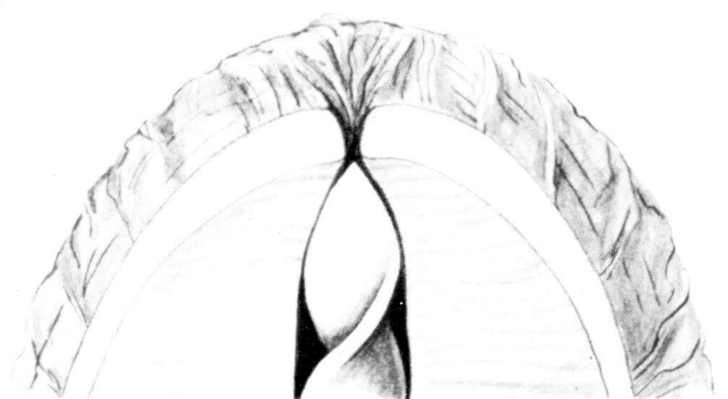

Fig. 3–12. Instruments and filling material should terminate at cementodentinal junction, narrowest width of canal and its termination at foramen. This point is often 0.5 mm. from apex; however, canal need not terminate at exact root end.

The fact must also be established that the apical ***foramen*** does not always lie at the exact apex of the root. Often, canals exit laterally, short of the apex seen in the roentgenogram. This may be revealed by careful scrutiny of the film with a magnifying glass, or by placing a curved exploratory instrument to the exact ***canal*** length and repeating the x-ray examination.

Extension for Prevention

Seidler has described the ***ideal*** endodontic cavity as a round, evenly tapered space with a minimal opening at the foramen.[16] Because one is working with round tapered materials, one would think this ideal is easily achieved, particularly when one thinks of root canals as naturally round and tapered. As we have seen from the anatomic drawings in this chapter, however, few canals are round throughout their length. Thus we usually must compromise from the ideal, attempting to prepare the round tapered cavity, but knowing that filling techniques must be used to make up for the variance from ideal. This is why single-point fillings, be they of silver or gutta percha, are seldom used now.

The ***extension*** of the cavity preparation throughout its entire length and breadth is necessary, however, to ensure ***prevention*** of future problems. Peripheral enlargement of the canal, to remove all the debris, followed by total obturation is the primary preventive method. Techniques that achieve less than this are doomed to oblivion. The recent popularization of a technique dependent on root cavity preparation with power-driven instruments, followed by a paste filling squirted or whipped into a partially prepared canal, is forecast for failure—not this year or next—but long-term failure. The slipshod perversion of proper methods is compared to toy manufacture. A toy made of papier mâché or cheap plastic will last for only a while, but the properly made steel toy may be passed to the next generation. We owe our patients at least this—longevity of our dental services.

Instruments and Methods for Radicular Cleaning and Shaping

Before launching into a detailed or even a broad discussion of the methods and shapes of canal cavity preparation, a description of the instruments and methods used in cleaning and shaping the canal is necessary. "The order of their appearance" during preparation will also be discussed: basic endodontic instruments; irrigation; exploration for canal orifices; pulpectomy; exploration of the canal; and length of tooth determination. The techniques of intraradicular cavity preparation will follow in detail.

Basic Endodontic Instruments

Endodontic instruments are manufactured in carbon or stainless steel and produced in four basic types: reamers, files, drills, or broaches. They can be powered by two sources: hand-powered or engine-driven. The hand-powered instruments come with two types of handles: short handles (style B) in plastic or metal, and long handles (style D) in metal. The engine-driven instruments fit a contra-angle handpiece.

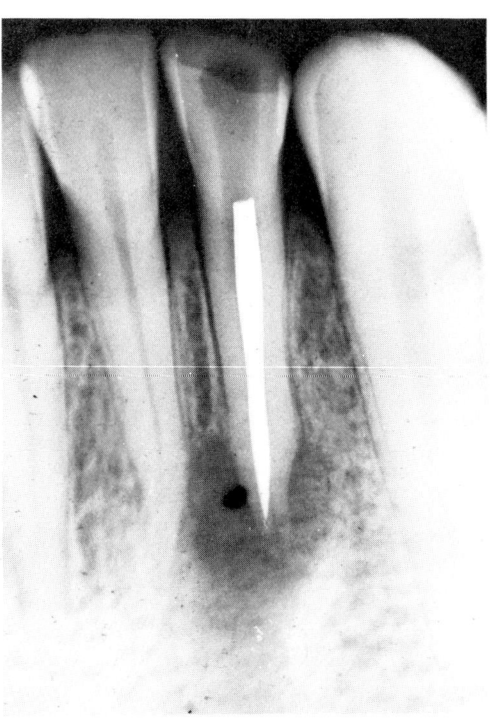

Fig. 3–13. Peeso drill fractured in canal. If drill is impossible to remove but loose in canal, foramen should be closed with a retrofilling. (Courtesy Dr. Enrique Garcia, Bogota, Columbia.)

Despite the recent flurry of interest in the engine-driven instruments, few situations arise in which these dangerous instruments may be used safely (Fig. 3–13). First, they are less flexible than the hand-powered instruments and generally can only be used in perfectly straight canals. Second, there is a loss of tactile sensation with engine-powered instruments. Working "blind" in the canal, the dentist must depend upon sensation transmitted through his fingers, as instruments encounter unexpected curves or obstructions. In addition, the engine-powered instruments only drill down through the center of the ovoid part of the canal, ignoring the surrounding debris and bacteria.

In short, the canals most apt to have a round lumen throughout their length, where these high-powered drills might be used, are curved, and the uncontrolled drill would probably perforate the root. On the other hand, the perfectly straight canals in which these instruments might be used are usually ovoid, and the perfectly round drill does not reach the mass of debris around the perimeter of the ovoid canal. This toxic debris is best removed by filing, and engine-driven instruments only ream or drill.

A different type of engine-powered handpiece, with a reciprocating quarter-turn motion, has also been highly touted of late. Using conventional broaches or Hedstrom style files, great claims are made for the ***speed*** of operation afforded by this instrument.[17] Dihn has shown that cavities prepared into perfect roundness by means of hand instruments used in a reaming action will be converted to an irregular shape (Fig. 3–14),[18] if the cavity is reworked with a power-driven Hedstrom file as recommended by Sargenti.[17] O'Connell and his associates also found that "conventional ***hand*** instrumentation proved to be superior and required approximately the same amount of time as automated instrumentation."[19]

More recently, K-style reamers have been recommended for endodontic handpieces.[20] Again, this handpiece drills and does not file. The claim is made that this instrument will drill out the apical third of the canal in preparation for immediate filling. The ovoid portion of the canal is then to be debrided with a conventional reamer spinning full circle in a regular handpiece. The contention that the reamer functions by side cutting action is not borne out by fact. More investigation needs to be done on these latest

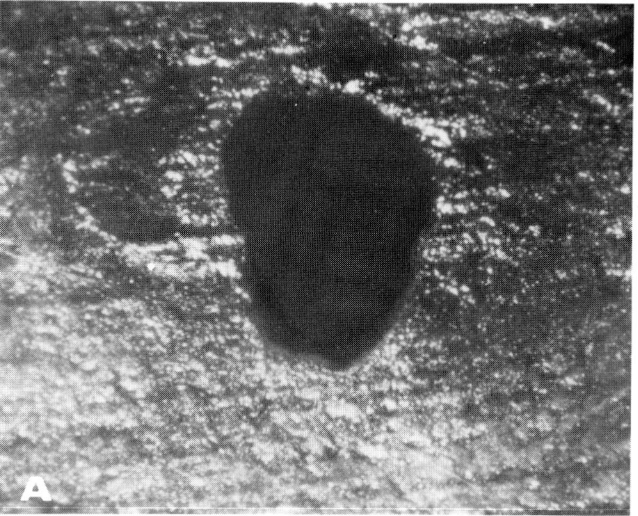

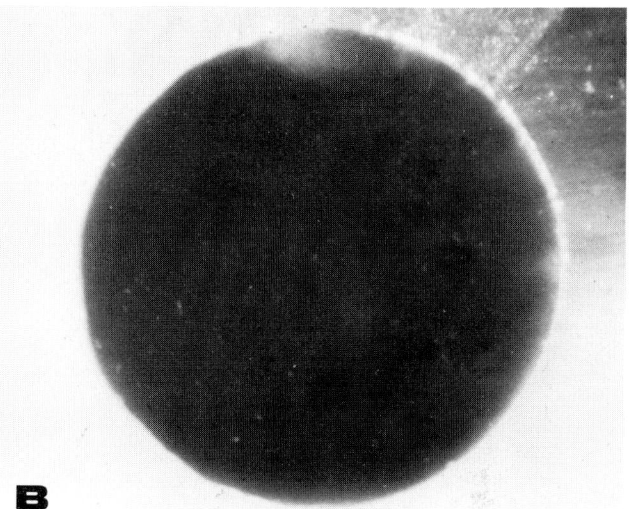

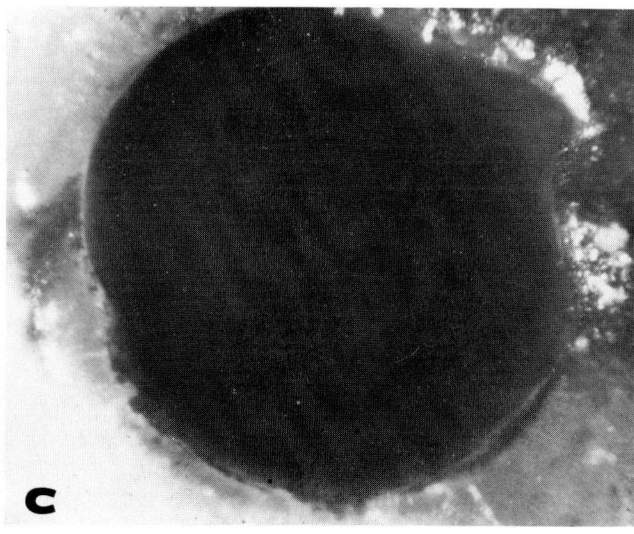

Fig. 3–14. *A,* Cross section of tooth exposing lumen of canal 2 mm. from apex. Uninstrumented lumen is here 0.32 × 0.48 mm. *B,* Lumen of canal prepared by hand reaming 0.70 × 0.70 mm. *C,* Same lumen after continued preparation with Giromatic instruments is now 0.70 × 0.75 mm. Development of perfect round shape with hand instruments and loss of roundness from power-driven instruments is dramatic. (Courtesy Dr. Quan Dihn, Master's Degree Thesis, University of Minnesota, 1972.)

recommendations for the use of power-driven instruments.

The secret, of course, of using hand-powered instruments is to use sharp instruments and to be organized in their use. Working with an assistant, the accomplished dentist can cleanse and shape a root canal in a matter of minutes. Most of the time lost in endodontics does not relate to the slowness of hand-powered energy as compared to engine-powered energy, but rather to disorganization. In fact, endodontics was one of the first disciplines in dentistry to recognize the importance of four-handed dental care, prepackaged and sterilized trays set-up for any situation, and the time value of disposable supplies, including files and reamers.

Files and Reamers. Most reamers are manufactured by pulling and twisting a ***triangular*** wire into a ***sharpened*** tapered instrument of gradual spirals (Fig. 3–15). Most files are produced by twisting ***square*** wire into a tapered pointed instrument of much tighter spirals than the reamer (Fig. 3–15). Reamers can only be used for reaming, but files can be used for both reaming and filing. These conventional instruments are made with sharp points, but are available "bull-nosed" as well. Many dentists report the use of ***files only***, but use these instruments alternately with a filing and reaming action.

The ***reaming*** action from both reamers and files is accomplished by three motions: (1) penetration, (2) rotation, and (3) retraction.[21] ***Penetration*** is accomplished by ***forcibly*** pushing and gradually rotating the instrument down the canal until it is tightly in place at the full depth at which it is to be used. For the second step, ***rotation***, the instrument is "set" in the dentin by rotating the handle clockwise one-quarter to one-half turn. While under this tension the

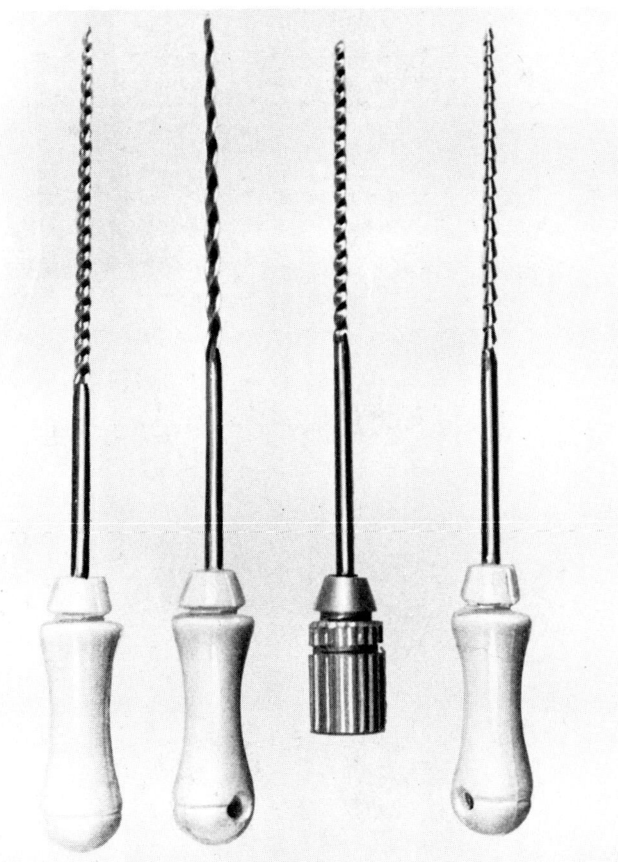

Fig. 3–15. Endodontic instruments, "K-type," style B (short handle), stainless steel with plastic and conventional handles. *Left to right:* file, reamer, batt file (bull-nosed), and Hedstrom file. (Courtesy Star Dental Manufacturing Co.)

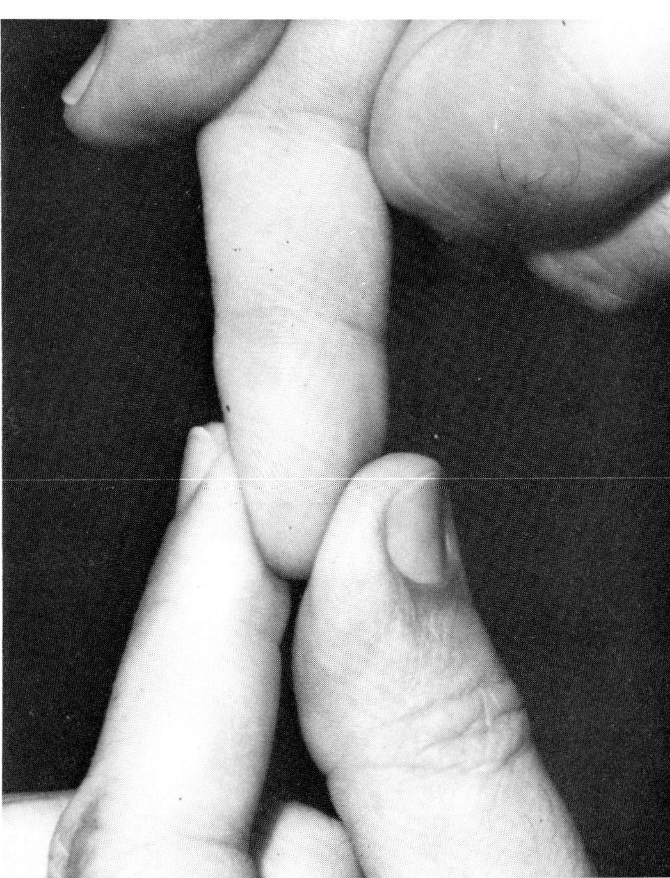

Fig. 3–16. Demonstration of sensation of endodontic instrument which is "set" into dentin walls during reaming action.

instrument is then forcibly withdrawn. This is the ***retraction*** stage, when the cutting blades, locked in the dentin wall, remove the dentin. The tactile sensation of an endodontic instrument "set" into the dentin walls in the canal may be gained by pinching one index finger between the thumb and forefinger of the opposite hand and then rotating the extended finger (Fig. 3–16).

Initially rotating the instrument more than one-half turn while it is locked in place may break the instrument. As it loosens, it may be safely turned a full turn or more, serving as a drill. Luks has shown that the smaller reamers and files may be easily broken by twisting the blades beyond the limits of the metal until the metal separates.[22] Gutierrez, of Concepcion, Chile, has evaluated instruments as they arrived from the United States manufacturer, and as they were used.[23] He found that, in general, new instruments, except for some minor manufacturing burs along the blades, were well made and sharp (Fig. 3–17*A*). Using the instruments, on the other hand, caused great change related to locking and twisting. Since instruments are made by twisting the square steel in a *counter-clockwise* direction, locking the instrument in dentin and twisting clockwise could cause what he termed "elongation" from unwinding (Fig. 3–17*B*). Locking and twisting counter-clockwise, on the other hand, only tightens the fluting and causes "roll-up" and shortening* (Fig. 3–17*C*). The illustrations also show the loss of blade cutting edge and the blunting of the tip, both of which attest to the futility of continued instrument use after dulling. Eventually, cracks developed in the metal (Fig. 3–17*D*) which would finally lead to breakage and all its attendant problems. If the instrument is loose enough to be twisted in the canal, it cannot be broken by this action; on the other hand, neither is it functioning.

In a subsequent study,[24] Gutierrez also demonstrated the destructive effect sodium hypochlorite, the most commonly used root canal irrigating solution, has upon carbon steel endodontic instruments. Starting with new instruments, Gutierrez observed under magnification the rapid destruction of carbon steel by the sodium hypochlorite. Within 20 seconds deterioration had started. In 20 minutes huge rust

*Researchers at Northwestern University recently demonstrated that "endodontic files twisted in a counterclockwise manner were extremely brittle in comparison to those twisted in a clockwise manner." They warned that dentists "should excercise caution when 'backing-off' embedded root canal instruments during the cleansing and shaping of the root canal." Chernick, L. B., Jacobs, J. J., Lautenschlager, E. P. and Heuer, M. A.: Torsional failure of endodontic files. J.O.E., *2*:94, April, 1976.

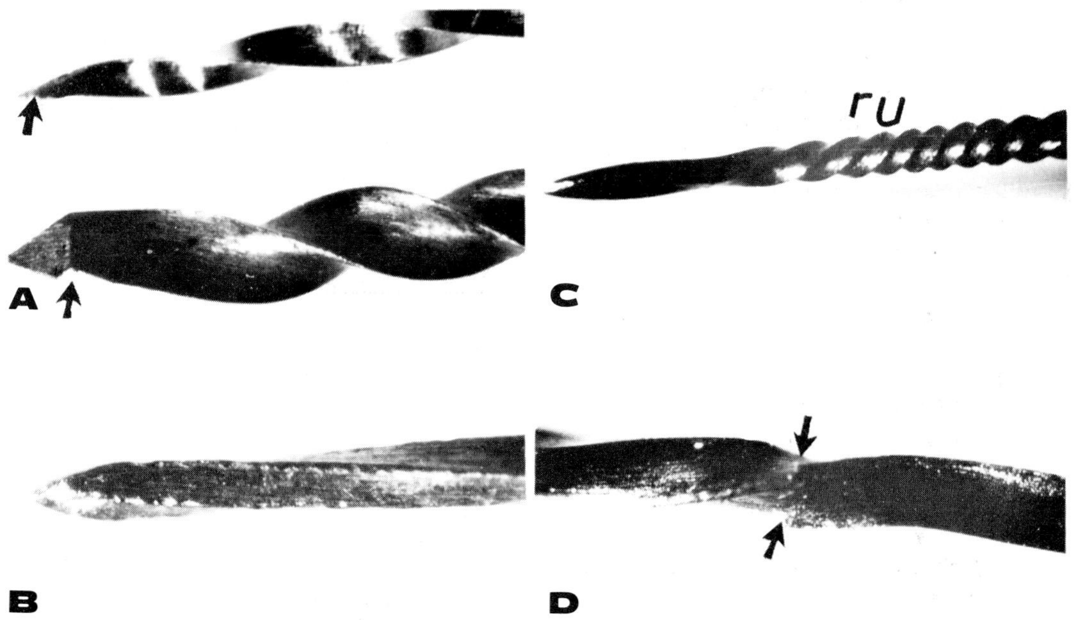

Fig. 3–17. *A,* New instruments are well made and sharp with only minor burs present. *B*, Elongation and unwinding caused by locking and twisting clockwise., Note blade dullness. *C*, Roll-up at "ru" caused by locking and twisting counter-clockwise. Roll-up tightens fluting and shortens instruments. Note dullness of blade. *D*, Crack in blade of reamer caused by stress from incorrect use. Instrument is ready to separate. (From Gutierrez, J. H., Gigoux, C., and Sanhueza, I.: Oral Surg., *28*:394, Sept., 1969.)

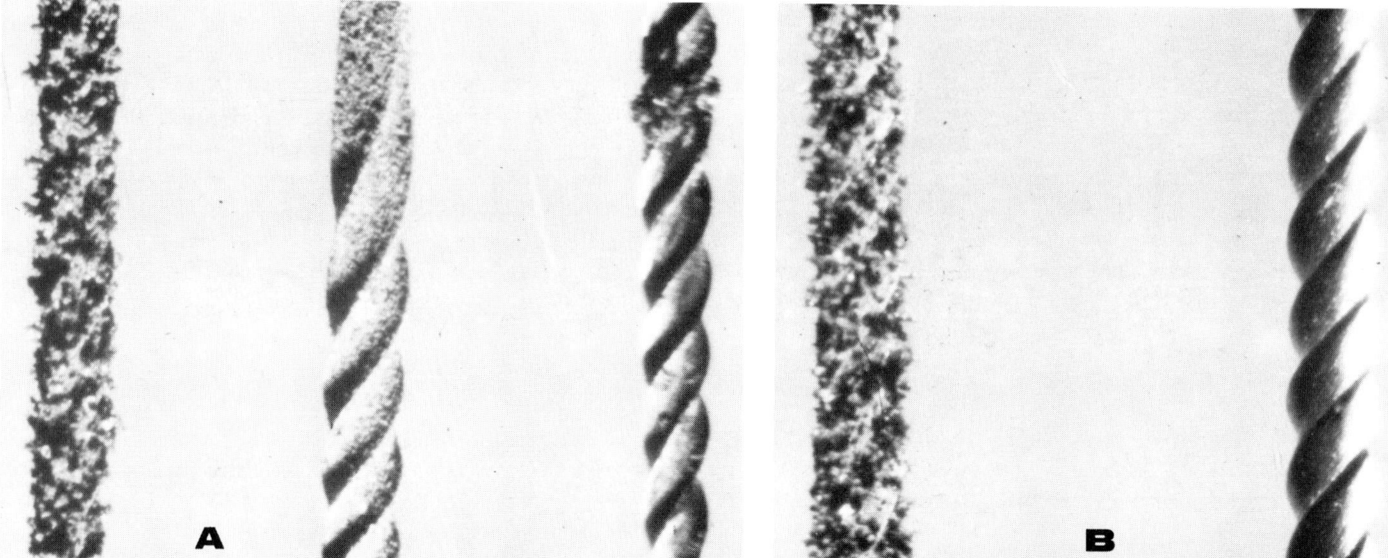

Fig. 3–18. *A,* Carbon steel endodontic instruments corroded by irrigating solution. *Left:* 5% sodium hypochlorite plus collagen. *Middle:* 1.6% sodium hypochlorite plus collagen. *Right:* 5% sodium hypochlorite alone. *B,* Instruments immersed in 5% sodium hypochlorite plus collagen. *Left:* carbon steel instrument. *Right:* stainless steel instrument. (Courtesy Dr. Marvin Eichner and Dr. David Schoen, submitted for publication, April, 1975.)

blisters had formed, and in 120 minutes the instrument was totally destroyed as such. Eichner and Schoen have shown the corrosive effect of sodium hypochlorite to be alarmingly increased within the root canal.[25] Research showed it was a combination of the sodium hypochlorite plus the collagen from the dentin that produced the violent reaction (Fig. 3–18). Corrosive material from the instruments was often left behind in the canal. Stainless instruments did not corrode. Again, the reader is urged to throw away used carbon steel instruments.

The penetration of the instrument down the canal by forcibly ***pushing*** and gently rotating the instrument back and forth deserves emphasis, for this is one aspect of instrument use which is grossly overlooked. The instrument may have to cut its way down the canal, but usually it is a matter of ***pushing*** the instrument to full depth before making the cut. This action will greatly reduce the formation of ledges or steps in the canal, so conducive to failure.

The endodontic ***file*** may be used in the reaming or drilling action, as described, or it may be used as files and rasps have always been used, that is, in a push-pull motion with the blades set to cut on either the push or the pull. In the ***filing action*** the instruments are used in the ovoid portion of the canals, where reamers do not adapt nor function.

Files are produced in two different designs: either the Kerr-type (K-type) file with narrow spirals, or the Hedstrom file which has the blades cut to resemble an inclined screw (Fig. 3–15). Because of its design the Hedstrom file requires more finesse in handling. In addition, it is difficult to ream or drill with the instrument, for it becomes "set" so completely in the dentin walls it cannot be removed with a pull stroke, but must be "backed-off" as a screw and then removed. In this situation it does not cut. Because of these objections, the K-type instrument is more universally used, although for wide uncomplicated canals the Hedstrom file is the more aggressive instrument.

Files used in rasping have generally the disadvantage of packing dentin filings ahead of the instrument, thus blocking the canal. Filing must therefore be followed by irrigation and reaming to clear the canal. Because of their closely packed blade design, files are more apt to force debris from the apical foramen when used as a rasp or drill in the apical one-third of the canal (Fig. 3–19).

The delicate Kerr type ***files,*** on the other hand, ***have a definite advantage over reamers as a pathfinding*** instrument in fine canals. Because of the closely packed spirals, fine files have more stability and are less apt to roll-up or bend as they are forced down the

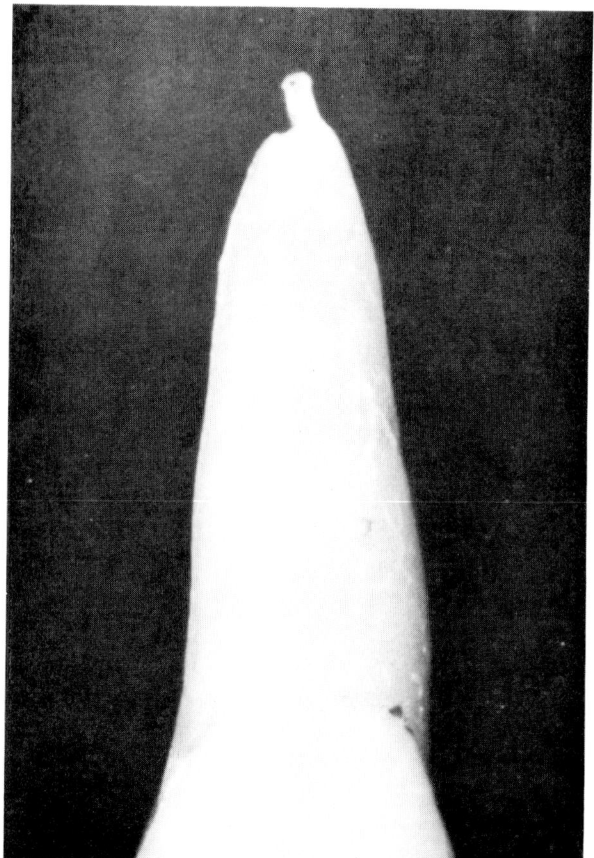

Fig. 3–19. "Worm" of necrotic debris which has been forced from apex during canal enlargement. This mass of material could contain millions of bacteria which would act as nidus for acute apical abscess.

canal. Furthermore, files will cut their way while penetrating the tight canal, whereas reamers have to be twisted to function, an action that may cut a ledge in the canal wall or break the fine instrument.

To summarize the basic action of files and reamers, it may be stated that ***either*** files or reamers are used to ream out or drill the round, tapered apical cavity, and that files, in addition, are used as a push-pull instrument to enlarge certain curved canals as well as the ovoid portion of large canals.

It goes without saying that instrumentation coupled with irrigation is much more effective than instrumentation alone. In addition, constant cleansing of the instruments in a moist cotton roll is necessary to clear the blades and prevent packing through the foramen. The dentist should develop the habit of working with the instrument in one hand and the cotton roll in the other. If the coronal preparation is accurate, the mouth mirror is not needed, and the left hand is thus free for holding the cotton roll.

Endodontic Instrument Standardization. Until recently, endodontic instruments, like most dental instruments, were not standardized in size or shape. Actually, the problem was more severe than this, for the instrument numbering system was entirely arbitrary: there was little uniformity in quality control of manufacture; no uniformity existed in progression from one instrument to the next; and there was no correlation of ***instruments*** and ***filling materials*** in terms of size and shape.

Beginning in 1955 a serious attempt was made to correct these abuses, and a new line of standardized instruments and filling material was introduced to the profession:[26–29]

1. A formula for the diameter and taper in each size instrument and filling material was agreed upon.
2. A formula for a graduated increment in size from one instrument to the next was developed.
3. A new instrument-numbering system based on instrument diameter was established.

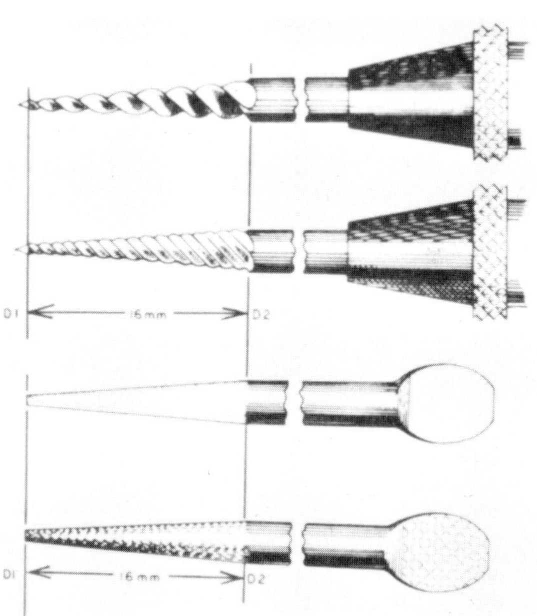

Fig. 3–20. Standardized instruments with cutting blades 16 mm. in length are same size and numbers as standardized filling points. Number of instrument is determined by diameter size at D_1 in tenths of millimeters. Diameter 2 (D_2) is uniformly 0.32 mm. greater than D_1. (From Ingle, J. I.: *Transactions of the Second International Conference on Endodontics.)*

A new numbering system, using numbers from 10 to 100, was developed. The new numbers of the instruments and filling points were not just arbitrary figures, but were based on the diameter of the instruments in tenths of millimeters at the beginning of the tip of the blades, a point called D_1—diameter 1 (Fig. 3–20), and extending up the blades to the end point of the blades at D_2—diameter 2—16 mm. in length. Initially, only one manufacturer-distributor would produce the standardized instruments which called for a "considerable investment in new dies and machinery to produce them."[30] Eventually all manufacturers, worldwide, accepted the new sizing, but great variance continued to exist in standards and quality control.

In order to maintain standards, the American Association of Endodontists urged the American Dental Association and the United States Bureau of Standards to appoint a committee on Endodontic Instrument Standardization, and this was done. This pioneering effort was followed by a worldwide committee formed by the *Federation Dentaire Internationale* in collaboration with the World Health Organization. As an outgrowth of the work of these national and international committees, international

Table 3–1. Dimensions (in mm.)[31]

Size	*Dimension D_1 (Tolerance ± 0.020 mm.)*	*Dimension D_2 (Tolerance ± 0.020 mm.)*
10	0.100	0.420
15	0.150	0.470
20	0.200	0.520
25	0.250	0.570
30	0.300	0.620
35	0.350	0.670
40	0.400	0.720
45	0.450	0.770
50	0.500	0.820
55	0.550	0.870
60	0.600	0.920
70	0.700	1.020
80	0.800	1.120
90	0.900	1.220
100	1.000	1.320
110	1.100	1.420
120	1.200	1.520
130	1.300	1.620
140	1.400	1.720

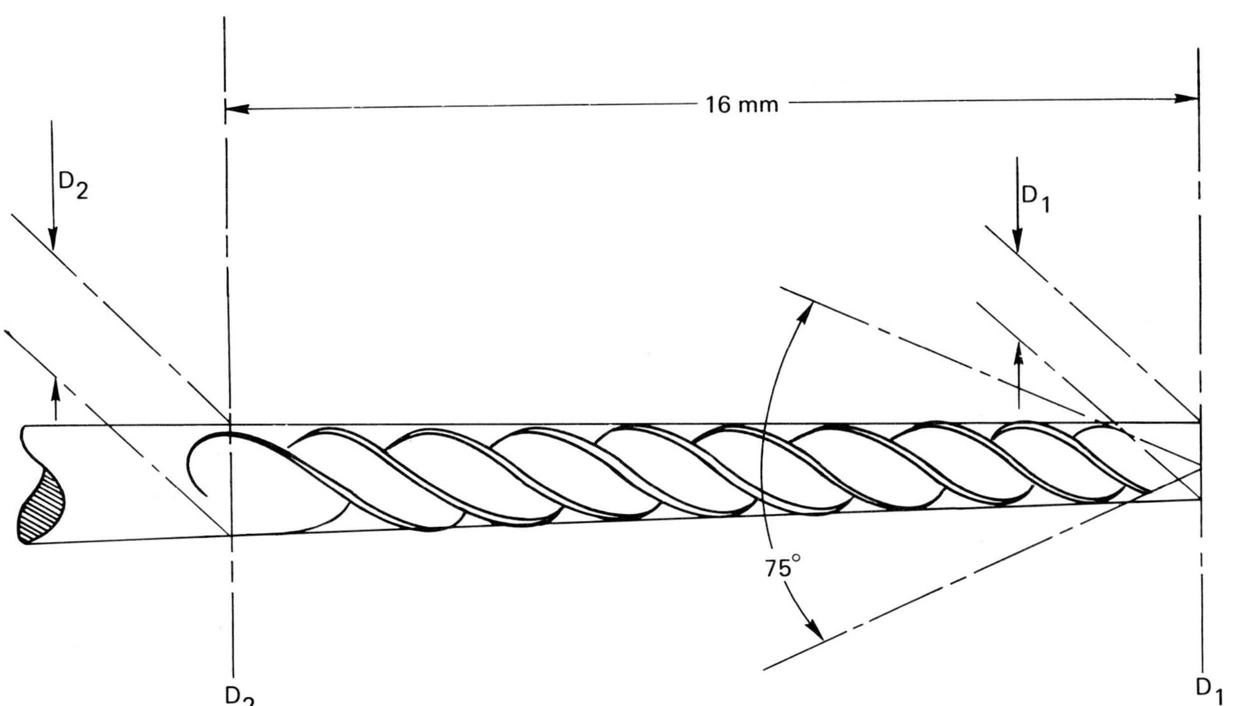

Fig. 3–21. Official endodontic instrument specifications drawn up by FDI–WHO–ADA–AAE standardization committee. Tip of instrument shall be ground at 75-degree angle. There shall be gain in diameter of 0.02 mm. per mm. of shaft.

specifications have been developed by slightly modifying Ingle's original standardization.[28]

Requirements for standardized instruments have been established for: diameter, length, resistance to fracture, stiffness, and resistance to corrosion. These "specs" apply only to "K" type instruments, not to Hedstrom files or to rasps, broaches, or filling materials.

"The dimensions for ***diameter*** are shown in Table 3–1. Manufacturing tolerances of plus or minus 20 microns were allowed. The ***taper*** of the spiral cutting section of the file or reamer shall be a gain of 0.02 mm. per mm. of shaft length. The ***tip*** of the instrument shall be an included angle of 75 degrees with an allowable tolerance of plus or minus 15 degrees (Fig. 3–21). The length of the spiral cutting section of the instrument shall be not less than 16 mm."[31]

The standard instrument length is 25 mm. from the tip of the instrument to the hub. Some teeth, particularly canines, and occasionally maxillary incisors, will be much longer than this standard length. For this additional length, instruments as long as 31 mm. are available. It is highly advisable not to attempt treatment with inadequate instrument lengths, even though it may be necessary to order and wait for new instruments.

In some instances, particularly in treating second molars, there is inadequate intermaxillary space to perform instrumentation easily with standard-length reamers and files. For these situations, 21 mm. instruments are indicated even though, again, ordering them might entail a temporary delay in treatment.

In addition to establishing international standards for dimensions, the FDI-WHO-ADA collaborative committee developed the standards, testing equipment, and tests for resistance to fracture-by-twisting for every size instrument. Standards and tests to measure stiffness for each size have also been established, along with standards for resistance to corrosion using copper sulfate solution and potassium ferricyanide as corrosive agents. International standards for packaging, lot numbers, length of instrument from handle to tip, and handle color coding for size identification were also set down (Table 3–2).[31] No corrosion of steel instruments is allowable, although it was accepted that carbon steel would corrode and rust under virtually all chemicals. No tests for sharpness were devised, although this is being considered.

Some individual attempts have been made to determine the cutting efficiency of endodontic instruments. Oliet and Sorin evaluated endodontic reamers from four different manufacturers and found "considerable variation in the quality, sharpness of the cutting edges, cross-sectional configuration, and number of flutes" of the 147 different reamers tested.[32] They further found that "***triangular*** cross-sectional reamers cut with greater efficiency than do the ***square*** cross-sectional reamers," but the failure rate of the triangular instruments was considerably higher. Carbon steel instruments also outperformed stainless steel instruments.

In making their tests they found that frequent cleaning and debriding (recapitulation) of the test holes (in bovine bone) were necessary in order to maintain the cutting efficiency of the instruments. They found further that "wear does not appear to be a factor in instrument function, but rather instruments generally fail because of deformation or fracture of the blades. Once an instrument became permanently distorted, additional rotation only caused additional distortion, with minimum cutting frequently leading to fracture." Jungmann et al. found that K-style files used in a reaming action produced the roundest preparations in the apical third of the canal.[33]

No attempt has been made by the FDI-WHO-ADA Task Force to establish specifications for filling materials. However, several manufacturers under-

Table 3–2. Color Coding[31]

Size	*Color*	*Abbreviation*
10	Purple	Pur
15	White	Wh
20	Yellow	Yel
25	Red	Red
30	Blue	Blu
35	Green	Grn
40	Black	Bkl
45	White	Wh
50	Yellow	Yel
55	Red	Red
60	Blue	Blu
70	Green	Grn
80	Black	Blk
90	White	Wh
100	Yellow	Yel
110	Red	Red
120	Blue	Blu
130	Green	Grn
140	Black	Blk

took matching silver points to standardized instrument size following the original recommendations by Ingle.[28] The overall diameter of the silver points was made about 9 microns (0.009 mm.) smaller than the enlarging instruments. This difference in size compensates for the thickness of the cementing medium, for dentin compressibility, and for the common failure on the part of the operator to utilize the instrument to the utmost.

Later attempts have been made to standardize gutta percha points, but these are less exact because of the compressibility of the material (which is one of its virtues). Standardization, according to instrument size, of endodontic implants as well as restorative dowels was a natural development.

Although instruments throughout the world are now manufactured to these specifications, there is no agency responsible for maintenance of standards or quality control. This will be the next step in the quest for international standardization.

Barbed Broaches. Barbed broaches are short-handled instruments used primarily for extirpation of the vital pulp. They are also occasionally used to loosen debris in necrotic canals or to remove paper points or cotton pellets from within the root canal. They are manufactured from a round wire whose smooth surface has been notched to form barbs bent at an angle from the long axis. These barbs are used to engage the pulp as the broach is carefully rotated within the canal until it begins to meet resistance against the walls of the canal. The broach should never be forced into a canal beyond the length where it first begins to bind. The proper use of this instrument will be described in the section to follow on pulpectomy.

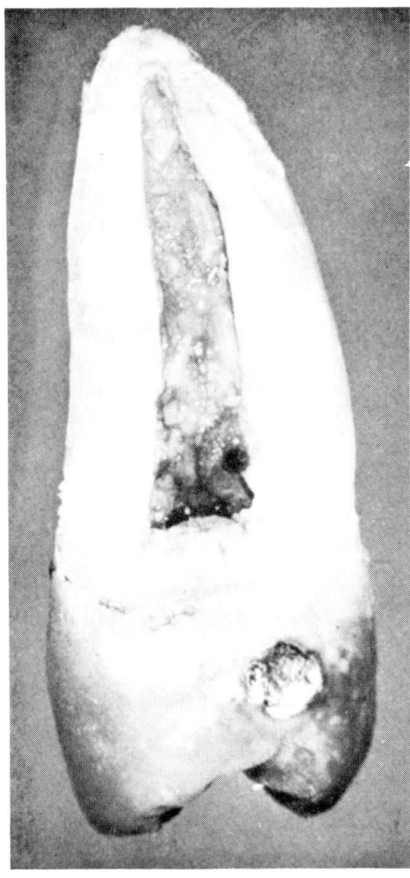

Fig. 3–22. Gelatinous mass of necrotic debris should be eliminated from pulp canal before instrumentation is started. Forcing this noxious material through apical foramen might lead to acute apical abscess.

Irrigation

Chemical Debridement

The pulp chamber and root canals of untreated nonvital teeth are filled either with a gelatinous mass of necrotic pulp remnants and tissue fluid (Fig. 3–22), or with shreds of dry mummified tissue. An instrument thrust into the canal is likely to force some of this noxious material through the apical foramen, and periapical infection or apical periodontitis may result. For that reason, prior to and at frequent intervals during instrumentation, the canals are washed out or irrigated with a solution capable of disinfecting and dissolving organic matter. If a bacteriologic culture is desired, a specimen must be taken before irrigation, since the microbial flora of the canal will be materially reduced by this action. Irrigation serves the additional purpose of facilitating instrumentation by lubricating canal walls and by removing dentin filings from the canals. Total debridement of the pulp chamber and canals is a most important aspect of endodontic treatment.

Any acceptable irrigating solution is used. None provides the spectacular pyrotechnics observed by Schreier (1893), who removed necrotic tissues by introducing potassium and sodium crystals into root canals.[34] Aqueous hydrogen peroxide (3%) will effectively "bubble" out debris and mildly disinfect the canal.[35] Alternating solutions of hydrogen peroxide and sodium hypochlorite (5% or less) causes a violent release of nascent oxygen. This combination is especially useful when much debris has accumulated in the pulp cavity. Hydrogen peroxide is sometimes combined with lubricating and chelating agents (Glyoxide and RC Prep), which are used to facilitate instrumentation. It must be remembered that preparations containing hydrogen peroxide must not be sealed into the canals. They must be neutralized with sodium hypochlorite irrigation or a severe pericementitis may result from the continued release of oxygen bubbles.

Chloramine-T is often used in endodontic treatment, but has little ability to dissolve necrotic tissues.[36] Solutions of quaternary ammonium compounds and antibiotics show promise,[37,38] but probably will not be widely accepted until they can be combined with more effective tissue solvents. Martin has compared potentiated acid 1,5 pentanedial with sodium hypochlorite and found that, against four test organisms, it was more germicidal than NaOCl in the presence of serum proteins.[39] He claimed that "a 1% solution of potentiated acid 1,5 pentanedial would be an efficient bactericidal irrigating solution," but he did not speak to its capability of dissolving necrotic tissue, only that it would coagulate blood.

Loel has suggested the use of 50% citric acid as an irrigating solution.[40] He believes that it opens the dentinal tubules to permit chlororosin penetration in the gutta percha diffusion filling technique. Alcohol, isopropyl or ethyl, in concentrations of 70% to 95% can be used as an irrigating solution. It is a mild disinfectant and fat solvent, and is favored by those who use the gutta percha diffusion technique since it dehydrates the dentin and theoretically facilitates bonding of the filling material to the canal walls.

McComb and Smith have shown that a commercial form of EDTA (REDTA) produced the "cleanest walls," particularly if it was sealed in the canal for 24 hours.[40a]

For general use, sodium hypochlorite solution is still considered the irrigating solution of choice. It is a necrotic tissue solvent: by virtue of its halogen content it is effective as a disinfectant[41] and bleach; and it is readily available, since it is widely used as a household bleach and disinfectant. Household bleaches such as Clorox contain approximately 5.25 sodium hypochlorite in water. They may be used directly from the bottle, but are usually diluted with one or two parts of water to reduce the chlorine odor. Baker et al. have some evidence that a 1% solution of sodium hypochlorite may not be significantly better than a simple saline solution for irrigation; therefore the solution should not be diluted to that level.[42]

Method

The technique for irrigation is simple, fast, and effective. From the towel kit a glass Luer syringe and ¾″ needle are used. One of the dappen dishes from the kit is kept filled with sodium hypochlorite by the dental assistant. She fills the syringe by immersing the syringe hub in the solution while withdrawing the plunger. The bent needle is then placed on the

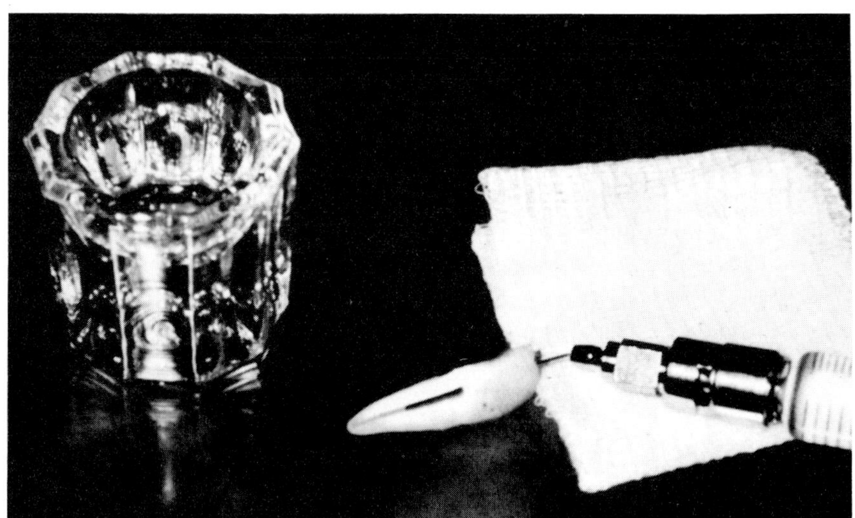

Fig. 3–23. Irrigation armamentarium. Dappen dish filled with sodium hypochlorite, 3-ml. Luer syringe with bent 25-gauge needle, and surgical sponge to catch solution as it flows from tooth.

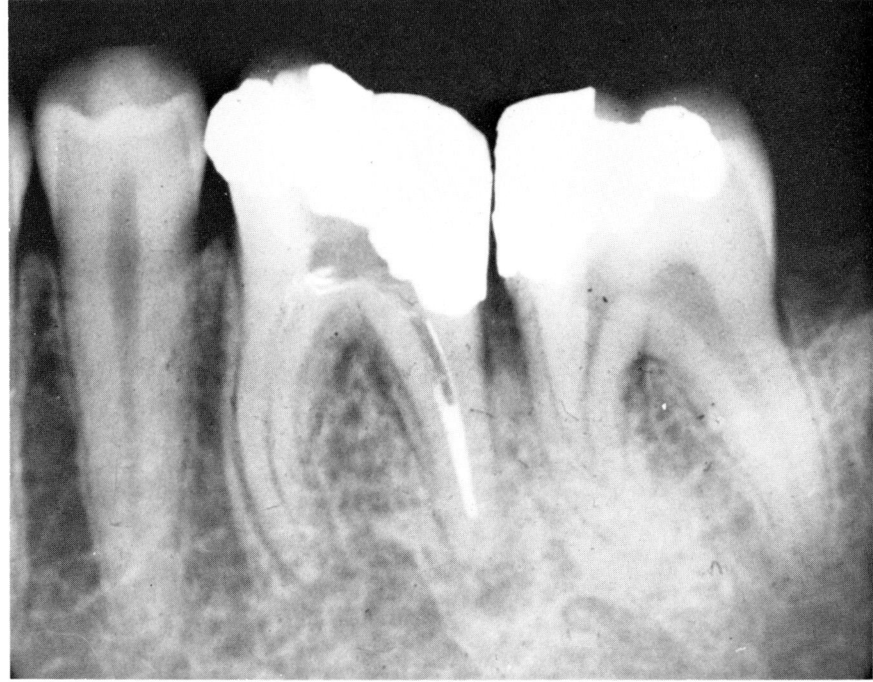

Fig. 3.–24. Amalgam filings totally obstructing canal of lower molar. Repeated irrigation during cavity preparation would have prevented this unfortunate happening.

syringe and inserted loosely in the root canal. The irrigating solution is slowly ejected, and the overflow is caught on a surgical sponge (Fig. 3–23), or with the high-speed evacuator. Sodium hypochlorite is a bleach and will injure fabric if permitted to drip on the patient's clothing.

Care must be taken not to seat the needle tightly in the canal or the solution may be forced through into the periapical tissues. Becker et al.[43] and Bhat[44] have emphasized the importance of not injecting irrigants beyond the apical foramen. They reported severe and lasting pain, swelling, ecchymosis, and tissue emphysema as sequelae to the accidental injection of irrigant into the periapex.

The bulk of the irrigant is removed from the canal by withdrawing the plunger of the syringe with the needle still in the canal. The balance is then absorbed on cotton pellets and paper points. The efficiency of this combined mechanical washing and chemical dissolution will be apparent from the collection of debris on the sponge.

The importance of frequent irrigation cannot be overemphasized. Enamel, gold, or amalgam fragments dropped into the pulp chambers of teeth during access preparation and driven into the canals with an instrument spell disaster, for they rarely can be removed (Fig. 3–24). Thorough irrigation following access preparation not only guards against this occurrence, but also facilitates location of the canal orifices. The bleaching action of the sodium hypochlorite accentuates the contrast between the dark lines in the dentin connecting the canal orifices, and the remainder of the floor of the pulp chamber (Fig. 3–25).

Instrumentation is made easier by frequent irrigation and recapitulation* with fine instruments. Dentin shavings and soft-tissue fragments are kept from accumulating in the canal. There is also less likelihood that debris will be packed into the constricted apical third of the canal or forced through the apical foramen during canal enlargement.

Finally, the disinfecting potential of the irrigation process should not be minimized. Adequate instrumentation and careful irrigation with germicidal solutions have been shown to disinfect a significant number of canals without the aid of other medication.[45,46]

Unless they are disposable, the syringe and needle must be washed well at the completion of the appointment, or crystallized sodium hypochlorite will

*Term suggested by Dr. Herbert Schilder.

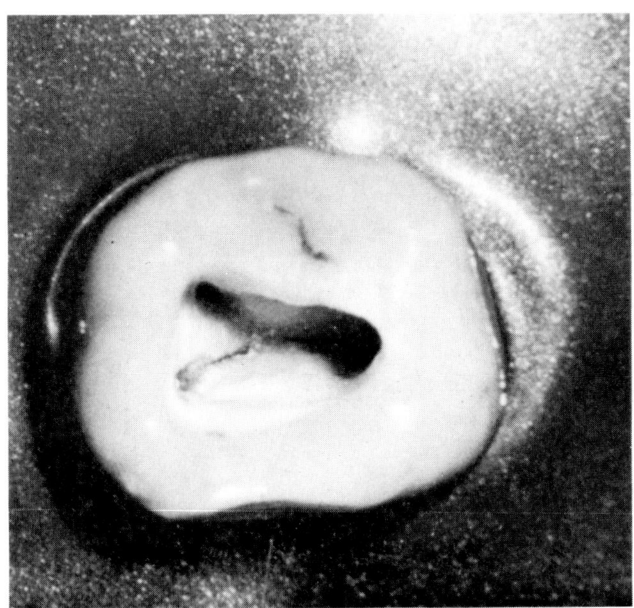

Fig. 3–25. Debris removal and bleaching action of sodium hypochlorite accentuates dark lines and orifices of molar triangle.

permanently block the needle lumen and seal the plunger to the syringe barrel.

The following are the stages in a series of endodontic procedures at which thorough irrigation (2 ml.) of the pulp chamber and canals is indicated:

1. ***Prior to instrumentation of a pulp cavity previously opened for drainage.*** The irrigant will remove food particles and saliva.
2. ***During access preparation,*** following the culture, when the pulp chamber is sufficiently open to permit flow of the irrigating solution.
3. ***At completion of the access preparation,*** prior to the use of intracanal instruments.
4. ***Following pulpectomy*** to remove the blood that can stain the tooth.
5. ***At intervals during instrumentation*** when reamers and files are cutting dentin fragments from canal walls.
6. ***At the completion of canal instrumentation*** prior to placement of the medicament.

In summary, irrigation is preceded by culturing and is followed by a detailed search for the orifices of the canals. This in turn is followed by exploration of the full length of the root canals.

Exploration for the Orifice

Before the canals can be entered, their orifices must be found. In the older patient, finding a canal orifice may be ***the*** most difficult and time-consuming operation.

Quite obviously, a knowledge of pulp anatomy—knowing where to look and expect to find the orifices—is of first importance. Perseverance is the second requirement, followed by a calm resolve not to become desperate and decimate the internal tooth when the orifice does not appear.

The endodontic explorer is the greatest aid in finding a minute canal entrance (Fig. 3–26). As soon as the pulp chamber is perforated, the explorer should be used with a poking action, feeling along the walls and into the floor of the chamber in the area where the orifices are expected to be. Extension toward these points forms the perimeter of the preparation.

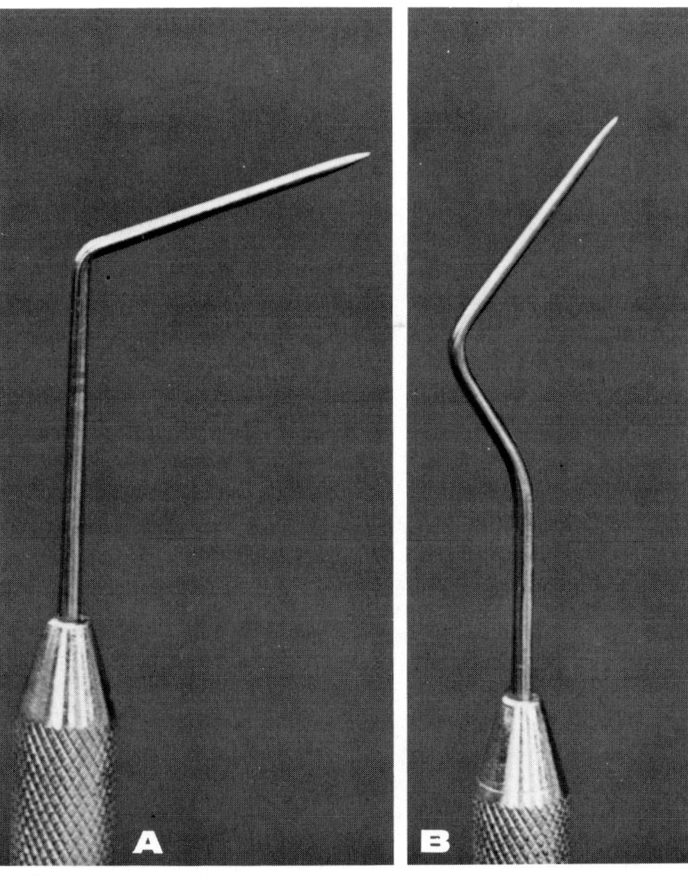

Fig. 3–26. Opposite ends of endodontic explorer. *Left:* binangle; *Right:* right angle. (Courtesy Star Dental Manufacturing Co.)

The roentgenogram is invaluable in determining just where and in which direction canals enter into the pulp chamber. This is especially true in the maxillary molars (see Fig. 1–24). The initial roentgenogram is one of the most important aids available to the clinician, but unfortunately one of the least used during cavity preparation. A bite-wing radiograph is particularly helpful in providing an undistorted view of the pulp chamber. The handpiece and bur may be held up to the radiograph to estimate the correct depth of penetration and direction to the orifices.

Color is another invaluable aid in finding a canal orifice. The ***floor*** of the pulp chamber and the continuous anatomic line that connects the orifices (the so-called molar triangle) are dark (Fig. 3–27*A*)—dark gray or sometimes brown in contrast to the white or light yellow of the ***walls*** of chamber (Fig. 3–27*B*). Using a No. 2 bur, and "following out" the colored pathway from one orifice often leads to the elusive second, third, or even fourth orifice.

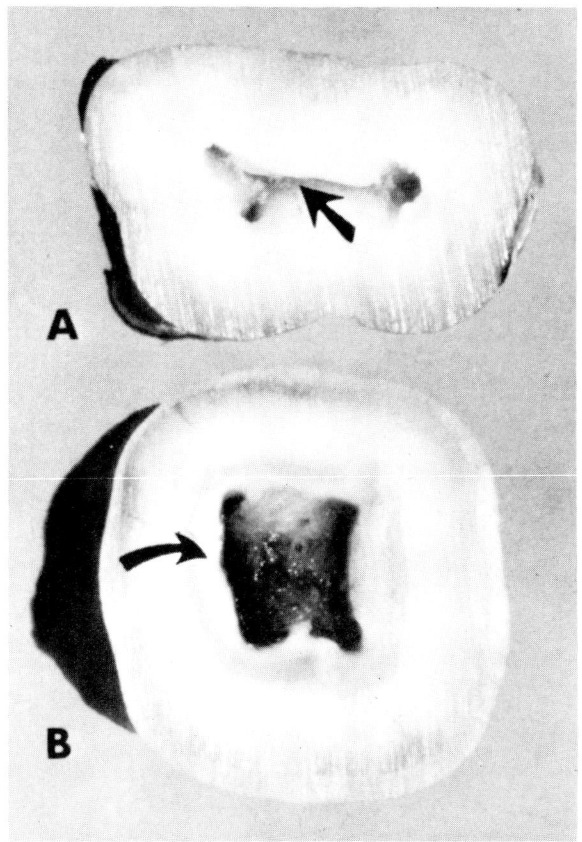

Fig. 3–27. *A*, Dark line of molar triangle is obvious in this cross section of mandibular second molar. *B*. Dark color of floor of pulp chamber contrasts markedly to light color (arrow) of side walls of preparation.

Sometimes a greatly receded pulp has to be followed well down into the root to find the orifice to the remaining canal. Measurements on the roentgenogram indicate how many millimeters to drill before the orifice is encountered. The use of surgical-length burs, even in a miniature handpiece, will extend the depth of cut to well beyond 15 mm. It is most important to enlarge the occlusal opening so that complete authority over the direction of the bur can be maintained (Fig. 3–28). Repeated roentgenograms to verify depth and direction of cut are also invaluable.

Axioms of Pulp Anatomy

Remembering the axioms of pulp anatomy can be most helpful:

1. The two orifices of the maxillary first premolar are further to the buccal and the lingual than is usually suspected (Plate XIII).

2. The orifices of the mesiobuccal canals in both the maxillary and mandibular molars are well up under the mesiobuccal cusp, and the outline form must often be widely extended into the cusp (Plates XXI and XXII).

3. The orifice to the lingual canal in the maxillary molars is ***not far*** to the lingual, but is actually in the center of the mesial half of the tooth (Plates XXI and XXII).

4. The orifice to the distobuccal canal of the maxillary molars is ***not far*** to the distobuccal, but is actually almost directly buccal from the lingual orifice (Plates XXI and XXII).

5 The orifice to the distal canal in mandibular molars is ***not far*** to the distal canal, but is actually in almost the exact center of the tooth (Plates XXV and XXVI).

6. The orifice to the mesiolingual canal of the mandibular molars is not far to mesial lingual, but is actually almost directly mesial from the distal orifice (Plates XXV and XXVI).

7. Certain anatomic variations occur with enough frequency to warrant mention here:

a. The mesiobuccal root of the maxillary first molar may have an extra mesiolingual canal just lingual to the mesiobuccal orifice (Fig. 3–29). It is found in the groove that comes off the mesiobuccal orifice like the tail on a comma. This entire groove should be explored for the mesiolingual canal; 38%

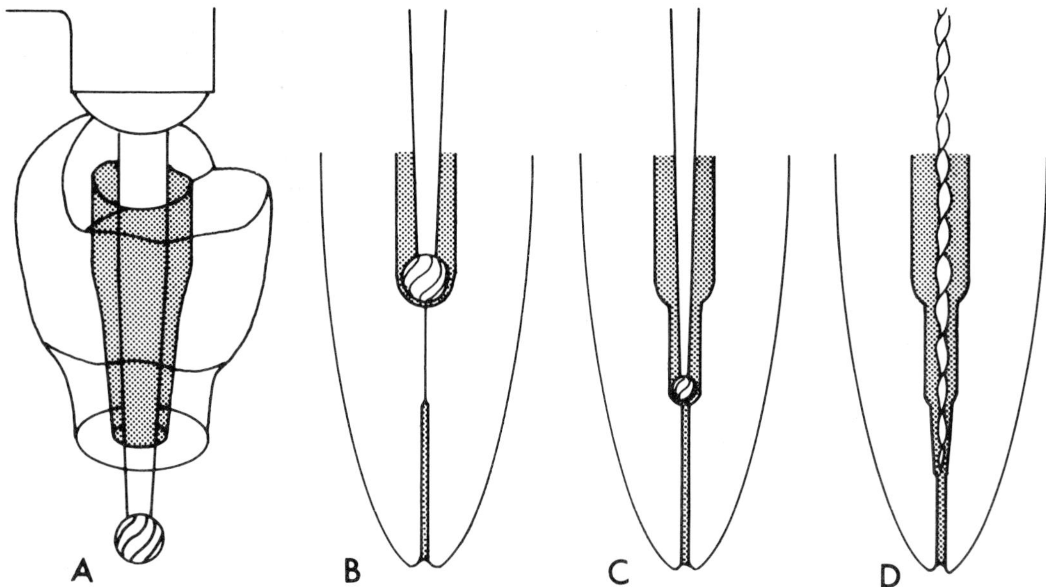

Fig. 3–28. Necessity of maintaining control over burs and endodontic instruments in following out advanced pulpal recession. *A*, Coronal cavity is enlarged sufficiently to accommodate shaft of #4 surgical-length bur which must function without touching cavity walls. *B*, Freely operating #4 surgical-length bur following out receded pulp. *C*, #2 surgical-length bur used in depths of preparation. Repeated roentgenograms may be necessary to judge progress of instrument, *D*, Fine root canal reamer used to explore and finally enlarge patent portion of canal.

of the time the two mesial root canals join into one foramen, but 25% of the time the ***two mesial canals exit through two separate foramens.***[10]

b. Mandibular ***second*** molars frequently have a common mesial orifice which divides about 1 mm. below the floor of the pulp chamber into a mesiobuccal and mesiolingual canal.

c. Mandibular first and second molars may have two ***distal*** canals, either with separate orifices or with a common orifice as described for the mesial.

d. Mandibular ***first*** premolars frequently have a second canal branching off the main canal to the buccal or lingual, several millimeters below the pulp chamber floor.

e. Mandibular incisors frequently have two canals. The mesiolingual canal is hidden beneath the ***internal*** "shoulder" that corresponds to the lingual cingulum. This "shoulder" prominence must be removed with a No. 2 long-shank round bur to permit proper exploration.

In summary, the unexpected should always be anticipated, and the operator must be prepared to expand the access cavity for convenience in enlarging one of these canals, or even just to increase visual examination of the pulp chamber floor in searching for such anatomic variance.

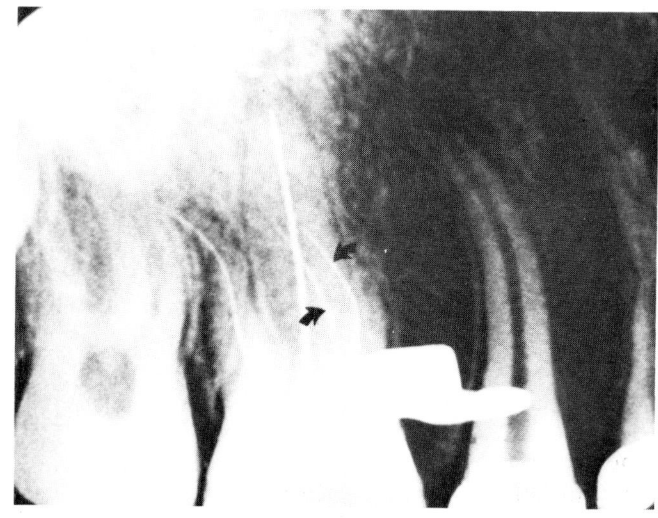

Fig. 3–29. Two canals in mesial root clearly discernible by radiograph. Both canals apparently have separate apical foramen. (Courtesy Dr. James D. Zidell.)

Exploration of the Canal

Use of a curved fine reamer or file as a pathfinder is by far the best method available to determine curvature in canals. Exploration of the canals will also reveal the presence of vital pulp tissue, which will require special removal by pulpectomy. This is described in detail on pages 210–213.

If just the tip of the exploring instrument is curved, the operator may truly explore the walls and direction of the canal. The curved tip of the instrument will scribe a circle when the instrument is turned on its axis, whereas the perfectly straight instrument will only rotate on the central axis of the instrument (Fig. 3–30). Exploring the ***uneven*** and curved walls of the canal with a ***straight*** instrument will only lead to failure, for the instrument will hang up at the curve, or pivot on a catch on the walls (Fig. 3–31). The ***curved, pathfinding*** instrument, on the other hand, can be rotated away from a catch or curve in the wall, and advanced down the canal to the apical region (Fig. 3–31*B* and *C*). From the initial pathfinding instrument, length of tooth may be established (p. 186). By controlling probing, poking, twisting, and turning, the fine pathfinder can almost always be penetrated to working length. This complex rolling-rotating motion is called *vaivén* in Spanish, the pitching, yawing motion of a ship in a high sea.[21]

Fig. 3–30 When turned on its axis, tip of curved instrument (left) scribes circle. Tip of straight instrument (right) turns on its own axis, which reduces control of tip of instrument.

When working depth is reached by *vaivén,* the operator must then know which direction the canal takes. This may be learned by withdrawing the instrument in a straight line and observing the direction in which the tip of the instrument is pointing. This is a valuable clue, for now the clinician knows the direction in which to aim the curve of the instrument. Valuable time is saved by eliminating exploration each time the instrument is placed in the canal.

If there were only one piece of advice that could be given to the neophyte endodontist, it would relate to the curved instruments: ***Always use a curved instrument as an initial explorer, and always use a curved instrument in a curved canal.*** The inexperienced hesitate to take this advice for fear of breaking the instrument at the curve. Again instruments are usually not broken but are twisted off while locked in the canal. However, they will break if a sharp angular bend is made in the blade, a point which may act as a fracture line.

The best method to curve an instrument is to insert the tip into the end of a sterile cotton roll and bend the instrument under the pressure, through the cotton, of the thumb nail (Fig. 3–32). This method is preferable to bending the instrument in the bare fingers for two reasons: (1) the cotton roll is sterile and the fingers are not, and (2) the padding of cotton allows for a gradual bend rather than a sharp bend. Pulling the instrument through cotton pliers, another method of placing a bend, will dull the instruments. Furthermore, pliers will place a sharp bend which may act as a fracture line. When large instruments must be curved, however, the handle of the pliers may be used to make the curve. This method is also used to place the gradual, overall curve in large files. The operator must constantly bear in mind not to contaminate instruments, hence the use of sterile cotton rolls and pliers rather than fingers.

In exploring a canal with a curved instrument, the clinician should always expect the worst. He should probe with the point toward the buccal and lingual,

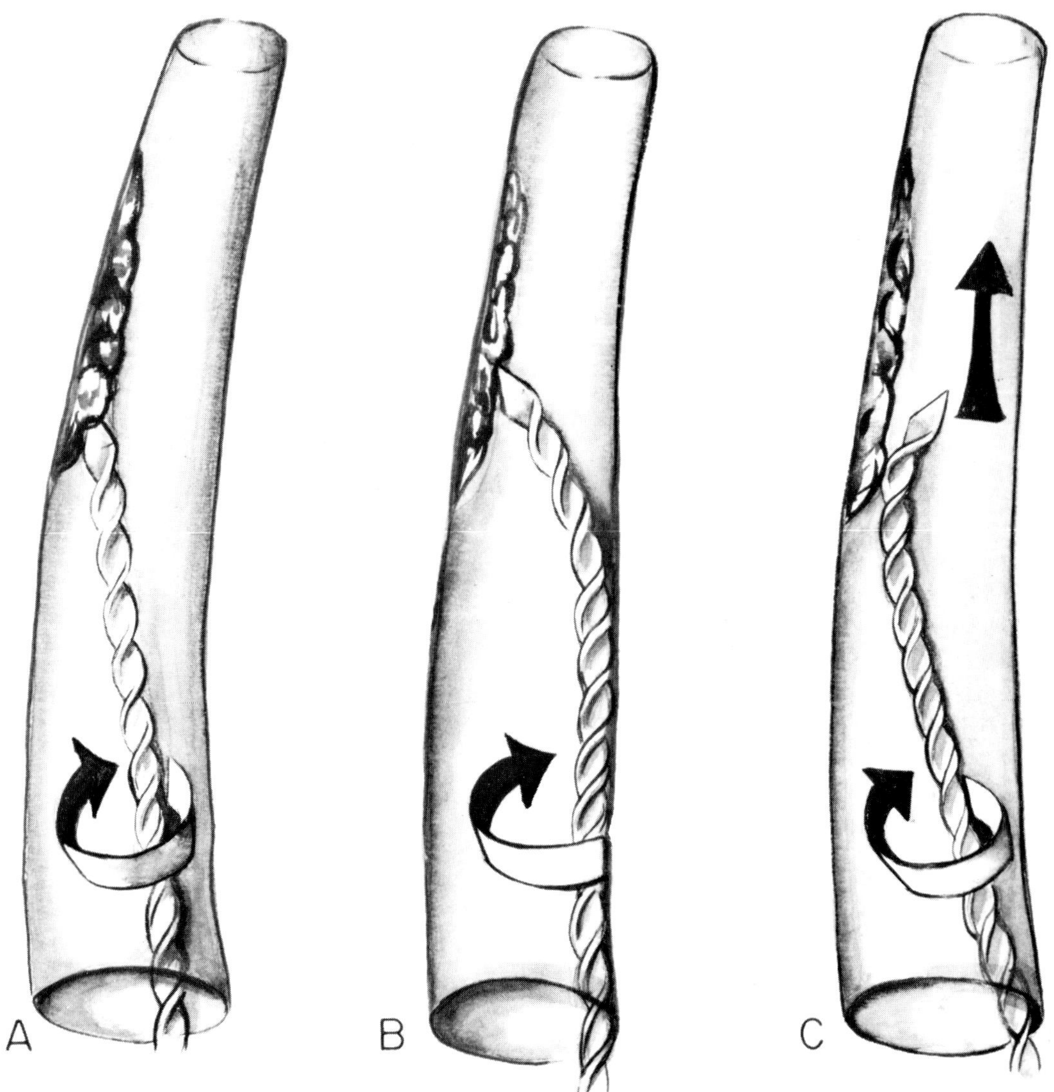

Fig. 3–31. *A,* When straight instrument catches on canal obstruction, turning instrument merely drives point deeper into obstruction. *B* and *C,* When curved instrument catches on obstruction, rotating point of instrument will detach it from obstruction so that instrument may be moved up canal.

that is, toward the direction of the x-ray beam, always searching for the unusual curvature which does not show on the roentgenogram. As mentioned previously, the palatal canals of ***maxillary*** molars, and the ***maxillary*** lateral incisors and canines are always suspect. In mandibular ***premolars,*** curvature of the canal toward the buccal or lingual is a common occurrence as well. In these teeth, particularly the ***mandibular*** first premolar, anomalies of the canals frequently exist; double canals, bifurcated canals, and apical delta are common. This also applies to the ***mandibular*** anterior teeth, where a search with the curved pathfinder should always be made for two canals, toward the labial and the lingual (Plates IX, F and XI, D).

Extra canals, such as three canals in the maxillary first premolar, two canals in the maxillary second premolar, or two canals in the mesiobuccal root of the maxillary first molar should also be searched for (Plates VIII, XIV, XXI). The fourth canal toward the distal in a mandibular molar will occasionally be found by careful exploration with first the endodontic

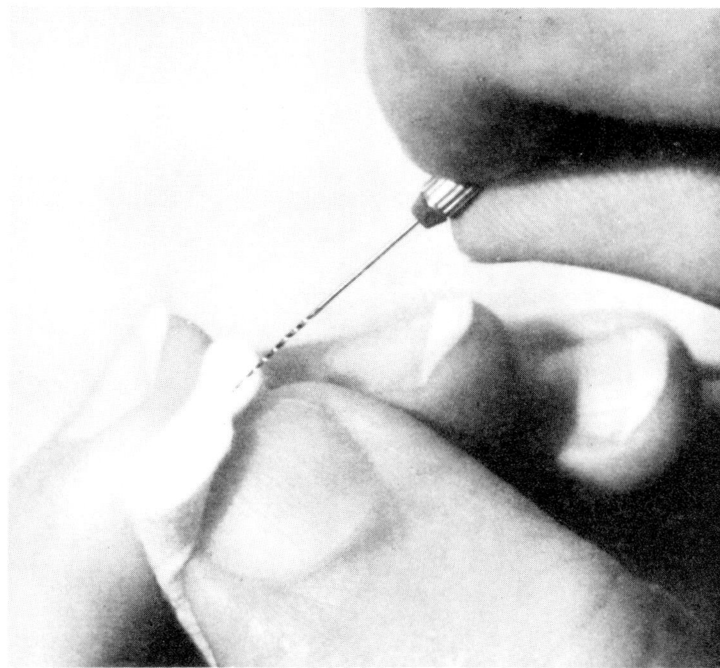

Fig. 3–32. Curving point of instrument. Tip is introduced into end of sterile cotton roll and is bent under thumbnail padded by cotton.

explorer and then the curved instrument (Plate XXV, G and H). Finding the extra or unusual canal spells the difference between success and failure.

Determination of Length of Tooth

Following the completion of adequate coronal access, and canal exploration, the most critical act in assuring success of therapy is the ***accurate determination of the length of the tooth*** prior to radicular preparation.

The length-of-tooth procedure establishes the apical extent of instrumentation and the ultimate apical level of root canal filling. Failure to accurately determine the length of tooth may lead to apical perforation and overfilling with increased incidence of postoperative pain. In addition, one might expect a prolonged healing period and increased failure due to the incomplete regeneration of cementum, periodontal ligament, and alveolar bone.

Failure to determine length of tooth accurately may also lead to ***incomplete*** instrumentation and underfilling with attendant problems. Among them should be noted persistent pain and discomfort from inflamed shreds of retained pulp tissue as well as the possibility of a persistent positive culture due to the failure to debride ***all*** of the canal. In addition, ledge formation may be developed, short of the apex, making adequate treatment or retreatment extremely difficult or often impossible. Finally, apical percolation may develop into the unfilled "dead space" at the apex. This could result in a continued periapical lesion and an increased incidence of failure.

The requirements of a method for determining the length of tooth are: (1) it must be accurate; (2) it should be easily and readily performed; and (3) it must be easily confirmed.

Methods requiring formulas to remember or devices to use in determining length of tooth have been found wanting. Some methods require the ***total*** length of the tooth and the instrument to show in the roentgenogram—a demand that is frequently difficult to fully attain. Other methods involve complex devices that are clumsy, bulky, time-consuming, inaccurate, and frustrating. Conversely, it has been suggested by some that a precise length-of-tooth procedure is not necessary; instead, these authors rely on the tactile appreciation of canal constriction present in the apical 2 mm. of most teeth. This may satisfy the experienced endodontist, but does not suit the needs and level of skill of a student or practitioner inexperienced in root canal therapy. It also gives no consideration to the incompletely developed root canal, the canal that is narrow and constricted throughout its entire length, or the canal of an excessively curved root where the instrument contacts the canal walls at many sites.

Length-of-tooth roentgenograms are often not taken because of a clumsy, frustrating technique of taking a roentgenogram with the rubber dam in place as well as the time-consuming x-ray, developing and fixing procedures. The sections on the rubber dam and roentgenology suggest solutions to these problems.

The method that will be here presented has been compared by Bramante with three other methods of determining tooth length.[47] According to Bramante, this method proved to be "superior to the others."

Materials and Conditions

The following items are essential to perform this procedure.

1. A good, undistorted, preoperative roentgenogram showing the total length and all roots of the involved tooth.
2. Adequate coronal access to all canals.
3. An adjustable endodontic millimeter ruler.
4. Working knowledge of the average length of all the teeth.
5. A definite, repeatable plane of reference to an anatomic landmark on the tooth, a fact that should be recorded on the patient's record. For intact or well-restored teeth, the most common site of reference is the incisal edge of anterior teeth and the cusp height on posterior teeth.

It is imperative that teeth with fractured cusps or cusps severely weakened by caries or restoration be reduced to a flattened surface, supported by dentin. Failure to do so may result in cusps or weak enamel walls being fractured between appointments (Fig. 3–33). Thus the original site of reference is lost. If this fracture goes unobserved there is the probability of overinstrumentation and overfilling, particularly if anesthesia is used.

In order to establish length of tooth, a style B reamer or file with a rubber instrument "stop" on the shaft will be needed. The exploring instrument size must be small enough to negotiate the total length of the canal, but not so small as to be loose in the canal. A loose instrument may unknowingly move in or out of the canal after the roentgenogram, and be the cause of serious error in determination of the length of the

Average Lengths of Teeth (in mm.)[3]

	Average	*Maximum*	*Minimum*
Maxilla			
Central incisor	23.7	27.3	21.5
Lateral incisor	23.1	26.0	19.2
Canine	27.3	33.3	22.3
First premolar	22.3	25.8	18.8
Second premolar	22.3	26.4	16.7
First molar	22.3	25.0	19.6
Second molar	22.2	25.2	20.1
Mandible			
Central incisor	21.8	25.1	19.4
Lateral incisor	23.3	25.0	21.0
Canine	26.0	27.4	24.6
First premolar	22.9	24.2	21.2
Second premolar	22.3	25.0	19.3
First molar	22.0	25.0	19.3
Second molar	21.7	25.8	19.0

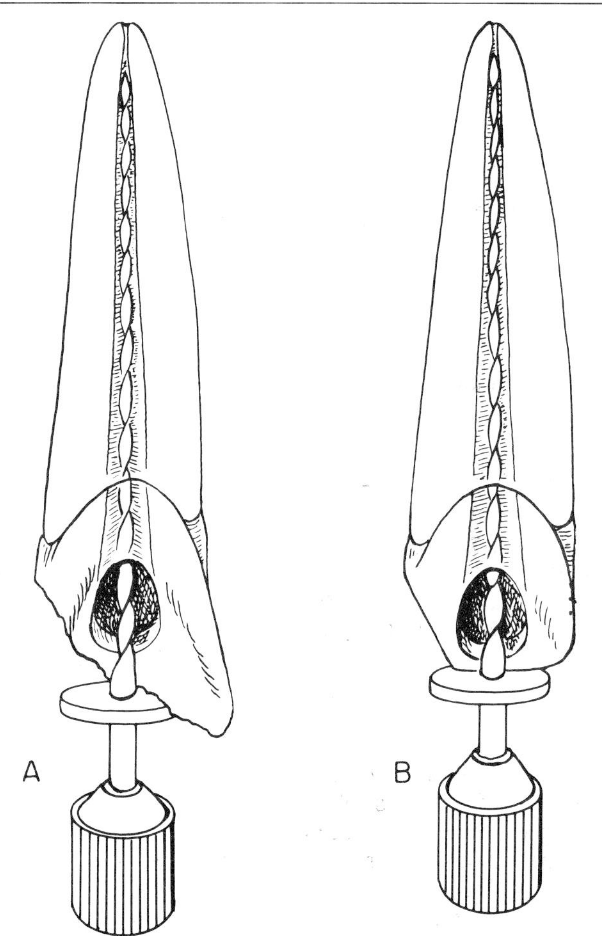

Fig. 3–33. *A,* Do not used weakened enamel walls or diagonal lines of fracture as site of reference for length-of-tooth measurement. *B,* Weakened cusps or incisal edges are reduced to well-supported tooth structure. Diagonal surfaces should be flattened to give accurate site of reference.

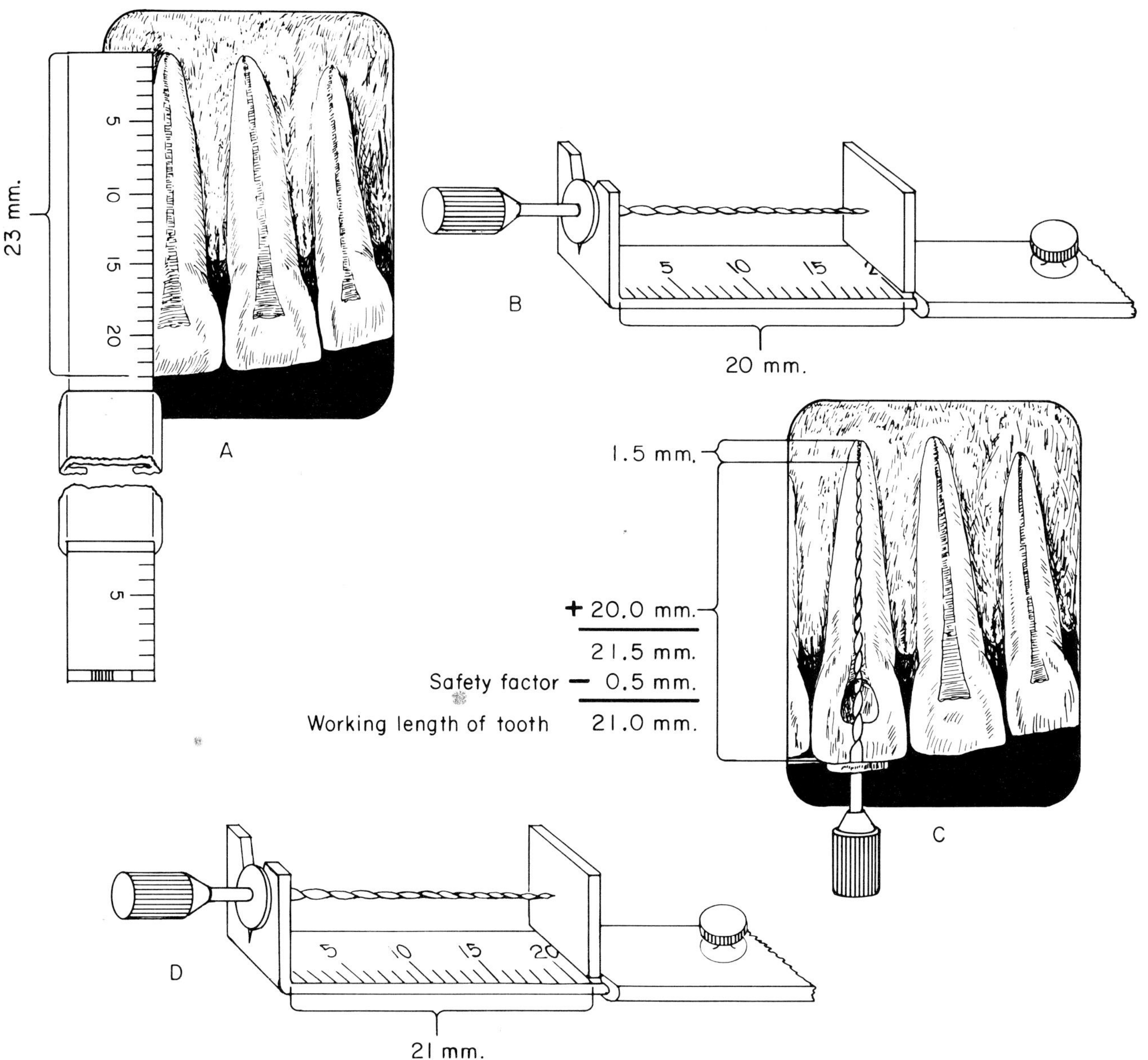

Fig. 3–34. Steps in establishing accurate length-of-tooth measurement: *A,* Shadow of tooth is measured on good preoperative roentgenogram. In this case tooth appears to be 23 mm. long. Reverse, or unsterile, end of endodontic measuring gauge is used on roentgenograms. *B,* As safety precaution, 3 mm. are subtracted from initial length-of-tooth measurement. Measuring gauge is set at this new length, and rubber stop attachment is positioned on initial instrument at this length. *C,* Insert instrument in canal to stop, and expose and process roentgenogram. Measurement may then be made from end of instrument to end of root. Adding length of instrument in canal (in this case 20 mm.) to amount instrument was short of apex (in this case 1½ mm.) will establish accurate length of tooth (in this case 21½ mm.). A 0.5 mm. safety factor is subtracted to establish working length (in this case 21 mm.) of tooth at cementodentinal junction. *D,* Working length of tooth (in this case 21 mm.) is set on endodontic measuring gauge. All instruments subsequently inserted in canal are set at this length.

tooth. In ***all*** instances of a curved canal, a ***curved instrument*** must be used.

Method

1. Measure the tooth on the preoperative roentgenogram (Fig. 3–34*A*).

2. Subtract 2 or 3 mm. "safety allowance" for measuring error and possible image distortion.

3. Set the endodontic ruler at this measurement and adjust the rubber stop on the instrument at that level (Fig. 3–34*B*).

4. Place the instrument in the canal until the rubber stop is at the plane of reference unless pain is

felt, in which case the instrument is left at that level and the rubber stop readjusted to this new point of reference.

5. Expose, develop, and clear the roentgenogram.

6. On the roentgenogram, ***measure the difference between the end of the instrument and the site where the canal leaves the root.*** Add this amount to the original measured length the instrument extended into the tooth (Fig. 3–34*C*). If through some oversight, the exploring instrument has gone beyond the apex, subtract this difference.

7. From this adjusted length of tooth subtract 0.5 mm. for a "safety factor" to conform with the apical termination of the root canal (p. 167) at the cementodentinal junction (Fig. 3–34*C*).

8. Set the endodontic ruler at this new corrected length and readjust the stop on the exploring instrument (Fig. 3–34*D*).

9. Because of the possibility of roentgenographic distortion, sharply curving roots, and operator measuring error, a confirmatory roentgenogram of the adjusted length is highly desirable. In many instances this added investment of a few minutes will prevent the discomfort and failure that stem from inaccuracy.

10. When the length of tooth has been ***accurately*** confirmed, reset the endodontic ruler at this measurement.

11. ***Record*** this measurement and the enamel ***point of reference*** on the patient's record.

12. Even though accurately determined and confirmed, the length-of-tooth measurement may shorten as ***curved*** canals are enlarged. Since "a straight line is the shortest distance between two points," the length-of-tooth measurement may shorten by as much as 1 or 2 mm. as the curved canal is straightened out by instrumentation. It is therefore recommended that the "length of tooth" in a curved canal be reconfirmed after instrumentation of three or four sizes.

Variations. When the two canals of a maxillary first premolar appear to be superimposed, much confusion and lost time may be saved by several simple means. Occasionally it is advantageous to take individual roentgenograms of each canal with its length-of-tooth instrument in place. Another method is to place a file in one canal and a reamer in the other and take a single roentgenogram. The spiral blades of the reamer and file may be differentiated in the film. A preferable method is to expose the roentgenogram from a ***mesial*** horizontal angle. This causes the lingual canal to always be the more mesial one in the image (MLM, Clark's rule), or conversely MBD.

The mesial canals of the mandibular molars usually appear to have a common foramen, or appear to be of equal length. In this case, only one length-of-tooth roentgenogram is necessary. An instrument will be seen in the distal canal and in either mesial canal.

When a mandibular molar appears to have two mesial roots or apices of different lengths or position, two mesial instruments can be used and again the tooth can be examined radiographically from the mesial and Clark's rule (MLM) applied.

The Japanese have recently developed battery powered electrical devices for measuring tooth length. Based on the difference in electric potential between two electrodes, one applied to the lip or cheek and the second placed in the canal as a probe, these "electroconductometers" either give off a characteristic sound or record 40 microamperes on a dial when the tissue at the apical foramen is approached.

Bramante[47] found the method and device suggested by Sunada[48] to be particularly accurate for the lingual roots in maxillary premolars and molars. On the other hand, he found the radiographic method presented in this text, to which he refers as the "Ingle method," to be more consistently accurate.

O'Neill, using an electric root canal probe, measured the length of 53 canals and was perfectly accurate 83% of the time.[49] In the remaining 17%, the instrument measured the tooth length short, but only by 0.5 mm.

Seidberg et al.,[50] on the other hand, were disappointed in the outcome using the Sono-Explorer introduced by Inoue.[51] Comparing results of determining the length of tooth by means of this electronic probe with results of determining the foramen constriction by "digital-tactile" sense, they found the Sono-Explorer to be less reliable than their own digital-tactile sense.

Both methods were highly inaccurate, however, short measurements being recorded nearly one-half the time with the electronic probe and one-third the time by digital-tactile sense. They concluded that "the electronic device should not replace radiographic control . . . as a measuring device." One might say the same for digital-tactile sense. Endodontic specialists in the United States Navy tested both the Sono-Explorer (sound) and the Endometer (voltmeter). Both devices were approximately 87% accurate.

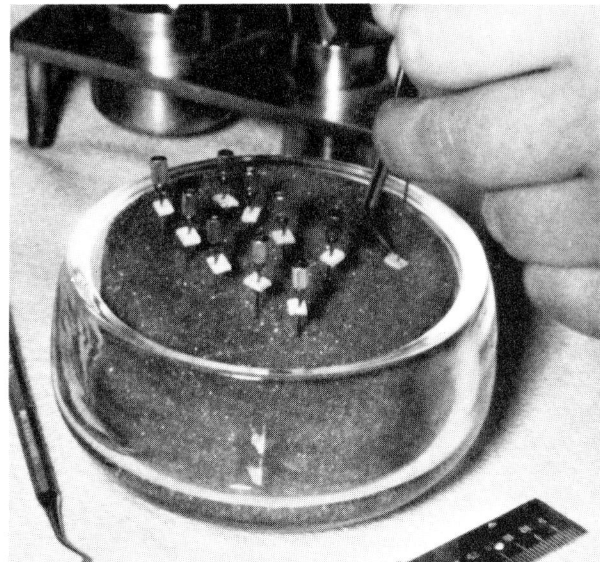

Fig. 3–35. Instrument may be inserted through stop attachment at right angle by holding rubber stop on surface of banker's sponge and forcing instrument through rubber stop perpendicular to its surface. Assistant has already arranged two rows of instruments in numerical order.

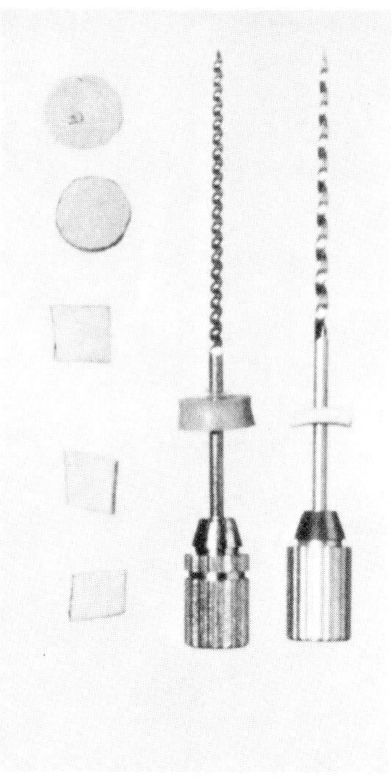

Fig. 3–36. Stop attachments made from rubber or silicone. Round silicone "rubber" stops are made with leather punch. Flat square rubber stops are cut from 2 mm. wide rubber band.

The Endometer was more consistent and less complicated to use.[52]

Stop Attachments. When tooth length has been established, the operator is ready to proceed with canal instrumentation. The assistant selects all reamers and files of appropriate sizes and uses the endodontic ruler to adjust the instrument stops on them. The instruments are then arranged in order of size in a banker's sponge soaked with tincture of Zephiran (Fig. 3–35).

A variety of stop attachments are available; however, the least expensive and simplest to use are the rubber "stops." The rubber "stops" may be 2 × 2 mm. pieces cut from a flat rubber band, or better, 2 mm. circles cut from silicone "rubber" with a leather punch (Fig. 3–36).

The length adjustment of the stop attachment on the blade may be made against the edge of a sterile metric ruler or a gauge made specifically for endodontics. The rubber stop attachment is grasped in the operating pliers placed on top of the banker's sponge, and the instrument is pushed at a right angle through the rubber (Fig. 3–37, *left*). It is important that the rubber stop be perpendicular and not oblique to the shaft of the instrument (Fig. 3–37, *right*). The length is then adjusted against the gauge.

The disadvantage of these particular "stops" is that

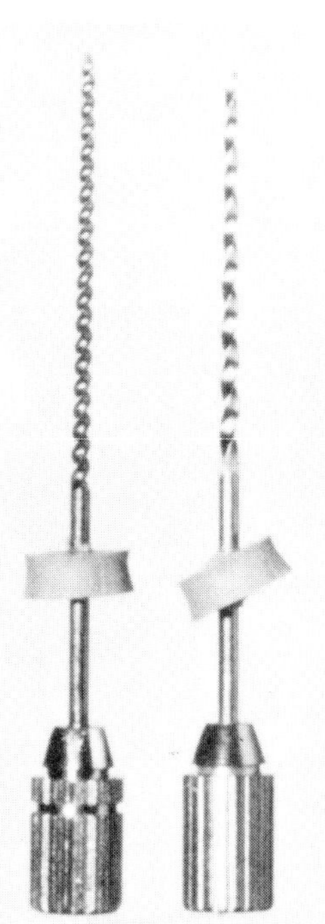

Fig. 3–37. *Left,* Rubber stop attachment should be placed perpendicular to long axis of instrument. *Right,* Obliquely placed stop attachment will vary length of tooth measurement over 1 mm.

they may get pushed up the blade during use, thus elongating the working length of the instrument, which in turn may lead to apical perforation. The clinician should develop a mental image of the position of the stop attachment on the blade in relation to the base of the handle, and any movement from this position should be immediately detected. The operator should also develop the habit of looking directly at the stop attachment where it meets the tooth. For point of reference, the same cusp or position of the "stop" against the incisal edge should always be used. For future reference a note should be made on the patient's chart of the point of contact of the "stop," e.g., "MB canal—ML cusp."

Both Guldener[53] and Rowe and Forrest[54] have perfected a device that assists in adjusting stop attachments at the proper measured level. The device consists of a block with holes drilled to varying depths, from 15 mm. to 31 mm. (Fig. 3–38). If the length of tooth is, say, 21 mm., a rubber stop attachment is placed on the instrument which is then plunged into the hole marked "21." This would be particularly helpful when completing a "telescoping"

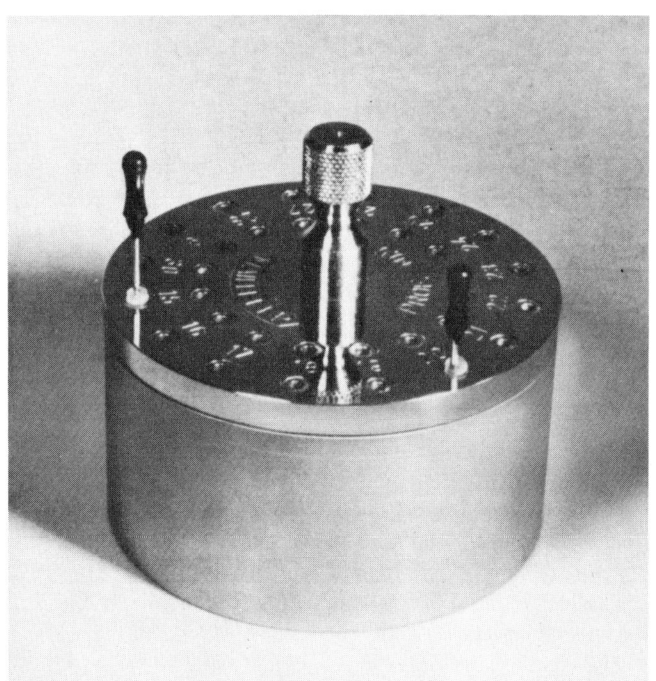

Fig. 3–38. "Endo-M-Bloc" used to set working length of instruments. After instrument stop is placed on blade, instrument is inserted into hole marked with length needed. Pushing blade to depth positions "stop." (Courtesy Star Dental Manufacturing Co.)

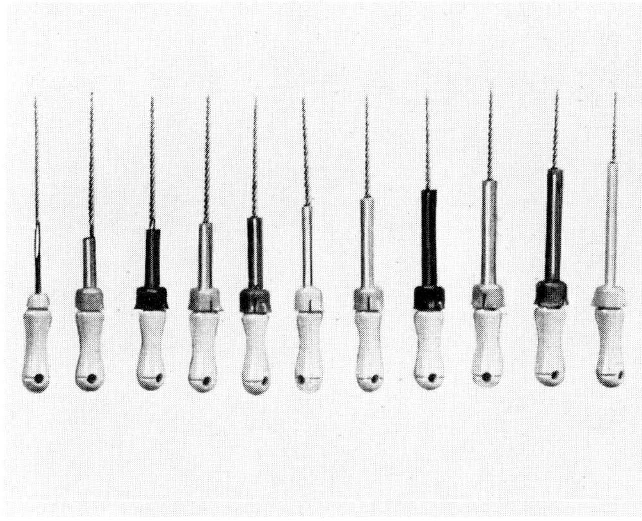

Fig. 3–39. Plastic reusable instrument stops, color coded as to length. Plastic strikes floor of chamber. Other plastic stops are available which strike margin of cavity. (Courtesy Star Dental Manufacturing Co.)

cavity preparation as one "steps back" 1 mm. at a time (see pp. 199–200).

Fixed stop attachments, both in metal and colored plastic, are available which have the advantage of not shifting, but take longer to apply (Fig. 3–39).

Anatomic Considerations in Radicular Cavity Preparation

The primary objective of all this precise measuring and confirming of the length of tooth is to limit instrumentation and subsequent filling to the root canal. As previously stated, the apical termination of the canal is the junction of the internal dentin and the external cementum—the cementodentinal junction at the foramen. Kuttler,[15] Green,[55] and others[56,57] have demonstrated that this CD junction is often found about 0.5 mm. from the external surface of the root seen in the radiograph. Although this point is usually suspected of being at the very apex of the root, it need not be; in fact, the location of the foramen may vary as much as 2 mm. from the apex (Fig. 3–40). For this reason it is advisable to reconfirm tooth length, once it has been established, by placing an instrument at this position and repeating the roentgenographic examination.

Once a good deal of experience is gained, the operator may be able to "feel" the foramen, but again, the neophyte is warned that many foramens stand

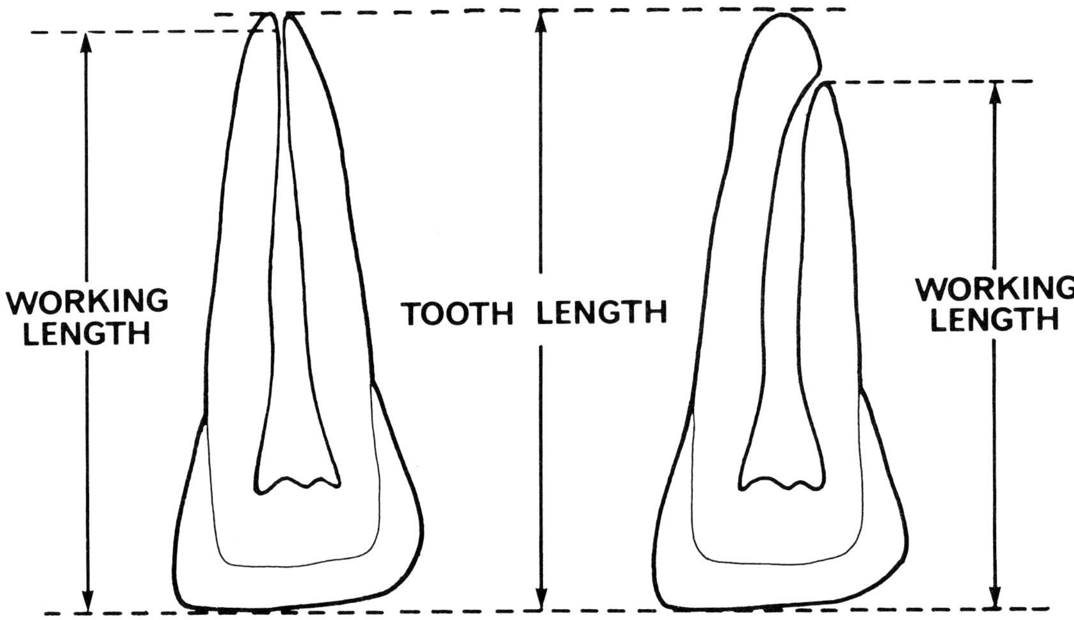

Fig. 3–40. Care should be exercised to establish position of foramen. Normally it appears at apex and 0.5 mm. is subtracted from that tooth length as safety factor. Lateral exit of canal can sometimes be seen in radiograph or discovered by instrument placement and re-examined radiographically. Even patient reaction to instrument is warning of "early exit," especially toward labial or lingual unseen in radiograph. (From Serene, T., Krasny, R., Zeigler, P., Higginbotham, T., and Longhurst, G.: Principles of Preclinical Endodontics. Dubuque, Iowa, Kendall/Hunt Publishing Co., 1974.)

wide open to allow small instrument passage, or conversely, a canal may be so restrictive that an instrument binds throughout its length. The patient's reaction may often be counted upon if he is not anesthetized. There is a decided difference in discomfort reaction between the instrument touching or even approaching the periapical tissue at the CD junction and an instrument touching a shred of remaining vital pulp. Pulp remnants evoke a sharp instantaneous response, whereas the reaction at the CD junction ranges from a mild awareness to possibly no reaction at all. The latter reaction is common when a periapical lesion is present because this tissue is not as richly innervated with sensory nerves as is the tissue of the periodontal membrane or pulpal remnants.

Any warning at all by the patient calls for a reconfirmation of the tooth length. First, the average length of the tooth may be checked against the figures given here in this text, knowing full well these figures are averages and variations must be expected. Second, the radiograph should provide a clue, and this calls for magnification and a study of the root end to see if the foramen can be detected short of the apex. Finally, placing the instrument at the point of patient complaint and repeating the x-ray examination should indicate whether the tip of the instrument is well short of the foramen or is in fact at or past the CD junction. If the instrument appears somewhat short and the patient is subjected to an electrifying shock each time the tissue is touched, one is undoubtedly dealing with vital pulp remnants, and their removal must be done under local anesthesia.

Classification of Root Canal Systems

Planning intraradicular preparation and filling begins with an analysis of the anatomic configuration of the root canal, as seen in the initial roentgenograms or discovered by exploration with a fine endodontic instrument. Thus, root canals may be classified, and for each class there is an optimum method of cleaning, shaping, and filling.

Class I. Uncomplicated, mature root canal (Fig. 3–41*A*)—straight or gradually curved with constriction at the foramen.

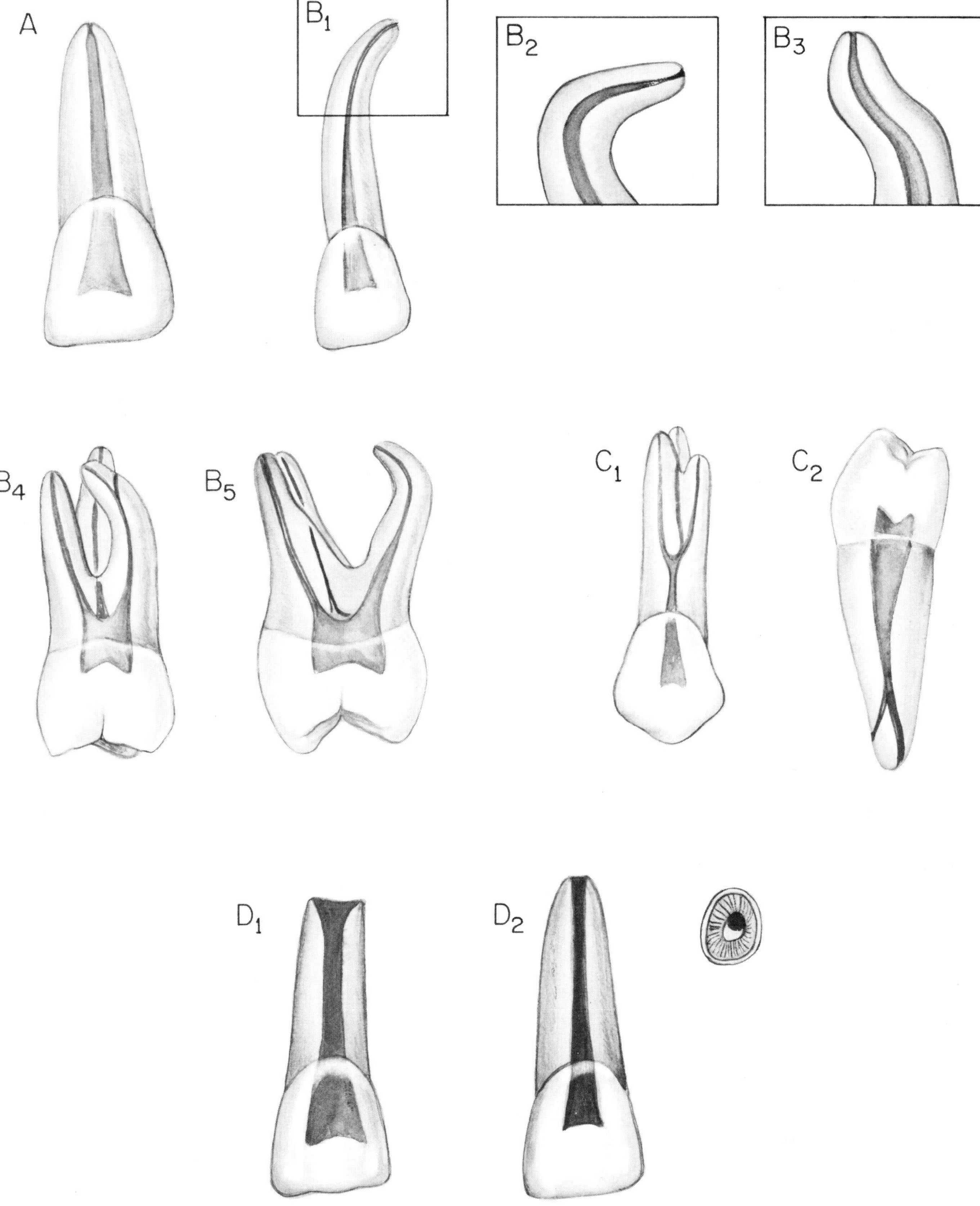

Fig. 3–41. Classification of root canal systems. *A,* Class I, uncomplicated with constricted foramen. *B* and *C,* Class II, complicated with constricted foramen. *B1,* Severe curve. *B2,* Dilacerated curve. *B3,* Bayonet curve. *B4,* Apical bifurcation. *B5,* Apical curve. *C1,* Additional canals. *C2,* Lateral or accessory canals. *D,* Class III, Immature root canal. *D1,* Blunderbuss apex. *D2,* Open apex, tubular canal. (Courtesy Dr. James D. Zidell.)

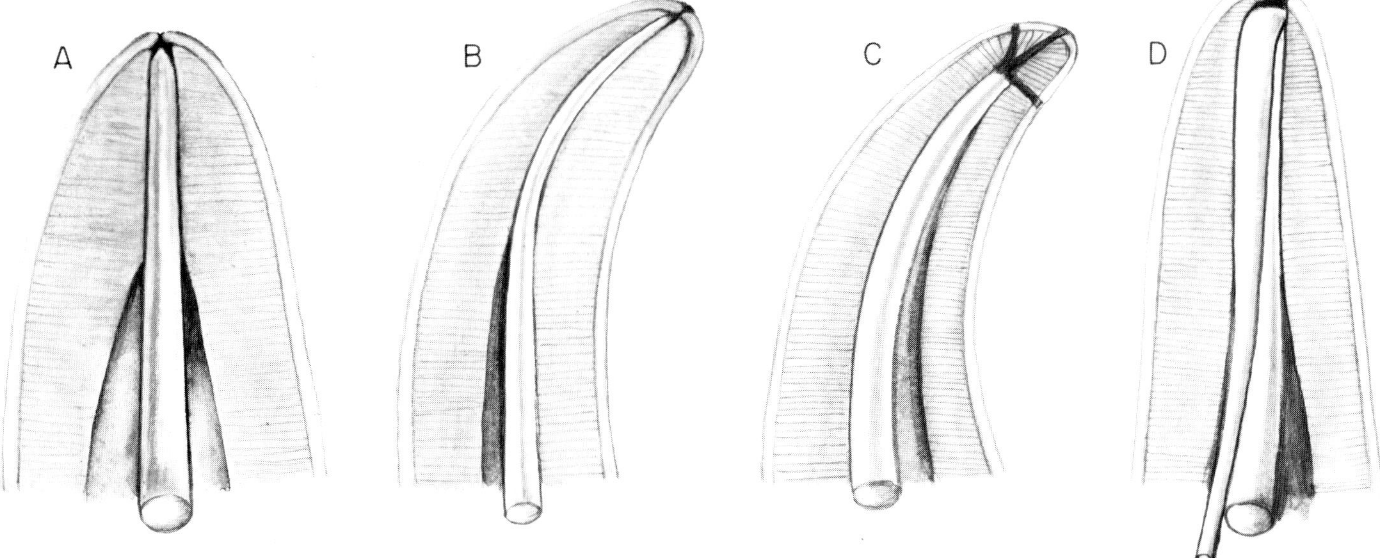

Fig. 3–42. Choosing filling material prior to canal cavity preparation based upon classification of canal anatomy. *A,* Class I, straight canal obturated with gutta percha and lateral condensation technique. *B,* Class II, curved canal which in some cases can be filled with silver point and gutta percha or with laterally condensed gutta percha. *C,* Class II, curved canal with multiple foramens enlarged by telescope preparation and filled with softened gutta percha. *D,* Class III, tubular canal, open foramen filled by inverted or custom-rolled gutta percha plus lateral condensation. (Courtesy Dr. James D. Zidell.)

Class II. Complicated, mature root canal (Fig. 3–41B_{1-5}) —severely curved or dilacerated, or with apical bifurcation (Fig. 3–4$C_{1,2}$), or auxiliary, lateral or accessory canals, but all with constriction of the foramen (or foramens).

Class III. Immature root canal either flaring at the apex in the so-called blunderbuss apex (Fig. 3–41D_1), or the open foramen (Fig. 3–41D_2).

Class IV. Primary tooth undergoing resorption.

For each of these shapes and sizes there is an optimum preparation and an optimum filling material (Fig. 3–42).

Techniques of Radicular Cavity Preparation

Preparation of the round, tapered endodontic cavity specifically to receive the preformed filling materials, occupies the majority of the operative time devoted to root canal treatment. Ideally, this round, tapered apical "seat" can be developed with a reamer or file used in a reaming action in a straight canal. This action will drill out the uneven dentin walls to an even bore the approximate size and shape of the filling materials (Fig. 3–43).

In addition to preparing the ***retention form*** of the apical seat by reaming, most root canals require some filing. The shape of most root canals is a greater flare than the taper of the instrument used in apical-third

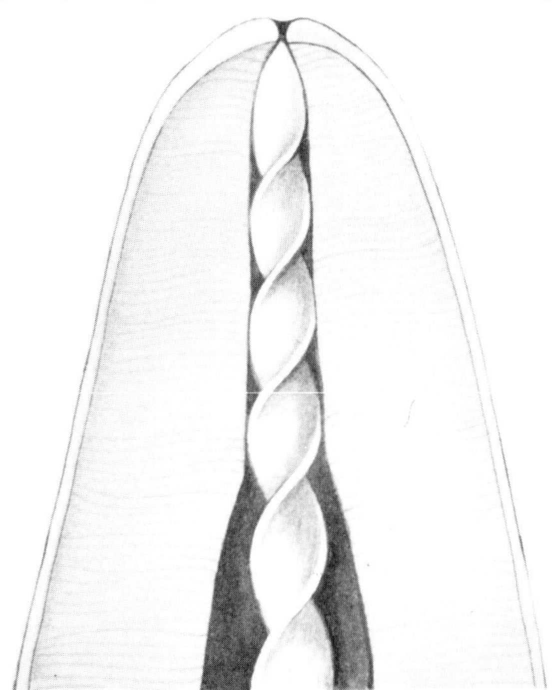

Fig. 3–43. Apical third of straight canals in anterior teeth and large canals in posterior teeth are reamed into round tapered preparation into which round tapered filling materials should accurately seat. Ideally, this apical portion of canal should be obturated completely by primary filling point. Remaining ovoid portion of canal must be filled by lateral or vertical condensation of additional gutta percha points into space.

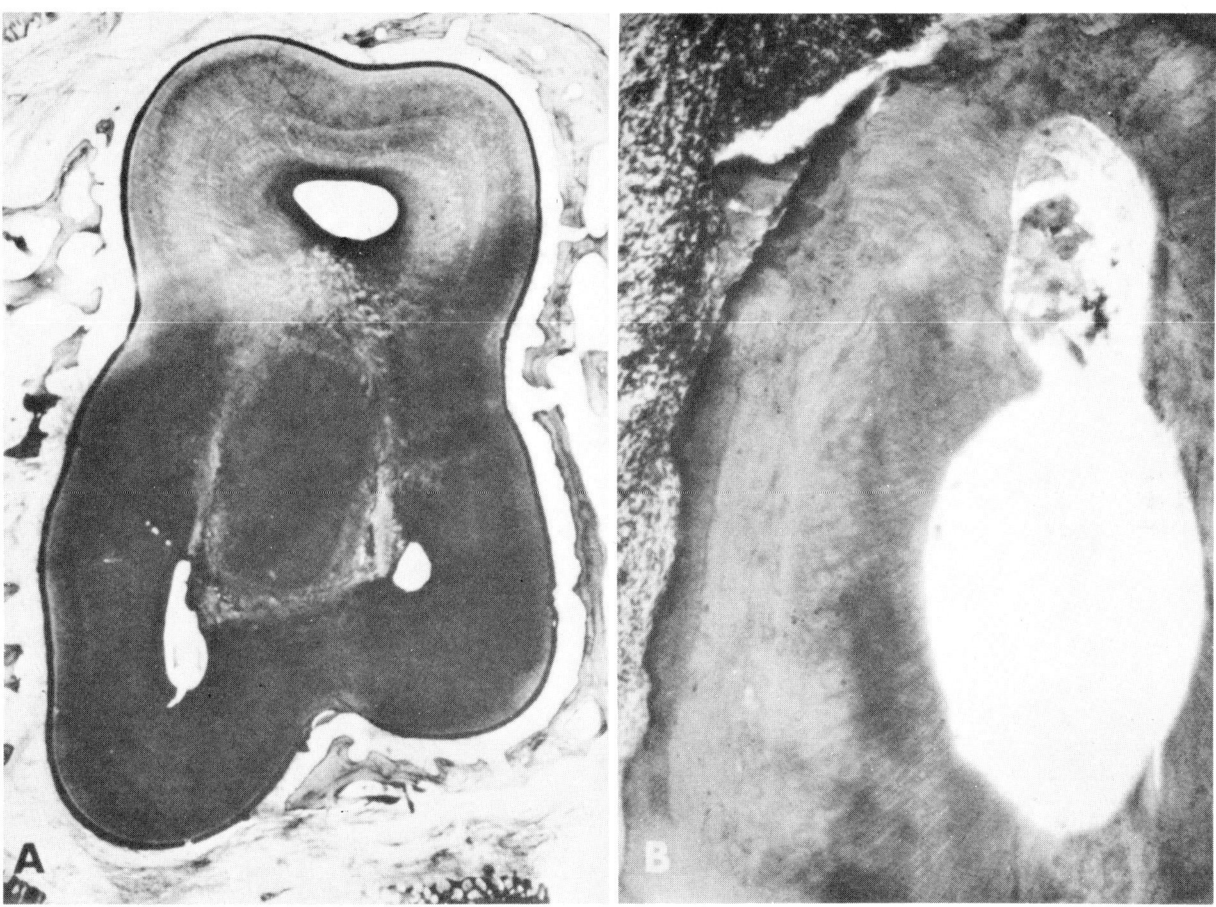

Fig. 3–44. *A,* Ovoid canal shape in "young" mandibular molar sectioned just below floor of pulp chamber. Distal canal *(top)* and mesiobuccal canal *(lower left)* will both require filing to complete their preparation. Reaming action alone would accurately shape mesiolingual canal *(lower right)* into round tapered preparation. *B,* "Dumbbell" shaped canal which could not accurately be enlarged into round tapered preparation. Filing action and multiple gutta percha point filling would be required to accurately shape and obturate this shape canal. Tactile sensation with curved exploring instrument would inform operator that he was not dealing with round tapered canal.

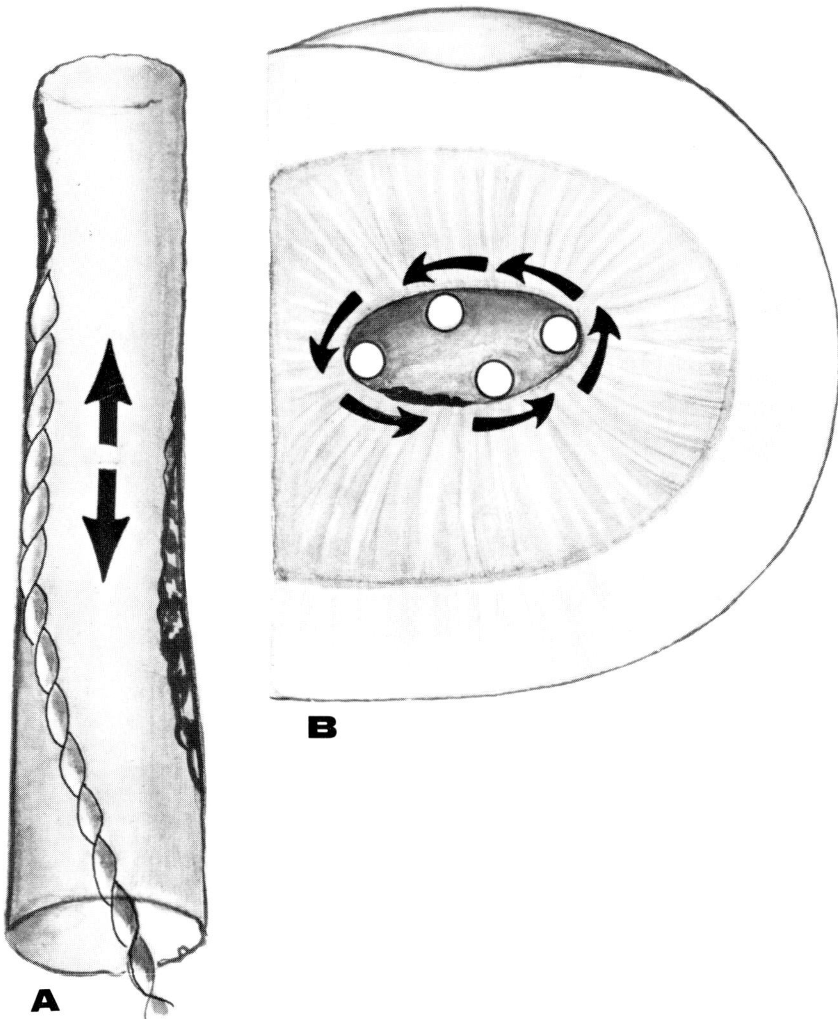

Fig. 3–45. *A,* Perimeter filing action used to debride and shape larger ovoid portions of canal. File is used in up-and-down rasping action with pressure exerted cross-canal against all walls. *B,* Cross sections showing shaping of ovoid canal. This "multiple exposure" illustration shows how file is used as rasp against walls around entire perimeter of canal. Only small area remains to be cleaned and shaped.

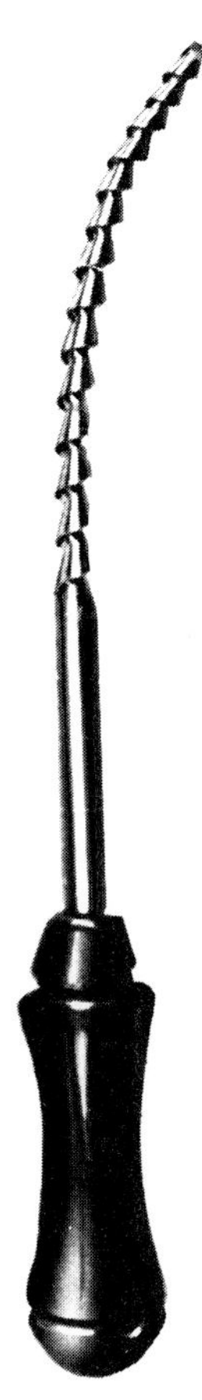

Fig. 3–46. Heavy Hedstrom file curved to better engage walls of ovoid canal. Blunted tip prevents encroachment into Retention Form cavity. (Courtesy Star Dental Manufacturing Co.)

preparation. Therefore, filing action must be used to enlarge the ovoid portion of the canals where reaming is ineffective (Fig. 3–44). The file cannot be merely worked up and down in the canal as a piston, but rather should be forced against the walls in all directions (Fig. 3–45). If the file is curved gradually, it may be more easily manipulated in this operation (Fig. 3–46).

Enlargement of the Straight Canal—Class I

The uncomplicated, mature root canal with restriction at the foramen, is easy to enlarge with hand instruments and requires only minutes of operating time. Speed of operation and caution not to force debris out the foramen go hand-in-hand.

After the length of the tooth has been established (p. 186) and the canal thoroughly irrigated of debris (p. 176), canal enlargement by reaming is begun. Selecting the initial reamer or file of optimum size will save operating time. This should be an instrument that will ***penetrate*** the canal to within 0.5 mm. of the apical foramen, yet cut into the walls when ***rotated*** and ***retracted.*** One may select the initial instrument by first judging the size of the canal in the roentgenogram, then choosing an instrument of this approximate width. By holding the instrument up to the roentgenogram, one may check the silhouette of the instrument against the canal size in the film.

As soon as the size of the initial instrument is established, the assistant may then prepare the subsequently numbered instruments by positioning stop attachments at the point of the working length on the blades, and then lining up the instruments in numerical order in a banker's sponge soaked in a germicide.

Resistance and Retention Form. In the presence of the sodium hypochlorite irrigating solution, the first instrument is ***penetrated*** into the canal to full length, is ***rotated*** a half turn, and is forcibly ***retracted.*** If the instrument was the proper size and caught in the wall, it returns with debris and discolored dentin filings. Thus begins the development of the ***retention form*** in the apical third of the canal (Fig. 3–47*A* and *B*) and the ***resistance form*** at the apical foramen (Fig. 3–47*C*). The instrument is cleaned on the depressed end of a cotton roll moistened in germicide, and is reintroduced, rotated, and retracted until it no longer cuts. This initial instrument is then set aside for ***recapitulation,*** which is the follow-up cleaning action of returning full-length with this smaller sized instrument to remove the dentinal debris that forms as the body of the canal is being shaped with the larger instruments.

To complete the ***retention form,*** files of consecutively increasing size are used to develop the ideal round preparation in the apical third. Clean white dentin chips indicate that the debris has been removed and that the instruments have properly "machined" the cavity walls. To achieve the round shape, one may need larger instruments than expected. Gutierrez and Garcia found that mandibular incisors were ***not*** adequately enlarged if the nonstandardized No. 6 (equal to standardized No. 50) instruments were used, nor were canines adequately prepared with No. 100 instruments.[58] In both cases, considerably larger instruments were needed.

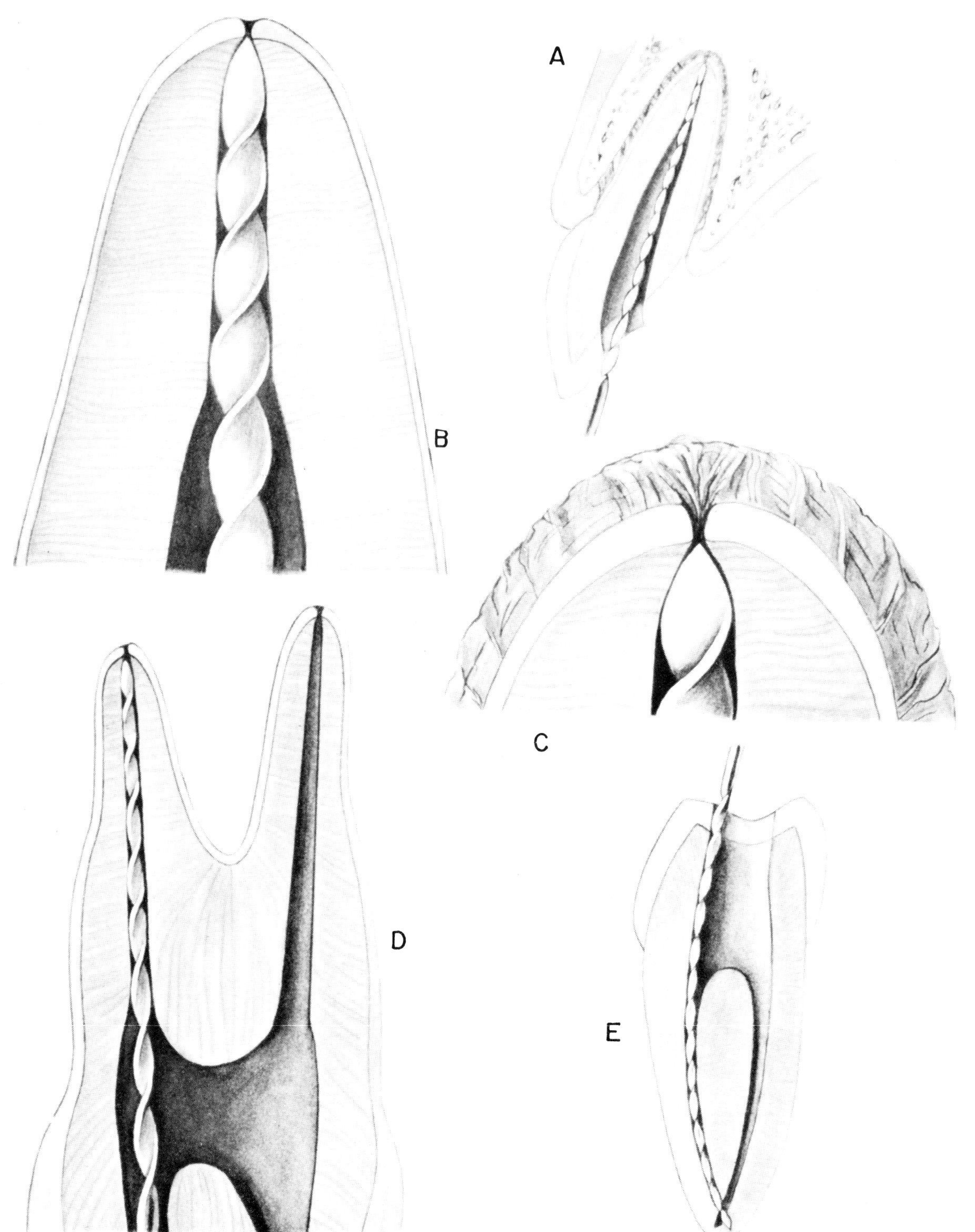

Fig. 3–47. *A,* Round, tapered apical seat for preformed filling materials is established by reaming action when instrument reaches apex unobstructed by interfering cavity walls. *B,* Apical third of straight canals in anterior teeth and large canal in molars and mandibular premolars is reamed into round tapered preparation into which round, tapered filling materials should accurately seat. Ideally, this apical portion of canal should be obturated completely by primary filling point. Remaining ovoid portion of canal must be filled by lateral or vertical condensation of additional gutta percha into the space. *C,* Apical limitations of instrumentation should be at cementodentinal junction, which is about 0.5 mm. from anatomic end of root. *D.* Fine canals of maxillary first premolar can often be reamed throughout their length to round tapered preparation and each canal subsequently filled with preformed filling point. *E,* In older patients, mesial canals in mandibular molars and buccal canals in maxillary molars may often be prepared throughout their length to receive round, tapered filling materials.

Haga also found it inadequate to enlarge canals only "two sizes larger than the first instrument that started to bite 5 to 6 mm. from the apex" (files smaller than No. 35).[59] For files larger than No. 35, the canals were prepared three sizes larger and were still inadequate. Haga was particularly disappointed in his failures to achieve round preparations 2 mm. from the apex in the mesiobuccal canals of maxillary molars (very broad buccolingually), the mesial canals of mandibular molars, and mandibular incisors and premolars. He pointed out that many of the mesial canals of mandibular molars are ribbon shaped and must be enlarged to the size of a "No. 50 file in order to be rid of all irregularities." He felt that enlargement must go beyond "bringing up 'white dentin' chips," even though preparations "feel" adequate during enlargement.

Vessey found that both reamers and files, ***when used in a reaming action,*** produced a circular canal preparation.[60] Files used as files, however, produced ovoid preparations as one might expect. Jungmann, Uchin, and Bucher evaluated the effectiveness of various methods of instrumentation on the shape of preparation in curved molar canals.[33] As did Haga, they considered instrumentation complete when the canal was enlarged two sizes beyond the first effective instrument. This did not prove adequate, however. The roundest preparations were produced with a K-style file used in reaming action, but only 55% of the time. Using a No. 5 Giromatic reamer, only 30% were round.

Owing to their anatomic shape, a few canals may sometimes be enlarged entirely by reaming action. These canals are (1) the two canals in the maxillary first premolar (Fig. 3–47*D*) and (2) the small canals in the molars (buccal canals in the maxillary and mesial canals in the mandibular, Fig. 3–47*E*), particularly in older patients in whom secondary dentin has narrowed the lumen of the canals.

If the initial instrument is No. 50 or larger, it is virtually impossible to break the instrument, and so more force and greater rotation may be used. The smaller sizes, however, must be handled with care. Fine instruments—tight in the canal—should be lubricated by a liquid soap, Septisol or R-C Prep which is a mixture of urea, EDTA, and glycerated hydrogen peroxide. All necrotic canals, large and small, should also be enlarged in the presence of sodium hypochlorite. First the lubricant is introduced; instrumentation follows; and then irrigation with sodium hypochlorite is carried out.

The clinician must be careful in developing the cavity in the apical third of the canal, for it is during this preparation that noxious and/or infected canal contents are forced out of the foramen into the periapical tissue. In this action, files are more apt to be the culprits than are reamers; however, it is usually the operator who is at fault, not the instruments.

In the event the canal cannot be prepared by reaming throughout its length (and this usually is the case), the dentist must return to filing the remainder of the canal. To repeat, this has been referred to as the ***toilet of the cavity,*** the perimeter filing to solid "white" dentin. In filing the coronal two-thirds of the preparation, one must carefully avoid the apical one-third, which has just been prepared into the round, slightly tapered preparation to receive the initial filling material. The instrument stop should be moved up 3 to 4 mm. to prevent the file from invading the apical third. Of course copious irrigation should accompany the filing, as should ***recapitulation*** with the smaller apical instrument, to ensure that this part of the cavity is not clogged with debris.

The shape of the final preparation has often been likened to the ***Washington Monument****—the silhouette of an obelisk, tapered to end in a pyramid at the apex reflecting the 75-degree point of the preparatory instruments.

The Class I canals, straight, uncomplicated, and mature with a constrictive foramen, have been prepared with the indicated filling material and method in mind. In most cases, for the larger tapered preparations gutta percha will be used, condensed with lateral or vertical force. In a few cases, primarily in elderly patients, single silver-point fillings can be used. These are the narrow-lumen canals which have been reamed to the round tapered shape throughout their entire length. The techniques of filling these canals will be discussed in the following chapter.

The variance in straight canals ranges from the uncomplicated, already described, to the enormous class III canals with the open or flaring apex. Another variant is the canal so constricted by calcification that great difficulty is encountered in exploring or enlarging. In such cases, chelation may be of some help.

Chelation and Enlargement. A straight canal that is almost totally calcified or blocked by a pulp stone or point of calcification may still be enlarged. Chelation by means of ethylene diamine tetra-acetic acid (EDTA) buffered to pH 7.3 has been advocated

*Dr. Dudley Glick has been credited with this concept.

by Nygaard-Ostby,[61] and appears to help in preparation. When the mineral salts have been removed from the obstructing dentin by chelation, only the softened matrix remains,[62,63] and this may then be removed by reamers or files used to "drill past" the obstruction.

Contrary to popular belief, Fraser has shown that chelating agents "do not soften dentin in the narrow apical parts of the root canal," although softening can occur in the cervical and middle portions, allowing more space for instrumentation in the unchelated apical portion. Although the lumen of the canal may be very fine, a stronger heavier instrument must be used to drill past the calcification. A No. 20 to 30 reamer or file is indicated. This straight, drilling action ***cannot*** be done in a curved canal, however, or a ledge will be developed. EDTA can be carried into the chamber in the beaks of cotton pliers.

Enlargement of the Curved Canal—Class II

Complications of the mature root canal vary, ranging from curved canals to accessory canals to apical bifurcations. With all these complications, however, there is still a natural constriction of the apical foramen. During the preparation of class II root canals most of the endodontic accidents occur—ledge or shelf formation, perforations, and broken instruments.

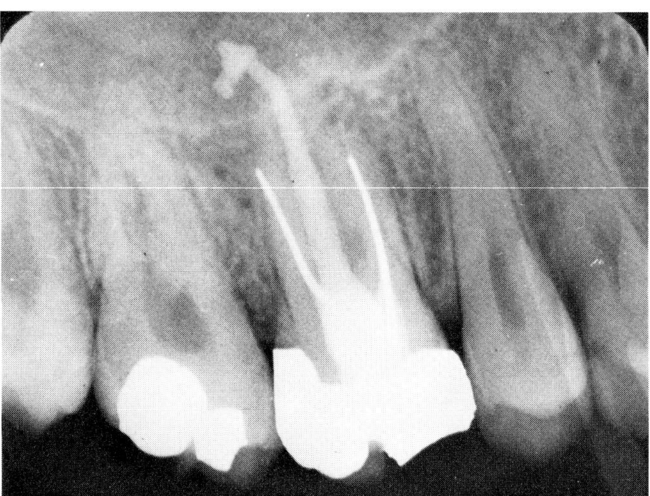

Fig. 3–48. Apical curve to buccal of palatal root went undetected and was perforated by heavy instruments and then overfilled. Right-angle radiographs fail to reveal buccal or lingual curves. Telescopic preparation could have prevented perforation. (Courtesy Dr. Richard E. Walton.)

Curved roots, and hence curved canals, may be any of five types: (1) the apical curve, (2) the gradual curve, (3) the defalcation or sickle-shaped curve, (4) the dilaceration or sudden angular bend, and (5) the bayonet or double curve. Pucci has presented a similar classification.[65]

The curved root often can be seen in the radiograph and taken into account during treatment. However, roots that curve toward the central beam of the x-ray, that is, toward the buccal or lingual, are much more difficult to discover. The frequent finding (55%) of buccal curvature of the lingual root of the maxillary first molar (Fig. 3–48), and the labial or lingual curvature of the maxillary central incisor or canine are the most exasperating examples (Plates IV, VI, XXI).

Occasionally, the curvature in line with the central beam will show up as a "bulls-eye" or "target" at the apex of the root returning upon itself. These radiographic characteristics may be subtle and easily missed.

Resistance and Retention Form. ***Always use a curved instrument in a curved canal*** (an endodontic axiom). Use of the curved instrument *per se* will not necessarily ensure success. However, it can be stated categorically that ***straight instruments used in curved canals will ensure failure.*** The clinician must know that a curved instrument will not remain curved during reaming, but will be straightened as it is forcibly withdrawn from its locked position. The retraction that makes the cut also unbends the instrument. ***It is imperative that the curve be restored*** after each use; hence the operator should acquire the habit of always working with a cotton roll in the left hand, to clean and restore the bend to each instrument each time it is withdrawn.

Initially, a curved No. 10 or 15 file must be carefully worked down the canal, frequently aided by the chelation of EDTA, often pushing and rotating the tip in two or three directions according to the complexity of the curve—***impulsion*** and ***vaivén.*** Not until the instrument is completely to depth is it ***retracted*** to make the primary cut. If ***rotation*** is used to "set" a small instrument in the dentin, it must be held to a minimum of a half turn, for more tension leads to breakage. Recurving the instrument before it is re-introduced reduces the chance of ledge formation.

Another cause of ledge formation is the use of too large an instrument in the confining lumen of the curved canal. Curved canals are often fine in caliber, and it is rarely necessary to enlarge the terminus of these apical-third cavity preparations beyond a size 35 to 45 instrument. There are exceptions to this observation, primarily in young teeth; however, the ***large*** curved canals are not the problem the ***fine*** curved canals can be. The wide lumen of the large canal encourages instrumentation across the width of the space, whereas in the fine canal, the instrument is held tightly against the entire wall surface.

Returning again to the thesis that the preparation of the root canal cavity is related to the filling material to be used, one easily visualizes the difference in instrumentation for silver point or gutta percha obturation. Two basic types of preparation will be presented, to be followed by the use and modifications of these preparations related to the five different curves in root canals.

Silver Point Preparation, Class II Canals. The properties of a firm but flexible silver point permit it to be guided around the curvature of a canal and inserted with a great amount of pressure into the seat of the apical preparation. It is this firmness that recommends it over gutta percha for ***fine*** curved canals. If the dentist believes, however, that a preparation other than a perfectly round one is being produced, the idea of using a silver point should be abandoned and the preparation modified, as described in the next section, to receive gutta percha.

Silver point preparation and cementation are somewhat faster than gutta percha, and the selection of silver is often made on this basis alone. Totality of obturation rather than expediency, however, should be the deciding factor. As the larger files (size 35 and above) are reached for a silver point preparation, one should begin re-evaluating the outcome of the preparation and consider the use of gutta percha.

Silver point preparation is done by reaming action. The instrument should fit the constrictive canal throughout its length. Starting with a No. 10 or 15 instrument tight in the canal, one advances the sizes upward, but rarely past No. 25 or 30. At this point, clean white dentin is removed with each cutting, and the round tapered preparation is being formed. Remember ***recapitulation***—returning frequently with the first instrument to break up and remove any chips or debris forming in the apical curve. The final preparation should resemble that illustrated in Figure 3–47*D* and *E*).

Gutta Percha Point Preparation, Class II Canals. A step-back method of cavity preparation, particularly adaptable for curved canals, has been described by Martin as a telescopic filing technique,[66] but will be referred to here as ***telescopic preparation.*** Walton has best detailed telescopic preparation as a special method of reaming (and terminally, filing) to permit resistance and retention form preparation of a curved tapered canal while minimizing the risk of

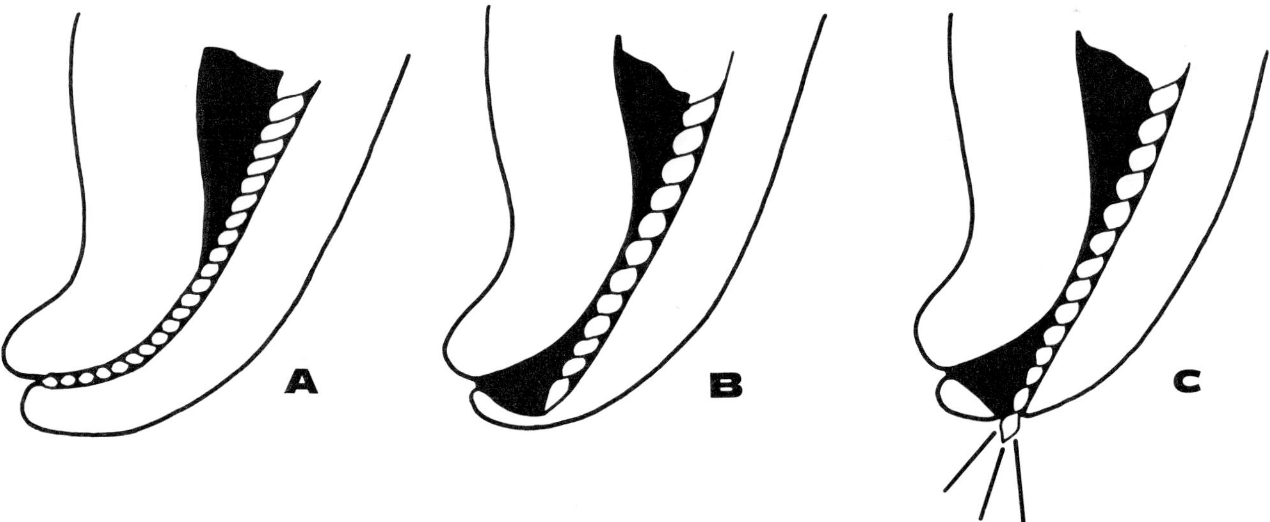

Fig. 3–49. Hazards of overenlarging apical curve. *A,* Small flexible instruments readily negotiate curves. *B,* Larger instruments, #40 and above, markedly increase in stiffness and cutting efficiency, causing fan-shaped preparation as they are turned. *C,* Persistent enlargement with larger instruments will result in perforation and impossible obturation situation. (Courtesy Dr. Richard E. Walton.)

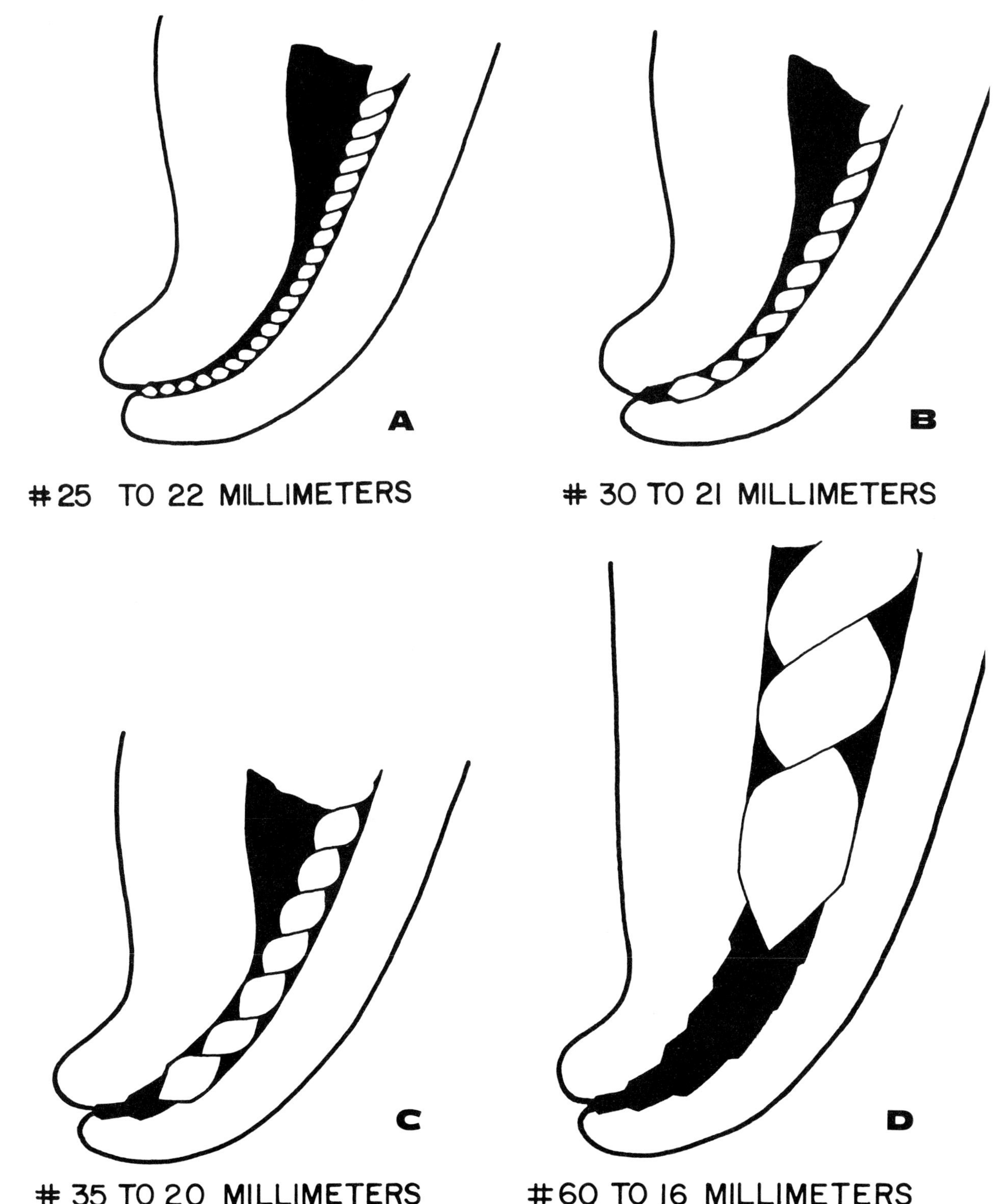

Fig. 3–50. *Telescopic Preparation* to properly enlarge apical curve. *A,* Working length of example tooth is 22 mm. Starting with #10 file, Resistance and Retention Form cavities are optimally enlarged to size 25 (for example). *B,* When advancing to next size, #30, working length is shortened 1 mm. to 21 mm. *C,* Next size file is shortened to 20 mm. and so on up through sizes. *D,* Size 60 instrument is being used at 16 mm, and curve has been properly enlarged, cleansed, and straightened without perforation. Frequent recapitulation with #25 file and irrigation removes dentinal debris and smooths "steps" of preparation. (Courtesy Dr. Richard E. Walton.)

apical perforation.[67] The cavity preparation ultimately resembles an open telescope, its size increasing, section by section, from apex to chamber.

A frequent dilemma is that of a canal that is large and ovoid in its middle space, but curving and tapering rapidly in its apical portion. In an attempt to prepare this curve properly, and at the same time to develop adequate space for gutta percha, the operator often works with increasingly larger instruments. Smaller flexible instruments are preferable, for they readily deform as they adapt to the curvature of the canal (Fig. 3–49*A*). When No. 35 instruments are reached, however, the degree of stiffness increases, and these larger instruments do not easily deform to match the curve.[68] Straight instruments will remove dentin only from the outside of the curve, shaving a straight pathway (Fig. 3–49*B*). If enlargement is continued, the root will eventually be perforated (Fig. 3–49*C*).

Telescopic preparation resolves many of the aforementioned problems and affords additional advantages. The basic technique is as follows:

1. The curved apical portion of the canal is enlarged by reaming to a No. 25, No. 30 or No. 35

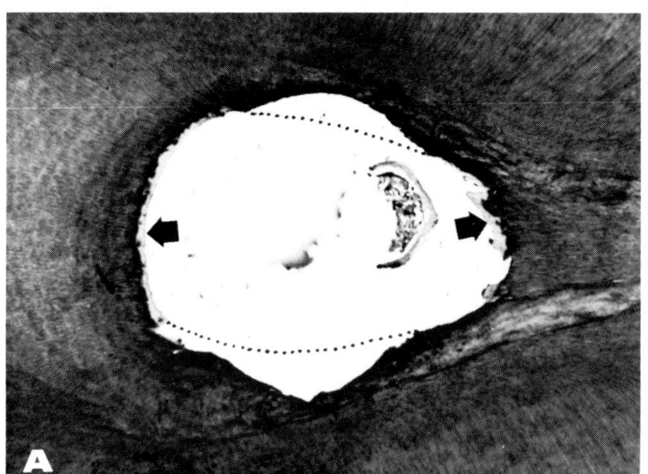

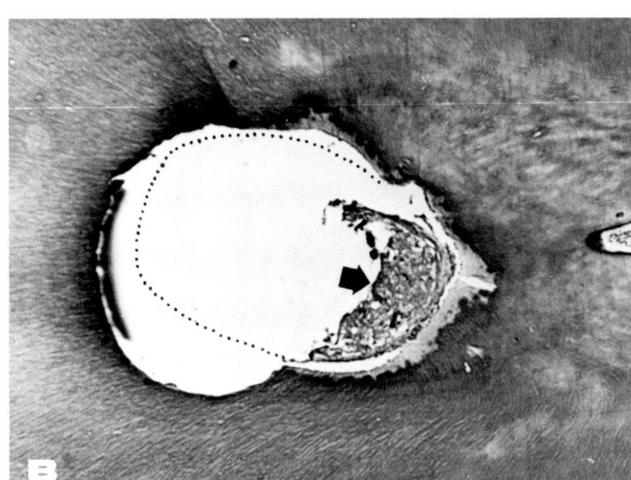

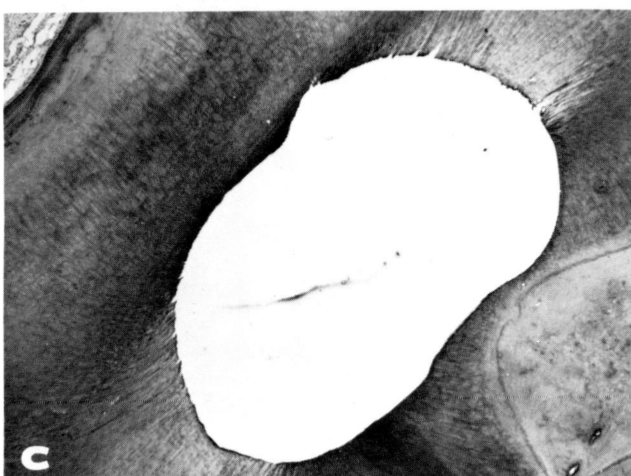

Fig. 3–51. Evaluation of three different methods of curved canal enlargement done *in situ* in patients. *A,* Canal preparation by reaming alone to size 45 produces clean white dentin and "smooth" walls. Dotted line indicates outline of original canal. Reamer shaved round hole in center of ovoid canal, as evidenced by remaining predentin (arrows). *B,* Filing to size 45 produces clean shavings and smooth walls. Only portion of original walls (dotted line) were planed by the files, leaving debris (arrow) pressed into untouched portion of canal. *C,* Canal enlarged by telescopic preparation. Begun with size 25 instrument at apex, canal is thoroughly debrided through size 70 only a few millimeters from apex. (Courtesy Dr. Richard E. Walton.)

instrument—the greater the curvature, the smaller the instrument (Fig. 3–50*A*).

2. When the ***resistance form*** preparation is complete at the foramen, successively larger files are then employed (as reamers) at decreasingly shorter lengths. In other words, as each larger instrument is employed, the "length-of-tooth" measurement is shortened by 1 mm. A series of concentric steps (telescoping) is thus created (Fig. 3–50*B* and *C*).

3. This operation is continued until the entire curved portion of the canal has been prepared (Fig. 3–50*D*). Weine has described a similar technique.[69]

4. By ***recapitulation***, the initial instrument used in apical preparation is used frequently to full depth to smooth off the "steps" and break up the dentin chips and debris to be eliminated by copious irrigation.

The advantages of this technique are: (1) less possibility of perforation or ledging, (2) uniform enlargement of irregularly shaped canals, (3) better debridement, (4) savings in operating time, and (5) obturation with gutta percha in severely curved canals, with the exaggerated taper permitting greater compression of the gutta percha in the apical portion of the canal.

Walton has histologically demonstrated the superiority of the telescoping preparation of curved canals when compared to straight reaming or filing of this space (Fig. 3–51).[67]

This technique requires precision teamwork, with an assistant carefully measuring and applying the stop attachments to the succession of instruments. Using progressively larger and larger files speeds up operation as they become progressively more efficient. This method is most certainly not recommended if a silver point is to be used.

Apical Curve. The most common root curve encountered is the apical curve, found in all types of teeth but occurring most frequently (53%) in maxillary lateral incisors. The enlarging instrument of choice is a file. The necessary curve placed in the file should approximate the curve in the canal. It should resemble the curve placed in the exploring instrument, that is, the bend should be near the tip of the instrument, but the shaft should be straight (Fig. 3–52). In the presence of Septisol or R-C Prep, the curved instrument is carried up the canal with the curve aimed in the same direction as the curve in the canal. When the instrument is completely to depth, the handle is rotated one-half turn to lock the blades into the dentin, and the file is retracted. This action

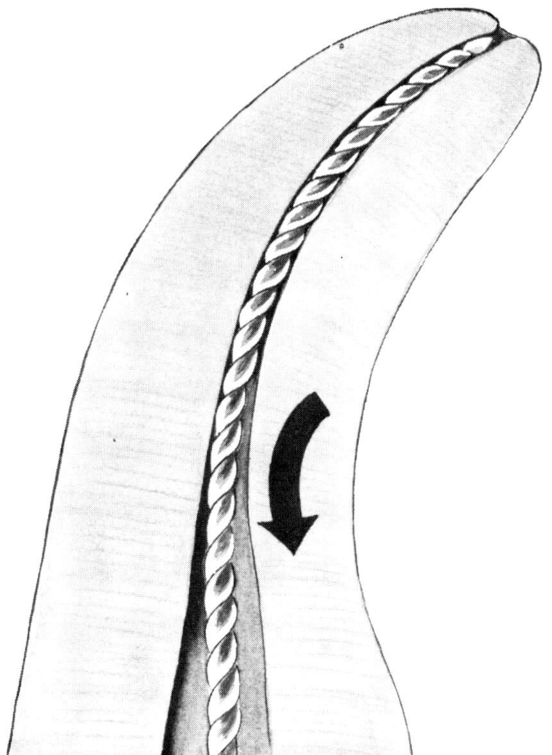

Fig. 3–52. Correct placement of initial curved instrument. It is introduced to full working length, set by a half rotation and retracted. Repeating this action with successively larger files establishes Resistance and Retention Forms.

produces the termination of the tapered cavity in the ***apical*** portion of the canal, the ***resistance form.*** The details of the development of the telescoped ***retention form*** of the cavity and the remaining tapered but straight part of the cavity are well described and illustrated in the previous sections.

When the curved tip instrument is used, caution must be exercised not to hollow out or cavitate a preparation. This error develops from rotating or spinning a curved instrument, which might be loose in the canal, through complete rotation rather than "locking" the instrument and retracting with half rotations. The curved tip of the instrument, turning in a full arc, tends to gouge out the apical cavity into a hollow cavern-like preparation rather than to machine-out an optimum round shape (Fig. 3–53).

Access to the curved apical region may be greatly improved by skewing the ***coronal*** access cavity preparation toward the side of the tooth opposite the curve (Plate V, E–H). This approach often presents a straightened trajectory up to the curved apex.

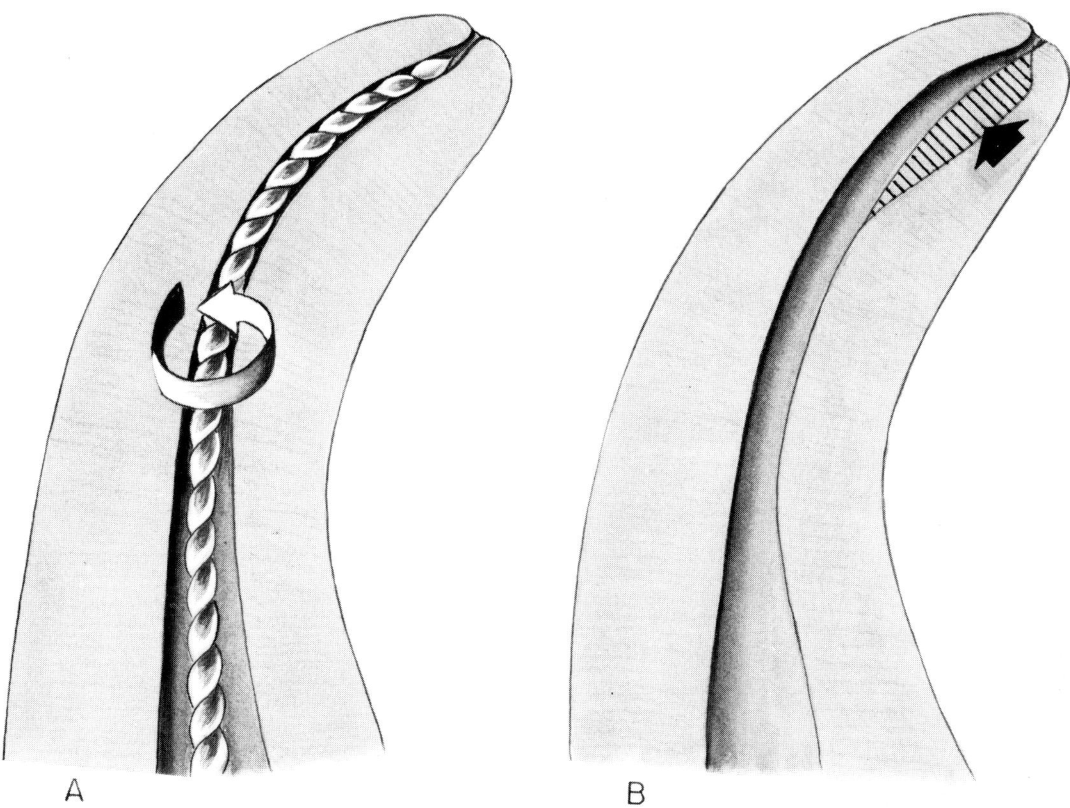

Fig. 3–53. *A,* Incorrect enlargement of apical curve will lead to cavitation. If larger curved instruments are spun in canal, curved tip will gouge cavity. *B,* Ovoid cavity (arrow) which has been developed by incorrect reaming action.

Gradual Curve and Defalcated Curve. These two curves are similar in trajectory but vary only in degree. The suggested approach to preparation is therefore the same. In the presence of EDTA, a small file (No. 10 or No. 15) with a full curve in the blade, is passed down the canal with the tip aimed in the direction of the curve. When the tip is down to full depth, the handle of the file is forced laterally away from the curve, thus placing the blade under tension. While the handle is held in this position, the instrument is forcibly withdrawn (Fig. 3–54*A*). It is essential that the tip of the instrument is at full working length when the cut is made. When the file can be easily slipped to full length and is no longer cutting, the next size file is curved and used, but at a 1-mm. shorter length. Each successive file must be eliminating clean white dentin before the apical preparation is considered complete by ***"telescoping."***

If the remaining straight portion of the canal is ovoid in shape, it may be filed smooth by pressing the file against all walls. The continued filing may deposit dentin chips and block the canal. ***Recapitulation*** with the initial instrument removes any of the filings packed ahead of the instruments.

Occasionally decuspation is necessary in order to reach along unobstructed lines into the defalcated canal; this procedure leaves the chamber at a severely obtuse angle (see Fig. 1–24). Decuspation allows the instrument to be placed into the canal along a straighter trajectory than was previously possible.

Dilaceration or Sudden Angular Bend. The file used to prepare the ***resistance form*** cavity in the dilacerated canal must have a ***severe*** curve ***near the tip.*** The major problem in these cases is the exploration, hence the ***pathfinder curve*** in the instrument.

Again, EDTA may be used to soften the dentin walls. The fine file (No. 10) penetrates the canal to the apex, with the tip aimed to hug constantly the inside wall of the canal. Slight twisting, pushing, and "jiggling" of the instrument are often required to clear the area of severe curvature. The cut should not be made until the tip of the instrument is in full position, then the handle is forced in the opposite direction of the curve and the instrument forcibly withdrawn while under tension (Fig. 3–54*B*).

The fine file will enlarge the canal to the point where it is no longer cutting. Successively larger instruments are then used in ***telescoping*** the preparation, each one shortened by 1 mm., until clean white dentin is being removed and the ***retention form*** cavity is complete.

The remainder of the cavity is then finished by vertical filling. ***Recapitulation*** and irrigation must be used to remove dentin chips packed ahead of the files. Skewing of the coronal access cavity may also be an essential to success.

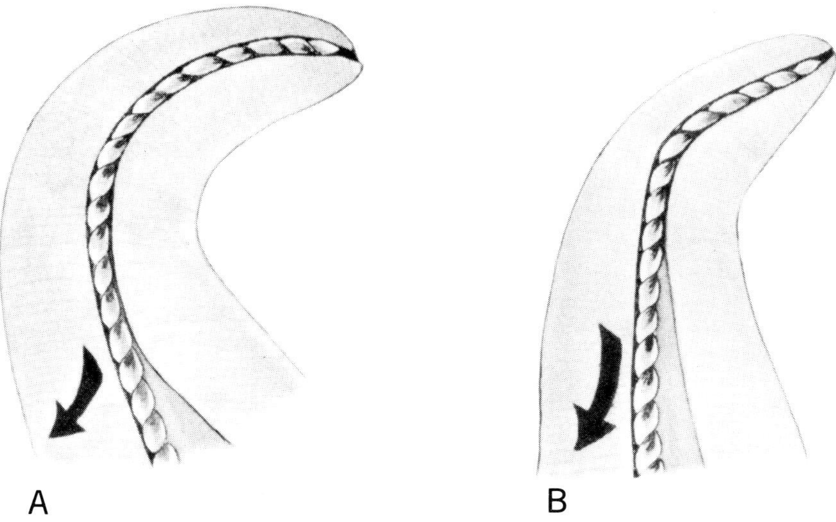

Fig. 3–54. Correct resistance and retention form preparations of defalcated and dilacerated canals. *A*, Defalcated (sickle shape) canal is best enlarged by introducing fine curved file to full depth, locking instrument into dentin by slight rotation, and forcibly retracting instrument. Using successively larger flexible files to full depth establishes resistance form terminal preparation. *B*, Correct enlargement of dilacerated canal. Resistance form is developed as described in *A*. Retention form for both preparations is done by telescoping—step-back reaming with successively larger and shorter instruments.

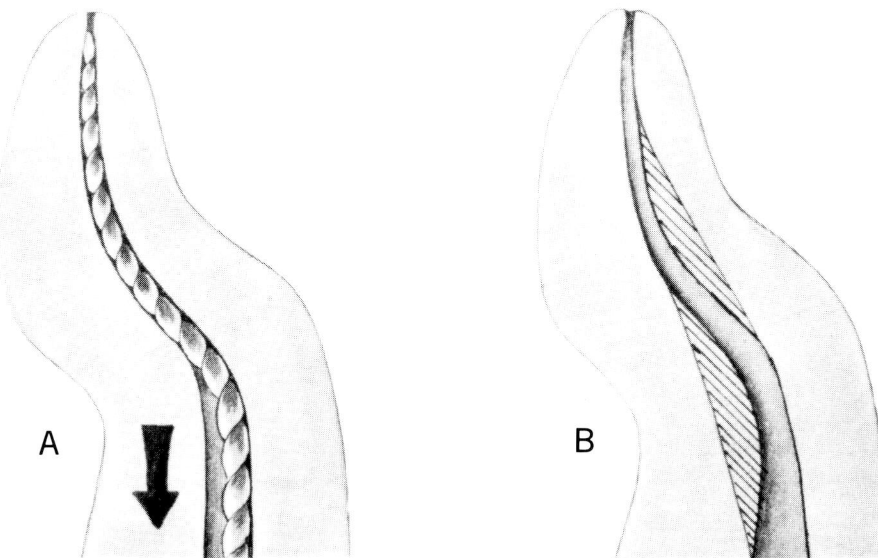

Fig. 3–55. *A*, Correct enlargement of bayonet or "S" shaped canal. Small curved file is introduced to full depth and forcibly retracted vertically. *B*, Filing action debrides and shapes entire canal and removes bulk of dentin from inside and outside of the curves. Apical third cavity is then prepared by telescoping.

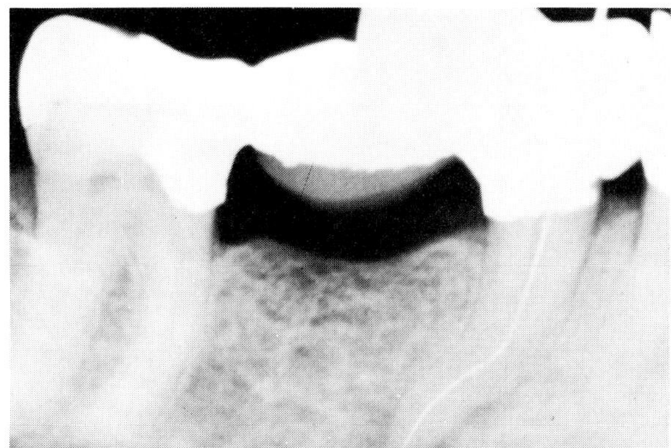

Fig. 3–56. Exploration and instrumentation of bayonet canal. Fine curved exploring file is introduced to full depth in canal. This instrument is used to full capacity and is following by progressively larger files. Lubrication with Septisol and repeated irrigation is necessary to prevent blockage of canal.

Bayonet or Double Curve. The S-shaped curve of the bayonet canal is best explored with a fine file (No. 10) in the presence of EDTA. The gently curved instrument is passed up the canal aimed in the direction of the first curve. When this curve is passed, the sharp point of the instrument can be felt against the inside dentin wall, and at this point the instrument is given a one-half turn to aim the point in the direction opposite that of the second curve. By pushing, the instrument makes two cuts—the ***resistance form*** preparation at the foramen and the vertical planing of the opposite walls at the point of "bayonet" (Fig. 3–55). Apical ***retention form*** is then completed by "telescoping," while the S curvature is filed into a gentle trajectory, which can then be dealt with as a gradual curve (Fig. 3–56).

It is imperative that the curve constantly be replaced in the instruments during use. Forcibly retracting an instrument from a bayonet canal will completely straighten the blade. If this straight instrument is then replaced in the curved canal and nicks the wall beyond the curve, a ledge will be started at this point. Every instrument that is subsequently placed in the canal will "hang-up" on the ledge.

Iatrogenic Errors in Endodontic Cavity Preparation

1. *Correction of the Error of Ledge Formation.* The best correction for ledge formation is its prevention. Most ledges in canals are formed by inattentive or careless operation; that is, the access cavity is not sufficiently or correctly prepared to allow direct access down the canal to the apex, or straight instruments are used in curved canals, or too large an instrument is used. Occasionally, even the skilled and careful clinician develops a ledge in a canal, usually owing to some unsuspected aberration in canal anatomy or direction (Fig. 3–57).

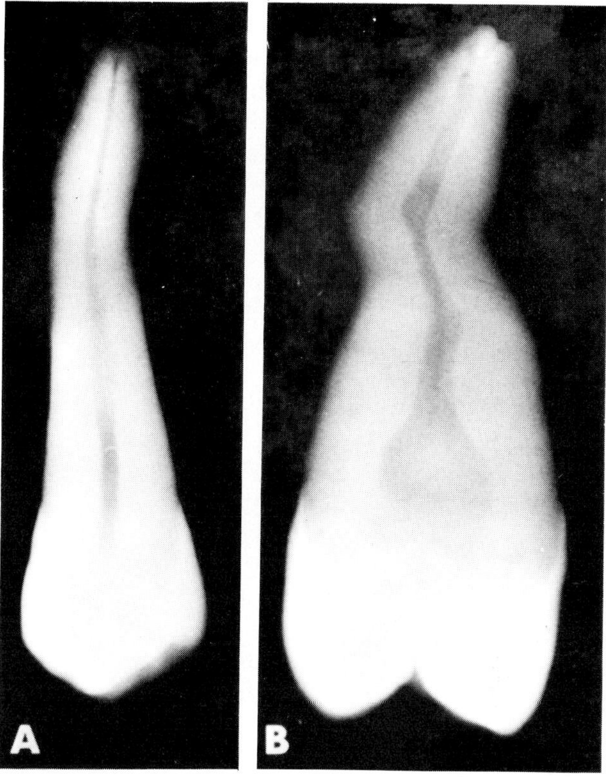

Fig. 3–57. *A,* Unsuspected aberration in canal anatomy is not apparent in standard buccolingual roentgenogram. *B,* Severe bayonet shape of canal shown here in mesiodistal roentgenogram would be determined by careful exploration. Instrumentation would terminate at apical delta.

Ledge formation is suspected when the enlarging instrument no longer can be passed down the canal to full working length. There is also a loss of the normal tactile sensation of the tip of the instrument passing through the lumen. This feeling is supplanted by the feeling that the point of the instrument is hitting against a blank wall—a loose feeling with no tactile sensation of tensional binding (Fig. 3–58*A*).

Rather than foolishly continue with enlargement, the operator should immediately examine the tooth roentgenographically with the instrument in place.

The central x-ray beam should be directed exactly through the involved area. If the roentgenogram shows the instrument point apparently leaving the lumen of the canal, an entirely different approach must be employed to remove the ledge and yet complete enlargement.

First, the fine ***file***, No. 10 or 15, is selected to explore the canal to the apex. A ***severe curve*** is set in the ***point*** of this instrument, and it is carried down the canal with the very tip hugging the wall opposite the ledge. The *vaivén* motion (p. 182) often helps in advancing the instrument. If the exploring instrument can be introduced to full working length, a larger file is selected, one that will reach to the apex yet fill the lumen of the canal. Again, the point is severely curved in this instrument, and by accurate alignment of the point and *vaivén* motion, it is carefully worked down the canal to full depth. It is wise to take a roentgenogram at this time to confirm one's tactile sense.

Filing should begin when the clinician is absolutely certain that the point of the instrument is correctly placed. The filing is done in the presence of a lubricant or irrigant and should be in a vertical stroke, always maintaining the point against the inside wall and pressing the blades against the ledge area (Fig. 3–58*B*). The canal should be constantly irrigated to wash out dentin filings. The tip of the file must be checked repeatedly to be certain the curve is maintained. If the instrument is allowed to straighten, it will again catch on the ledge and repeated filing might well lead to deepening the ledge, or worse, to perforation. The possibility of perforation is enhanced by chelation from the EDTA; hence it is not advised for the novice.

2. *Perforation.* There are two locations of iatrogenic perforations. The first is the ***lateral*** perforation, an outgrowth of the ledge or shelf formation already described. The second is the ***apical*** perforation.

Perforations in both these locations may be caused by two errors of commission: (1) starting a ledge and

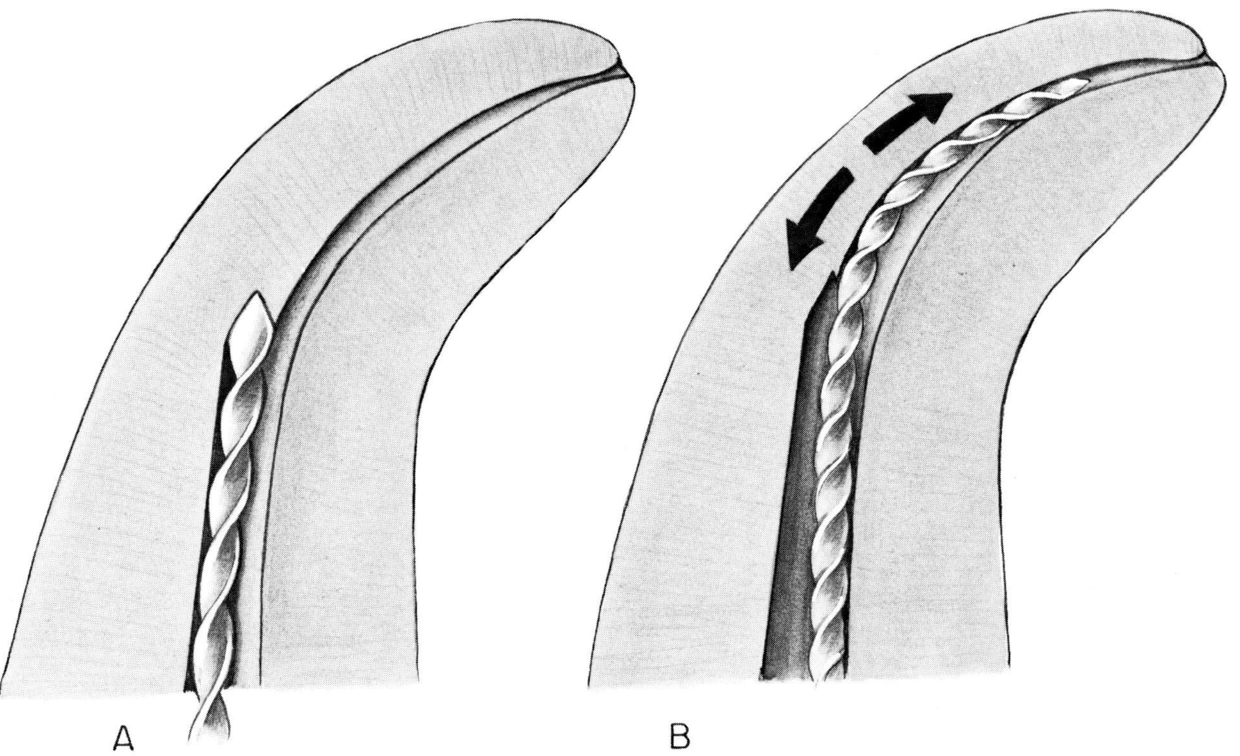

Fig. 3–58. Cause and correction of ledge formation in curved canal. *A,* Large straight instrument has been used in curved canal and immediately cuts ledge at curve. *B,* This ledge may be painstakingly removed with severely curved file, rasping against ledge in presence of sodium hypochlorite or Septisol. In order to bypass ledge, tip of correcting instrument must be severely curved so it will hug inside wall of curve.

then drilling out through the side of the root at a point of canal obstruction or root curvature (see Fig. 1–47), and (2) using too large or too long an instrument and either perforating directly out through the apical foramen or "wearing" a hole in the lateral surface of the root by overinstrumentation.

Apical Perforations. Failure to follow the apical curvature of a canal leads to the frequent perforations of maxillary lateral incisors or the palatal roots of maxillary molars. Throughout the sections on cavity preparation, the importance of using curved and proper sized instruments in curved canals has been stressed. Failure to do so inevitably leads to perforation at the curve (Fig. 3–59*A*). Once the accident has happened, it is important to return to the natural canal in order to complete the debridement and a ***telescopic*** preparation. This is done by bypassing the perforation with severely curved instruments. The curve in the instrument and the proper placement in the canal must coincide with the canal curvature. Confirmation by x-ray examination is important.

One is now dealing with two foramens—one natural, the other iatrogenic (Fig. 3–59*A*). Obturation of both of these foramens and of the main body of the canal requires the vertical compressive techniques with softened gutta percha or chloropercha (Fig. 3–59*B*), described in Chapter 4.

Apical perforation also occurs in a perfectly straight canal owing to incorrect tooth length. This invariably causes discomfort to the patient, if not an apical abscess. The cause is failure to establish a ***resistance form*** cavity, or foramen, at the cementodentinal junction. Filling will be difficult.

It can be corrected in part by re-establishing tooth length to the former CD junction and then enlarging the canal with ***much*** larger instruments to this point. In this way, the initial gutta percha placed in the

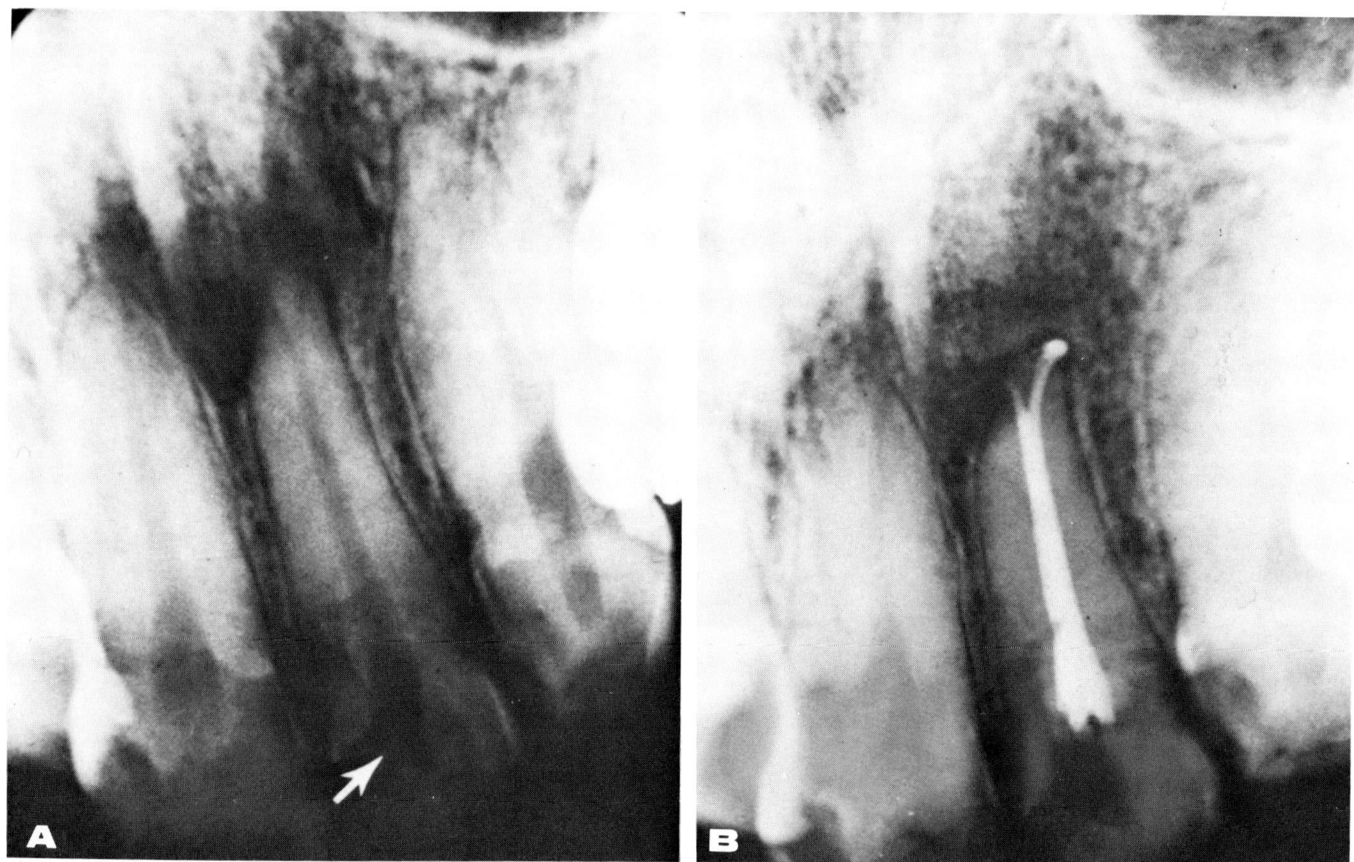

Fig. 3–59. *A,* Inadequate access preparation in crown (arrow) has diverted enlarging instruments and caused perforation and two open foramens. *B,* Using softened gutta percha technique, perforations are obturated. (Courtesy Dr. James D. Zidell.)

retention form cavity will not be forced out the apex, even though some cement might be. The solution is a compromise, but is usually preferable to a surgical correction.

Lateral Wall Perforation. Perforations part way up the canal, at a point of canal obstruction or ledge formation, can best be overcome with severely curved instruments correctly oriented in the curved canal as already described. The location of the perforation can be learned by placing a paper point in the canal until it is removed with a bloody tip, and measuring this distance on the point.

The lateral perforation caused by overinstrumentation and "wearing" through a thin wall is most likely to happen on the "inside" curve of a severely curved canal. In another case, overzealous enlargement with an instrument whose diameter exceeds the width of the canal at its narrowest point leads to perforation (Fig. 3–60). This is most common in the mesial roots of mandibular molars or in the area of mesial concavity in maxillary first premolars.

Obturation of canals with lateral perforations can best be accomplished with gutta percha condensed by lateral pressure. Surgical correction of perforations may be necessary in refractory cases.

3. *Broken Instruments.* Once again, the best correction for broken instruments is prevention. Prevention is best accomplished by being willing to discard any file that has been bent more than 45 degrees or shows signs of stress along its spiral surface. When the spacing becomes uneven between the cutting edges of a reamer or file, it means the instrument has been stressed at that point and should be discarded.

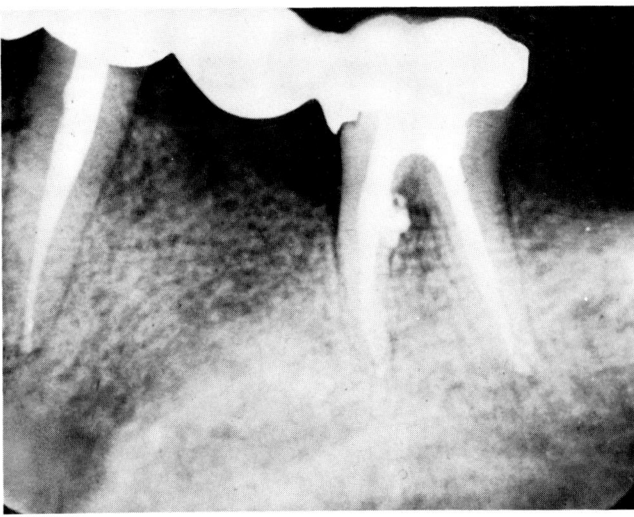

Fig. 3–60. Lateral perforation by wearing through thin wall at furcation. (Courtesy Dr. James D. Zidell.)

Certain instruments, such as Nos. 8, 10, and 15, should never be reused and are often discarded, even during use on one patient. These smaller instruments, Nos. 8, 10, and 15, must never be forced or wedged into a canal: rather, they must be teased gently. If they do not pass to the desired depth, the instrument must be removed, the curvature or the deflection of the tip of the instrument modified slightly, and the instrument reinserted again as a pathfinder. This process may be repeated many times before the pathway down the canal is located.

Often, these instruments break along the walls of the canal, being stuck between irregularities of secondary dentin or calcifications. Usually these instruments can be bypassed if the canals are oval and irregular in shape. Bypassing these instruments is made easier with EDTA, if used with great care. The broken fragment has a "nasty habit" of diverting the bypass instrument, producing a perforation.

Why all this fuss about the retrieval of broken instruments? Crump and Natkin,[70] as well as Fox,[71] have shown that success following instrument fragmentation is as good as success from a properly filled canal. These are the cases in which the instrument was twisted off at the apex, and being locked tightly in the dentin, served to prevent apical percolation. Chapter 4 deals with the subject of obturating canals with "broken" instruments.

If an instrument is broken and ***loose*** within the canal, it may lie in a "sea of debris." This is hardly conducive to success, and it is this kind of fragment that should be removed.

In addition to the aforementioned bypassing, attempts have been made to ensnare the fragment with a broach or a broach with cotton fibers, in the hope that the cotton would entangle the fragment. Another method, which may work if the fragment is visible in the chamber, involves drilling around the fragment with a small round bur to develop some space and then grasping the fragment with splinter forceps. Wide and destructive access must often be prepared, however, to accommodate the splinter forceps.

Recently, Feldman et al. described a specific technique designed to retrieve broken instruments.[72] It consists of enlarging the canal to accommodate an Extractor specially designed to clamp and remove the fragment.

The first step is to enlarge the canal down to the

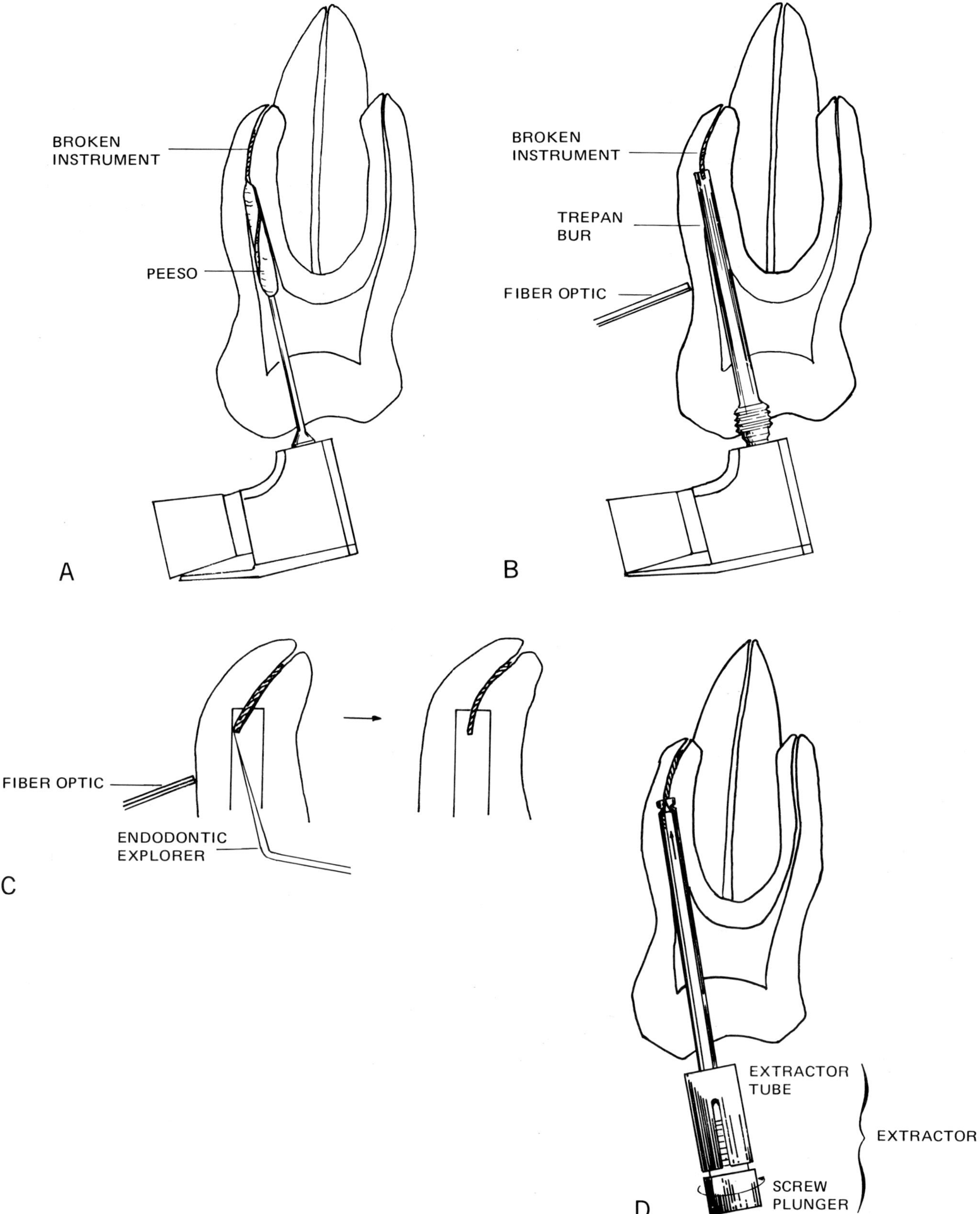

Fig. 3–61. Method suggested by Feldman to recover broken instruments. *A,* Canal is ***carefully*** enlarged with peeso drill to provide access to instrument. *B,* Special end-cutting trepan bur prepares space around instrument. Fiberoptic shining through tissue will illuminate canal to show broken instrument. *C,* Strong endodontic explorer used to center instrument in canal. *D,* Special Extractor is placed around broken instrument and vice grip tightened by turning screw plunger. Instrument is removed in Extractor. (From Feldman, G., et al.: J.A.D.A., *88*:588, Mar., 1974.)

broken piece with a Peeso drill (Fig. 3–61*A*). This is followed with trepan burs—hollow tube burs that cut only on the leading edge (Fig. 3–61*B*). Since the ability to see the fragment is essential to success, a fiber optic light source is used to shine through the tissue and the root, or through the root alone, if placed properly at the cervical (Fig. 3–61*B* and *C*). Finally, the Extractor is placed directly over the fragment, and the vise grip is tightened by means of two pairs of serrated pliers on the handle. Theoretically, when the Extractor is removed it is accompanied by the fragment (Fig. 3–61*D*).

Obviously, great skill and care are required, in addition to these specialized instruments, to successfully remove a fragmented instrument without perforating the root. Occasionally, the fragment extends out into the periapical tissue and has to be removed surgically (see Fig. 15–15).

PULPECTOMY

Pulp ***extirpation*** or ***pulpectomy*** is the surgical removal of a vital pulp from a tooth. These terms are reserved for living pulps only. ***Total pulpectomy,*** extirpation of the pulp to or near the apical foramen, is indicated when the root apex is fully formed and the foramen sufficiently closed to permit obturation with conventional filling materials. If the pulp must be removed from a tooth with an incompletely formed root and an open apex, ***partial pulpectomy*** is preferred. This technique leaves the apical portion of the pulp intact with the hope that the remaining stump will encourage completion of the apex. The necrotic or "mummified" tissue remaining in the pulp cavity of a ***nonvital*** tooth has lost its identity as an organ, hence its removal is called ***pulp cavity debridement.***

Indications. Pulp "mummification" with arsenic trioxide, formaldehyde, or other destructive compounds was at one time preferred to extirpation.[73] With the advent of effective local anesthetics, pulpectomy has became a relatively painless process, and superseded "mummification" with its attendant hazards of bone necrosis (Fig. 3–62) and prolonged postoperative pain. ***Pulpectomy is indicated in all cases of irreversible pulp disease.*** With pulpectomy, dramatic relief is obtained in cases of acute pulpitis resulting from infection, injury, or operative trauma. Pulpectomy is usually the treatment of choice where

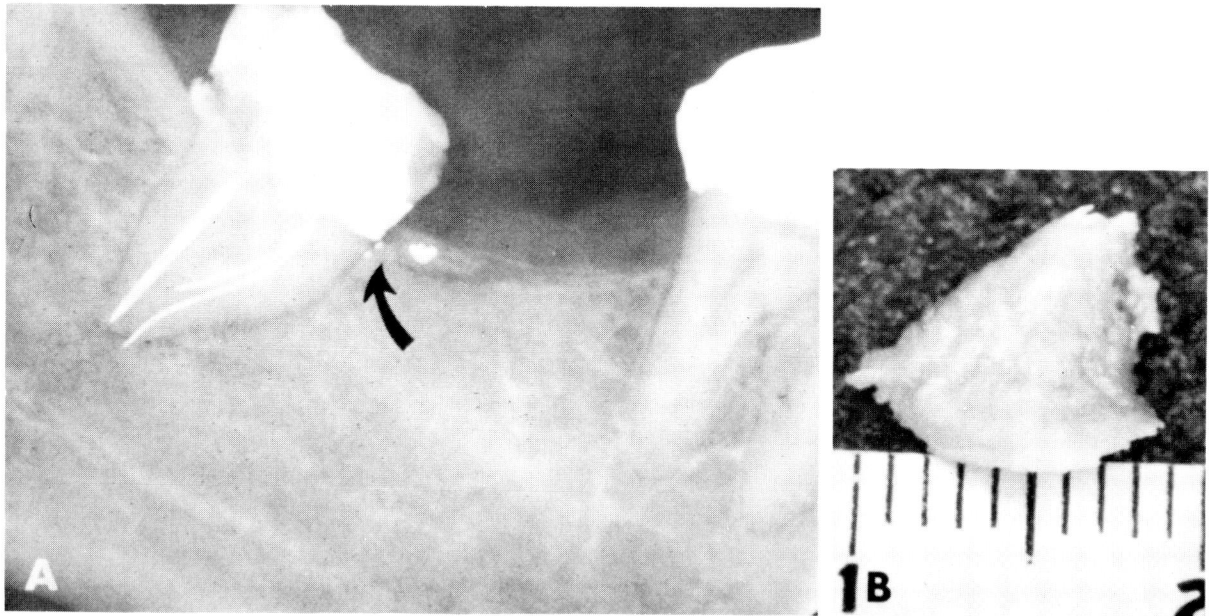

Fig. 3–62. Destruction of alveolar process by arsenic trioxide. *A,* In attempting to open into pulp chamber of severely tilted, mandibular third molar bridge abutment, dentist perforated through mesial of tooth. Mistaking tissue of gingival sulcus for the pulp, dentist introduced arsenic trioxide to "mummify" the pulp. Arrow indicates area where perforation occurred and crestal bone has sloughed. *B,* Large piece of crestal bone which sloughed from action of arsenic trioxide. Patient experienced excruciating pain for over two weeks.

carious or mechanical exposure has occurred. In a number of instances, restorative and fixed prosthetic procedures require intentional extirpation.[74]

Technique. The following are the steps in the performance of a well-executed pulpectomy:

1. Obtain regional anesthesia.
2. Prepare a minimal coronal opening and test the pulp for depth of anesthesia.
3. If necessary, inject anesthetic intrapulpally.
4. Complete the access cavity.
5. Excavate the coronal pulp.
6. Extirpate the radicular pulp.
7. Control bleeding and debride the canal.
8. Place medication or the final filling.

Each of these steps must be completed carefully before the next is begun, and each requires some explanation.

Profound Anesthesia. Methods for obtaining profound infiltration and conduction anesthesia have been considered earlier. One aspect of the subject deserves repetition: its unusual importance in endodontics! From the era when pulps were extirpated by driving wooden pegs, red-hot wires, or crude broaches into the living tissues without benefit of anesthesia,[75] there has persisted a profound and widespread dread of "having a nerve taken out of a tooth." The popular misconception that endodontic treatment invariably involves suffering will not be completely dispelled until all practitioners employ effective anesthesia techniques while completing procedures as potentially painful as pulpectomy.

Minimal Coronal Opening and Intrapulpal Anesthesia. It is wise to anticipate that in spite of apparently profound anesthesia, an intrapulpal injection may be required to obtain total anesthesia, particularly with an inflamed pulp. If the patient experiences pain during the initial stage of access preparation, there is no question that manipulation of the pulp will be a painful process. The success of the intrapulpal injection will be assured if the initial penetration of the pulp chamber is made with a bur just slightly larger than the injection needle. Since the needle fits the small opening tightly, the anesthetic can be forced into the pulp under pressure. Total anesthesia follows immediately.

Completion of the Access Preparation. Coronal access must be adequate and complete to allow for thorough excavation of the tissue from the pulp chamber. Because intrapulpal injection with 2% lidocaine with 1:50,000 epinephrine promotes excellent hemostasis, it can be used during the completion of the access cavity to prevent interference from hemorrhaging tissue.

Excavation of the Coronal Pulp. All the tissue in the pulp chamber should be removed before extirpation of the radicular pulp is begun. All pulp tissue which has not been removed by the round bur should be eliminated with a small sharp spoon excavator (Fig. 3–63). The tissue is carefully curetted from the pulp horns and other ramifications of the chamber. Failure to remove all tissue fragments from the pulp chamber may result in discoloration of the tooth. At this point, the chamber should be irrigated well to remove blood and debris.

Extirpation of Radicular Pulp. The instrument used for this procedure is determined by the size of the canal and/or the level at which the pulp is to be excised.

Large Canal, Total Pulpectomy. If the canal is large enough to admit a barbed broach (Fig. 3–64) and a total pulpectomy is desired, the approach is as follows:

1. A pathway for the broach to follow is created by sliding a reamer or file along the wall of the canal to the apical third. If the pulp is sensitive or bleeding, the anesthetic syringe needle may be used as the "pathfinder." A drop of anesthetic deposited near the apical foramen will stop the flow of blood and all pain sensations. At the same time, the needle displaces the

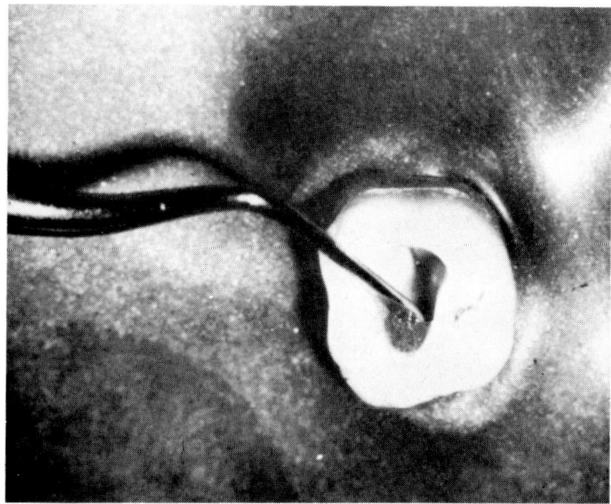

Fig. 3–63. Long spoon excavator is used to remove coronal portion of molar pulp.

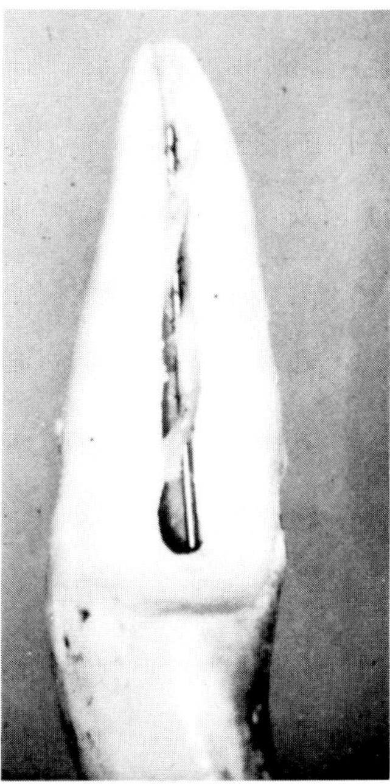

Fig. 3–64. Total pulpectomy accomplished with a large barbed broach which fits loosely in canal. By rotating broach, pulp has become entwined and will be removed upon retraction.

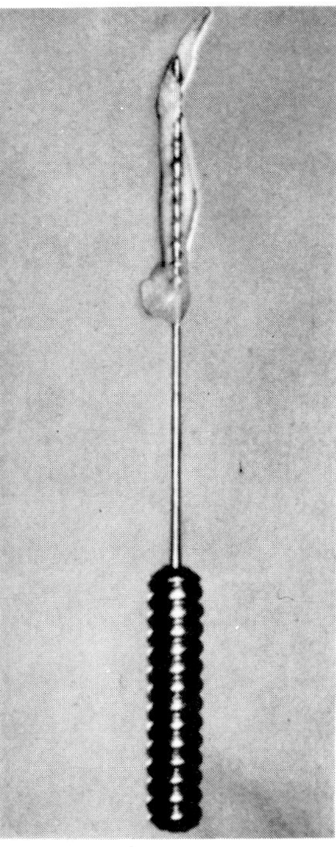

Fig. 3–65. Total pulpectomy by barbed broach. Young, huge pulps will require two or three broaches inserted simultaneously to successfully entwine pulp.

pulp tissue and creates the desired pathway for a broach.

2. A broach, just small enough not to bind in the canal, is passed to the apex. The instrument is rotated ***slowly*** to engage the fibrous tissue of the pulp, then slowly withdrawn. Hopefully, the entire pulp organ will be removed with the broach (Fig. 3–65). If not, the process is repeated. If the canal is large, it may be necessary to insert two broaches simultaneously to entwine the pulp on a sufficient number of barbs to ensure its intact removal.

3. If the pulp is not removed intact, small broaches are used to "scrub" the canal walls from the apex outward to remove adherent fragments. ***A word of caution!*** The barbed broach is a friable instrument and must never be locked into the canal. Handle with care!

Small Canal, Total Pulpectomy. If the canal is slender, and a total pulpectomy is indicated, extirpation becomes a part of canal preparation. A broach need not be used. Small files are preferred for the initial instrumentation because they cut more quickly than reamers. In such a canal, the first few will remove all the pulp tissue as ***telescopic preparation*** removes the dentin walls. Pulp in the larger or ovoid part of the canal is removed by filing down to clean white dentin.

Partial Pulpectomy. When a partial pulpectomy is planned, a technique described by Nygaard-Ostby is employed.[76] From a good radiograph, the width of the canal at the desired level of extirpation is determined. A Hedstrom file of correct size is ***blunted,*** so that the flattened tip will bind in the canal at the predetermined point of severance (Fig. 3–66). The Hedstrom file has deep fluting and makes a cleaner incision than can be expected from other intracanal instruments. Enlargement of the canal coronal portion is then carried out with a series of larger instruments trimmed to the same length.

Control of Bleeding and Debridement of Canal. Incomplete pulpectomy will leave in the canal fragments of tissue that may remain vital if their blood supply is maintained through accessory foramens or along deep fissures in the canal walls. These remnants of the pulp may be a source of severe pain to the patient, who will return seeking relief as soon as the anesthesia wears off. This is a desperately painful condition and requires immediate re-anesthetization and extirpation of all tissue shreds. Any overlooked tissue shreds will also interfere with proper obturation during immediate filling procedures.

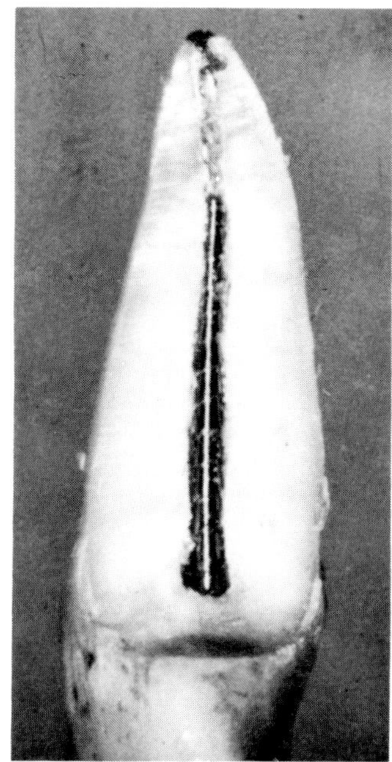

Fig. 3–66. Partial pulpectomy accomplished with blunted Hedstrom file after the method suggested by Nygaard-Ostby. Spiral blades of file will neatly amputate pulp at desired level, leaving apical portion of vital pulp tissue.

Persistent bleeding following extirpation is usually a sign that "tags" of pulp tissue remain. If the flow of blood is not stopped by scrubbing the canal walls with a broach, as described earlier, it may originate in the periapical area. A paper point soaked in epinephrine can be carried to the apex and held in place until the blood flow is stemmed.[77] A blunted paper point carrying phenol or formaldehyde-cresol, held at the apex of the canal for three or four minutes, will accomplish the same end by cauterizing the periapical tissues.[78] The canal should then be well irrigated and dried with cotton pellets and ***blunted*** absorbent paper points.

Placement of Medication or Root Canal Filling. If pulpectomy was necessitated by a pulpitis resulting from operative or accidental trauma, or planned extirpation of a normal pulp for restorative purposes was done, enlargement and obturation of the canal can be completed immediately. If a delay is necessary, a mild antiseptic-obtundant, such as eugenol, should be sealed in the chamber. The sedative qualities reduce postoperative periapical discomfort, yet maintain the sterility of the canal. The final canal filling should never be placed, however, unless all pulpal shreds are removed and hemorrhage has stopped.

Immediate filling is contraindicated if the possibility of pulpal infection exists. In cases of pulpitis resulting from deep carious lesions or with traumatically exposed pulps that have been exposed to the saliva for more than a few hours, it is wise to medicate the canal conventionally before filling.

REFERENCES

1. Black, G. V.: *Operative Dentistry.* Vol. II. Chicago, Medico-Dental Pub. Co., 7th Ed., 1936, p. 137.
2. Pucci, F. M. and Reig, R.: *Conductos Radiculares.* Vol. II. Buenos Aires, Editorial Medico-Quirurgica, 1944, p. 289-295.
3. Bjorndal, A. M., Henderson, W. G., Skidmore, A. E., and Kellner, F. H.: Anatomic measurements of human teeth extracted from males between the ages of 17 and 21 years. Oral Surg., *38*:791, Nov., 1974.
4. Dempster, W. T., Adams, W. J., and Duddles, R. S.: Arrangements in the jaws of the roots of teeth. J.A.D.A., *67*:779, Dec., 1963.
5. Benjamin, K. A., and Dowson, J.: Incidence of two root canals in human mandibular incisor teeth. Oral Surg., *38*:122, July, 1974.
6. Vertucci, F. J.: Root canal anatomy of the mandibular anterior teeth. J.A.D.A., *89*:369, Aug., 1974.
7. Carns, J. E., and Skidmore, A. E.: Configurations and deviations of root canals of maxillary first premolars. Oral Surg., *36*:880, Dec., 1973.
8. Vertucci, F. J., Selig, A. and Gillis, R.: Root canal morphology of the human maxillary second premolar. Oral Surg., *38*:456, Sept., 1974.
9. Zillich, R. and Dowson, J.: Root canal morphology of mandibular first and second premolars. Oral Surg., *36*:783, Nov., 1973.
10. Seidberg, B. H., Altman, M., Guttuso, J., and Suson, M.: Frequency of two mesiobuccal root canals in maxillary permanent first molars. J.A.D.A., *87*:852, Oct., 1973.
11. Pineda, F.: Roentgenographic investigation of the mesiobuccal root of the maxillary first molar. Oral Surg., *36*:253, Aug., 1973.
12. Pomeranz, H. H., and Fishelberg, G.: The second mesiobuccal canal of maxillary molars. J.A.D.A., *88*:119, Jan., 1974.
13. Green, D.: Double canals in single roots. Oral Surg., *35*:689, May, 1973.
14. Ingle, J. I., and Zeldow, B. J.: An evaluation of mechanical instrumentation and the negative culture in endodontic therapy. J.A.D.A., *57*:471, Oct., 1958.
15. Kuttler, Y.: Microscopic investigation of root apexes. J.A.D.A., *50*:544, May, 1955.
16. Seidler, B.: Root canal filling: an evaluation and method. J.A.D.A., *53*:567, Nov., 1956.
17. Sargenti, A.: *Endodontics.* Locarno, Switzerland, Angelo G. Sargenti, 1973.

18. Dihn, Q.: An *in vitro* Evaluation of the Giromatic Instrument in the Mechanical Preparation of Root Canals. Master's Thesis, University of Minnesota, Dec., 1972.
19. O'Connell, D. T., and Brayton, S. M.: Evaluation of root canal preparation with two automated endodontic handpieces. Oral Surg., *39*:298, Feb., 1975
20. Sargenti, A.: Engined Powered Canal Preparation. Addendum to Sargenti *Endodontics,* Locarno, Switzerland, 1974.
21. Pucci, F. M.: Op. cit., p. 312.
22. Luks, S.: An analysis of root canal instruments. J.A.D.A., *58*:85, March, 1959.
23. Gutierrez, J. H., Gigoux, C., and Sanhueza, I.: Physical and chemical deterioration of endodontic reamers during mechanical preparation. Oral Surg., *28*:394, Sept., 1969.
24. Gutierrez, J. H.: Personal communication. June, 1972.
25. Eichner, M. and Schoen, D.: Endodontic Instruments React. Presented to American Association of Endodontics, April 25, 1975.
26. Ingle J. I.: The need for endodontic instrument standardization. Oral Surg., *8*:1211, Nov., 1955.
27. Ingle, J. I., and Levine, M.: The Need for Uniformity of Endodontic Instruments, Equipment and Filling Materials. Presented to the 2nd International Conference on Endodontics, June, 1958.
28. Ingle, J. I.: A standardized endodontic technique using newly designed instruments and filling materials. Oral Surg., *14*:83, Jan., 1961.
29. Green, E. N.: Microscopic investigation of root canal file and reamer width. Oral Surg., *10*:532, May, 1957.
30. Annual Catalog. Star Dental Manufacturing Co., Conshohocken, Pa., 1975.
31. Proposed F.D.I.-W.H.O.-A.D.A. Specifications for Root Canal Files and Reamers. 7th draft, March 1, 1974.
32. Oliet, S. and Sorin, S. M.: Cutting efficiency of endodontic reamers. Oral Surg., *36*:243, Aug., 1973.
33. Jungmann, C. L., Uchin, R. A., and Bucher, J. F.: Effect of instrumentation on the shape of the root canal. J. Endodont., *1*:66, Feb., 1975.
34. Schreier, E.: The treatment of infected root canals with kalium and natrium. Dental Cosmos, *38*:863, Sept., 1893.
35. Stewart, G., Cobe, H., and Rappaport, H.: A study of a new medicament in the chemomechanical preparation of infected root canals. J.A.D.A., *63*:33, July, 1961.
36. Grossman, L: Accepted Dental Remedies. Chicago, American Dental Association, 1964, pp. 108-109.
37. Grahnen, H., and Krasse, B.: The effect of instrumentation and flushing of non-vital teeth in endodontic therapy, I. Odontologisk Revy, *14*:167, 1963.
38. Grahnen, H.: The effect of instrumentation and flushing of non-vital teeth in endodontic therapy, II. Odontologisk Revy, *114*:361, 1963.
39. Martin, H.: Quantitative bactericidal effectiveness of an old and a new endodontic irrigant. J. Endodont., *1*:64, May, 1975.
40. Loel, A. D.: Use of acid cleanser in endodontic therapy. J.A.D.A., *90*:148, Jan., 1975.

40*a*. McComb, D., and Smith, D.C.: A preliminary electron microscopic study of root canals after endodontic procedures. J. Endodont., *1*:238, July, 1975.

41. Senia, S. E., Marraro, R. V., Mitchell, J. L., Lewis, A. G., and Thomas, L.: Rapid sterilization of gutta percha cones with 5.25 per cent sodium hypochlorite. J. Endodont., *1*:136, Apr., 1975.
42. Baker, N. A., Eleazer, P. D., Averbach, R. E., and Seltzer, S.: Scanning electron microscopic study of the efficacy of various irrigating solutions. J. Endodont., *1*:127, Apr., 1975.
43. Becker, G. L., Cohen, S., and Borer, R.: The sequelae of accidentally injecting sodium hypochlorite beyond the root apex. Oral Surg., *38*:633, Oct., 1974.
44. Bhat, K. S.: Tissue emphysema caused by hydrogen peroxide. Oral Surg., *38*:304, Aug., 1974.
45. Auerbach, M. B.: Antibiotics vs. instrumentation in endodontics. New York St. Dent. J., *19*:325, May, 1953.
46. Stewart, G.: Importance of chemomechanical preparation of the root canal. Oral Surg., *8*:993, Sept., 1955.
47. Bramante, C. M., and Berbert, A.: A critical evaluation of some methods of determining tooth lengths. Oral Surg., *37*:463, Mar., 1974.
48. Sunada, I.: New method for measuring the length of the root canal. J. Dent. Res., *41*:375, 1962.
49. O'Neill, L. J.: A clinical evaluation of electronic root canal measurement. Oral Surg., *38*:469, Sept., 1974.
50. Seidberg, B. H., Alibrandi, B. V., Fine, H., and Logue, B.: Clinical investigating of measuring working lengths of root canals with an electronic device and with digital-tactile sense. J.A.D.A., *90*:379, Feb., 1975.
51. Inoue, N.: Dental "stethoscope measures root canal." Dent. Surv., *48*:38, Jan., 1972.
52. Blank, L. W., Tenca, J. I., and Pelleu, G. B.: Reliability of electronic measuring devices in endodontic therapy. J. Endodont., *1*:141, Apr. 1975.
53. Guldener, P., and Imobersteg, C.: Neu Methode Zur Exakten Langeneinstellung von Wurzelkandinstrumenten. Schweiz. Mschr. Zahnheilk., *82*:280, 1972.
54. Rowe, A. H. R., and Forrest, J. O.: The Endo-Meter. Brit. Dent. J., *134*:437, May 15, 1973.
55. Green, D.: Stereoscopic study of 700 root apices of maxillary and mandibular posterior teeth. Oral Surg., *13*:728, June, 1960.
56. Burch, J. G., and Hulen, S.: The relationship of the apical foramen to the anatomic apex of the tooth root. Oral Surg., *34*:262, Aug., 1972.
57. Pineda, F., and Kuttler, Y.: Mesiodistal-buccolingualroentgenographic investigation of 7,275 root canals. Oral Surg., *33*:101, Jan., 1972.
58. Gutierrez, J. H., and Garcia, J.: Miscroscopic and macroscopic investigation on results of mechanical preparation of root canals. Oral Surg., *25*:108, Jan., 1968,
59. Haga, C. S.: Microscopic measurements of root canal preparations following instrumentation. J. Brit. Endodont. Soc., *2*:41, 1969.
60. Vessey, R. A.: The effect of filing vs. reaming on the shape of the prepared root canal. Oral Surg., *27*:543, Apr., 1969.

61. Nygaard-Ostby, B.: Chelation in root canal therapy. Sartryck ur Odontologisk Tidskrift, *65*:1, 1957.
62. Patterson, S. E.: In vivo and in vitro studies of the effect of the disodium salt of ethylenediamine tetraacetate on human dentine and its endodontic implications. Oral Surg., *16*:83, Jan., 1963.
63. Von der Eehr, F. R., and Nygaard-Ostby, B.: Effect of EDTAC and sulfuric acid on root canal dentin. Oral Surg., *16*:199, Feb., 1963.
64. Fraser, J. G.: Chelating agents: their softening effect on root canal dentin. Oral Surg., *37*:803, May, 1974.
65. Pucci, F. M.: Op. cit., p. 319.
66. Martin, H.: A telescopic technique for endodontics. J. Dist. Columbia Dent. Soc., *49*:12, Summer, 1974.
67. Walton, R. E.: J. Endodont. In press.
68. Craig, R. C., and McIlwain, E.: Bending and torsion properties of endodontic instruments. Oral Surg., *25*:239, Feb., 1968.
69. Weine, F.: *Endodontic Therapy.* C. V. Mosby Co., St. Louis, 1972, pp. 209-11.
70. Crump, M. C., and Natkin, E.: Relationship of broken root canal instruments to endodontic case diagnosis: a clinical investigation. J.A.D.A., *80*:1341, June, 1970.
71. Fox, J., et al.: Filling root canals with files: Radiographic evaluation of 304 cases. N.Y. State Dent. J., *38*:154, Mar., 1972.
72. Feldman, G., et al.: Retrieving broken endodontic instruments. J.A.D.A., *88*:588, Mar., 1974.
73. McQuillen, J. H.: Dr. Maynard's method of extirpating the pulp. Dental Cosmos, *1*:312, Jan., 1860.
74. Bohannan, H. M., and Abrams, L.: Intentional vital pulp extirpation in periodontal prosthesis. J. Pros. Dent., *11*:781, July-Aug., 1961.
75. McQuillen, J. H.: Review of dental literature and art. "Who first filled nerve cavities?" Dent. Cosmos, *3*:556, May, 1862.
76. Nygaard-Ostby, B.: Personal communication.
77. Grossman, L.: *Endodontic Practice.* Philadelphia, Lea & Febiger, 1974, 8th ed.
78. Sommer R., Ostrander, F. D. and Crowley, M.: *Clinical Endodontics.* Philadelphia, W. B. Saunders Co., 1962, p. 215.

Chapter 4

Obturation of the Radicular Space

JOHN I. INGLE, RAYMOND G. LUEBKE, RICHARD E. WALTON, and JAMES D. ZIDELL

The Washington study of endodontic success and failure suggests percolation of periapical exudate into the incompletely filled canal as the greatest cause of endodontic failure. Nearly 60% of the failures in the study were apparently caused by incomplete obliteration of the radicular space (p. 43).

Dow and Ingle demonstrated *in vitro* the possibility of apical percolation using a radioactive isotope.[1]

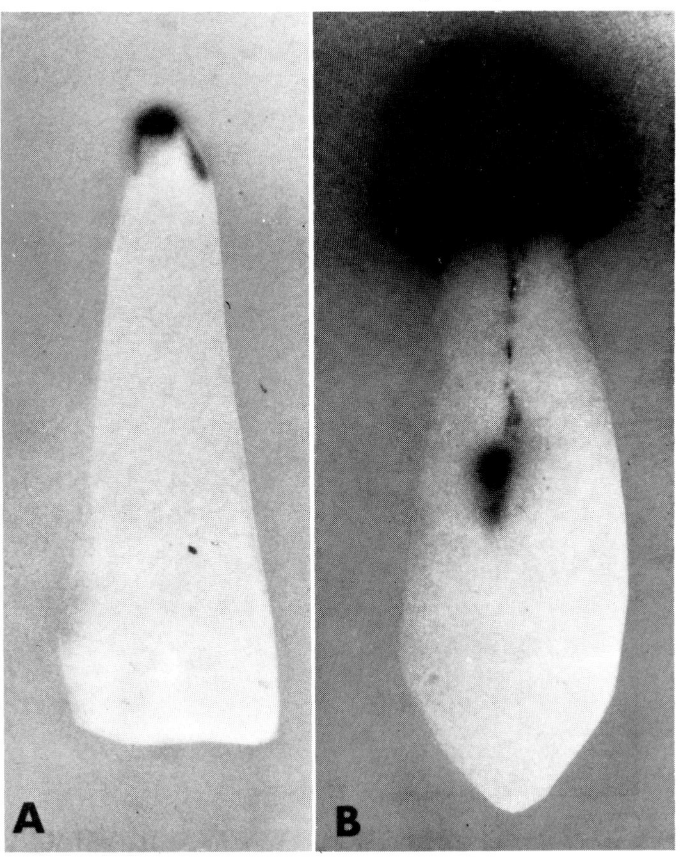

Fig. 4–1. *A,* Failure of radioactive iodine (^{131}I) to penetrate into well-filled canal. Only periapical cementum which was not coated with sticky wax has absorbed isotope. *B,* Massive reaction to penetration of radioactive iodine (^{131}I) into poorly filled canal. Violent response at periapex is comparable to *in vivo* response to toxic canal products. (Dow, P. R., and Ingle, J. I.: Oral Surg., 8:1100, 1955.)

After filling the root canals of extracted teeth, Dow placed the teeth in radioactive iodine, ^{131}I. In those teeth with a fluid-tight seal of the apical foramen and a well-obliterated canal space, there was no penetration of the radioactive iodine (Fig. 4–1*A*). In the poorly filled canals—filled so by design—a deep penetration into the canal by the ^{131}I was apparent in the radioautographs (Fig. 4–1*B*).

On the basis of this study, one might hypothesize that the penetration of radioactive iodine into a poorly-filled root canal *in vitro* is analogous to fluid percolation into the canal of *in situ* pulpless teeth with incomplete canal obliteration (Fig. 4–2). Apical percolation may be considered a logical hypothesis. However, the role of the end products of percolation in the production of periapical inflammation is open to speculation. It would seem safe to assume that the noxious products from the apical foramen act as an inflammatory irritant. The unanswered question relates to the production of irritants in the canal. At the present time it is speculated that the exudate constantly leaking into the unfilled or partially filled canal arises indirectly from the blood serum, and consists of a number of water-soluble proteins, enzymes, and salts. It is further speculated that the serum is trapped in the *cul-de-sac* of the poorly filled canal, away from the influences of the blood stream, and there undergoes degradation. Later, when the degraded serum slowly diffuses out to the periapical tissue, it acts as a physicochemical irritant to produce the periapical inflammation of chronic apical periodontitis.

Such a sequence of events might well explain the paradox of the periapical lesion associated with a ***non***-infected pulpless tooth. Periapical inflammation will presumably persist under the influence of any noxious substance. Bacteria certainly play a major role in the production of toxic products in the root canal. However, in the absence of bacteria, degraded serum *per se* may well assume the role of the primary tissue irritant. The persistence of periapical inflammation in the ***absence*** of bacterial infection can thus be attributed to the persistence of apical percolation of serum and its breakdown products.

Objectives. In light of the foregoing discussion, it is apparent that the primary objective of operative

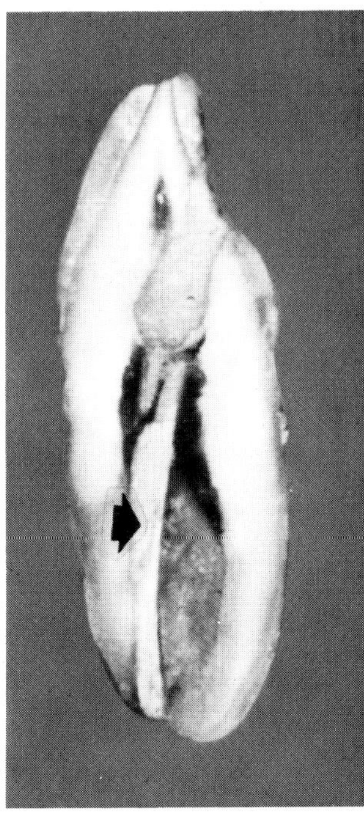

Fig. 4–2. Lateral section of endodontic failure. Gutta percha point (*arrow*) in no way obliterates foramen. Unfilled canal space contains necrotic debris, severe irritant.

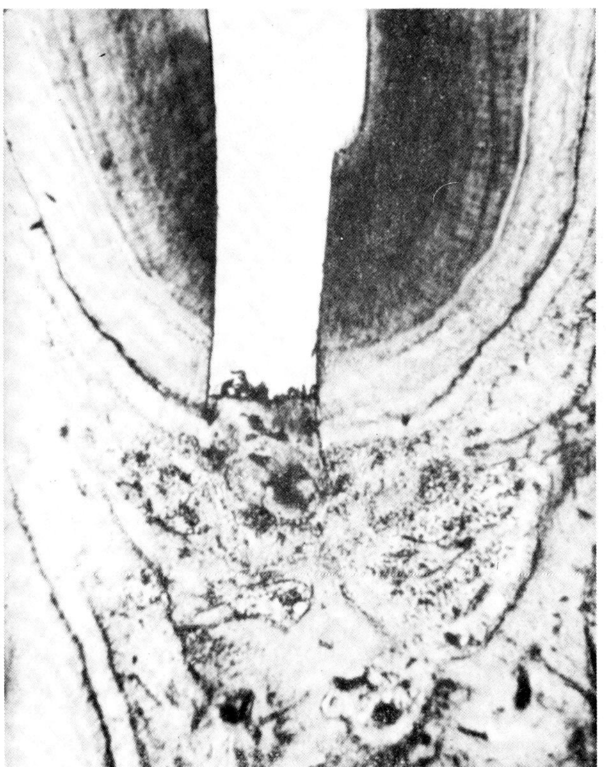

Fig. 4–3. Total repair at periapex by "osteocementum" formation. Limitation of cementodentinal junction has been bypassed in instrumentation. At this point pulp tissue is transformed into connective tissue of periodontal space. (Courtesy Dr. Seiichi Matsumiya.)

endodontics is the development of a fluid-tight seal at the apical foramen, and total obliteration of the root canal space. The anatomic limits of this space are the dentinocemental junction apically, and the pulp chamber coronally. Debate persists, however, with regard to the ideal apical limit of the root canal filling.

Extension of the Root Canal Filling. Canals that are filled to the apical dentinocemental junction are filled to the anatomic limit of the canal. Beyond this point the periodontal structures begin (Fig. 4–3). The dentinocemental junction is about 0.5 mm. from the external surface of the apical foramen as clearly demonstrated by Kuttler.[2] It is this point that should limit canal instrumentation and filling. Not only is the dentinocemental junction the anatomic limit of the root canal, it is usually the narrowest diameter of the apical foramen, and as such, is the major factor in limiting filling material to the canal (Fig. 4–4).

A number of authors are in disagreement with this point of limitation, preferring rather to fill to the end

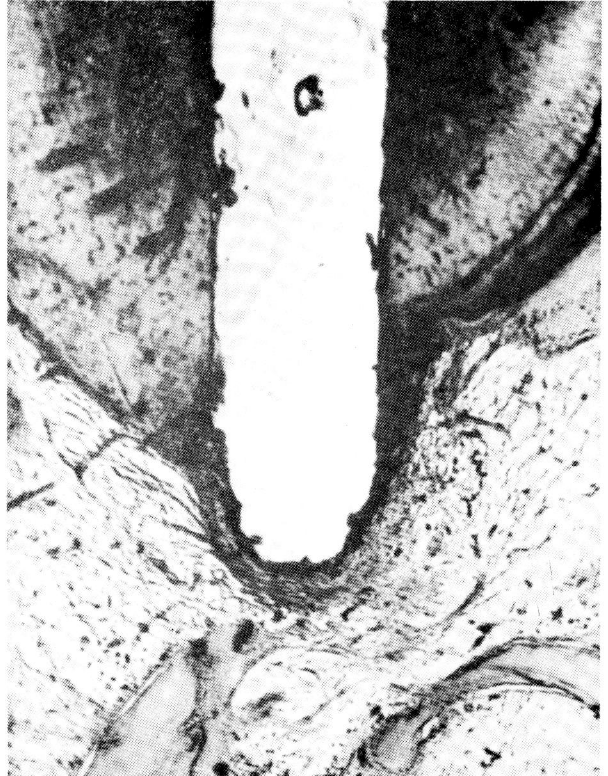

Fig. 4–4. Instrumentation and root canal filling beyond apical limitation. Minor inflammatory and foreign body reaction has developed in response to irritant. (Courtesy Dr. Seiichi Matsumiya.)

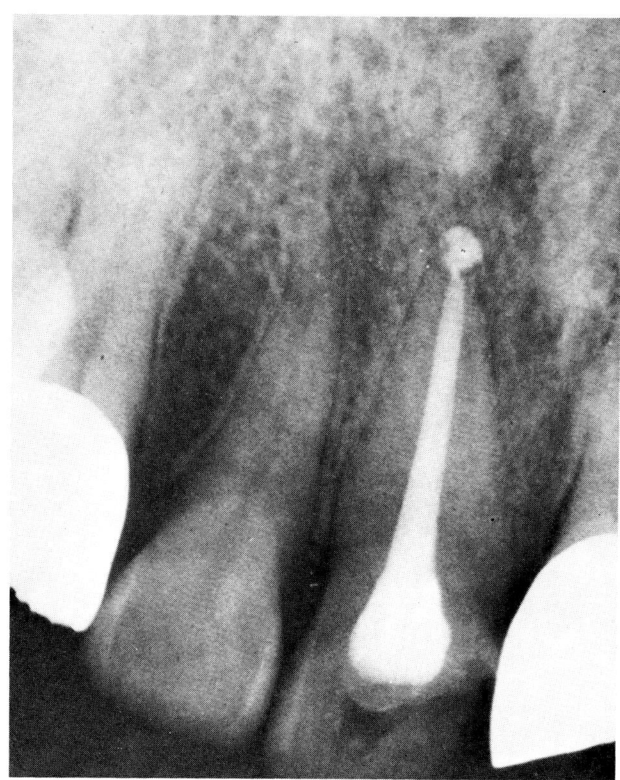

Fig. 4–5. Periapical "button" is considered by some to provide adequate assurance that apical foramen has been sealed.

of the root or purposely to overfill with a periapical "button" (Fig. 4–5). Filling to the roentgenographic end of the root is actually overfilling, for as Figure 4–6 shows, the apical flare of the foramen is filled with periodontal tissue. Purposely overfilling to produce a periapical "button" is advocated primarily by the proponents of the diffusion technique or the softened gutta percha technique. Ostensibly the "button" is designed to compensate for shrinkage of the filling by pulling down tightly against the apex. Although no proof exists that this is true, the advocates of softened gutta percha fillings interpret the apical "button" as an indicator that the filling material has been densely packed into the apical preparation and has completely obturated all the aberrations as well as the lateral and accessory canals of the root canal system. No accounting is given of postoperative discomfort.

In any case, the overfilled canal tends to cause more postoperative pain than do those filled to the dentinocemental junction. Writing from Israel, Shochat and Garfunkel reported "an unusual case of

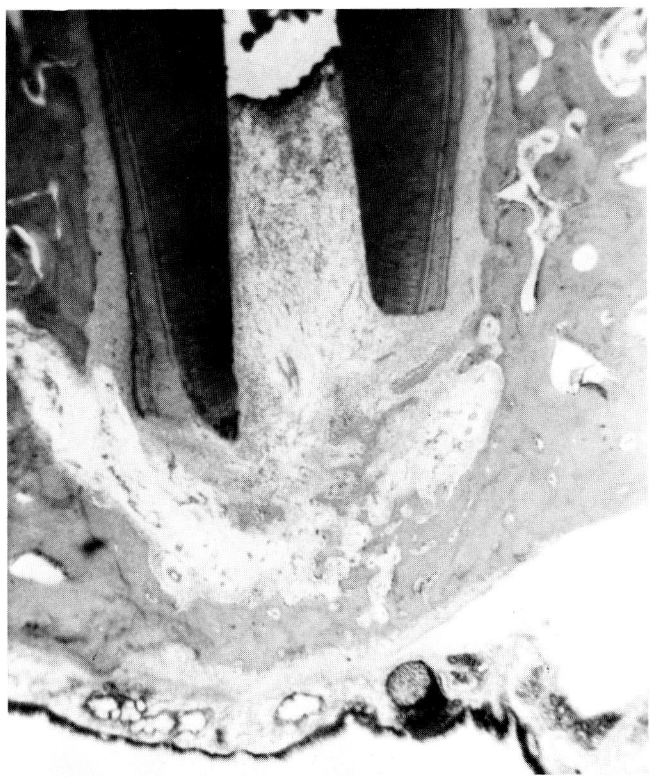

Fig. 4–6. Partial pulpectomy adequately obliterated to point of amputation. Even though root canal filling is short of apex, perfect healing has developed as evidenced by normal pulp and periapical tissue. (Courtesy Dr. Seiichi Matsumiya.)

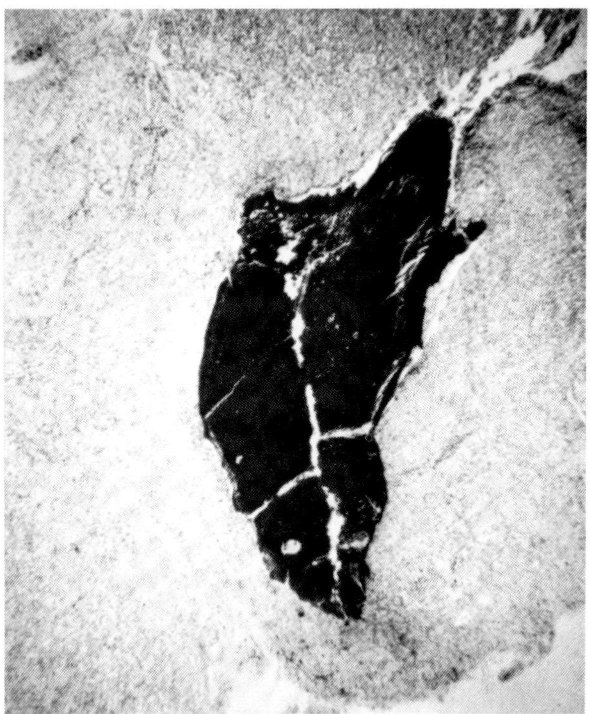

Fig. 4–7. Tissue reaction to foreign body such as gutta percha. (Courtesy Dr. S. N. Bhaskar and U. S. Army Institute of Pathology.)

neurologic complications following overfilling of the root canals of two mandibular premolars."[3] After one year of neuralgia, the region was surgically explored and the endodontic filling material was found to be in contact with the "mental nerve sheath." Since no improvement followed its removal, a neurectomy was performed to give relief.

A number of authors believe that filling just short of the apex is greatly preferred to overfilling. Filling short of the apex is especially recommended following pulpectomy by Nygaard-Ostby,[4] Blayney,[5] and more recently Strindberg.[6] In addition to these authors, the Washington study attributed no failures among those ***well-obliterated*** cases in which the filling terminated slightly short of the apex (Fig. 4–6), whereas 3.85% of the failures were due to overfilling.

In spite of this, a high degree of success is still achieved if overfilling occurs. Fortunately, most of the root canal sealers currently used, as well as the solid core filling materials, gutta percha and silver, are tolerated by the periapical tissues once the cements have set. The tissue reaction that does occur can be a fibrous walling off of the foreign body (Fig. 4–7). On the other hand, fewer stormy postoperative reactions can be expected if canal instrumentation and filling are limited by the apical foramen.

When to Obturate the Canal. The root canal is ready to be filled when: (1) the canal is enlarged to an optimum size, (2) the tooth is comfortable, (3) a negative bacteriologic culture has been obtained, and (4) the canal is dry. The dry canal may be obtained with absorbent points except in those cases of suppurative apical periodontitis or apical cyst in which "weeping" into the canal persists.

The exception to the aforementioned criteria is the case in which ***mild*** discomfort persists, but bacteriologic culture is ***negative.*** Experience has shown that filling the root canal in such cases usually alleviates the symptoms. Filling a known infected root canal is chancy. Ingle and Zeldow have shown the increase in discomfort that developed postoperatively from filling infected root canals.[7] They also have shown that the degree of success in a group of infected cases was 11.2% less than that in an *a priori* group of cases with a negative bacteriologic culture.[8]

Materials Employed in Obturation

The number of materials used to fill root canals is legion, running the gamut from gold to feathers. Grossman groups acceptable filling materials into plastics, solids, cements, and pastes.[9] He also delineates 10 requirements for an ideal root canal filling material that apply equally to the metals, plastics, and cements: (1) it should be easily introduced into a root canal; (2) it should seal the canal laterally as well as apically; (3) it should not shrink after being inserted; (4) it should be impervious to moisture; (5) it should be bacteriostatic, or at least not encourage bacterial growth; (6) it should be radiopaque; (7) it should not stain tooth structure; (8) it should not irritate periapical tissue; (9) it should be sterile, or easily and quickly sterilized immediately before insertion; and (10) it should be removed easily from the root canal if necessary. Both the plastic gutta percha point and the solid silver point admirably meet these requirements. If the gutta percha point has a fault, it lies in its inherent plasticity, for it requires special handling to position it. The major fault with the silver point is its lack of plasticity—its inability to be compressed. Both must be cemented to place, however, to be effective.

Solid Core Materials

Gutta percha is by far the most universally used solid core root canal filling material and may be classified as a plastic. To date, modern plastics such as Teflon have been disappointing endodontic filling materials. However, new plastics are on the horizon. Silver amalgam, used in the retrosurgical technique wherein the canal is filled from the apex, must also be considered a "plastic" filling material.

Because, to date, the modern petrochemical plastics have proved so disappointing for canal obturation, a new interest has developed in old fashioned gutta percha. First shown as a curiosity in the mid seventeenth century, gutta percha escaped notice as a practical product for nearly 200 years. The first successful use of this curious material seems to have been as an insulation for underseas cables. This was in 1848, and was followed by patents for its use in the manufacture of "corks, cement thread, surgical instruments, garments, pipes, and sheathing for ships. Even boats were wholly made of gutta percha. Gutta percha golf balls were introduced by the latter part of the nineteenth century, and until 1920, golf balls were called 'gutties.' Gutta percha has been known to dentistry for over 100 years."[10]

Chemically, gutta percha is a naturally occurring polymer of isoprene and, as such, is a close relative of natural rubber and of chicle used in chewing gum. A "trans" polyisoprene gutta percha has a more linear chemical bonding than the "cis" bonding of rubber and therefore crystallizes more readily than the kinked elastometric rubber. Consequently, it is harder, more brittle, and less elastic than natural rubber.[10] Gutta percha has also been produced synthetically. It compares to natural gutta percha as a mild tissue irritant.[11]

At high temperatures, gutta percha forms an "amorphous rubbery melt in which the linear molecular chains can be envisioned as random coils, continually changing orientation as a result of thermal excitation. At sufficiently low temperatures the same polymer is a rigid solid with its chains locked in position" by crystallization or vitrification.[10]

Gutta percha exists in two distinctly different crystalline forms (alpha and beta) which can be converted into each other. The "alpha" form comes directly from the tree, whereas most commercial gutta percha is the "beta" crystalline form. There are no differences in physical properties between the two forms, merely a difference in the crystalline lattice related to the different rates of cooling from melt. The "beta" dental form of gutta percha has a melting point of 64° C.[10] The effect of heating on the volumetric change of gutta percha is most important to dentistry. Gutta percha was found to expand slightly upon heating, a desirable trait for an endodontic filling material.[12] This physical property manifests itself as an increased volume of the material which may be compressed into a root canal cavity.

"Volumetric studies show that it is possible to 'overfill' a root canal preparation when heat and vertical condensation are applied, because the volume of the gutta percha filling is greater than the space the filling occupies."[13] Although thought to be compressed with force which would reduce its volume, the material, studies have shown, is actually compacted, not compressed, and increased volumetric changes are due to heating.[14]

Silver points are the most widely used solid core ***metallic*** filling material, although points of gold, iridio platinum, and tantalum are also available. Whereas gutta percha was a product of the

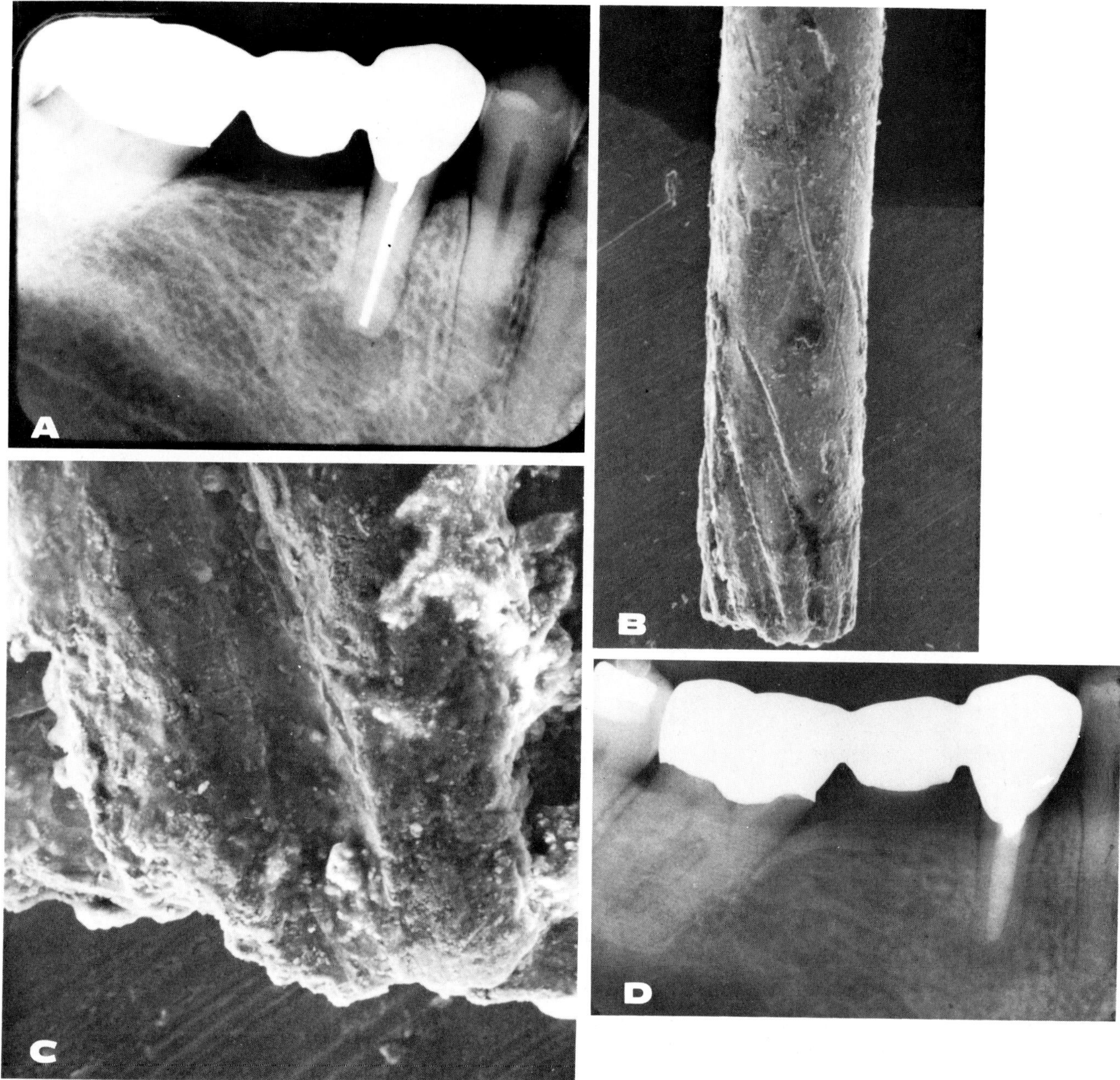

Fig. 4–8. Root canal filling failure after 20 years. *A,* Silver point incorrectly used in mandibular premolar. Pain and swelling were first indications of periapical inflammation. *B,* Electron photomicrograph (×60) of corroded silver point removed from canal seen in *A.* Moisture and broken down cement were found in canal as well. *C,* Electron photomicrograph (×300) of point in *B.* Corrosive deposits are apparent. *D,* Osseous repair one year following retreatment of failure case *(A)* with gutta percha condensed laterally. (Electron photomicrographs courtesy Dr. Samuel Seltzer.)

nineteenth century, silver points are a twentieth century development. As previously stated, they are often indicated in ***mature*** teeth with small or well-calcified round tapered canals—maxillary first premolars with two or three canals, or the buccal roots of ***mature*** maxillary molars and mesial roots of mandibular molars. In youngsters, even these canals are too large and too ovoid for single silver point use. Silver points are also ***not*** indicated for filling anterior teeth, single canal premolars, or large single canals in molars. They often fail when misused in these situations (Fig. 4–8). These failures in judgment have given silver points a bad name. Seltzer et al. have dramatically shown that failed silver points are always black and corroded when removed from the canal.[15] The assumption has developed, therefore, that silver points always corrode. This need not be true if the round tapered point truly fits the round tapered cavity, sealing the foramen as a cork seals a bottle (Fig. 4–9). The only cement depended upon is that "flashing" between the silver and the dentin wall. Silver has more rigidity than gutta percha and hence can be pushed into the tightly fitting canals and around curves, where it is difficult to place gutta percha.

The Sealers

In addition to the basic requirements for filling material, Grossman has listed 11 requirements and characteristics of a good root canal sealer:[16] (1) it should be tacky when mixed to provide good adhesion when set between it and the canal wall; (2) it should make a ***hermetic*** seal; (3) it should be ***radiopaque*** so that it can be visualized in the radiograph; (4) the particles of powder should be very fine so that they can ***mix easily*** with the liquid; (5) it should ***not shrink*** upon setting; (6) it should ***not stain*** tooth structure; (7) it should be ***bacteriostatic*** or at least not encourage bacterial growth; (8) it should ***set slowly***; (9) it should be ***insoluble*** in tissue fluids; (10) it should be ***tissue tolerant,*** i.e., non-irritating to periapical tissue; and (11) it should be ***soluble*** in a common solvent if it is necessary to remove the root canal filling.

Cements, Pastes, and Plastics. The ***cements*** with wide American acceptance are primarily zinc oxide–eugenol cements, the polyketones, and epoxy. The ***pastes*** currently in worldwide vogue are chloropercha and eucapercha, as well as the iodoform pastes, which include both the rapidly absorbable and

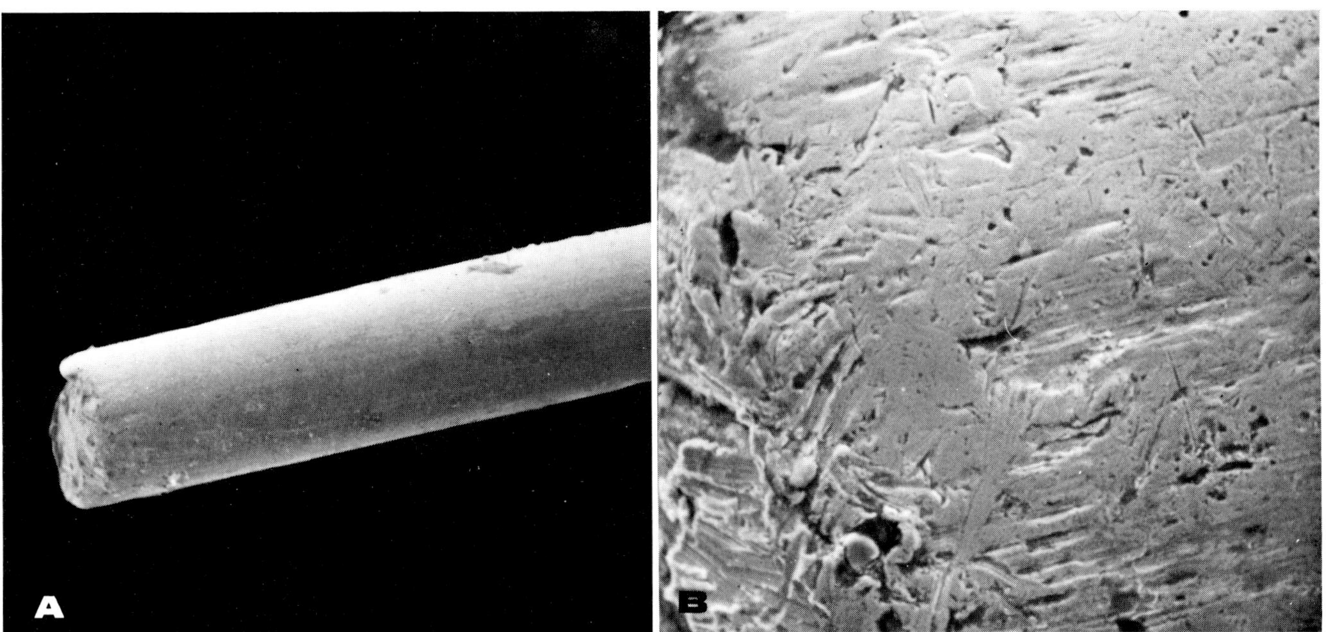

Fig. 4–9. Silver point removed from palatal canal of successfully treated molar, seven years after treatment. No corrosive deposits are apparent. Magnifications: *A*, ×60; *B*, ×600. (From Seltzer, S., Green, D., Weiner, N., and DeRenzis, F.: Oral Surg., *33*:589, Apr. 1972.)

the slowly absorbable types. Despite their disadvantages, pastes have application in certain cases. The ***plastics*** are still in the experimental stage but show great promise.

At present the methods most frequently used in filling root canals involve the use of solid core points, which are inserted in conjunction with cementing materials. Gutta percha and silver *per se* are not considered adequate filling materials ***unless*** they are cemented in place in the canal. The sealers form a fluid-tight seal at the apex by filling the minor interstices between the solid material and the wall of the canal, and by filling as well patent accessory canals and multiple foramens. Dye immersion studies have shown the necessity of cementation, without which dye penetrates back into the canal after condensation; this occurs with ***all*** known solid core root canal filling techniques.[13,14]

Cements and Plastics. The original zinc oxide–eugenol cement developed by Richert was the standard for the profession for years. It admirably met the requirements set down by Grossman except for severe staining. The silver, added for radiopacity, caused discoloration of the teeth, thus creating an undesirable public image for endodontics. Removal of all the cement from the crowns of teeth would have prevented these unfortunate incidents.[17]

In 1958, Grossman recommended a nonstaining ZO-E cement as a substitute for Richert's formula.[18] It has since become the standard by which other cements are measured in that it reasonably meets Grossman's own requirements for a cement.

The formula for Grossman's nonstaining cement is now:[16]

Powder		*Liquid*
Zinc oxide, reagent	42 parts	Eugenol
Staybelite resin	27 parts	
Bismuth subcarbonate	15 parts	
Barium sulfate	15 parts	
Sodium borate, anhydrous	1 part	

This cement is available commercially as Procosol Nonstaining Sealer. All ZO–E cements have an extended working time, but will set faster in the tooth than on the slab. If the eugenol used in the above nonstaining cement becomes oxidized and brown, the cement sets too rapidly for ease of handling. If too much sodium borate has been added the setting time is overextended.

The main virtue of such a cement is its plasticity and slow setting time in the absence of moisture, together with good sealing potential because of the small volumetric change on setting. Zinc eugenate has the disadvantage, however, of being decomposed by water through a continuous loss of the eugenol. This makes ZO–E a weak unstable material and precludes its use for any bulk use, such as a retrofilling placed apically through a surgical approach.[19]

Although cements are usually used as sealers for solid core materials, Goerig and Seymour have advocated the use of ZO–E cement as a total obturating medium.[20] It is injected into place with a disposable tuberculin syringe and needle, and the authors claim a 10-year success rate "equal to other endodontic filling techniques." Unfortunately, no proof to substantiate this claim is given.

Other cements enjoy favor with American dentists. Diaket was first reported in 1952 as a chemically similar type of material to ZO–E, again being a resin reinforced chelate formed between zinc oxide and a diketone. The epoxy AH–26, on the other hand, is a good deal different. First reported about 1957, it is essentially a simple type of epoxy resin formed from bisphenol diglycidyl ether and hexamethylene tetramine. "All these root canal cements differ widely in setting times, plasticity, and physical properties. None of the materials show hermetic (sic) sealing in the literal sense."[19]

Effectiveness of the Sealers. Using radioactive isotopes, Kapsimalis and Evans tested the sealing properties of eight endodontic filling materials. Only Proco-Sol Silver Cement (staining) and AH–26 showed no leakage.[21] Using dye penetration, Curson and Kirk "found to be satisfactory" Grossman's nonstaining sealer, Richert's Root Canal Sealer, Diaket, Tubliseal and AH–26.[22] Weiner and Schilder, on the other hand, tested the available marketed sealers (except Diaket) and found statistically significant shrinkage at room temperature and humidity.[23] Interestingly, AH–26 apparently expanded, cracking the glass testing tubes, and had not shrunk within seven days.

Because of the failure potential inherent in all endodontic cements, Smith, in 1972, suggested polycarboxylate cements as root canal sealers, even though they are generally too quick-setting and too viscous for sealers.[19] Composed of a zinc oxide powder and a liquid of polyacrylic acid, the polycarboxylates have the advantage of bonding to tooth structure (enamel better than dentin) and setting in a moist milieu. A thinner mix and modified zinc oxide allows for the adequate setting time needed for endodontic sealers. Tissue reaction was less with the polycarboxylates than for ZO–E, and the cement even inhibited bacterial growth.

Sanders reported on the use of polycarboxylate cements as a sealer for silver points. He concluded "that the polycarboxylate cement was an inferior root canal sealer, and, therefore, not indicated for clinical use with a silver point technique at this time."[24] Barry and Fried also concluded that polycarboxylate cement was unsatisfactory as a root canal sealer in addition to being difficult to manipulate.[25]

In spite of these negative reports, Smith has not given up on the polycarboxylate cements for root canal obturation. Working with McComb, Smith has continued to modify the polycarboxylate formula and then compare the results with commercial sealers.[21a] They stated that, "the polycarboxylate formulations showed definite advantages over the commercial root canal sealers in properties of strength, adhesion, and solubility. The tensile bond strength of polycarboxylate to root dentin was twice that of AH–26" (the next most adhesive material). The flow properties of the polycarboxylates were good, but the radiopacity was less than that of the commercial sealers. These, of course, were all *in vitro* tests.

McComb and Smith tested other physical properties of the commerically available cements.[26] They found that setting times varied from 17 minutes (Kerr Tubli Seal) to 630 minutes (AH–26). They found also that only AH–26 and 5 TD polycarboxylate adhered to dentin in the presence of water, and for the ZO–E cements and Diaket, adhesion was nonexistent. In addition, solubility tests proved Diaket and the polycarboxylate 5 TD to be the least soluble and Kerr Pulp Canal Sealer to be the most (Fig. 4–10).

More recently, research with other petrochemicals has proved both encouraging and discouraging. Using "specially devised endodontic cones fabricated of silicone rubber," Yee and his associates tested a cyanoacrylate, a polycarboxylate, and a silicone adhesive as canal sealers.[27] They found they could achieve "proper obliteration of the root canal space . . . comparable to those fillings of gutta percha and zinc oxide and eugenol." On the other hand, they found microscopic gaps between the polycarboxylate cement and the filling material, but not between the cement and the dentin wall. In addition, the unpolymerized silicone rubber (Silastic) solid core material and the cyanoacrylate cementing medium both caused "extensive reactions" in implanted tibias. The authors believed Silastic, in its polymerized state, to be biocompatible. "Cyanoacrylate was judged too toxic for use as an endodontic filling material," they said.

Rising and his colleagues also tested silicone rubber (Silastic 382) as a filling material sealed into incisor

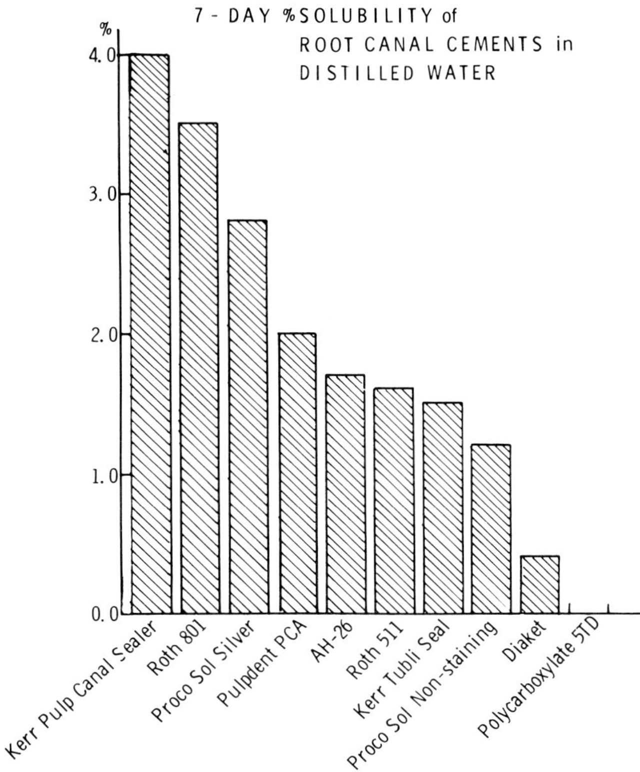

Fig. 4–10. Solubility of root canal cements. Zinc oxide-eugenol cements were most soluble, and polyketones and polycarboxylates least soluble. (From McComb, D., and Smith, D.: J.O.E., *2*: July, 1976.)

Fig. 4–11. *A,* Hydron model of prepared root canal. Notice irregularities in canal walls, presence of lateral canals, and large fin near apex. *B,* Photomicrograph of Hydron (*left*) tightly adapted to canal wall and penetrating into dentinal tubules. (*A* and *B* from Benkel, B. H., Rising, D. W., Goldman, L. B., Rosen, H., Goldman, M., and Kronman, J. H.: J.O.E., *2*: July, 1976.) *C,* Comparable tubule penetration by zinc oxide-eugenol cement. Canal was obturated with gutta percha and ZO–E based sealer. Thin layer of sealer remains pressed against entire inner surface of walls. *D,* High power of area framed in "C" demonstrates that ZO–E sealer is occasionally forced into dentinal tubules *(arrows)*. (From Walton, R.: J.O.E., *2*: Oct., 1976.)

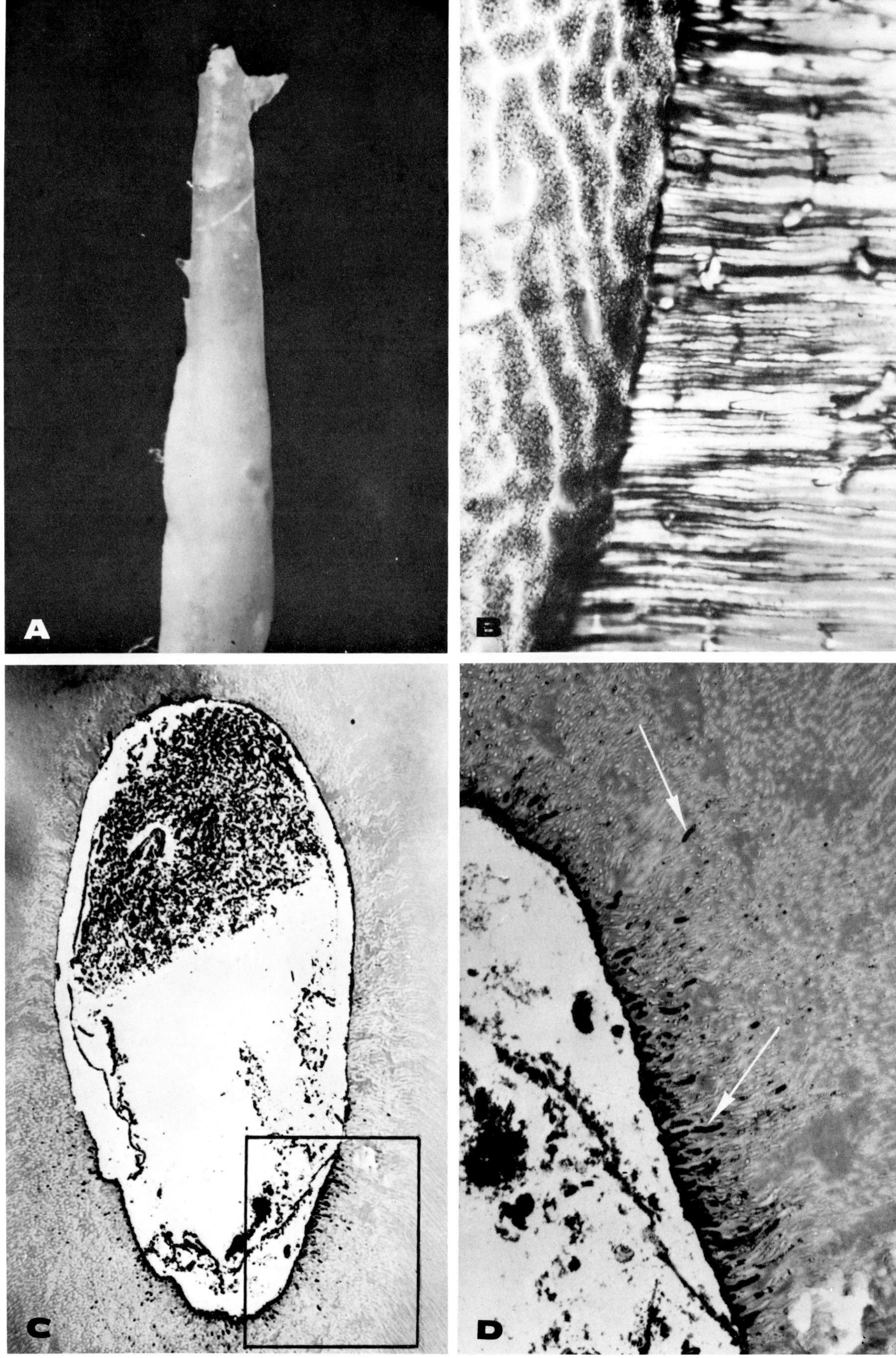
A
B
C
D

canals of monkeys with the Silastic Medical adhesive.[28] Against vital pulp tissue, "only a mild inflammatory response was seen." However, when the material escaped apically into existing periapical lesions, "there did not appear to be any significant healing." They called for additional study.

Hydron, on the other hand, a hydrophilic acrylic resin, "was well tolerated in the vital teeth as well as the pulpless teeth . . . there was not one case of persisting periapical inflammation" in spite of intentional overfilling. They reported, furthermore, that Hydron "adapts well to the walls of the canal since it is hydrophilic"[28a] (Fig. 4–11). In spite of these early encouraging results, Rising and his associates widely recommended research on long-term effects.[28a]

In recent years a cement "N2," along with a technique, the "Sargenti method," has enjoyed great popularity in both this country and abroad. The method and Sargenti have been imported from Switzerland, but the cement, N2, has been barred by the United States Food and Drug Administration. This is not to prevent its manufacture, however, and the N2 proponents distribute a formula which can be used by any pharmacist.

There are a number of formulations for N2 (or its American counterpart RC–2B), but for this purpose, only the latest will be listed,[29] which is modified but slightly from Sargenti's latest formula.[30]

Powder	%	*Liquid*
Prednisolone	0.21	Eugenol
Hydrocortisone	1.20	
Phenylmercuric borate	0.09	
Barium sulfate	3.00	
Titanium dioxide	4.00	
Bismuth subnitrate	4.00	
Paraformaldehyde	6.50	
Bismuth subcarbonate	9.00	
Lead tetroxide	11.00	
Zinc oxide	61.00	

In spite of the heated discussions centering around N2, it is only right that the product be given a full airing. Analyzing the ingredients of N2 and the paucity of literature concerning its actual contents, one finds that each ingredient is there for a specific purpose.

The corticosteroids, prednisolone and hydrocortisone, are anti-inflammatory agents in the event some of the material escapes into the tissue. Most of the metals—barium sulfate, bismuth subnitrate and subcarbonate, and lead tetroxide—are presumably included to act as radiopacifiers so that the filling can be seen radiographically. The titanium dioxide is supposed to cause "adhesion." A remaining metal, phenylmercuric borate, evidently serves as an antiseptic and, according to Sargenti,[30] is "not absolutely necessary," although the borate may act to slow the setting time. The final metal salt, zinc oxide, which makes up 61% of the formula, reacts with the liquid, eugenol, to give the product its traditional cementing qualities.

The most important constituent of N2 is evidently the paraformaldehyde. Sargenti allows for the removal of any ingredient from the powder except the paraformaldehyde.[30]

A good deal of investigation has been undertaken to evaluate the effects of N2 on ***living*** tissue. As Sargenti has stated, the most significant research should be *in vivo* with the release of the material into the tissue of the periapex or placement against the vital pulp. Significant *in vitro* studies, however, should be noted. Spangberg, using HeLa cells, compared N2 with two American products that also contain paraformaldehyde—Triolin and Oxpara.[31] He found that "all three had too strong a toxic effect to justify their use," but that N2 was the least toxic of the three.

In an animal study outside of the oral cavity, Spangberg and Langeland injected mice with radioactive phenylmercury and 12 hours later found the mercury dispersed in the bone marrow, liver, kidney, and digestive tract.[32] The researchers reasoned that phenylmercury would be released from N2 cement because the cement is resorbable.

Both Guttuso[33] and Rappaport et al.[34] tested numerous root canal sealers including the original formula of N2. Suturing implants of the mixed material (Guttuso using a fresh mix and Rappaport a "set mix") into the subcutaneous connective tissue of the ventral surface of rats, Rappaport found N2 provoked the "most severe inflammation elicited by any of the test materials." This was the only material, out of the ten sealers tested, "that did not produce a moderate response in the 35-day group" of rats. One of the sealers (AH–26) elicited no response at 35 days. Barker and Lockett, on the other hand, overfilled dogs' premolars and found N2 caused a degree of inflammation "in no way as severe as that observed by Rappaport."[45]

In vivo studies conducted in and about the oral cavity have also shown N2 to be toxic. Again, Spangberg implanted freshly prepared N2, as well as Riebler's paste, in the mandibles of guinea pigs.[35]

Histologic examination revealed maximum necrosis within one week with N2, which persisted for two weeks, but was largely resorbed and replaced by granulation tissue ***without*** bone regeneration in 12 weeks. Friend and Browne implanted, in the tibias of rabbits, polythene tubes loaded with various root canal filling materials. Although initial bone necrosis developed under all the sealers, "with N2 Normal there was evidence to suggest that the area of dead bone showed some increase up to 4 weeks. . . . There were occasions when vital trabeculae of new bone were found close to, though not up against, the material." The authors concluded, "It would seem that N2 Normal may be used safely provided that it is kept within the root canal."[36]

Another systemically toxic metal of course is lead, which is contained in N2. Grossman used N2 in primates and observed a rise in the levels of lead in the blood for several weeks thereafter.[37] Reporting further on this study, Shapiro et al. substituted radioactive lead nitrate, 210Pb, in otherwise lead-free N2 cement, and filled pulpless canals in monkeys.[37a] "Radiographs of the obturated teeth verified that all filling materials were confined to the root canal and did not extend beyond the apex . . ." In spite of this confinement of N2, radioactive lead in the blood of two monkeys increased significantly, more than doubling in one animal from 2.65 ug./100 ml. of blood to 6.32 ug./100 ml. Oswald and Cohn mixed radioactive lead with RC–2B sealer, which contains 11% lead tetroxide, and filled cats' incisors.[38] Alpha emissions from the lead nucleotide "were significant" in liver, kidney, and adrenal gland 72 days later.

Sargenti advocates the use of N2 in both vital pulp and necrotic pulp.[39] Evidently recognizing the destructive action of the paraformaldehyde, however, he recommends that his material not be used against large pulp surfaces.[30] On the other hand, he describes how N2 can be used in retrofilling open apex cases, which also present large tissue surfaces.

It is the claim that "fundamental to a successful outcome" with N2 is the formation of a "scurf" at the interface between the cement and the tissue. The scurf is said to be a sclerotic zone,[40] but Crabb[41] and Nygaard-Ostby[42] point out that this interface tissue is ***necrotic*** not sclerotic, and as such, is no different from other necrotic pulp tissue which eventually leads to chronic apical inflammation.

The essentiality of the paraformaldehyde in N2 is claimed to be its antiseptic quality continually released.[30] Continued release for antisepsis, however, would also spell continuing necrosis. Snyder et al. noted that in dogs, pulp tissue in all vital canals filled with N2 became necrotic.[43] No "sclerotic zone" was evident at the site of amputation, and a mild to moderate periapical inflammatory reaction also occurred (Fig. 4–12). Barker and Lockett, also using dogs, noted total necrosis in 9 out of 10 vital pulps.[45] In contrast to the "permanent antiseptic state is guaranteed" quality of N2,[44] Barker and Lockett found bacteria in roots filled with N2.[45] The proponents of N2 have experimented with the product. Rowe claims that in three cases the pulp remained normal despite tissue damage adjacent to the N2.[46]

As far as overfilling with N2 is concerned, Sargenti claims that overfills are "reasonably well tolerated," that overfilling "seems" to stimulate periapical healing, and that a small quantity of the extruded cement is to be "considered favorably" in the cases of "gangrenous pulps."[30] The first point might well be confirmed by Snyder.[43] Rappaport, however, observed that N2 "produced the most severe inflammatory response" of ten root canal sealers tested.[34] Langeland et al., using pigs, monkeys, and humans and observing them for over a year, concluded that N2 is far from nonirritating in periapical tissues.[47]

Reports[45,48] of N2 extruded into the maxillary sinus and mandibular canal with resultant pain and paresthesia have been countered by Sargenti who, in discussing similar instances, asserted that the outcome is without permanent harm.[30] He stated further that only "transitory occasional paresthesia" resulted.

As far as the sealing and obturation qualities of N2 and its technique of placement are concerned, Sargenti has asserted that ***obliteration*** along with disinfection are important for success.[30] On the other hand, he has also stated that it is "not mandatory to have a compact root canal filling."[30] One must ask if a noncompact root canal filling truly obliterates the canal space deemed important for success by Sargenti and others.

One must also ask if N2 is soluble in the canal. If it is not soluble, how can it continue to exert its permanent antiseptic activity deemed so important by its proponents? Sargenti claims his sealer is not resorbed from the canal, but is slowly absorbed from the periapical tissues; he calls it "semi-resorbable."[49] At another time, however, he modifies this statement by saying that N2 is "practically" nonresorbable from the canal.[30]

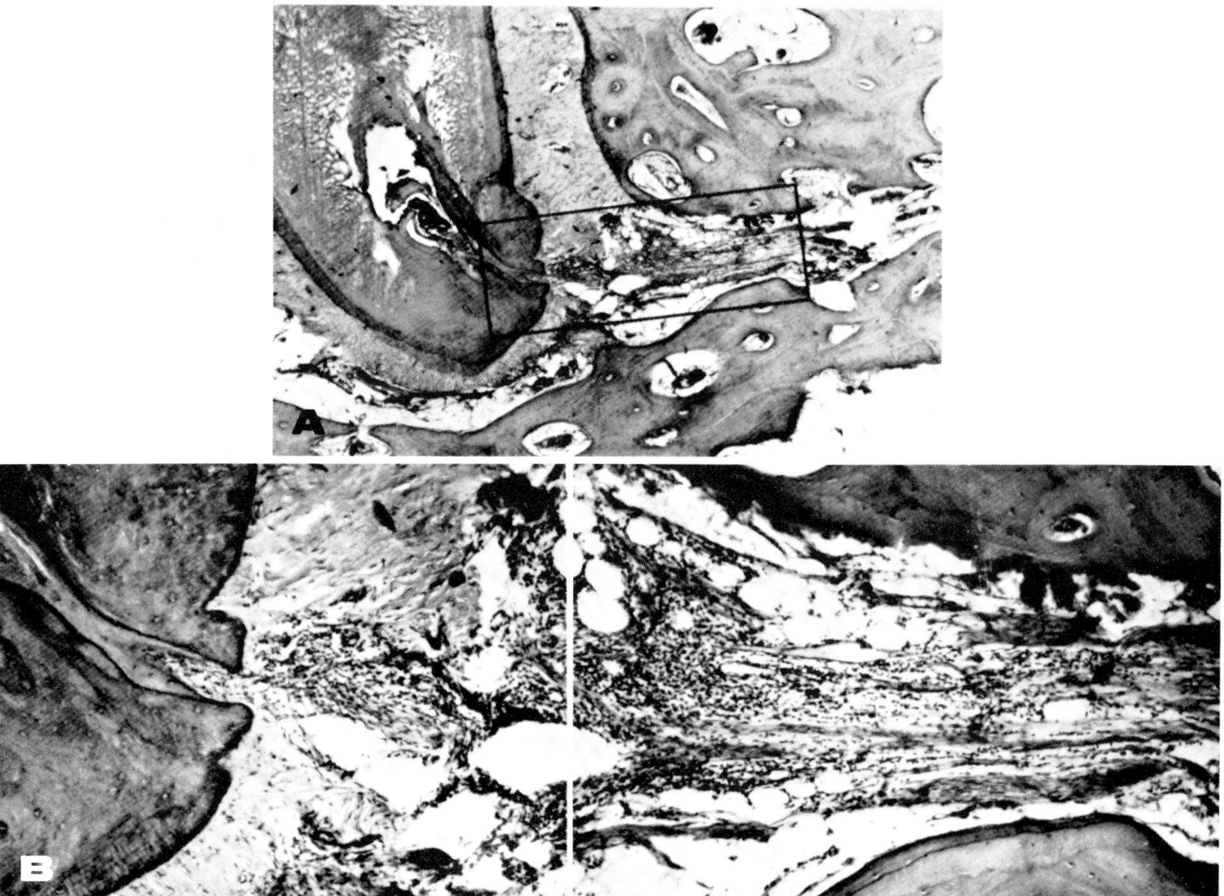

Fig. 4–12. Dog tooth filled with N2 after vital pulp extirpation 1.5 to 2 mm. from apex according to Sargenti method. Observation period—four months. *A,* Overview of root (*left*) and periapical tissue. *B,* Frame in *A* showing chronic inflammation caused by irritants from root canal (*left*). (From Spangberg, L., and Langeland, K.: Oral Surg., *35*:402, Mar., 1973.)

As far as placement of N2 is concerned, it is recommended that it be spun or whipped into the canal by means of a Lentulo spiral. This is a perfectly reasonable method of insertion, but evidently voids remain if it is considered "not mandatory to have a compact filling."[30] Sargenti does warn, however, that without great care overfilling with this technique is likely.[30]

Weine has been unable to find a suitable solvent for Sargenti's sealer, so necessary in retreatment cases.[50]

As far as staining qualities of N2 are concerned, Goerig found N2 to be in the middle range of sealers.[51] In his text, Sargenti shows how to hide the sealer so that it will not show through thin walls.[30]

Sargenti, in his texts, presents a rather straightforward, traditional, three-appointment approach to treating necrotic pulp cases; on the other hand, he also appears to agree with his American followers who advocate the rapid, one-appointment approach, what has been called "one-stop" endodontics. With this one-appointment procedure, there is no rubber dam, no tooth measurement, power-driven canal instrumentation, and no irrigation. Instrumentation is followed immediately by a rapid-filling of the canal with N2 alone (or RC–2B) as a "sealer."

The rationale for this rather imprecise approach was given by Sargenti at a meeting of the American Dental Association in 1974. "In my opinion," he said in discussion, "it is about time to introduce some compromise in endodontics—between the extreme position of extraction of the tooth or a perfect, exact root canal treatment."[52] Earlier, however, Sargenti had

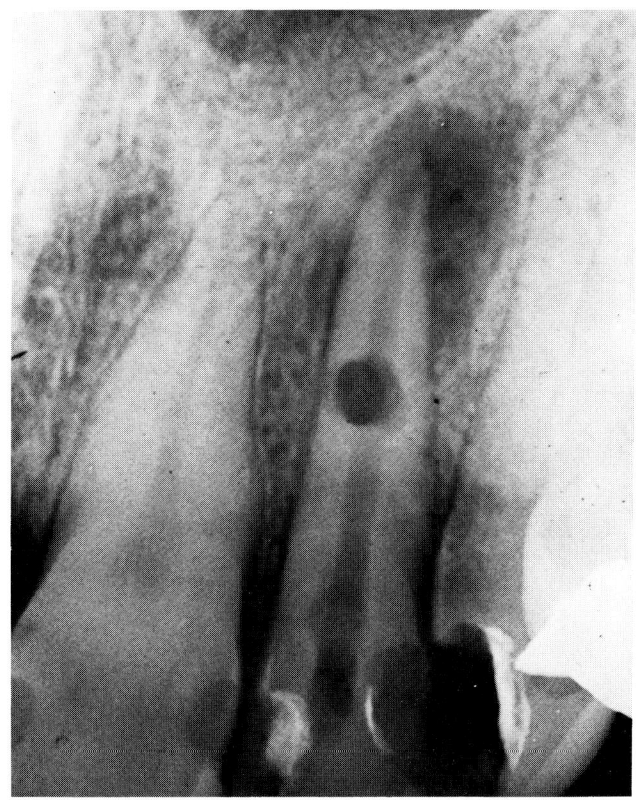

Fig. 4–13. Perforation of maxillary incisor through use of Fistulator. (Courtesy Dr. Alfred L. Frank.)

spoken to a double standard of quality when he stated, "If I had endodontic problems myself and if I wished to have an exact endodontic treatment, I should certainly ask Dr. Schilder* to treat me."[52]

In summary, the material N2 (as well as RC–2B, Oxpara and Triolin) has been shown to be severely irritating to vital tissue. This along with the imprecise method of preparation and root canal filling, appears to have resulted in postoperative problems frequently enough to cause N2 proponents to recommend apical trephination. For this exigency, the dentist is supplied with a "Fistulator" to trephine to the periapex to relieve the pressure and pain that might follow treatment with N2 (Fig. 4–13). A survey conducted by the American Endodontic Society, of 48,134 cases treated by 411 dentists, shows 9910 cases of trephination.[30] This indicates that the method is used in 20.5% of cases. "One-appointment treatment can be performed with any technique if one disregards the postoperative pain sequelae."[53]

Tissue Reaction to Other Cements. With the emphasis upon, or warnings against, overfilling, one must be concerned about the possible toxic effects from any of the sealers escaping the foramen. *In vitro* studies by Spangberg and Langeland have shown that all the cements tested against HeLa cells were highly toxic.[54] Within one hour the HeLa cell–cement interaction resulted in total cell lysis. This included Richert's and Grossman's sealers, Tubli-Seal, N2, and AH–26. Testing the cements after they had set for 24 hours gave essentially the same results. For controls, gutta percha points were used and, in contrast to the sealers, produced little cell lysis. These points are not purely gutta percha, mind you, but contain in addition zinc oxide, barium sulfate, and a pink coloring agent. These secondary contents are bound by the gutta percha.

In vivo studies of the effects upon live tissue of root canal sealers were conducted by Erausquin and Muruzabal.[55] Performing root canal therapy in the mandibular molars of rats, these researchers conducted hundreds of tests of techniques and materials. They concluded that all the commercial root canal sealers were toxic, causing extensive to moderate tissue damage as soon as they escaped through the foramen (Fig. 4–14). In all honesty, however, the authors did believe that periapical necrosis may be due in part to an infarct caused by pressure obstruction of the region's vessels.[56] Necrosis of the periodontal ligament provoked necrosis in the adjacent cementum and alveolar bone as well (Fig. 4–15). In the rat, the PDL regenerated within seven days if toxic irritation did not continue.

In comparing the various sealers, Erausquin and Muruzabal found that straight zinc oxide–eugenol cement was "highly irritating to the periapical tissues and caused necrosis of the bone and cementum."[57] Inflammation persisted for two weeks or more. Finally, the ZO–E became encapsulated.[57] In contrast, Curson and Kirk,[22] and Barker and Lockett,[58] all felt that ZO–E was better tolerated in the periapex than the other root canal sealers.

In a further study, Erausquin and Muruzabal studied other ZO–E based cements. All the cements, if the canal was overfilled, "showed a tendency to be resorbed" by phagocytes. Grossman's Sealer and N2 both provoked severe inflammatory reactions, and Richert's sealer caused moderate infiltration. The most severe destruction of the alveolar bone, how-

*Dr. Herbert Schilder of Boston University has an international reputation for a meticulous technique, which includes obturation with softened gutta percha compacted with vertical force.

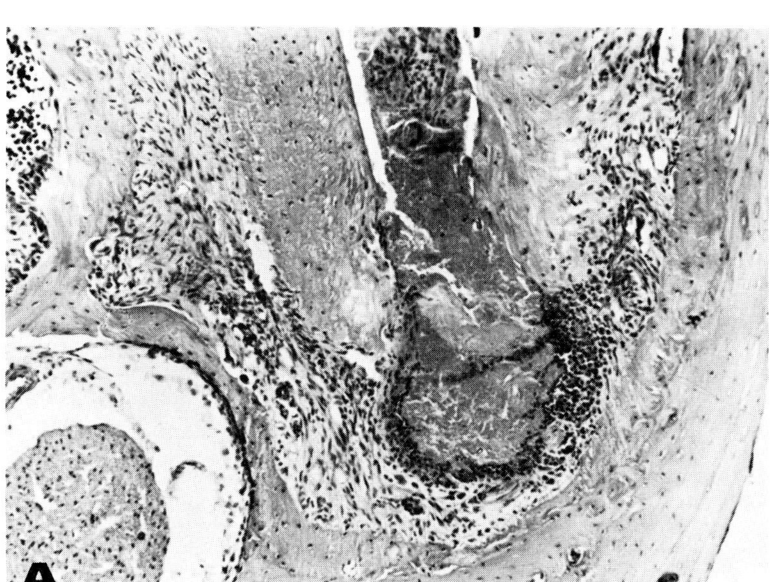
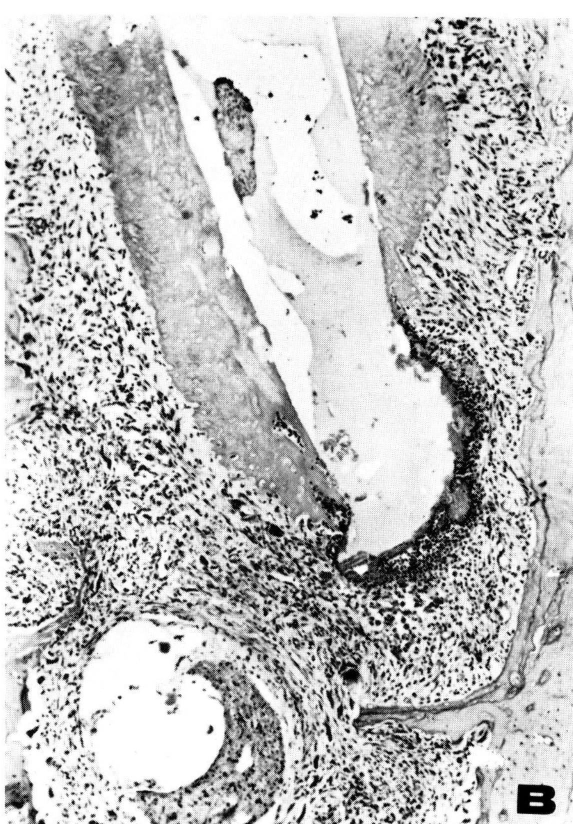

Fig. 4–14. Periapical tissue reaction to overfilling of rat's teeth. *A*, Filling with Procosol Nonstaining Sealer one day postoperative. Polymorphonuclear leukocytes have invaded even crack in cement. *B*, Filling with zinc oxide-eugenol cement four days postoperative. Early PMNL infiltration, in reaction to material, is apparent. (From Erausquin, J., and Muruzabal, M.: Arch. Oral Biol., *11*: 373, 1966.)

ever, was caused by poor debridement and poor filling of the canals. The least reaction was found when the canal was not overfilled.[55]

The least irritating of the cements tested by Erausquin and Muruzabal were Diaket and AH–26. Following overfilling with these sealers, the "inflammation was generally very mild." Diaket, which showed a marked tendency to be projected beyond the apex, became readily encapsulated (Fig. 4–16). AH–26, on the other hand, was resorbed instead (Fig. 4–17). The researchers observed, "when a foreign body is not too irritating, it becomes either resorbed or encapsulated by the body. Both of these processes occurred in teeth filled with Diaket and AH–26."[59]

The tissue reactions to overinstrumentation and overfilling noted by Erausquin and Muruzabal were confirmed by Seltzer and Soltanoff.[60] Using human beings and monkeys as subjects, these researchers purposely filed and reamed beyond the apex in all cases; then in half the cases they filled just short of the apex and in the other half overfilled. In all cases, they found immediate periapical inflammation in response to overinstrumentation. When the root canals were ***filled short*** of the foramen, the reactions tended to subside within three months and complete repair eventually took place. In contrast, the teeth with overfilled root canals exhibited persistent chronic inflammatory responses. There was also a greater tendency toward epithelial proliferation and cyst formation in the overfilled group.

One must conclude that periapical tissue reaction to all the cements will at first be inflammatory, but as the cements reach their final set, cellular repair takes place unless the cement continues to break down, releasing one of its toxic components.

The Pastes. The pastes used in root canal fillings differ greatly in content as well as in the purposes for which they are used. Chloropercha and eucapercha are made by dissolving gutta percha in either chloroform or eucalyptol. The resulting thick, tacky

Fig. 4–15. Periapical tissue reaction to overfilling with N2 one day postoperative. N2 protruding beyond apical foramen has caused compression of periodontal ligament. (From Erausquin, J., and Muruzabal, M.: Arch. Oral Biol., *1*:373, 1966.)

paste is then used primarily as a cement in combination with gutta percha points. Both pastes harden by the evaporation of the chloroform or eucalyptol. The evaporation, of course, leads to shrinkage, which has been a deterrent from routine use. Chloropercha, as a sealer for solid core gutta percha, has been returning to favor in the softened gutta percha technique.

Spangberg and Langeland tested irritant qualities of chloropercha against that of other root canal sealers.[54] They pointed out that the rate of chloroform evaporation in a sealed root canal is not known, but it is reasonable to believe it is slow as it is eliminated through the tissue fluids. During this period, chloropercha is as toxic as the cements. When set, however, it is far less toxic, particularly Moyco chloropercha. Somewhat more toxic, but with more adhesive quality and more volume stability, is Kloropercha N-O (Nygaard-Ostby). In addition to the chloroform, it also contains Canada balsam, rosin, and zinc oxide added to the powdered gutta percha.

The iodoform-type pastes are used extensively in Europe and Latin America as the sole canal filling. They have the reported advantage of being resorbed by the tissue if the canal is overfilled.[61] This resorbable quality, on the other hand, can be a great disadvantage, as shown by Nygaard-Ostby, who demonstrated that resorption is not confined to the excess paste extruded periapically, but may extend into the canal, thus breaking the apical seal and allowing percolation.[62] Maisto has modified the typi-

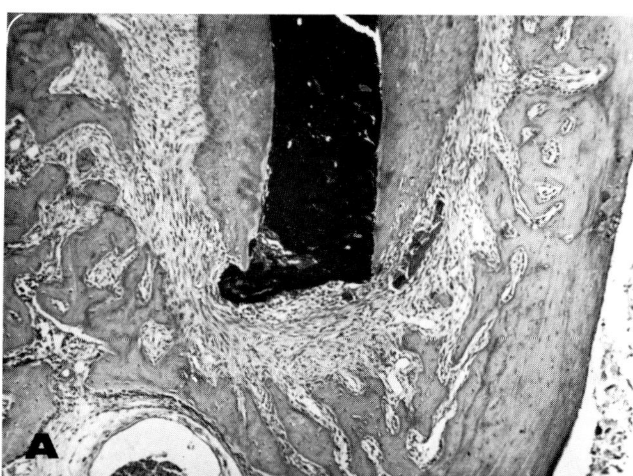

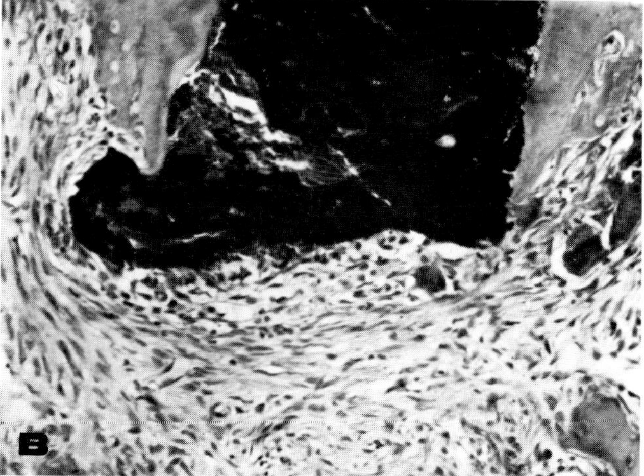

Fig. 4–16. *A,* Moderate overfilling with Diaket 15 days postoperative. Debris from instrumentation is to right of apex and black filling. *B,* High-power (×22) view of Diaket and periapex. Loose connective tissue, abundance of fibroblasts, and some macrophages and giant cells are apparent. Dentinal debris *(right border)* is also being attacked by macrophages. (From Erausquin, J., and Muruzabal, M.: Oral Surg., *21*:786, 1966.)

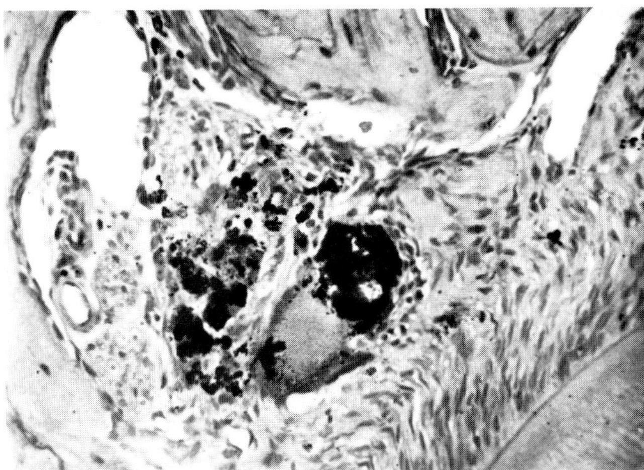

Fig. 4–17. Fragments of AH–26 scattered throughout periapical tissue 30 days postoperative, indicating resorption of sealer. Giant cells surround large fragment of AH–26. (From Erausquin, J., and Muruzabal, M.: Oral Surg., *21*:786, 1966.)

cal iodoform paste formula by adding zinc oxide, which slows resorption.[63] He also used the paste as a cementing vehicle with gutta percha points. The iodoform pastes, generally speaking, have not found great favor in the United States.

METHODS OF OBTURATING THE ROOT CANAL SPACE

Today the various techniques for obturating the root canal range from injections of cements or pastes ***only*** to obliteration with solid core materials, introduced under some pressure and sealed there with cements. Under the latter rubric falls the single-point insertion with silver points; the multiple-point insertion usually of gutta percha points condensed with lateral force; or the sectional insertion of softened gutta percha condensed with vertical force.

As previously emphasized, selection of the filling material and associated technique was made prior to cavity preparation, and was based upon the anatomic configuration of the canal. The cavity was then prepared specifically to receive the filling materials selected (Fig. 4–18). Dentists today employ a combination of materials often in filling one canal—silver, gutta percha, and cement for example. The rigidity of being "married" to one particular method or material will not only limit the cases acceptable for treatment, but will materially limit success.

Class I Canal Anatomy

The Class I canal is the mature ***uncomplicated*** canal, straight or slightly curved, with constriction at the apical foramen. The mature uncomplicated root canal is usually filled with gutta percha. A primary point is first positioned, and obturation is completed by compacting additional gutta percha points against this initial point by using lateral pressure. Final compaction is by vertical pressure. Some mature Class I canals may be filled with a single silver point and some with a combination of silver and gutta percha. In all cases, a cementing sealer must be used.

In any event, the fit of the primary point is most important. Both gutta percha and silver points have been standardized in size and shape to match the standardized instruments. Presumably, a primary point the same size as the file or reamer which prepared the apical third of the cavity will fit exactly. Leaving nothing to chance, however, the point must be tested in place. This is known as the ***trial point measurement.***

Trial Point

Before trial insertion, the initial point should be sterilized. Gutta percha points may be stored in a germicide, such as tincture of Zephiran, or held with cotton pliers and wiped with a sponge soaked in a germicide. Silver points are held in cotton pliers and heated over a low bunsen flame, care being taken not to melt the fine points. The point should be immersed at once in a germicide, which cools the point and also anneals it, making it more flexible in negotiating canal curvatures.

Either gutta percha or silver points should be tested by three methods to be certain that they fit properly: (1) visual test, (2) tactile test, and (3) roentgenographic test.

To test visually, the point should be measured and grasped with the cotton pliers at a position 1 mm. short of the working length of the tooth. The point is then carried into the canal until the cotton pliers touch the morsal surface of the tooth. If the working length of the tooth was correct and the point goes completely to position, the ***visual test*** has been passed unless the point can be pushed beyond this position. This can be determined by grasping 1 mm. further back on the point and attempting to push it apically. If the point can be pushed to the root end, it might well be pushed beyond into the tissue. Either the foramen was originally large or it has been perfo-

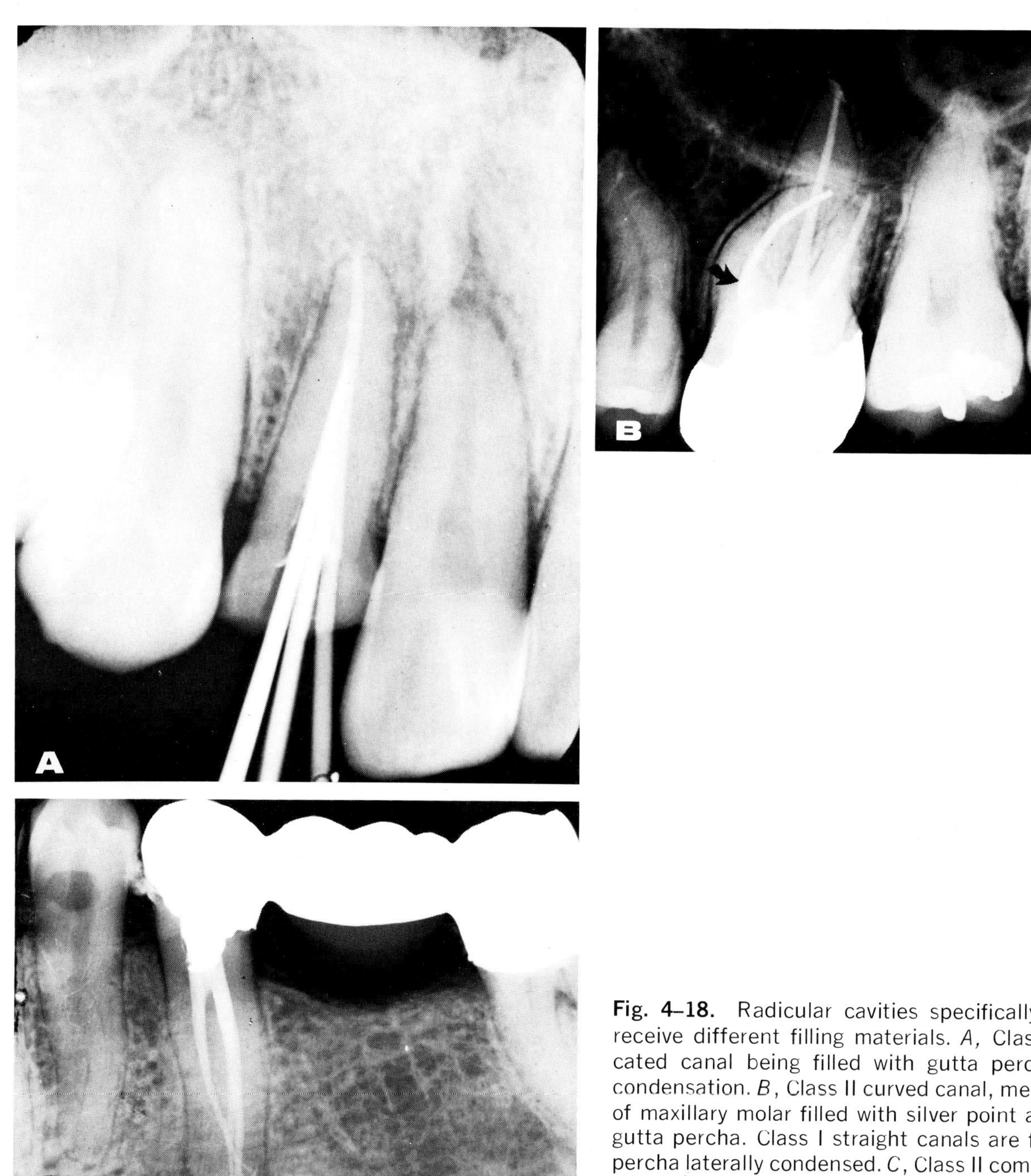

Fig. 4–18. Radicular cavities specifically prepared to receive different filling materials. *A,* Class I uncomplicated canal being filled with gutta percha by lateral condensation. *B*, Class II curved canal, mesiobuccal root of maxillary molar filled with silver point and additional gutta percha. Class I straight canals are filled by gutta percha laterally condensed. *C*, Class II complicated canal filled with softened gutta percha vertically condensed. (Courtesy Dr. James D. Zidell.)

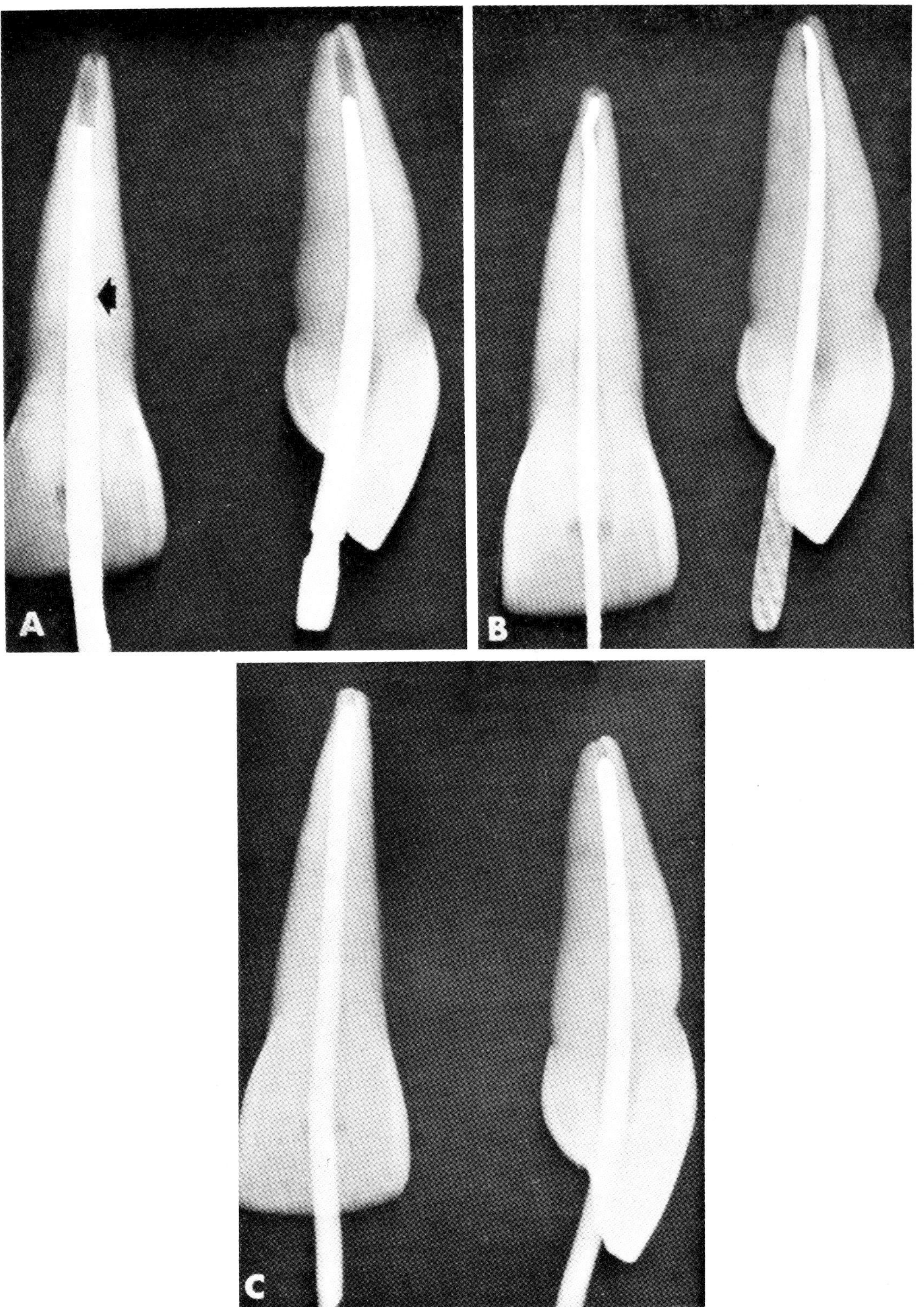

Fig. 4–19. Importance of trial point roentgenogram. *A*, Gutta percha point which binds in canal (arrow) short of apical third. Canal needs more filing at this position. *B*, Gutta percha point to full depth, but far too fine as indicated by buckling. *C*, Gutta percha trial point which goes to depth and will totally obliterate apical third of canal with vertical condensation.

rated. If the point can be extended beyond the apex, the next larger size point should be tried. If this larger point does not go to place, the original point should be used by cutting 2-mm. pieces off the tip end. Each time the tip is cut back, the diameter is larger. By trial and error the point should be retried in the canal until it goes to the correct position and fits tightly.

The second method of testing the trial point is by ***tactile sensation*** and will determine whether the point tightly fits the canal. Some degree of force should be required to seat the point, and once in position, a good deal of pulling force should be required to dislodge it. This is known as ***"tugback."*** Again, if the point is ***loose*** in the canal, the next larger size point should be tried, or the method of snipping segments from the tip of the initial point, followed by trial and error positioning, should be used.

After the visual and tactile tests for the trial point have been completed, its position must be checked by the third test, the ***roentgenogram.*** The film must show the point extending to within one mm. from the sharply tapered tip of the preparation (Fig. 4–19). The blunted or ***"bull-nosed"*** tightly fitting point is less apt to be forced through the apical foramen. If the operator prefers, square end points may be rounded to reach the apex of the preparation.

The trial point roentgenogram presents the final opportunity to check all the operative steps of therapy completed to date. This roentgenogram will show whether the working length of the tooth was correct. It will also show whether instrumentation followed the curve of the canal or whether a perforation developed. It will, of course, show the relationship of the initial filling point to the preparation (Fig. 4–19). Occasionally the roentgenogram will show the point forced well beyond the apex. If this is the case, the incorrect length of tooth was used during instrumentation, and the operator has probably been wondering why the patient has complained of discomfort. The overextended point should ***always*** be shortened from the fine end and then carefully returned to proper position. In this new position it should again pass the tactile and roentgenographic tests of the trial points. It should never be manipulated so that it just appears to fit in the film. ***It must fit tightly and come to a dead stop.***

Occasionally the initial point will not go completely to place even though it is the same number as the last enlarging instrument. This condition may arise because: (1) the enlarging instrument was not used to its fullest extent or (2) the instrument was untwisted by force during use and thus is not of full diameter, (3) debris remains in the canal, or (4) a ledge exists in the canal upon which the point is catching.

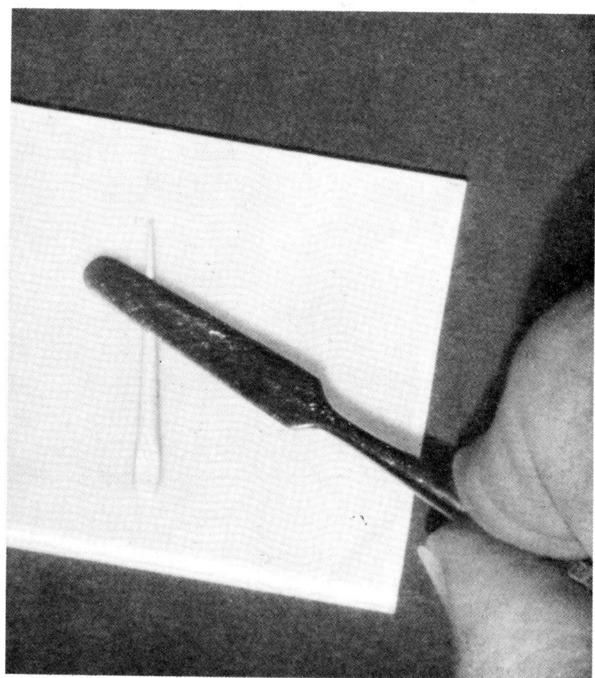

Fig. 4–20. "Cold-rolling" to reduce slightly oversized gutta percha point. Tip should be blunted before insertion.

In any case, the problem can be solved by one of two methods: by selecting a new file and reinstrumenting the canal to full working length until the file is loose in the canal, or, in the case of gutta percha, by cold-rolling to thin down the point with a sterile spatula on a sterile glass slab (Fig. 4–20). Trial and error will determine when the point is seated. If a ledge has been developed in the canal wall, it must be removed by the method suggested on page 206.

Preparation of the Initial Point

After the initial point has passed the trial point tests, it should be removed. In the case of a gutta percha point, it is removed with a pair of cotton pliers which scar the soft point at the incisal edge (Fig. 4–21). Silver points should be removed with a hemostat, which grasps the point at a right angle while resting against the height of the cusp. The point is locked in the hemostat, which is not unlocked until

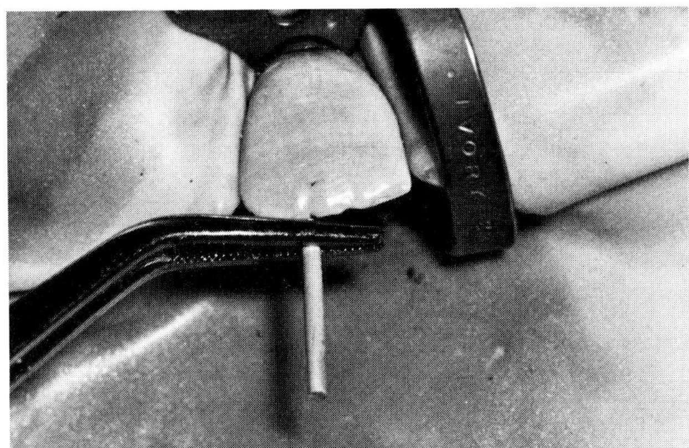

Fig. 4–21. Removal of measured and tested initial gutta percha point. Cotton pliers mark gutta percha at incisal edge.

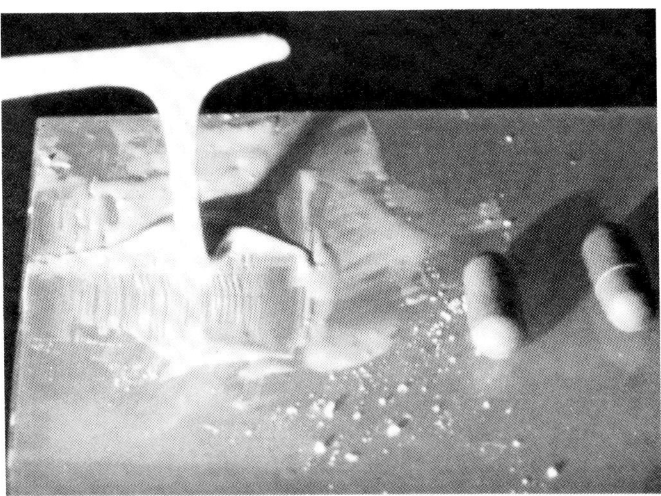

Fig. 4–22. Root canal cement should be mixed to thick creamy consistency, which may be strung off slab for one inch.

it is cemented into place. To prevent slippage, a second hemostat or pair of pliers should be used to help remove the point.

Cementation of the Primary Point

While preparations are being made to cement the filling point, be it silver or gutta percha, an absorbable paper point should be present in the canal to absorb moisture that might accumulate. To determine the presence of moisture in the canal, the absorbent point is removed and the tip drawn along the surface of the rubber dam. If the point is moist, it will leave a mark as it removes the powder from the dam. When this procedure has been repeated with fresh points that no longer streak the dam, the canal is considered ready to receive the cement.

A sterile slab and spatula are removed from the instrument case or are sterilized by wiping with a gauze sponge soaked in germicide and dried with a sterile sponge. One or two drops of liquid are used and the cement is mixed according to the manufacturer's directions. The cement should be creamy in consistency but quite heavy, and should string out at least an inch when the spatula is lifted from the mix (Fig. 4–22).

Root canal cement may be placed in the canal with either a Lentulo spiral or a reamer. The former instrument is made of fine wire spiraled into the shape of a reverse auger. When the spiral is turned ***clockwise,*** by either the fingers or the handpiece, it carries the cement apically (Fig. 4–23*A*). Although the spiral is an efficient instrument, the neophyte seems to have trouble with it. It is not effective in narrow canals, and if inadvertently locked in the canal, it will break (Fig. 4–24). In addition, it tends to "throw" cement past the apex if used in the handpiece and may also cause cement to set too rapidly as a result of its whipping action. In some "cement only" filling techniques, the spiral alone is used, presumably to condense the cement in the canal cavity. Whether the cement is compacted, however, is under question.

To carry cement apically the use of a reamer turned ***counterclockwise*** in the canal has been suggested. Reversing the action of the reamer produces an effect similar to that of the Lentulo spiral (Fig. 4–23*B*). To use this method, a new sterile reamer, one size smaller than the last instrument used for enlargement is selected. The safest approach is to place a stop attachment on the blade of the instrument just short of the working length of the tooth. A small amount of cement is then gathered on the blades of the instrument and carried up the canal by rapidly twirling the handle counterclockwise. The procedure is repeated until the canal appears to be liberally coated with cement. The canal preparation is now ready to receive the primary or initial gutta percha point, which is placed in the same manner for either the lateral condensation method of filling or the softened gutta percha technique.

The ***initial point*** is coated with cement, inserted in the canal, and slowly forced to place with the hemostat. The patient may experience some minor discomfort from this procedure as ***air is evacuated***

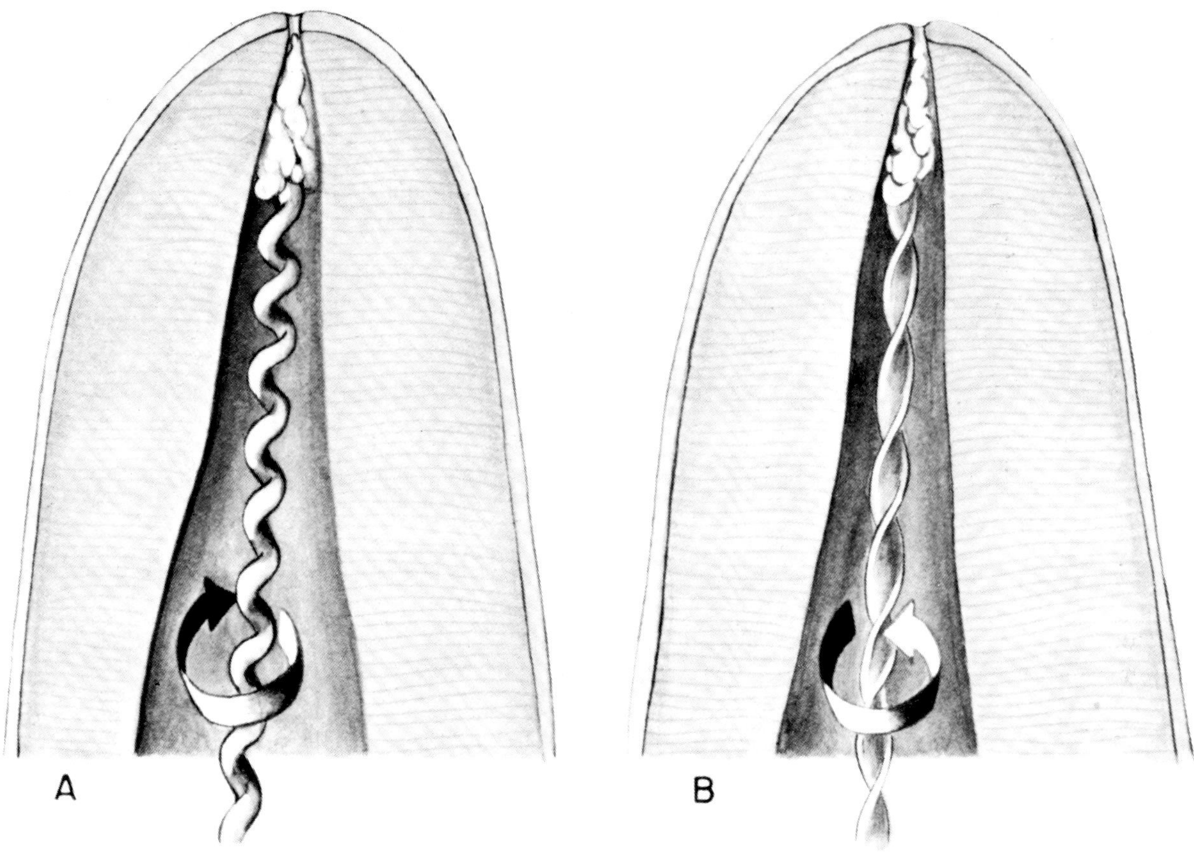

Fig. 4–23. *A,* Lentulo spiral operated in *clockwise* action will spin cement into apical portion of canal. *B,* Reamer smaller than canal lumen will carry cement into apical canal when operated in *counterclockwise* motion.

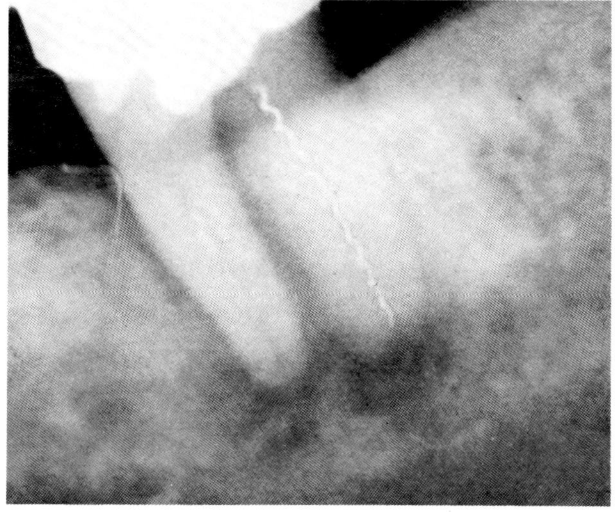

Fig. 4–24. Lentulo spiral fractured in distal canal of lower molar. Careful observation reveals spiral also fractured in mesial canal as well as broken reamer in mesial gingiva. (Retouched for clarity.)

from the canal through the foramen. If the resistance form has been correctly instrumented, so that a "minimal opening" exists at the foramen, no more than, and usually not as much as, a tiny "worm" of cement will be forced from the apex. When the hemostat strikes the morsal surface, the point should be in position at the apex.

The question is frequently asked why the well-fitting initial point does not force a great quantity of cement through the apical foramen. The answer lies in the tapered shape of the point and corresponding shape of the canal. One should not think of the point as a plunger, for a plunger has straight walls. The tapered point does not actually touch the walls of the prepared canal until just that moment when it reaches its final seat. It will thus not force quantities of cement ahead of it, but will rather displace cement coronally as it is slowly forced into position. Thus one need not fear that there is an excessive amount of cement in the canal prior to placement of the point.

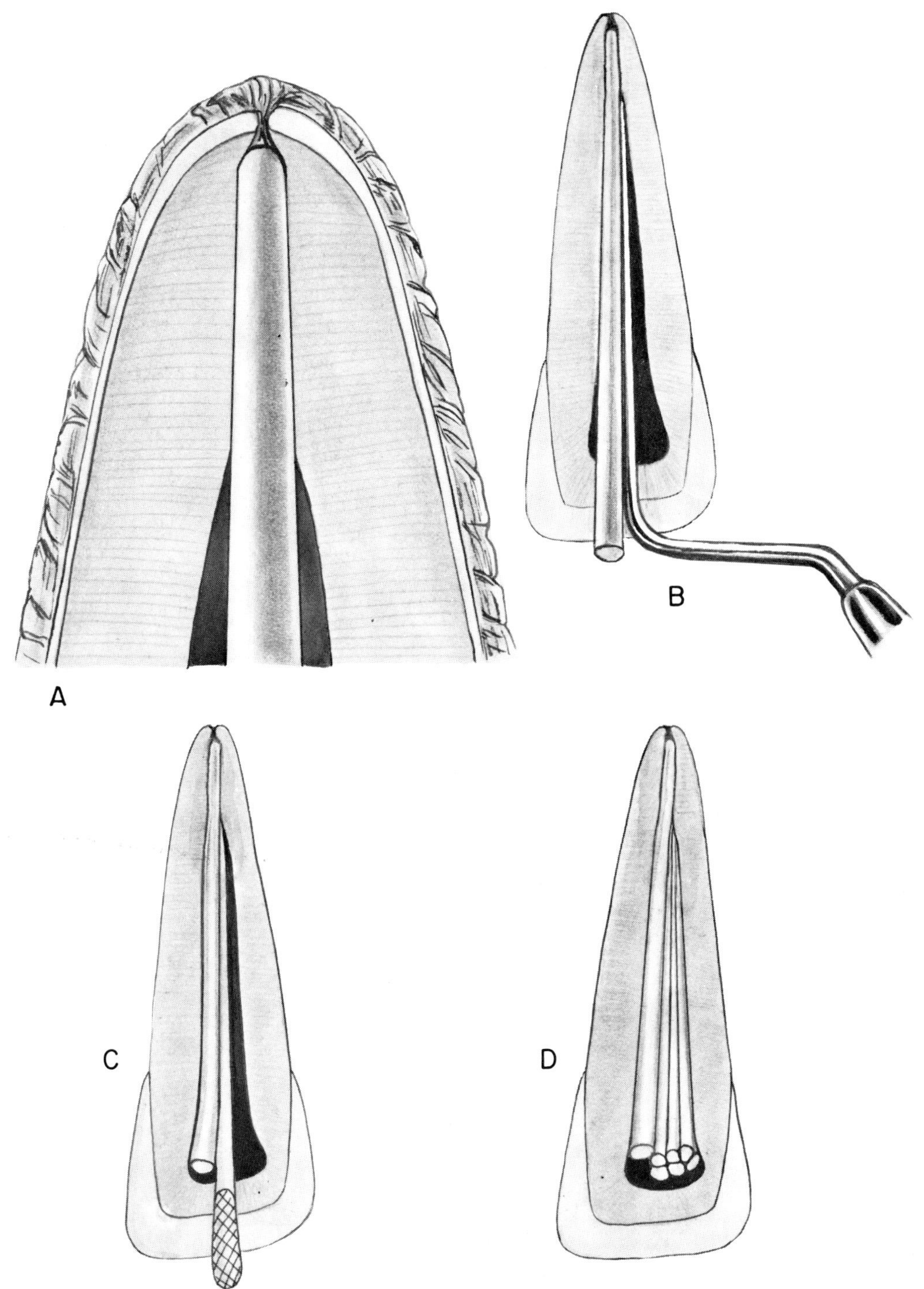

Fig. 4–25. Multiple point filling procedure. *A,* Primary filling point accurately fits round, tapered apical cavity prepared by reaming. This point when cemented to place should completely obliterate apical third of canal. *B,* No. 3 spreader is forcibly worked up canal as far as apical third. This instrument moves primary point aside forming pathway for additional points. Rotary motion is used to remove spreader, which is immediately followed by additional point. *C,* First added point goes to full depth formed by No. 3 spreader. *D,* By constantly spreading and adding additional points, entire canal space is totally obliterated. All excess gutta percha and cement in pulp chamber should be removed to below gingival level. Finally, vertical compression with blunt plugger is used to compact gutta percha and cement into solid mass.

Multiple Point Obturation with Lateral Condensation

Candidates for laterally condensed gutta percha fillings are all those with class I canal anatomy. These canals are also ovoid, at least in part, and typify the majority of the endodontic cases. Laterally condensed gutta percha fillings are applicable to all the anterior teeth, most of the premolars, and the large single canals of the molars—palatal of the maxillary and distal of the mandibular.

There are exceptions, of course, in which a single silver point has been used successfully in such cases—for example, when the apical foramen stands open, and a flexible compressible filling is forced beyond the apex. Nonetheless, if a high success rate is to be achieved, gutta percha obturation is ideal if the canal is other than round and tapered for its entire length.

The initial phases of multiple point obturation have been discussed, *i.e.,* the primary point is selected, positioned, tested visually, tactilely, and roentgenographically to ensure optimum fit in the apical one-third of the canal, and cemented to place. The primary point should obliterate the apical one-third

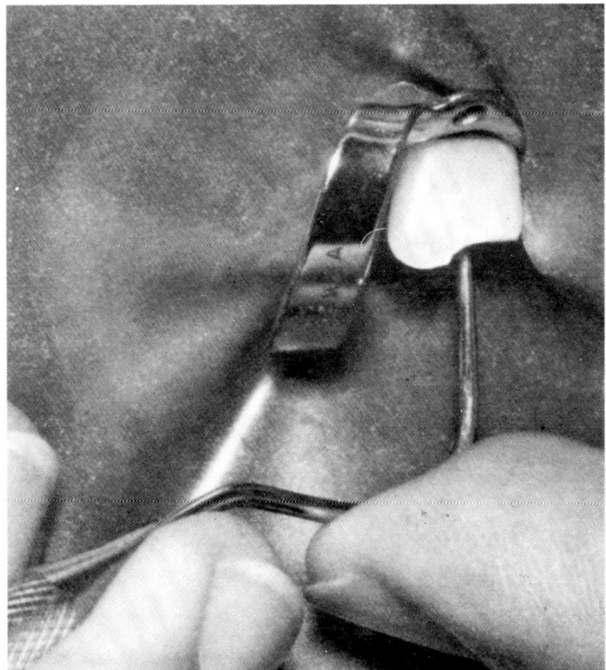

Fig. 4–26. Use of root canal spreader to prepare pathway for additional gutta percha points. As spreader is rotated from side to side with right hand, pressure is applied with index finger of left hand. Spreader must be removed with same rotary motion.

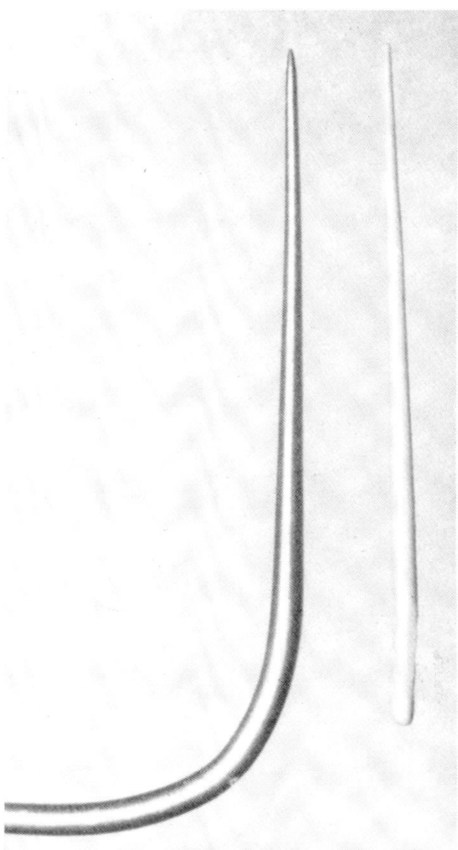

Fig. 4–27. Fine, style "A" gutta percha points are same size and taper as No. 3 spreader.

of the canal (Fig. 4–25). When the fit of the primary point is ensured, the butt end extending into the coronal cavity should be removed to allow room for the spreader which is to follow.

Because the width of the ***coronal*** two-thirds of the ovoid canal is larger than that of the primary point, the point must be displaced laterally with a sharp-pointed tapered instrument, a ***No. 3 spreader*** (Fig. 4–25*B*). Additional gutta percha points are then added (Fig. 4–25, *C* and *D*). The spreader is forced apically by pressure from the left index finger as the spreader is rotated from side to side (Fig. 4–26). Care must be used not to force the spreader past the apical foramen. This may be controlled by placing a rubber stop on the spreader short of the length of the tooth. The spreader is removed from the canal by the same reciprocating motion.

The additional points used in lateral condensation are the same size and taper of the No. 3 spreader (Fig. 4–27). These are "fine-style A" gutta percha points. Note their shape. They are not the same as the gutta percha points standardized to instrument size, which are used as primary points. Rather, they are sharply tapered and pointed as the spreader. Often four or five additional "fine" gutta percha points may be added to the canal when the lateral condensation method is used. Some dentists will place 25 to 30 "***extra*** fine" additional points in the canal by lateral condensation. This is a time-consuming practice and can be improved upon by use of the "fine" size point rather than the "extra fine." Obliteration by this method is considered complete when the spreader can no longer penetrate the filling mass beyond the cervical line (Fig. 4–25*D*).

There is some question whether the condensation of gutta percha by lateral force will produce a truly compacted filling. To be dense, of course, the additional gutta percha points must be forced to the depth of the tapered space prepared for them with the spreader. They should also be coated with

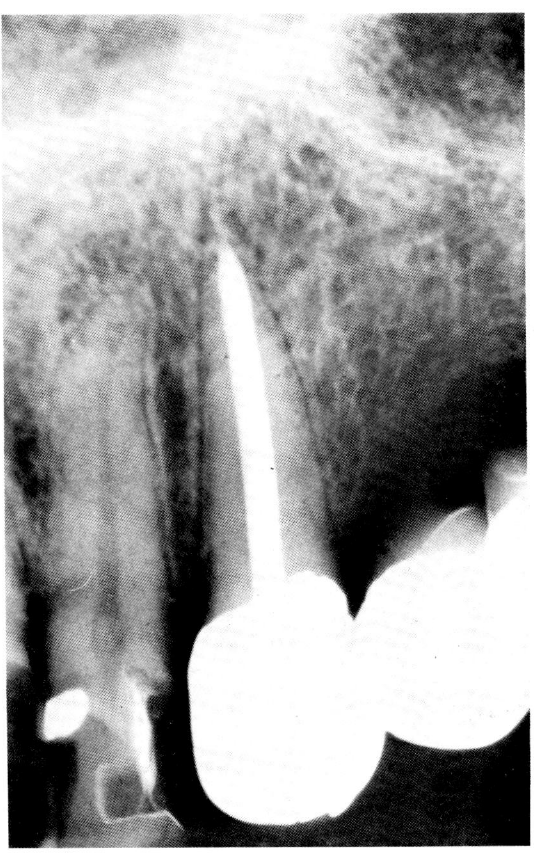

Fig. 4–28. Complete root canal obliteration using multiple point technique. Notice density of gutta percha mass. Filling conforms exactly to size and shape of last endodontic instrument used.

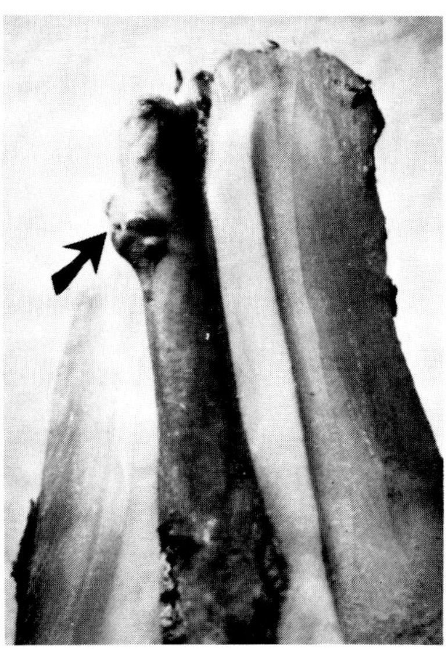

Fig. 4–29. Prepared root canal obturated by lateral condensation of gutta percha and sealer. Note extension of gutta percha into depression in canal *(arrow)*. (Courtesy Dr. J. H. Gutierrez and Dr. C. Gigoux, Concepcion, Chile.)

additional sealer, which fills any slight voids. Finally, the ***vertical*** compaction with heavy pressure ensures dense obturation, which is the keystone to success (Fig. 4–28). Using lateral condensation, Gutierrez and Gigoux have demonstrated the movement of gutta percha into the variances in canal anatomy and the denseness of the filling (Fig. 4–29).[64]

Because the silver points fit the well-prepared, round tapered apical third cavity so perfectly, they are sometimes used as the initial or primary point. As with gutta percha, annealed silver also may be moved aside with a spreader and additional gutta percha points compressed to totally obturate the canal. The situations in which silver points are found wanting, however, are canals that are initially ovoid in the apical third and cannot be shaped to be perfectly round to match the silver point.

Single Point Obturation with Silver Points

The teeth with class I canal anatomy—mature, uncomplicated, relatively straight, and with a constricted foramen—which lend themselves to obturation with a single silver point are generally the two canals in maxillary first premolars (Fig. 4–30) and the small canals in molars—buccal roots in the maxilla and mesial roots in the mandible. Large straight

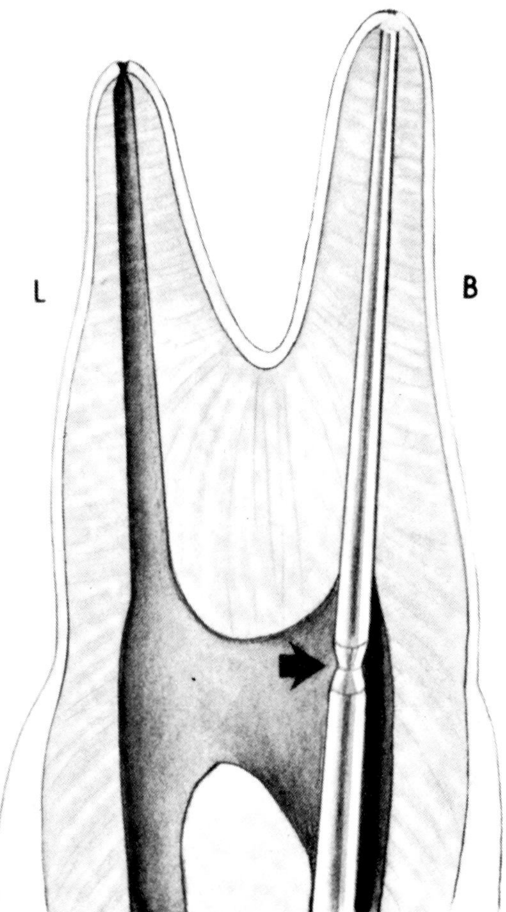

Fig. 4–30. Single point filling of maxillary first premolar with straight canals. Lingual canal (L) has been perfectly shaped into round tapered preparation to receive preformed round tapered filling material. Buccal canal (B) is totally obliterated with single silver point cemented to place. Point will separate where partially severed (*arrow*).

molar canals in older patients also may occasionally be obturated with silver. Silver also may be preferred if the foramen is open from perforation or external resorption—class III canal anatomy. Well-fitting silver points may be placed without the gross overfilling that might result from compacting gutta percha.

In a number of other cases, silver points are preferred to gutta percha because of their accuracy of fit and stiffness, which allows for easier insertion. Use of silver points in class II and III canals will be discussed later under those titles.

If a silver point fits the preparation too tightly and will not go fully to place, the canal will have to be reamed with a ***new*** instrument. In canals difficult to enlarge, one must remember that as instruments bind they tend to unwind, thus becoming smaller in diameter. Conversely, if the point is too loose, the next size is used or 2-mm. sections are cut from the tip of the first point until it fits.

The silver point is forced to the full measured length of the canal (less 0.5 mm. to compensate for the square or "bull nosed" shape of the point) and is checked visually, radiographically, and for "tug-back." If the point checks out perfectly, it is grasped at the cusp height with a hemostat and removed with both the hemostat and an extra pair of pliers so that the hemostat does not slip (Fig. 4–31).

Arrangements must now be made to break off the butt end of the point after the terminal portion has been cemented in the canal. The first step in this procedure is to measure the length of crown (Fig. 4–32). From this length, which is usually 7 to 9 mm., 2 mm. is subtracted; the latter is the amount the butt of the point should extend into the pulp chamber. This will facilitate the subsequent removal of the point if necessary.

The ruler is then placed against the beaks of the hemostat opposite the number of millimeters to be removed (Fig. 4–33). When the sharp edge of the ruler is dragged across the point, it will leave a mark. It is here a cut is made with a carborundum disk, which ***almost*** severs the point, leaving only enough silver to maintain control of the point during

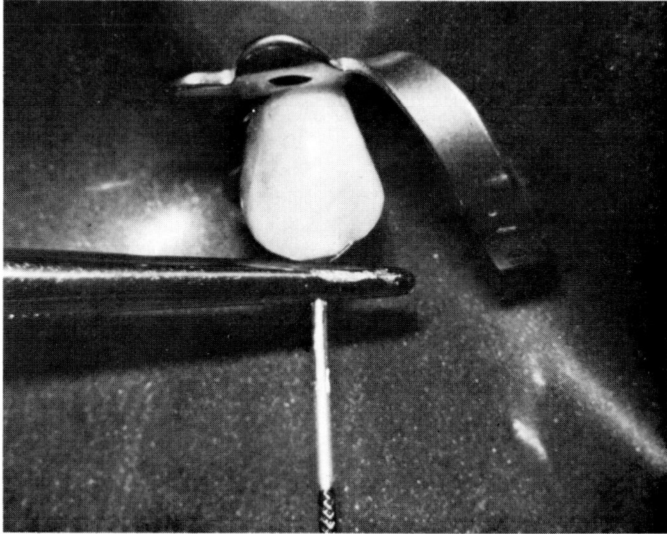

Fig. 4–31. Measured silver point should be marked at point of cusp by locking in hemostat. To prevent slippage, point should be removed with second pair of pliers.

cementation (Fig. 4–34). Weine has suggested using toenail clippers, modified so that they will notch but not completely cut through the point.[65]

After the silver point is prepared for separation, it should be resterilized by flaming over a low bunsen flame, and care is taken not to melt the fine points. It is then set aside on the tray, still locked in the hemostat, while the cement is prepared and the canal dried.

A word should also be said concerning the utilization of single points in the canals of multiple canal teeth such as molars. Each of the trial points should be removed, locked in an individual hemostat. The hemostats should then be placed at widely separated positions on the working tray. To prevent confusion, the letters designating the canal MB for mesiobuccal, ML for mesiolingual, and so on, should be printed on the surface of the towel opposite each hemostat.

The canal is liberally coated with cement, as previously described, and the point itself is thoroughly covered. Carefully and slowly the point is inserted in the canal; time is allowed for the cement to flow back as it is displaced. When the hemostat strikes the cusp of the tooth, the point should be in perfect position at the apex (see Fig. 4–30). If additional canals are being filled with silver, all the points should be placed before a radiograph is taken. By varying the horizontal angle of the central beam, one can separate the image of the points in the film and ascertain that the points are perfectly positioned. A small triangle of cement should be apparent at the tip of the point sealing the foramen (Fig. 4–35).

After radiographic assurance of obturation, the butt end of the point is removed by twisting and "worrying" the silver until it separates. Apical pressure must be exerted throughout this procedure so that the point will not be unseated.

In an occasional case the canal may be filled with a single point, separated in the apical third of the canal. Preparing a canal to receive a retention dowel is an indication for this approach. Obliteration of the apical third of the canal, followed by a filling of a nonperforating defect remaining after internal resorption is another indication for the apical third filling (Fig. 4–36). In any case, one must be certain

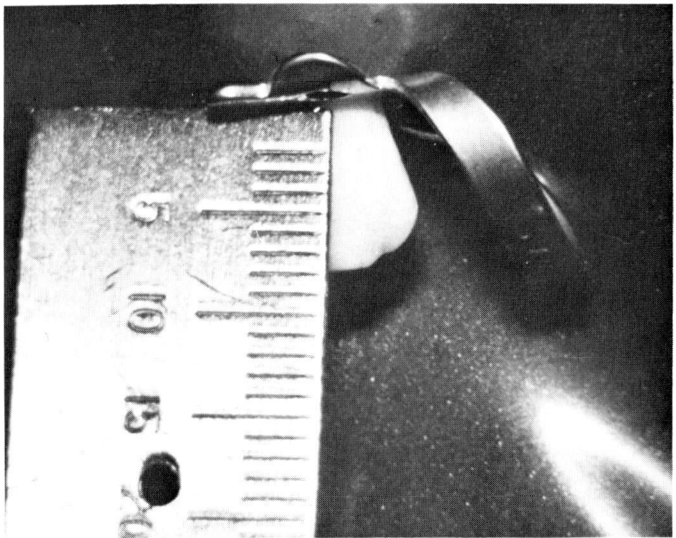

Fig. 4–32. Length of crown must first be established to determine point to separate silver point.

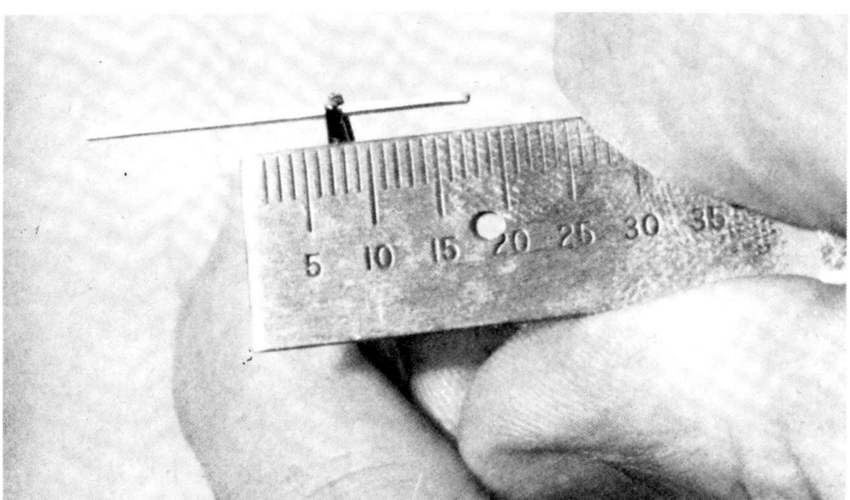

Fig. 4–33. Crown length less 2 mm. is marked on soft silver with sharp edge of ruler.

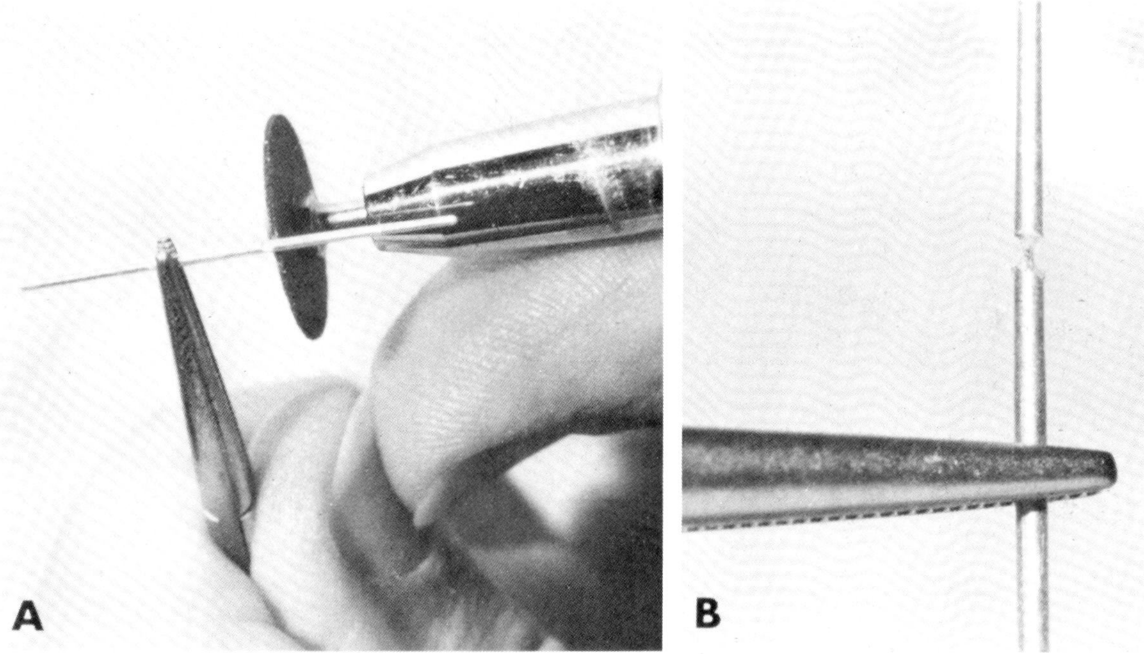

Fig. 4–34. *A,* Silver point locked in hemostat is notched with carborundum disc. Note stability of thumb against thumb in this operation. *B,* Carborundum disc almost severs silver to establish point of breakage after cementation.

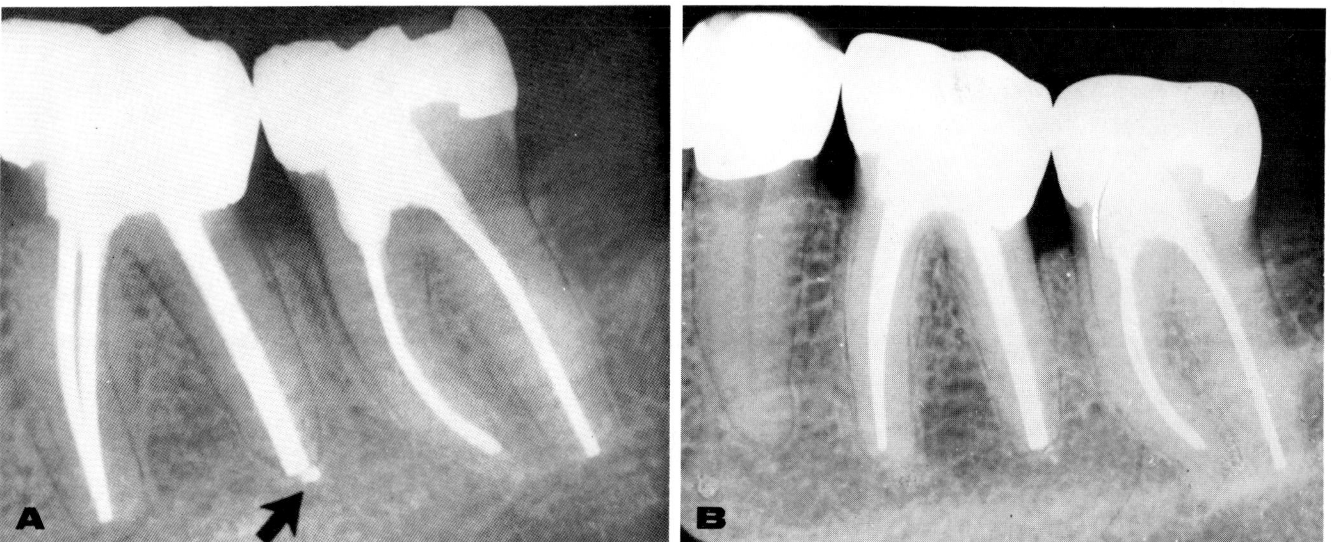

Fig. 4–35. *A,* Use of silver points to fill mature canals and combination of silver and condensed gutta percha to obturate distal canal in first molar. Tiny extrusion of cement *(arrow)* demonstrates how well open foramen may be filled without gross overfilling. *B,* ***Twenty-year*** recall radiograph, which proves the longevity of treatment with silver points in properly prepared and obturated canals.

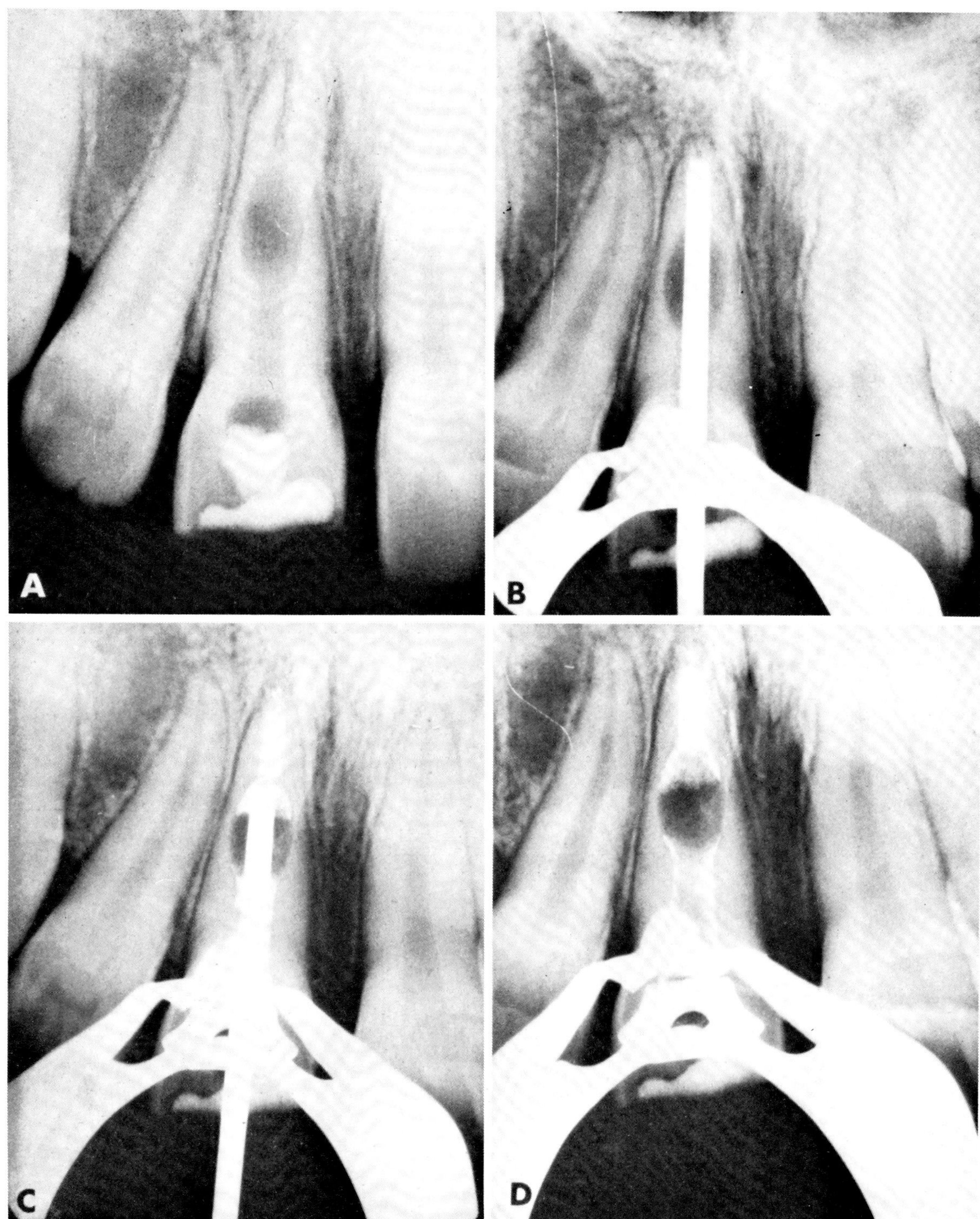

Fig. 4–36. *(Continued on opposite page.)*

that the single point will totally obliterate the apical third, for once cemented and separated, the split point is irretrievable.

When total obturation of the canal has been ascertained, the excess cement should be cleaned from the chamber and a provisional filling placed to cover the points and temporarily close the cavity. If the occlusal cavity is extensive or the crown has been previously weakened by caries or filling, no time should be lost in placing a final protective restoration.

To remove the excess cement from the chamber, cotton, excavators, and solvent are used. Any alcohol-acetone combination will rapidly clear away the excess cement. If a ***tincture*** germicide (Zephiran) is used in the tray top sterilizer, it is excellent for removing excess cement as well as cleaning the mixing slab and spatula.

The filling placed immediately over the stump of the points should be soft in case later removal of the points is necessary. Zinc oxide-eugenol cement may be used, and should subsequently be covered by a more permanent filling material as outlined in Chapter 18, Restoring the Pulpless Tooth.

Class II Canal Anatomy

In this category falls the mature complicated canal—curved or dilacerated; or with apical bifurcation; or lateral or accessory canals, but with constriction of the apical foramen (or foramens).

Endodontic cavity preparations in canals with class II anatomy can be obturated with any number of filling techniques using solid core materials plus cements or pastes.

Curved or Dilacerated Canals

Apical Curve. Over 40% of the maxillary lateral incisors exhibit a "breaking curve" in the apical third of the root. The same applies to over 50% of the

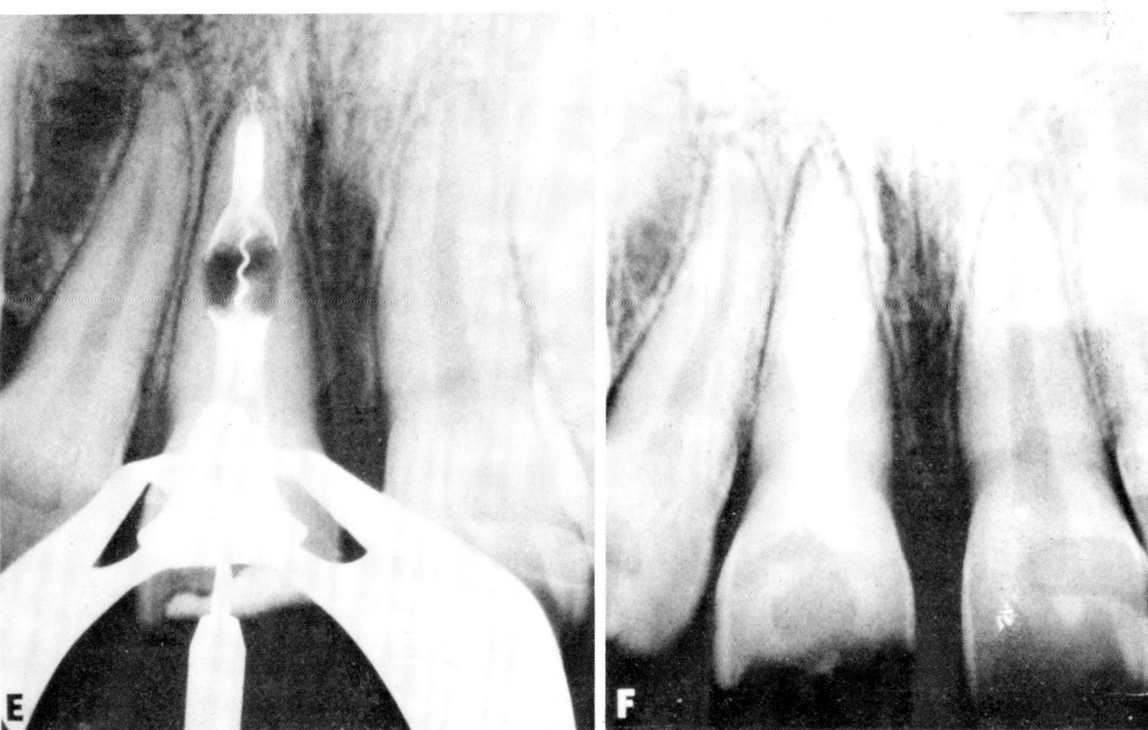

Fig. 4–36. Step-by-step procedure to prepare and fill maxillary central incisor with nonperforating internal resorption. *A,* "Before" roentgenogram. Extensive internal resorption following calcium hydroxide pulpotomy. *B,* Following pulpectomy and canal enlargement, single silver point is tested. Perfectly fitting point is notched for separation at depth of resorptive lesion. Apical third cavity must be enlarged to enormous size to ensure preparation of perfectly round cavity. *C,* Notched silver point is cemented to place. *D,* Point is separated at depth of resorption. *E,* Additional cement is carried into canal and void with Lentulo spiral. *F,* Additional gutta percha points are added to completely obliterate remaining portion of canal as well as resorptive lesion. (Courtesy Dr. William Clem.)

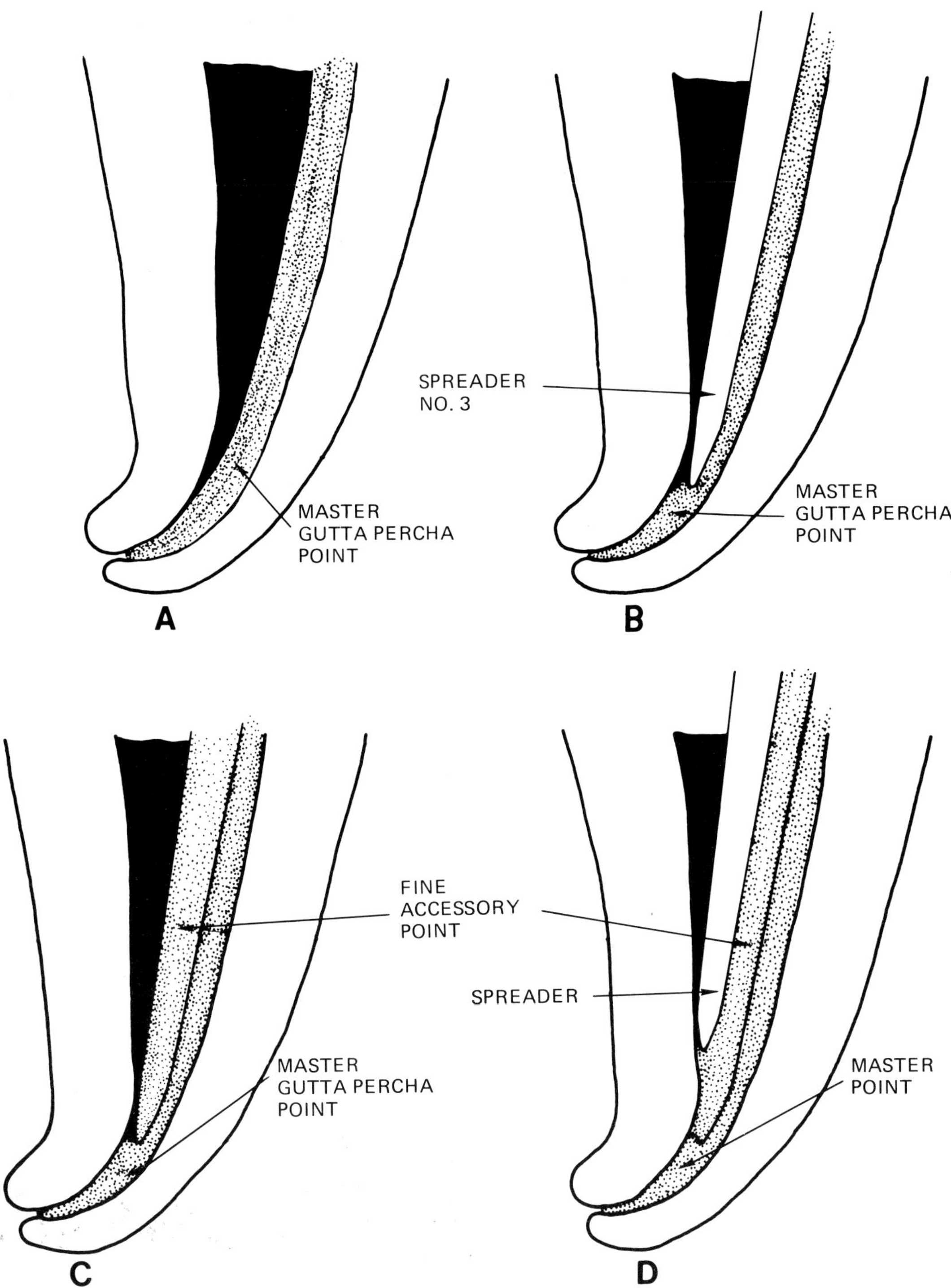

Fig. 4–37. Obturation by lateral condensation of telescopic preparation. *A*, Master gutta percha point (with sealer) fits canal in apical portion of Resistance Form preparation. *B*, Measured No. 3 spreader with instrument stop in place is forced close to apex condensing gutta percha laterally as well as apically. *C*, "Fine" accessory points are added after each use of spreader. *D*, Obturation is built up from apex into well-condensed filling. Final compaction is by vertical plugging. (Courtesy Dr. Richard E. Walton.)

palatal roots of maxillary first molars. For this type of special case, "telescopic" preparation and filling with gutta percha, either laterally or vertically compressed, provides optimum obturation. The same applies to any canal that is ovoid in part and cannot be properly filled with a single point.

Lateral Condensation of Gutta Percha. The method of filling a ***curved*** canal with multiple gutta percha points condensed by lateral pressure is essentially the same as filling a ***straight*** canal. The major difference lies in the shape of the preparation. In the straight canal the apical third of the cavity has fairly parallel walls into which the standardized point fits snugly, exhibiting "tugback." The canal with apical curvature, on the other hand, has been prepared by "telescoping," which produces a widely flaring preparation, curved at its terminus but with a straightened canal up to the curve. In the telescopic preparation, the gutta percha point fits only at the terminus of the cavity—at the apical foramen, that is. Hence, when tested by withdrawal, there will be no feeling of "tugback." Nonetheless, the first point snugly fits the final millimeter or two of the cavity. The standardized point used is the same size and shape as the instrument used to develop resistance and retention forms. The point should effectively block the foramen (Fig. 4–37*A*).

If there is any doubt about the perfect placement of the primary point, that is, if the operator feels the point might have buckled or hung-up on the walls, it should be checked by radiograph. In the film, one should see the tip of the point, surrounded by cement, at the terminus of the cavity, i.e., 0.5 mm. to 1 mm. from the outside of the root, usually the apex.

Following the cementing of the primary point to place, it is compressed laterally with a No. 3 spreader marked just short of the working length of the tooth (Fig. 4–37*B*), and a second point with cement is added (Fig. 4–37*C*). The final filling is built up by the addition of more points and cement (Fig. 4–37*D*) until the spreader will no longer penetrate the mass. The gutta percha is excised with a hot instrument at the canal orifice, and final compaction is completed with vertical pressure with a plugger that tightly fits the canal.

Softened Gutta Percha Technique. Schilder[66] has suggested a variation of the Coolidge sectional gutta percha technique,[67] which has proved most effective in filling the canals of severely curved roots and roots with accessory canals, lateral canals, or multiple foramens. Since the first indication of such anatomic variation may be observed during the filling procedure, the proponents of this technique recommend its use for all cases.

The widely flaring endodontic cavity is prepared much the same as described for the lateral condensation technique. Proper resistance form must be maintained or created to permit the application of vertical pressure against the gutta percha, which is to be softened with heat and packed into the apical preparation. Also, to allow for the larger rigid plugger, convenience form may need to be extended far enough beyond the outline to permit lateral condensation with a spreader. The extension may

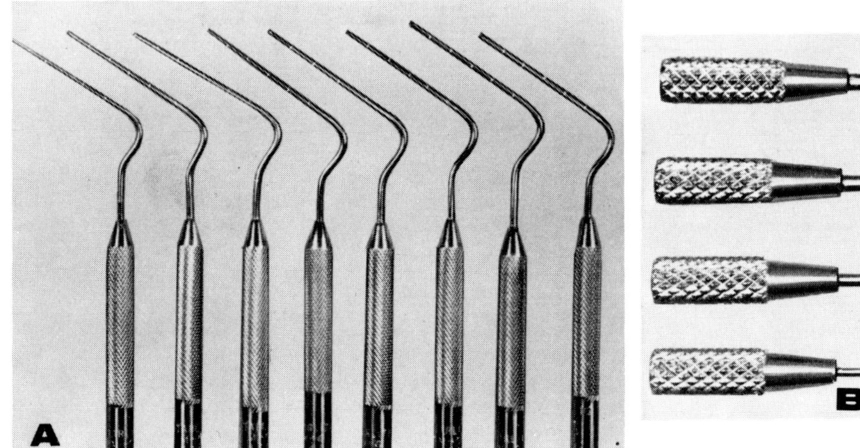

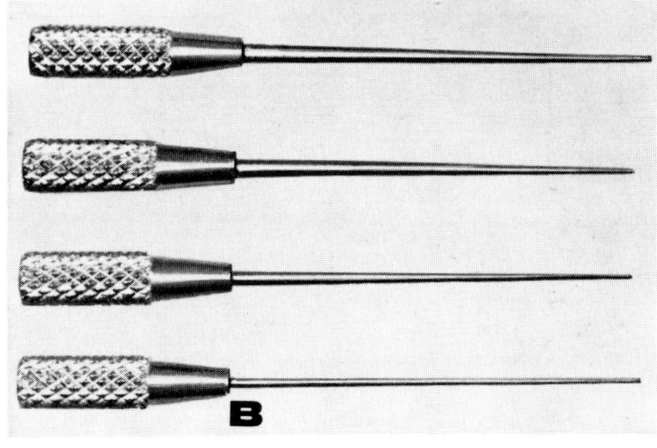

Fig. 4–38. Graduated size pluggers used for vertical condensation. *A*, "Hand" pluggers sizes (*left to right*) 8, 9, 9½, 10, 10½, 11, 11½, 12. Shafts are marked at 5 mm. intervals. *B*, "Finger" pluggers sizes (*bottom to top*) A to D. (Courtesy Star Dental Manufacturing Co.)

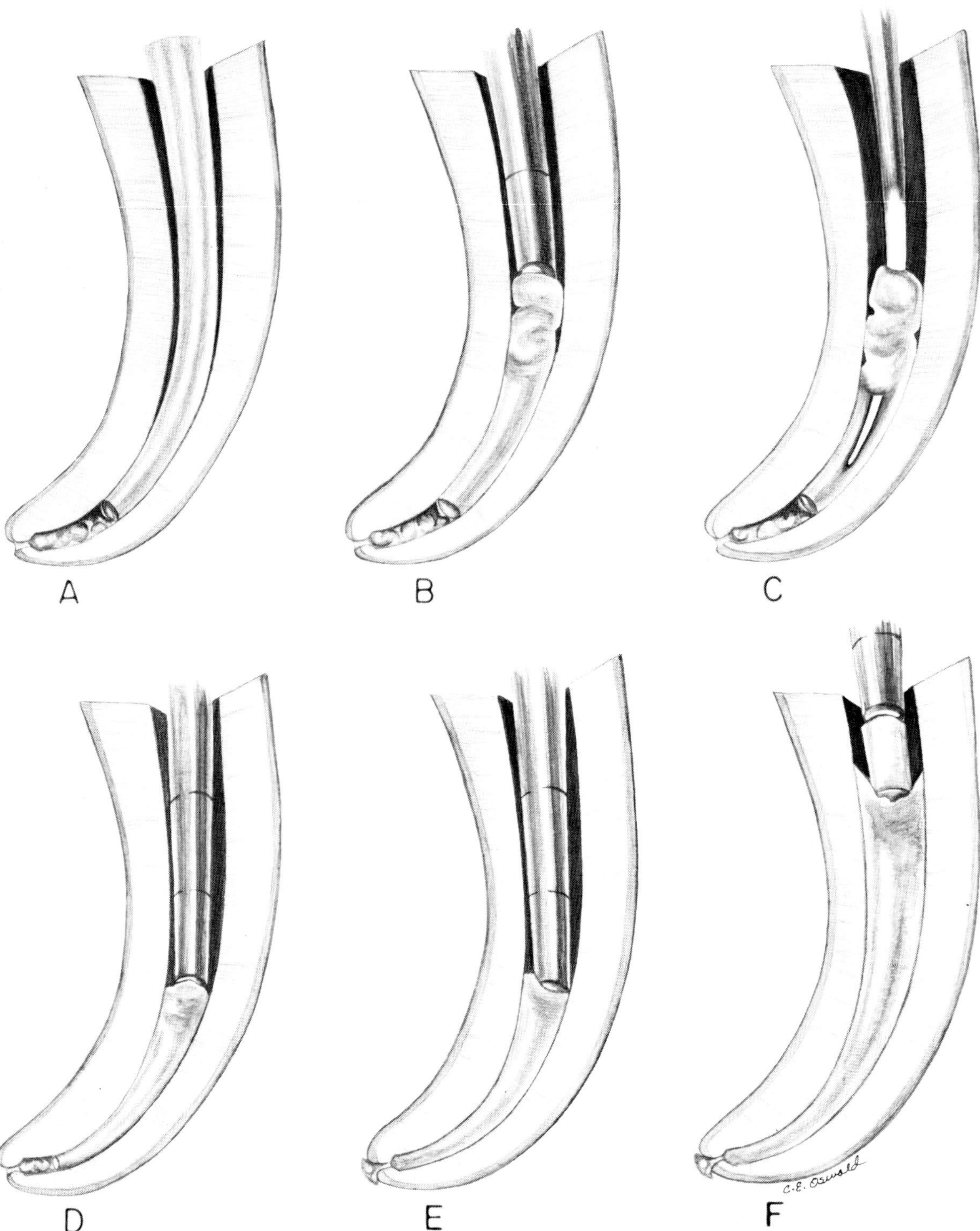

Fig. 4–39. Technique for vertical condensation of heat-softened gutta percha. *A,* Blunted, nonstandardized gutta percha point, with sealer, fits tightly in canal 2 to 3 mm. short of apical foramen. Coronal excess is cut off with hot plastic instrument. *B, Cold* root canal plugger crushes point into well-flared canal. *C, Hot* No. 3 spreader is plunged into mass and quickly withdrawn. *D,* Cold plugger immediately condenses mass of gutta percha. *E,* Alternate use of hot spreader and cold plugger moves softened gutta percha mass apically. *F,* Small pieces of heat-softened gutta percha build up mass to obturate entire canal space. (Courtesy Dr. James D. Zidell.)

require the enlarging of the access cavity and the telescoping of the body of the canal to create a greater flare from the apical preparation to the access cavity. This convenience extension is made necessary because condensation is done with a series of root canal pluggers (Fig. 4–38), which are more rigid and which have a greater diameter than the No. 3 spreader used for lateral condensation. Proper vertical condensation may occasionally require that the small plugger be used in each canal to fit to within 3 to 4 mm. of the apical preparation.

Standardized gutta percha points are ***not*** used in this technique for two reasons. First, the canal usually has been prepared by telescoping, and the points made to match instrument size do not match the canal shape. The objective of the technique is to obliterate the canal with a filling material softened by heat and packed with sufficient vertical pressure to force it to ***flow*** into the root canal system, whatever that may be. Second, the ***non***standardized gutta percha points are manufactured with a greater flare from the tip to the butt end, providing a greater mass of gutta percha to absorb the heat and vertical pressure.

The tip of the primary point is cut away until it reaches a diameter that ***fits to within 2 to 3 mm.*** of the length of tooth measurement. At this point the diameter of the cut end of gutta percha should exceed the diameter of the root canal, so that it cannot be inserted beyond that length (Fig. 4–39*A*). Since the body of the canal is deliberately flared more than the taper of the gutta percha point, there will be minimal "tugback" or resistance to withdrawal of the point.

Root canal sealer is prepared and placed into the canal as described previously. The primary point is inserted to full depth and should come to a definite stop. If the lubricating effect of the root canal sealer permits the primary point to pass beyond its measured length, a larger point must be selected before vertical condensation begins.

Once the primary point is properly fitted in the canal ***2 to 3 mm. short of the length*** of tooth, a hot plastic instrument is used to cut off the length of gutta percha coronal to the orifice of the canal. A ***cold*** root canal plugger is immediately used to apply vertical pressure against the cut end of gutta percha within the canal. As the body of the canal has been flared to exceed the taper of the gutta percha, this vertical pressure will force the gutta percha point to fold up upon itself within the canal (Fig. 4–39*B*).

The fit of the apical end of the gutta percha into the narrowed apical preparation will act as a stop, so that the mass of gutta percha is folded into the middle portion of the root canal preparation without permitting that mass to move in an apical direction.

A No. 3 spreader is then heated cherry red and carried quickly into the cold mass of gutta percha and immediately withdrawn (Fig. 4–39*C*). If the spreader is hot enough, the gutta percha should not stick to it and be withdrawn. A cold plugger is then forced into the canal against the warmed mass of gutta percha and vertical pressure is created (Fig. 4–39*D*). The cold plugger should be dipped in zinc-oxyphosphate cement powder to prevent its sticking to the gutta percha.

This procedure is repeated alternately with the hot spreader followed immediately by the cold plugger. Each time the spreader is removed a small amount of gutta percha adheres to its surface and must be wiped away before the spreader is reheated. The first series of heating and plugging acts to soften and unite the mass of gutta percha in the body of the canal. As the series is repeated, the spreader penetrates and heat is carried to the apical end of the gutta percha.[13] As this initial mass of gutta percha is softened, it begins to move apically as the vertical force is applied (Fig. 4–39*E*). Tremendous pressure is built up in the apical mass of gutta percha, owing to the narrowing of the endodontic cavity and the vertical pressure placed against it.* The heat-softened gutta percha and sealer are forced to flow around curves and into the irregularities of the root canal system (Fig. 4–40). The apical movement of the gutta percha is observed by x-ray examination during the vertical condensation. The heating and condensation are repeated until the gutta percha is packed to the desired length. The entire mass of gutta percha has been moved apically, and the apical portion of the filling is now complete. The body of the canal now remains to be filled. This is accomplished by carrying 3 to 4 mm. segments of gutta percha into the canal with cotton pliers. The ***tip*** of each gutta percha segment is passed lightly through a flame prior to insertion into the canal. If properly flamed, the ***tip*** will become soft and adhere to the gutta percha sealed within the canal, but at the same time, the end of the gutta percha

*A Temple University group recently observed that "when the canals were filled by the vertical condensation method, more cracks in the dentin were discernible than were seen in the teeth filled by lateral condensation." Wollard, R. R., Brough, S. O., Maggio, J. and Seltzer, S.: Scanning electron microscopic examination of root canal filling materials. J.O.E. *2*:98, April, 1976.

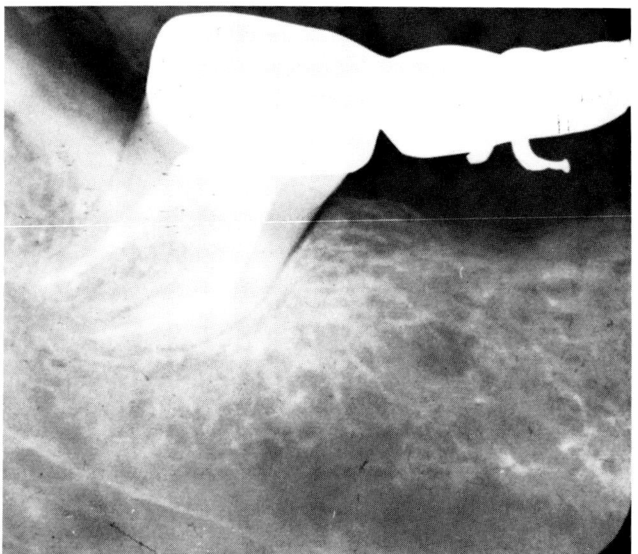

Fig. 4-40. Telescopic preparation of curved canals is obturated by heat-softened gutta percha. (Courtesy Dr. James D. Zidell.)

segment that is held in the cotton pliers must remain firm so that it can be released from the pliers and condensed with a cold plugger. Segmented pieces of gutta percha are repeatedly compacted into the canal in this fashion until the body of the canal has been obliterated (Fig. 4-39*F*). The softened gutta percha has other uses in the obturation of canals with Class II anatomy, and these will be discussed.

Modification of the Softened Gutta Percha Technique. A modification combining the softened gutta percha technique and the chloropercha technique should be considered. For this technique the canal is prepared, and a blunted primary point is prepared as described for the heat-softened gutta percha filling procedure. This point is immersed in a mixture of chloropercha (p. 267) for a period of three to eight seconds, depending on the degree of softening required. The point is inserted fully into the canal. Vertical and lateral pressure is then applied with a ***No. 3 spreader*** to create space ***alongside*** the master point for insertion of one or two auxiliary gutta percha points. These points are cut off at the orifice with a hot instrument, and additional vertical pressure is applied with a No. 3 spreader or root canal plugger. The mass of gutta percha should have moved apically to obturate the apical space.

A roentgenogram is taken at this time and evaluated. If the length of tooth has not been reached, additional vertical pressure is applied with the spreader or plugger. Heat may also be used to soften the gutta percha if necessary. When the apical portion of the cavity has been completed, the body of the canal is filled by means of the spreader and lateral condensation of additional gutta percha points. Compaction is completed with vertical pressure with a plugger that tightly fits the canal (Fig. 4-41).

Although this technique is similar in concept and procedure to the softened gutta percha method, its advantage lies in the fact that it softens the apical end of the gutta percha directly rather than by the time-consuming procedure of heat softening the gutta percha from the apical end first.

Goldman compared endodontic fillings produced by the chloroform softened technique (as detailed here) with the lateral condensation technique in which cement is used as a sealer (previously described).[68] Using both Kloraperchа N-O and Moyco Chloropercha as softening-sealing agents, Goldman concluded that "the Kloropercha models showed more homogeneity than the models made with the lateral condensation technique." By the same token, chloropercha fillings demonstrated greater porosity and change in volume than Kloropercha fillings or lateral condensation, even though initially it appeared to better replicate the irregularities of the canals. Goldman attributed this porosity to the fact that chloropercha is merely powdered gutta percha dissolved in chloroform, and as soon as the chloroform evaporates the gutta percha returns to its former powdered state. Kloropercha, on the other hand, also

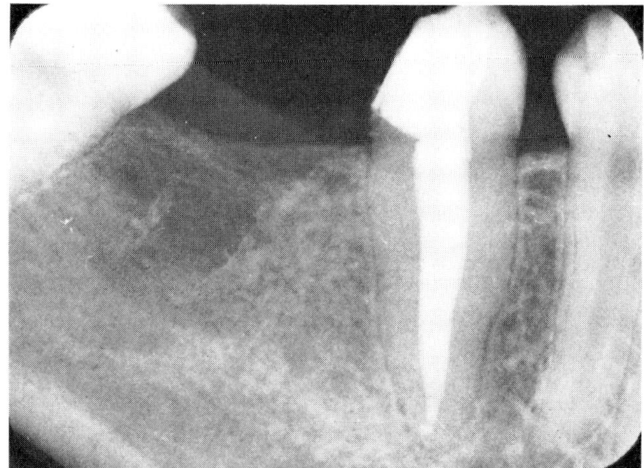

Fig. 4-41. Telescopic preparation is obturated by gutta percha softened in chloropercha. (Courtesy Dr. Richard E. Walton.)

contains rosin, zinc oxide, and Canada balsam, which dissolve in the chloroform to form a more homogeneous mass when the chloroform evaporates.

Severely Curved, Dilacerated, or Bayonet Canals

The complicating anatomy of root canals with severe curves precludes their obturation by multiple gutta percha points and lateral condensation. First of all, it is difficult to tease the flexible primary gutta percha point to place at the apex. Second, the stiff spreader cannot be forced and rotated down the curved canal to the apical area. A filling method must therefore be used which employs a rigid point, or in which the condensing instruments do not have to negotiate the curve or the "elbow" of the curve. These requirements may be satisfied either by the softened gutta percha technique, by silver point insertion, by a combination of silver point and gutta percha, or by filling with new root canal instruments purposely broken off in the canals.

Softened Gutta Percha Technique. Severely curved or dilacerated canals may be obturated with heat-softened gutta percha, as described in the previous section. The spreader, used to carry the heat, loses its temper and becomes pliable. Thus it fits quite easily around curves to extend the heat apically. The result achieved by alternate heating and plugging can be most satisfactory (Fig. 4–42). Modification of this technique using chloropercha as the softening agent also leads to satisfactory obturation (Fig. 4–43).

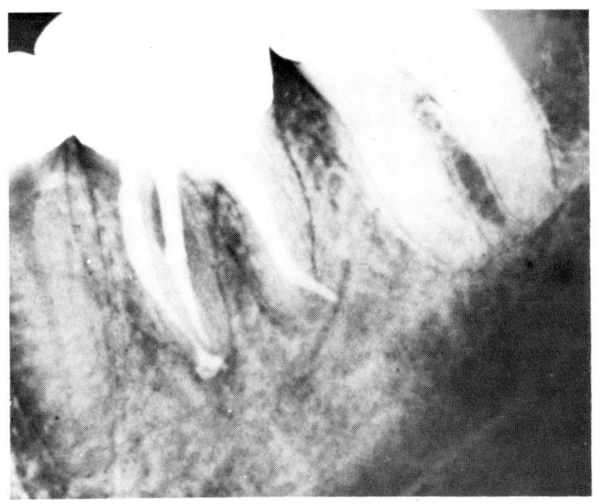

Fig. 4–42. Heat-softened gutta percha obturates dilacerated distal canal. (Courtesy Dr. James D. Zidell.)

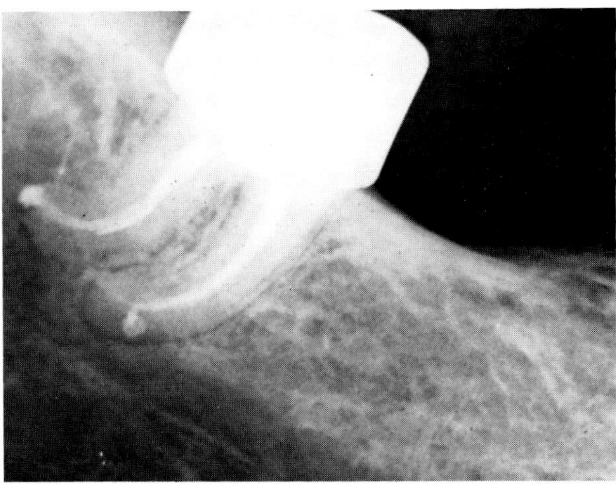

Fig. 4–43. Chloropercha-softened gutta percha filling of severely curved canals. "Button" at apical foramen is quite typical of softened gutta percha fillings. (Courtesy Dr. James D. Zidell.)

These techniques of course are indicated for ovoid or large curved canals or cases with suspected extra foramens at the apex.

Silver Point Technique. Some curved canals can be filled entirely by silver points if the mature round canal can be shaped throughout its entire length into the round tapered preparation that can be fully obturated by the single silver point or a combination of silver and gutta percha. The flexibility of silver, coupled with its rigidity, enables the point to be inserted with great pressure to provide the apical seal. Most cases of curved canal in which silver points can be used are found in older patients with considerable secondary calcification. The buccal roots of maxillary molars or the mesial roots of mandibular molars are the favorite sites (Fig. 4–44). These canals are entirely prepared by reaming.

The bayonet-shaped canal, which has been prepared by both reaming and filing, may well be filled with silver as the primary point, followed by spreading and the addition of gutta percha points. The selection of the silver point depends on maintaining the round shape of the apical third preparation. The gutta percha obturates the curved spaces that develop as the bayonet is "straightened" out (Fig. 4–45).

To maintain better control over silver points being placed in curved canals, silver point pliers are often a help. If they are to be used, the point is cut off exactly at the height of the nearest cusp for future reference.

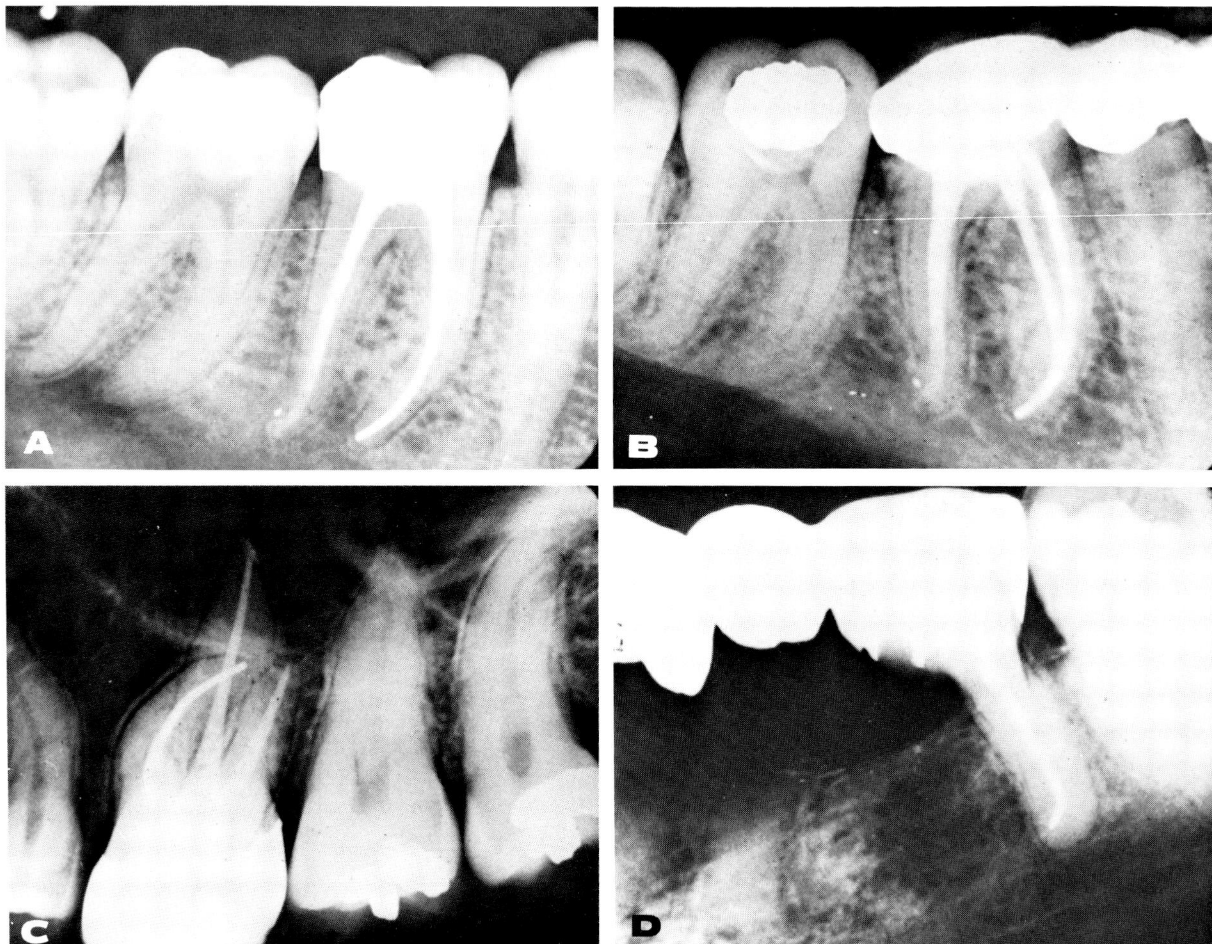

Fig. 4–44. Silver points used to fill curved canals in mature molars. *A,* Mesial canals filled with silver and gutta percha added by lateral condensation. *B,* Severely curved canal obturated with silver. Softened gutta percha used in other canals. *C,* Curved mesiobuccal root of maxillary molar filled with primary silver point and additional gutta percha. *D,* Dilacerated distal canal of mature molar, root amputated, filled with silver and gutta percha. (Courtesy Dr. James D. Zidell.)

Then the point is notched so that following cementation it will separate above the floor of the pulp chamber. The point is then grasped by the beaks of the silver point pliers ***beyond the notch***. This returns the rigidity to the point needed to force and guide it to place in a tortuous canal (Fig. 4–46). After cementation, when the pliers are released, the butt end of the point should coincide with the cusp height against which it was measured. When it is confirmed radiographically, the butt end is then separated.

Occasionally a canal is so fine and so tortuous that a silver point or gutta percha cannot be carried to the apex. In these cases, a broken instrument may be cemented into place to serve as a root canal filling (Fig. 4–47).

"Broken Instrument" Obturation. Although the routine filling of canals with broken instruments is to be ***highly*** discouraged, particularly in view of the success achieved in similar cases using the softened gutta percha technique, one cannot ignore those complicated situations in which the "broken" instrument is the last resort. The tortuous dilacerated canals of a mandibular third molar come to mind; in this area it is most difficult if not sometimes impossible to use spreaders and pluggers for filling compaction.

One has every right to question the long-term success of the "broken instrument" filling. Crump and Natkin did just that.[69] They evaluated 53 cases in which root canal instruments had been inadvertently

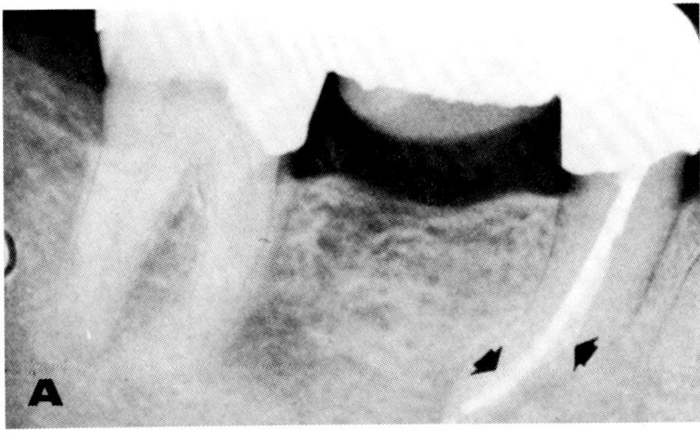

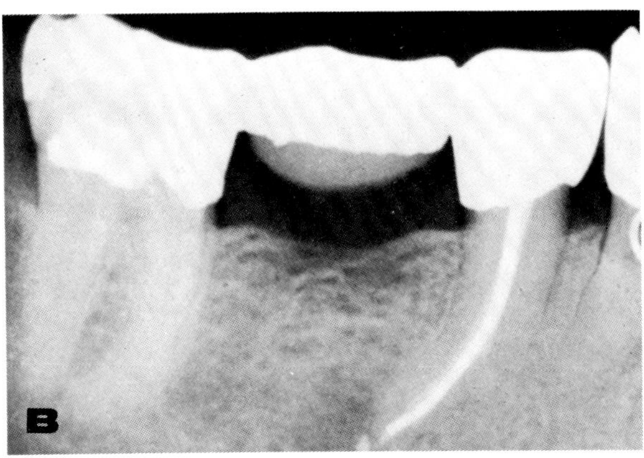

Fig. 4–45. *A*, Introduction of cement and primary filling point shows bayonet shape of canal has been changed into gradual curve. Former shape of canal is outlined by radiopaque cement (*arrows*). *B*, Total obliteration of bayonet canal is accomplished with primary silver point followed by spreading and multiple gutta percha points.

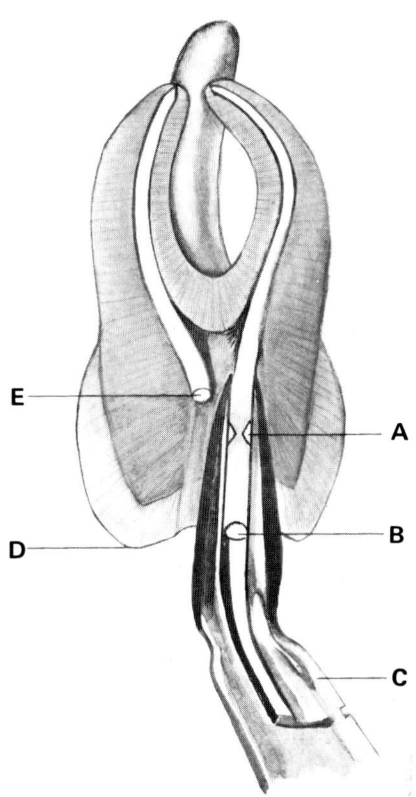

Fig. 4–46. Special silver point pliers used to give rigidity to placement of points. *A*, Silver point notched to separate. *B*, Butt end silver point. *C*, Pliers. *D*, Reference point—tip of cusp. *E*, Cemented point separated. (Courtesy Dr. James D. Zidell.)

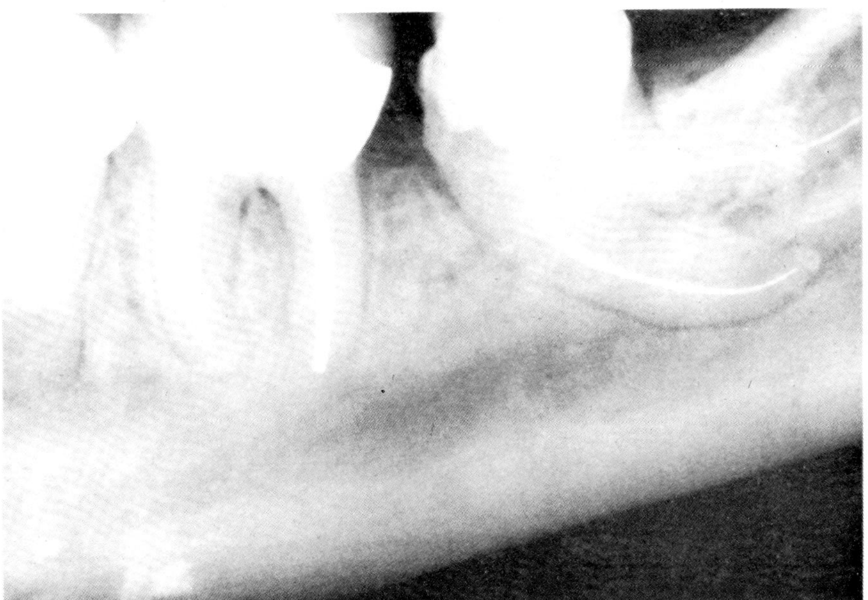

Fig. 4–47. Intentional use of "broken" instruments to fill severely curved canals. Gutta percha and silver points could not be positioned in these canals. New endodontic files were readily cemented to place. (Courtesy Dr. Adrian J. Sampeck.)

broken and then carefully matched these cases with 53 controls. All the cases had been completed at least two years. Using clinical and radiographic criteria to judge success and failure, they found no statistical difference in failure rates between the control and "broken instrument" groups.

When one thinks about it, such a high success rate should not be unexpected in these cases. Most instruments are fragmented by locking the blades in the dentin and inadvertently twisting off the shaft of the instrument. This mechanical union of metal to dentin evidently serves to obturate the space as shown

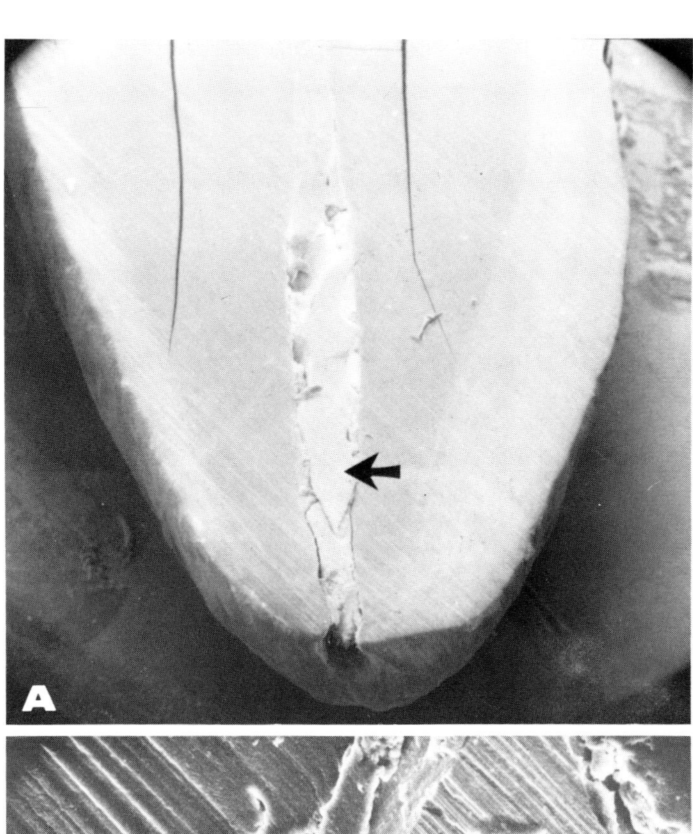

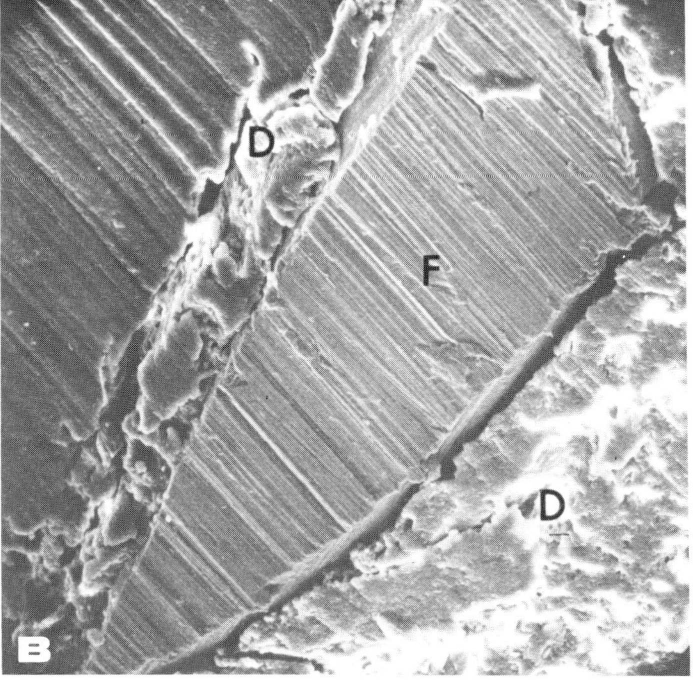

Fig. 4–48. Successful "broken instrument" filling. *A,* Instrument in place (*arrow*) surrounded by dentinal debris. *B,* High-power photomicrograph showing instrument fragment and dentinal debris blockage of apical foramen. Space is caused by microscopic preparation method. (Courtesy Dr. William R. Adams, 1974.)

by Sampeck.[70] Adams has shown obturation with broken instruments when dentinal debris blocks the foramen (Fig. 4–48).[71]

The inadvertently broken instrument ***which is loose*** in the canal with no cement around it frequently rusts within six months to a year and is no longer apparent in the recall roentgenogram. Even the so-called stainless instruments may rust away (Fig. 4–49). When a broken instrument has rusted, the canal should be reinstrumented and a new root canal filling placed.

After canal instrumentation and medication is complete, a ***file*** of the size last used to enlarge the canal is selected and curved to match the curve of the canal. After a reamer is used to coat the canal liberally with cement, the prepared file, coated with cement, is carried to position and literally "screwed" into place

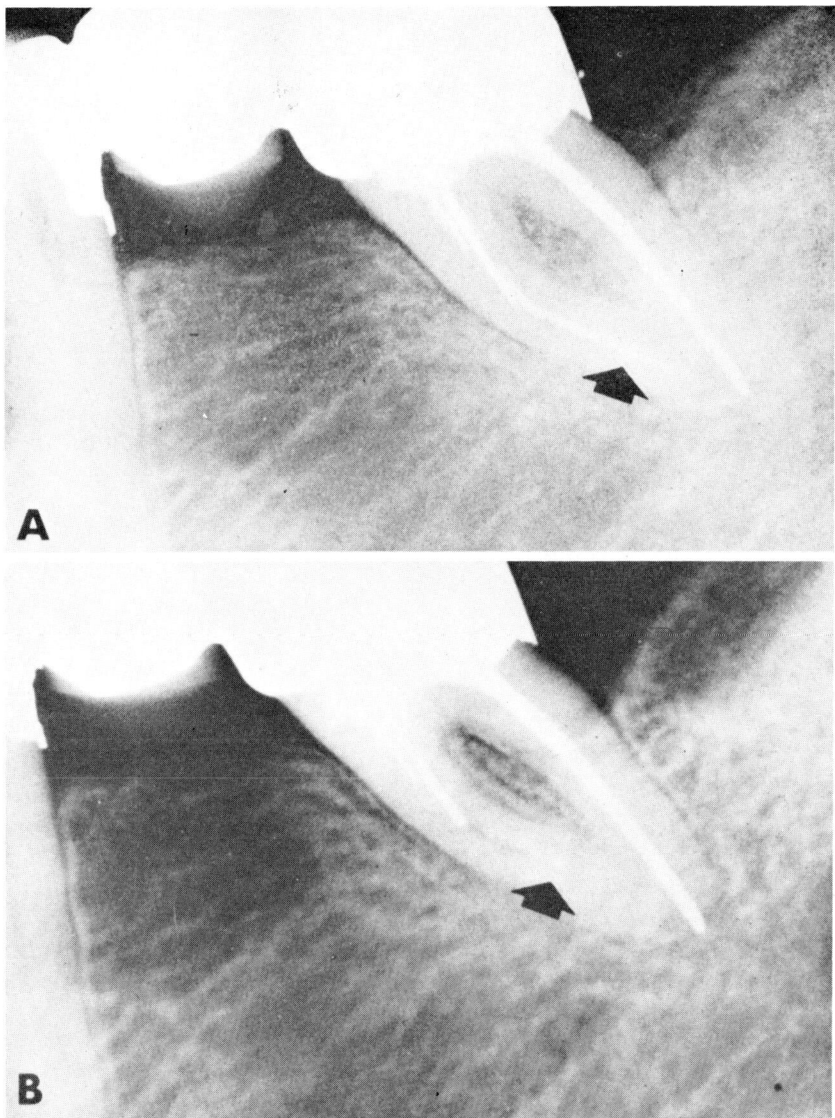

Fig. 4–49. Loose, fragmented instrument will "rust" away in canal. *A,* Endodontic instrument fragmented in canal by overzealous action. Incorrect occlusal cavity preparation put instrument under severe stress leading to breakage. *B,* In six-months' recall roentgenogram, loose instrument is clearly missing. Evidence that instrument has "rusted" away is substantiated by rust-like material removed from canal.

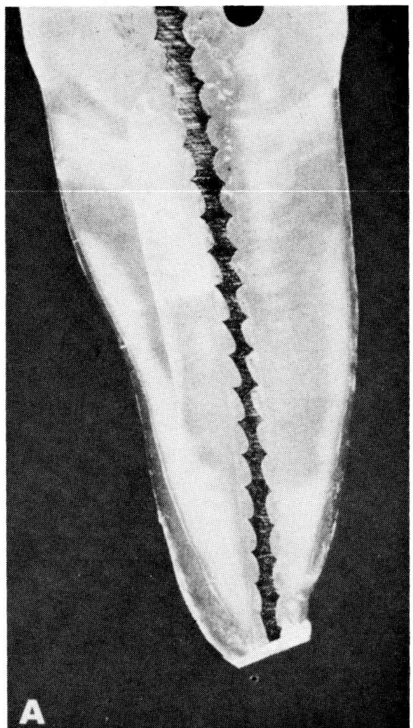

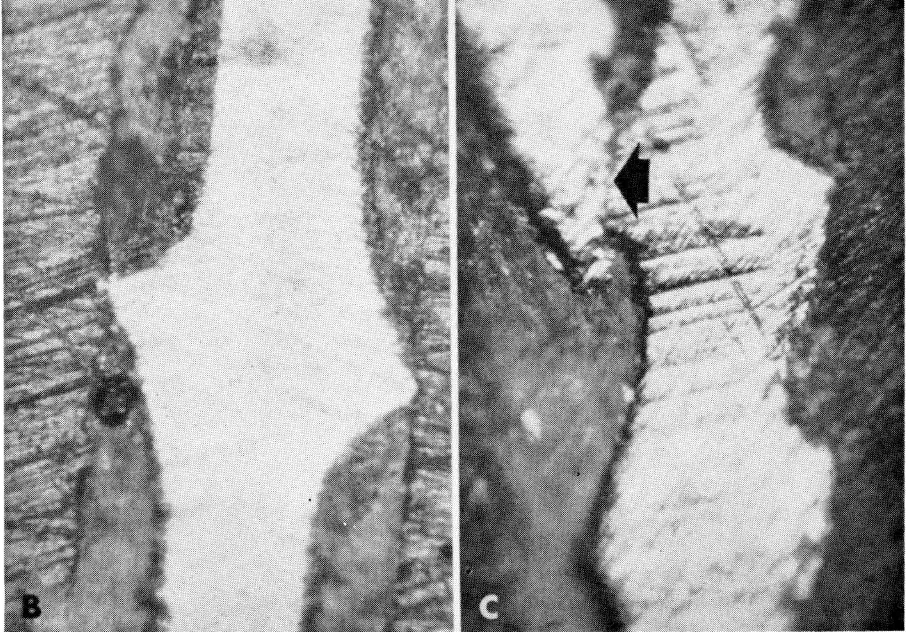

Fig. 4–50. *A,* Low-power photomicrograph of endodontic file used to obliterate well-calcified canal. *B,* High-power photomicrograph of root canal file (*white*) totally obliterating lumen of canal. File has cut through secondary dentin and is firmly lodged in primary dentin. *C,* Point of contact (*arrow*) between two files used to obliterate two canals which coalesce. (Courtesy Dr. Adrian J. Sampeck.)

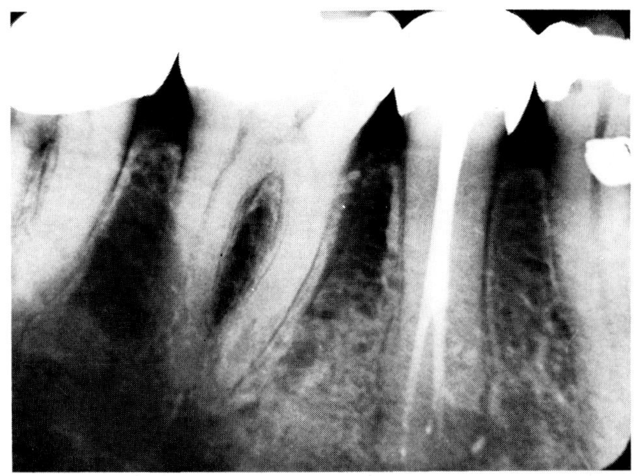

Fig. 4–51. Auxiliary canal, obturated with softened gutta percha. (Courtesy Dr. James D. Zidell.)

(Fig. 4–50). This may require some force. The position should be confirmed roentgenographically. To remove the excess instrument, a diamond point in an accelerated contra-angle is used to cut off the shaft of the instrument down in the cavity.

Apical Bifurcations of Lateral or Accessory Canals

Auxiliary canals (Fig. 4–51) or obvious apical bifurcation (Fig. 4–52*A,B*) or lateral canals (Fig. 4–53 *A,B,C*) pose serious problems in obturation. A pulpless lateral canal can often be determined before treatment by observing an osseous lesion ***lateral*** to the root rather than periapical. All too frequently, however, these canals are noticed only by hindsight after they are secondarily filled. It stands to reason, therefore, that obturating methods employing filling

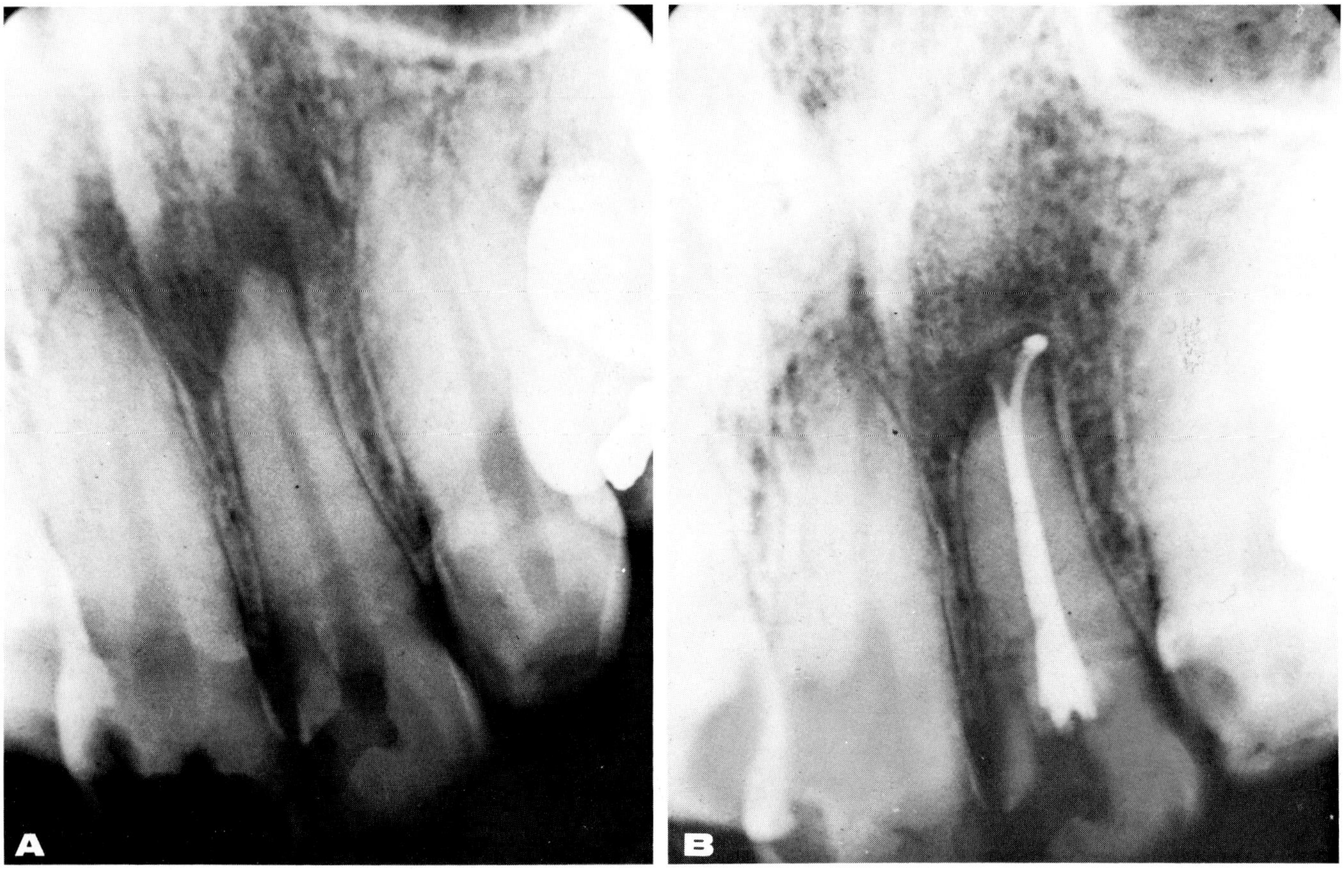

Fig. 4–52. *A*, Apical perforation causing bifurcated open foramens. *B*, Obturation by softened gutta percha is basis for periapical healing. (Courtesy Dr. James D. Zidell.)

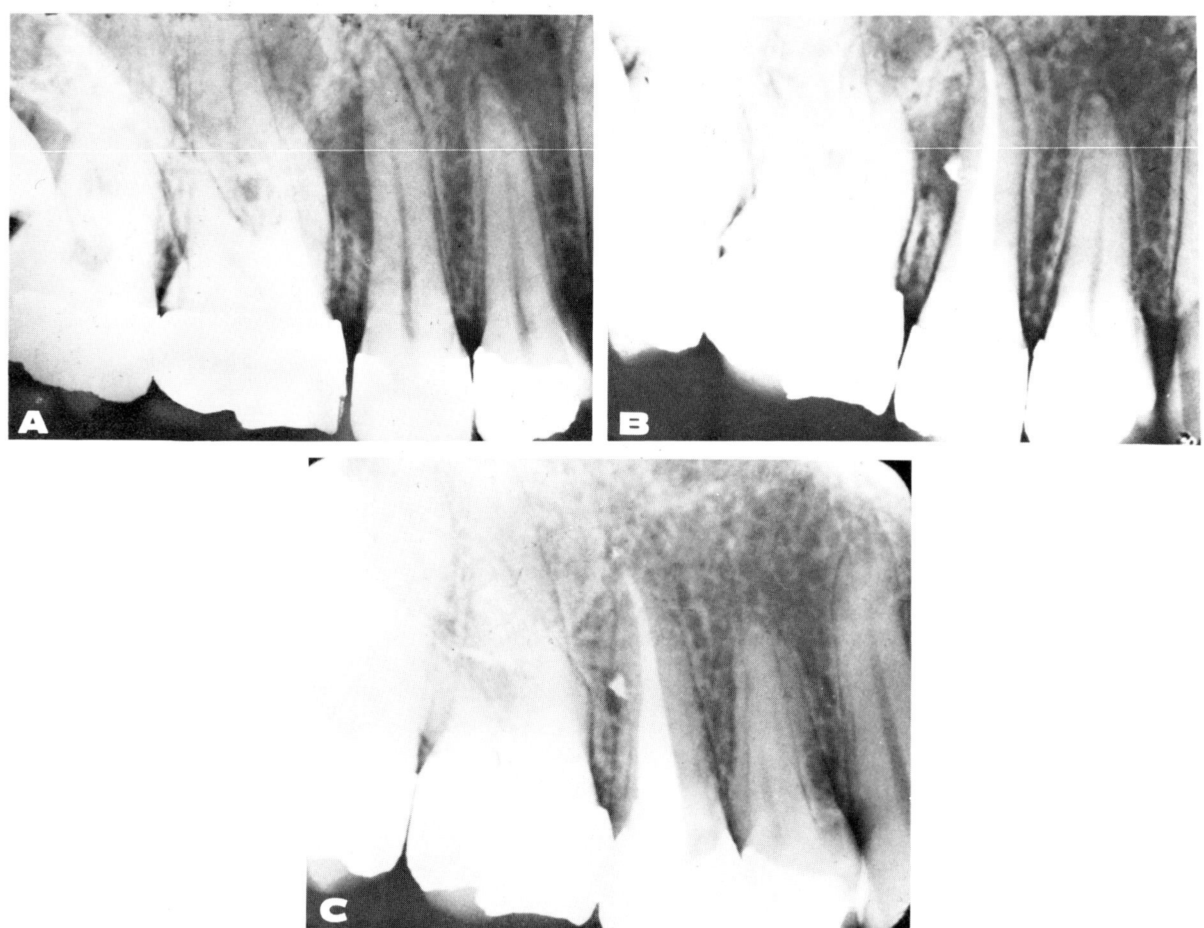

Fig. 4–53. *A,* Lesion distal to second premolar indicates presence of pulpless lateral canal. *B,* Softened gutta percha obturates entire canal space as well as lateral canal. *C,* Healing of lateral lesion is apparent in 10-month recall radiograph. (Courtesy Dr. James D. Zidell.)

materials that flow under pressure will best serve these needs.

Lateral condensation of gutta percha in straight canals sometimes forces cement out patent lateral canals, forming a "button" on the root surface (Fig. 4–54*A*). Vertical condensation of gutta percha softened by heat or chloropercha sometimes gives the same result, often to the surprise of the operator (Fig. 4–54*B,C*).

Because lateral and accessory canals are filled inadvertently, it behooves the dentist to use a filling technique that ensures their obturation in the event they are patent rather than filled with vital tissue.

The same can be said of second or auxiliary canals—canals that join before they exit. Usually these are discovered before or during treatment, either on the roentgenogram or during instrumentation. In these cases the canals may be properly prepared, but filling them is something else—access to one canal may be blocked while another is being obturated. If both canals are to be filled, they can be filled simultaneously with softened gutta percha by applying vertical pressure down both canals from the common orifice (Fig. 4–55*A,B,C*). Sometimes the dentist is surprised to learn that more than one canal exists and has been filled.

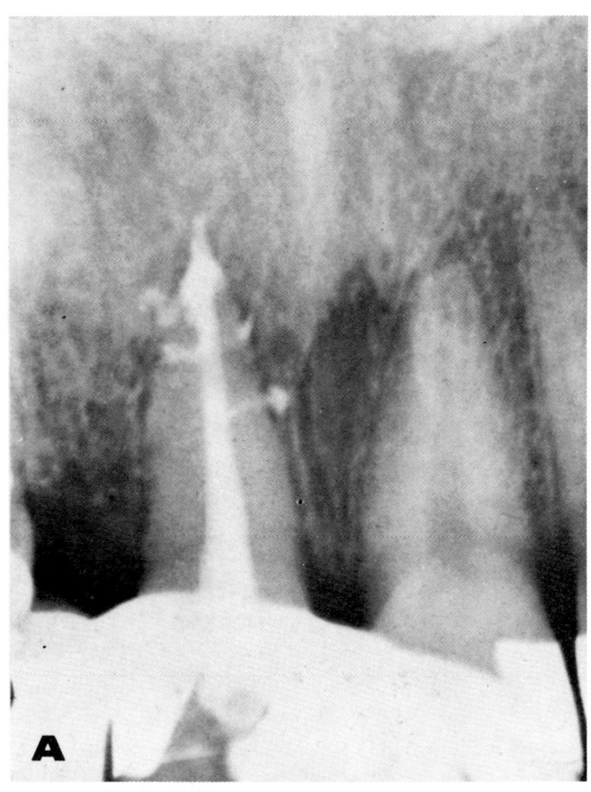

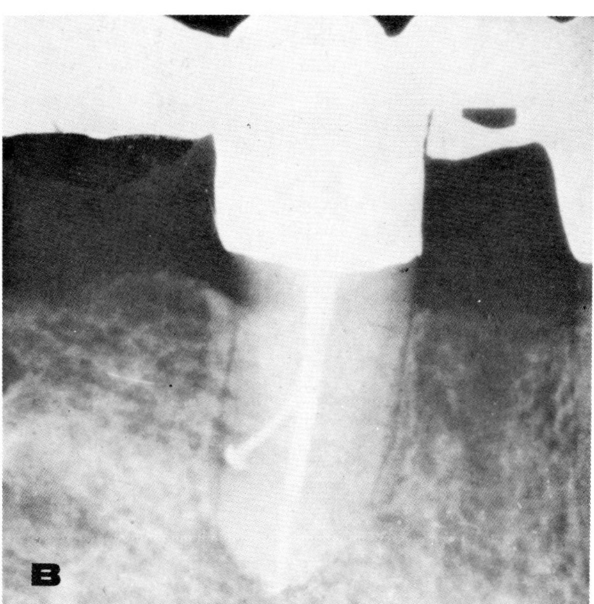

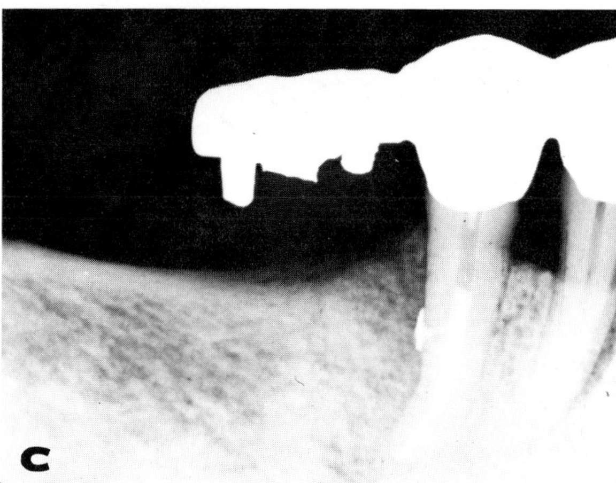

Fig. 4–54. *A,* Gross overfilling using spreading and multiple gutta percha point technique. Foramen has been perforated either during instrumentation or by external resorption. Lack of minimal opening at foramen allowed escape of excess filling material. Cement has also extruded through accessory canals. *B,* Outstanding example of obliteration obtained by softened gutta percha technique which fills accessory and severely curved canals. Premolar is abutment tooth for fixed prosthesis. (Courtesy Dr. Herbert Schilder.) *C,* Softened gutta percha used to obturate an obvious lateral canal. (Courtesy Dr. James D. Zidell.)

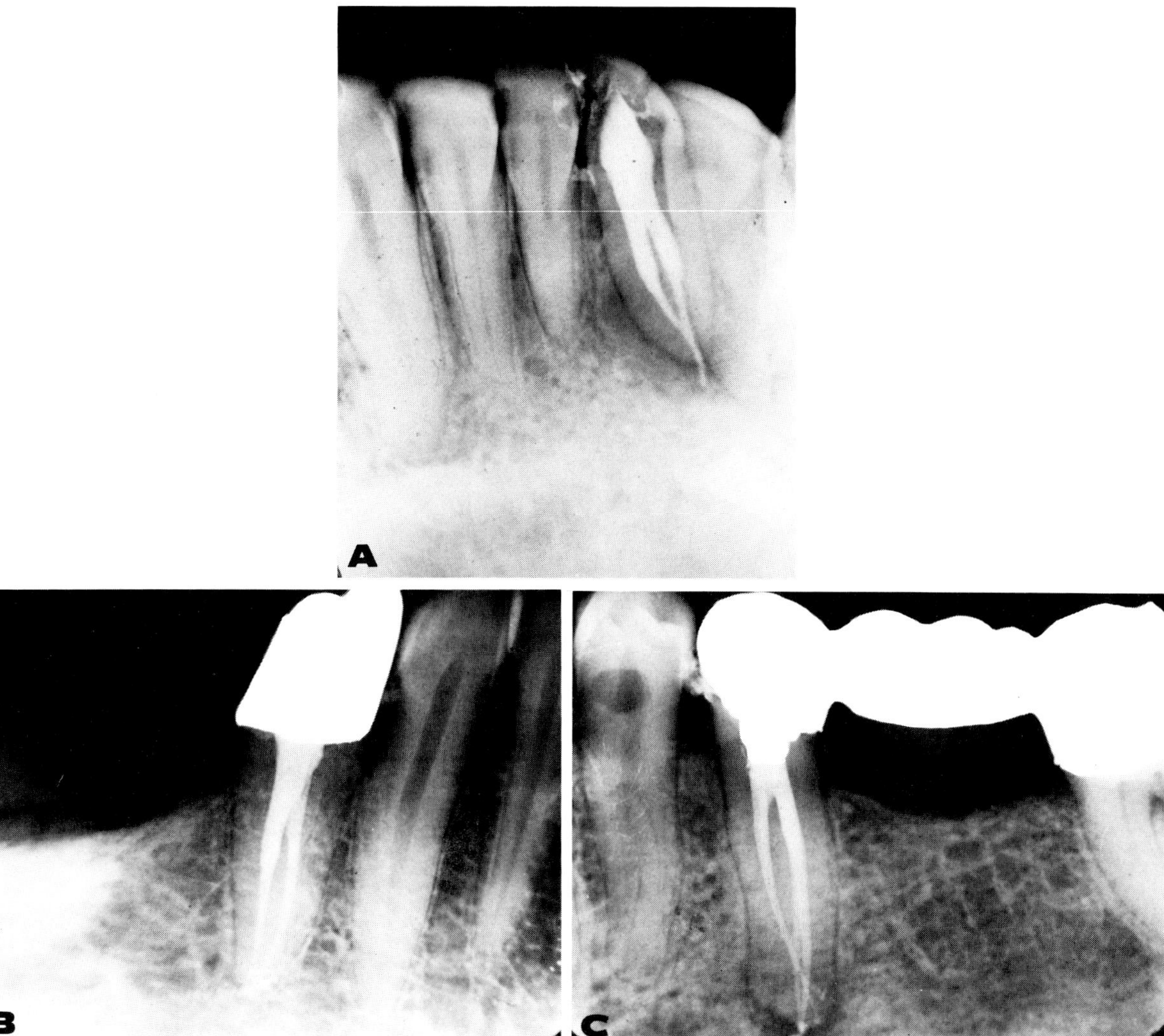

Fig. 4–55. Three examples of auxiliary canals filled by softened gutta percha. *A,* Canine with two canals, one foramen. *B,* Premolar with two canals and two foramens. *C,* Premolar with multiple canals, multiple foramens. (Courtesy Dr. James D. Zidell.)

Class III Canal Anatomy

In this category the immature canal is complicated by a gaping foramen. The apical opening is either a nonconstrictive terminus of a tubular canal or a flaring foramen of a blunderbuss shape.

Every effort should be made to attain the genetically programmed closure of the foramen remaining open because of early pulp death. This can be accomplished by ***apexification***, a method of recharging the growth potential and restoring root growth and foramen closure. Apexification is discussed thoroughly in Chapter 16, pages 689–699.

In the event apexification fails or is inappropriate, special methods must be employed to obturate the canals without benefit of the constrictive foramen's serving as a confining matrix against which to condense. Fortunately, in most of these cases, pulps of straight-rooted maxillary incisors have been devitalized by impact trauma. In other cases, the foramen has either been trephined to allow for abscess drainage or has been destroyed by the erosion of external root resorption. Occasionally an immature first molar with pulp necrosis from early caries will be a candidate.

These rather straightforward cases respond well to the use of an enormous primary gutta percha point condensed by lateral pressure to add additional gutta percha. Occasionally, however, the canal may be prepared so perfectly that a silver point may be used for obturation. Rarely would the softened gutta percha technique with heavy vertical pressure be used. This would lead to gross overfilling.

It goes without saying that the canal preparation is shaped to receive the filling material best suited for total obliteration of the space.

Lateral Condensation of Gutta Percha

Coarse, Blunted Primary Point. The large tubular canal with little constriction at the foramen may best be filled with a "coarse" primary gutta percha point which has been blunted by cutting off the tip. Sometimes the canal is so large a "tailor made" point must be used (p. 263). In either case, the "trial point" should pass the tests of proper fit.

The objective of the primary point is to block the foramen, insofar as possible, while auxiliary points are condensed to complete the filling (Fig. 4–56). The length of tooth must be marked on the spreader so it will not be forced out the apex. With care a well-compacted filling may be placed without gross overfilling of either cement or gutta percha.[72]

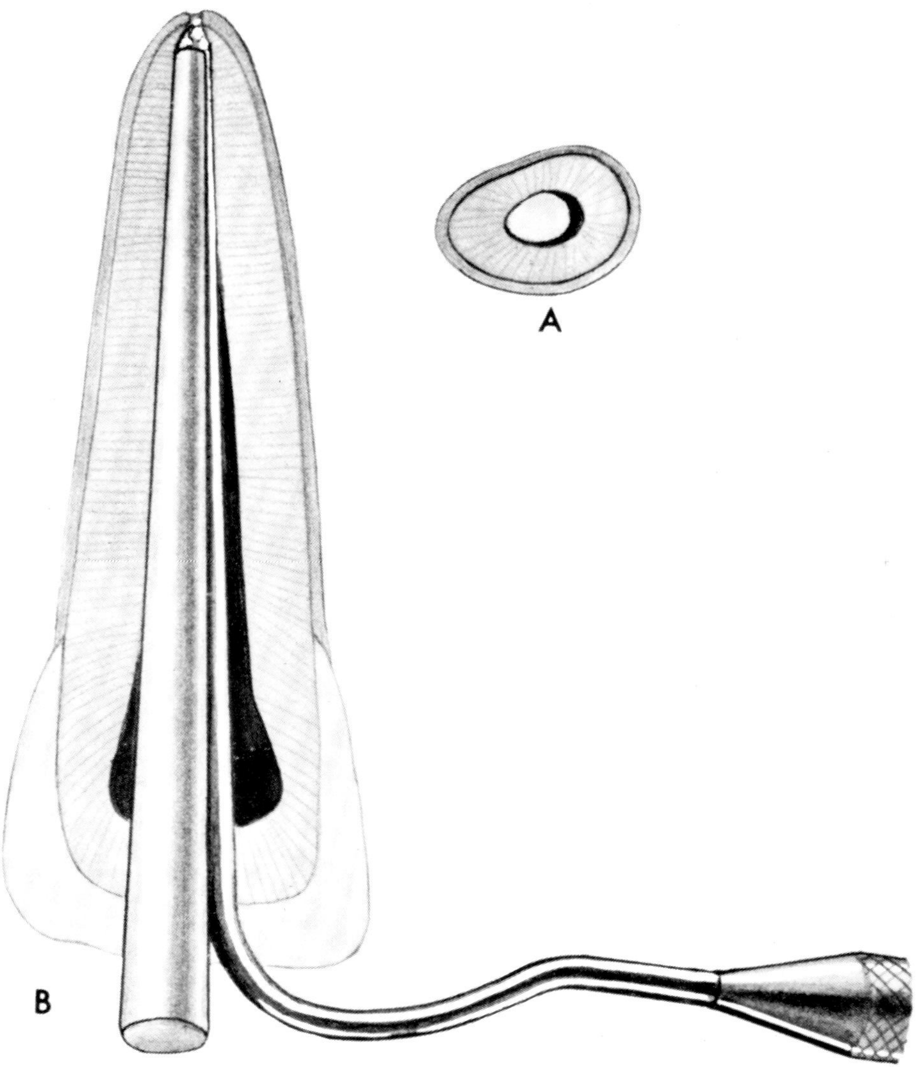

Fig. 4–56. *A,* Cross section of tubular canal in "young" tooth which is ovoid in shape and should not be filled with single point technique nor with initial silver point. *B.* Blunted, coarse gutta percha point or tailor-made gutta percha point should be used as primary filling point. This is followed by spreading and additional points, which will totally obliterate ovoid space. Final compaction is done with large blunt plugger using vertical force.

Inverted Point Technique. The particular type of canal for which this method of filling is most applicable is the tubular canal found in the tooth that has suffered early death of the pulp.

As the primary point, a "coarse" gutta percha point is selected and the serrated butt-end of the point is removed with scissors. The point is ***inverted*** and tried in the canal, ***butt-end first***. It should pass the three tests of a trial point, *i.e.,* it should visibly go to full depth, but stop dead just short of the apex; it should exhibit "tugback" when an attempt is made to remove it; and finally, it should appear in the roentgenogram to be in optimum position to obliterate the foramen area of the canal.

If the inverted point is deemed to fill correctly the requirements of a primary point, the canal is liberally coated with cement and the cement-coated point is slowly pushed to full position. This point may act as a plunger because of the shape of the canal and the tight fit of the point. The patient may complain of the

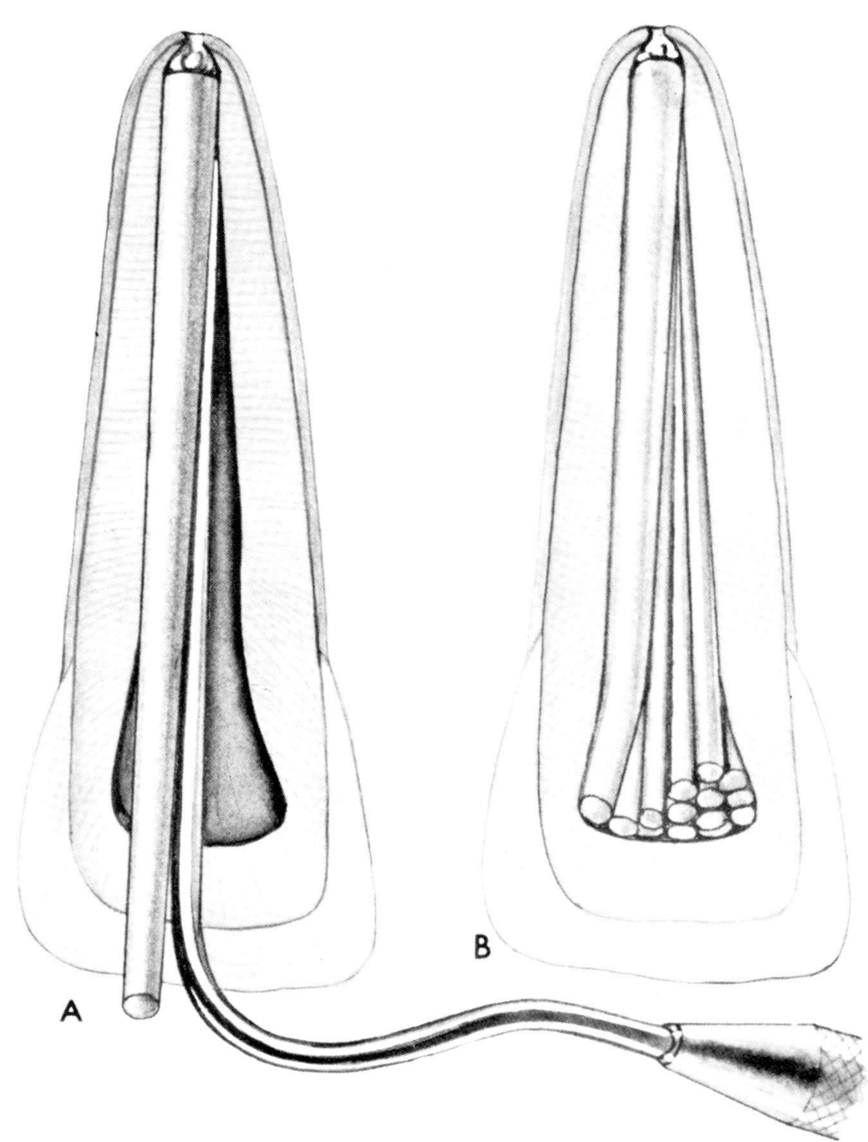

Fig. 4–57. Root canal filling technique for large canal using inverted, primary gutta percha point. *A,* Inverted point should adequately fill apical canal space. Using spreader, multiple gutta percha points are added. *B,* Total obliteration of large canal with inverted primary and additional gutta percha points. Excess gutta percha should be removed from crown of tooth with hot instrument and followed by vertical compression with large plugger.

discomfort of air evacuation; however, if the point is placed slowly, relatively little cement will be forced into the periapical tissue.

When the primary inverted point is in place, additional gutta percha points should be carefully added by lateral condensation with the spreader (Fig. 4–57*A*). It is most important at this time to mark the length of the tooth on the spreader, so that the instrument will not penetrate into the periapical tissue. The spreader is used repeatedly, followed by "fine" gutta percha points until the canal is totally obliterated (Fig. 4–57*B*). The common error in this technique is an outgrowth of fear of overfilling. Insufficient pressure is applied during lateral condensation, resulting in a poorly condensed filling. This in turn allows subsequent leakage and invites failure.

Tailor-Made Gutta Percha Roll. If the tubular canal is so large that the largest inverted gutta percha point is still loose in the canal, a tailor-made point must be used as a primary point. This point may be prepared by heating a number of gutta percha points and combining them, butt-to-tip, until a roll has been developed much the size and shape of the canal (Fig. 4–58). The roll must be chilled with a spray of ethyl chloride or Fluori Methane to stiffen the gutta percha before it is fitted in the canal. If it goes to full depth easily but is too loose, more gutta percha must be added. If it is only slightly too large, the outside of the gutta percha can be flash heated over the flame and the roll forced to proper position. By this method, an impression of the canal is actually secured (Fig. 4–59).

The rolled gutta percha should be tested for tugback and by means of the roentgenogram. If satisfactory, it should be cemented to place. The gutta percha protruding from the crown should then be severed at the base of the pulp chamber with a hot spoon excavator so that the spreader may be introduced. The spreader should be marked just short of the working length of tooth as described above. Lateral condensation is necessary in conjunction with the tailor-made gutta percha roll to ensure obliteration of the canal space (Fig. 4–60).

Simpson and Natkin have suggested a specialized filling technique for those teeth with tubular canals but closed apices.[72] These are the roots that were originally blunderbuss in shape, but have been induced to complete their growth by the introduction of a biologically active chemical, such as calcium hydroxide, into the root canal.

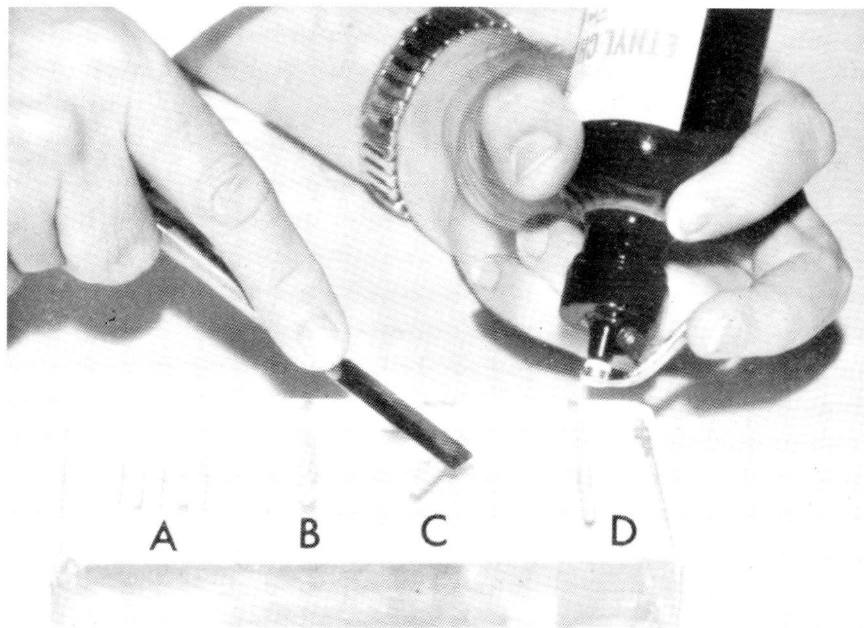

Fig. 4–58. Preparation of "tailor-made" gutta percha roll. *A,* Number of heated, coarse, gutta percha points are arranged butt-to-tip on sterile glass slab. *B,* Points are rolled with spatula into rod-shaped mass. *C,* By repeated heating and rolling the roll of gutta percha is formed to approximate size of canal to be filled. No voids should exist in mass. *D,* Before trial point testing of tailor-made roll, gutta percha should be chilled with ethyl chloride or Fluori Methane spray.

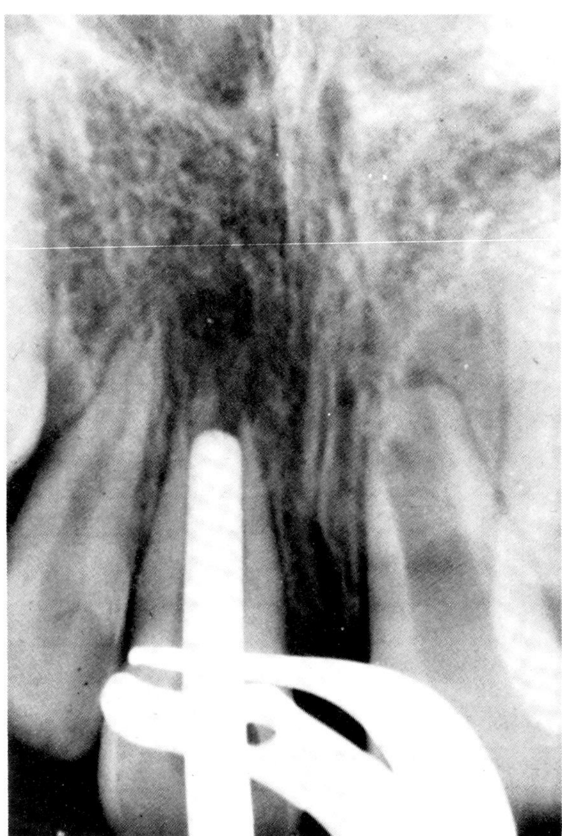

Fig. 4–59. Trial point roentgenogram of tailor-made gutta percha point. Space exists alongside of this roll which indicates it should be enlarged and retested.

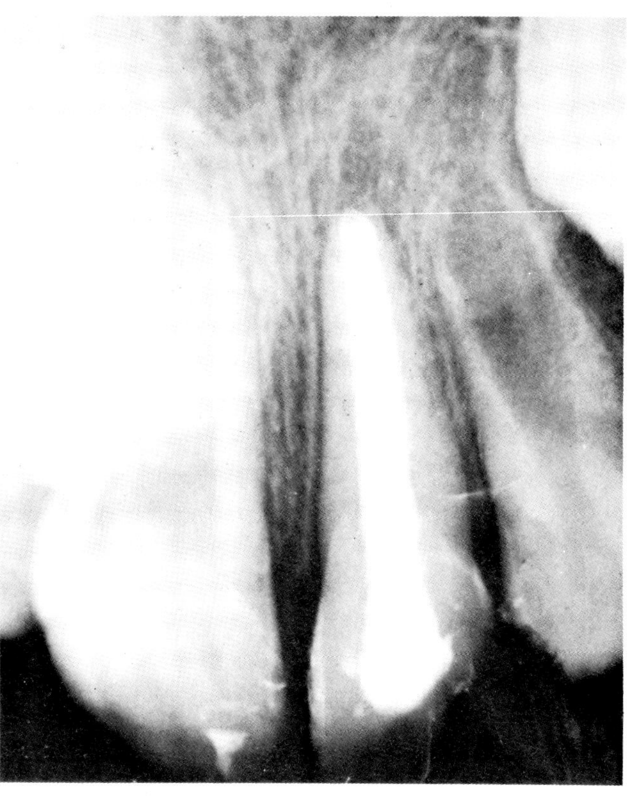

Fig. 4–60. Final obliteration of tubular canal with open apex. Inverted primary gutta percha point was spread aside and multiple gutta percha points added to completely seal canal.

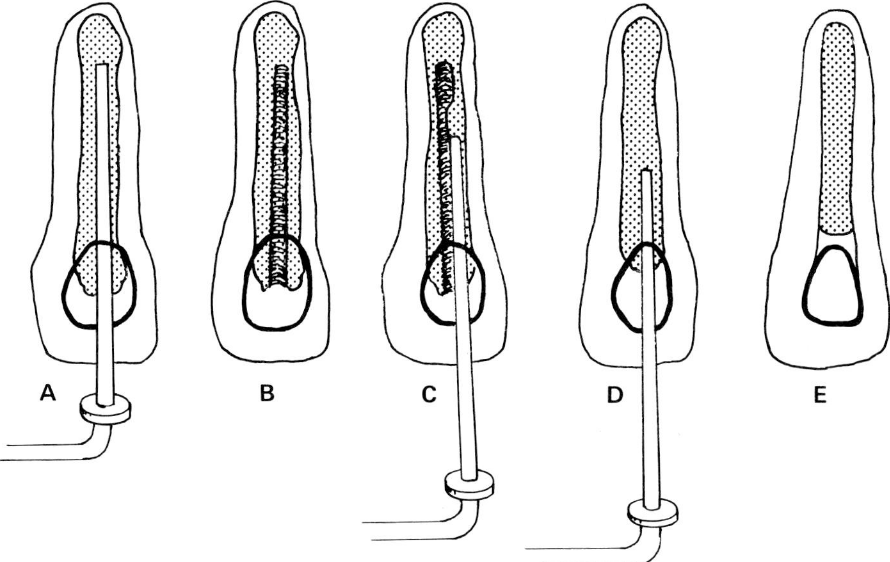

Fig. 4–61. Special method of obturating tubular canals with closed apex. *A,* Large cold plugger is used to force softened tailor-made gutta percha to apex. *B,* Twisting removal of plugger leaves central void. *C,* Plugger is used to collapse gutta percha into void. *D,* Heated plugger may be used to further compact filling. *E,* Final obturation by adding sections of gutta percha with vertical compression. (From Simpson, T., and Natkin, E.: J. Brit. Endodont. Soc. 3:59, Summer, 1972.)

The canal is initially filled with a warmed and softened tailor-made gutta percha roll cemented to place and severed at the canal orifice with a hot spoon excavator. Using a heavy plugger, the gutta percha is forced to the apex and compacted to place (Fig. 4–61*A*). Pressure with the plugger will leave a void in the center of the mass when the plugger is removed with a twisting motion (Fig. 4–61*B*). It may be necessary to hold the gutta percha in place with an explorer when removing the plugger. The plugger is dipped in oxyphosphate of zinc powder to prevent sticking and is then used to collapse the gutta percha into the space created by the initial plugging (Fig. 4–61*C*). If the gutta percha begins to set, the plugger is heated to better compact the filling (Fig. 4–61*D*). With heavy vertical pressure, the entire canal is obturated and the excess gutta percha seared off at the gingival level (Fig. 4–61*E*).

The Silver Point Technique. Occasionally one encounters a rather mature canal with associated loss of constriction at the foramen. Such cases are the result of apical root resorption or of trephination through the apex with a large instrument to establish abscess drainage through the canal.

These cases may be filled with single silver points (Fig. 4–62) or with a silver point at the apex followed by lateral condensation and additional gutta percha.

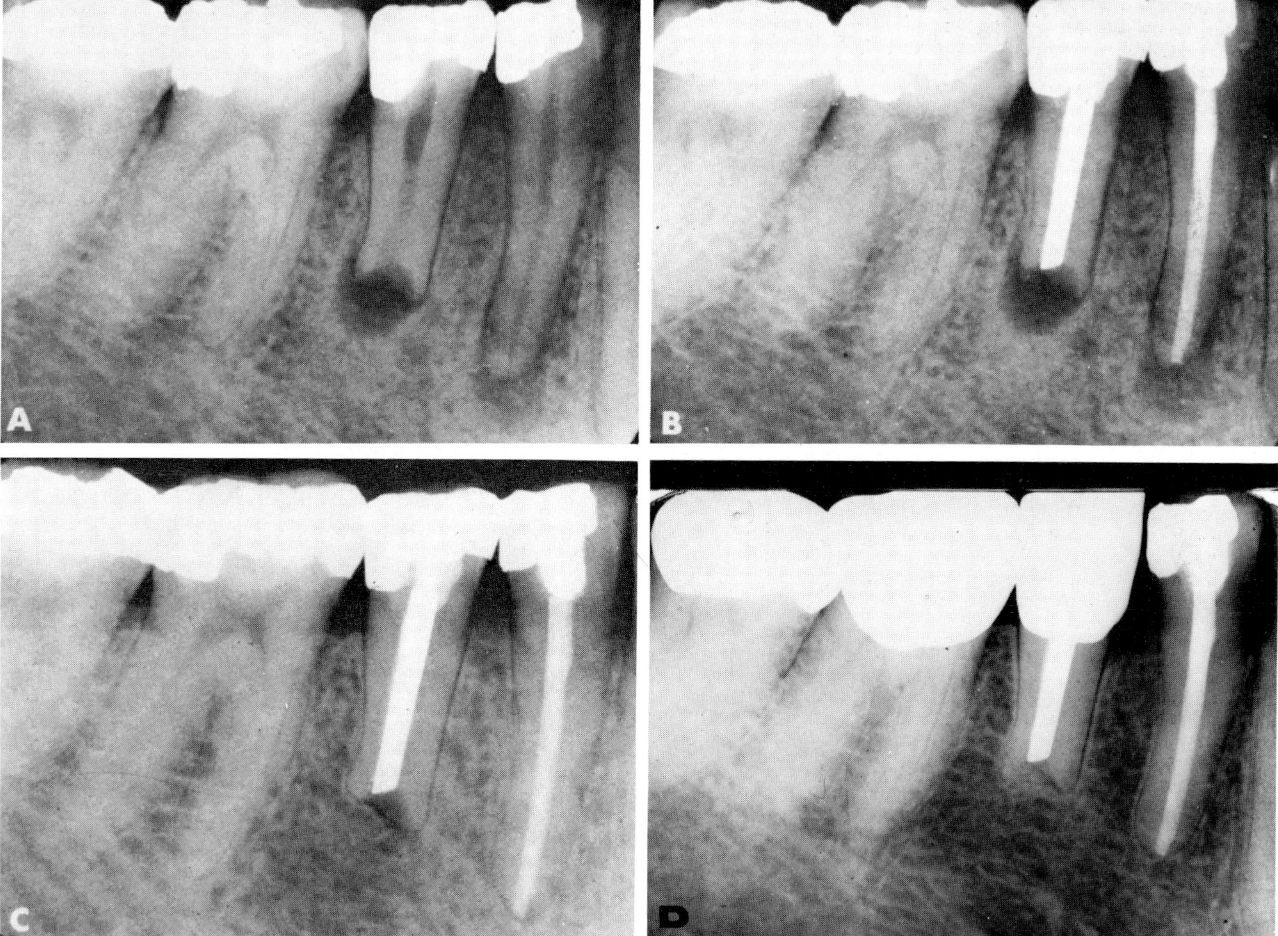

Fig. 4–62. *A,* Unusual external root resorption and dumbbell-shaped canal in mandibular second premolar. Careful canal preparation into perfect round tapered shape will prevent gross overfilling. *B,* Root canal filling with single silver point cemented into perfectly prepared canal. Canal of first premolar has been filled with multiple gutta percha points. *C,* Total healing two years after root canal obliteration with single silver point. External resorption has stopped. Periapical healing of first premolar is also evident. *D,* ***Twenty-year*** recall radiograph. The wise choice of gutta percha for the first premolar and silver for the second premolar is proven by time. Superb execution of therapy is an obvious important component of long-term success. (Courtesy Dr. Clifford Ames.)

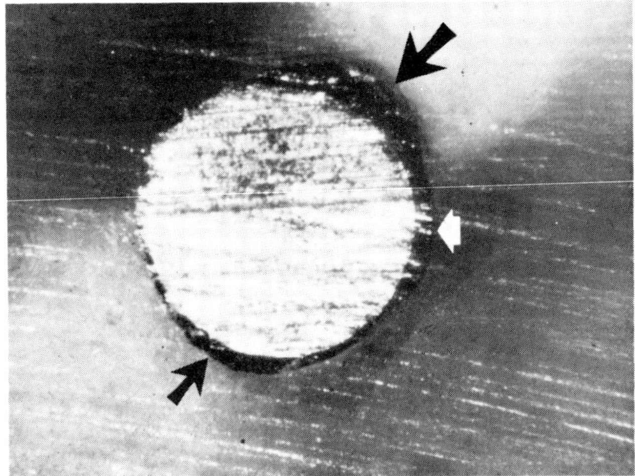

Fig. 4–63. Cross section of silver point used to fill prepared canal. Black border partially surrounding silver point is cement proving that preparation was not round. Gradual decomposition of cement would lead to leakage and failure. (Courtesy Dr. Quan Dihn.)

In either case, meticulous preparation of the canal to establish a round, tapered cavity is necessary. In order to work right to the lip of the foramen, the tips of the enlarging instruments must be blunted by grinding.

To be successful, the silver point must occlude the canal as well as a cork closing a bottle (Fig. 4–63). This calls for great care in establishing the proper size of the trial point—cutting back the silver until the point fits the canal so tightly it is difficult to remove with a hemostat. Examine the point carefully to be sure the silver is scarred by the dentin walls all around the perimeter, not in just one or two places. The cement must be carefully placed in the canal and the point slowly inserted to allow the cement to flow back. Remember these tubular walls are nearly parallel and the point could serve as a plunger if rapidly forced to place. Success can be achieved with this technique without gross overfilling.

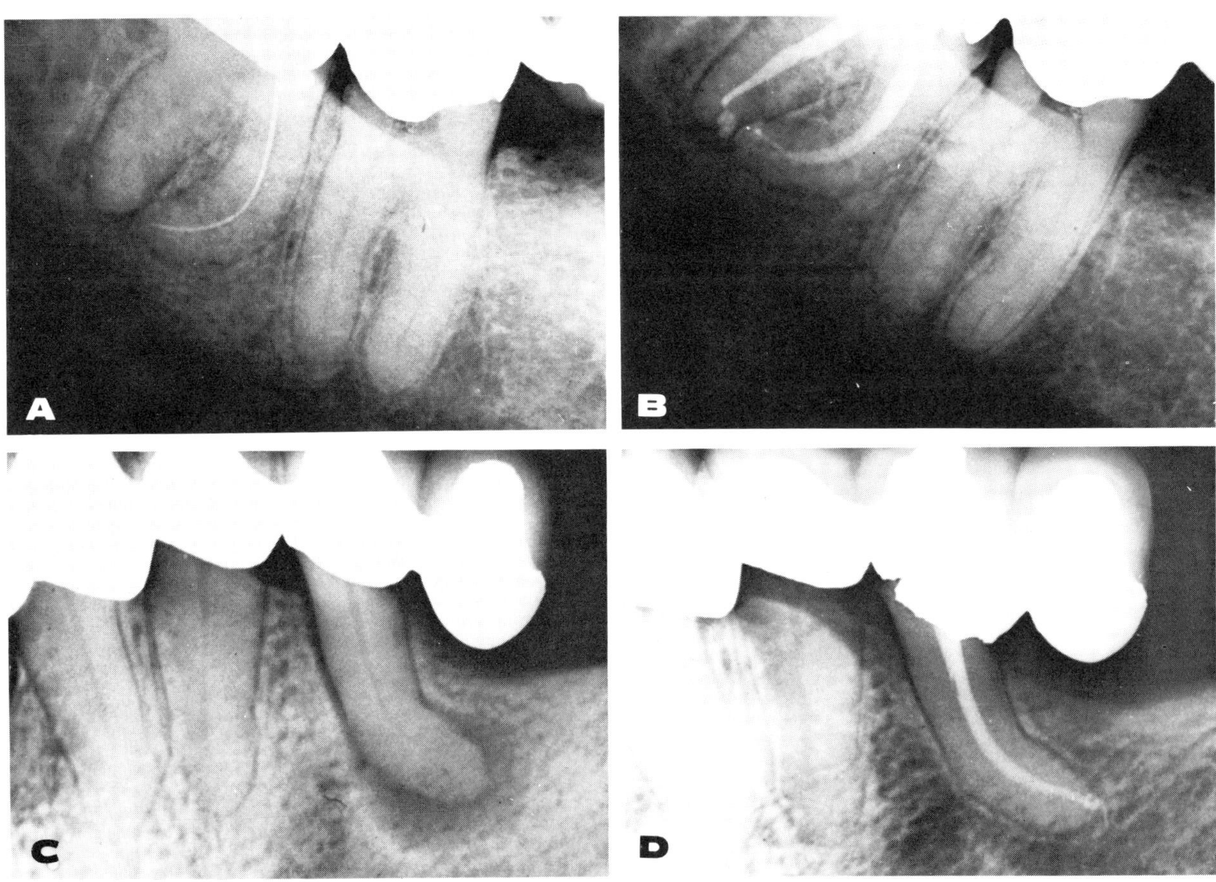

Fig. 4–64. Severely curved canals to be filled by diffusion technique. *A*, Instrument proving severity of curvature. *B*, Diffusion technique filling with chloropercha. *C*, Large periapical lesion associated with pulpless bridge abutment. *D*, Healing of lesion one year following obturation with diffused chloropercha. (Courtesy Dr. Jack Weichman.)

Paste or Cement-Only Methods of Filling

Chloropercha Diffusion Technique. Chloropercha, made by dissolving gutta percha in chloroform, was advocated in 1914 by Callahan as a primary filling material for the root canal space.[73] Callahan's method was later modified by Johnston,[74] whose technique used chloropercha as a cementing medium for gutta percha points which form the bulk of the filling (Fig. 4–64). The Johnston-Callahan technique is still used extensively today, and a modification of this technique has already been discussed under the "softened gutta percha technique."

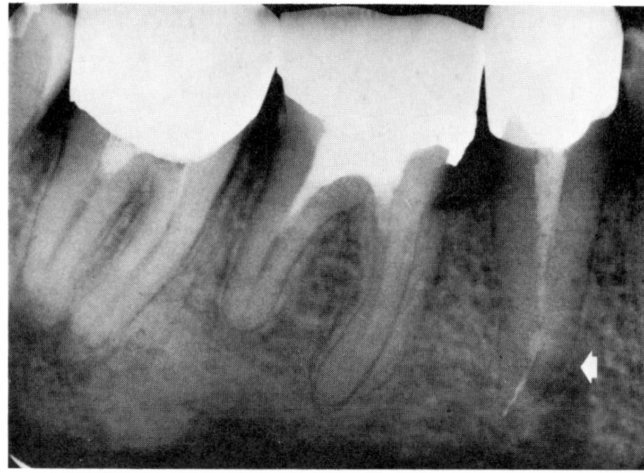

Fig. 4–65. Three failures of teeth with paste filled canals. *Left to right,* Second molar shows periapical lesion and root resorption as well as osteosclerosis indicating chronic inflammation. First molar has distal root resorption indicative of chronic inflammation. Premolar has broken Lentulo spiral at apex and mesial lateral periapical lesion associated with porous root canal filling. (Courtesy Dr. Worth Gregory.)

Chloropercha "sets" as the chloroform volatilizes, leaving the mass of gutta percha. Quite obviously the volatilization reduces the total volume of the filling. ***Chloropercha*** *per se* ***as a filling material is unacceptable*** because of the apical percolation that would follow the shrinkage of the filling. As a cementing medium it is perfectly acceptable with multiple gutta percha points, but would be unacceptable when used with a single silver point because of its shrinkage. The silver point cannot be compacted in the apical third of the canal.

Cements Only. Filling root canals with cement only, that is, without a solid core material forming the bulk of the filling, has been advocated by Sargenti,[30] and by Goerig and Seymour.[51] There has been a paucity of ***proof*** as to the effectiveness of cement-only obturation, "proof" usually consisting of testimonials (Fig. 4–65). Sargenti recommends that the cement N2 be positioned in the canal with a Lentulo spiral used in a slow turning handpiece or by a reamer turning counterclockwise.[30] Goerig and Seymour, on the other hand, recommend that regular zinc oxide-eugenol cement be injected into the canal by means of

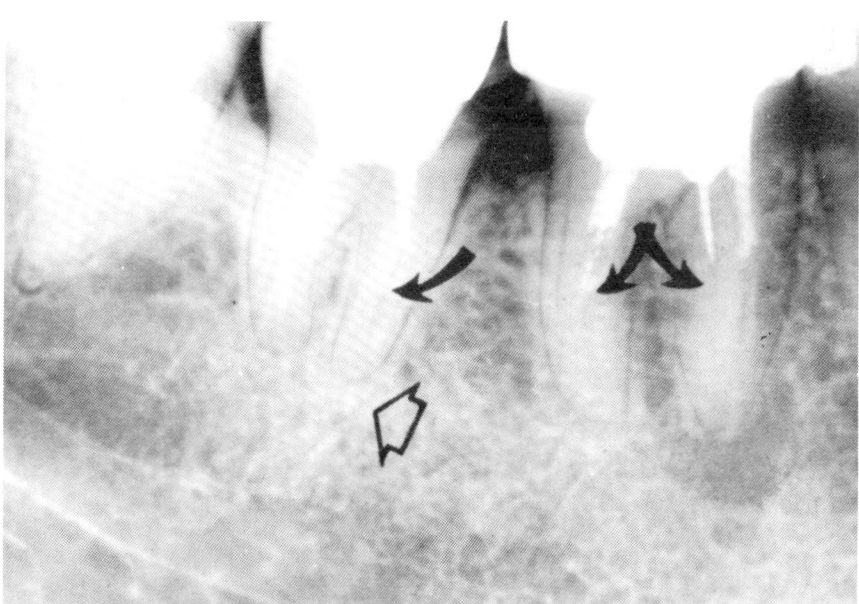

Fig. 4–66. Endodontic failure following use of resorbable paste as root canal filling material (*arrows*). Lesion periapical to mesial root of first molar is readily apparent. Open arrow indicates osteosclerosis developing from chronic low-grade inflammation.

a disposable tuberculin syringe and needle.[51] Wallentin has suggested the use of Cavit to obturate canals.[75] Moisture must be utilized to provoke the Cavit to "set."

For a more detailed description of these cements and their effect upon periapical tissue in the event the cement escapes the foramen, the reader is referred back to the section on cements and sealers, page 223.

Resorbable Pastes. The resorbable pastes were developed to obliterate the canal of the pulpless tooth with a periapical lesion. Iodoform, which is radiopaque and resorbable, is the basic ingredient in the paste. Gross overfilling was advocated, for the overfilled paste rapidly resorbed away from the periapex. Practically, however, the rapid resorption leads to failure in many cases so treated.

Nygaard-Ostby has demonstrated this unfortunate drawback of the material—the fact that the paste continues to be resorbed from the canal, thus resulting in percolation and possible failure.[76] The proponents of the technique, in their enthusiasm over the successes they enjoyed, neglected to notice the nearby failures (Fig. 4–66).

Maisto has modified straight iodoform paste and has used it with gutta percha points.[77] His modified paste is more slowly resorbed from the tissue, and by addition of gutta percha points, the continued resorption of paste from the canal tends to be eliminated.

With any ***overfilling***, the patient is likely to experience discomfort. If the periapical area is completely encapsulated in bone with no draining sinus, the pain is apt to be excruciating until resorption takes place. This would be a major complaint expressed by the patient.

Class IV Canal Anatomy

Primary Tooth Undergoing Physiologic Resorption. Filling Class IV anatomy canals will be dealt with in Chapter 17, Pediatric Endodontics.

Temporary Filling Materials

It was the endodontist who made popular the immediate temporary filling materials, the type squeezed from a tube. Prior to their arrival on the market, endodontic cavities were sealed between appointments with the so called double-seal fillings, usually a base of zinc oxide and eugenol covered with the more permanent oxyphosphate of zinc cement. This procedure was time-consuming and not altogether satisfactory. For this reason Cavit was a welcome endodontic cavity temporary cement. It is set by the presence of moisture

TABLE 4–1. AVERAGE LEAKAGE VALUES

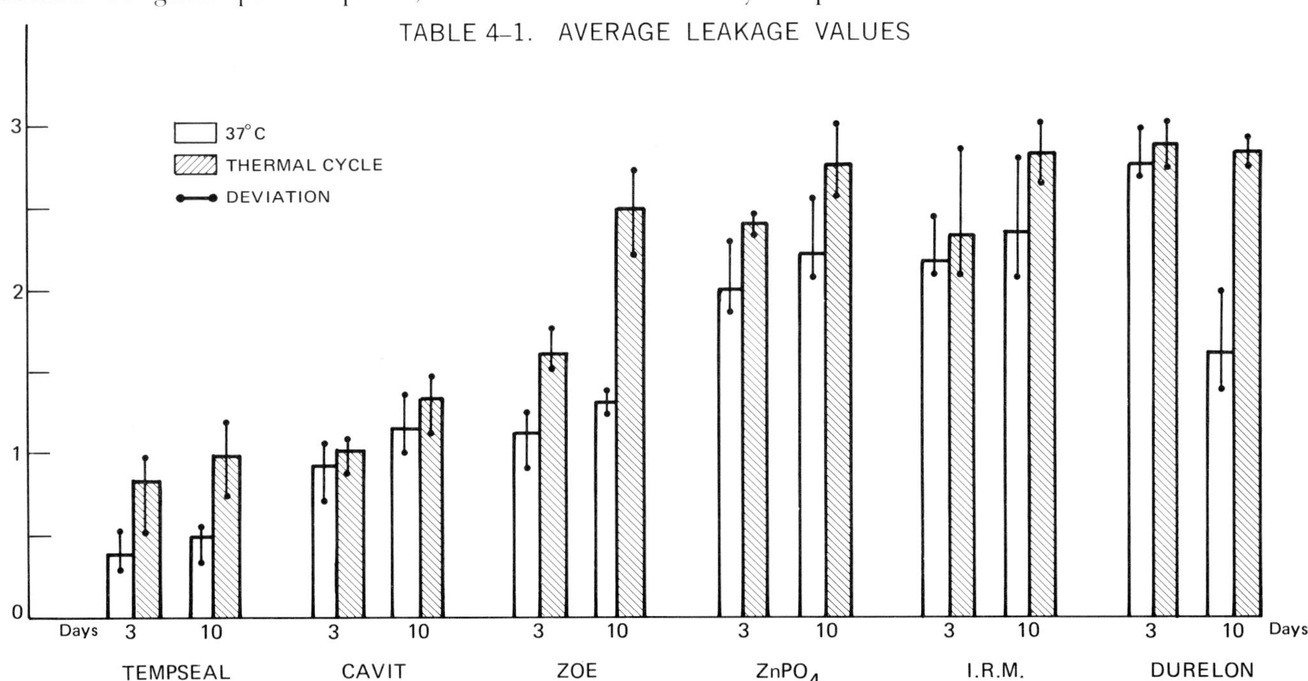

Leakage around six temporary cements. At both 3 days and 10 days there is a dramatic increase in leakage when cements other than Tempseal and Cavit are used. (From Marosky, J. F.: To be published.)

The efficacy of Cavit was first tested by Serene et al.,[78] who reported favorably about its sealing qualities. Using Cavit in both vital and pulpless monkey and human teeth *in vivo*, they found Cavit caused some discomfort in vital teeth, probably from dentin desiccation. Although Cavit contains zinc oxide, it does not contain eugenol, which acts as an anodyne in ZO–E fillings. Serene found that Cavit expanded nearly twice as much as ZO–E when exposed to moisture and even had the quality to "repair" itself if a piece broke away. Since it can be dissolved by the intracanal medicaments, it should be separated from them by dry cotton. Cavit was well recommended as a temporary filling material for pulpless teeth.

Recently Marosky has tested a number of temporary cements over periods of 3 days and 10 days, using Calcium 45 to produce autoradiographs.[79] He reported the least microleakage around Temp-Seal, with Cavit a close second. Following in order of ever-increasing leakage was zinc oxide-eugenol, oxyphosphate of zinc, I.R.M. and Durelon (Table 4–1). Further studies of other physical properties are needed.

Removal of Defective Root Canal Fillings

Occasionally it is necessary to remove a defective root canal filling so that the canal can be reinstrumented and refilled. Fortunately, both the zinc oxide-eugenol cements and gutta percha may be dissolved to facilitate their removal. Silver points, on the other hand, require a more mechanical method of removal. Oxyphosphate of zinc cement cannot be removed by any method and should not be used as a root canal sealer. Weine has also stated he has not found an effective solvent for N2 cement.[65]

For removal of gutta percha–zinc oxide–eugenol fillings, both xylol and chloroform may be used as a solvent, although chloroform is preferred. The gutta percha and cement in the canal are exposed through the standard endodontic cavity preparation in the crown of the tooth. With a syringe and needle the canal is flooded with chloroform. This is followed by a medium-size reamer, which is forced into the softened gutta percha. The reamer breaks up the gutta percha, allowing the solvent to flow into the spaces. As the material is removed and the apex approached, smaller reamers are used to conform to the size of the canal. Solvent is repeatedly added.

The gutta percha is dissolved in the chloroform and removed from the canal on the reamers, which are then cleaned with cotton rolls. Near the apex, care must be used to avoid forcing the pieces of gutta percha and solvent through the foramen and to avoid perforation or development of a ledge in the canal. Even a small piece of gutta percha may divert a reamer against the wall of the canal, and if the operator does not recognize the difference in tactile sensation, a perforation might result (Fig. 4–67).

Removal of the filling is completed with a file used in the dry canal. Frequently, small remaining pieces of gutta percha and cement will be finally removed. The canal should be meticulously reprepared and should then be medicated. At a subsequent appointment a new trial point is tested and the canal refilled.

The removal of a cemented silver point is usually more difficult than the removal of gutta percha. If the cone is broken off down in the canal, a method suggested by Feldman,[80] in 1914, and recently modified by Glick[81] may be used. Glick forces three fine Hedstrom files down alongside the point as far as

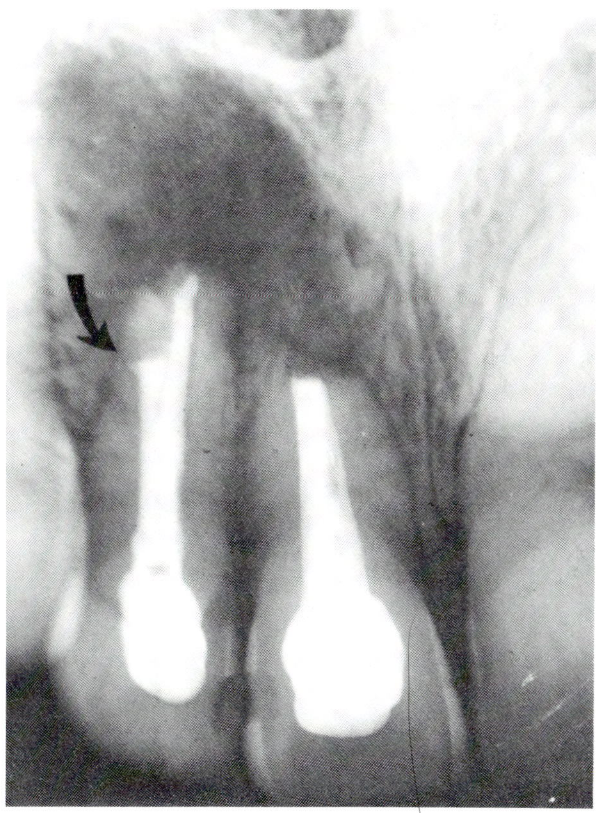

Fig. 4–67. Perforation (*arrow*) developed during attempt to remove old gutta percha filling. Small pieces of gutta percha will divert endodontic instruments leading to perforation.

they will go (Fig. 4–68*A*). The three files are then twisted around one another, thus entangling the soft silver point in a grip much like that exerted by a broach holder (Fig. 4–68*B*, *C*). This method has also been compared to the grip exerted by the trick Mexican straw finger "cot" which becomes tighter the harder one pulls. The gradual pull on the files often loosens the silver point. This procedure may be repeated a number of times, each time loosening the silver point a bit more.

If the point has fortunately been left protruding into the pulp chamber, a sharp spoon excavator or

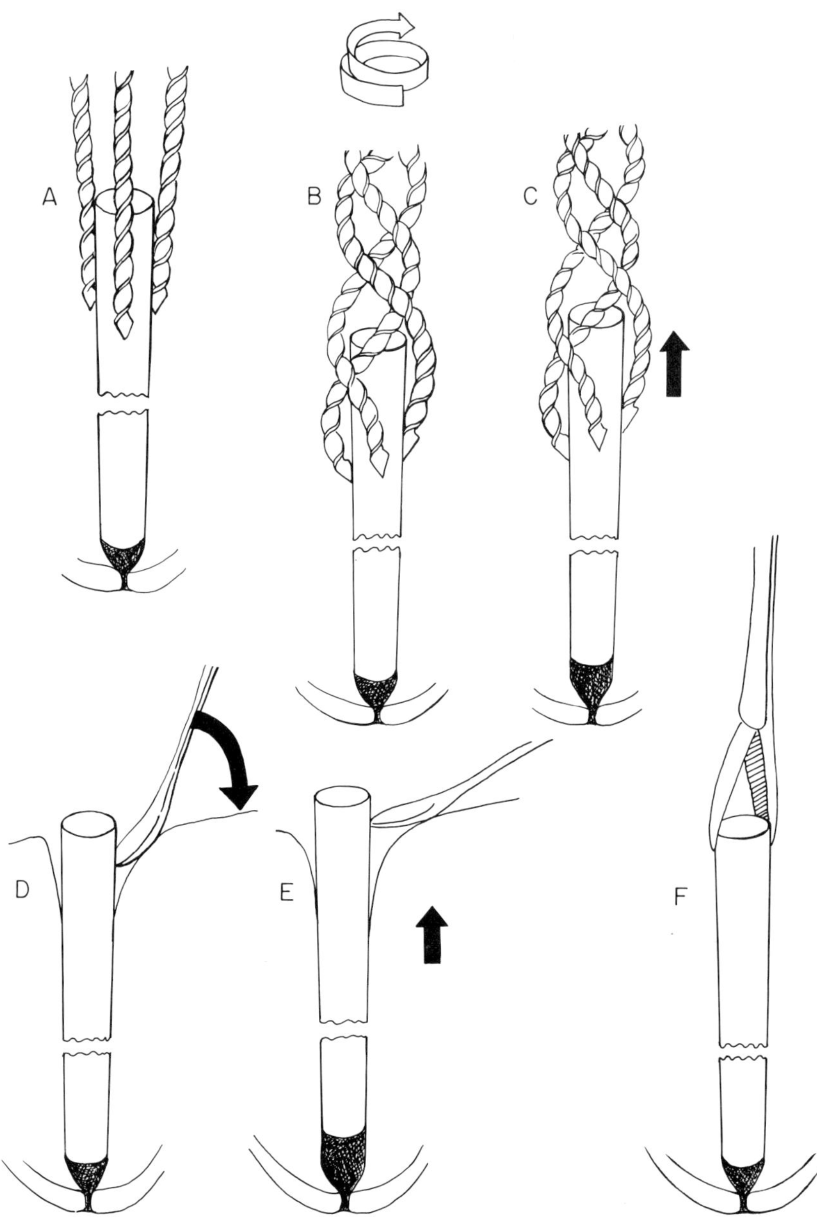

Fig. 4–68. Methods for removing silver point. *A,* In method advocated by Glick, three fine files are worked down alongside silver point. *B,* By clockwise motion three files are wound around each other forming vise-like grip on the soft silver. *C,* Gradual pull will often dislodge point from its seat. Repetition may be necessary before point is loosened. *D,* If point protrudes into chamber, sharp spoon excavator may be used to pry point from position. *E,* Repeated attempts with excavator will often loosen point from its seat. *F,* If space exists in occlusal cavity, point may be loosened with twisting motion using alligator ear forcep or hemostat.

curette also may be used to pry the point from its seat (Fig. 4–68 *D, E*). A more efficient spoon excavator has been marketed by Stardent with a triangular notch cut out in the tip of the blade. By this modification the blade grips the silver from two sides rather than just by the curve of the blade. Silver points may sometimes be grasped with an alligator ear forcep, broken loose from the cement by twisting, and removed (Fig. 4–68*F*). If the point can be removed, the canal is reinstrumented, sterilized, and filled at a subsequent appointment. If the point cannot be removed, the operator must consider the possibility of the retrosurgical approach.

A NEW ENDODONTIC PARADIGM*

More than a quarter century ago, Coolidge illustrated, with a series of excellent microphotographs, the ideal apical seal for the filled pulpless tooth—a layer of cementum deposited over and into the apical foramen (Fig. 4–69).[82] It has long been clear to thoughtful researchers and clinicians that only where cementum covers the entire root surface of the pulpless tooth can the integrity of the attachment apparatus be assured. In years past, the only method known for encouraging the formation of an apical cementum seal was to terminate root canal fillings at the cementodentinal junction and hope that nature would oblige.

Then, in 1962, Kaiser presented before the annual meeting of the American Association of Endodontists a method whereby the open apex of a pulpless immature tooth could be closed with calcified tissue through the process now termed "apexification."[83] The technique involved the placement of a paste of calcium hydroxide mixed with camphorated parachlorophenol in the canal of the tooth. Frank refined and popularized the technique as shown in Chapter 16. Steiner and Van Hassel concluded from animal studies that the calcified material deposited at the root apex could most accurately be described as cementum.[84]

Visionary and practical clinicians soon began extending the use of this technique in an effort to close resorptive and iatrogenic root perforations, halt apical resorption, repair root fractures, and prevent or reduce replantation resorption. Generally speaking, it was found that any unwanted orifice in the root

*Abstracted from a manuscript submitted for publication by Raymond G. Luebke, 1975.

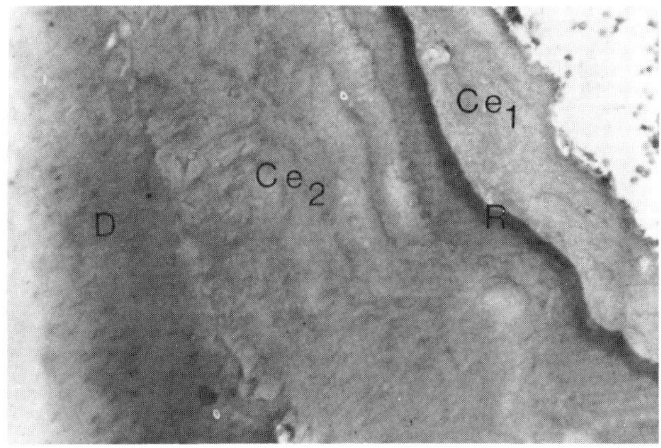

Fig. 4–69. Photomicrograph (×400) of cemental repair closing apex. Ce_1, Cellular cementum. Ce_2, Acellular cementum. *R,* Resting line separating two layers of cementum. *D,* Dentin. (From Klein, S., and Levy, B.: Oral Surg., *38*: Dec., 1974.)

surface could be closed with cementum by the technique. If unwanted orifices could be closed, why not the apical foramen?

The remarkable success of these efforts created a wave of excitement which has led to promising new materials and methods. The most extensive research activities have been carried out with calcium hydroxide combined with disinfectants, but reports of new materials capable of inducing cementogenesis are appearing monthly. A form of tricalcium phosphate ceramic has shown promise in animal studies performed by Koenigs and others.[85] Nevins and his associates have reported dramatic success in producing apical and intracanal cementification in animals with a gel made up of collagen and biologically active chemicals (Fig. 4–70).[86]

It requires little foresight to visualize the result of these research efforts. Clearly the ideal apical cementum seal for the pulpless tooth is now predictably attainable. A functional fibrous attachment of this cementum to bone has been demonstrated.[86] The sealing potential of induced cementification is easily demonstrated (Fig. 4–71). Age, once considered a possible limitation to the effectiveness of the process, has been shown to be irrelevant (Fig. 4–72). Posterior teeth are as responsive as anterior teeth. Indeed, the calcium hydroxide mixture has been found to be a remarkably effective long-term canal disinfectant (Fig. 4–73), and has already been used by a number of clinicians as a semi-permanent root canal filling material.

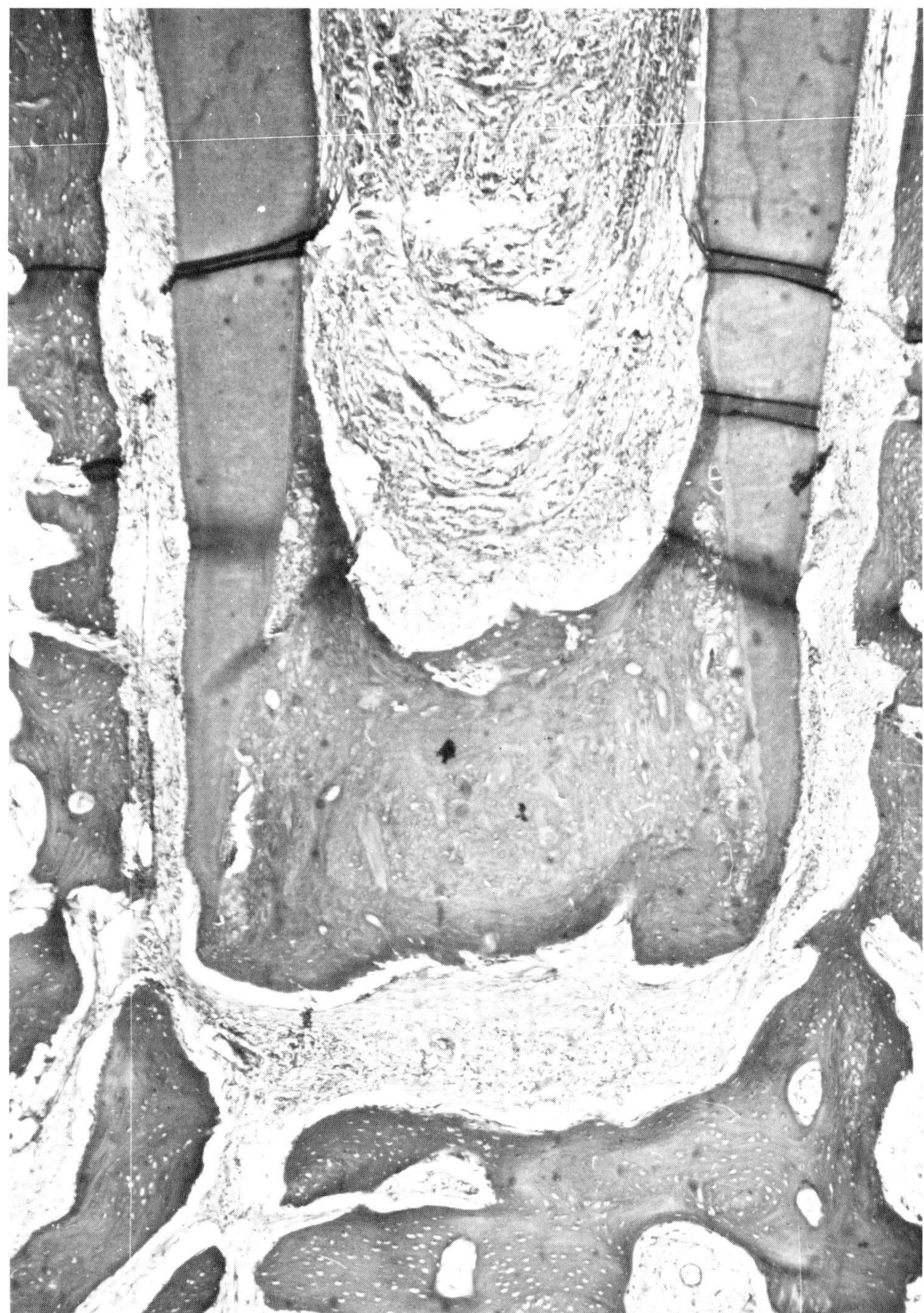

Fig. 4–70. Apical closure achieved after 12 weeks in infected mandibular incisor with open apex in Rhesus monkey. Canal was filled with mixture of collagen gel, 1.0 ml.; $CaCl_2$, 0.05 ml. (2.0 M); K_2HPO_4, 0.05 ml. (1.8 M); and KI 5%, 0.05 ml. (Courtesy Dr. Alan J. Nevins.)

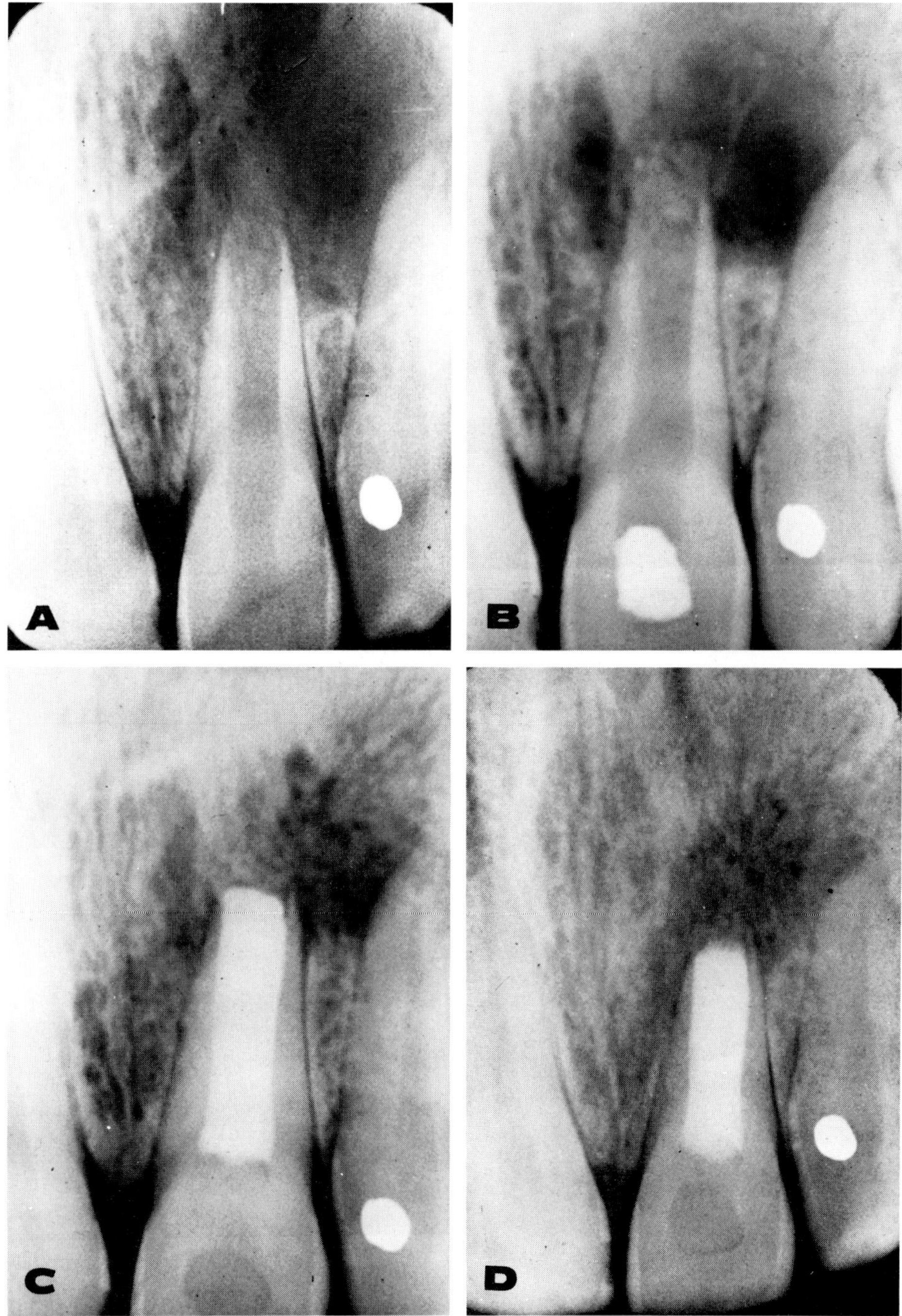

Fig. 4–71. Apexification of pulpless incisor with periapical lesion. *A,* Preoperative film. *B,* Calcium hydroxide and camphorated monochlorophenol filling canal and extruded through apex. *C,* Nine months later, canal filled with sealer, softened gutta percha, and heavy vertical condensation. No overfilling. *D,* Two-year recall. (Courtesy Dr. Raymond G. Luebke.)

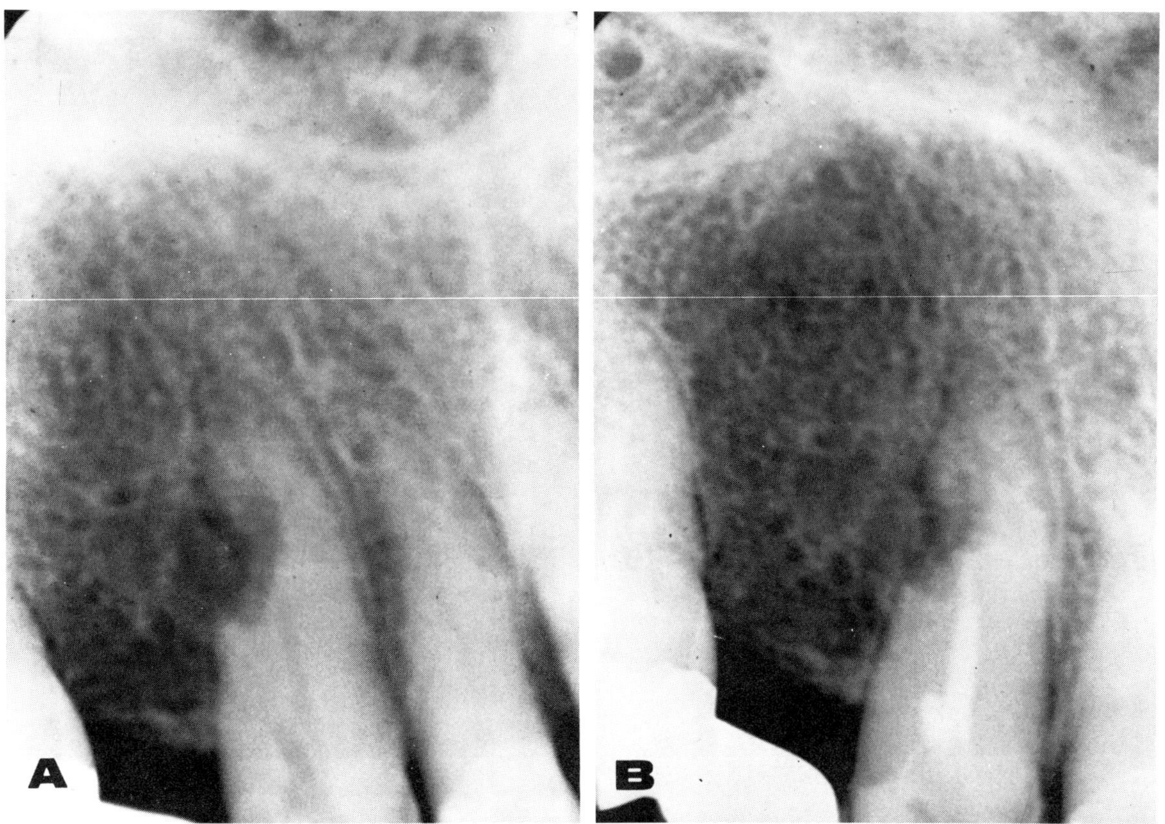

Fig. 4–72. Age is no deterrent to healing. Patient in this case was 65-year-old woman. *A,* Canine gouged and devitalized during surgery on adjacent incisor. *B,* Canal was filled with calcifying agent for nine months and then filled with gutta percha. Cementum and bone have filled in defect. (Courtesy Dr. Raymond G. Luebke.)

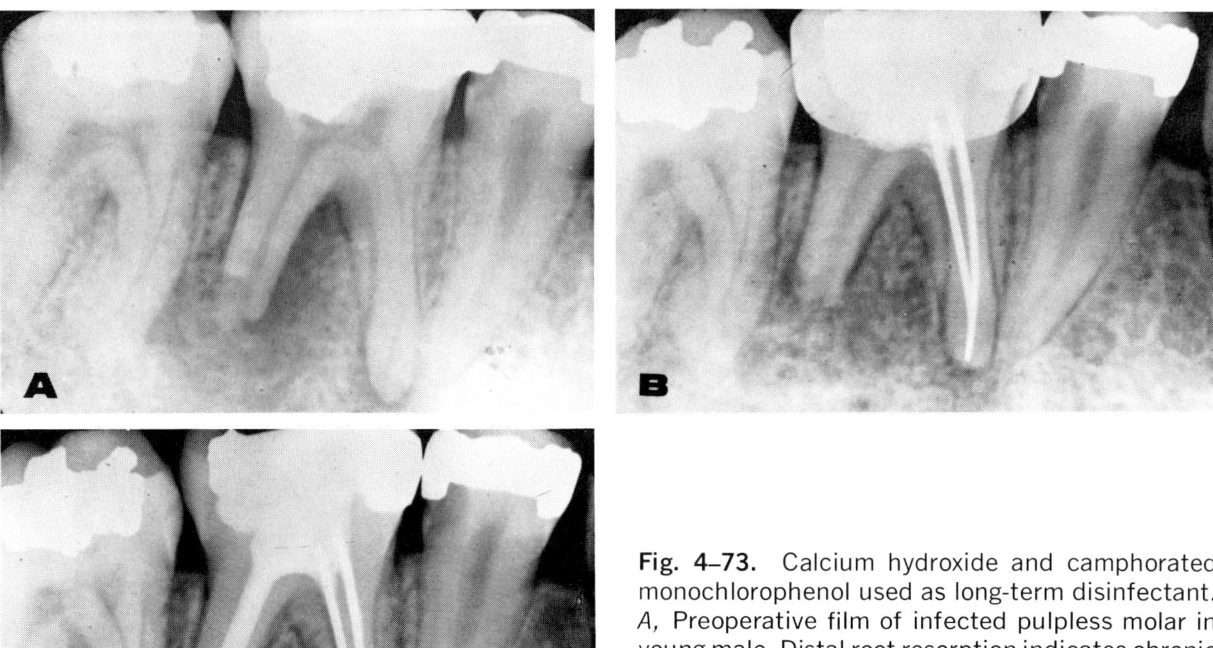

Fig. 4–73. Calcium hydroxide and camphorated monochlorophenol used as long-term disinfectant. *A,* Preoperative film of infected pulpless molar in young male. Distal root resorption indicates chronic inflammation. *B,* Fine mesial canals filled with calcium hydroxide—CMCP sealed in distal canal. *C,* After mixture was in place six months, canal was instrumented and filled. Heavy vertical pressure was used in obturation. (Courtesy Dr. Raymond G. Luebke.)

Unfortunately, the calcium hydroxide pastes are rapidly resorbed from the root canal so that complete cementification of root orifices requires paste replacement at intervals of three months for approximately one year. The obvious next development will be a biologically active "paste" with ***controlled*** resorbability that, when placed into clean canals, will induce cementification of the apical foramen, lateral canals, and any other root orifices, as it is slowly resorbed from those areas. The resorption will stop, of course, when the orifices are closed, and the bulk of the material will remain as a permanent root canal filling. It may even resume its function of cementogenesis if additional avenues of communication with the periodontal tissues appear as a result of resorption or fracture.

When this "dream" root canal filling material becomes a reality, all other materials may be abandoned. The simplicity of its use should terminate the use of the potentially dangerous pastes now being touted and eventually eliminate the tedious obturating techniques which have plagued the profession for a century.

REFERENCES

1. Dow, P., and Ingle, J. I.: Isotope determination of root canal failure. Oral Surg., *8*:1100, Oct., 1955.
2. Kuttler, Y.: Microscopic investigation of root apexes. J.A.D.A., *50*:544, May, 1955.
3. Shochat, S., and Garfunkel, A.: Neurologic complications arising from overfilled root canals. Oral Surg., *35*:684, May, 1973.
4. Nygaard-Ostby, B.: The role of the blood clot in endodontic therapy. Acta Odont. Scand., *19*:323, No. 3–4, 1961.
5. Blayney, J. R.: The medicinal treatment and the filling of root canals. J.A.D.A., *15*:239, Feb., 1928.
6. Strindberg, L. Z.: The difference in the results of pulp therapy on certain factors. Acta Odont. Scand., *14*, Supplement 21, 1956.
7. Ingle, J. I., and Zeldow, B. J.: An evaluation of mechanical instrumentation and the negative culture in endodontic therapy. J.A.D.A., *57*:471, Oct., 1958.
8. Zeldow, B. J., and Ingle, J. I.: Correlation of the positive culture to the prognosis of endodontically treated teeth: a clinical study. J.A.D.A., *66*:23, Jan., 1963.
9. Grossman, L. I.: *Endodontic Practice*. 8th Ed., Philadelphia, Lea & Febiger, 1974, p. 283.
10. Goodman, A., Schilder, H., and Aldrich, W.: The thermomechanical properties of gutta percha. II. The history and molecular chemistry of gutta percha. Oral Surg., *37*:954, June, 1974.
11. Nicholson, R. J., Casanova, F., Greenspan, J., and Stark, M.: Comparison of tissue response between a synthetic gutta percha and a natural gutta percha endodontic filler. Oral Surg., *39*:802, May, 1975.
12. Gurney, B. F., Best, E. J., and Gervasio, G.: Physical measurements of gutta percha. Oral Surg., *32*:260, Aug., 1971.
13. Marlin, J., and Schilder, H.: Physical properties of gutta percha when subjected to heat and vertical condensation. Oral Surg., *36*:872, Dec., 1973.
14. Schilder, H., Goodman, A., and Aldrich, W.: The thermomechanical properties of gutta percha. I. The compressibility of gutta percha. Oral Surg., *37*:946, June, 1974.
15. Seltzer, S., Green, D. B., Weiner, N., and De Renzis, F.: A scanning EM exam of Ag cones removed from endo treated teeth. Oral Surg., *33*:589, April, 1972.
16. Grossman, L. I.: Op cit. p. 299.
17. Richert, V. G., and Dixon, C. M.: The control of root surgery. Transactions 8th International Dent. Congress. Sec. III A, No. 9, p. 15–22, 1931.
18. Grossman, L. I.: An improved root canal cement. J.A.D.A., *56*:381, Mar., 1958.
19. Smith, D.C.: Some Observations on Endodontic Cements. Presented at meeting of Canad. and Amer. Assoc. Endodont., April, 1972.
20. Goerig, A. C., and Seymour, F. W.: Comparison of common root canal filling techniques and sealers with the simplified pressure injection method and zinc oxide eugenol as the sealing agent. J.A.D.A., *88*:826, April, 1974.
21. Kapsimalis, P., and Evans, R.: Sealing properties of endodontic filling materials using radioactive isotopes. Oral Surg., *22*:386, Sept., 1966.
22. Curson, I., and Kirk, E. E. J.: An assessment of root canal sealing cements. Oral Surg., *26*:229, Aug., 1968.
23. Weiner, H., and Schilder, H.: A comparative study of important physical properties of various root canal sealers. Oral Surg., *32*:928, Dec., 1971.
24. Sanders, S. H., and Dooley, R. J.: A comparative evaluation of polycarboxylate cement as a root canal sealer utilizing roughened and nonroughened silver points. Oral Surg., *37*:629, April, 1974.
25. Barry, G. N., and Fried, I. L.: Sealing quality of two polycarboxylate cements used as root canal sealers. J. Endodont., *1*:107, Mar., 1975.
26. McComb, D., and Smith, D. C.: Some physical and mechanical properties of root canal sealers. J.O.E., July, 1976.
27. Yee, F. S., Lugassy, A. A., and Peterson, J. N.: Filling of root canals with adhesive materials. J. Endodont., *1*:145, Apr., 1975.
28. Rising, D. W., Goldman, M., and Brayton, S. M.: Histologic appraisal of three experimental root canal filling materials. J. Endodont., *1*:172, May, 1975.

28a. Benkel, B. H., Rising, D. W., Goldman, L. B., Rosen, H., Goldman, M., and Kronman, J. H.: The use of a hydrophilic plastic as a root canal filling material. Part I. J.O.E., *2*: July, 1976.

29. TDC Laboratories, Woodland Hills, Calif. Formula for Use in Rational Endodontic Technique, 1974.
30. Sargenti, A. G.: Fifth International Conf. on Endo. Transcript, Philadelphia, 1973.

31. Spangberg, L.: Studies on root canal medicaments. Swedish Dent. J., *64*:1, 1971.
32. Spangberg, L., and Langeland, K.: Biologic effects of dental materials. Oral Surg., *35*:402, Mar., 1973.
33. Guttuso, J.: Histopathologic study of rat connective tissue response to endodontic materials. Oral Surg., *16*:7, 1963.
34. Rappaport, H. M., Lilly, G. E., and Kapsimalis, P.: Toxicity of endodontic filling materials. Oral Surg., *18*:785, Dec., 1964.
35. Spangberg, L.: Biologic effects of root canal filling materials. Oral Surg., *38*:934, Dec., 1974.
36. Friend, L. A., and Browne, R. M.: Tissue reactions to some root filling materials implanted in the bone of rabbits. Arch. Oral Biol., *14*:629, 1969.
37. Grossman, L. I., Shapiro, I. M., and Iaquinta, S.: Lead Blood Levels After Use of N2. Presented at meeting Amer. Assoc. Endodont., Apr. 18, 1974.
37a. Shapiro, I. M., Iaquinta, S., Mitchell, G.,. and Grossman, L. I.: Blood-lead levels of monkeys treated with a lead-containing (N2) root canal cement: a preliminary report. J.O.E., *1*:294, Sept., 1975.
38. Oswald, R. J., and Cohn, S. A.: Systemic distribution of lead from root canal fillings. J. Endodont., *1*:59, Feb., 1975.
39. Sargenti, A.: *Endodontics*. Locarno, Switzerland, Angelo G. Sargenti, 1973.
40. Rowe, A. H. R.: Treatment with N2 root canal sealer. Histological report of three teeth. Brit. Dent. J., *117*:27, 1964.
41. Crabb, H. S. M.: The basis of root canal therapy. Dent. Pract. and Dent. Rec., *15*:397, 1965.
42. Nygaard-Ostby, B.: Fifth Internat. Conf. on Endo., Philadelphia, 1973.
43. Snyder, D. E., Seltzer, S., and Moodnik, R.: Effects of N2 in experimental endodontic therapy. Oral Surg., *21*:635, 1966.
44. American Endodontic Society. Transactions of the A.E.S. Conf., Atlantic City, N.J., 1971.
45. Barker, B. C. W., and Lockett, B. C.: Periapical response to N2 and other paraformaldehyde compounds confined within or extruded beyond the apices of dog root canals. Dent. Pract. and Dent., Rec., *22*:370, June, 1972.
46. Rowe, A. H. R.: Treatment with N2 root canal sealer. Histological report of three teeth. Brit. Dent. J., *117*:27,
47. Langeland, K., Guttuso, J., Langeland, L., and Tobon, C.: Methods in the study of biologic responses to endodontic materials. Tissue responses to N2. Oral Surg., *27*:522, 1969.
48. Friend, L. A., and Browne, R. M.: Tissue reactions to some root canal filling materials. Brit. Dent. J., *125*:291, 1968.
49. Sargenti, A.: Cassette tape that accompanies Sargenti *Endodontics*. Locarno, Switzerland, Angelo G. Sargenti, 1973.
50. Weine, F.: Presentation to the Northwest Academy of Endodontists. Seattle, Wash., 1973.
51. Goerig, A. C., and Seymour, F. W.: Comparison of common root canal filling technique and sealers with simplified pressure injection method and zinc oxide-eugenol as the sealing agent. J.A.D.A., *88*:826, 1974.
52. Sargenti, A.: Transcript of Panel Discussion: Endodontic Sealing Techniques. Annual Meeting A.D.A., Nov. 10, 1974.
53. Gell, J., Hoepfinger, L., Steiner, D., and Yavorsky, J. D.: A Position Paper on the Sargenti Technique: Methods and Materials. Seattle, Wash., Univ. of Washington, Dept. of Endodontics, 1974.
54. Spangberg, L., and Langeland, K.: Toxicity of root canal filling materials on HeLa cells *in vitro*. Oral Surg., *35*:402, Mar., 1973.
55. Erausquin, J., and Muruzabal, M.: Tissue reactions to root canal cements in the rat molar. Oral Surg., *26*:360, Sept., 1968.
56. Erausquin, J., and Muruzabal, M.: Necrosis of the periodontal ligament in root canal overfilling. J. Dent. Res., *45*:1084, Jul.-Aug., 1966.
57. Erausquin, J., and Muruzabal, M.: Root canal filling with zinc oxide-eugenol cement in the rat molars. Oral Surg., *24*:548, Oct., 1967.
58. Barker, B. C. W., and Lockett, B. C.: Reaction of dog tissue to immediate root filling with zinc oxide-eugenol cement and gutta percha. Aust. Dent. J., *17*:1, 1972.
59. Erausquin, J., and Muruzabal, M.: Response to periapical tissues in the rat molar to root canal fillings with Diaket and AH–26. Oral Surg., *21*:786, 1966.
60. Seltzer, S., Soltanoff, W., and Smith, J.: Periapical tissue reactions to root canal instrumentation beyond the apex and root canal fillings short of and beyond the apex. Oral Surg., *36*:725, Nov., 1973.
61. Castagnola, L., and Orlay, H. G.: Treatment of gangrene of the pulp by the Walkhoff method. Brit. Dent. J., *93*:92, Aug., 1952.
62. Nygaard-Ostby, B.: Uber die gewebsveranderungen im apikalen paradentium des menschen nach verschiedenartigen eingriffen in den wurzelkanalen. Skritter utgitt av det Norske Videnskaps-Akademi 1 Oslo. I. Mat.-Nat. Klasse. 1939. Nr. 4.
63. Maisto, O. A.: Personal communication.
64. Gutierrez, J. H., and Gigoux, C.: Macroscopic and microscopic investigations on results of mechanical preparation on root canals of first permanent molars. Personal communication, 1972.
65. Weine, F.: *Endodontic Therapy*. St. Louis, C. V. Mosby Co., 1972.
66. Schilder, H.: Filling root canals in three dimensions. Dent. Clin. No. Amer., pp. 723–44, Nov., 1967.
67. Coolidge, E.D.: Clinical pathology of treatment of the dental pulp. In *Dental Therapeutics*. 2nd Ed., Philadelphia, Lea & Febiger, 1946, p. 134.
68. Goldman, M.: Evaluation of 2 filling methods for root canals. J. Endodont., *1*:69, Feb., 1975.
69. Crump, M. C., and Natkin, E.: Relationship of broken root canal instruments to endodontic case prognosis: a clinical investigation. J.A.D.A., *80*:1341, June, 1970.
70. Sampeck, A. J.: Personal communication, 1965.
71. Adams, W. R.: Broken Instruments: A Study in Leakage. Master's Thesis, Indiana University, 1974.
72. Simpson, T. H., and Natkin, E.: Gutta percha techniques for filling canals of young permanent teeth after induction of apical root formation. J. Brit. Endodont. Soc., *3*:59, Summer, 1972.
73. Callahan, J. R.: Resin solution for the sealing of the

dental tubuli and as an adjuvant in the filling of root canals. J. Allied Dent. Soc., *9*:53, Mar., 1914.
74. Johnston, H. B.: The principle of diffusion applied to the Callahan method of pulp canal filling. Dent. Summary, *43*:743, Sept., 1927.
75. Wallentin, R.: Presented at meeting of Amer. Assoc. Endodont., San Diego, 1974.
76. Nygaard-Ostby, B.: Om vevsforandringer i det apikale paradentium hos mennesket ved notbehandling. Skrifter Utgitt av det Norski Videnskaps-Akademi I Oslo. I Mat.-Naticov. Klasse. 1944. No. 2, p. 58.
77. Maisto, O. A.: Personal communication.
78. Widerman, F. H., Eames, W. B., and Serene, T. B.: The physical and biologic properties of cavit. J.A.D.A., *82*:378, Feb., 1971.
79. Marosky, J. E.: *In Vitro* Studies on Marginal Leakage of Temporary Sealing Materials Assessed by Ca45. Presented at meeting of Amer. Assoc. Endodont., Apr. 25, 1975.
80. Feldman, M. H.: To remove broken reamer or bur from a root. Outlook, *1*:254, 1914.
81. Glick, D.: Personal communication.
82. Coolidge, E. D., and Kesel, R. G.: *Endodontology*. 2nd Ed., Philadelphia, Lea & Febiger, 1956.
83. Kaiser, J. H.: Root End Closure by Calcification. Presented at meeting of Amer. Assoc. Endodont., 1962.
84. Steiner, J. C., and Van Hassel, H. J.: Experimental root apexification in primates. Oral Surg., *31*:409, Mar., 1971.
85. Koenigs, J. F., Heller, A. L., Brilliant, D. J., Melfi, R. C., and Driskell, T. D.: Induced apical closure of permanent teeth in adult primates using a resorbable form of tricalcium phosphate ceramic. J. Endodont., *1*:102, Mar., 1975.
86. Nevins, A. J., Finklestein, F., Borden, B. G., and Moodnik, R.: Revitalization of pulpless open apex teeth in Rhesus monkeys using collagen-calcium phosphate gel. J.O.E., *2*:159, June, 1976.

Chapter 5

Plan of Treatment

Previous chapters have provided details of endodontic cavity preparation and filling, as well as the preliminary and ancillary steps necessary to achieve success. The neophyte in endodontics can easily become lost in the wealth of detail necessary in total treatment.

In order to follow a treatment plan systematically, an outline for ***conventional*** endodontic therapy is presented. For the beginner, this outline should serve as a checklist, each point reminding him of the detail necessary to execute that step. The clinician then moves on to the next step; and the next.

Just as any other technique is ingrained by repetition, endodontic procedures also become second nature by constant practice. This outline of treatment will then no longer be needed. It is recommended that one week be allowed between appointments.

FIRST APPOINTMENT

History and Examination

1. History
   a. chief complaint
   b. present illness
   c. past history of oral problems
   d. past medical history
2. Examination
   a. visual
   b. percussion and palpation
   c. roentgenographic
   d. electric vitality testing
   e. thermal vitality testing
   f. if necessary, the test-cavity and anesthetic testing

Initial Treatment

1. Anesthetize if necessary
2. Place the rubber dam
3. Lay out equipment:
   a. arrange the towel kit contents
   b. position the instrument case
   c. place appropriate burs in the contra-angles
4. Disinfect the operating field
5. Prepare the access cavity

If the Pulp is Vital:

6. Establish the length of the tooth
7. Perform a pulpectomy
8. Cleanse and shape the canals to appropriate size, irrigate
9. If time permits:
   a. test the trial point
   b. fill the canal(s)

If the Pulp is Necrotic or Canal is Open to Saliva:

6*a.* Take a bacteriologic culture
7*a.* Irrigate repeatedly with sodium hypochlorite
8*a.* Carefully remove the canal contents with paper points
9*a.* *DO NOT ROUTINELY ENLARGE THE CANAL WITH INSTRUMENTS*
10*a.* Place intracanal medicament
11*a.* Insert temporary filling
12*a.* Remove rubber dam and reappoint the patient in seven days

SECOND APPOINTMENT

1. Anesthetize if necessary
2. Place rubber dam

3. Lay out equipment
4. Disinfect the operating field
5. Remove the temporary filling
6. Examine the previous bacteriologic culture

If the Culture is Positive:

7. Reculture the canal contents
8. Irrigate, leaving the irrigant in the canal
9. Enlarge the canal(s) to appropriate size
10. Re-irrigate
11. Place intracanal medicament
12. Insert temporary filling
13. Remove rubber dam and reappoint the patient in seven days

If the Culture is Negative:

7b. Irrigate, leaving the irrigant in the canal
8b. Enlarge the canal(s) to appropriate size
9b. Re-irrigate and dry the canal(s)
10b. Select and test the primary filling point(s)
11b. Fill the canal(s) and place the final restoration

THIRD APPOINTMENT (IF NECESSARY)

1. Anesthetize if necessary
2. Place rubber dam
3. Lay out equipment
4. Disinfect the operating field
5. Remove the temporary filling
6. Examine the previous bacteriologic culture

If the Culture is Positive:

7. Check the walls of the preparation or remaining restorations to determine if leakage of saliva has caused contamination. Correct if necessary.
8. Reculture the canal contents
9. Irrigate with sodium hypochlorite and dry with paper points
10. If possible, enlarge the canal(s) to a larger size
11. Change to a different intracanal medicament
12. Insert a new temporary filling
13. Remove the rubber dam and reappoint the patient in seven days.

If the Culture is Negative:

7c. Irrigate with sodium hypochlorite and dry with paper points
8c. Select and test the primary filling point(s)
9c. Fill the canal(s) and place final restoration

FOURTH APPOINTMENT (IF NECESSARY)

1. Anesthetize if necessary
2. Place rubber dam
3. Lay out equipment
4. Disinfect the operating field
5. Remove the temporary filling
6. Examine the previous bacteriologic culture

If the Culture is Positive:

7. Re-examine the tooth for saliva leakage
8. Irrigate with sodium hypochlorite
9. "Freshen" the walls with instruments
10. Re-irrigate
11. Remedicate with a different intracanal medicament
12. Replace all of the coronal fillings
13. Remove the rubber dam and reappoint the patient in seven days.

If the Culture is Negative:

7d. Irrigate with sodium hypochlorite and dry with paper points
8d. Select and test the primary filling point(s)
9d. Fill the canal(s) and place the final restoration

It is obvious that the most common cause of repeated positive bacteriologic cultures is salivary leakage through a defective temporary filling or failing proximal restoration. It is imperative that the pulpless tooth be properly restored following root canal therapy. The reader is referred to Chapter 18 for a discussion of restoration procedure.

The step-by-step outline of periradicular surgery is thoroughly discussed in Chapter 15.

Chapter 6

Histology and Physiology of the Dental Pulp

ALFRED L. OGILVIE and L. DANIEL SCHAEFFER

As the principal source of pain within the mouth and as the major site of attention in endodontic treatment, the pulp warrants direct inspection. By its very location it defies this in the usual course of events. There are exceptions. Occasionally when required to deal with the problem of an accidentally fractured cusp, the dentist will be afforded a glimpse of the normal pulp. He will note a pink, coherent soft tissue, obviously dependent on its normal hard dentin shell for protection and hence, once exposed, extremely sensitive to all contact (Fig. 6–1).

When such tissue is removed en masse from a tooth in the course, say, of vital pulpectomy, the dentist gains a reinforced view of the pulp. Here is connective tissue obviously rich in fluid and highly vascular. In a matter of moments after exposure to air, the

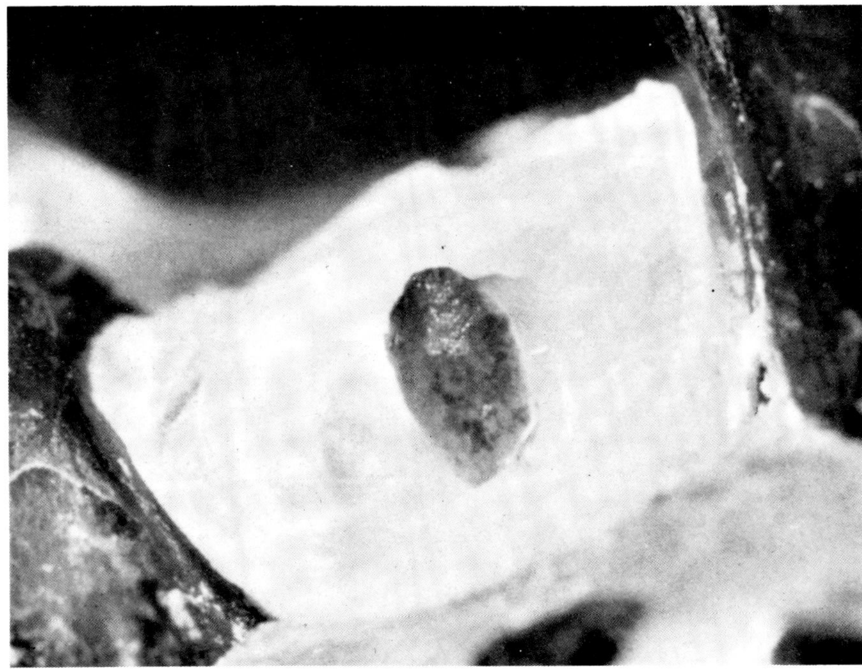

Fig. 6–1. Exposed pulp of right human mandibular premolar. Living coronal pulp is seen after removal of overlying enamel and dentin. (From Beveridge, E. E.: Oral Surg., *19*:655, May, 1965.)

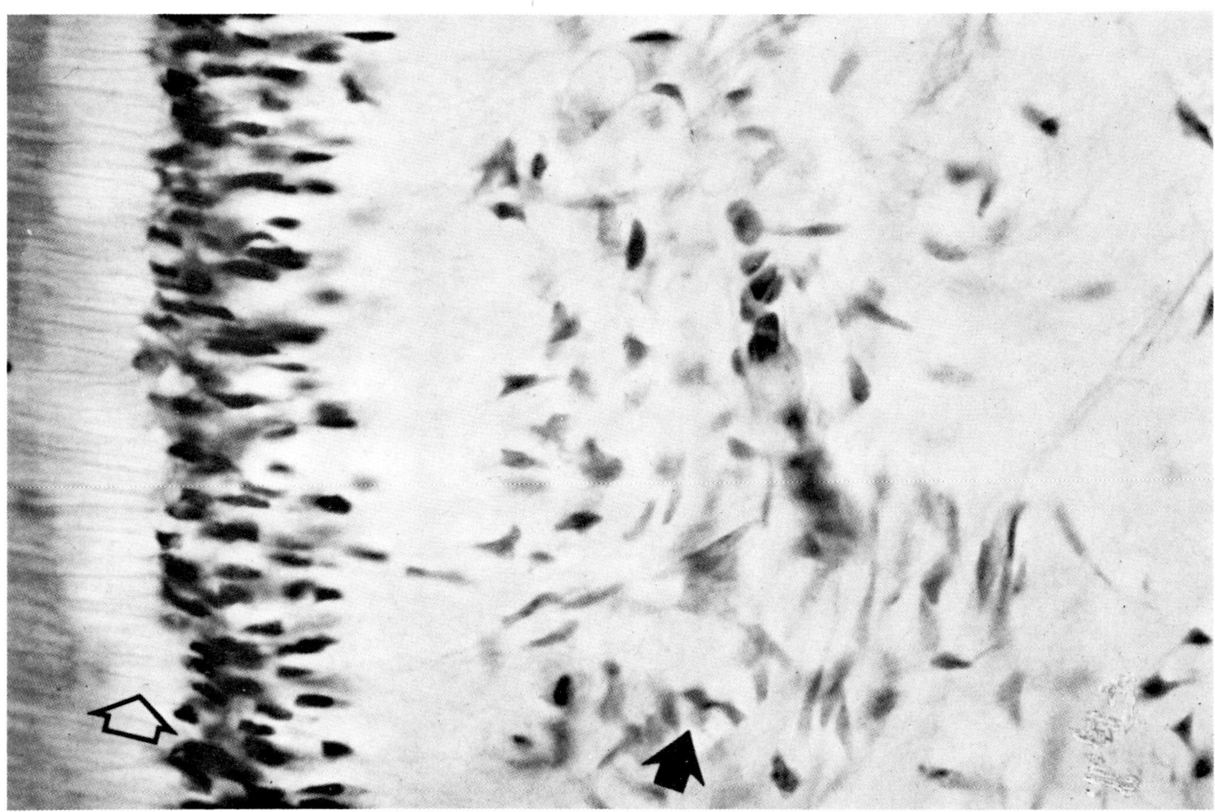

Fig. 6–2. Structural "layers" on periphery of normal human pulp. From left to right are calcifying dentin, predentin (*open arrow*), columnar odontoblast cells, "cell-free" zone of Weil, "cell-rich" zone (*black arrow*) and dominant stroma of pulp. (Orban collection.)

appearance and volume of the tissue change as the fluid evaporates. It is apparent that this is a tissue adapted, therefore, to live in health in one locale and that alone—the protected interior of the tooth.

As the price of this protection, the pulp contributes to a close symbiosis. The way in which the normal pulp relates to its immediate environment can be best explained by a review of its own morphology and that of the tissues with which it is confluent, namely the dentin and the periodontal ligament. In general perspective, the pulp demonstrates a homogeneity in its blend of cells, intercellular substance, fiber elements, vessels, and nerves. On the periphery, however, structural "layers" are apparent. These are usually evident in a medium-power photomicrograph (Fig. 6–2). Next to the predentin lies the palisade of columnar odontoblast cells. Central to these is the subodontoblastic layer termed the "cell-free" zone of Weil.[1,2] Plexuses of capillaries and nerve fibers ramify in this subodontoblastic layer. Deep to it again is the "cell-rich" zone, which blends in turn with the dominant stroma of the pulp. The "cell-rich" zone consists primarily of undifferentiated mesenchymal cells, which sustain the population of odontoblasts by proliferation and differentiation.[3]

These zones vary in their prominence from tooth to tooth and from area to area on the pulp margin of the same tooth. The ***"cell-free" zone of Weil,*** for instance, is usually indistinct or absent in the embryonic pulp and at any time when dentin formation is active.[2] It tends to become increasingly prominent as the pulp ages. Both the "cell-free" zone and the deeper "cell-rich" zone are less constant and less prominent near the root apex.

FUNCTIONS

The pulp lives for the dentin and the dentin lives by the grace of the pulp. Few marriages in nature are marked by a greater affinity. Thus it is with the pulp and the four functions which it serves, namely: the formation of dentin, the nutrition of dentin (and

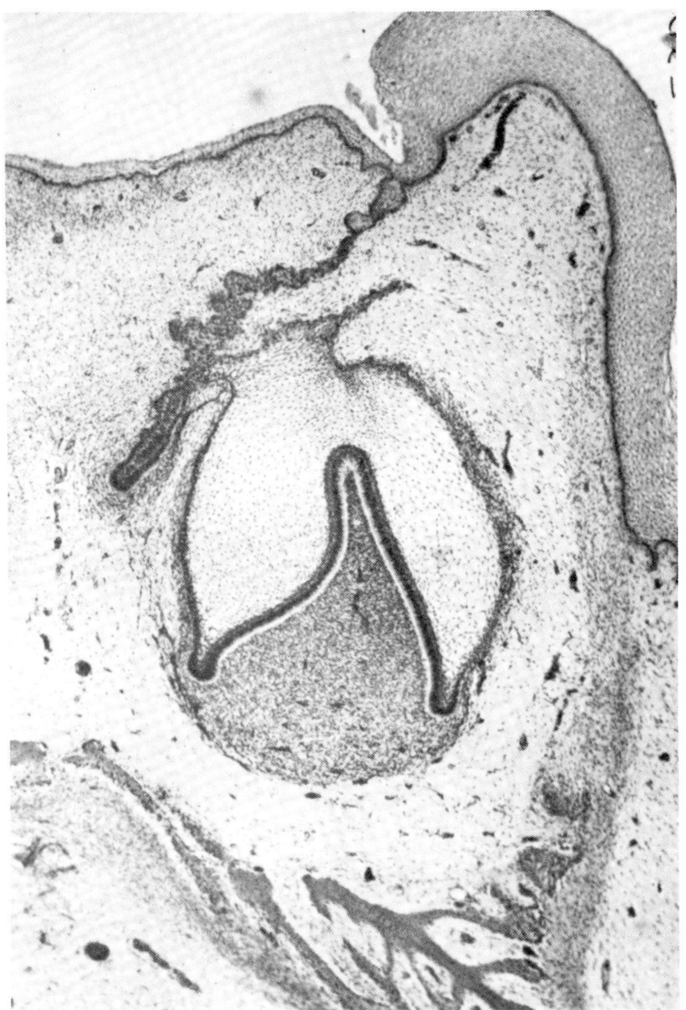

Fig. 6–3. Interaction of ectoderm with mesoderm which initiates process of dentin formation. Ectodermal cells of inner dental (enamel) epithelium stimulate odontoblasts at incisal edge of dental papilla to production of first dentin. Anteroposterior section through lower anterior tooth germ. Bell stage of tooth development. Human fetus—105 mm., 14 weeks. (Orban collection.)

enamel), the innervation of the tooth, and the defense of the tooth. ***Formation of the dentin*** is the primary task of the pulp in both sequence and importance. From the mesodermal aggregation known as the dental papilla arises the specialized cell layer of odontoblasts, adjacent and internal to the inner layer of the ectodermal enamel organ. Ectoderm interacts with mesoderm,[4] and the odontoblasts initiate the process of dentin formation (Fig. 6–3). Once under way, dentin production continues rapidly until the main form of the tooth crown and root are created. Then the process slows, though seldom to a complete halt. The ***nutrition*** of the dentin is a function of the odontoblast cells in the aggregate. It is established through the network of tubuli within the dentin which the odontoblasts have created to contain their terminal processes. ***Innervation*** of the tooth is linked to the dentinal tubuli, to the odontoblast processes within them, to the cell bodies of the odontoblasts in turn, and thus to the sensory nerves of the pulp proper.

Defense of the tooth and the pulp itself is served basically by the creation of new dentin in the face of irritants. This the pulp can do well by galvanizing odontoblasts into action or by producing new odontoblasts to form the needed hard tissue barrier (Fig. 6–4). Characteristics of the defense are several. The dentin formation is localized. The dentin is produced at a rate faster than that seen at sites of nonstimulated secondary dentin formation. Microscopically, too, this dentin is often different from secondary dentin and has earned several designations (irritant dentin, ***reparative dentin,*** irregular dentin, osteodentin). The type and amount of dentin created during this defensive response appear to depend on numerous factors. How urgent is the assault? Is it chemical, thermal, or bacterial? How long has the irritation been applied? What is the status of the pulp at the time of response and during it? A second defensive reaction, namely inflammation within the pulp at the site of injury, should not be ignored. This phenomenon will be explored in more detail in Chapter 8.

DEVELOPMENT

The pulp of a given tooth develops in response to the presence of the tooth bud of that tooth along the course of the dental lamina. Ectodermal lamina gives rise to ectodermal bud. Each bud promotes a mesodermal cell concentration called the ***dental papilla*** at the genetically determined site. The sequence is a familiar one throughout mammalian embryology.[5,6]

Ectoderm also determines the ***form*** of the central mesodermal mass, a pattern well illustrated by the growing tooth. The ectodermal tooth bud first changes its own form into a more specialized cap-shaped ***dental*** organ (enamel organ). The mesoderm beneath is shaped in turn to fit this ectodermal mold and thereby becomes the true ***dental papilla.*** Maturation of the dental papilla proceeds

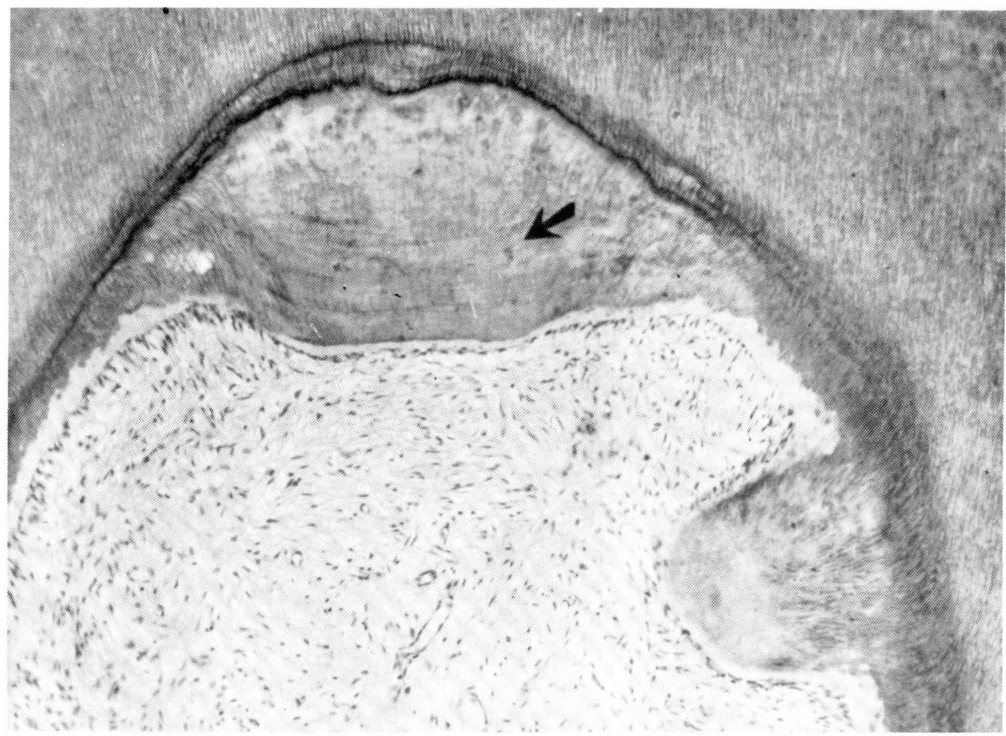

Fig. 6–4. Reparative dentin (*arrow*) on coronal aspect of pulp. Human primary tooth. (Orban collection.)

only slightly behind that of the enamel organ. By the time the enamel organ at its most coronal level can be recognized as a four-layered structure, the papilla is also greatly altered. A rich network of embryonic blood vessels appears. Reticular fibrils abound and are increasingly supplemented by collagen bundles. More mature cells, like those that can synthesize collagen, are present in growing numbers. However, the entry of nerves into this future pulp is delayed[7] (Fig. 6–5).

The lag in structural specialization of the dental papilla, as contrasted to the development of the enamel organ, is only evident up to a certain stage. Once the inner enamel epithelium is formed, the odontoblasts outreach their ectodermal neighbors, produce dentin at the cusp tip, and thereby become the first cells to produce calcified tooth structure. Only when dentin has been formed do the ameloblasts appear and produce enamel. Likewise, in the forming root, it is the presence of the first dentin against the epithelial root sheath that signals the retreat of the ectoderm. These phenomena are basic to the establishment of the dentinoenamel and dentinocemental junctions. They implement the genetic message with regard to both the external shape of the tooth and the form of the pulp.

Maturation of the dental papilla moves like a tide from the tooth's most coronal levels to its apex. The lateral presence of the enamel organ or root sheath precipitates the differentiation of odontoblasts and, before long, the formation of dentin by them. At this stage the cellularity and vascularity of the subodontoblastic plexus are noteworthy. Nerve fibers are absent in the vicinity of the forming dentin. Gradually, as the coronal and root dentin thicken, sensory nerve elements enter the papilla and approach the coronal dentin.[8] Concurrently, autonomic vasomotor fibers enter the papilla and establish their linkages with the different vessels. By the time a tooth erupts, the pulp within could arbitrarily be termed "mature." The predominance of cell over fiber has disappeared, the bulk of the coronal dentin and much of the root dentin have been formed, and the adult nerve-blood vessel pattern has been established.

ANATOMY

The living pulp, as we have seen, creates and shapes its own locale in the center of the tooth. We call this home of the pulp the ***pulp cavity*** and speak of its two main parts as the ***pulp chamber*** and the ***root canal.*** Clinical implications of pulp form and varia-

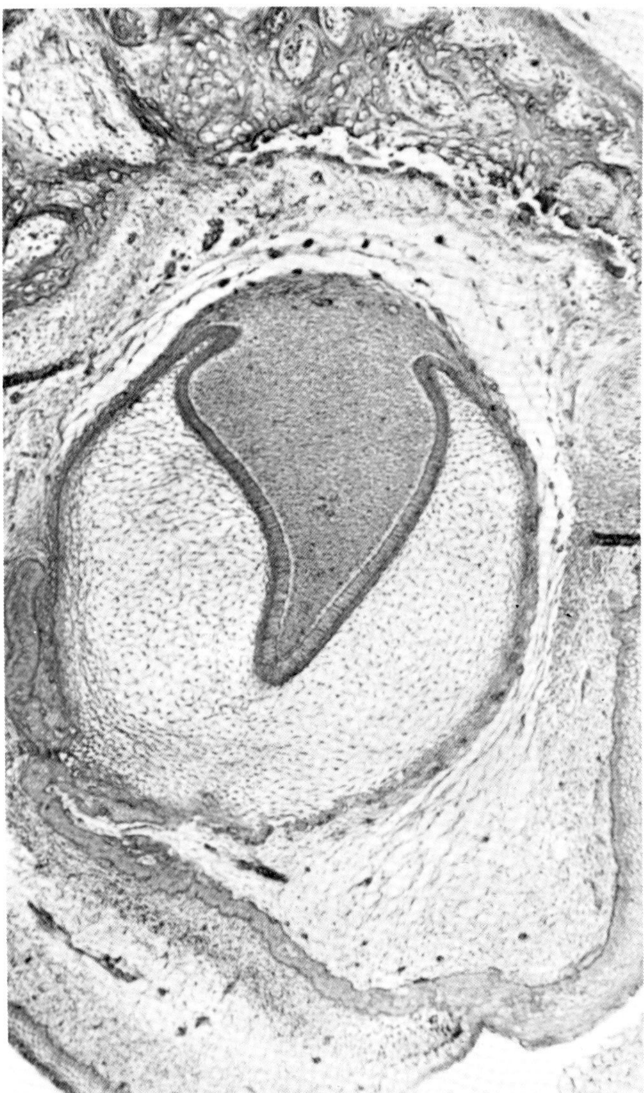

Fig. 6–5. Absence of nerve fiber bundles in early dental pulp (dental papilla). Primary *maxillary* canine tooth. Nerve fiber bundles are evident in cross section as dark bodies apical to dental papilla yet within dental follicle. Below, in dental papilla itself, no nerve elements are stained. Human fetus: 19 weeks. Palmgren nerve stain. (From Arwill, T., and Haeggstrōms, I.: Innervation of the Teeth, Tr. Royal School of Dentistry (Stockholm), *3,* 1958.)

tion have been extensively covered in Chapter 3. Indeed, the key word in an understanding of the gross anatomy of the pulp is ***variation.*** Equally evident in any study of the pulp is the ***reduction in size*** of the chamber and canals with ***age.*** Soon it becomes apparent that aging supplements the size, creating new variations.

Pulp Chamber

The pulp chamber of a tooth at the time of eruption reflects the external form of the enamel. Anatomy is less sharply defined, but the cusp form is there. Often the pulp will suggest its original perimeter (and threaten its future) by leaving a filament of itself, the ***pulp horn,*** within the coronal dentin. A specific stimulus such as caries will lead to the formation of reparative dentin on the roof or wall of the chamber adjacent to the stimulus (Fig. 6–6). The chamber undergoes steady reduction in size, of course, on all surfaces as secondary dentin is produced. Where permanent posterior teeth are con-

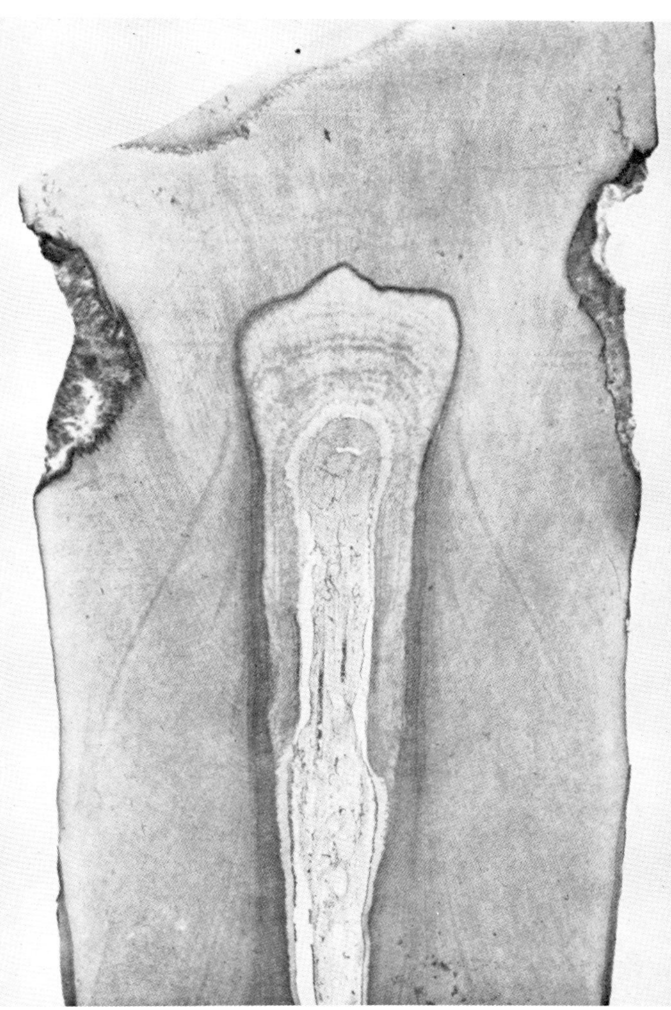

Fig. 6–6. Extensive formation of reparative dentin on roof and walls of pulp chamber in response to specific stimuli. There is deep carious penetration of dentin on both mesial and distal surfaces. Marked wear of incisal portion of crown is also evident. Elongated clear spaces on margin of pulp are artifacts. (Orban collection.)

cerned, at least one investigator has observed either an equal distribution of secondary dentin on all walls of the chamber or a maximum on the roof.[9] The prevailing view has been that dentin forms most rapidly on the pulp floor and roof.[10,11]

The ***pulp stone*** provides the most unpredictable factor in the reduction of pulp size. The potential size, form, and numbers of this calcified body which may arise cannot be predicted with certainty. Stones may reach such proportions that they replace all but a minimum of the original soft tissue. Infrequently they may merge with secondary or reparative dentin and thereby become, in effect, an outgrowth of the wall.

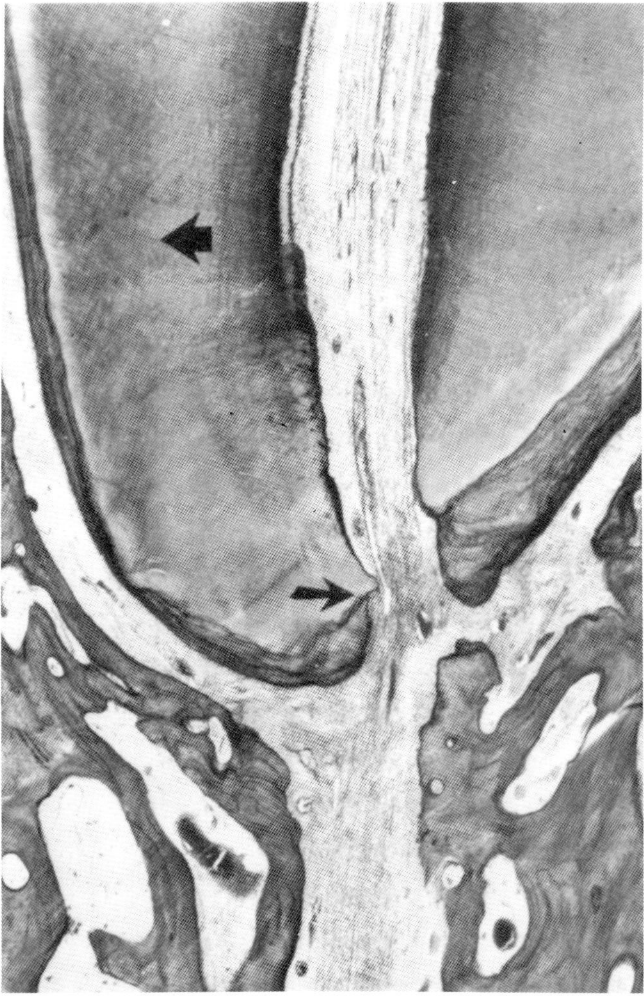

Fig. 6–7. Features often noted in normal yet aging tooth: deviation of apical foramen as result of mesial physiologic migration of the tooth (*top arrow*) (selective resorption and apposition of root structure have changed position of the apex); narrowing of apical third of root canal by increments of secondary dentin; flaring of apical foramen from its smallest diameter at dentinocemental junction (*bottom arrow*) to its greatest diameter at cemental surface; abundance of collagen fibers in the radicular pulp. (From Matsumiya, S.: *Atlas of Oral Pathology,* Tokyo Dental College Press, 1955.)

Root Canal

An unbroken train of connective tissue passes from the periodontal ligament through the root canal(s) to the pulp chamber. Each root is served by at least one such pulp corridor. Actually the root canal is subject to the same pulp-induced changes as the chamber. Its diameter becomes narrowed, rapidly at first as the foramen takes shape in the post-eruptive months, but with increasing slowness once the apex is defined. A root canal of an old tooth is seldom completely occluded. Dentin apposition or a discrete pulp stone may obliterate the entrance to the canal. Apical to this obstruction, the canal remains patent; much reduced from its initial diameter but still discernible as it follows the curvature of the root.

The shape of a canal, "to a large degree, conforms to the shape of the root. A few canals are round and tapering, but many are elliptical, broad and thin."[12] A curve at the end of the root means almost invariably that the canal follows this curve.[13]

"Roots that are round and cone-shaped usually contain only one canal, but roots that are elliptical and have flat or concave surfaces more frequently have two canals than one."[14]

As both Orban and Meyer have described, the foramen can change in shape and location because of functional influence on the tooth (*e.g.,* tongue pressure, occlusal pressure).[15,16] The pattern that develops is the reverse of the changes in the alveolar bone around the tooth. Resorption occurs on the wall of the foramen farthest from the force, apposition on the wall nearest. The net result is a deviation of the foramen ***away*** from the true apex (Fig. 6–7).

Foramens

The anatomy of the root apex is determined by the location of blood vessels. When the tooth is young and just erupting, for example, the foramen is an open delta. Islands of dentin may have appeared within the main stream of connective tissue where the root sheath has induced them, but these islands are widely separated. Progressively the main channel narrows. The primary vessels and nerves, though never directly threatened, come to have a restricted passage. Increments of cementum contribute to this continuous modeling. So varied are the possibilities of vascular branching at the apex that prediction of the number of foramens in a given tooth becomes impossible.

We do know that the incidence of multiple foramens is high.[13,17] The majority of single-rooted teeth have a single canal which terminates in the single foramen.[18] Less often they possess an apical delta, which terminates in a major channel and one or more collateral exits. Occasionally the delta has several channels of equal magnitude. Root canals of the multirooted teeth, on the other hand, tend to

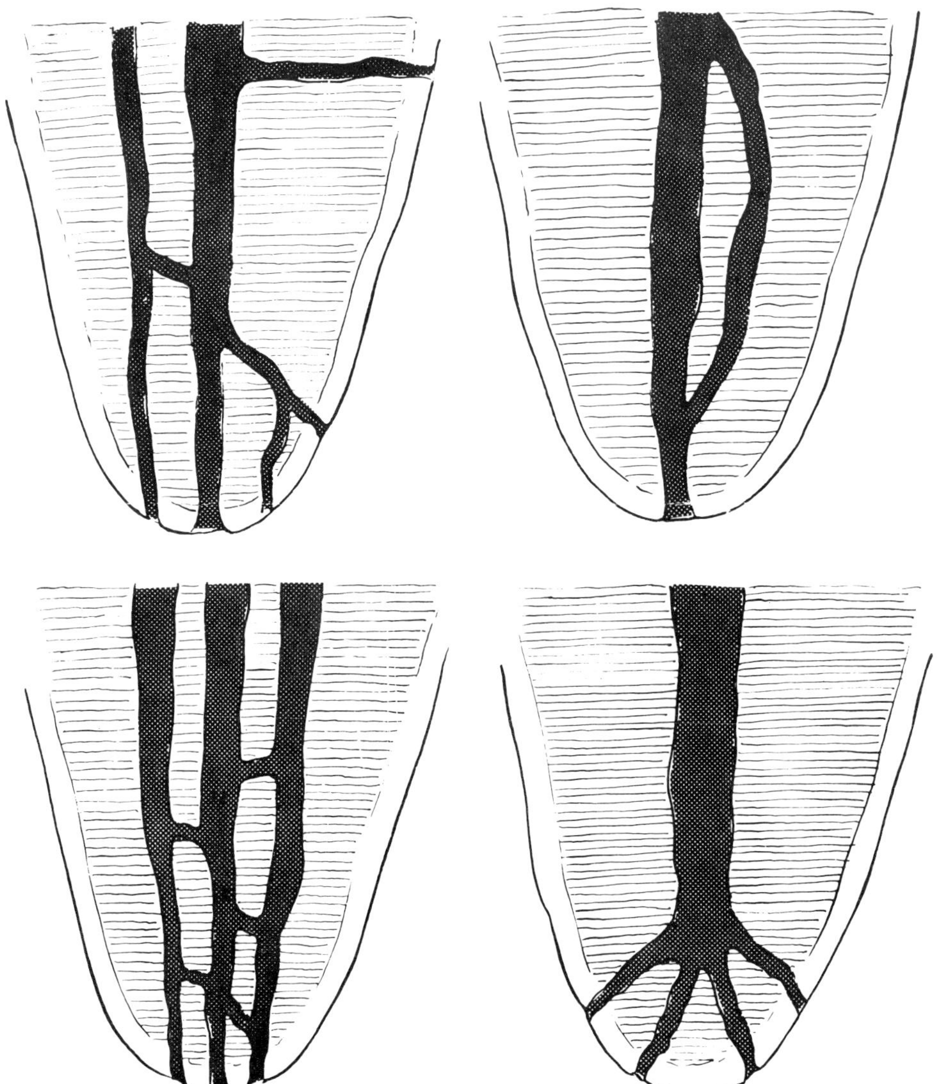

Fig. 6–8. Some patterns of root canal distribution in human tooth.

Upper Left: Two vertical root canals, wider one being principal canal, the other a minor canal. Principal canal gives off two accessory canals to root surface and link to minor canal. Both vertical canals make independent exit at apex.

Upper Right: Single branching of principal canal. Minor branch rejoins principal canal near apex. There is one apical foramen.

Lower Left: So-called "reticular canals." Three vertical canals are present with lateral interconnections.

Lower Right: Wide branching of principal canal near apex, thereby forming distinct delta. When several branches terminate on curved apex, as in this case, they all make somewhat lateral exit. (From Pucci, F. M., and Reig, R.: *Conductos Radiculares,* Vol. 1, Montevideo, Uruguay, Casa Barriero y Ramos S. A., 1944.)

have a more complex apical anatomy. Multiple foramens are the rule rather than the exception. When accessory foramens are found in one root of a multirooted tooth, the other roots usually have similar conditions.[13] Moreover, because the individual roots of such teeth often contain two or even three canals, a new factor is introduced. These canals can merge but they need not and often do not merge before making their exit. Instead, each may leave the root independently. Lateral branching of the emergent canals within the apical area is a common finding, again because the pre-existing vessels were so linked. It is well to recall that the outer surface of the root apex is convex. Consequently, when there are multiple foramens, most of these make a somewhat lateral exit. The drawings of Pucci illustrate these aspects well[19] (Fig. 6–8).

It is also well to recall that cementum forms in abundance at the root apex. Because of the apposition of new layers of cementum, the foramen anatomy is by no means constant. The center of the foramen tends to deviate increasingly from the apical center.[20] Many root canals have two apical diameters. The minor diameter at the level of the dentinocemental junction can be as small as one-half that of the major diameter at the surface.[13,21] Cementum deposit, one can readily see, tends to produce an apical funnel of increasing divergence.[20] Contributing to this is the secondary dentin formation which narrows the dentinal orifice of the canal to an irreducible minimum (see Fig. 6–7).

Stereomicroscopic analysis of some 700 posterior root apices showed that at least half of the major foramens take eccentric positions which deviate as far as 2 mm. from the apex. Accessory foramens, on the average, were found to be located twice the distance of the major foramens from the vertex[63] (Fig. 6–9).

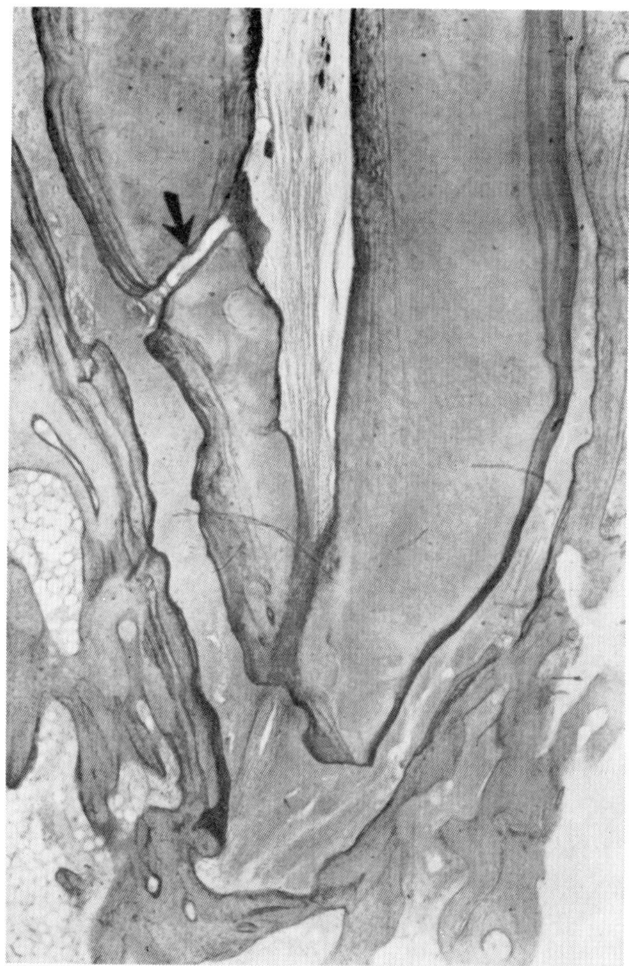

Fig. 6–9. Accessory foramen (*arrow*) in mandibular anterior tooth. On the average, accessory foramens are at least twice as far as major foramen is from vertex of tooth. (Orban collection.) (From Sicher, H.: *Oral Histology and Embryology,* 5th Ed., St. Louis, C. V. Mosby Co., 1962.)

Accessory Canals

Communication of pulp and periodontal ligament is not limited to the apical region. ***Accessory canals*** are found at every level. Recent vascular perfusion studies have demonstrated vividly how numerous and persistent these tributaries are[22,23] (Fig. 6–10). A certain number in time become sealed off by cementum and/or dentin, but many remain. The majority appear to be encountered in the apical half of the root (Fig. 6–11). Some have been observed to pass directly from pulp chamber to periodontal ligament (Fig. 6–12).

One of the common areas in which accessory canals appear is the furcation area of molar teeth. Burch and Hulen found that 76% of all molars presented openings in the furcation areas—2.5 foramens per furcation in maxillary molars and 2.14 in mandibular molars.[24] They did not state how many of these accessory canals were patent from pulp to PDL.

Vertucci and his associates injected dye into the pulp space of molars, and in 46% of the cases, the dye came through the furca canals.[25] Lowman and his colleagues did essentially the same thing under vacuum and found that the dye appeared in 59% of the furcas.[26]

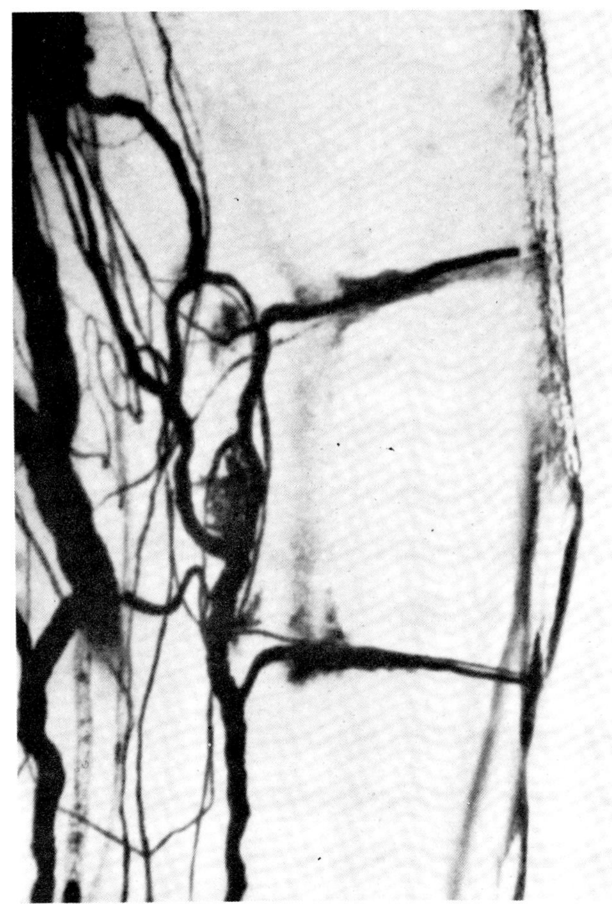

Fig. 6–10. Two accessory canals in buccal root of human permanent molar tooth. Canals can be seen extending from main root canal on left to root surface on right. Each accessory canal carries pair of vessels, one larger than the other. Smaller vessel resembles artery and larger vessel resembles vein. Vascular perfusion. (From Kramer, I. R. H.: Arch. Oral Biol., *2*:177, 1960.)

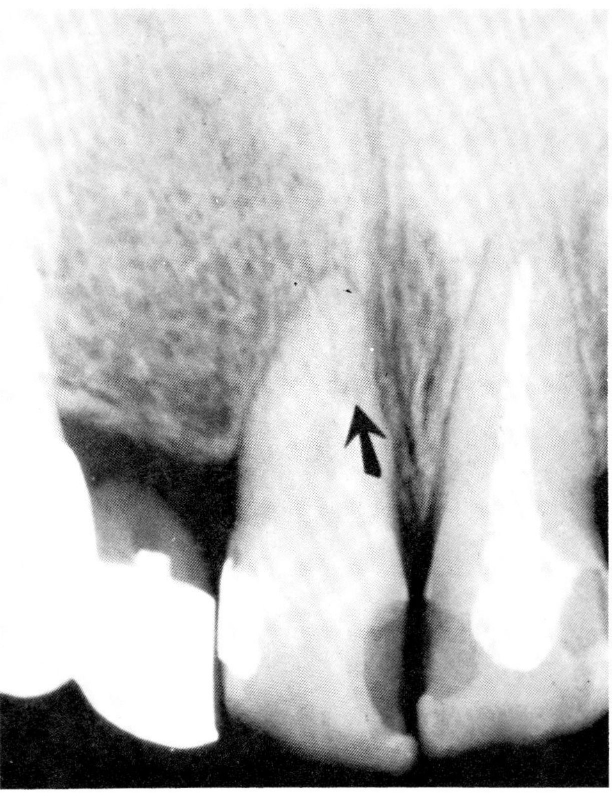

Fig. 6–11. Radiograph of untreated maxillary central incisor. Accessory canal (*arrow*) in apical half of root.

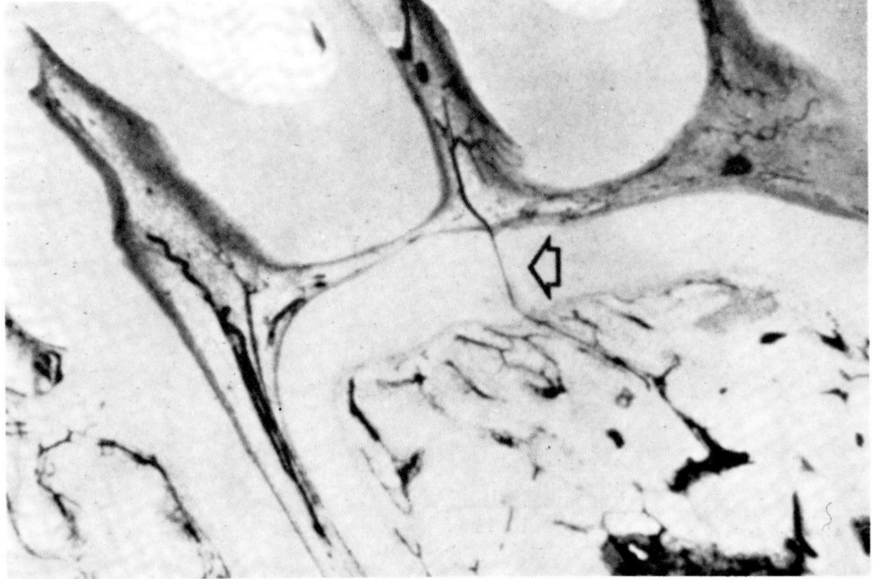

Fig. 6–12. Accessory canal (*arrow*) providing communication between coronal pulp (*above*) and periodontal ligament (*below*) in bifurcation area. Vascular perfusion. Lower molar of rat. (Courtesy Dr. D. Walter Cohen and Dr. Jack Piekarsky.)

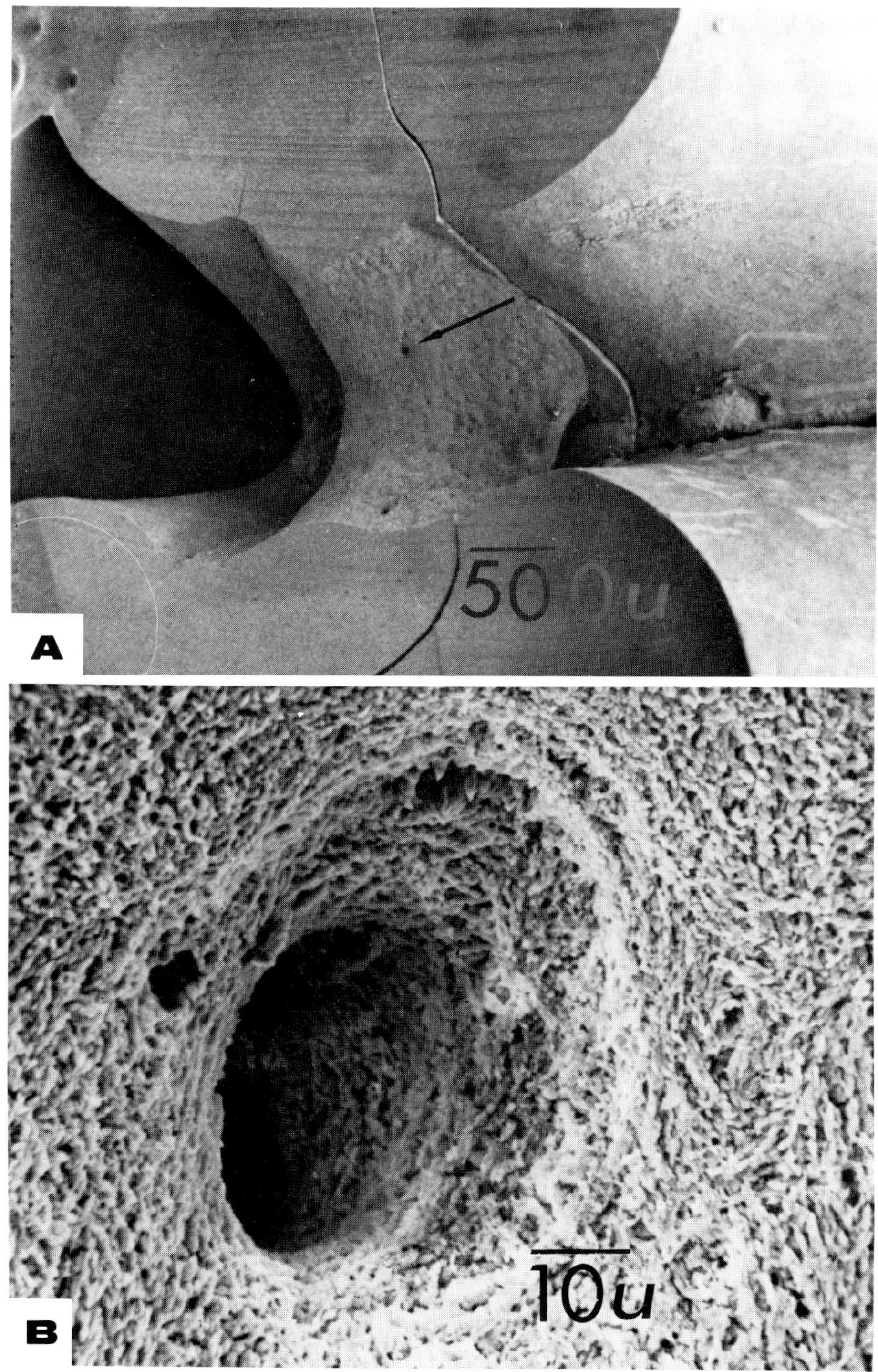

Fig. 6–13. Foramens of accessory canals in molar furcation. *A,* Cross section amputation of molar roots. Looking down into furca. Foramen of accessory canal indicated by arrow (× 20). *B,* Foramen seen in *A,* magnified × 1000. Canal is about 35 microns across, flaring to 60 microns at surface. Note two peripheral foramens on rim. (From Koenigs, J. F., Brilliant, J. D., and Foreman, D. W.: Oral Surg., *38*:773, Nov. 1974.)

Koenigs and Brilliant did a scanning electron microscopic study of the furca area of molars and discovered a frightening array of accessory canals[27] (Fig. 6–13).

Unfortunately for the vitality of the pulp, the accessory canals do not at any time provide an adequate collateral circulation. At the most, their contribution to the total blood supply of the pulp is a minor one. Encased as they are by dentin, they can add little when the pulp tissue is denied its apical blood supply.

Structural Elements

The dental pulp resembles in structure the other loose connective tissues of the body more closely than it differs from them. On the one hand are connective tissue ***cells*** of various types. On the other hand lies an ***intercellular component*** made up of ground substance and fibers, through and among which ramify an incredible network of blood vessels, lymphatics, and nerves. The location, function, and immediate environment of the pulp are, of course, unique. As will be noted, these come to limit greatly its resilience. From the standpoint of major component elements, however, the only unique inhabitant is the odontoblast cell. Even here the similarities to the osteoblast of periosteum or endosteum are numerous.

Fibroblasts and Fibers. The fibroblasts (fibrocytes) are the most prevalent cell in the healthy, mature pulp. Their morphology is characteristic, only the long ovoid nucleus being visible in routine section (Fig. 6–14). In recent electron microscopic studies they are seen to be active cells directly concerned with the production of collagen.[28] Connective tissue fibrils lie everywhere throughout the pulp stroma. Under the influence of the fibroblasts the collagen fibrils appear (Fig. 6–15), aggregate to become fibers, and in time physically replace some of the ground substance and many of the cells of the young pulp (Fig. 6–16). The distribution of ***collagen fibers*** may be widely diffuse or somewhat compact (diffuse *vs.* bundle collagen). A true fibrosis does not appear in the normal pulp.

Stanley was able to study the influence of age upon the quantity of collagen fibers in teeth and determined that (1) ***anterior teeth*** have more collagen in their pulps than do posterior teeth, (2) bundle-type collagen is common in the pulps of young anterior teeth (Fig. 6–17), (3) coronal pulps of older ***intact*** posterior teeth have surprisingly little collagen (Fig. 6–18) and (4) ***root pulp tissue*** contains more collagen than coronal pulp tissue after the age of twenty years. It may very possibly be that increased pulp collagen stems not so much from age *per se* as from previous irritation. A tooth that has been stimulated sufficiently to produce irregular dentin should therefore contain more collagen.[29]

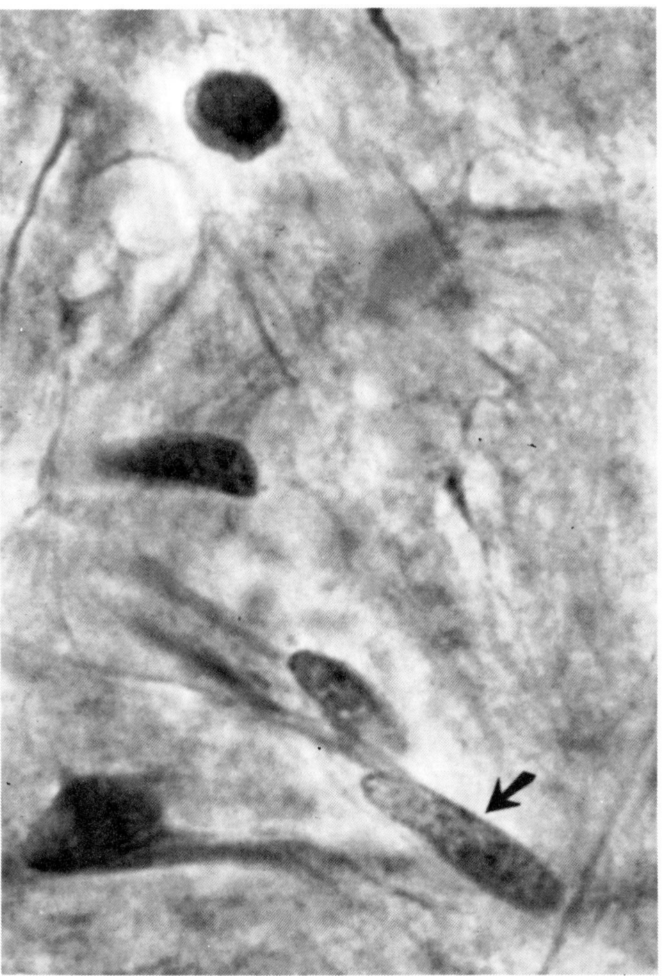

Fig. 6–14. Fibroblast (fibrocyte) in healthy mature pulp. Only long ovoid nucleus (*arrow*) of fibroblast is visible in routinely stained section such as this. Cellular processes and cell membrane are invisible. Human tooth. (Orban collection.)

Like the elastic connective tissue fiber, the oxytalin fiber of Fullmer has not been demonstrated so far in the pulp.[30] Evidence grows, however, to support the belief that ***oxytalin fibers*** are actually present in both dental papilla and mature pulp. They may be the forerunners of the elastin-like component of dentin.[31]

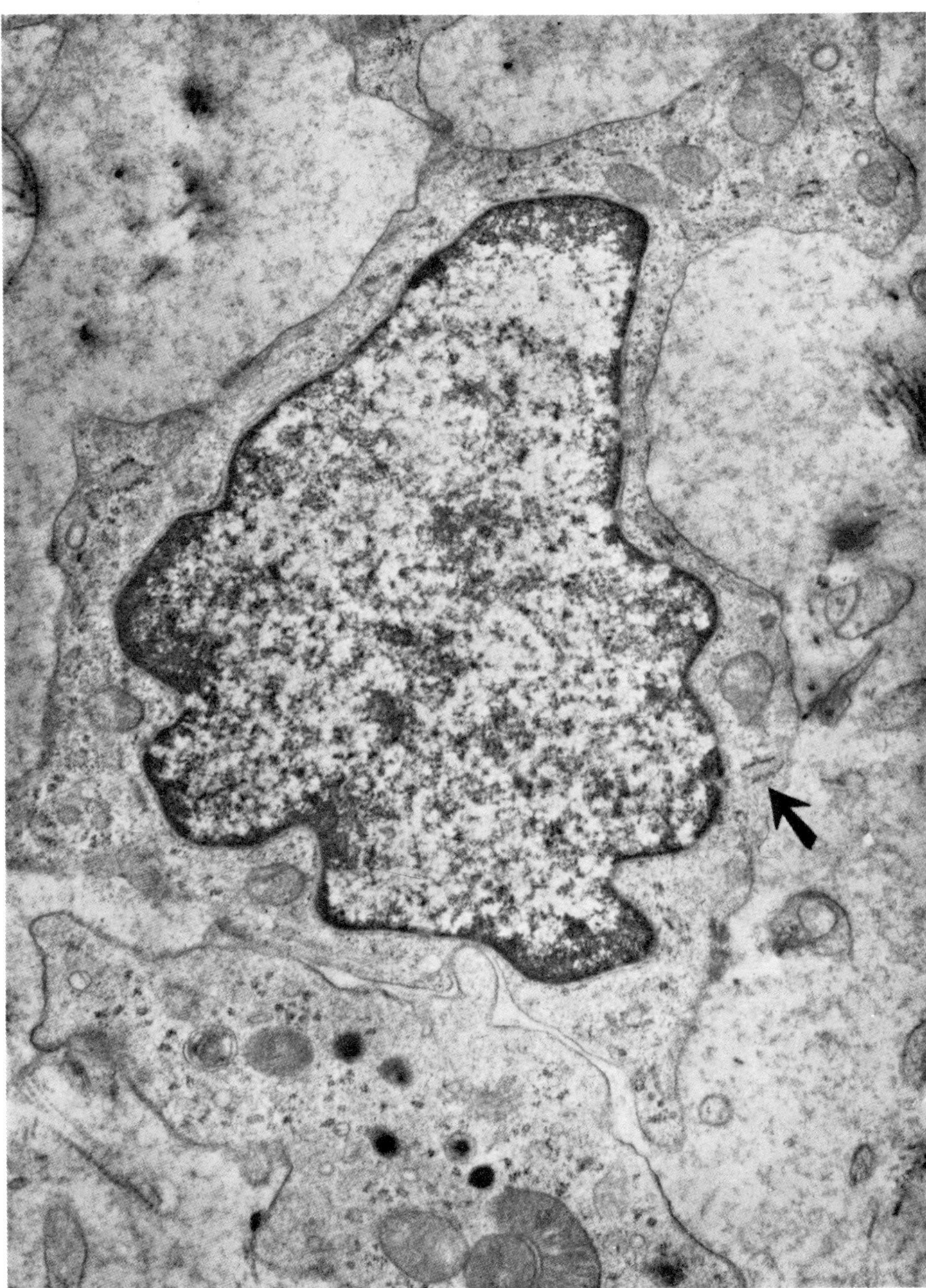

Fig. 6–15. Fibroblast (fibrocyte) from dental pulp. Cell is inactive, as can be judged by small amount of perinuclear cytoplasm and by inconspicuous organelles. Few profiles of endoplasmic reticulum can be seen. These appear as electron-dense paired structures (*arrow*) between nucleus and cell membrane. Endoplasmic reticulum is linked to protein synthesis. Collagen fibrils with characteristic 640 A banding are evident outside fibroblast in upper left and lower left. Many such fibrils grouped together make up single collagen fiber. Electron micrograph. Guinea pig. × 16,000. (Courtesy Dr. Seong S. Han.)

Korff's Fibers. Reticular fibers, of course, abound in the loose connective tissue stroma of the pulp. As long as dentin is forming, many fibers of this type (more truly, fibrils) are found just deep to the odontoblast cell layer (Fig. 6–19). There is little doubt that this particular concentration of fibers is closely related to the process of dentinogenesis and hence to the odontoblast cells. The path of these fibers between

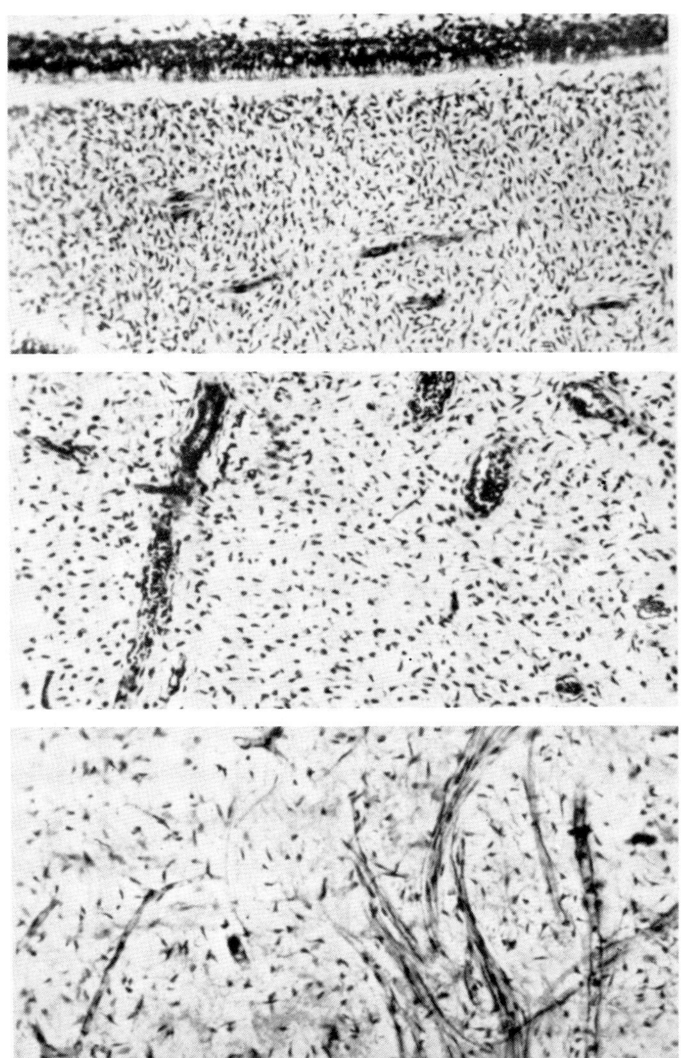

Fig. 6–16. Progressive changes in normal human pulp with advancing age. *Top,* pulp in human newborn. Preponderance of cellular elements. *Center,* pulp in human infant of nine months. *Bottom,* pulp in human adult. As pulp ages, fibrous collagenous elements replace some of ground substance and many cells of young pulp. (Orban collection.) (From Sicher, H.: *Oral Histology and Embryology,* 5th Ed., St. Louis, C. V. Mosby Co., 1962.)

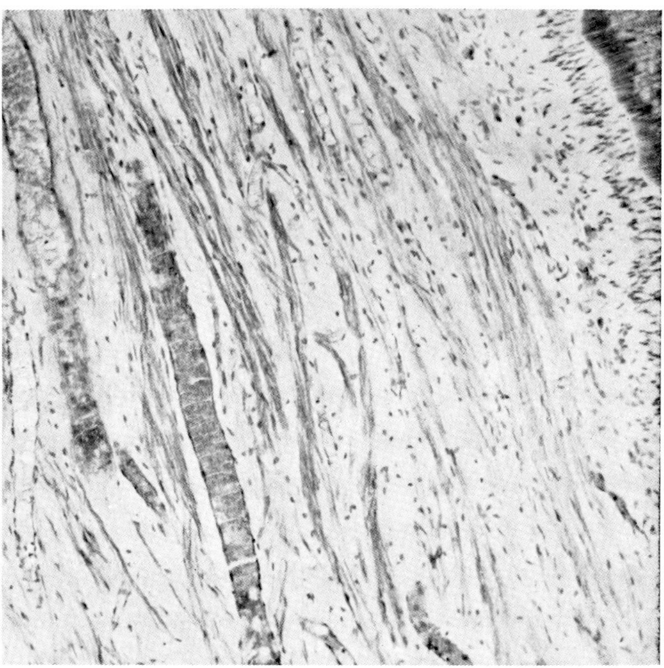

Fig. 6–17. Pulp tissue in root of anterior tooth. Collagen fibrils are numerous and are arranged in prominent "bundles." It is believed that anterior teeth have more collagen in their pulps than do posterior teeth at same age. (From Stanley, H. R.: Oral Surg., *15*:1396, Nov., 1962.)

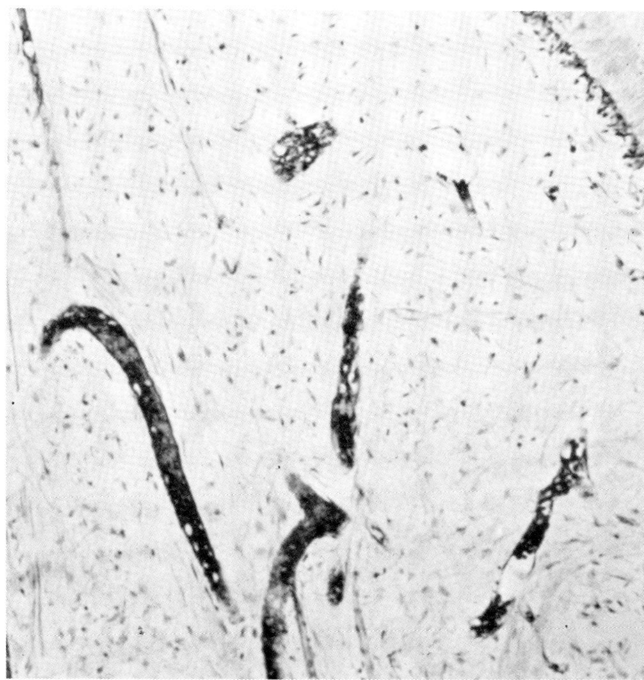

Fig. 6–18. Surprisingly small amount of collagen present in pulp of older, intact posterior tooth. This is pulp from 39-year-old patient. Collagen fibers are few. (From Stanley, H. R.: Oral Surg., *15*:1396, Nov., 1962.)

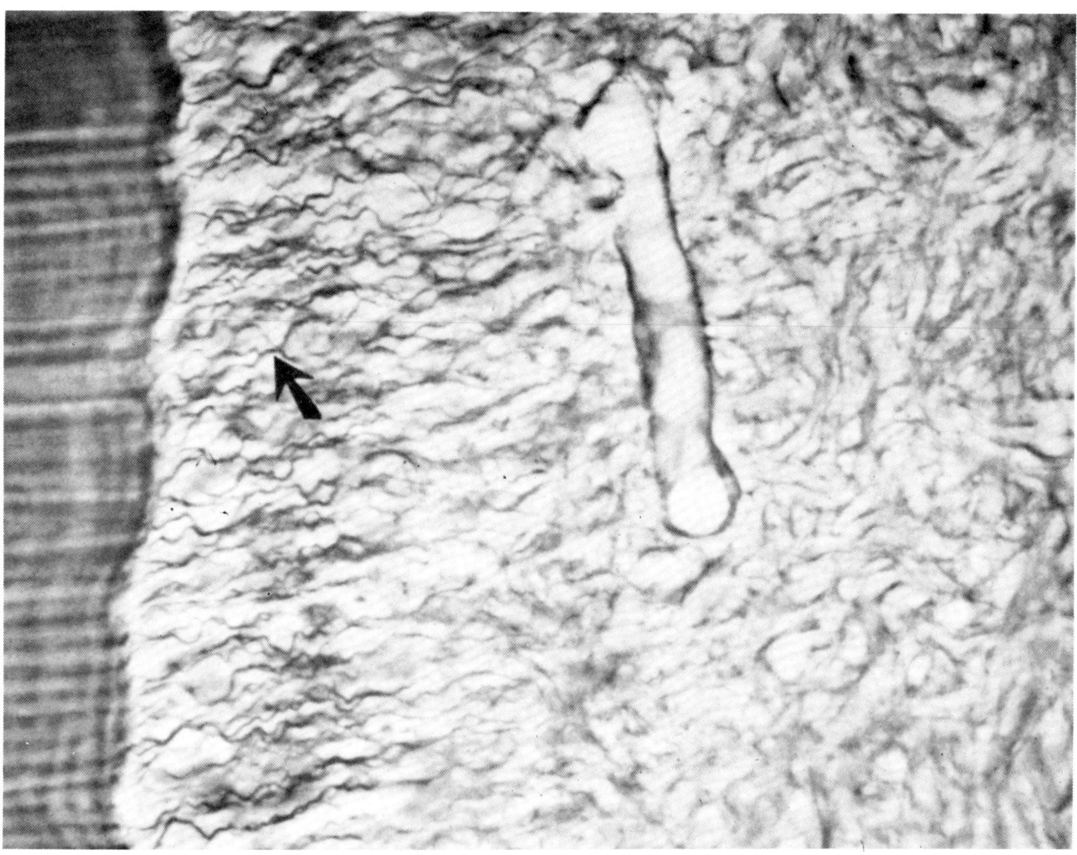

Fig. 6–19. Reticular fibrils in pulp of human tooth. Fibrils are concentrated near forming dentin and are prominent between odontoblast cells (*arrow*). Here they are known as Korff's fibers and have a part to play in dentin formation. Silver stain. (Orban collection.) (From Sicher, H.: *Oral Histology and Embryology,* 5th Ed., C. V. Mosby Co., 1962.)

the odontoblast cells and into the predentin zone has often been traced.[32] It now appears probable that Korff's fibers are either continuous with, or become transformed into, certain of the collagen fibrils within (calcifying) dentin.[33]

Ground Substance. If the cells of a loose connective tissue are thought of as the inhabitants of the sea, and the abundant fibers as their product, then the ground substance is the sea water, the all-pervading intermediary, rich in dissolved material. From the chemical standpoint the ground substance is a loosely aggregated, negatively charged molecular complex of water, carbohydrates, and protein.[34] Physically it provides a gelatinous bond, supplementing the fiber mesh. Every biologic process affecting the cells of the pulp is mediated by this complex. Leukotaxine traverses it when departing the injured cell. It is the highway upon which the summoned phagocytes journey in response to chemotaxis.[35]

Actually the ground substance does more than mediate. While implementing change, it, too, is changed. The edema created during inflammation, for example, means that an already loose aggregate has "loosened" even further, that some negative charge has been dropped, and that the molecules of the carbohydrate-protein complex have amassed further water at the expense of colloid content.[34,36]

Odontoblasts. The odontoblasts are cells of singular character and interest. They owe allegiance to two tissues, pulp and dentin, and actually are a part of both. Dependent on the pulp for their existence and perpetuation, these cells in turn are the key to growth of dentin and its maintenance as a vital tissue. (How these cells respond to remote daily stimuli, to direct therapeutic contact, and to the actual invasions of disease is the very substance of dentistry.)

In the developing tooth, and certainly in the young formed tooth, they should be thought of as forming a continuous sheet on the perimeter of the chamber and root canal. Their prominence in the pulp of the healthy tooth is related to dentin formation taking place. Along the roof of the pulp chamber of a young tooth, for example, the cells are arranged in a tight palisade. By contrast, a section taken from the margin of the root canal of an aging person would show few, if any, odontoblasts. It should also be noted that as go the odontoblasts, so goes the predentin. Columnar prominent odontoblasts, being active, have adjacent to them a definite predentin zone. In their absence predentin is a most uncommon finding.

An unfortunate concept about the odontoblast plagues the thinking of the profession today. Those who hold this view consider the odontoblast, for all practical purposes, to end where the predentin begins. The portion of the cell that is discrete and visible within the pulp and happens to contain the prominent nucleus is taken as the whole cell. When such a concept underlies the approach to a tooth, the pulp of the tooth is in jeopardy.

The confusion may arise first from the knowledge that the odontoblast ***is*** a low columnar cell when it begins its active life and from the observation that the ***pulp*** part of a mature odontoblast is of similar shape. It is a natural step then to assume that the

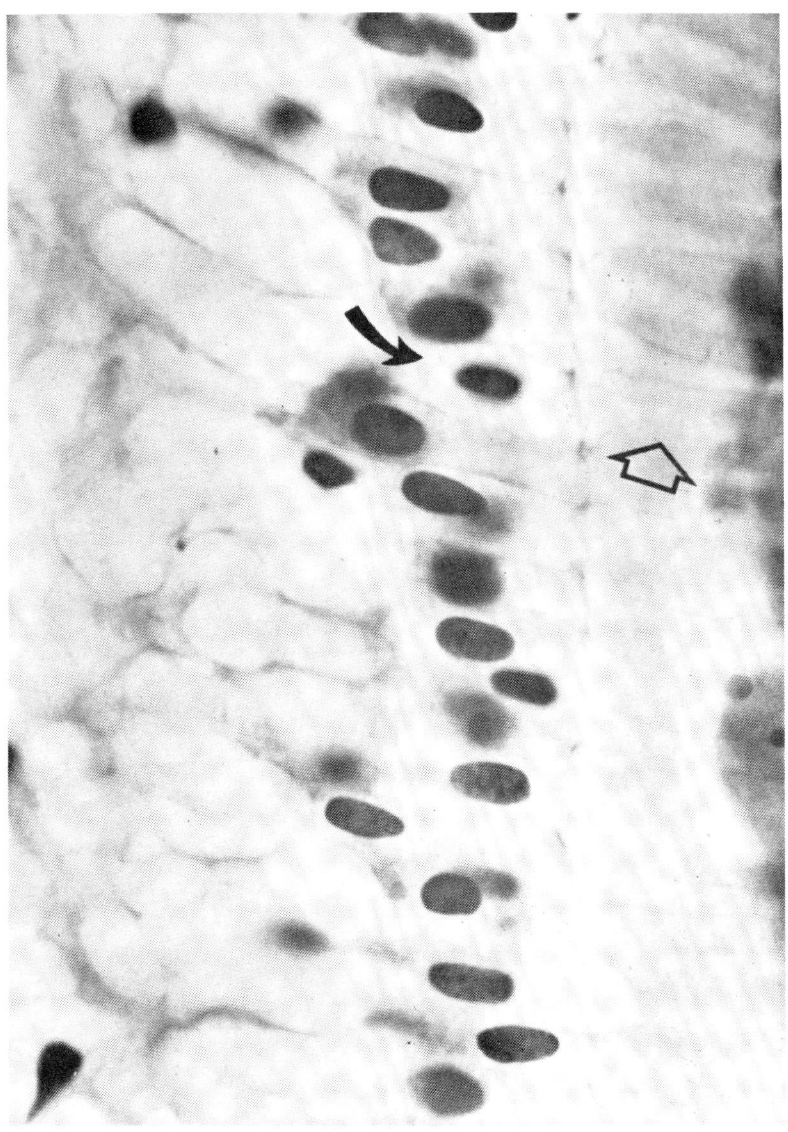

Fig. 6–20. Basal portion of odontoblast cell with its contained nucleus (*curved arrow*). Trunk of cell continues outward through predentin (*open arrow*) and beyond to dentinoenamel junction. Human tooth. (Orban collection.)

shape of the entire cell never changes. Actually, there is great change, and this continues as long as the cell remains active.

Established odontoblasts are long cells that extend from the ***enamel*** or the ***cementum*** to the zone of Weil. They are as profusely equipped with branched processes as they are long. Their terminal arborization in the dentin immediately adjacent to enamel or cementum is especially rich. Lateral or secondary branches create anastomoses at all levels. At the level of the predentin, one main trunk blends with the basal portion of the cell (Fig. 6–20).

Several important phenomena can be better understood in the light of this cellular continuum within dentin. For example, the deposit of new dentin on the walls of the tubuli must connote odontoblast activity similar to that responsible for the incremental deposit of secondary dentin at the pulp margin. The progressve mineralization of all dentin ***after*** it has been defined in matrix and partially calcified is also a case in point. The sensitivity of dentin to contact is another. In this respect it is enough for the moment to know that nerve endings make contact with odontoblast cells in the pulp and that the cell cytoplasm is "everywhere" in the dentin, especially where terminal twigs arborize near cementum and enamel. The drying of dentin upon exposure to air, the extreme dehydration which follows pulpectomy, and the swift passage of dentin by bacteria and injurious chemicals (orthophosphoric and other acids, silver nitrate, and phenol) find partial explanation on the same basis.

Defense Cells (undifferentiated mesenchymal cells, histiocytes, lymphoid wandering cells). The loose connective tissues of the body respond, of course, to a provoking stimulus with inflammation, and the pulp is no exception. In common with many another loose connective tissue, the normal pulp contains representatives of three types of cells which are particularly active in the inflammatory response. Orban gave them classic description years ago.[37,38] All are located in close proximity to blood vessels. This increases their defensive usefulness because they are thereby positioned where they may act locally or, by moving into the capillary, travel to a more distant site of inflammation.

The ***undifferentiated mesenchymal cells*** of the pulp are of great interest. They are the cells of multiple potential, the reserve force. Much of the "cell-rich zone" is comprised of them and with good reason. When replacement of odontoblasts does occur, it is

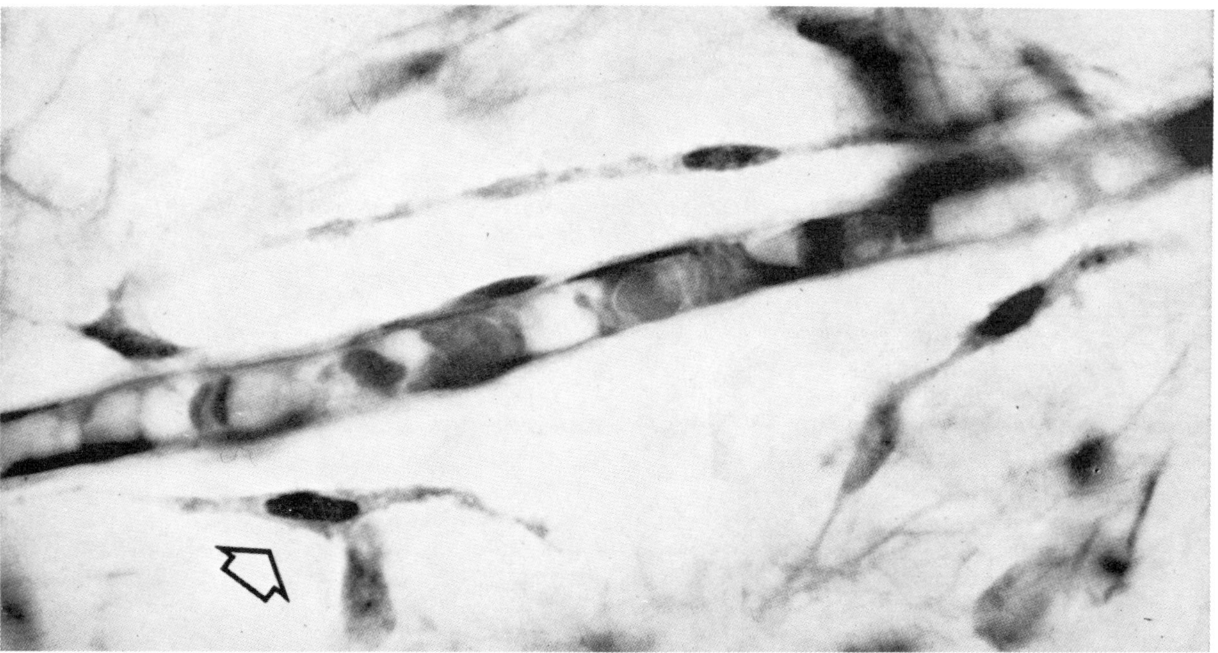

Fig. 6–21. Histiocytes or resting wandering cells in adult human pulp. Cells are near capillary, but are distinct from actual wall of vessel. Each is elongated branching cell (*arrow*) with prominent granular cytoplasm and nucleus packed with chromatin. (Orban collection.)

through the proliferation and differentiation of these cells.[1,39] When even more extensive pulp repair is necessary, the new cells of all sorts are, to a large extent, similarly derived.

The ***histiocytes,*** or resting wandering cells, share with the undifferentiated mesenchymal cells an important capability. Both cells can and do become macrophages.[1] Through their active phagocytosis, the macrophages in turn remove bacteria, foreign bodies, and dead cells and thus set the stage for repair.[40] Without them many a minor inflammation of the pulp would progress.

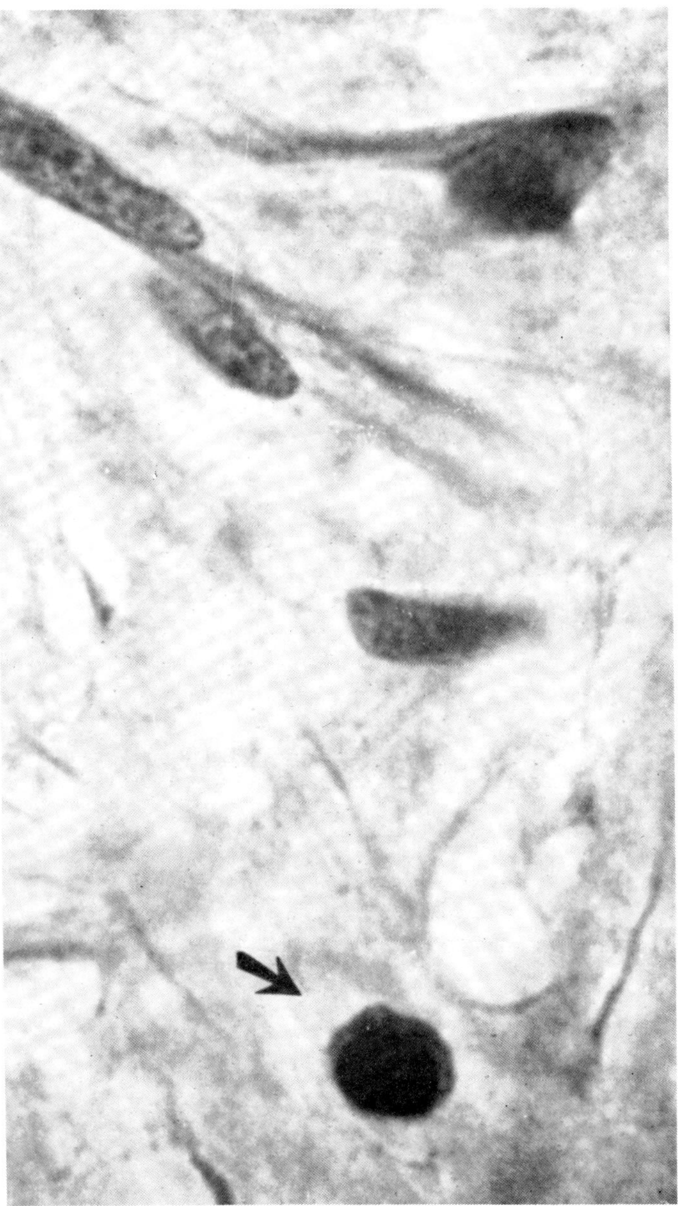

Fig. 6–22. Lymphoid wandering cell of adult human pulp. Cell (*arrow*) closely resembles small lymphocyte of circulating blood. It stands out in sharp contrast to fibroblast cells whose nuclei are visible in upper left-hand corner. (Orban collection.)

Identification of the histiocytes in an adequately fixed and stained section is no problem. Again, this cell is near the capillary but well removed from the actual wall of the vessel. The morphology is unique—an elongated, branching cell, prominent granular cytoplasm, a nucleus densely packed with chromatin (Fig. 6–21).

The ***lymphoid wandering cells*** (or tissue lymphocytes) of pulp tissue closely resemble the small lymphocytes of blood (Fig. 6–22). They also migrate to the site of injury. Plasma cells of an inflamed pulp are thought to come from them.[41] If any specific role can yet be ascribed to the lymphoid cell it would be as an antibody source.[42,43]

When the extent of the intermingling of cells and hard dentin is considered, it should come as no surprise that the odontoblasts respond sharply to stimuli (direct or indirect) which are applied to dentin. The response is extremely critical. Many of the early microscopic features of this response, moreover, are observable only in the pulp. The chapter on pulp pathoses (Chapter 8) will cover this subject.

Blood Vessels and the Pulp Circulation

It is convenient to examine in passive fashion the blood vessels, the nerve plexuses, and the lymphatic system of the pulp as separate entities. It is also important to remember that they exist to function and to function together. Their *raison d'être* is to maintain the pulp as a responsive tissue, to link the dentin to the body at large.

Fortunately, blood vessels and pulp circulation have become better understood in recent years. One should keep in mind the small size of the pulp. Even in a young central incisor the widest diameter of the chamber does not exceed 3 mm., and the apical lumen measures approximately 0.4 mm.[18,44] Within these dimensions lie a host of vessels (Fig. 6–23). Under normal circumstances, much of this network lies dormant and collapsed.[45,46]

The vascular profusion can best be explained by the fact that the pulp has the dentin to nourish as well as itself. Multiple, rather than single, arterial and venous trunks pass through the apical foramen.[23,47,48] Within the pulp there are many arteriovenous

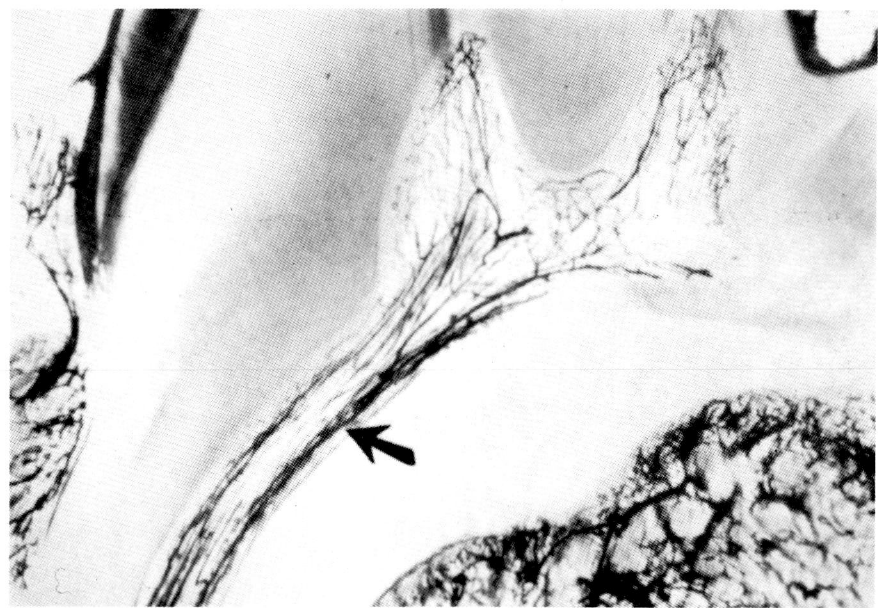

Fig. 6–23. Dense aggregation of blood vessels within dental pulp of dog. Vessels from each root anastomose within coronal pulp. Coronal pulp also contains final subdivision of vessels into terminal (subodontoblastic) plexus. Larger vessels are concentrated within root canal (*arrow*) and central portion of coronal pulp. Greatest branching occurs in peripheral zone of coronal pulp. Vascular perfusion. (Courtesy Dr. D. Walter Cohen.)

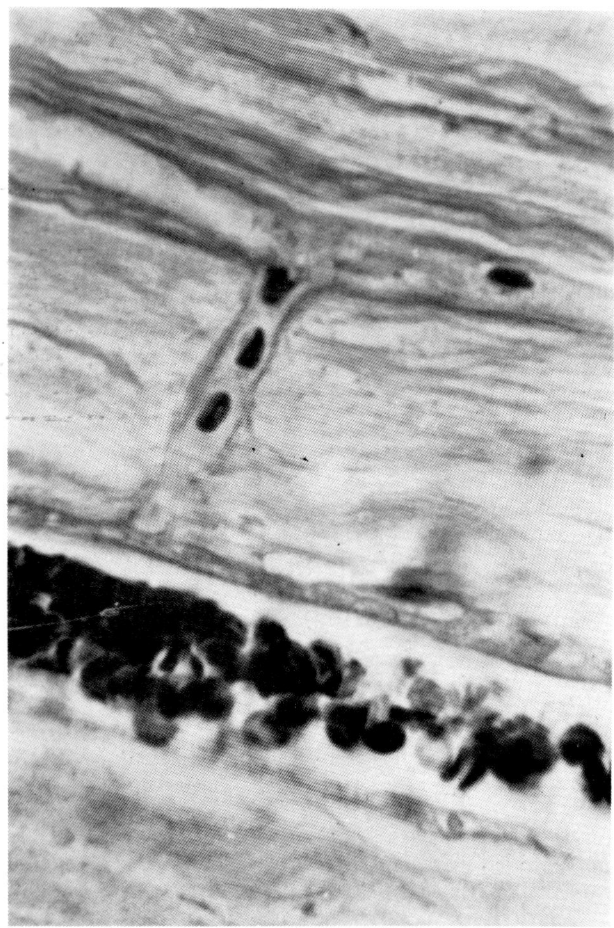

Fig. 6–24. Arteriovenous connection (arteriovenous anastomosis) within human pulp. Three erythrocytes are seen passing through anastomosis from artery to vein in lower half of photomicrograph. (From Provenza, D. V.: *Oral Histology*, Philadelphia, J. B. Lippincott Co., 1964, p. 276.)

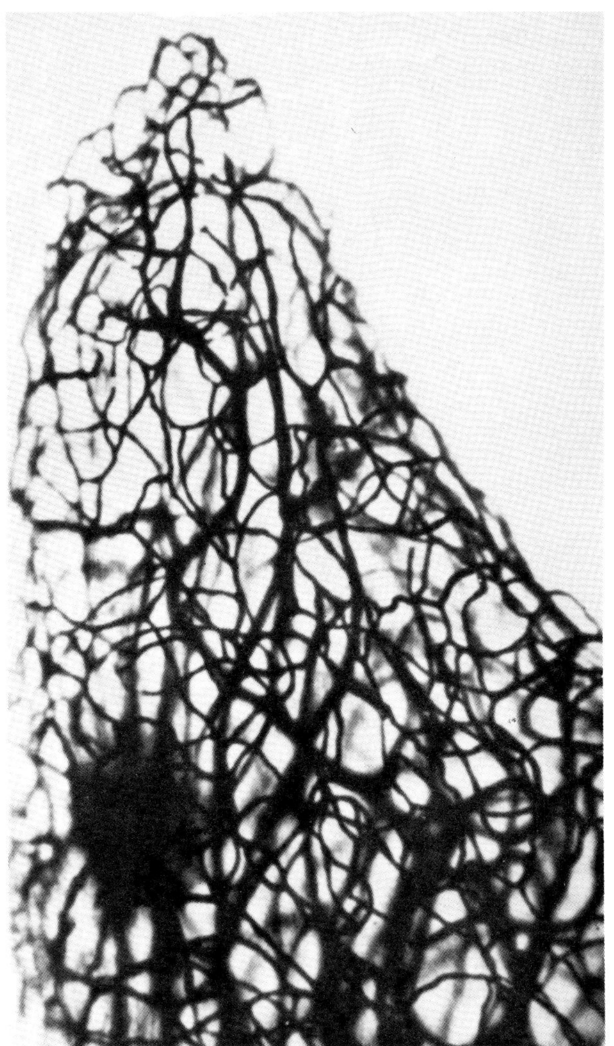

Fig. 6–25. Subodontoblastic capillary plexus in zone of Weil. This superficial plexus of vessels is particularly rich just deep to odontoblasts on periphery of pulp. Coronal pulp of human mandibular first permanent molar. Vascular perfusion. (From Kramer, I. R. H.: Arch. Oral Biol., *2*:177, Aug., 1960.)

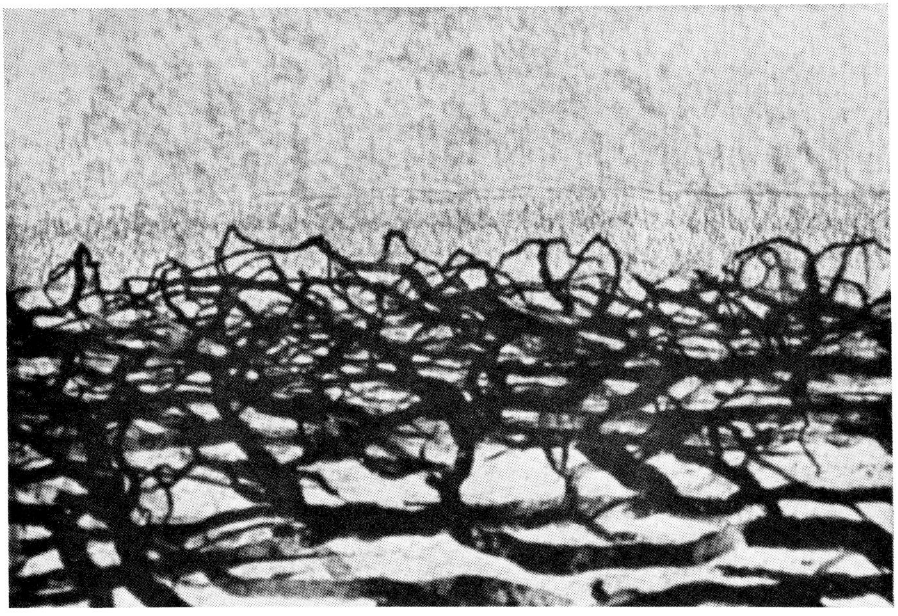

Fig. 6–26. Typical view of peripheral capillary plexus. Although plexus is mainly subodontoblastic, few loops penetrate odontoblast layer and lie among odontoblast cells close to inner aspect of predentin. Odontoblast nuclei are invisible. Coronal pulp of human tooth. Vascular perfusion. (From Kramer, I. R. H.: Arch. Oral Biol., *2*:177, Aug., 1960.)

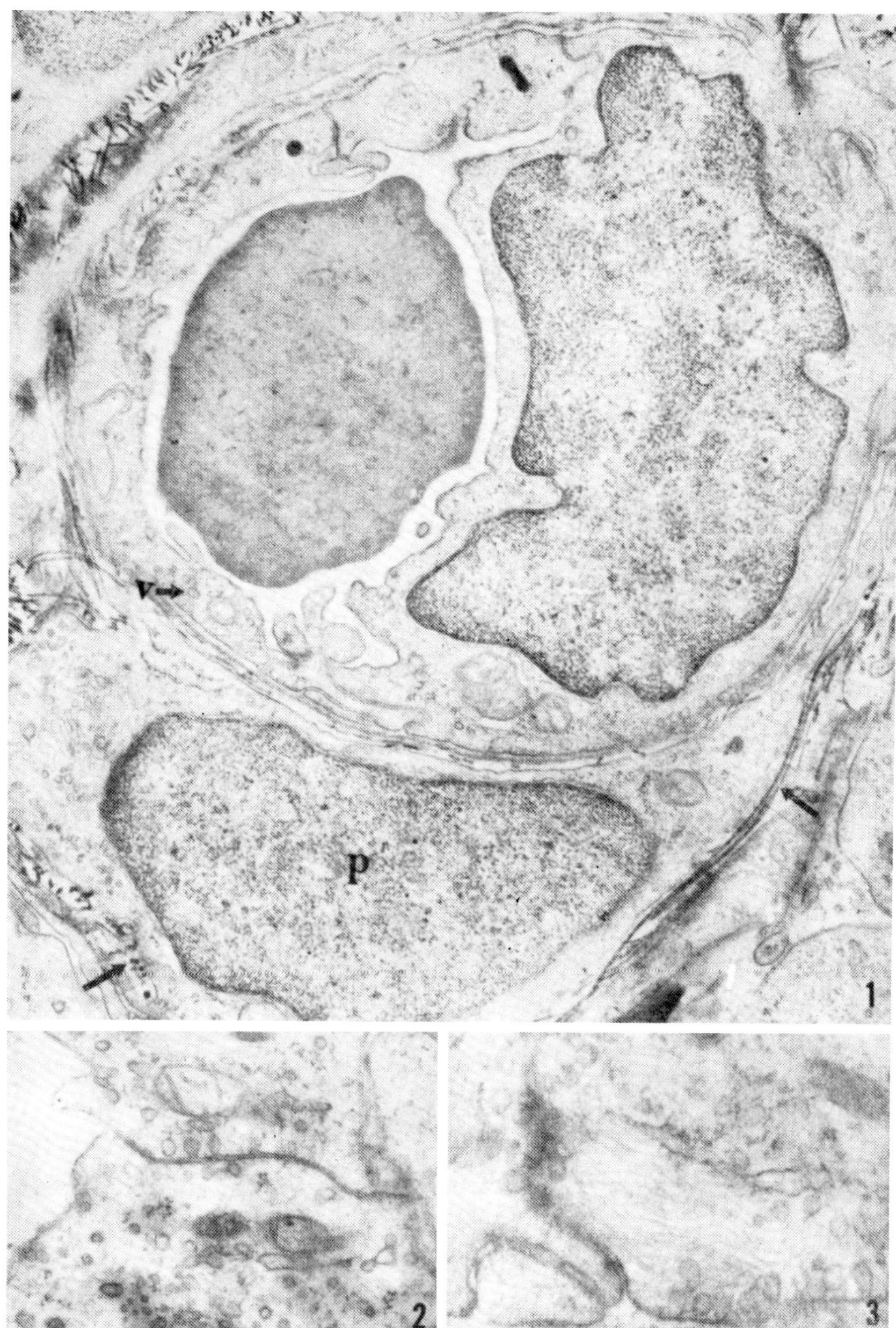

Fig. 6–27. *1,* Transversely sectioned capillary from incisor pulp of hamster showing portions of several endothelial cells, basement membrane, and extravascular pericyte (p). Red blood cell is prominent in lumen and endothelial cell nucleus with wrinkled contour is prominent to right of it. There are numerous micropinocytosis vesicles (v). Notice collagen fibrils (*arrows*) seen along surface of pericyte. This capillary is in no way different from capillaries found elsewhere in body. × 15,200.

2, Simple contact made by relatively thick cytoplasmic ends of adjoining endothelial cells. Several micropinocytosis-vesicles and inpocketings are seen along apposing plasma membranes. × 24,000.

3, Attachment zone which is sectioned obliquely. Many intracytoplasmic fibers appear to converge into this zone of junction of two endothelial cells. × 38,000. (From Han, S. S., and Avery, J. K.: Anat. Rec., *145*:549, Apr., 1963.)

connections (A-V shunts) to facilitate blood flow to areas of greatest need (Fig. 6–24).[23,49,50] On the pulp margin, where the major work of the pulp must be done, *i.e.*, the supplying of blood to the odontoblasts, the capillary bed (subodontoblastic plexus in the zone of Weil) is particularly rich[23,51,52] (Figs. 6–25 and 6–26).

Recent perfusion studies have added much to our understanding of the circulation peculiar to ***multirooted teeth.*** "In the pulp chamber, for instance, there appears to be a full anastomosis between the vessels of each root, rather than separate closed vascular systems. Where the roots are flat and have more than one canal, as in lower molars, or where they are fused, a complex of vessels is seen passing from one root to the other across the dentine

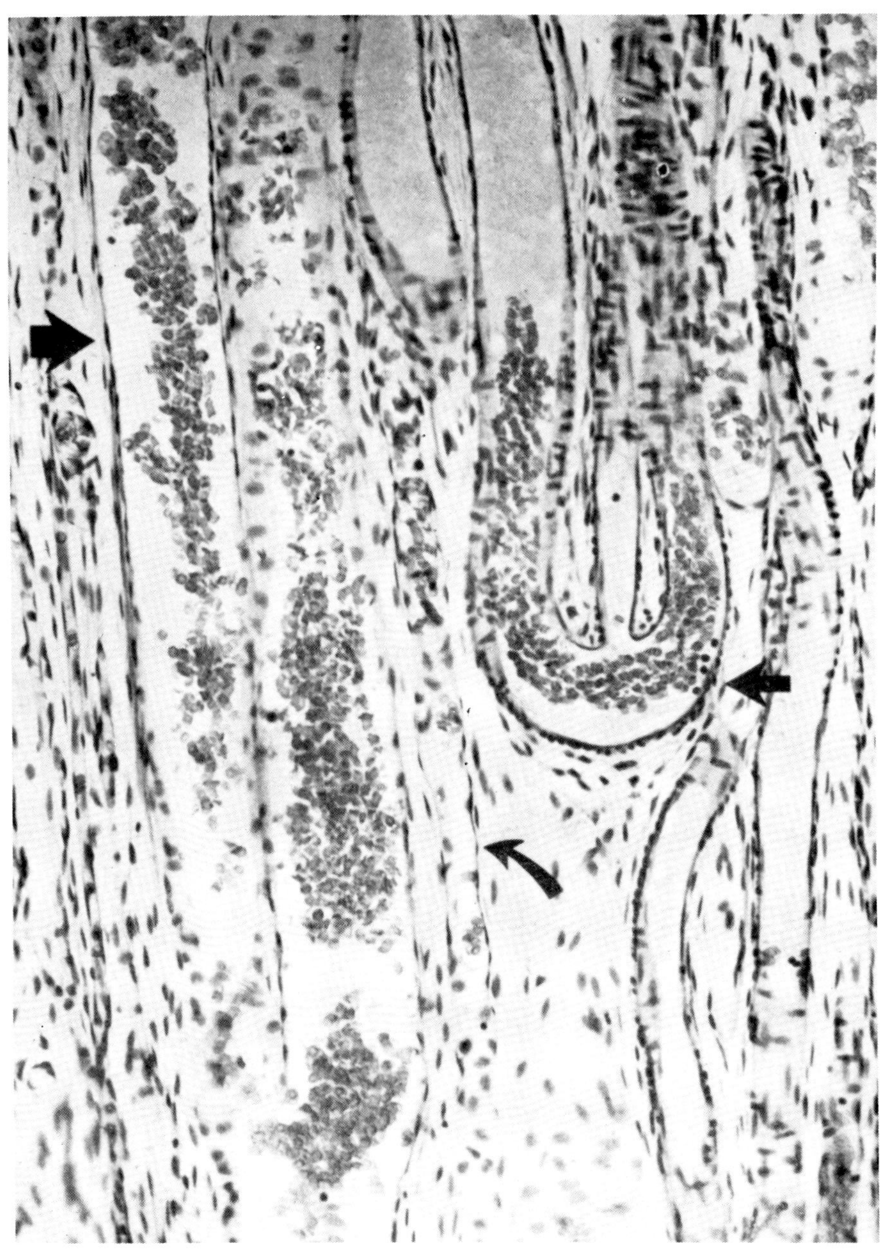

Fig. 6–28. Veins, arteries, and capillary within human pulp. Vein (*left arrow*); artery (*right arrow*); capillary (*curved arrow*). Walls of pulp veins and arteries are more delicate than those seen in vessels outside pulp. This is particularly true of their tunica media. (Orban collection.)

bridge."[48] Finally, there is strong evidence of collateral venous drainage in many multirooted teeth, the exits often being in the region of the furca or high on the axial root surface.[23]

Electron microscopy is now clarifying the status of the pulp capillary. The vessel is in no way different from capillaries elsewhere in the body. There is some evidence to suggest that the ***endothelial cells*** are themselves contractile[53,54] (Fig. 6–27). The ***pericyte,*** at very high resolution, resembles known collagen fibril-producing cells (fibroblasts) (Fig. 6–27). It appears capable of contributing more to the substance of the perivascular connective tissue sheath than to the restriction of the vessel lumen.[53]

Veins and ***arteries*** in the pulp exhibit several peculiarities. Reversal of flow has been observed.[60] Both have walls more delicate than are found in vessels of comparable diameter almost anywhere else in the body. The central layer of the wall (tunica media) is particularly thin in both[55] (Fig. 6–28). Strangely enough the major veins become narrower rather than wider as they near the foramen.[67]

Intrapulp pressure has recently been explored with increasing refinement.[56–58] There is no question now but that this pressure varies during the normal pulse wave and more widely during physiologic and pathologic change (Fig. 6–29).

Lymph Vessels

Logic dictates that the pulp should possess a lymphatic meshwork equally as elaborate as that of the blood capillaries.[59,60] So far, however, the existence of a widely distributed plexus of lymphatics can only be deduced. Lymphatic drainage from the pulp into lymphatics beyond the teeth does occur.[61]

Nerves

"If only my teeth did not ache." Teeth do ache, however, and nerves are responsible. More often than

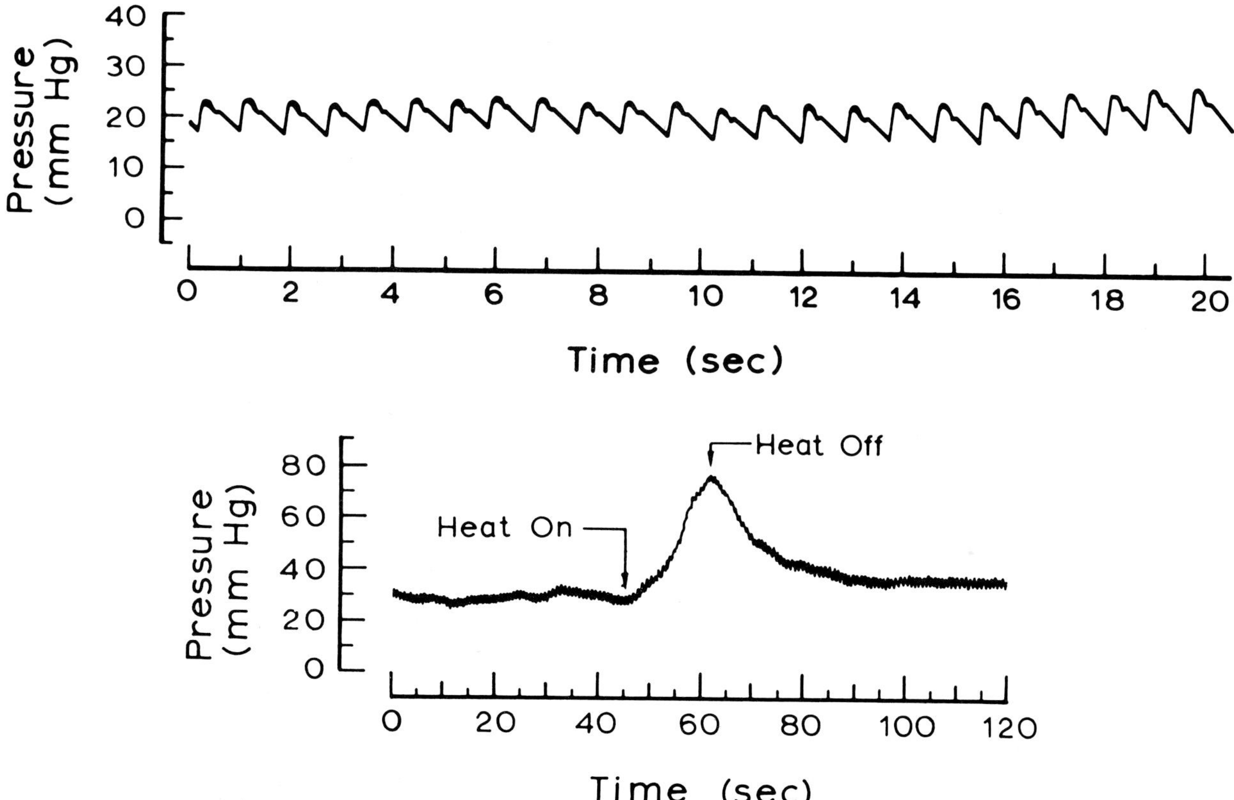

Fig. 6–29. *Top,* Typical pulse wave recording from right human maxillary first premolar. *Bottom,* Effect of heat upon intrapulpal pressure. Hot gutta percha was applied to occlusal surface of left human maxillary first premolar. A 45-mm. Hg rise in pulp pressure was noted. Pressure remained amplified with passage of time, even though it fell from maximum level attained some seconds after application of heat. (From Beveridge, E.: Oral Surg., *19*:655, May, 1965.)

not the nerves concerned are those within the pulp. At other times, nerves within the periodontal ligament generate pain indistinguishable from that of pulp origin. In the pulp, free nerve endings of the central nervous system are responsible for the sensation. Sicher[62] describes these endings:

> ". . . we know today that the receptors of painful stimuli are the very simplest sensory nerve endings, known as free nerve endings. They are almost ubiquitous, but they are the only nerve endings found in the cornea, the eardrum, and the dental pulp. The fact that these organs register pain only, no matter what the applied stimulus may be, is evidence for these free nerve endings being the receptors for pain. Their simplicity compared to the complexity of other nerve endings is of paramount importance. Other nerve endings are, because of their complex structure, both highly specific and highly sensitive. . . . The free nerve endings, devoid of any auxiliary (and therefore sensitive and specific) structures, have neither specificity nor great sensitivity. They register pain under high pressure, intense cold, or heat, but only when these stimuli are strong enough to transcend the high threshold of the free nerve endings. This lack of specificity for certain stimuli and this high threshold explains the well-known facts and still is not in contradiction to the law of specificity of nerve endings: not the quality of the stimulus, but the reaction to any stimulus, namely, the sensation of pain, is specific for the free nerve endings and the fibers arising there."

Indirectly, other nerves of the pulp, those of the autonomic group, contribute to the pain we feel. These fibers are believed to exert vasomotor control over the arterioles.[63,64] When they permit an increased blood flow to the pulp through relaxation of the muscle cells of the arterial wall, they are in effect increasing the hydraulic pressure on the free nerve endings. This can only mean pain.

Nerve fibers of both sensory and autonomic purpose enter the adult pulp with the blood vessels. Often the nerve trunks surround the vessels. Comparatively little branching occurs in the root canal.[65,66] In the coronal pulp chamber, however, the distribution becomes complete. While some of the sensory nerve fibers ramify on their own, others accompany the unmyelinated autonomic fibers and therefore the vessels (Fig. 6–30). For the sensory fibers the primary

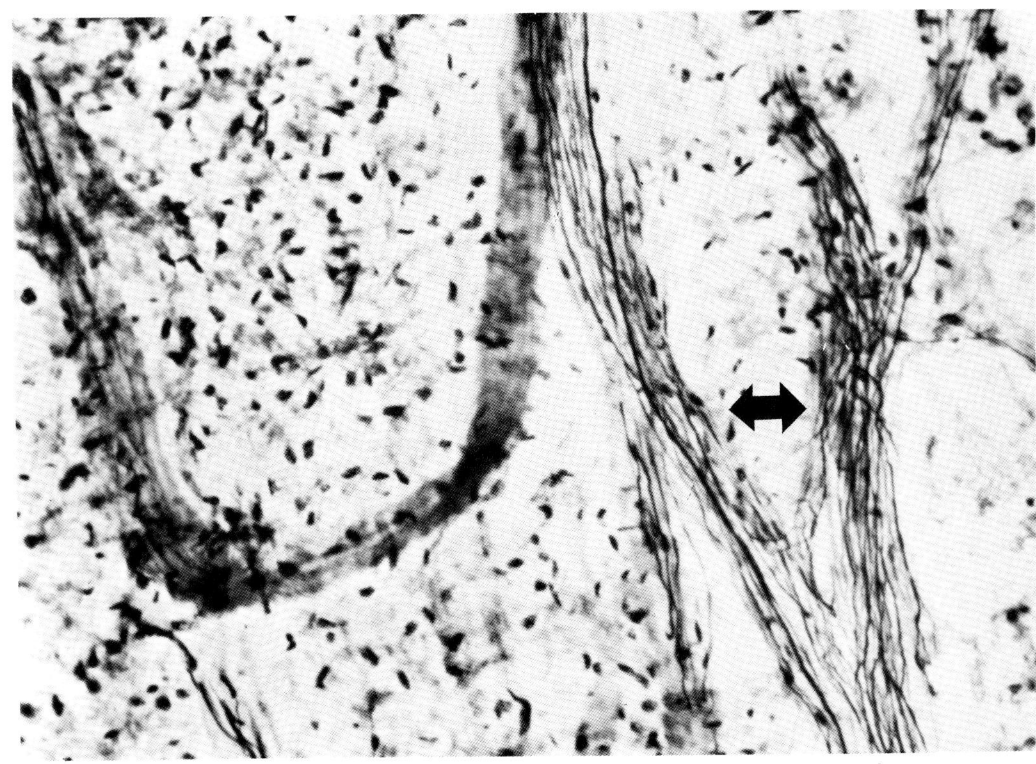

Fig. 6–30. Peripheral nerve fiber bundle accompanying vessels in coronal pulp. Nerve fibers (*arrow*) follow branching of vessels as seen to right. Upper left first premolar. Human, 15 years old. Palmgren nerve stain. (Courtesy Dr. Tore Arwill.)

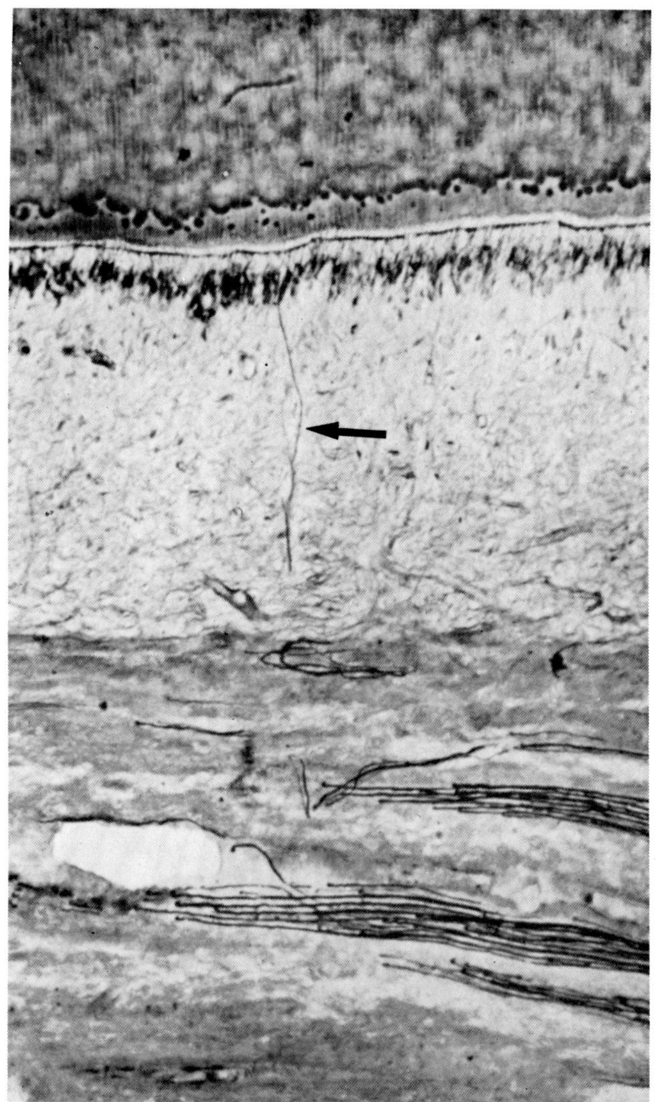

Fig. 6–31. Terminal branch of sensory nerve fiber on periphery of human pulp. Single fiber can be traced (*arrow*) in center of photomicrograph, passing from left to right to end in odontoblast cell layer. Palmgren nerve stain. (From Arwill, T., and Haeggströms, I.: Innervation of the Teeth. Tr. Royal School of Dentistry (Stockholm), *3,* 1958.)

destination is the very periphery of the pulp. Here their myelinated sheaths are lost and the final branchings are made[67] (Fig. 6–31). Many terminate in the "cell-free zone." Many others terminate in apparent contact with the odontoblasts,[68,69] and a few loop into the predentin only to turn back[70,71] (Fig. 6–32). The innervation of fully formed dentin still is not completely understood.[72–75,89]

REGRESSIVE CHANGES

The connective tissues of the pulp demonstrate regression and aging in several ways. (1) Discrete calcifications of the pulp stone variety, for example, are commonplace (Fig. 6–33). They are a daily encounter during endodontic treatment. (2) The continuous laying down of secondary dentin, and even reparative dentin, also is related to aging. (3) The phenomenon of sclerosis of the tubules of aging teeth has had excellent verification[76] (Fig. 6–34). (4) Fibrosis of the pulp has long been considered as an inevitable feature of aging. For the radicular pulp this still appears to be valid.[29,77] Here the odontoblasts disappear, the cell population dwindles, and collagen fibers loom large. For the coronal pulp of any given tooth, however, the picture changes. Stanley and Ranney, and Seltzer, Bender and Ziontz stress that, for the latter, the determining factor is the history of insult suffered by the pulp.[29,77] The healthy pulp of an older tooth (intact and uninflamed) is surprisingly free of fibrosis (see Fig. 6–18).

So-Called "Degenerative Changes"

Degenerative change as it is known in the literature of the pulp must now be totally re-evaluated. Within the past decade, important new techniques of fixation, embedding, and sectioning the pulp have been developed. There is much to be revised, as a result.[3,45,53,78] Through errors of fixation the well-documented "reticular atrophy" and "vacuolation of odontoblasts" can be developed in what is actually a normal pulp. Later, in Chapter 8, the importance of standard technique in the evaluation of pulp change will be re-emphasized.

PULP STRUCTURE AND INFLAMMATION

Factors that contribute to the vulnerability of the pulp are well known. Nonetheless they deserve reiteration, because when they are kept in mind by an alert dentist they can favorably influence his actions. Necrosis following inflammation—this is the threat to which the pulp is uniquely susceptible. Inflammation implies a prompt vascular response, bringing increased blood flow to the part and an increase in the fluid content of the ground substance. Unfortunately, the pulp does not tolerate major inflammation well. But for the narrow foramen, it is rigidly encased by dentin. There is no substantial collateral circulation.

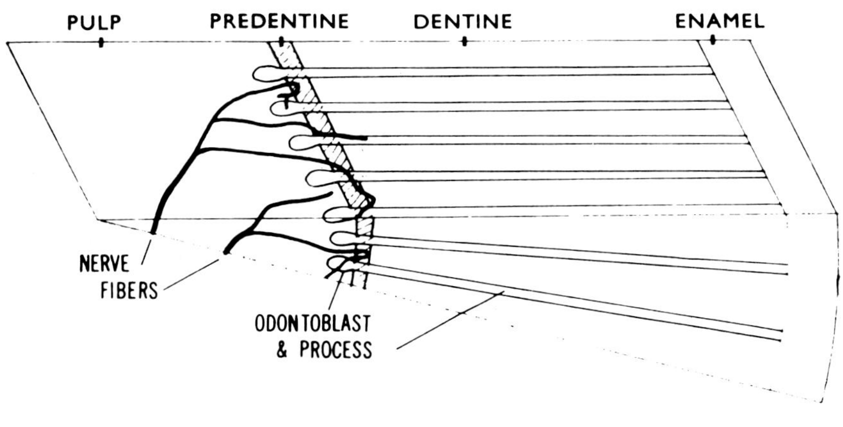

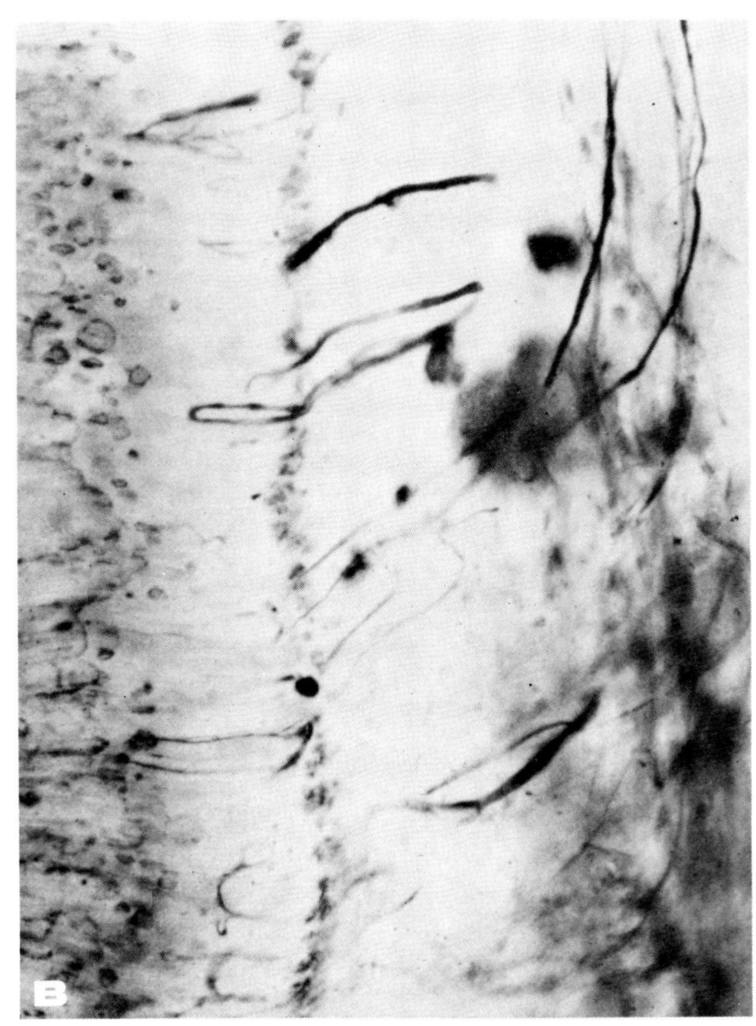

Fig. 6–32. *Top,* Peripheral innervation of tooth. Sensory nerve endings are known to terminate between odontoblast cells in pulp, on odontoblast cells (basal part) in pulp, and in predentin. It is possible that some terminal fibers may extend into more peripheral portions of odontoblast cells. (From Scott, D.: *Sensory Mechanisms in Dentine.* New York, Macmillan Company, 1963.) *Bottom,* Nerve fibrils entering predentin zone, where they form loops. Human tooth, older age (50 to 70 years). Palmgren nerve stain. (From Arwill, T.: Oral Surg., *13*:743, June, 1960.)

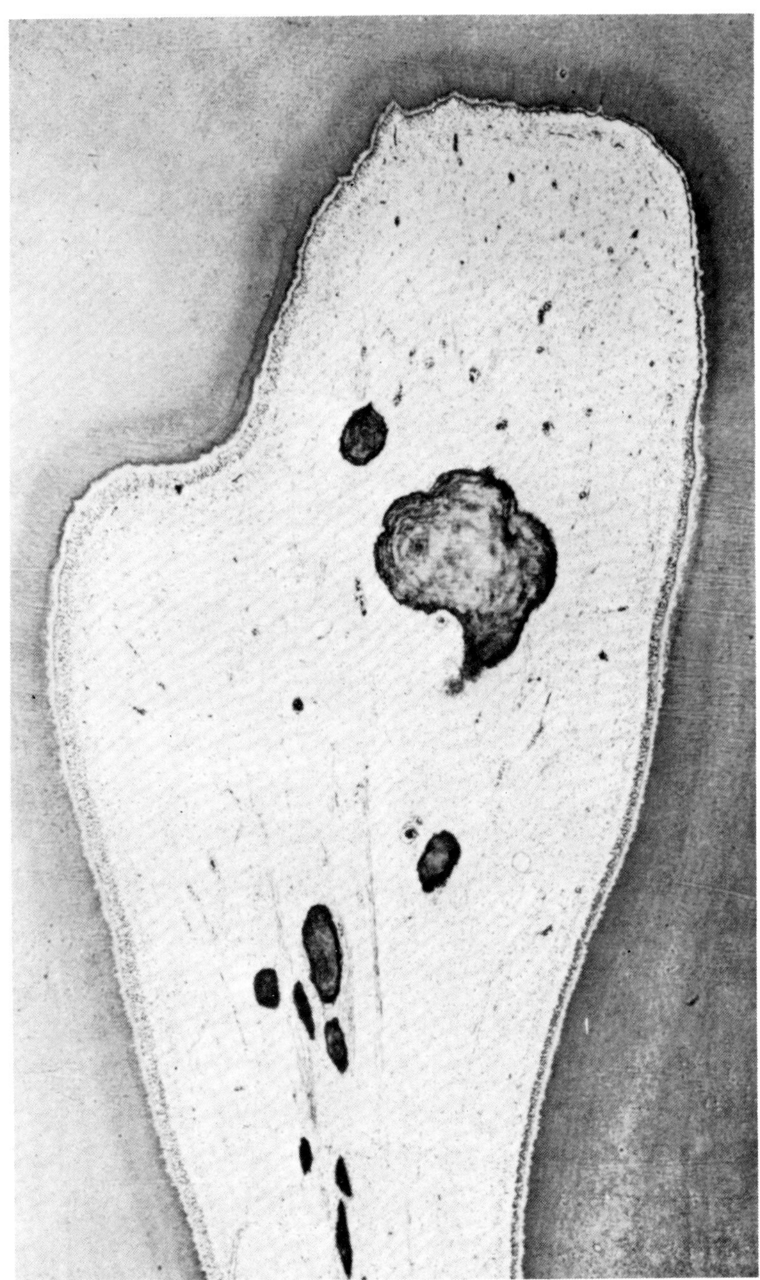

Fig. 6–33. Pulp stones toward center of normal pulp. Calcifications in root canal tend to be more diffuse and to be near larger nerve fibers and blood vessels. Young adult human tooth. (Orban collection).

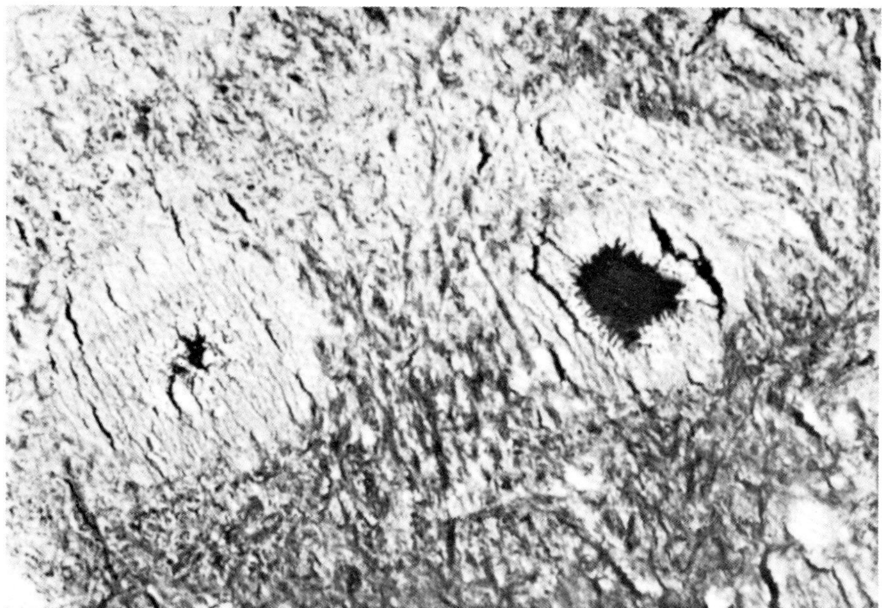

Fig. 6–34. Sclerosis of dentinal tubules of aging human tooth. Electron micrograph of transparent root dentin from 45-year-old individual. More densely mineralized peritubular dentin is white and tubule itself is black. Two tubules are visible in cross section. Tubule on left is almost completely occluded. Progressive nature of sclerosis is evident in tubule on right. × 10,260. (Courtesy Dr. John Nalbandian.)

Rising hydraulic pressure develops, and the walls of the afferent arterioles at the foramen are pressed closer and closer together. In many cases the vascular flow to a pulp becomes so restricted that the tissue dies.

HISTOLOGY OF THE PERIAPICAL REGION

The periapex is of unusual interest to the student of endodontics. Here the connective tissues of root canal, foramen, and periapical zone form a continuum that is inseparable. One has merely to reflect on how frequently disease in the pulp incites disease beyond the tooth to see this confirmed. When both the pulp and periapex are jointly involved by disease, therapy often must focus not on the pulp but on the periapical region. Even in the more common encounters, in which only pulp therapy is necessary, cardinal principles of instrumentation and obturation indicate how necessary it is to respect the periapical connective tissues.

Actually the tissue at the immediate apex of the tooth is more akin to the content of the root canal than to the periodontal ligament (periodontal membrane). The concentration of nerves and vessels there is such, in fact, that supportive fibers normally associated with the ligament space are well-nigh excluded. The connective tissue sheaths of vessel and nerve groups lie close together. A close analogy can be drawn to the foramens of the vertebral column. It is small wonder that inflammatory change is found concentrated at this zone of vessel egress. As we know, inflammation selects the connective tissue sheaths of vessels as a pathway of spread.[79,80]

The true periodontal ligament, of course, encroaches closely upon the confluence of pulp and periapical tissue. Sharp contrasts set this fibrous attachment apparatus off from pulp tissue: (1) It is, for example, an organ of the finest tactile reception. The lightest of contact upon the tooth will stimulate its numerous pressor receptors. (2) Collateral blood supply, so lacking within the pulp, is a vital reality in this area (Fig. 6–35). (3) Cords of ectodermal cells derived from the original root sheath form a tight network in this narrow zone between tooth and bone. These cells, the epithelial rests of Malassez, may serve a constructive function, and several such functions have been postulated.[81–83] However, interest has long focused on their capacity to spring to life when periapical inflammation touches them. As will be seen in Chapter 9, it is these cells that provide the epithelial "seed" for the lining sheet of the apical cyst.

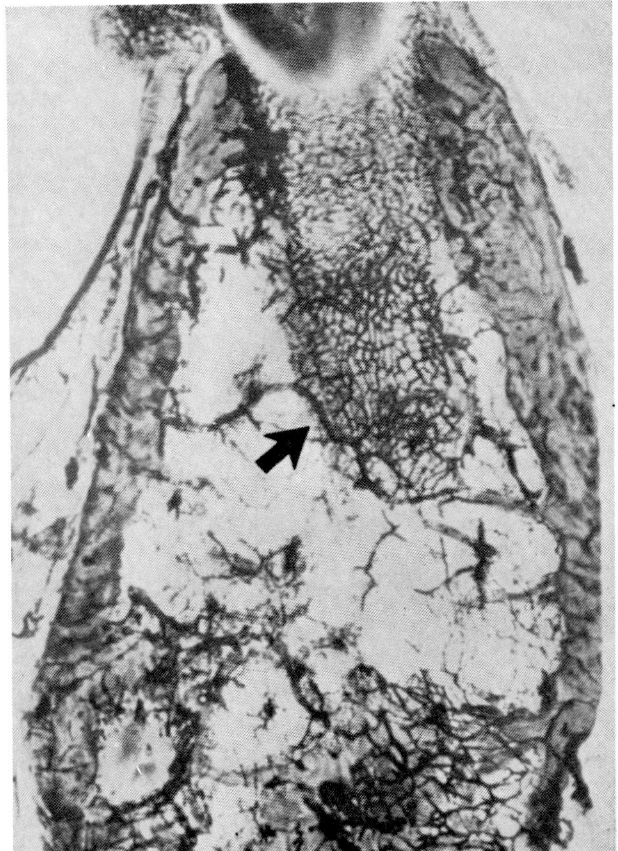

Fig. 6–35. Vessels of periodontal ligament. Continuity (anastomosis) of these vessels with those of alveolar bone and marginal gingiva is evident. Arrow indicates vascular network on proximal surface of root of mandibular tooth. Vascular perfusion. Dog. (Courtesy Dr. D. Walter Cohen.)

Beyond the ligament is the alveolar bone with its associated marrow. One image of the alveolar bone worth retaining is that of still another connective tissue, merging smoothly with the periodontal ligament just as the latter did with the pulp tissue of the root canal. The transition is made among the myriad perforations of the alveolar bone proper. This bone, at the periapex as much as on the lateral walls of the socket, is truly a cribriform plate (Fig. 6–36). Interstitial connective tissue of the periodontal membrane passes through it, carrying vessel and nerve, to blend with the fatty marrow of the alveolar supporting bone.

The potentials of this marrow are rich and significant. The mesenchymal and other cells of the marrow are what make possible nature's debridement and repair in the periapical zone following adequate pulp therapy.

DENTAL PULP PHYSIOLOGY

To properly evaluate symptoms arising from the dental pulp, one must be aware of recent developments in its physiology. At first blush, one thinks of the "nerve" in the pulp. Actually, pulp vitality is associated with its circulation, not its sensory mechanism. Moreover, the circulation of the pulp is unique, being enclosed in a rigid dentin capsule that limits changes in its blood volume.[57,58,84–86] It is generally believed that increasing the pressure within

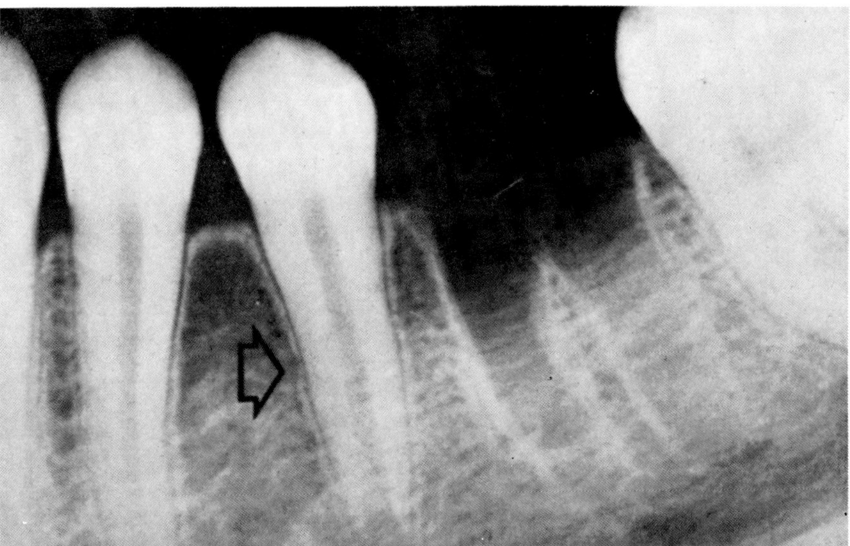

Fig. 6–36. Roentgenographic appearance of human alveolar bone proper. Perforations of alveolar bone proper (cribriform plate) are evident on mesial aspect of second premolar (*arrow*). Socket of recently removed first molar is clearly outlined.

the dental pulp induces dental pain.[87–90] Conversely, elimination of "increased" pulp pressure is accepted as reasonable dental treatment because it relieves the symptoms of acute pulpalgia.[91–93] Both presumptions bear scrutiny.

One of the earliest studies of dental pulp pressure was reported by Yankowitz.[94] Using a clever method developed by him and Brown (Fig. 6–37), he recorded an intrapulp blood pressure, in dogs, of 35 to 85 mm. Hg with a mean of 62 mm. Hg. To record systemic pressure, an indwelling catheter was placed in the left internal thoracic artery as well (Fig. 6–37). Refining the technique and equipment, Brown and Yankowitz later reported a pressure of 57 mm. Hg in the canine teeth of the dog.[57]

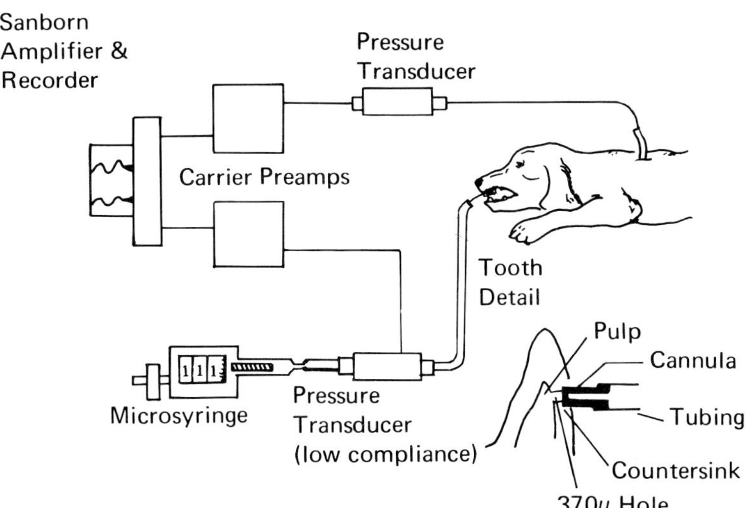

Fig. 6–37. Experimental arrangement for simultaneously measuring tooth pulp pressure and systemic arterial pressure. Lower right inset: method of tapping into tooth pulp. (From Brown, A. C., and Beveridge, E. E.: Arch. Oral Biol., *11*:1181, Nov., 1966.)

Modifying the same equipment for use in human beings, Beveridge reported a pulp pressure of 28 mm. Hg for the maxillary first premolar[58] (Fig. 6–38). Since these initial findings, Van Hassel has reported an average pulp pressure of 25 mm. Hg.[86] This figure was based on several hundred experiments.

Methods other than pressure transducer measurement have been used to observe the viable dental pulp. Pohto and Scheinin, using a "dentin window" technique of microcinematography, recorded blood flow variations in rat incisors and demonstrated the potent effects of epinephrine, norepinephrine, and local anesthetics on pulp blood flow.[49] Van Hassel and Brown, using similar techniques, found a positive correlation between pulp blood flow and the "appearance" of interstitial fluid from exposed dentinal tubules.[95]

The results of these basic studies in dental pulp pressure may be summarized as follows: (1) Pulp pressure shows rhythmic changes coinciding with heartbeats. (2) Pulp pressure exhibits a close relationship with the blood flow to and from the dental pulp, *i.e.*, pulp pressure falls when the common carotid

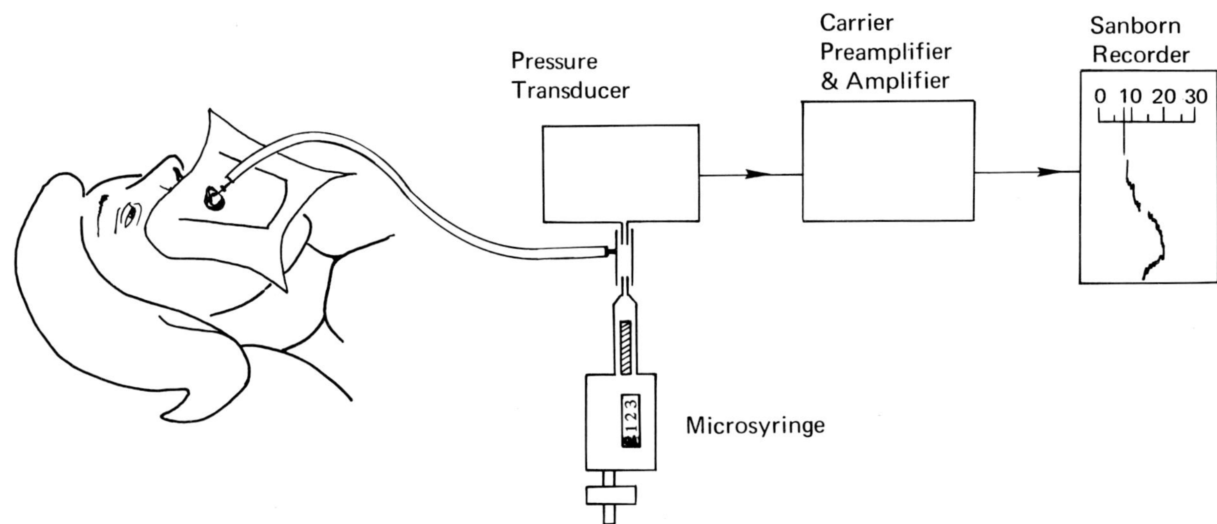

Fig. 6–38. Schematic diagram of system used by Beveridge to measure human pulp tissue fluid pressure. The tap-in to the tooth is the same as illustrated in Fig. 6–37. (From Beveridge, E. E., and Brown, A. C.: Oral Surg., *19*:655, May, 1965.)

artery is ligated, but rises if the jugular vein is ligated. (3) Pulp pressure is affected by vasoactive drugs, which would control systemic blood flow to the pulp—the vasoconstrictor, epinephrine, decreases the pressure whereas the vasodilator, acetylcholine, increases the pressure. (4) Pulp pressure is directly correlated to temperature fluctuations—lowering pulp temperature leads to lower pulp pressure and *vice versa*.

Following the establishment of this baseline information on intrapulp pressure, new techniques have been developed to further study the pulp and its peculiarities. Using photoconductive cells, Burnette and Hohn have studied pulps of dogs after most of the enamel and dentin had been removed.[56] They found a rhythmic pulsating change in pulp circulation. Through further refinements in this technique,[96,97] direct correlations of optical density to pulsatile variations in pulp blood flow were made in the intact tooth. The "pulsatile" waves of optical density were found to be synchronized with the electrocardiogram, pulsation being produced by the inflow of blood during each systolic blood pressure rise.

Photoplethysmography also has a singular advantage over photoconductive cells for studying vasomotor changes in the tooth pulp.[97–99] With this procedure, the enamel and dentin "capsule" are not removed, thus eliminating the unphysiologic exposure of the dentinal tubules and irritation of the pain fibers located in the predentin. By means of this method, recent studies in human beings have shown that definite changes in pulp blood flow can be observed in response to various respiratory maneuvers such as the Valsalva test (holding the nose and blowing) and deep breathing, both known to exhibit reflexive vascular reactions.[99] Application of local anesthesia to the tooth did not abolish these induced vascular reflex actions. Subsequent studies have shown that stimulation of the cervical sympathetic nerve had an interesting biphasic response on pulp pressure—initially it rose and then fell from normal baseline patterns.[99] After cessation of the stimulus, however, there was an "overshoot," gradually returning to control levels. Periapical injection of lidocaine, on the other hand, caused a disappearance of the changes induced by cervical sympathetic nerve stimulation.

Miscellaneous Aspects of Pulp Physiology. Other aspects of pulp physiology have attracted considerable research efforts in recent years. The role of the flow of dentinal interstitial fluid, the tooth's analogue of lymph, in eliciting pain responses in the dentin has been determined and reported by many researchers.[100–103] Brannstrom and others conducted several *in vivo* human being studies showing how noxious stimuli (chemical, thermal, dehydrating agents and drilling in the dentin) are all transformed into osmotic or hydrostatic pressures and thereby elicit pain impulses. From these experiments, Brannstrom has formulated a hydrodynamic theory of dental pain, involving the movement of the dentinal interstitial fluid, to explain the initiation and transmission of pain-producing stimuli through the dentin.

A number of investigators have studied the sensory mechanisms in dentin and nerve impulse transmission of the pulp.[104–111] Yet, in 1971, Seltzer was moved to conclude, "Complete knowledge and understanding of the mechanism underlying dentin sensitivity are yet to be attained."[93]

Another interesting area of dental pulp research has been the endogenous oxygen uptake measurement as an index of respiration and glycolysis—overall indicators of pulp metabolism.[112–117] In these experiments, standard Warburg manometric determinations of oxygen uptake of bovine, rat, and rabbit incisor pulps were made. In general, findings indicate that the pulp has a high level of ***anaerobic*** glycolysis (in comparison to other tissues) and that both respiration and glycolysis proceed at higher rates in pulps actively producing dentin. Similar experiments were performed on human dental pulps,[118] and the oxygen uptake was found to be increased approximately 20% following sequential additions of epinephrine. Rosett has also found that the mitochondrial membrane in bovine pulp is highly selective, admitting only succinates of all the Krebs cycle acids.[119] Before extrapolation of these *in vitro* pulp metabolism studies can be applied clinically, a more satisfactory explanation of the aforementioned effects awaits further study.

Finally, a research finding with direct clinical application is that of Page, Trump and Schaeffer, who found that radioactive tetracycline placed on the exposed molar pulp was rapidly absorbed by the pulp circulation and could be monitored in the general circulation almost immediately.[120] Thus we are presented with another avenue for developing drug sensitivity in our patients.

REFERENCES

1. Sicher, H.: *Orban's Oral Histology and Embryology.* 5th Ed., St. Louis, C. V. Mosby Co., 1962, p. 152.
2. Schour, I.: *Noyes' Oral Histology and Embryology.* 8th Ed., Philadelphia, Lea & Febiger, 1960, p. 145.
3. Stanley, H. R.: The cells of the dental pulp. Oral Surg., *15*:849, July, 1962.
4. Gray, G. W.: The organizer. Sc. Amer., *197*:79, Nov., 1957.
5. Arey, L. B.: *Developmental Anatomy.* 6th Ed., Philadelphia, W. B. Saunders Co., 1954, pp. 176–178.
6. Patten, B. M.: *Human Embryology.* 2nd Ed., New York, Blakiston, 1953, p. 67.
7. Arwill, T.: Innervation of the teeth. Tr. Royal Schools of Dentistry, Stockholm, *3*:1, 1958.
8. Ibid., pp. 36 and 61.
9. Green, D.: Morphology of the pulp cavity of permanent teeth. Oral Surg., *8*:743, July, 1955.
10. Sicher, H.: Op. cit., p. 139.
11. Provenza, D. V.: *Oral Histology.* Philadelphia, J. B. Lippincott Co., 1964, p. 246.
12. Coolidge, E. D., and Kesel, R. G.: *A Textbook of Endodontology.* 2nd Ed., Philadelphia, Lea & Febiger, 1956, p. 139.
13. Green, D.: Stereomicroscopic study of 700 root apices of maxillary and mandibular posterior teeth. Oral Surg., *13*:728, June, 1960.
14. Coolidge, E. D., and Kesel, R. G.: Op cit., p. 129.
15. Orban, B.: Op. cit., p. 145.
16. Meyer, W.: Ist das Foramen apicale stationär? Deutsche Monatschr. f. Zahnk., *45*:1016, 1927.
17. Pucci, F. M., and Reig, R.: *Conductos Radiculares.* Vol. 1, Montevideo, Uruguay, Casa A. Barreiro y Ramos S. A., 1944, p. 167.
18. Green, D.: A stereomicroscopic study of the root apices of 400 maxillary and mandibular anterior teeth. Oral Surg., *9*:1224, Nov., 1956.
19. Pucci, F. M., and Reig. R.: Op. cit., p. 160.
20. Kuttler, Y.: Microscopic investigation of root apices. J.A.D.A., *50*:544, May, 1955.
21. Green, E. N.: Microscopic investigations of root canal diameters. J.A.D.A., *57*:636, Nov., 1958.
22. Cohen, D. W.: Personal communication.
23. Kramer, I. R. H.: The vascular architecture of the human dental pulp. Arch. Oral Biol., *2*:177, Aug., 1960.
24. Burch, J. G., and Hulen, S.: A study of the presence of accessory foramina and the topography of molar furcations. Oral Surg., *38*:451, Sept., 1974.
25. Vertucci, F. J., and Williams, R. G.: Furcation canals in the human mandibular first molar. Oral Surg., *38*:308, Aug., 1974.
26. Lowman, J. V., Burke, R. S., and Pellen, G. V.: Patent accessory canals: incidence in molar furcation region. Oral Surg., *36*:580, Oct., 1973.
27. Koenigs, J. F., Brilliant, J. D., and Foreman, D. W.: Preliminary scanning electron microscope investigations of accessory foramina in the furcation areas of human molar teeth. Oral Surg., *38*:773, Nov., 1974.
28. Avery, J. K., and Han, S. S.: The formation of collagen fibrils in the dental pulp. J. Dent. Res., *6*:1248, Nov.–Dec., 1961.
29. Stanley, H. R., and Ranney, R. R.: Age changes in the human dental pulp. I. The quantity of collagen. Oral Surg., *15*:1396, Nov., 1962.
30. Fullmer, H. M., and Lillie, R. D.: The oxytalin fiber, a previously undescribed connective tissue fiber. J. Histochem. & Cytochem., *6*:425, Nov., 1958.
31. Fullmer, H. M.: The use of histochemistry in oral histology. In Provenza, D. B.: *Oral Histology.* Philadelphia, J. B. Lippincott Co., 1964, p. 517.
32. Bevelander, G.: The development and structure of the fiber systems of dentin. Anat. Rec., *81*:79, Sept., 1941.
33. Nylen, M. U., and Scott, D. B.: Electron microscopic studies of the early stages of amelogenesis. J. Dent. Res., *37*:22, Feb., 1958, Abstract.
34. Engel, M. B.: The structure and reactivity of connective tissues. In *Biology of the Pulp.* Symposium conducted by the Amer. Assoc. of Endodontists, Chicago, Illinois, Feb. 2, 1961.
35. Menkin, V.: *Biochemical Mechanisms in Inflammation.* 2nd Ed., Springfield, Charles C Thomas, 1956.
36. Engel, M. B.: Water-soluble mucoproteins of the gingiva. J. Dent. Res., *32*:779, Dec., 1953.
37. Orban, B.: Contribution to the histology of the dental pulp and periodontal membrane, with special reference to the cells of "defense" of these tissues. J.A.D.A., *16*:965, June, 1929.
38. Sicher, H.: Op. cit., p. 138.
39. Stanley, H. R.: The cells of the dental pulp. Oral Surg., *15*:849, July, 1962.
40. Zander, H. A.: Phagocytes in the dental pulp. J. Endodont., *1*:26, Sept., 1946.
41. Orban, B.: *Oral Histology and Embryology.* 4th Ed., St. Louis, C. V. Mosby, 1957, p. 150.
42. Coolidge, E. D., and Kesel, R. G.: Op. cit., p. 100.
43. Bloom, W., and Fawcett, D. W.: *A Textbook of Histology.* 8th Ed., Philadelphia, W. B. Saunders Co., 1962, p. 314.
44. Mueller, A. H.: Anatomy of the root canals of the incisors, cuspids, and bicuspids of the permanent teeth. J.A.D.A., *20*:1361, Aug., 1933.
45. Langeland, K.: Histologic evaluation of pulp reactions to operative procedures. Oral Surg., *12*:1235, Oct., 1959.
46. Scheinin, A.: Flow characteristics of the pulpal vessels. J. Dent. Res., *42*:438, Jan.-Feb., 1963.
47. Boling, L.: Blood vessels of the dental pulp. Anat. Rec., *82*:25, Jan., 1942.
48. Russel, L. H., and Kramer, I. R. H.: Observations on the vascular architecture of the dental pulp. J. Dent. Res., *35*:957, Dec., 1956. Abstract.
49. Pohto, M., and Scheinin, A.: Microcinematography of the Living Dental Pulp. (16 mm., sound, color presentation, 38 min., Bureau of Audiovisual Service, Am. Dent. Assoc., DT 178.) Filmed at University of Helsinki, Finland, 1957.
50. Provenza, D. V.: *Oral Histology.* Philadelphia, J. B. Lippincott Co., 1964, p. 275.

51. Saunders, R. L. de C. H.: X-ray microscopy of human dental pulp vessels. Nature, *180*:1353, 1957.
52. Provenza, D. V.: The blood vascular supply of the dental pulp with emphasis on capillary circulation. Circ. Res., *6*:213, Mar., 1968.
53. Han, S. S., and Avery, J. K.: The ultrastructure of capillaries and arterioles of the hamster dental pulp. Anat. Rec., *145*:549, Apr., 1963.
54. Fawcett, D. W.: The fine structure of capillaries, arterioles and small arteries. In *Microcirculation.* Edited by S. R. M. Reynolds and B. Zweifach, University of Illinois Press, Urbana, 1959, pp. 1–27.
55. Schour, I.: Op. cit., p. 146.
56. Burnette, E. W., and Hohn, W. O.: Investigation of possible circulatory changes in pulp. J. Dent. Res., *42*:1038, July–Aug., 1963.
57. Brown, A. C., and Yankowitz, D.: Tooth pulp tissue pressure and hydraulic permeability. Circ. Res., *15*:42, July, 1964.
58. Beveridge, E. E., and Brown, A. C.: The measurement of human dental intrapulpal pressure and its response to clinical variables. Oral Surg., *19*:655, May, 1965.
59. Yoffey, J. M., and Courtici, F. C.: *Lymphatics, Lymph and Lymphoid Tissue.* 2nd Ed., Cambridge, Harvard University Press, 1956.
60. Ham, A. W., and Leeson, T. S.: *Histology.* 4th Ed., Philadelphia, J. B. Lippincott Co., 1961, p. 152.
61. Noyes, F. B., and Dewey, K.: Lymphatics of the dental region. J.A.M.A., *71*:1179, Oct., 1918.
62. Sicher, H.: Problems of pain in dentistry. Oral Surg., *7*:149, Feb., 1954.
63. Uchizono, K., and Homma, K.: Electron microscopic studies on nerves of human tooth pulp. J. Dent. Res., *38*:1133, Nov.–Dec., 1959.
64. Schour, I.: Op. cit., pp. 152–153.
65. Arwill, T.: Op. cit., p. 36.
66. Engstrom, H., and Ohman, A.: Studies on the innervation of human teeth. J. Dent. Res., *39*:799, July–Aug., 1960.
67. Sicher, H.: Op. cit., p. 156.
68. Rapp, R., Avery, J. K., and Rector, R. A.: A study of the distribution of the nerves in human teeth. J. Canad. Dent. A., *23*:447, Aug., 1957.
69. Bernick, S.: Differences in nerve distribution between erupted and nonerupted human teeth. J. Dent. Res., *43*:406, May–June, 1964.
70. Bernick, S.: Innervation of teeth and periodontium after enzymatic removal of collagenous elements. Oral Surg., *10*:323, Mar., 1957.
71. Arwill, T.: Some morphological aspects of the dentinal innervation. In *Sensory Mechanisms in Dentin.* Symposium edited by D. J. Anderson. New York, The Macmillan Co., 1963, pp. 3–14.
72. Wassermann, F.: The innervation of teeth. J.A.D.A., *26*:1097, July, 1939.
73. Powers, M. M.: The staining of nerve fibers in teeth. J. Dent. Res., *31*:383, June, 1952.
74. Avery, J. K., and Rapp, R.: An investigation of the mechanism of neural impulse transmission in human teeth. Oral Surg., *12*:190, Feb., 1959.
75. Fearnhead, R. W.: The histological demonstration of nerve fibres in human dentin. In *Sensory Mechanisms in Dentin.* Symposium edited by D. J. Anderson. New York, The Macmillan Co., 1963, pp. 15–26.
76. Nalbandian, J., Gonzales, F., and Sognnaes, R. F.: Sclerotic age changes in root dentin of human teeth as observed by optical, electron and x-ray microscopy. J. Dent. Res., *39*:598, May–June, 1960.
77. Seltzer, S., Bender, I. B., and Ziontz, M.: The dynamics of pulp inflammation: correlations between diagnostic data and actual histologic findings in the pulp. Oral Surg., *16*:846, July, 1963.
78. Langeland, K.: *Tissue Changes in the Dental Pulp.* Norweg. Institute Dent. Res., Oslo, Oslo University Press, 1957, p. 57.
79. Weinmann, J. P.: Progress of gingival inflammation into the supporting structures of the teeth. J. Periodont., *12*:71, July, 1971.
80. Glickman, I., and Smulow, J. B.: Alterations in the pathway of gingival inflammation into the underlying tissues induced by excessive occlusal forces. J. Periodont., *33*:7, Jan., 1962.
81. Wentz, F. M., Weinmann, J. P., and Schour, I.: The prevalence, distribution and morphologic changes of the epithelial remnants in the molar region of the rat. J. Dent. Res., *29*:637, Oct., 1950.
82. Reitan, K.: Behavior of Malassez' epithelial rests during orthodontic tooth movement. Acta Odont. Scand., *19*:443, Dec., 1961.
83. Provenza, D. V.: *Oral Histology.* Philadelphia, J. B. Lippincott Co., 1964, p. 336.
84. Brown, A. C., and Beveridge, E. E.: The relation between tooth pulse pressure stimuli through the dentin. In *Sensory Mechanisms in Dentin.* Symposium edited by D. J. Anderson. New York, The Macmillan Co., 1963, pp. 73–79.
85. Van Hassel, H. J., and Brown, A. D.: Effect of temperature change on intrapulpal pressure and hydraulic permeability. Arch. Oral Biol., *14*:301, Mar., 1969.
86. Van Hassel, H.: Physiology of the human dental pulp. Oral Surg., *32*:126, July, 1971.
87. Stone, H. H.: *Oral and Dental Diseases.* 2nd Ed., Edinburgh, E. & S. Livingstone, 1951, p. 374.
88. Thoma, K. H.: *Oral Pathology.* 4th Ed., St. Louis, C. V. Mosby, 1954, p. 385.
89. Tiecke, R. W., Stuteville, O. H., and Calandra, J. C.: *Pathologic Physiology of Oral Disease.* St. Louis, C. V. Mosby, 1959, p. 382.
90. Sicher, H.: Op. cit., p. 138.
91. McGehee, W. H. O., True, H. A., and Inskipp, E. F.: *A Textbook of Operative Dentistry.* 4th Ed., New York, McGraw-Hill, 1956, p. 646.
92. Seltzer, S., and Bender, I. B.: *The Dental Pulp.* Philadelphia, J. B. Lippincott, 1965, p. 246.
93. Seltzer, S.: Hypothetic mechanisms of dentin sensitivity. Oral Surg., *31*:388, Mar., 1971.
94. Yankowitz, D., and Brenglemann, G.: Tooth-pulp pressure and hydrostatic permeability. Physiologist, *6*:30, Aug., 1963.
95. Van Hassel, H. J., and Brown, A. C.: Microcirculation

of the dental pulp. (16 mm sound, color, Bureau of Audiovisual Service, Am. Dent. Assoc.) Filmed, Dept. of Physiology, Univ. of Washington, Seattle, 1969.

96. Upthegrove, D. D., Bishop, J. G., and Dorman, H. C.: A method of detection of blood flow in the dental pulp. J. Dent., Res., *45*:1115, July–Aug., 1966.
97. Upthegrove, D. D., Bishop, J. G., and Dorman, H. C.: Indirect determination of the blood pressure in the dental pulp. Arch. Oral Biol., *13*:929, Aug., 1968.
98. Erb, A., and Sciaky, A.: Electronic registrations of the pulpal pulse. Refuat Hashinaim, *10*:32, 1961.
99. Shoher, I., Mahler, Y., and Samueloff, S.: Dental pulp photoplethysmography in human beings. Oral Surg., *36*:915, Dec., 1973.
100. Anderson, D. J., and Naylor, M. N.: Chemical excitants of pain in human dentin and dental pulp. Arch. Oral Biol., *7*:413, May–June, 1962.
101. Brannstrom, M. A.: Hydrodynamic mechanism in the transmission of pain-producing stimuli through the dentin. In *Sensory Mechanisms in Dentin.* Symposium edited by D. J. Anderson. New York, The Macmillan Co., 1963, pp. 73–79.
102. Brannstrom, M. A.: Sensitivity of dentin. Oral Surg., *21*:517, Apr., 1966.
103. Brannstrom, M. A., Johnson, G., and Linden, L. A.: Fluid flow and pain response in the dentin produced by hydrostatic pressure. Odont. Rev., *20*:15, 1969.
104. Bernick, S.: Innervation of the primary tooth and surrounding supporting tissues of monkeys. Anat. Rec., *113*:215, 1952.
105. Bernick, S.: Innervation of the teeth. In *Biology of the Dental Pulp Organ: A Symposium.* Edited by S. B. Finn. Birmingham, Univ. of Alabama Press, 1968.
106. Bernick, S.: Vascular and nerve changes associated with the healing of the human pulp. Oral Surg., *33*:985, June, 1972.
107. Pohto, P., and Antila, R.: Acetylcholinesterase and noradrenaline in the nerves of mammalian dental pulp. Acta Odont. Scand., *26*:641, Dec., 1968.
108. Pohto, P., and Antila, R.: Demonstration of adrenergic nerve fibers in human dental pulp by histochemical fluorescence method. Acta Odont. Scand., *26*:137, May, 1968.
109. Frank, R. M.: Ultrastructural relationship between the odontoblast, its process and the nerve fiber. In *Dentin and Pulp: Their Structure and Reactions.* Personal publication. London, 1968.
110. Mumford, J. M.: Pain perception threshold and adaptation of normal human teeth. Arch. Oral Biol., *10*:957, Nov.-Dev., 1965.
111. Mumford, J. M.: Pain perception threshold on stimulating human teeth and the histological condition of the pulp. Brit. Dent. J., *123*:427, Nov., 1967.
112. Fisher, A. K., Schumacher, E. R., Robinson, N. P., and Sharbondy, G. P.: Effects of dental drugs and materials on the rate of oxygen consumption in bovine dental pulp. J. Dent. Res., *30*:447, June, 1957.
113. Fisher, A. K.: Respiratory variations within the normal dental pulp. J. Dent. Res., *46*:424, Mar.–Apr., 1967.
114. Fisher, A. K., and Schwabe, C.: Respiration and glycolysis in bovine dental pulp. J. Dent. Res., *48*:439, May–June, 1969.
115. Kozam, G.: The oxygen uptake of the rat incisor pulp after adrenalectomy. J. Dent. Res., *47*:47, Jan.–Feb., 1968.
116. Kozam, G.: Oxygen uptake of rat incisor pulp after hypophysectomy. J. Dent. Res., *47*:214, Mar.–Apr., 1968.
117. Kozam, G.: Comparison of the exhaustion of the oxidative processes in rat and rabbit incisor pulp *in vitro.* J. Dent. Res., *48*:71, Jan.–Feb., 1969.
118. Schaeffer, L. D.: Unpublished material, 1972.
119. Rosett, T., Ashbridge, E., Belsky, A., Derenzo, G., Garner, P. S., Green, D., Pollack, R. L., and Tan, N. Y.: Respiration of homogenates and mitochondrial fractions of bovine dental pulp. Arch. Oral Biol., *17*:1961, Dec., 1972.
120. Page, D. O., Trump, G. N., and Schaeffer, L. D.: Passage of ^{3}H-tetracycline into the circulatory system through rat molar pulps. Oral Surg., *35*:555, Apr., 1973.

Chapter 7

Etiology and Prevention of Pulp Inflammation, Necrosis, and Dystrophy

JOHN I. INGLE and KAARE LANGELAND

The noxious stimuli responsible for pulp inflammation, death, or dystrophy are legion, ranging from bacterial invasion to hereditary dwarfism. Without question, bacterial invasion from a carious lesion is the most frequent cause of pulp inflammation. Paradoxically, an alarming amount of pulp involvement is induced by the very dental treatment designed to repair the carious lesion. An increase in automobile accidents and in body contact sports has also brought about an increase in pulp death due to trauma.

The causes of pulp inflammation, necrosis, or dystrophy may be arranged in a logical sequence, beginning with the most frequent irritant, microorganisms.

- I. Bacterial
  - A. Coronal ingress
    - 1. Caries
    - 2. Fracture
      - *a.* Complete
      - *b.* Incomplete
    - 3. Anomalous tract
      - *a.* Dens in dente
      - *b.* Dens invaginatus
      - *c.* Dens evaginatus
  - B. Radicular ingress
    - 1. Caries
    - 2. Retrogenic infection
      - *a.* Periodontal pocket
      - *b.* Periodontal abscess
    - 3. Hematogenic
- II. Traumatic
  - A. Acute
    - 1. Coronal fracture
    - 2. Radicular fracture
    - 3. Vascular stasis
    - 4. Luxation
    - 5. Avulsion
  - B. Chronic
    - 1. Adolescent female bruxism
    - 2. Attrition or abrasion
    - 3. Erosion
- III. Iatrogenic
  - A. Cavity preparation
    - 1. Heat of preparation
    - 2. Depth of preparation
    - 3. Dehydration
    - 4. Pulp hemorrhage
    - 5. Pulp exposure
    - 6. Pin insertion
    - 7. Impression taking
  - B. Restoration
    - 1. Insertion
    - 2. Fracture
      - *a.* Complete
      - *b.* Incomplete
    - 3. Force of cementing
    - 4. Heat of polishing
  - C. Intentional extirpation
  - D. Orthodontic movement
  - E. Periodontal curettage
  - F. Periapical curettage
  - G. Rhinoplasty
  - H. Intubation
- IV. Chemical
  - A. Filling materials
    - 1. Cements
    - 2. Plastics
    - 3. Cavity liners
  - B. Disinfectants
    - 1. $AgNO_3$
    - 2. Phenol
    - 3. NaFl

C. Desiccants
 1. Alcohol
 2. Ether

V. Idiopathic
 A. Aging
 B. Internal resorption
 C. External resorption
 D. Hypophosphatasia

BACTERIAL CAUSES

Coronal Ingress

Caries. Coronal caries is by far the most common means of ingress to the dental pulp for infecting bacteria and/or their toxins (Fig. 7–1). Long before the bacteria, *per se,* reach the pulp to actually infect it, the pulp has become inflamed from irritation by preceding bacterial toxins. Langeland reported pulp reactions, observed "with certainty," when superficial fissure caries was found clinically.[1] Seltzer and Bender have described these pulp changes from early reparative dentin formation under initial caries, through scattered macrophages and lymphocytes under moderately developed caries, to frank chronic inflammatory exudate under deep carious lesions.[2] Exposure of the pulp by caries is accompanied by chronic inflammation in the immediate area of the carious lesion, together with localized abscess formation.

Bacteria are an obvious formidable enemy of the pulp, but possibly not so formidable as once supposed. In a review of the clinical management of the deep carious lesion, Canby and Burnett discuss the wisdom of not exposing the pulp under deep caries.[3] "Removing ***all*** carious dentin and jeopardizing a ***vital pulp with no significant untoward history or reaction*** would seem to be a questionable method and a needless contribution to the complexity of treatment. . . ."

This approach is borne out by Muntz, Dorfman and Stephan,[4] and by Seltzer and Bender,[5] who predict the possibility of pulp recovery if its ability to produce reparative dentin keeps ahead of the carious process.

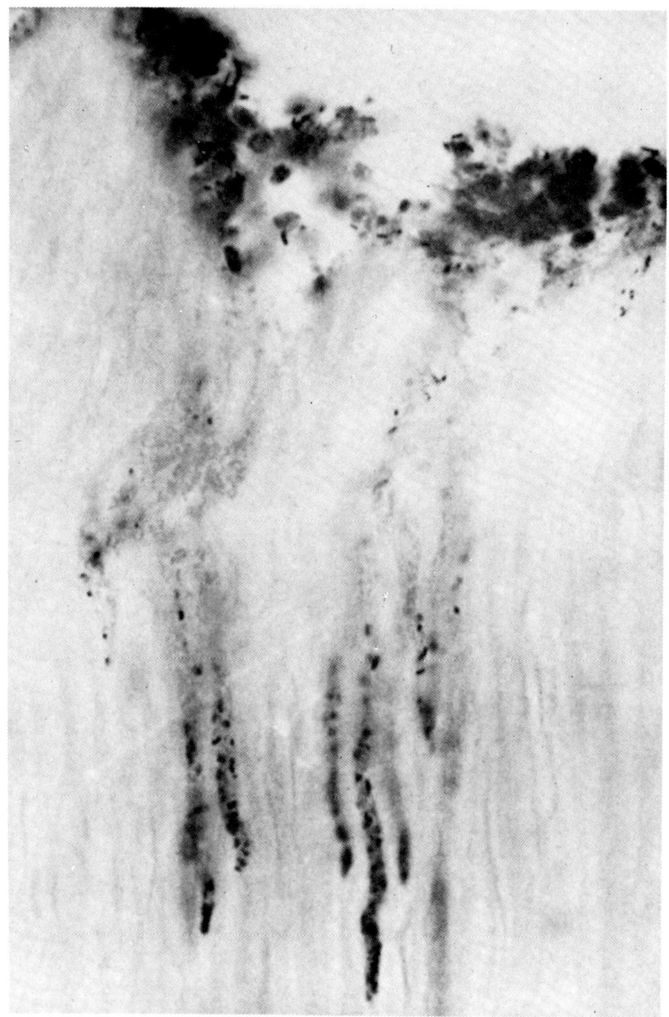

Fig. 7–1. Bacteria penetrating through dentinal tubules from carious lesion (*top*). Pulp inflammation is already established from toxins which precede bacteria (Orban Collection).

Fractured Crown. ***Complete Fracture.*** Accidental coronal fracture into the pulp seldom devitalizes the pulp at that instant. However, the inevitable pulp death of the untreated coronal fracture usually results from infection by oral bacteria gaining ready access to the pulp tissue. It matters not how extensive the fracture, but only that the pulp has been exposed to bacterial insult.

Most coronal fractures involve the maxillary anterior teeth, although posterior teeth are sometimes fractured in severe automobile accidents or sheared in half in boxing accidents. Classification of fractures and their treatment and restoration will be dealt with in detail in Chapter 16.

Incomplete Fracture. Incomplete fracture of the crown, often from mysterious causes, frequently allows ***bacterial entrance*** into the pulp. Ritchey and Orban reported 22 cases of toothache and pulp death associated with incomplete fracture in molars.[6] Pulp

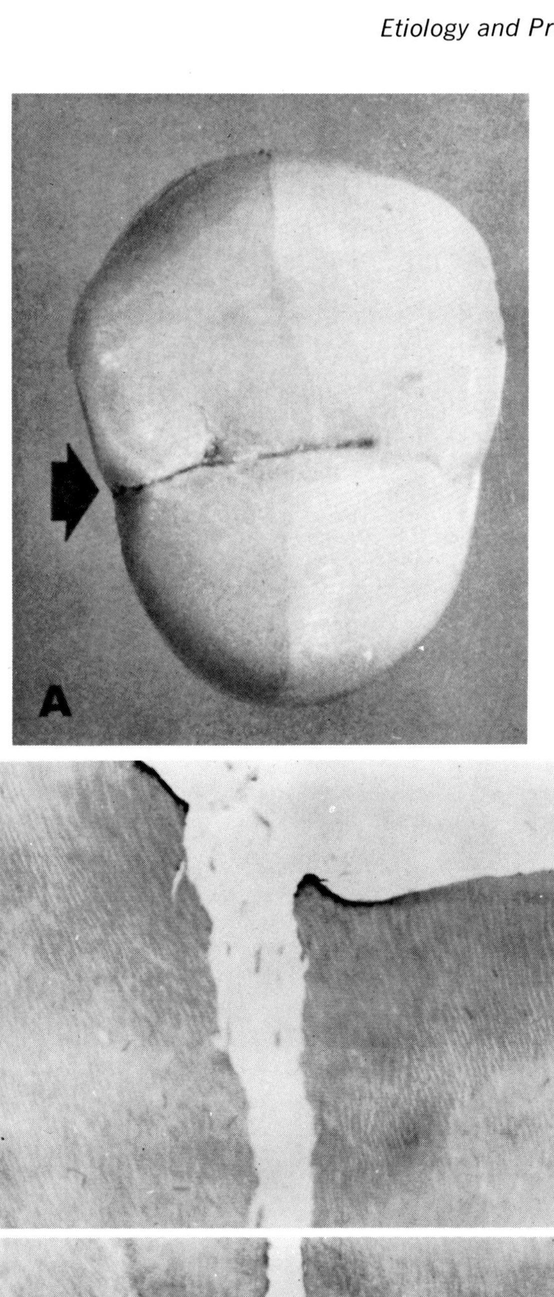

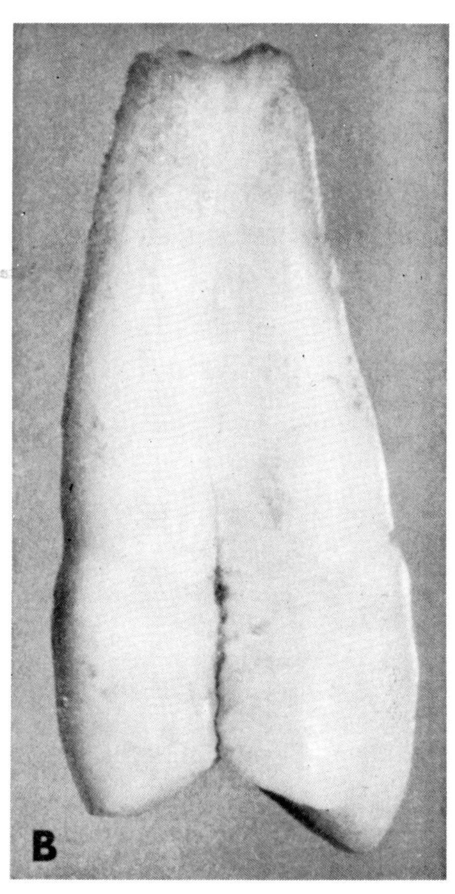

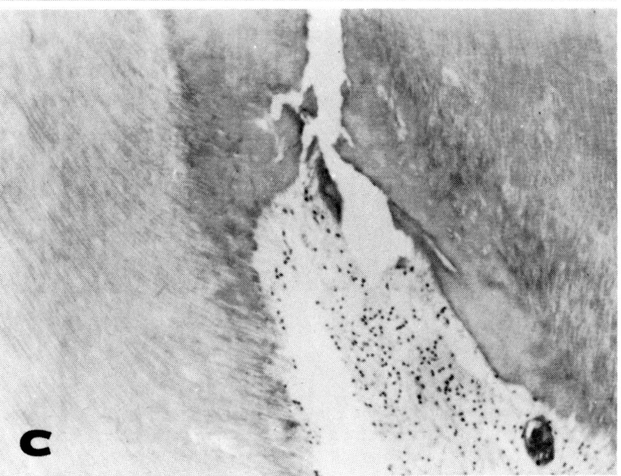

Fig. 7–2. Undetected fracture in otherwise sound premolar. *A*, Precipitated iodine discloses fracture (*arrow*). (Buccal-lingual fracture was caused by forceps.) *B*, Mesial view. Fracture extends into pulp which has become infected from invading bacteria. (Courtesy Dr. Dudley H. Glick.) *C*, Photomicrograph of undisclosed fracture from floor of cavity to pulp. Inflammatory degeneration of pulp is apparent. (Courtesy Dr. Harold Stanley.)

infection and associated inflammation depend on the extent of fracture, that is, whether the fracture is complete into the pulp chamber or is only through the enamel. In the former case pulpitis is certain to develop (Fig. 7–2); in the latter case the pulp will merely be hypersensitive to cold and mastication.

Anomalous Tract. Anomalous coronal development accounts for a substantial number of pulp deaths from ***bacterial invasion.*** In each case—*dens in dente, dens invaginatus* and *dens evaginatus*—the cause of pulp inflammation and eventual necrosis is the same—bacterial invasion of the pulp through an

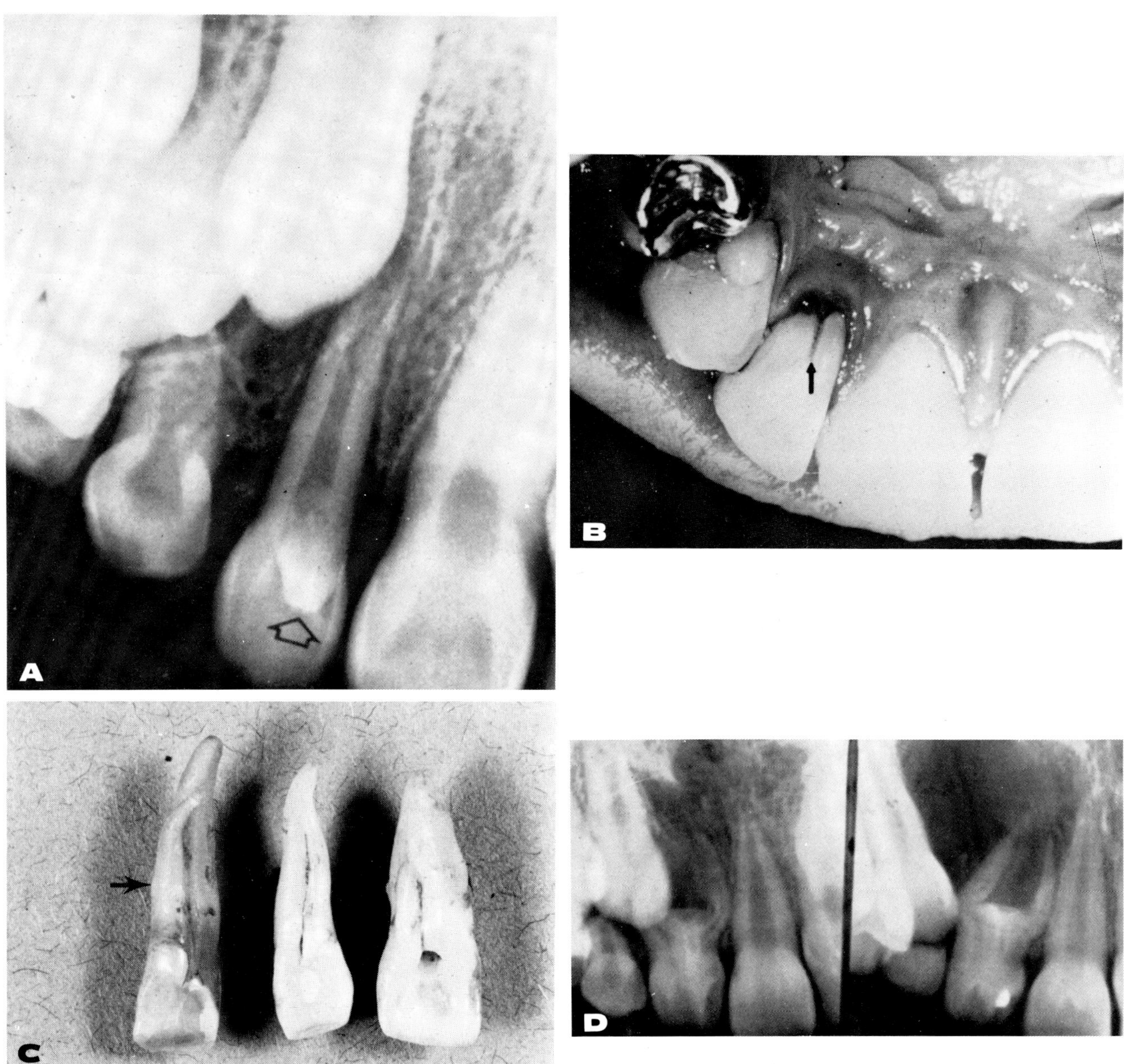

Fig. 7–3. Developmental anomalies of maxillary incisors. *A*, ***Dens invaginatus*** at cingulum (*arrow*) allows coronal bacterial ingress. *B*, Clinical appearance of ***dens invaginatus.*** Palatal periodontal pocket extends to apex. *C*, Three examples of lingual anomalies leading to tooth loss; *left*, invagination and accessory root (*arrow*); *middle*, ***dens invaginatus*** to the apex; *right*, ***dens invaginatus*** to midroot of central incisor. *D*, Bifid root formation. Bacteria have invaded through developmental tract not readily seen (*left*). Six months later (*right*) coronal defect has been filled but huge infected cyst has developed following pulp necrosis. (B and C from Simon, J. H. S., Glick, D. H., and Frank, A. L.: Oral Surg., *31*:823, June, 1971.)

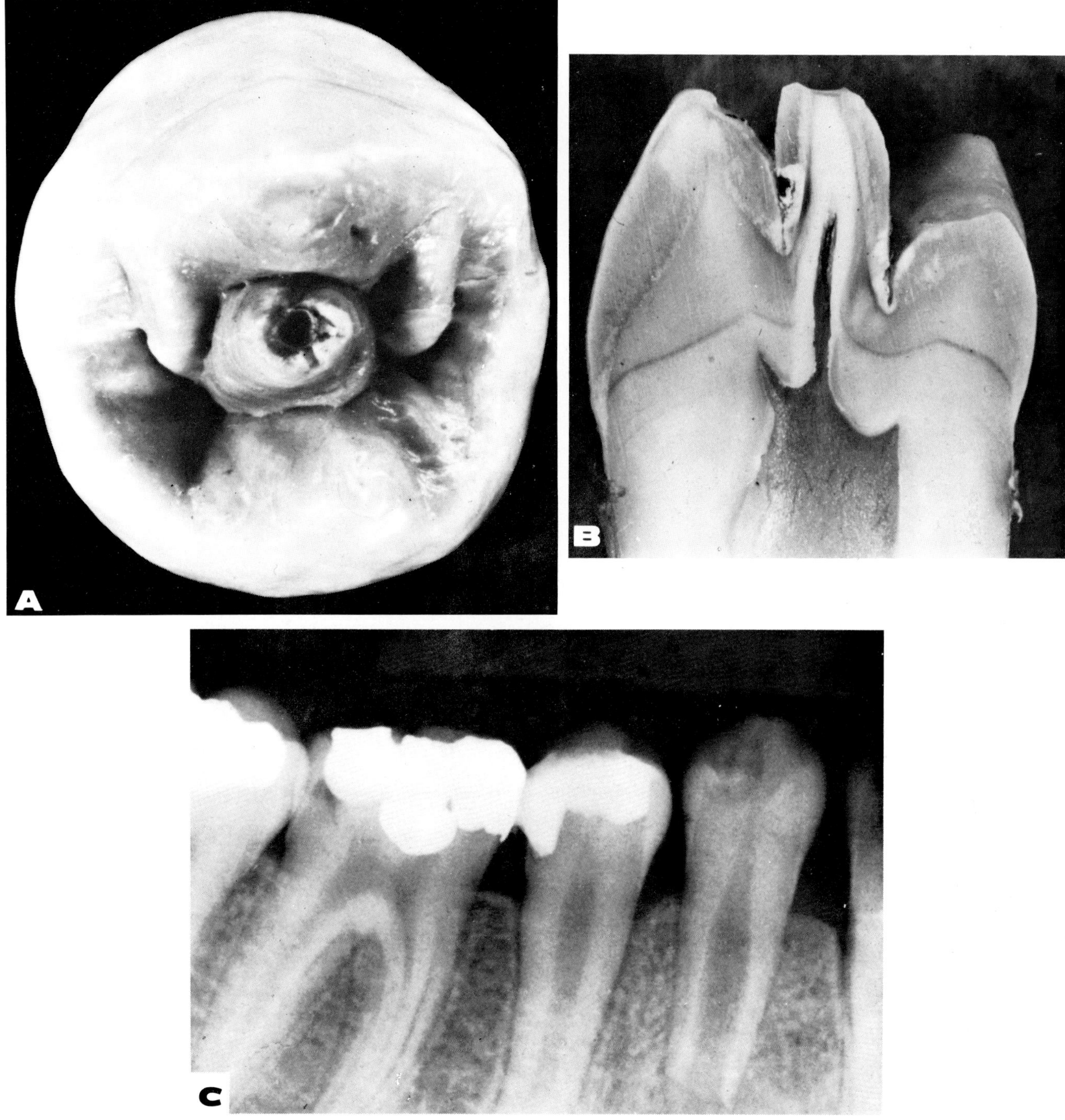

Fig. 7–4. ***Dens evaginatus.*** *A*, Volcanic appearance of extra cusp. Direct ingress of bacteria to pulp is possible. (Courtesy Dr. Ole Carlsen, Copenhagen, Denmark.) *B*, Extension of pulp into evaginated defect. (From Palmer, M. E.: Oral Surg., *35*:772, June, 1973.) *C*, Mandibular first premolar with necrotic pulp. Patient is Oriental with "extra cusp" and developmental tract through which bacteria invaded.

anomalous developmental tract extending from a "fault" in the enamel cap to the pulp tissue itself (Fig. 7–3). Almost all such tracts develop in maxillary lateral incisors and range from a slight lingual pit to a frank and obvious anomalous tract. The *dens evaginatus,* found usually on mandibular premolars, which has a tract to the pulp at its point of attachment, is a fairly common occurrence in Orientals.[7,8] Merrill also reports a high incidence (4.5%) of this anomaly in the Alaskan Eskimo, an observation that serves to illustrate the ethnic origin of the Eskimo.[9,10]

Wing-Kong Yip reports that 2.2% of 2,373 Singapore school children were afflicted with the condition, all of them of Oriental stock and none Indian in origin.[11] Senia reported the condition in a Filipino woman,[12] and Sykaras reported a case in the maxillary premolars of a Greek girl.[13] Carlsen reported a case from the Royal Dental College in Denmark,[14] and Palmer reported five evaginated odontomes in Caucasian children from England[15] (Fig. 7–4). Widerman and Serene also reported pulp death in a tauradontic tooth in a Caucasian boy[16] (Fig. 7–5).

It seems obvious that although ***in***vagination is found universally and primarily in maxillary lateral incisors, the ***e***vaginated tubercle of the mandibular premolars is primarily an Oriental, even Mongoloid, condition. *Dens evaginatus* is the antithesis of *dens* ***in****vaginatus* or *dens in dente.* It is "caused by the folding of a part of the inner enamel epithelium into the stellate reticulum . . . The evaginated enamel epithelium and the underlying cells of the dental papilla form an enamel tubercle with a dentin core which has a central canal connected with the pulp."[17] The tubercle gives the tooth a volcanic appearance.

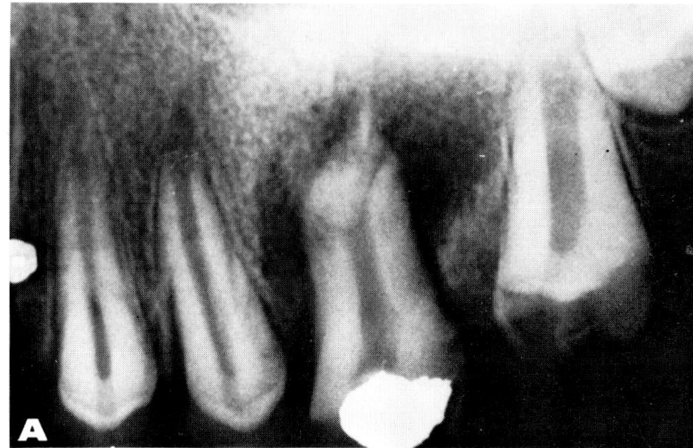

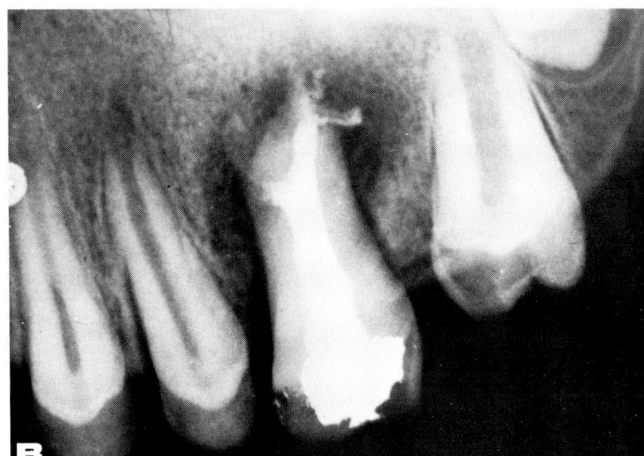

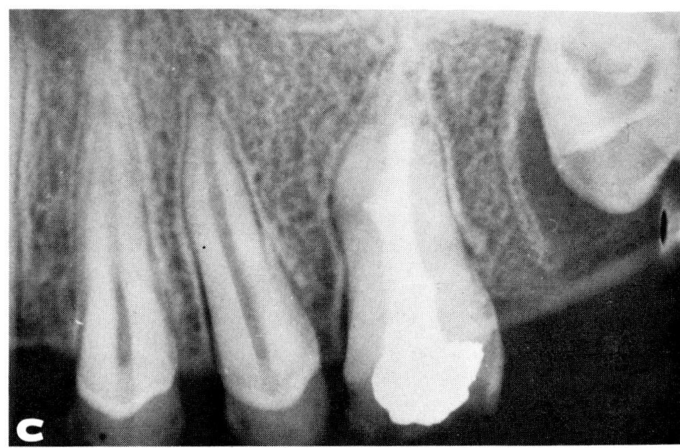

Fig. 7–5. Taurodontism. *A,* Preoperative radiograph of maxillary first molar. Large chronic abscess with draining fistula. *B,* Obturation by softened sectional gutta percha. *C,* Two year recall with healing of lateral and apical lesions. (Courtesy Dr. Fred. H. Widerman and Dr. Thomas P. Serene.)

Radicular Ingress

Caries. Root caries is, of course, a less frequent occurrence than coronal caries, but remains, nonetheless, a ***bacterial source*** of pulp irritation. Cervical root caries, particularly at the buccogingival, is a common sequela to gingival recession. Interproximal radicular caries often follow periodontal procedures if meticulous oral hygiene is not maintained. Caries in the furca also may follow periodontal involvement of this region (Fig. 7–6).

Retrogenic Infection. ***Periodontal Pocket.*** That the pulp does not frequently become infected through the apical foramen or lateral accessory canals as-

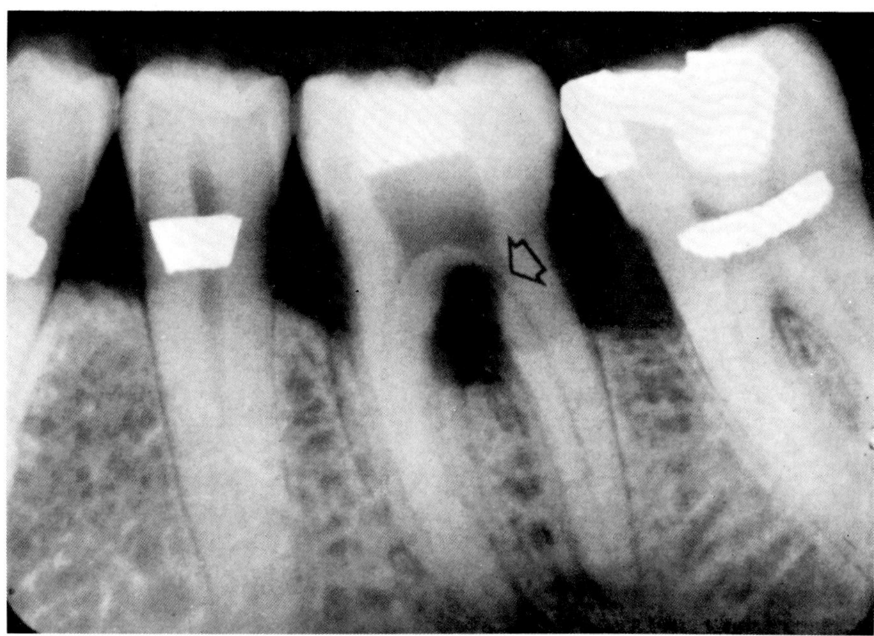

Fig. 7–6. Carious invasion of pulp (*arrow*) at furca of periodontally involved tooth.

sociated with a chronic periodontal pocket, attests to the inherent ability of the pulp to survive. Seltzer and Bender have shown increased atrophy and dystrophic calcifications in the pulps of periodontally involved teeth, but not necessarily infection.[18] Massler and Mazur, on the other hand, could not demonstrate these changes.[19]

The periodontist often encounters periodontal pockets that extend to and surround the apex (Fig. 7–7), as well as lateral accessory canals, or accessory canals in the furca area of molars (Fig. 7–8), which also extend into septic and infected pockets.[20] In view of the frequency of deep pocket occurrence, one is hard pressed to explain why retrogenic pulp infection is not more common. Nonetheless, it does occur and, in combination with the dystrophic changes observed,[18] might well serve to explain why these pulps become necrotic. Langeland et al. observed that "pathologic changes occurred in the pulp tissue when periodontal disease was present, but the pulp did not succumb as long as the main canal—the major pathway of the circulation—was not involved."[21] Involved lateral canals or root caries will damage the pulp, they said, "but total disintegration apparently occurs only when all main apical foramina are involved in the bacterial plaque" (Fig. 7–9).

Periodontal Abscess. *Retrogenic pulp infection,* either accompanying or immediately following an acute periodontal abscess, is also an infrequent cause of otherwise unexplained pulp necrosis.

Hematogenic Infection. ***Bacteria gaining access*** to the pulp through vascular channels is entirely within reason. The anachoretic attraction of bacteria to a lesion readily applies to injured pulp tissue.[22] Anachoresis of bacteria from the vessels of the gingival sulcus, or from a ***systemic transient bacteremia,*** also serves to explain the unusual number of infected pulp canals, following impact injury without fracture to 46 intact teeth, observed by MacDonald and Hare.[23]

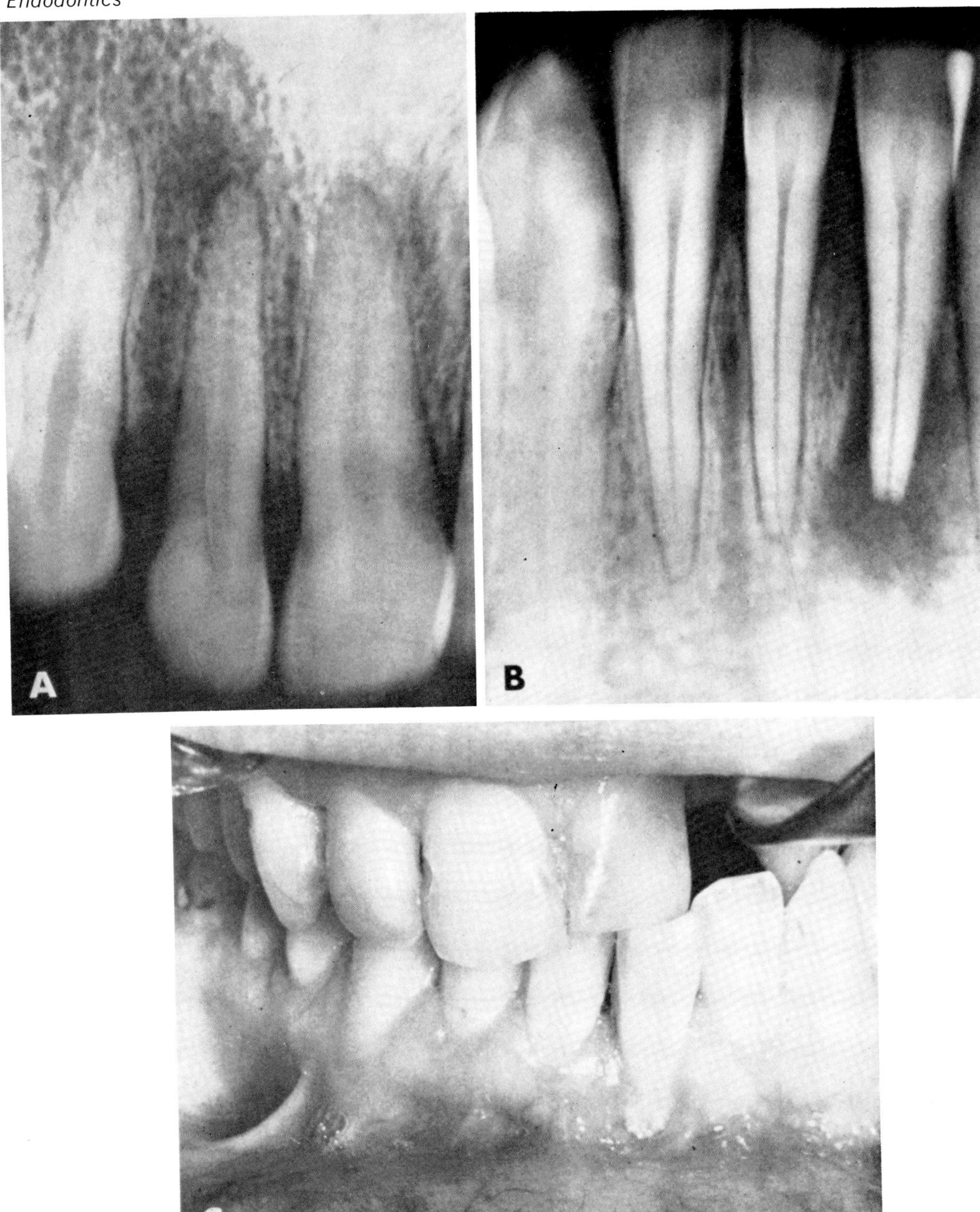

Fig. 7–7. Differential diagnosis of retrogenic pulp infection from periodontal pocket. *A*, Pulp of lateral incisor is infected and necrotic, and apparently related to distolingual pocket which extends to apex. Occlusal traumatism may be factor, although there was no history of impact trauma. *B*, Roentgenographic appearance mistakenly diagnosed as chronic apical periodontitis. Pulp is vital in involved central incisor. *C*, Orifice to labial periodontal lesion is seen as well as traumatic relationship between maxillary and mandibular incisors. Pulp is not involved in spite of extensive pocket.

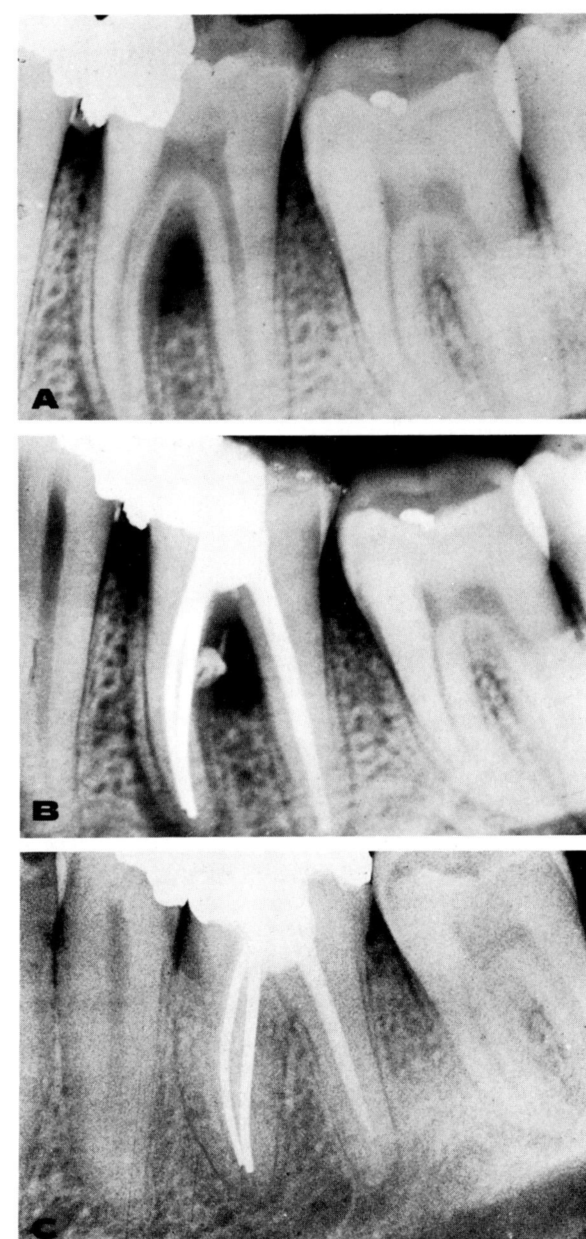

Fig. 7–8. *A,* Bony lesion in furcation draining through buccal gingival sulcus. Molar is pulpless. *B,* Obturation reveals lateral accessory canal. *C,* Three-year recall radiograph. Total healing is apparent. No surgery was used. (Courtesy Dr. Rafael Miñana, Madrid, Spain.)

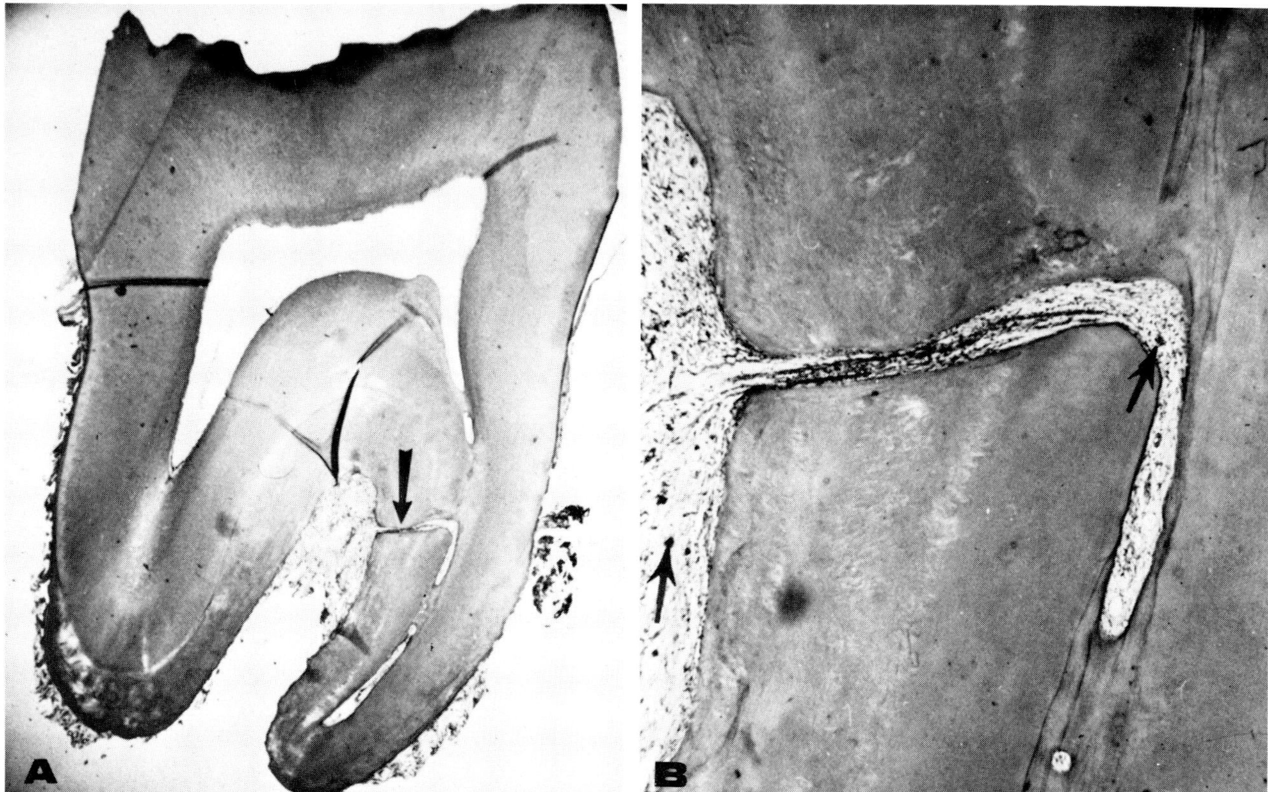

Fig. 7–9. *A,* Accessory canal (*arrow*) from vital pulp into inflamed tissue of molar bifurcation. *B,* Inflammation in accessory canal with only slight inflammation in canal pulp. Epithelial rests (*arrows*) are present in both bifurcation and pulp canal. (From Rubach, W. C., and Mitchell, D. F.: J. Periodont., *36*:34, Jan.–Feb., 1965.)

TRAUMATIC CAUSES

Acute Trauma

Coronal Fracture. Most pulp death following coronal fractures is incidental to the bacterial invasion which follows the accident. There is no question, however, that severe impact injury to the coronal pulp initiates an inflammatory attempt toward repair. Untreated, bacterial invasion negates any possibility of sustained vitality.

Radicular Fracture. Accidental fracture of the root so disrupts the pulp vascular supply that the injured pulp seldom remains vital. Severing the vessels usually supplies *le coup de grâce* to the remaining coronal pulp tissue, even though the tissue in the radicular fragment may retain its vitality.

One should not assume pulp death too soon following an accident. Complete repair of the fracture by callus formation of cementum has been known to occur (see Fig. 16–27*A*). Moreover, the blood supply may remain viable either through the apical vessels or through the ingrowth of new vessels through the fracture site (see Fig. 16–27*B*). In one paradoxic case, the ***coronal fragment remained vital*** and the fracture of the root repaired. The blood supply to the coronal pulp evidently was reestablished through the fracture, while the apical portion of the pulp became necrotic. The coronal pulp finally filled-in completely with reparative dentin (see Fig. 16–16*A*).

As with any other condition affecting the pulp, the younger the patient, the better the prognosis for pulp vitality. The extensive vascular supply through the incompletely formed root end provides a much greater opportunity for repair than the fractured root and disrupted blood supply of a fully formed tooth.

Vascular Stasis. The tooth that receives a severe impact injury, yet is not dislocated or fractured, is more apt to lose pulp vitality immediately than the tooth that fractures. Evidently the pulp vessels are either severed or smashed at the apical foramen.

Pulp canal calcification by reparative dentin is another pulp response to trauma. Thus the pulp may either die immediately from trauma or furiously eliminate itself by dentin formation.

Again, following trauma and depending upon the age of the patient, the possibility exists for pulp repair and returned pulp vitality. The developing tooth with open flaring apex is quite apt to remain vital or regain vitality. In the older patient, the prognosis for repair is limited.

Luxation. Partial avulsion or intrusion nearly always results in pulp death. The ***tooth*** should be given the benefit of the doubt even though the test shows the ***pulp*** to be nonvital. On the other hand, one is occasionally surprised to find a young but severely luxated tooth retaining pulp vitality (see Fig. 16–40).

Avulsion. It goes without saying that pulp necrosis is the obvious consequence of total avulsion of a tooth. In spite of pulp death, however, the tooth can still be replanted following root canal filling (see Chapter 16).

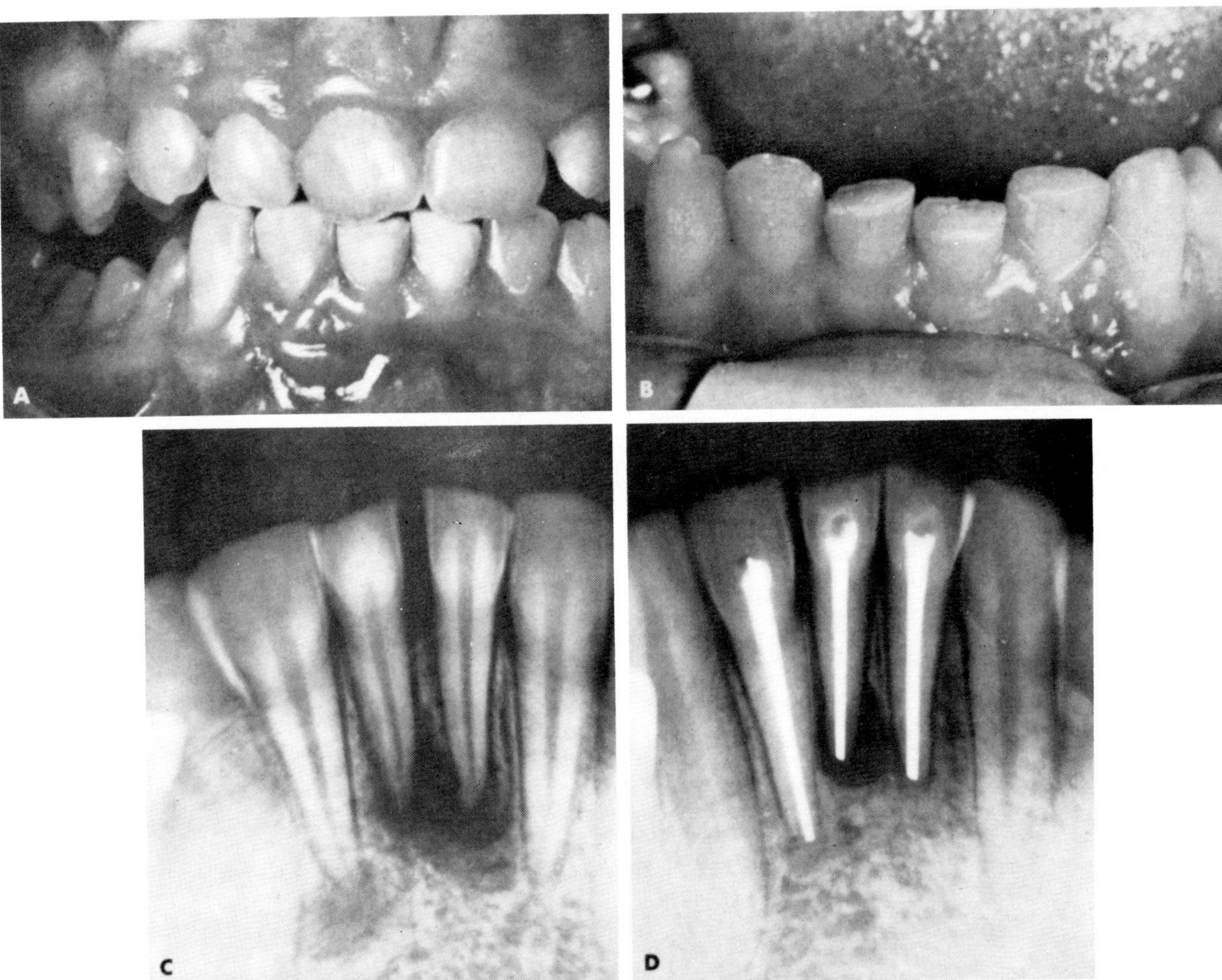

Fig. 7–10. Osteoporosis and pulp death of mandibular incisors in adolescent girl who compulsively grinds her teeth in protrusive excursion. *A,* Position assumed during bruxism by 14-year-old girl. *B,* Extensive wear of mandibular incisors caused by compulsive grinding. *C,* Pulps of three incisors have been devitalized by force of traumatic habit. Acute abscess has separated central incisors. *D,* One year following root canal therapy, some repair has occurred; however, persistent habit prevents complete healing. (From Natkin, E., and Ingle, J.: J. Amer. Soc. Periodont., *1*:260, Nov.–Dec., 1963.)

Chronic Trauma

Adolescent Female Bruxism. Ingle and Natkin have reported an unusual syndrome of osteoporosis and pulp death of mandibular incisors in adolescent females who compulsively grind their teeth in protrusive excursion.[24,25] Evidently the trauma is so severe and sustained that pulp necrosis eventually develops (Fig. 7–10). Gruchalla has reported a similar case—a girl who died of erythroblastosis at age 14[26] (Fig. 7–11).

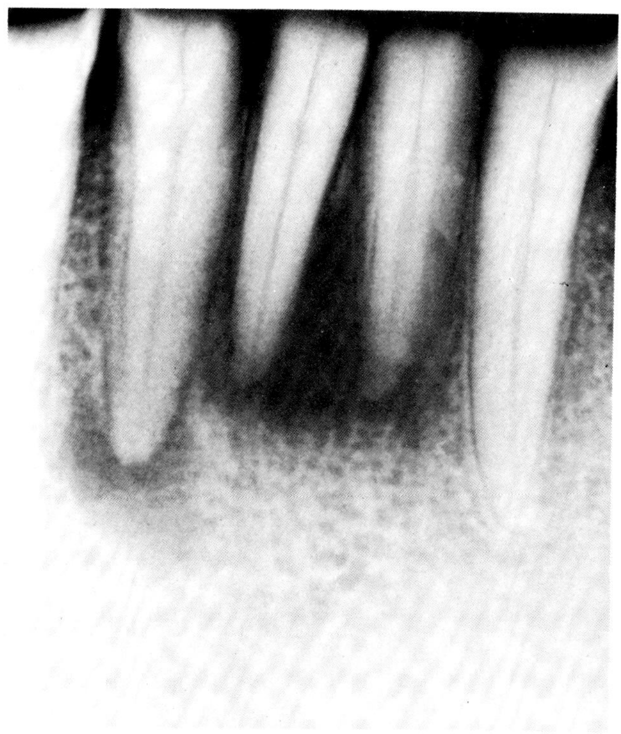

Fig. 7–12. Incisal abrasion into pulp, leading to pulp necrosis of three mandibular incisors.

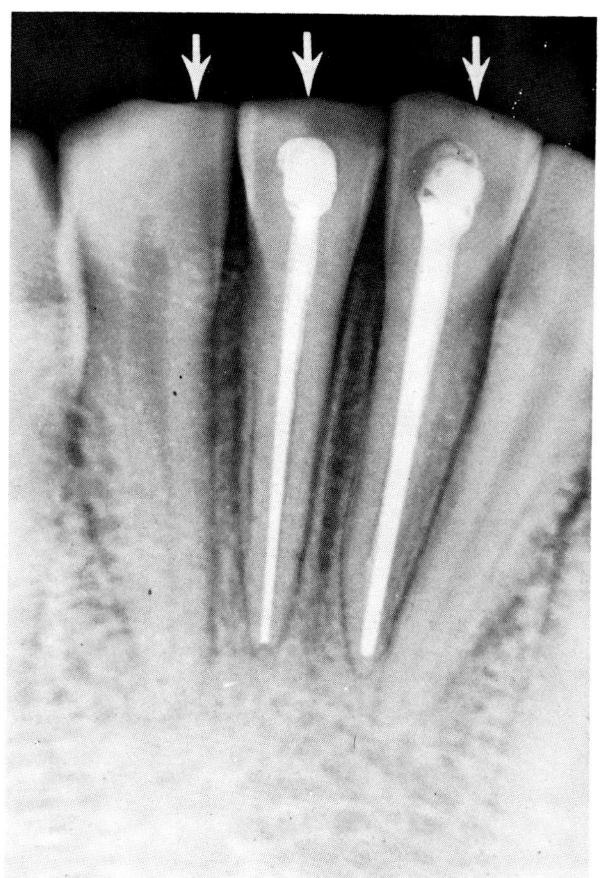

Fig. 7–11. Adolescent female bruxism. Note advanced incisal wear in 12-year-old girl. Patient died of Cooley's anemia two years later as did her twin. (Courtesy Dr. Frank Gruchalla.)

Attrition or Abrasion. Pulp death or inflammation related to incisal wear or gingival erosion is a rarity. The reparative power of the pulp to lay down dentin as it recedes ahead of this stimulus is phenomenal. Occasionally, however, a severely worn mandibular incisor is encountered, with a necrotic pulp and an observable incisal opening into the pulp chamber (Fig. 7–12). Quite possibly the pulp of this case was devitalized at an earlier time and attrition finally reached the chamber. Incisal attrition is more apt to develop opposite porcelain teeth. Seltzer and Bender noted retrogressive and atrophic pulp changes, but not total necrosis, in relation to the constant irritation of attrition or abrasion.[18] Sognnaes et al. have reported cervical erosion so severe that the pulps of maxillary incisors were invaded[27] (Fig. 7–13).

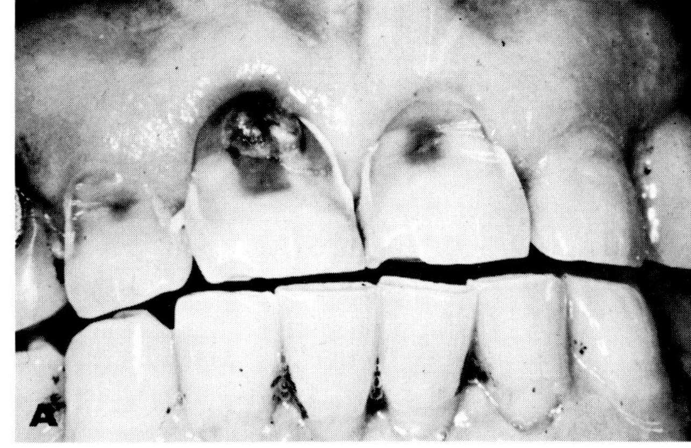

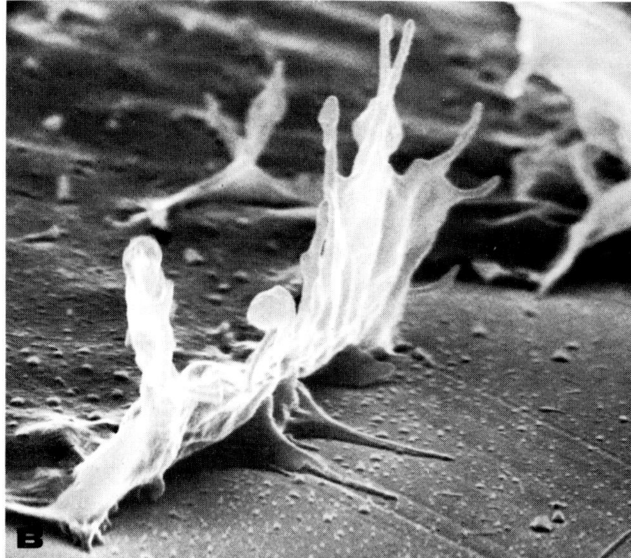

Fig. 7–13. *A,* Dental erosion has exposed pulps of maxillary central incisors. (From Sognnaes, R. F., Wolcott, R. B., and Xhonga, F. A.: J.A.D.A., *84*:571, Mar. 1972.) *B,* Possible cause of erosion. Fibroblastic cell perambulation by a process of "ruffling" may cause ablation of tooth or plastic surfaces. (From Revel, J.-P.: Engineering and Science, California Institute of Technology, Nov.–Dec., 1973.)

IATROGENIC CAUSES

Cavity Preparation

Heat of Preparation. The heat generated by grinding procedures on tooth structure has been shown to be the greatest single cause of pulp damage during cavity preparation. As Kramer has stated,[28] "If the use of these instruments today is not to provide a harvest for the endodontist tomorrow, it is essential that the development of these high-speed handpieces should be accompanied by the development of adequate cooling mechanisms" (Fig. 7–14). The inevitable inflammation following cavity preparation, ranging from reversible to irreparable changes, has been well documented by Stanley and Swerdlow,[29] Langeland,[1] Lefkowitz,[30] Brännström[31] and others. Swerdlow and Stanley[32] pointed out the basic factors in rotary instrumentation which cause temperature rise in the pulp. In order of their importance:

1. Force applied by the operator
2. Size, shape, and condition of cutting tool
3. Revolutions per minute
4. Duration of actual cutting time.

One would surmise that the ultra-speed (200,000 rpm) instruments of today are more traumatic to the pulp than the low-speed (6,000 rpm) instruments of the immediate past. Such is not the case if adequate air-water coolant is used. Stanley and Swerdlow concluded that speeds of 50,000 rpm and over were found to be less traumatic to the human pulp than techniques utilizing 6,000 and 20,000 rpm.[29] They point out, however, that the value of coolants becomes more significant at higher speeds. It was possible to "burn" the pulp in eleven seconds of preparation time if air alone was used as a coolant at 200,000 rpm. This concurs with findings of Vaughn and Peyton,[33] that the highest intrapulp temperatures were reached within the first ten seconds of grinding. Peyton and Henry also demonstrated a temperature rise up to 110° F at 15,000 rpm if no coolant was used while cutting with a No. 37 inverted cone diamond point at 0.5 pound load.[34]

Stanley and Swerdlow have stated that the degree of cellular displacement of odontoblastic nuclei into the cut dentinal tubules is the best indication of the severity of pulp inflammation.[35] They felt this displacement of the cells was due to a build-up of intrapulp pressure by an inflammatory response; that the edema, hyperemia, and exudation occurring in proximity to the pulp wall literally forced the odontoblasts and blood cells into the dentinal tubules (Fig. 7–15).

Using cellular displacement into the tubules as a criterion for pulp inflammation, Ostrom, in an ingenious experiment, was able to show that heat of preparation is one of the most logical causes of pulp inflammation during preparation, and that the cellular displacement into the tubules is the result of the pressure generated from intrapulp inflammation following the temperature rise.[36]

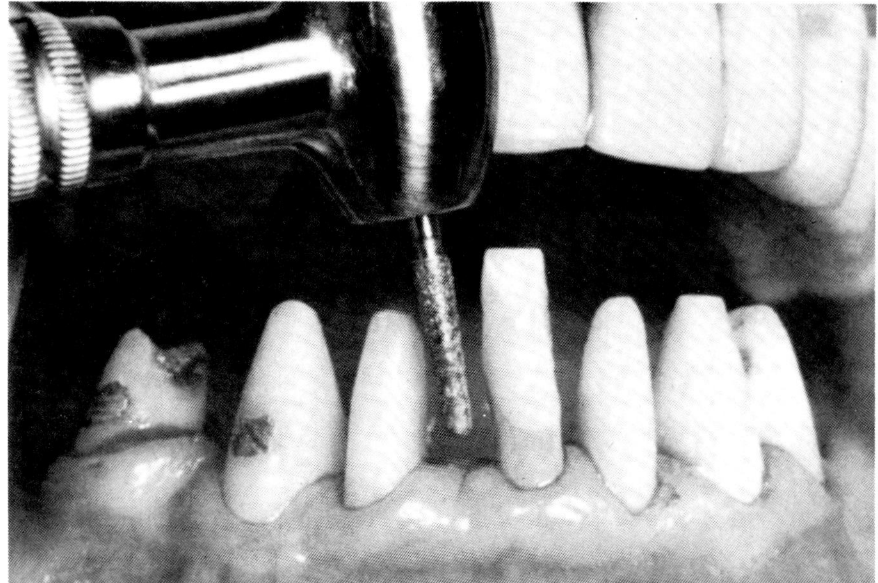

Fig. 7–14. Iatrogenic pulp death frequently occurs when teeth must be reduced to this extent. It is imperative that copious water coolant be used to protect pulp from heat damage and desiccation during preparation.

Pohto and Scheinin were also able to demonstrate arrested circulation and altered venule and capillary permeability by increasing pulp temperature with 46° C saline solution acting through 15 to 20 microns of dentin, thus showing inflammatory changes related to heat.[37]

Depth of Preparation. It can be stated categorically that the deeper the preparation, the more extensive the pulp inflammation that results. This has been shown by Seelig and Lefkowitz, who observed that the degree of pulp response is ***inversely*** proportional to the remaining thickness of dentin.[38]

Stanley and Swerdlow also point out the increased importance of air-water coolant as the dentin is thinned and the pulp approached.[35]

Seltzer and Bender noted "huge amounts" of reparative dentin under restorations; much more than under caries.[18] They also noted the reparative dentin under restorations to be more amorphous and irregular and the associated odontoblastic nuclei grossly altered in structure.

Dehydration. Brännström has well documented the damaging effects on the pulp by dehydration of the exposed dentin.[39,40] Constant drying and chip blowing with warm air during cavity preparation under the rubber dam could well contribute to pulp inflammation and possible necrosis, which sometimes follows restorative dentistry. Langeland demonstrated the first stage of inflammation "when the dentin of the floor of the cavity is blown dry, even if the preparation has been carried out under a water spray."[41]

Pulp Hemorrhage. Occasionally during cavity preparation, particularly full crown preparation of anterior teeth, the dentin is seen to suddenly "blush." Pulp hemorrhage has just taken place, quite possibly from an increase in intrapulp pressure so great as to rupture a pulp vessel and force erythrocytes past the odontoblasts out into the dentinal tubules. This phenomenon, which has also been seen during class V cavity preparation, must be similar to the hemorrhage into the dentin which often follows a severe traumatic blow to the tooth. In the latter case, however, it is surmised that the blood is driven into the dentin by the hydraulic pressure developed from the blow.

Pulps that have suffered a total hemorrhage into the dentin can hardly be considered candidates for longevity, although the "blushing" has been seen to disappear in time under zinc oxide and eugenol. At a later time, most pulps that appear clinically to have recovered have actually succumbed to the violence of their initial response. Microhemorrhages are probably a common occurrence during cavity preparation, a finding demonstrated by Orban in 1940.[42] Fortunately, recovery from these minor hemorrhages is the rule rather than the exception.

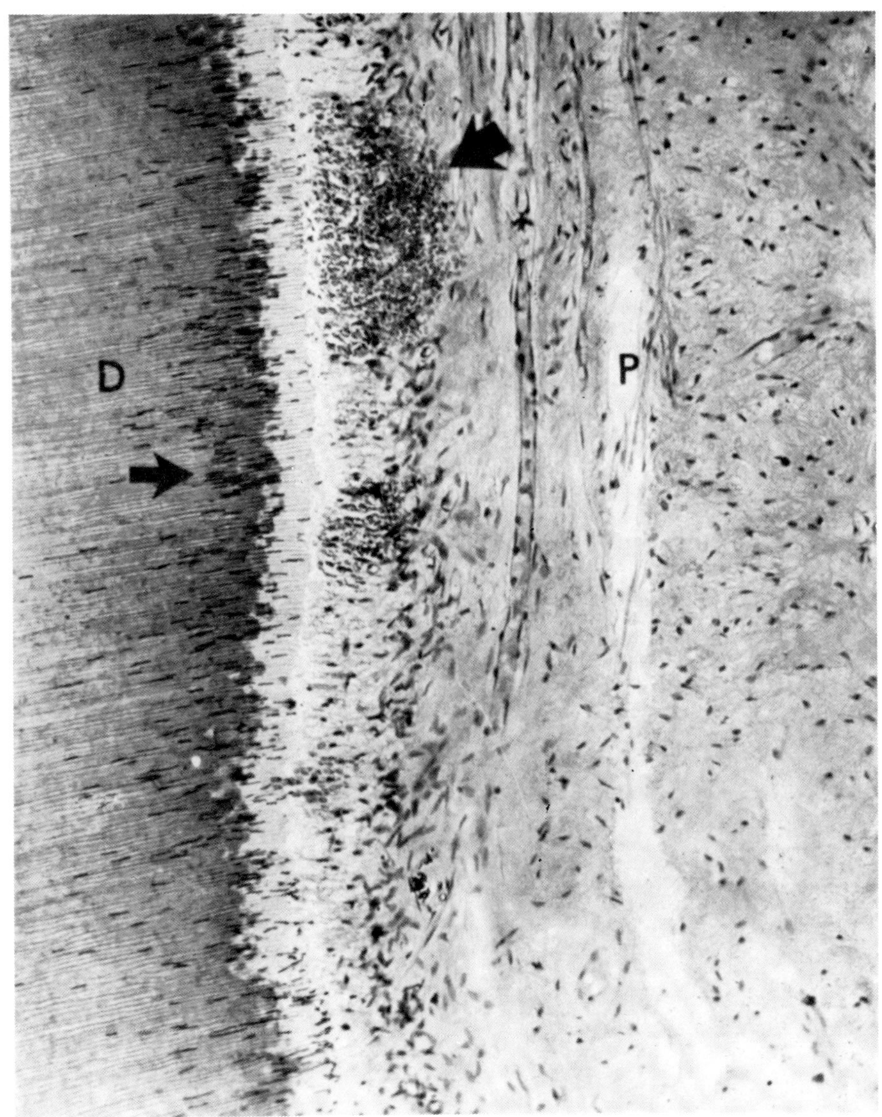

Fig. 7–15. Cellular displacement and microhemorrhage in pulp following cavity preparation. Odontoblast nuclei (*small arrow*) are displaced into dentin (*D*). Bleeding within pulp (*P*) is indicated by large arrow. (Orban Collection.)

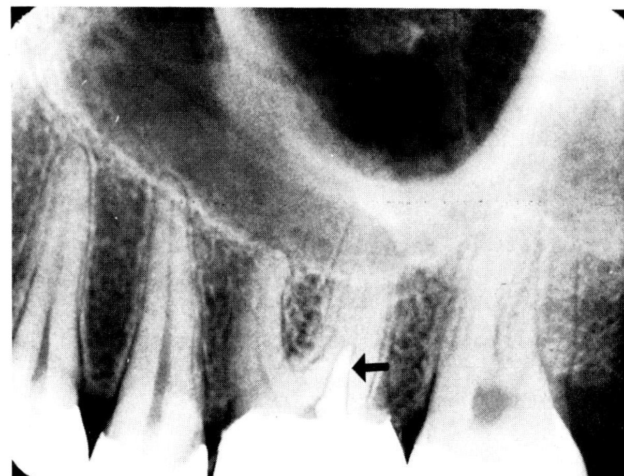

Fig. 7–16. Cement forced into pulp during cementation. Pulpitis and severe pulpalgia resulted.

Pulp Exposure. The increased incidence of pulp death following pulp exposure has been experienced by all dentists. If at all possible, a layer of dentin should be allowed to remain as pulp cover.[3] The numerous methods devised and drugs used to "cap" pulp exposures, and the discouraging results reported for pulp capping, verify the importance of maintaining pulp integrity.

On occasion a pulp exposure will be made unbeknownst to the dentist because there is no bleeding. The first indication of a problem is the patient's complaint of pulpalgia when the anesthesia "wears off." A radiograph reveals the exposure and cement forced into the pulp (Fig. 7–16).

Pin Insertion. Since the advent of pin placement into the dentin to support amalgam restorations, or as a framework for building up badly broken down teeth for full crown construction, an increase in pulp inflammation and death has been noted. Undoubtedly, in some cases, the trauma of preparing and inserting the pins is insult enough to finish off an already irritated pulp. In other cases, however, the pins may have inadvertently been inserted directly into the pulp or are so close that they act as a severe irritant. Suzuki et al. found pulp necrosis only in those experimental specimens in which pulp exposure had occurred, and in which the pins had been placed without the presence of calcium hydroxide.[43] In some cases, where preparation and placement were too close to the pulp, dentinal fractures occurred with resultant pulp inflammation just underneath (Fig. 7–17*A*). When preparation and placement were near the pulp, and in the presence of calcium hydroxide, irritant dentin formed to protect the underlying pulp, which remained normal (Fig. 7–17*B*).

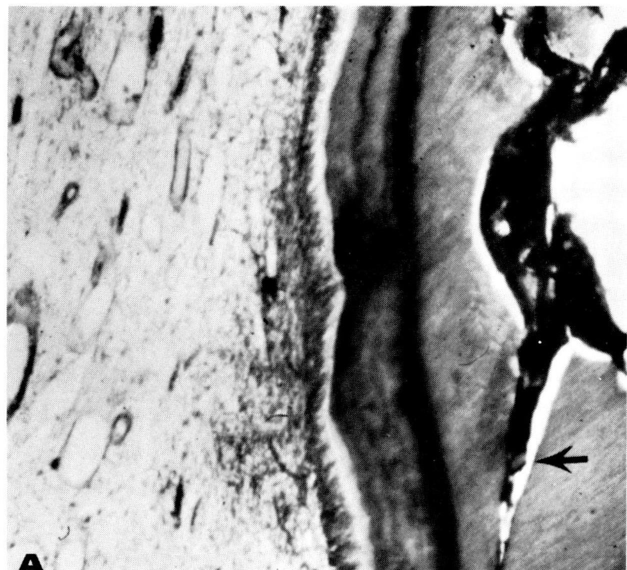

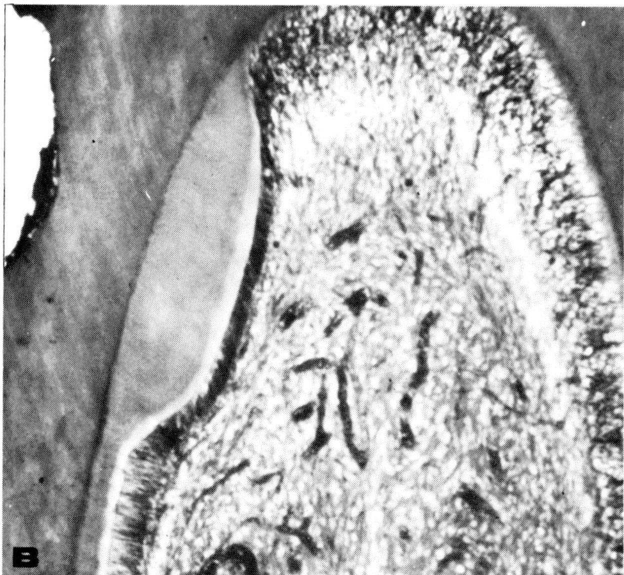

Fig. 7–17. *A,* Pin placement with calcium hydroxide. Note dentinal cracks from force of insertion (*arrow*). Cracks filled with calcium hydroxide. Moderate pulp inflammation under affected tubules. *B,* Pin placement with calcium hydroxide and no dentinal fracture. Reparative dentin response is apparent at 28 days. Remaining dentin thickness 0.08 mm. (From Suzuki, M., Goto, G., and Jordan, R. E.: J.A.D.A., *87*:636, Sept., 1973.)

Impression Taking. Seltzer and Bender have shown the damaging pulp changes that may develop from the act of taking impressions under pressure.[2] In one instance, bacteria placed into a freshly prepared cavity were forced into the pulp. One might well extrapolate these experimental findings to apply to impressions taken with force in deep cavities or full crown preparations. Moreover, the negative pressure created in removing an impression may also cause odontoblastic aspiration.

Restoration

Insertion. Severe hypersensitivity and pulpalgia, symptomatic of an underlying pulp inflammation and subsequent necrosis, have been noted following the insertion of gold foil and silver amalgam restorations. Foil insertion is evidently far more traumatic to the pulp than amalgam insertion in the ratio of 9:1, foil over amalgam.[44] James and Schour found gold foil to be the most irritating of eight filling materials, even more than silicate.[45]

Although the exact cause is not known, it is presumed that the force and direction of the blow from malleting foil may be traumatic to the vascular supply at the apical foramen. Kalnins and Millsop found following class V foil placement, "extensive hemorrhages . . . in the coronal pulp and root pulp . . . caused by rupture of the blood vessels."[46] If the teeth were splinted with acrylic, "hemorrhages due to malleting were less pronounced or absent."

Added to "malleting trauma" is the prolonged time spent in insertion of foil, and the trauma of separation procedures. When one considers the trauma to the pulp from cavity preparation, including the desiccating effect of chip blowing, plus the chemical irritation of a cement base, in addition to the trauma and prolonged operating time of insertion, as well as the heat generated in finishing, the number of pulps that survive the *rigors* of restoration is surprising.

Patients sometimes report protracted pulpalgia or hypersensitivity following the insertion of silver amalgam restorations. Again, this could be related to the force of insertion or possibly to the expansion of the amalgam after insertion. In any case, it seems reasonable to assume that the pulp pain is an outgrowth of pulp inflammation. Swerdlow and Stanley reported pulp changes when amalgam was condensed into fresh cavities prepared with high-speed equipment.[47] No significant differences in pulp response were noted, however, between hand or mechanical condensation.

Fracture. ***Complete.*** There is no question about pulp insult when a complete fracture into the pulp develops as a result of inlay or three-quarter crown placement or removal. In addition to the typical vertical fracture, a number of horizontal fractures have also been seen, developing at the gingival following a cleavage line set up in placing a class V foil restoration.

Incomplete. Incomplete fracture may be a sequela to restoration with either gold or silver. Patients sometimes complain of hypersensitivity or pulpalgia for months following the placement of a foil, inlay, or amalgam, only to gain relief when a cusp finally fractures away, or the crown fractures horizontally. Ritchey and Orban listed 22 cases of pulpalgia related to incomplete fracture of posterior teeth restored with "soft gold" inlays.[6] Incomplete fracture is further complicated by bacterial invasion through the microscopic fracture line (see Fig. 7–2*C*).

Force of Cementing. Unanesthetized patients invariably complain of pulp pain when an inlay or crown is finally cemented with oxyphosphate of zinc cement. Occasionally the pain does not "wear off" and the dentist realizes the final cementation was *le coup de grâce* to a sick pulp. Undoubtedly the chemical irritation of the cement liquid is a factor, but on the other hand, the tremendous hydraulic force exerted during cementation could not help but drive the liquid toward the pulp. The pressure exerted would be similar to the force exerted in taking a full-crown impression. Cavity liners have much to recommend their use.

Heat of Polishing. Finally, but by no means last in order of importance, one must consider the pulp damage caused by polishing restorations. This damage may be compounded by polishing with dry powders while the tooth is anesthetized. The subsequent temperature increase gives rise to the same pulp damage previously discussed under cavity preparation. Interproximal finishing of gold foils, silicates, or plastics with 18-inch finishing strips without a constant air coolant should be condemned.

Intentional Extirpation

A number of situations will arise in restorative dentistry, particularly periodontal prosthesis, where intentional extirpation of the pulp is indicated. Total root amputation or hemisection of periodontally involved roots requires intentional extirpation of the remaining pulps. A number of situations have been well documented by Bohannan,[48] who lists the following indications for intentional extirpation: reorientation of the occlusal plane of tipped, drifted, or elongated teeth; reduction of crown-root ratio in the face of advanced loss of bony support; and the establishment of parallelism of clinical crowns when a fixed prosthesis is being utilized. Added to these indications is the occasional necessity to utilize the root canal for dowel retention of a crown, plus intentional extirpation of a pulp of a tooth, badly drifted to the labial, which is now being restored with a jacket crown to a more esthetic relationship. The pulp must be entered in order to cut the preparation far enough back into the arch.

Orthodontic Movement

Although orthodontists may deny the possibility, dental pulps can be devitalized under orthodontic movement. Pulps have not only been devitalized, but they have also hemorrhaged, for when the patient presents himself for endodontic therapy, the tooth may be discolored. Paradoxically, the maxillary canine, which is seldom devitalized by other trauma, is the tooth most susceptible to pulp hemorrhage and necrosis under the forces of orthodontic movement.

Periodontal Curettage

Occasionally, during curettage of a periodontal lesion which extends entirely around the apex of a root, the pulp vessels are severed and the pulp devitalized. Pulp vitality is a small price to pay if the tooth can be retained by the periodontal curettage followed by root canal therapy.

Periapical Curettage

A not infrequent result of periapical surgery is the devitalization of the pulps of adjacent vital teeth during curettage of an extensive bony lesion (Fig. 7–18). This iatrogenic devitalization of normally vital pulps most frequently occurs in the mandibular incisor region. The possibility of this accident is good cause for the limitation of promiscuous periapical surgery in this region. If periapical surgery is absolutely indicated, accidental devitalization is less likely to occur if great care is exercised to avoid the tissue around adjacent teeth. A marsupial surgical technique has also been used.

Rhinoplasty

Nasal plastic surgery may be the cause of pulp death. Glick reports three cases of pulp death in maxillary anterior teeth following plastic reconstruction of the nose.[49] Root tips of maxillary central incisors have been fractured during this operation.

Intubation

A relatively common operating room accident, the luxation of the mandibular incisors, may be caused by the heavy retraction against these teeth with an

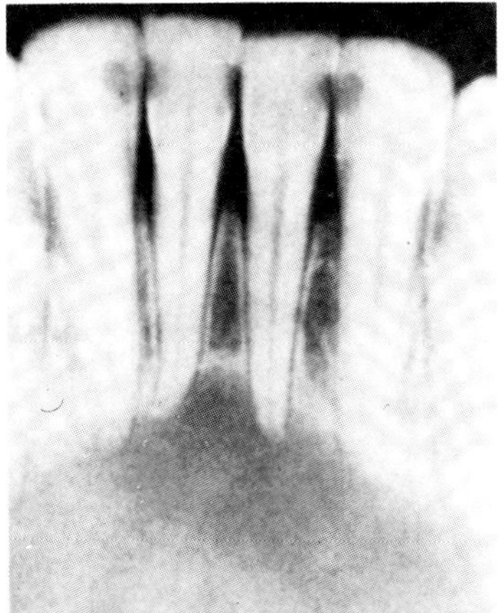

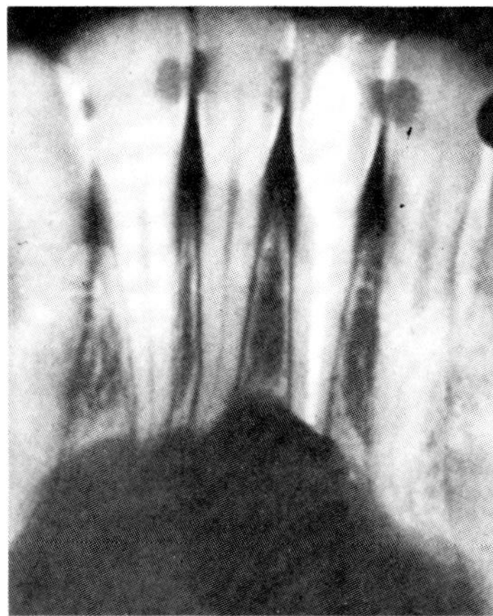

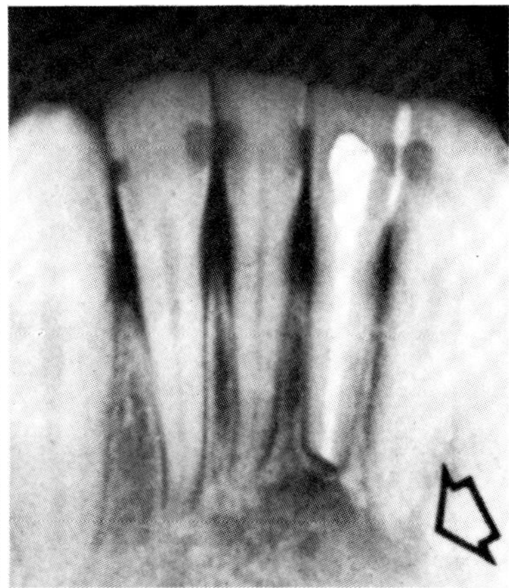

Fig. 7–18. Pulp death caused by periapical curettage during cyst enucleation. Huge apical cyst seen initially *(left)* is related to only one pulpless tooth which has been treated *(center)* and cyst carefully enucleated. Examination of one-year postoperative roentgenogram *(right)* reveals radiolucency *(arrow)* apical to lateral incisor which was devitalized during curettage.

inflexible endotracheal tube. Cases have been seen following tonsillectomy with all four mandibular incisors luxated.

CHEMICAL CAUSES

Filling Materials

Cements. To the severe insult to the pulp from bacteria of dental caries, plus the iatrogenic trauma from cavity preparation, must be added the chemical insult from the various filling materials. The commonly used cements are silicate, zinc phosphate, zinc oxide and eugenol, the polycarboxylates, and the immediate temporary cements.

Silicate cement has long been condemned as a pulp irritant (Fig. 7–19). Zander summarized an excellent investigation of the pulp effects of silicate by stating:

1. Silicate cement is highly irritating to the pulp.
2. Irregular dentin formation or a wide layer of primary dentin tends to minimize this irritation.
3. The pulps of younger persons are more likely to react severely to silicate cements than are the pulps of older persons.
4. Extension for prevention should be carried out with minimal dentin penetration.
5. A nonirritating base, such as zinc oxide-eugenol cement, should be used under silicates, especially in younger patients.[50]

Zander's work on silicates has more recently been confirmed by James and Schour,[51] Langeland,[41] and El-Kafrawy and Mitchell.[52]

Zinc phosphate cement has been both condemned[53,54] and praised[41] as a cementing medium and insulating and protective base. Langeland found zinc phosphate cement to be a good liner under the more irritating silicates.[63] More recently, Dubner and Stanley were not too concerned with pulp reaction under zinc phosphate cement.[55] James and Schour placed zinc phosphate cement about halfway between silicate as an irritant and zinc oxide–eugenol as a palliative.[51]

Langeland has pointed out that much of the earlier investigation of zinc phosphate cements was inaccu-

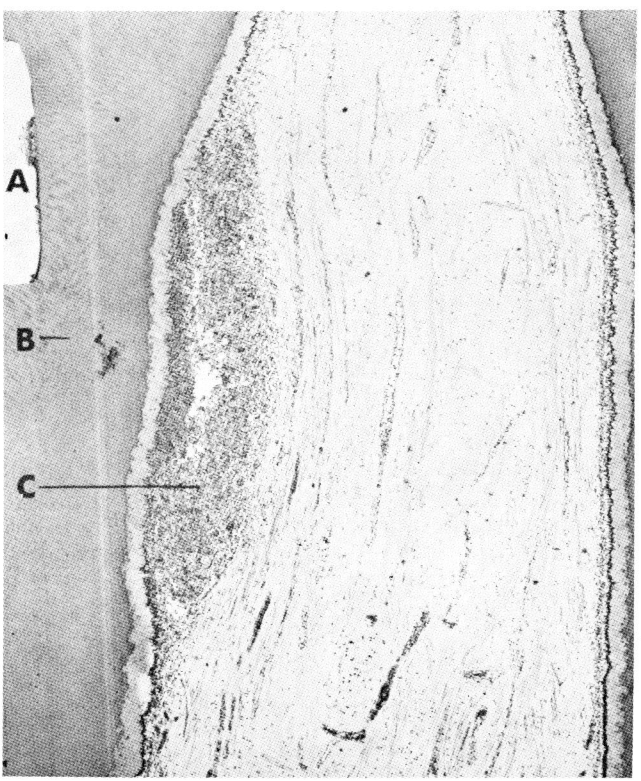

Fig. 7–19. Severe pulp inflammation related to silicate cement placement in sound tooth six weeks previous to extraction. Inflammatory reaction *(C)* is present adjacent to dentinal tubules *(B)* leading from cavity floor and wall *(A)*. (From Zander, H. A.: J.A.D.A., *33*:1233, Oct., 1946.)

rate in that the researchers were reading the effects of their experimental cavity preparations into their evaluation of the toxic effects of the cement.[56] Particularly damaging were the effects of dentin desiccation from the excessive cavity drying believed necessary. In experiments with drying performed without desiccation, oxyphosphate of zinc cements did not cause more than moderate reactions.

"Zinc oxide–eugenol still remains the most effective temporary filling material when prevention of pulpal injury is of prime concern." This statement by Dubner and Stanley[55] is echoed by all other investigators in the field. James and Schour have suggested that zinc oxide and eugenol "may even have exerted a palliative effect on the pulp."[51]

Red and black copper cements have been found to be quite irritating to the pulp and have practically passed from use.

Polycarboxylate cements, a mixture of resin and zinc phosphate cements, have been heavily advertised as adhesives. Evidently they do adhere to enamel and initially adhere also to dentin, although this latter bond is soon broken. Langeland et al. tested two polycarboxylates (PCA and Carboset) against pulp reaction in monkey teeth.[57] "In 14 cases polycarboxylate cement alone was used and there were 2 'none to slight' reactions, 2 'moderate' reactions, and 10 'repairs'. When used as a base under composite resins the variables were 10 'none to slight' reactions, 3 'moderate' reactions', 4 'severe' reactions and 1 'repair'."

The results indicate that polycarboxylate cements *per se* are relatively inert, but that care must be taken to secure full coverage of all exposed dentin to prevent reactions from the composite materials as in the case with all bases.

Plastic Filling Materials. The commonly used plastic filling materials are amalgam (which is not usually thought of as a plastic, although it is), the self-curing resins, and gutta percha or temporary stopping.

Amalgam. Silver alloy amalgam has been found to be a relatively nontoxic filling material, although Swerdlow and Stanley found twice as much inflammatory change under amalgam fillings than under zinc oxide and eugenol filled controls.[47] They attributed this difference to the "physical insertion of the amalgam . . . responsible for the greater responses than the toxic, chemical or thermal property of the restorative material itself." James and Schour found amalgam to be on a par with zinc oxide and eugenol.[51] Mitchell implanted 22 different filling materials into the subdermal tissue of rats.[58] He found silver amalgam to be a moderate to mild irritant but copper amalgam to be a consistently severe irritant.

Resins. When the self-curing resins were introduced following World War II, great hopes were expressed for these materials. Unfortunately, a flurry of reports appeared relative to the irritating effects of the resins on the pulp. Lefkowitz and Seelig, in animal experiments, first found self-curing acrylic to be less of an irritant than silicate, zinc phosphate, or zinc oxide and eugenol.[59] They stated that no cavity liner was necessary. In contrast to this report, Kramer and McLean reported adverse results with self-curing acrylic in 14 of 15 young patients;[60] however, they also used phenol and silver nitrate in the experimental cavities. Zander, using animals, tested five resins against controls of zinc oxide–eugenol and silicates.[61] He found the pulps under the resins to be not consistent in their reactions in comparison to the consistent inflammation from silicate and lack of inflammation from zinc oxide–eugenol.

Seelig, again reporting animal studies, suggested that pulp injury under plastics might be due to cavity preparation or salivary leakage around the plastic.[62]

In spite of the initial glowing reports on self-curing plastics, Grossman questioned 75 general dentists about their results with the resins.[63] These men had placed 11,050 plastic fillings and 9,086 silicate fillings in a six-month period. During this period 93 pulp deaths occurred under the plastics and 21 deaths under silicates. Grossman recommended cement bases under self-curing plastics.

Following this damaging report by Grossman, Nygaard-Ostby[64] tested the effects on pulp of five different plastics placed in 28 teeth of children and adults. The restorations were left in place as long as 14 months. All five plastics proved to be irritant, and in the case of adults, the most frequent microscopic observation was partial necrosis. In only one instance, however, were clinical symptoms observed. Langeland observed similar irreversible pulp changes under three plastics.[65]

More recently Spangberg et al., using HeLa cells, tested the toxic effects of cold-curing acrylics, the older silicate cements, and the newer composites.[66] Although silicate set the example as the most toxic material (both when freshly mixed and at four hours and 24 hours), the cold-cure acrylics matched silicate in toxicity in a freshly mixed state, but dropped to nearly control level in four hours. While silicate cement continues to release its chemical irritant throughout the day, the resins evidently set-up within four hours and no longer act as toxic agents. This initial toxic shock, however, is so severe, the extensive use of mouth curing plastics as fillings and temporary crowns might well account in part for the great number of pulp deaths in extensive restorative cases.

Composites. "Although when freshly prepared the composite materials cause less cell damage than the silicates or cold-curing plastics, the composites resemble the silicates in that they give off irritant components over a longer time than the cold-curing plastics."[66] The composites contain acrylic monomers in their catalyst system and it can be assumed that the monomer would cause damage, as in the case of the cold-curing resins. In *in vitro* testing, Dickey et al. found Adaptic as toxic as silicate.[67] Langeland also found no significant difference in pulp irritation between the silicates, cold-cure plastics, and composite materials.[56]

Cavity Liners. Again, testing a number of cavity liners against the viability of HeLa cells, Spangberg et al. observed "that the cytotoxicity of the liners is higher than that of the composite materials for which they are intended as liners."[68] The one exception appeared to be the 3M liner which caused relatively little cell lysis, whereas the 3M composite Addent 35 was the most toxic composite tested by the same method.[68] Although it is not implied that the results from *in vitro* tests may be directly applied to the *in vivo* behavior of the materials, the *in vitro* test gives an objective ranking of the materials according to their cytotoxicity.

Spangberg also pointed out that "the liners do not form a continuous film and there seems to be no rationale for their use for pulp protection."[68]

Gutta Percha. Gutta percha and temporary stopping have also been found to be severe pulpal irritants. Dubner and Stanley found gutta percha, heated and placed, to be twice as irritating as gutta percha placed with eucalyptol and eight times as irritating as zinc oxide–eugenol controls.[69] Temporary stopping was much less irritating than gutta percha, and about as irritating as zinc phosphate cement.

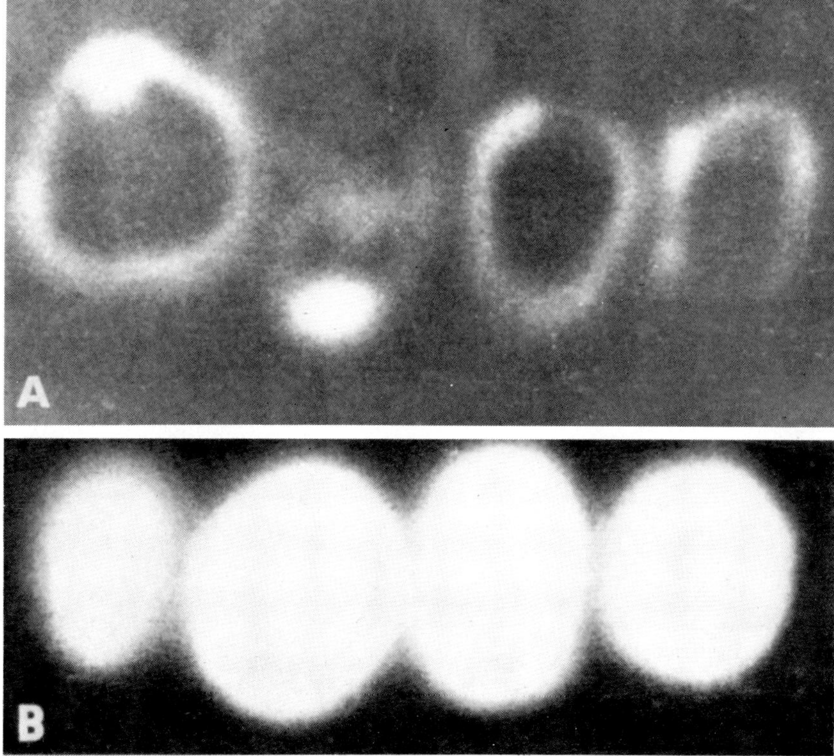

Fig. 7–20. Radioautographs of tooth cross sections in which is shown depth of penetration of radioactive NaCl, as substitute for NaFl, precipitated by electrolytic action. *A,* Two hours of electrolysis. *B,* Twelve hours of electrolysis. (Courtesy Briscoe, Monson, and Ingle, University of Washington, 1956.)

James and Schour also recommended zinc oxide–eugenol as a temporary filling material instead of gutta percha.[70] Somewhat later, Langeland found gutta percha to be very irritating but pointed out that a thick layer of zinc oxide–eugenol as a liner could prevent the reaction to gutta percha.[71] No repair of the pulp tissue was observed after gutta percha was used.

Disinfectants. The time-honored, empiric habit of dentists to attempt sterilization of prepared cavities before insertion of a restoration has been questioned for a great number of years. G. V. Black did not recommend that an antibacterial cavity agent be used although his contemporaries were using caustic drugs.[72] Dorfman, Stephan and Muntz also questioned the value of so-called cavity sterilization.[73,74]

More recently, Seltzer and Bender found silver nitrate to be "devastating" to the pulps of monkeys' teeth when applied to shallow cavities.[43] They also described pulps in a "severely disturbed condition" three months following the application of phenol to a deep cavity. As late as six months following the application of these drugs, recovery was questionable.

The irritating effects on the dental pulp of sodium fluoride have been noted by Lefkowitz and Bodecker[75] and by Rovelstad and St. John,[76] but denied by Maurice and Schour.[77] The use of the fluorides as a desensitizing agent on the external tooth surface is probably well within reason, even when precipitated by electrolytic action. Questionable, however, is the use of fluoride as a sterilizing agent or desensitizer when precipitated, particularly by electrolysis, upon a freshly cut dentin surface. By measuring beta ray emissions from preparations from teeth subjected to electrolytic action of radioactive sodium chloride, Briscoe, Monson and Ingle demonstrated the halogen driven completely to the pulp[78] (Fig. 7–20).

Desiccants. Time-honored desiccants, such as ethyl alcohol, ether or chloroform, are probably not damaging to the pulp by their chemical action but rather by upsetting the physiologic equilibrium of the dental ***interstitial fluid.*** Use of the desiccants is also invariably followed by a blast of air. The irritation of dehydration would have to be indicted as well.

IDIOPATHIC CHANGES

Aging

Inevitable retrogressive aging changes take place in the pulp as in all other body tissues. The decreased numbers and size of cells and increase in collagen fiber content has long been noted as an age change.[79] The constant recession of the normal pulp and its production of secondary and reparative dentin is as certain as death and taxes (Fig. 7–21).

Seltzer and Bender point out that atrophy of the pulp normally occurs with advancing age.[18] They describe these dystrophic changes as a "burned out" appearance of an "exhaustion atrophy." This aged pulp seems less likely to resist insult than the young "virile" pulp.

Internal Resorption

Although internal resorption is an inevitable microscopic finding in chronic pulpal inflammation, it also occurs as an idiopathic dystrophic change (Fig. 7–22). Trauma in the form of an accidental blow or traumatic cavity preparation can be indicted as a triggering mechanism for internal resorption. In this event, the metaplastic area of the pulp might develop from a localized hemorrhage. Dentin destruction follows (Fig. 7–23).

The metaplastic pulp involved in internal resorption seldom becomes necrotic *per se,* but later becomes infected when the dentin is completely perforated through the crown or into the sulcus, and oral organisms enter.

External Resorption

One cannot say that external root resorption is a pulp dystrophy, for its origin lies within the tissue of the periodontal membrane space. Chronic inflammatory tissue developing in periodontal pockets is the probable causative tissue. If for some reason the protective sulcular epithelial lining of the pocket is missing and chronic inflammatory tissue contacts the well-calcified cementum of the root, the calcified tissue will undergo decalcification.

When the external resorption destroys enough dentin to reach the pulp, pulp inflammatory changes begin. The same infection problem now exists that develops when internal resorption destroys enough tooth structure to reach the sulcus. Continued resorption is inevitable unless the process is interrupted, either by stimulation with a biologically active material such as calcium hydroxide introduced into the canal, or by surgery and retrofilling.

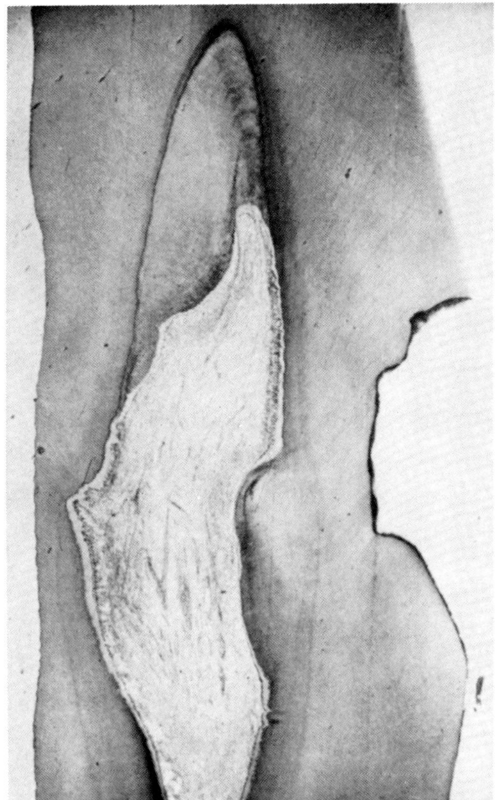

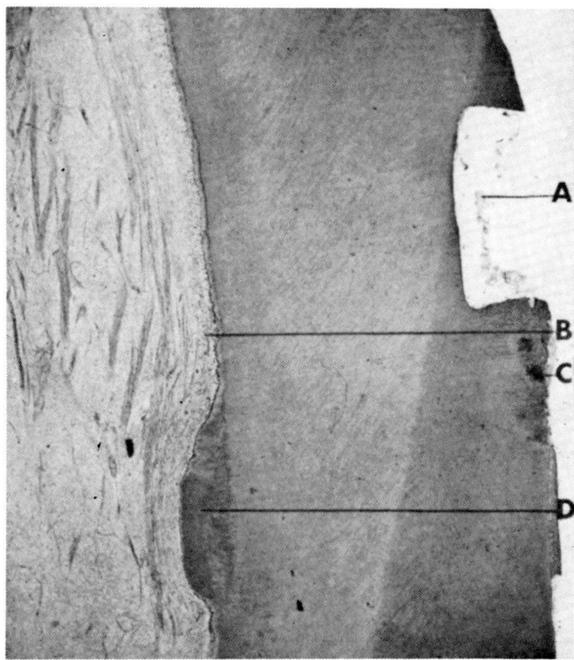

Fig. 7–21. *Left,* Pulp response to various irritant forces. Reparative dentin formation caused by incisal abrasion *(top)* and labial caries *(right).* Sweeping curvature of dentinal tubules leading from wall and floor of carious lesion causes reparative dentin formation at lower level (Orban Collection). *Right,* Cavity *(A)* extends into carious and sound dentin filled with silicate cement for five weeks. Mild inflammatory reaction *(B)* is adjacent to dentinal tubules leading to portion of cavity cut into sound dentin. No inflammation is adjacent to area of reparative dentin *(D),* which was formed as response to caries *(C).* (From Zander, H. A.: J.A.D.A., *33*:1233, Oct., 1946.)

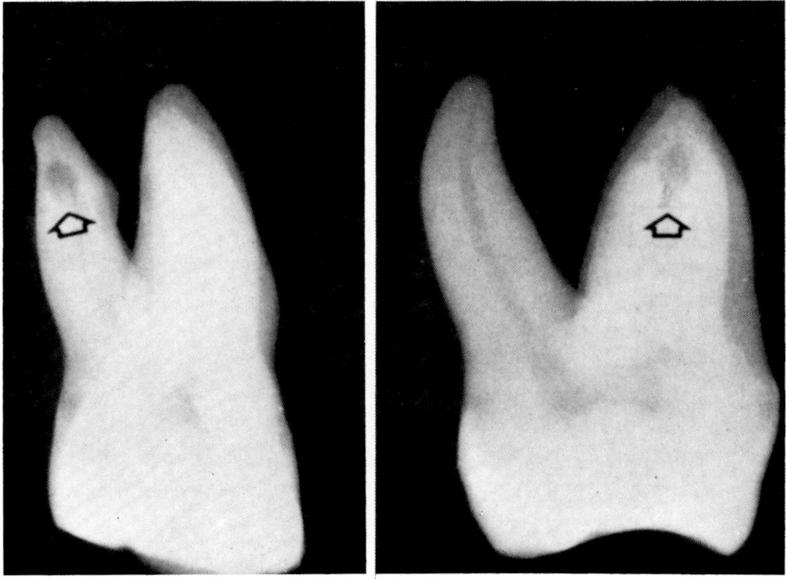

Fig. 7–22. Idiopathic internal resorption *(arrows)* was not detectable until this molar tooth was extracted.

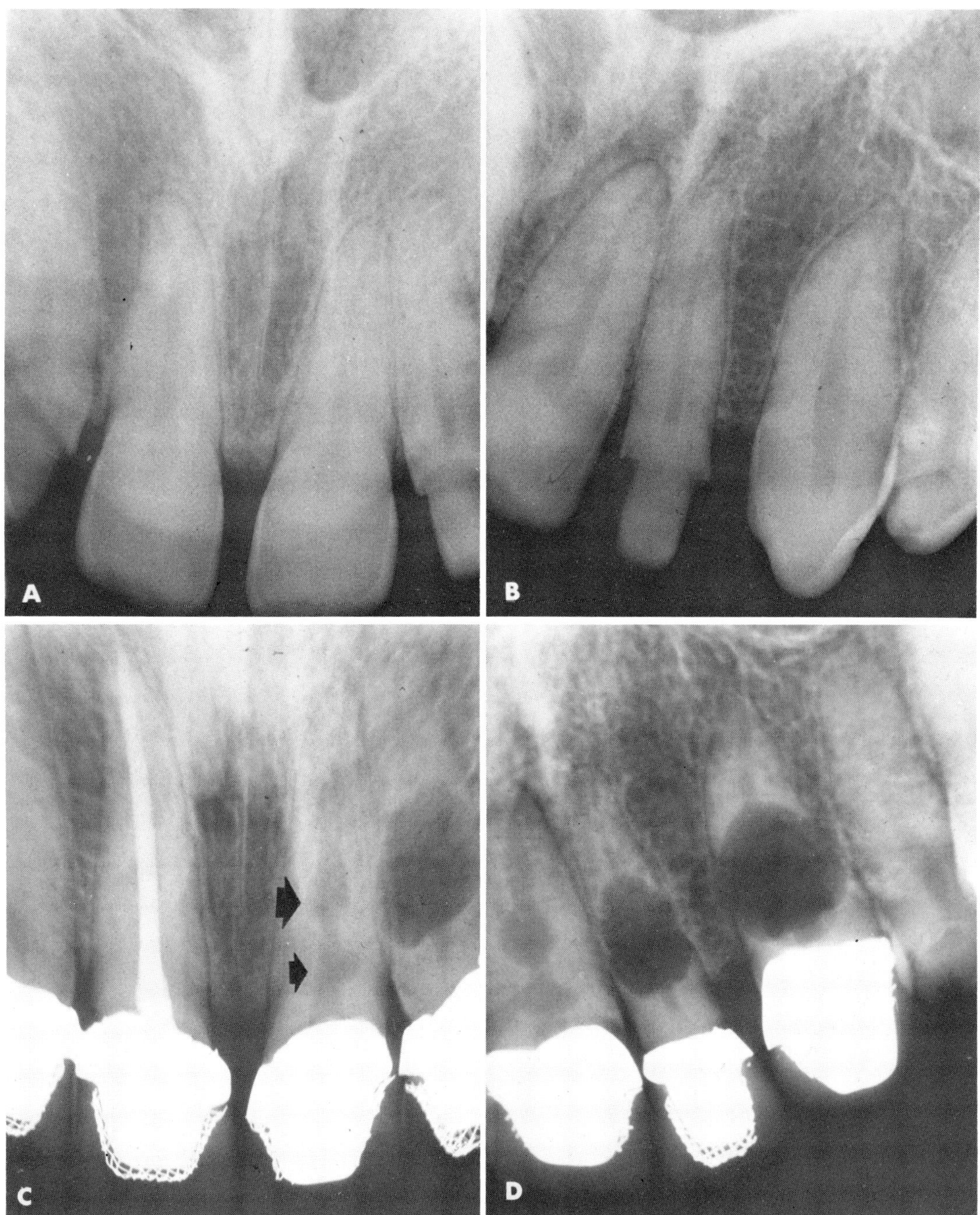

Fig. 7–23. Extensive internal resorption apparently triggered by iatrogenic causes. Normal condition of teeth prior to crown preparation is seen in "before" roentgenograms *(A* and *B).* Development of internal resorption from high-speed preparation without water coolant is seen one year later, *(C* and *D).* (Courtesy Dr. Dudley H. Glick.)

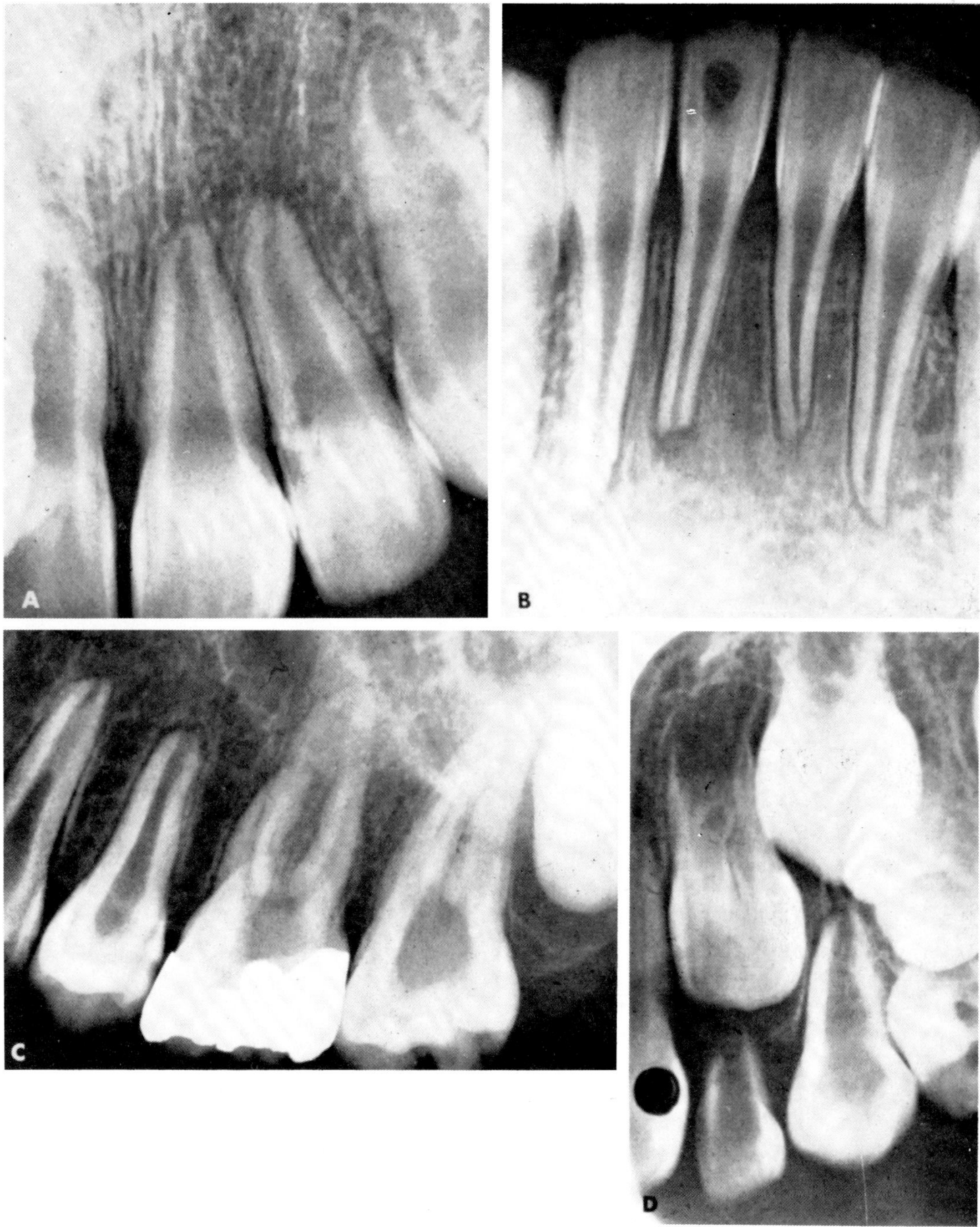

Fig. 7–24. Unusual pulp dystrophy seen with hereditary hypophosphatasia. Incomplete calcification of dentin and huge pulps leave these teeth vulnerable to pulp infection and necrosis. *A,* Adult maxillary incisors at age 13. Note huge pulp. *B,* Mandibular incisors, age 13. Right central and lateral incisors have been traumatized and pulp necrosis has developed. *C,* Huge pulp seen in premolar and molar teeth. Pulp of first molar later became necrotic. *D,* Same pulp size and shape is apparent in deciduous dentition. Diagnosis of condition could have been made at this stage from dental roentgenogram. Early vitamin D therapy might have prevented dwarfing.

Hereditary Hypophosphatasia

An unusual and rare cause of pulpal dystrophy occurs in those individuals afflicted with hereditary hypophosphatasia. This disease, which results in dwarfism and "tackle" deformity, was formerly called refractory rickets or vitamin D resistant rickets. It is characterized dentally by the huge pulps (Fig. 7–24) and incomplete calcification of the dentin. The pulps in the teeth of these dwarfs appear to be fragile and succumb to what would normally be minor irritating stimuli.

In one such case, the patient had 11 pulpless teeth that required endodontic treatment.

THE FUTURE

Pulp death seems to be on the increase, or perhaps only an apparent increase owing to an awareness of the value of the treated pulpless tooth.

By routine examination and early treatment, by a cautious, temperate approach to all restorative procedures, and by a sensible use of filling materials, the dentist can well ***prevent*** a great deal of the present pulp death.

PREVENTION OF PULP INJURY*

In 1969 the American Dental Association reported that American dentists extracted 56 million teeth, placed 213 million fillings, made 4 million bridges and 10 million complete and partial dentures, and completed 9 million root canal fillings. All of these 292 million cases of dental therapy had a direct relation to the dental pulp and are testimony either to its insult and injury or to its disease or loss.[80]

That some of this injury might have been prevented seems apparent. Caries alone probably accounted for most of this dental treatment. Impact trauma undoubtedly accounted for a large proportion, and that virtually unspoken third cause, iatrogenesis, accounted for an embarrassingly high percentage of the pulp injury and death reflected in the ADA report.

When one speaks of prevention of pulp injury there immediately comes to mind some obvious steps that might be taken: fluoridation of the communal water supply, programs for plaque control, reduction of sugar in the diet, the fastening of seat belts, the wearing of mouth guards in contact sports—the list is rather limited. As one critically reviews the list, however, one realizes that most preventive measures fall into the educational or political arena—measures that can be taken by the media, by educational institutions, or by municipalities. Most such measures require a change either in law or in life style, and to achieve this the people must act—in concert or as individuals.

Surely, everyone past infancy should be responsible for his or her own oral health. Personal plaque control, improved eating habits, and trauma avoidance should be the personal concern of each citizen. Motivating people to do this is not easy, as many dentists have learned to their disappointment. Development of a healthful life style will be the next big breakthrough in the prevention of all disease and disability, oral disease included.

There is something the dentist and his auxiliaries can do, of course, to motivate patients or directly prevent oral disease. Again plaque control and fluoridation come to mind, but this time on a one-to-one basis—an office plaque control program, nutritional counselling, oral prophylaxis, fluoride application, prophylactic filling of deep occlusal fissures, and construction of personalized mouthguards or night guards for contact sports and bruxism respectively. With care, pit and fissure sealant application should also be considered. It should not be applied, however, after fissural caries has begun. One must remember that bacteria may have already entered the peripheral ends of the dentinal tubules, and if they are facultative anaerobes, caries may progress beneath the sealant.[2]

But there is more. The dentist can take great care he does not personally contribute to the legion of irritants "out to get" the dental pulp. This means care in every operation upon the tooth and around its blood supply, for example, deep periodontal curettage. The dentist must be careful to avoid the pulp blood supply when curetting deep infrabony pockets.[2] During extractions or removal of impactions or cysts, injury to the adjacent teeth must be meticulously avoided. Orthodontic movement must be done with care and concern.

In larger measure, however, there are many more day-to-day insults levied against the pulp which must be ***prevented:*** (1) depth of cavity and crown preparation, (2) width and extension of cavity and crown preparation, (3) heat damage and desiccation during cavity preparation, (4) chemical injury through medi-

*Abstracted from Langeland, K.: Prevention of pulpal damage. Dent. Clin. N. Amer., *16*:709, Oct., 1972.

caments, (5) toxic cavity liners and bases, and (6) toxic filling materials.

Depth and Width of Cavity Preparation. Extreme pulp trauma results when the pulp is closely approached or the dentin is extensively removed. Overcutting cavity preparations, whether or not the pulp is exposed, is undoubtedly one of the greatest insults to the pulp. It should be quite obvious that full-crown preparations sever every single coronal odontoblast. Before one cavalierly decides upon full coverage for a tooth, if a less extensive restoration will do, the latter should be a standard preventive consideration. When elective, shallow preparations are always the wiser choice over deep preparations. The integrity of the pulp is affected as the rotary instruments approach the predentin, not just because of the immediate pulp damage, but because of the proximity of toxic filling materials as well. Udolph and Kopel, for example, found that composite filling materials would not irritate the pulp if 2 mm. of dentin remained between the pulp and the filling.[81] Although it is generally true that the risk of pulp damage diminishes with increasing distance[82] there is no sacred distance beyond which no damage occurs. The surface width of the cavity may be as important as the depth. In fact a cut into the dentin exposes the pulp to a variety of exogenous irritants.

Heat Damage and Desiccation During Cavity Preparation. The damage that results when high-speed rotary instruments are used without an adequate water coolant has been discussed. The obvious preventive measure is to use a water coolant, but in doing so, the dentist may be misled by his ineffective equipment (Fig. 7–25). In some high-speed contra-angles, the water jet is deflected away from the cavity by the air turbulence created by the bur and by the force of the air exhaust directed toward the point of operation. In addition to the problems caused by lack of water coolant, desiccation of the dentin and odontoblasts may be caused by the exhaust blast. In some handpieces, the spray outlets are misdirected, and the water bypasses the interface between the bur and the tooth. In others the water outlet is too far from the bur, so that an intervening cusp totally prevents the water coolant from reaching the interface.

Also damaging is the custom of preparing cavities under a constant blast of air directed by an assistant. Here again, the desiccation of the dentin (and eventually the pulp) is most damaging. Odontoblastic

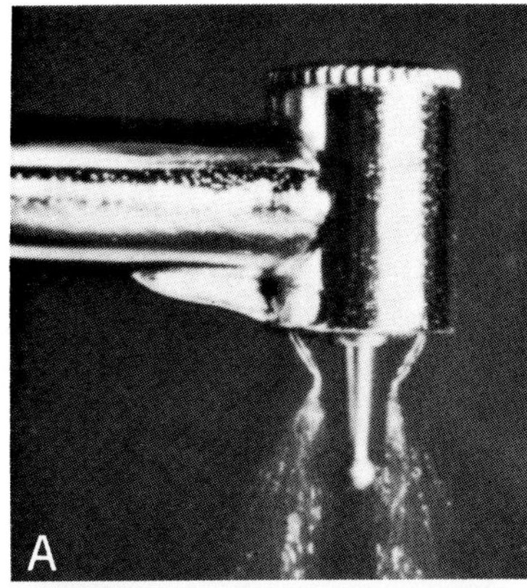

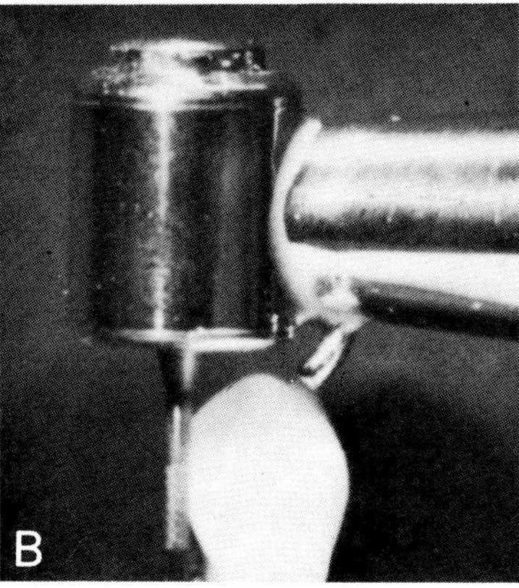

Fig. 7–25. Spray patterns from two air turbines. *A*, Water jet is deflected because of exhaust air and air turbulence created by bur. *B*, Water outlet is too far away from axis of bur. Cusp totally prevents water from reaching bur-tooth interface. (From Langeland, K.: Dent. Clin. N. Amer., *16*:709, Oct., 1972.)

nuclei and even erythrocytes can be seen microscopically, virtually "sucked up" into the desiccated tubules. Add to this damage the toxic effects of medicaments, liners, or bases and filling material to give the pulp *le coup de grâce.*

Chemical Injury Through Medicaments Applied to the Dentin. One could say that pulp injury from chemical irritants can be best prevented by not applying chemicals to the dentin. This prohibition refers to silver nitrate, phenol, alcohol, ether, acetone, thymol, fluoride, cyanoacrylate, or citric acid, to name a few irritants. Corticosteroids may be the exception to the rule. Van Hassel and McHugh reported the "ability of prednisolone to suppress inflammatory vascular changes can prevent pressure-induced venous collapse beneath deep cavity preparations."[83] On the other hand, one should not place false hope in cortisone to suppress all inflammation. It has been shown that inflammation will continue in the pulp despite the application of corticosteroids, alone or in combination with other medicaments,[84] if pulp inflammation has "passed that point of no return." Cortisone reduces pain, however, which may lull the dentist and patient into a false sense of security.

Toxic Cavity Liners and Bases. The very products made to protect the pulp might well be the toxins to bring about its demise. Spangberg et al. have shown that the commonly used cavity liners were more cytotoxic *in vitro* against HeLa cells than the composite filling materials they are to protect against.[85] "It is reasonable to believe," they said, "that the early irritation is caused by the solvent of the liner," which might soon dissipate by evaporation. In view of the fact that cavity liners have been shown to be ineffective as well as toxic, it follows that their use cannot be recommended as a preventive measure.

Cement bases, on the other hand, can serve to prevent the toxic and/or thermal damage which may be generated by filling materials. The most common bases are oxyphosphate of zinc cement, polycarboxylate cement, and zinc oxide and eugenol. All three have been shown to be only slight irritants to the pulp and may prevent great damage from other more toxic fillings.

Placing a cement base may lull one into a false sense of security. The usual thought is protecting the pulp ***floor*** of a cavity, but it is easy to forget that all open dentinal tubules, even those on the walls, are connected to the pulp and may serve as toxic conduits. Pulp floor cement bases were developed for thermal protection, but serve today as only partial protection against noxious chemical fillings. If in doubt, cover all the dentin. Baume and Fiore-Donno suggest that a base containing calcium hydroxide best protects beneath composite resin restorations.[86] These bases do not adapt well after curing, however, even if applied sufficiently thick to be immediately impenetrable. Through microleakage, irritants may then get around the calcium hydroxide bases to reach the open tubules.[87]

Cement bases have one other bonus—they block open tubules from bacteria and their noxious byproducts. Dickey et al. found severe pulp ***necrosis*** under a composite restorative material only when a bacterial plaque had formed on the cavity floors.[88] Bacterial entree was gained from marginal microleakage or cavity contamination prior to filling. The noxious role of bacterial plaque under restorations was confirmed by Brännström and Nyborg.[89] Spangberg et al. recommended a base for pulp protection from microleakage.[90] Unfortunately, bases of polycarboxylate cement, which is touted as being adhesive, allow bacterial plaque to form on the cavity floor under composite materials (Fig. 7–26).

Toxic Filling Materials. What more can be said about the noxious role toxic filling materials play in pulp inflammation. One cannot avoid them as a preventive measure, for they have no substitutes for esthetic anterior restorations. One can only say, "Use a proper protective base, one that covers all the exposed dentin surface in the cavity." Care must also be taken in drying the dentin even before placement of the base. If desiccation precedes the introduction of any cement base, the irritant components of the base will replace the tissue fluid, and the pulp reactions will be more severe than if care is taken during surface drying.

As previously stated, cavity liners themselves may be toxic. But they have another disadvantage. As they cure against the dentin surface, "pin holes" develop that lead directly to the open tubules. Attempts at building up layers of the liner by multiple applications do not solve the pinhole problem. The toxic chemical in the restorative material leaks directly through to the tubules to irritate the pulp (Fig. 7–27). Spangberg summarized it simply, "For pulp protection, a base is necessary."[90]

From this discussion one can readily see that there are a number of measures and programs that may be undertaken by the dentist and his staff to prevent insult and injury to the dental pulp. Most of all, he must follow the Hippocratic Oath—not to inflict through his ministrations additional trauma or irritation upon the patient (the pulp).

Caries Control. By not exposing the pulp, the dentist can avoid inflicting iatrogenic injury. Even in the face of deep caries, the dentin cover should be maintained if bacteria have not penetrated through to the pulp. Fauchard, in 1746, probably said it best ". . . exposing the nerve and making the cure worse than the disease."[91] Or Sir John Tomes, in 1859, voiced similar concern ". . . better to allow some carious dentin to remain over the pulp rather than run the risk of sacrificing the tooth."

The modern version of these warnings by Fauchard and by Tomes has developed a technique of caries control often mistermed "indirect pulp capping" which means leaving carious dentin permanently under the filling. In the modern version, carious dentin is not purposely left under a permanent restoration, but is left there only temporarily as the pulp is allowed to recover and protect itself with a layer of irritation dentin. To a great extent, the success of this procedure will depend on the genus of bacteria in the remaining dentin. If they are facultative anaerobes, continued breakdown may be the end result. On the other hand, if healing progresses, irritation dentin may be produced in amounts that may fill an entire pulp horn, but irritation dentin is still penetrable by microorganisms and medicaments.[92]

The technique is carried out in this manner: (1) The rubber dam is applied. (2) The soft carious dentin is removed along the walls of the cavity and as far pulpally as possible without exerting pressure up the pulp wall. (3) The cavity is washed with lukewarm water and is then carefully dried without desiccation. (4) A thick mix of zinc oxide–eugenol cement (chemically pure) is applied without pressure over the pulp floor. The ZO–E should be prepared by incorporating as much zinc oxide into the mix as possible and then removing excess eugenol with a squeeze cloth. (The suggestion has also been made that calcium hydroxide be placed against the carious dentin before the ZO–E base is inserted. No evidence exists, however, that this is an improvement over ZO–E alone.) (5) A good protective provisional

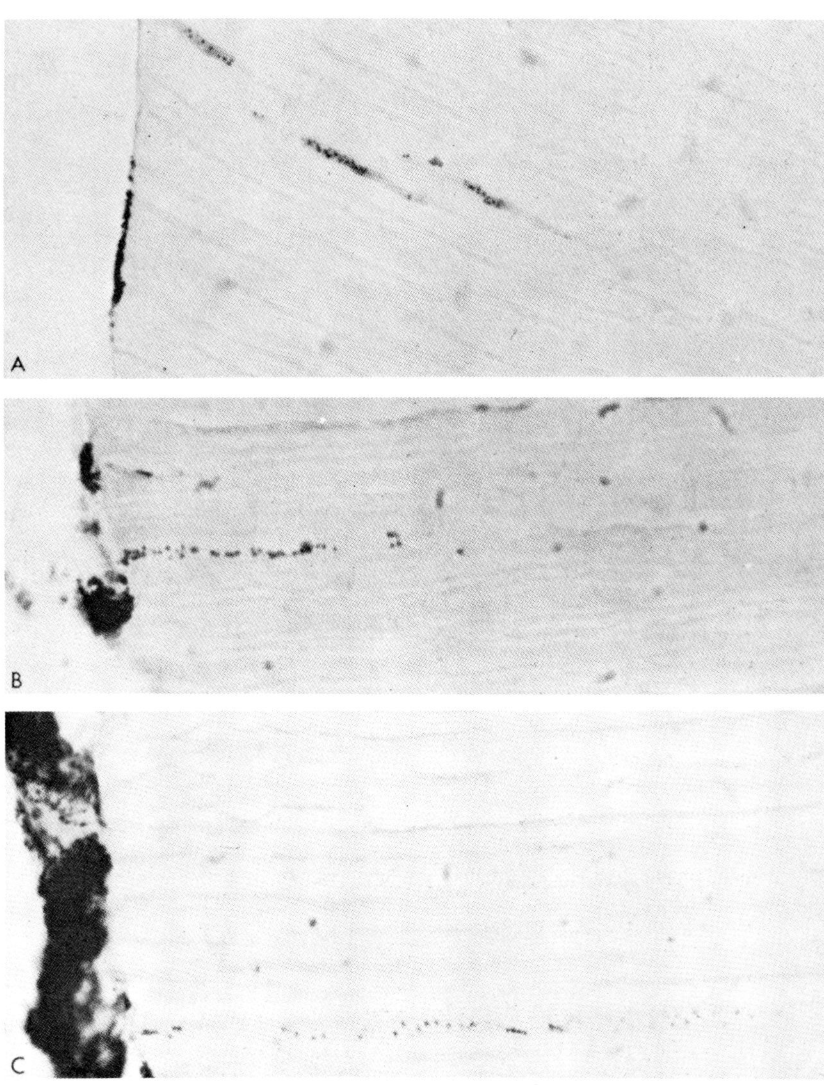

Fig. 7–26. Bacteria in dentinal tubules. Microleakage around and under three different composite materials and polycarboxylate cement. In all sections bacteria were found along filling margin, around entire filling and in subjacent dentinal tubules. (From Langeland, K.: Dent. Clin. N. Amer., *16*:709, Oct., 1972.)

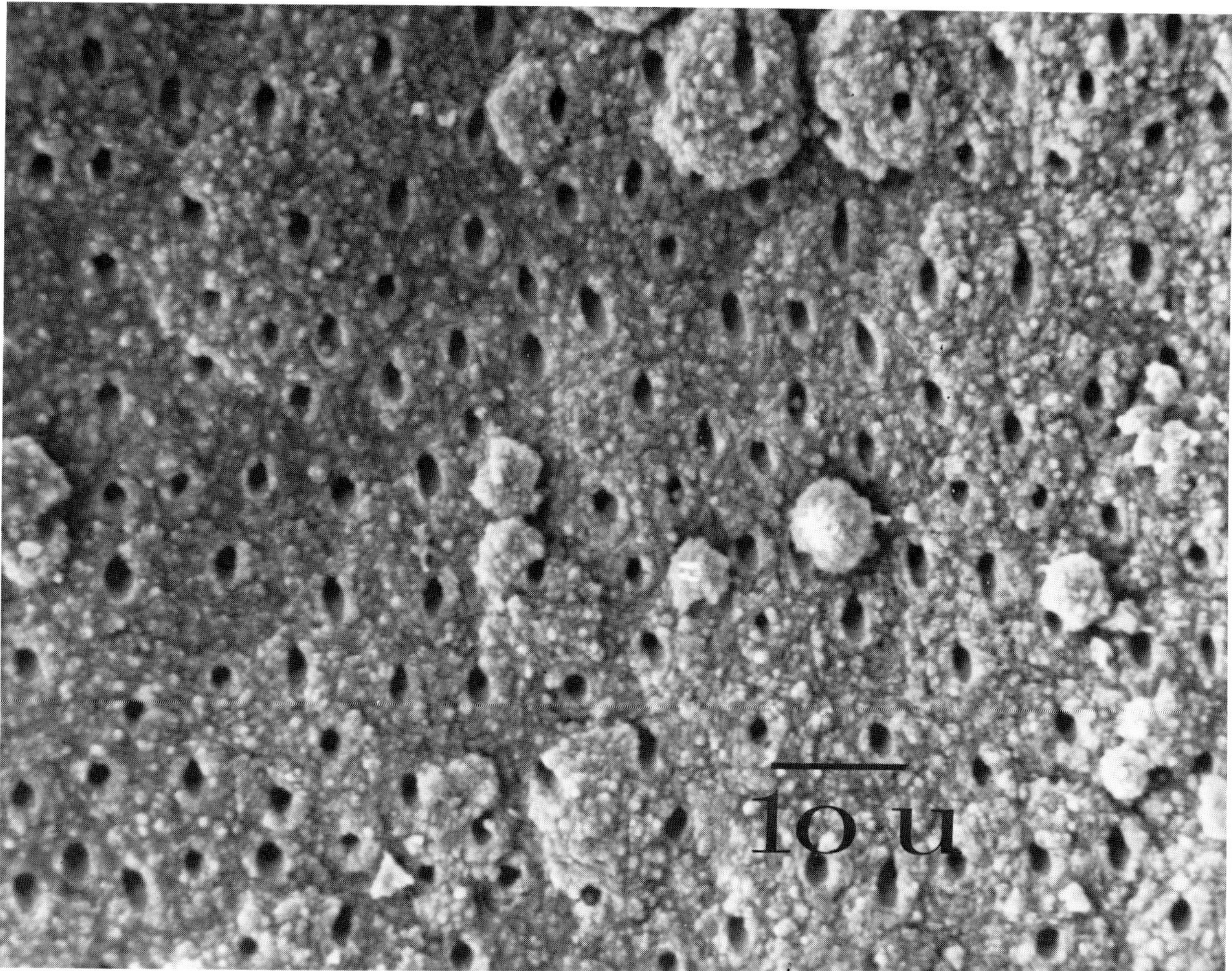

Fig. 7–27. Dentin wall magnified ×1000. Moisture-filled dentinal tubules cannot be sealed by cavity liners, and pin holes develop through which toxic filling materials penetrate to irritate pulp. (From Koenigs, J. F., Brilliant, J. D., and Foreman, D. W.: Oral Surg., *38*:573, Nov., 1974.)

filling is then placed. (6) Three to six months later the provisional filling and the ZO–E base are removed and the softened dentin is carefully excavated. (7) If hard dentin is found covering the pulp, a new thick ZO–E cement base is inserted and a permanent restoration is placed. (8) If an exposure is encountered, either from instruments or caries persisting under the ZO–E base, appropriate endodontic treatment is performed based upon the state of development of the pulp and the closure of the apical foramen.

High success rates are frequently reported based on clinical experimentation with "indirect pulp capping." The criteria used are lack of radiographically observable periapical lesions and lack of pain. Periapical radiolucency, however, takes longer to develop than the length of these studies, and lack of pain in the presence of inflammation is the rule rather than the exception. Thus histopathologic and microbiologic studies that show continued, although often slow, breakdown of the pulp under remaining caries should be accepted as a reflection of the factual clinical condition. Many of these teeth eventually are treated by the endodontist.

REFERENCES

1. Langeland, K.: Histologic evaluation of pulp reactions to operative procedures. Oral Surg., *12*:1235, Oct., 1959.
2. Seltzer, S., Bender, I. B., and Kaufman, I. J.: Histologic changes in dental pulps of dogs and monkeys following application of pressure, drugs and microorganisms on prepared cavities. Part II. Changes observable more than one month after application of traumatic agents. Oral Surg., *14*:856, July, 1961.
3. Canby, C. P., and Burnett, G. W.: Clinical management of deep carious lesions. Oral Surg., *16*:999, Aug., 1963.
4. Muntz, J. A., Dorfman, A., and Stephan, R. M.: *In vitro* studies on sterilization of carious dentin. I. Evaluation of germicides. J.A.D.A., *30*: 1893, Dec., 1943.
5. Seltzer, S., Bender, I. B., and Ziontz, M.: The dynamics of pulp inflammation: correlations between diagnostic data and actual histologic findings in the pulp. Oral Surg., *16*:969, Aug., 1963.
6. Ritchey, B., Mendenhall, R., and Orban, B.: Pulpitis resulting from incomplete tooth fracture. Oral Surg., *10*:665, June, 1957.
7. Kato, K.: Contributions to the knowledge concerning the cone shaped supernumerary cusp in the center of the occlusal surface on the premolars of Japanese. Nippon Shika Gaku Eassi, *30*:28, 1937.
8. Lau, T. C.: Odontogenesis of the axial cone type. Brit. Dent. J., *99*:219, Oct. 1955.
9. Merrill, R. G.: Occlusal anomalous tubercles on bicuspids of Alaskan Eskimos and Indians. Sr. Thesis. University of Washington, June, 1959.
10. Merrill, R. G.: Occlusal anomalous tubercles on premolars of Alaskan Eskimos and Indians. Oral Surg., *17*:484, Apr., 1964.
11. Wing-Kong Yip: The prevalence of *dens evaginatus*. Oral Surg., *38*:80, July, 1974.
12. Senia, E. S., and Regezi, J. A.: *Dens evaginatus* in the etiology of bilateral pathologic involvement of caries-free premolars. Oral Surg., *38*:465, Sept., 1974.
13. Sykaras, S. N.: Occlusal anomalous tubercle on premolars of a Greek girl. Oral Surg., *38*:88, July, 1974.
14. Carlsen, O.: Personal communication, June, 1972.
15. Palmer, M. E.: Case reports of evaginated odontomes in Caucasians. Oral Surg., *35*:772, June, 1973.
16. Widerman, F. H., and Serene, T. P.: Endodontic therapy involving a taurodontic tooth. Oral Surg., *32*:618, Oct., 1971.
17. Sykaras, S. N.: Op. cit.
18. Seltzer, S., Bender, I. B., and Ziontz, M.: The dynamics of pulp inflammation: correlation between diagnostic data and actual histologic findings in the pulp. Oral Surg., *16*:846, July, 1963.
19. Mazur, B., and Massler, M.: Influence of periodontal disease on the dental pulp. Oral Surg., *17*:592, May, 1964.
20. Johnston, H. B., and Orban, B.: Interradicular pathology as related to accessory root canals. J. Endodont., *3*:21, Apr., 1948.
21. Langeland, K., Rodrigues, H., and Dowden, W.: Periodontal disease, bacteria and pulpal histopathology. Oral Surg., *37*:257, Feb., 1974.
22. Robinson, H. B. G., and Boling, L.: The anachoretic effect in pulpitis. I. Bacteriologic studies. J.A.D.A., *28*:268, Feb., 1941.
23. MacDonald, J. B., Hare, G. C., and Wood, A. W. S.: The bacteriologic status of the pulp chambers in intact teeth found to be nonvital following trauma. Oral Surg., *10*:318, Mar., 1957.
24. Ingle, J. I.: Alveolar osteoporosis and pulpal death associated with compulsive bruxism. Oral Surg., *13*:1371, Nov., 1960.
25. Natkin, E., and Ingle, J. I.: A further report on alveolar osteoporosis and pulpal death associated with compulsive bruxism. J. Am. Soc. Periodont., *1*:260, Nov.–Dec., 1963.
26. Gruchalla, F.: Personal communication, 1972.
27. Sognnaes, R. F., Wolcott, R. B., and Xhonga, F. A.: Dental erosion. J.A.D.A., *84*:571, Mar., 1972.
28. Kramer, I. R. H.: Pulp changes of non-bacterial origin. Int. Dent. J., *9*:435, Dec., 1959.
29. Stanley, H. R., and Swerdlow, H.: Reaction of the human pulp to cavity preparation; results produced by eight different operative grinding technics. J.A.D.A., *58*:49, May, 1959.
30. Lefkowitz, W., Robinson, H., and Postle, H.: Interpretation of histologic sections of pulp. Ohio D. J., *31*:24, 1957.
31. Brännström, M.: Cavity preparation and the pulp. Dent. Progress, *2*:4, Oct., 1961.
32. Swerdlow, H., and Stanley, H. R.: Higher speeds in dentistry. J. Dist. Col. Dent. Soc., *34*:4, June, 1959.
33. Vaughn, R. C., and Peyton, F. A.: The influence of rotational speed on temperature rise during cavity preparation. J. Dent. Res., *30*:737, Oct., 1951.
34. Peyton, F. A., and Henry, E. E.: The effect of high speed burs, diamond instruments and air abrasives in cutting tooth tissue. J.A.D.A, *49*:426, Oct., 1954.
35. Stanley, H. R., and Swerdlow, H.: Aspiration of cells into dentinal tubules? Oral Surg., *11*:1007, Sept., 1958.
36. Ostrom, C. A.: Pulp damage by induced inflammation. Dent. Progress, *3*:207, July, 1963.
37. Pohto, M., and Scheinin, A.: Microscopic observations on living dental pulp. II. The effect of thermal irritants on the circulation of the pulp in the lower rat incisor. Acta Odont. Scand., *16*:315, 1958.
38. Seelig, A., and Lefkowitz, W.: Pulp response to filling materials. New York State Dent. J., *16*:540, Dec., 1950.
39. Brännström, M.: Dentinal and pulpal response. II. Application of an air stream to exposed dentin. Short observation period. Acta Odont. Scand., *18*:17, 1960.
40. Brännström, M.: Dentinal and pulpal response. III. Application of an air stream to exposed dentin. Long observation period. In *Sensory Mechanisms in Dentine.* Edited by D. J. Anderson. New York, The Macmillan Co. 1963, pp., 235–252.
41. Langeland, K.: Histologic evaluation of pulp reactions to operative procedures. Oral Surg., *12*:1357, Nov., 1959.
42. Orban, B.: Migration of leukocytes into the dentinal tubules. J.A.D.A., *27*:239, Feb., 1940.
43. Suzuki, M., Goto, G., and Jordan, R. E.: Pulpal response to pin placement. J.A.D.A., *87*:636, Sept., 1973.

44. Unpublished data. University of Washington.
45. James, V. E., and Schour, I.: Early dentinal and pulpal changes following cavity preparations and filling materials in dogs. Oral Surg., *8*:1305, Dec., 1955.
46. Kalnins, V., Millsop, R., and Natkevicius, G.: Pulpal injuries caused by placement of gold foil restorations and their prevention. Oral Surg., *18*:243, Aug., 1964.
47. Swerdlow, H., and Stanley, H. R.: Response of the human dental pulp to amalgam restorations. Oral Surg., *15*:499, Apr., 1962.
48. Bohannan, H. M., and Abrams, L.: Intentional vital pulp extirpation in periodontal prosthesis. J. Pros. Dent., *11*:781, July–Aug., 1961.
49. Glick, D. H.: Personal communication.
50. Zander, H. A.: The reaction of dental pulps to silicate cements. J.A.D.A., *33*:1233, Oct., 1946.
51. James, V. E., and Schour, I.: Early dentinal and pulpal changes following cavity preparations and filling materials in dogs. Oral Surg., *8*:1305, Dec., 1955.
52. El-Kafrawy, A. H., and Mitchell, D. F.: Pulp reactions to open cavities later restored with silicate cement. J. Dent. Res., *42*:874, May–June, 1963.
53. Gurley, W. B., and Van Huysen, G.: Histologic changes in teeth due to plastic filling materials. J.A.D.A., *24*:1806, Nov., 1937.
54. Massler, M.: Effects of filling materials on the pulp. New York J. Dent., *26*:183, May, 1956.
55. Dubner, R., and Stanley, H. R.: Reaction of the human pulp to temporary filling materials. Oral Surg., *15*:1009, Aug., 1962.
56. Langeland, K.: Prevention of pulpal damage. Dent. Clin. N. Amer., *16*:709, Oct., 1972.
57. Langeland, L. K., Walton, R. E., Rodrigues, H. H., Dowden, W. E., and Langeland, K.: Pulp response to polycarboxylate and composite resin. Abstract 383, J. Dent. Res., Mar., 1972.
58. Mitchell, D. F.: The irritational qualities of dental materials. J.A.D.A., *59*:954, Nov., 1959.
59. Lefkowitz, W., Seelig, A., and Zachinsky, L.: Pulp response to a self-curing acrylic filling material. New York State Dent. J., *15*:376, Aug.–Sept., 1949.
60. Kramer, I. R. H., and McLean, J. W.: Pulp response to the self-curing resins. Digest Dent. Sci., *2*:8, Jan., 1953.
61. Zander, H. A.: The effect of self-curing resins on the dental pulp. Oral Surg., *4*:1563, Dec., 1951.
62. Seelig, A.: The effect of direct filling resins on the tooth pulp. J.A.D.A., *44*:261, Mar., 1952.
63. Grossman, L. I.: Pulp reaction to the insertion of self-curing resin filling materials. J.A.D.A., *46*:265, Mar., 1953.
64. Nygaard-Ostby, B.: Pulp reaction to direct filling resins. J.A.D.A., *50*:7, Jan., 1955.
65. Langeland, K.: Pulp reactions to resin cements. Acta Odont. Scand., *13*:239, Nov., 1956.
66. Spangberg, L., Rodrigues, H., Langeland, L. K., and Langeland, K.: Toxicity of anterior tooth restorative materials on HeLa cells *in vitro*. Oral Surg., *36*:713, Nov., 1973.
67. Dickey, D. M., El-Kafrawy, A. H., and Mitchell, D. F.. Clinical and microscopic pulp response to a composite restorative material. J.A.D.A., *88*:108, Jan., 1974.
68. Spangberg, L., Rodrigues, H., and Langeland, K.: Effect of cavity liners on HeLa cells *in vitro*. Oral Surg., *37*:284, Feb., 1974.
69. Dubner, R., and Stanley, H. R.: Reaction of the human pulp to temporary filling materials. Oral Surg., *15*:1009, Aug., 1962.
70. James, V. E., Schour, I., and Spence, J. M.: Response of human pulp to gutta percha and cavity preparation. J.A.D.A., *49*:639, Dec., 1954.
71. Langeland, K.: Effect of various procedures on human dental pulp. Oral Surg., *14*:210, Feb., 1961.
72. Black, G. V.: *Black's Operative Dentistry*. Medico-Dental Pub. Co., South Milwaukee, Wisc., 9th Ed., Vol. II, p. 113.
73. Dorfman, A., Stephan, R. M., and Muntz, J. A.: *In vitro* studies on sterilization of carious dentin. II. Extent of infection in carious lesions. J.A.D.A., *30*:1901, Dec., 1943.
74. Stephan, R. M.: Consultant Symposium: Our Empiric Cavity Sterilization. Part III. New York State Dent. J., *26*:183, 1960.
75. Lefkowitz, W., and Bodecker, C. F.: Sodium fluoride; its effect on the dental pulp. Preliminary report. Ann. Dent., *3*:141, Mar., 1945.
76. Rovelstad, G. H., and St. John, W. E.: The condition of the young dental pulp after application of sodium fluoride to the freshly cut dentin. J.A.D.A., *39*:670, Dec., 1949.
77. Maurice, C. G., and Schour, I.: Effects of sodium fluoride upon the pulp of the rat molar. J. Dent. Res., *35*:69, Feb., 1956.
78. Briscoe, W. T., Monson, D. L., and Ingle, J. I.: Electrolysis in Tooth Structure. Senior Thesis, University of Washington, Seattle, 1956.
79. Sicher, H.: *Orban's Oral Histology and Embryology*. 5th Ed., St. Louis, C. V. Mosby Co., 1962, p. 160.
80. *Facts About the Dental Market*. Chicago, J.A.D.A. Press, Feb., 1975, Table 8. (Pamphlet.)
81. Udolph, C. H., Kopel, H. M., Melrose, R. J., and Grenoble, D. E.: Pulp response to composite resins with or without calcium hydroxide bases. J. Cal. Dent. Assoc., *3*:56, Mar., 1975.
82. Langeland, L. K., Guttuso, J., Jerome, D. R., and Langeland, K.: Histologic and clinical comparison of Addent with silicate cement and cold-curing materials. J.A.D.A., *72*:373, Feb., 1966.
83. Van Hassel, H. J., and McHugh, J. W.: Effect of prednisolone on intrapulpal pressure. Abstract 499, J. Dent. Res., Mar., 1972.
84. Langeland, K., Tobon, G., and Langeland, L. K.: The effect of corticosteroids on the dental pulp. Transactions of the Fourth International Conference on Endodontics. Edited by Louis Grossman, University of Pennsylvania, Philadelphia, Pa., 1968, pp. 15–45.
85. Spangberg, L., Rodrigues, H., and Langeland, K.: Effect of cavity liners on HeLa cells *in vitro*. Oral Surg., *37*:284, Feb., 1974.
86. Baume, L. J., and Fiore-Donno, G.: Response of the human pulp to a new restorative material. J.A.D.A., *76*:1016, May, 1968.
87. Langeland, K.: Criteria for biologic evaluation of

anterior tooth filling materials. Int. Dent. J., *17*:405, 1967.

88. Dickey, D. M., El-Kafrawy, A. H., and Mitchell, D. F.: Clinical and microscopic pulp response to a composite restorative material. J.A.D.A., *88*:108, Jan., 1974.
89. Brännström, M., and Nyborg, H.: Pulpal reaction to composite resin restorations. J. Prosthet. Dent., *27*:181, Feb., 1972.
90. Spangberg, L., et al.: Op. cit.
91. Fauchard, P.: The Surgeon Dentist or Treatise on the Teeth. Translated from the Second Edition (1746) by Lilian Lindsay. Milford House, Pound Ridge, New York, 1969, Chapt. 9, p. 57; Chapt. 5, p. 27.
92. Langeland, K., Dowden, W. E., Tronstad, L., and Langeland, L. K.: Human pulp changes of iatrogenic origin. In *The Biology of the Human Dental Pulp.* Edited by M. Siskin. C. V. Mosby Co., St. Louis, 1973, Chap. 9, pp. 122–159.

Chapter 8

Pulp Pathosis

ALFRED L. OGILVIE

A worthwhile point of departure in the study of pulp disease is the condition of normality. Can we define the normal pulp? To an extent we can. The vital symptom-free pulp is not necessarily normal at all from the standpoint of cellular integrity, nor from the standpoint of the microscopic norm is the pulp of a 15-year-old equivalent to that of an individual of 55. It becomes obvious right away that two definitions of the normal pulp exist. On the one hand, is the clinically normal pulp; on the other, the pulp judged normal after examination of serial microscopic sections. Given the placement and nature of the pulp within the tooth, it has not yet become possible (other than by extraction) to establish histologic normality in the presence of a clinical normality. Hence the two viewpoints and the need for qualification.

This much can be said. The ***clinically normal pulp*** is vital to testing procedures, responsive to a variety of excitations, but free of spontaneous symptoms. The ***microscopically normal pulp*** demonstrates only those histologic features that are compatible with its age. It is free of inflammatory change of any type.[1]

So beset is the human dental pulp with insults that the wonder lies in its remarkable capacity to remain healthy. The pulp does respond to the incessant stimuli which bear upon it. It is frequently involved in the hyperreactive phenomenon. Actually, as we know, the borderline between health and disease in any tissue is a shadowy one. Many, if not most, coronal pulps are fluctuating constantly between incipient inflammation and repair in some localized zone.[2]

Authors in the past have attempted to make pulp disease and pulp inflammation too clearcut. Rather than confirm the "all or none" view on pulp disease, it is possible on the basis of current knowledge to illustrate that ***pulp disease*** is either ***reversible or progressive.*** When the pulp is free of severe degenerative or age change, and when the stimulation applied to it is ***mild,*** it responds by a transitory hyperemia or by a reversible inflammation. When conditions are otherwise, however, the inflammatory response is marked by a progression from an incipient pulpitis (acute or chronic) to terminal necrosis[1] (Fig. 8–1).

THE HYPERREACTIVE PHENOMENON

The pulp changes that accompany the ***hyperreactive phenomenon*** (hypersensitivity and hyperemia) can be described today with reasonable exactness. Until recently it was possible merely to surmise the nature of these changes. Recent research has shown, however, that there is such a thing as a true hyperemia or elevated blood flow to the dental pulp under specific conditions.[3–5] The stimuli that give rise to this phenomenon are diverse in the extreme (*e.g.*, thermal change of hot or cold, acidic or touch stimulation through exposed dentin). Of the stimuli, all are mild in nature and brief in duration, and these facts override the diversity (Fig. 8–2). The vascular phenomenon is short-lived also, fading out to normality in a matter of minutes.

This true hyperemia represents the mildest of all

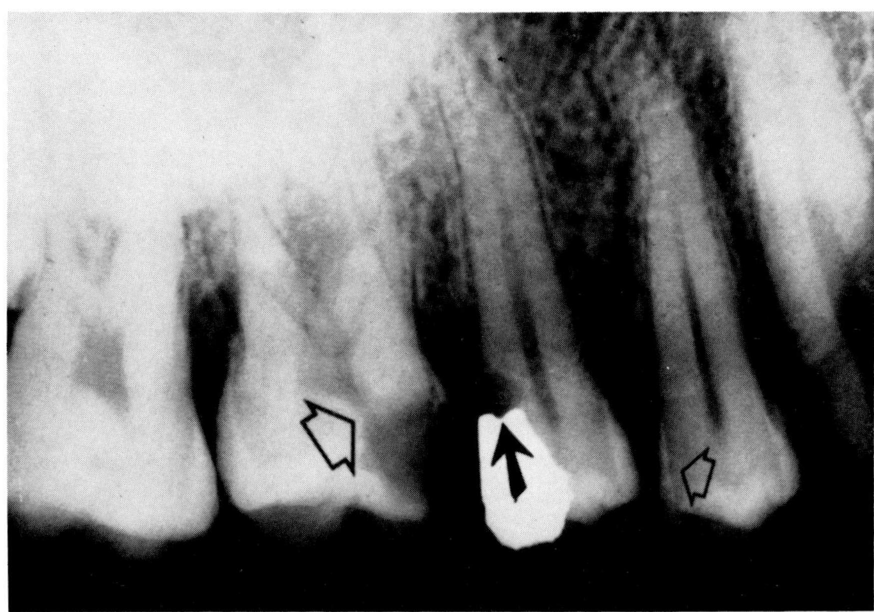

Fig. 8–1. Different degrees of clinical insult and resultant pulpitis. First premolar, second premolar, and first molar show progressive involvement by caries. Criteria other than roentgenographic were used to determine status of pulp: early dentin caries *(small arrow)* on distal of first premolar was accompanied by limited inflammation of coronal pulp; advanced dentin caries *(black arrow)* had led to more extensive pulpitis, but one that proved to be reversible; massive carious lesion *(large arrow)* had reached pulp of first molar, which demonstrated severe and irreversible pulpitis, leading to terminal necrosis.

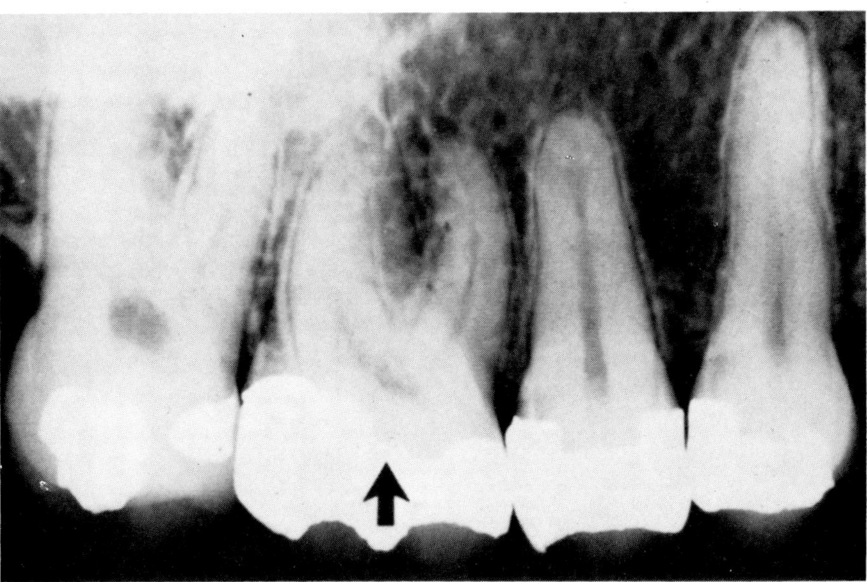

Fig. 8–2. First molar *(arrow)* with hyperreactive response to cold. Film was taken two months after placement of MOD amalgam restoration. No base was employed. Clinical symptoms gradually diminished until, six months after placement of restoration, hypersensitivity had disappeared.

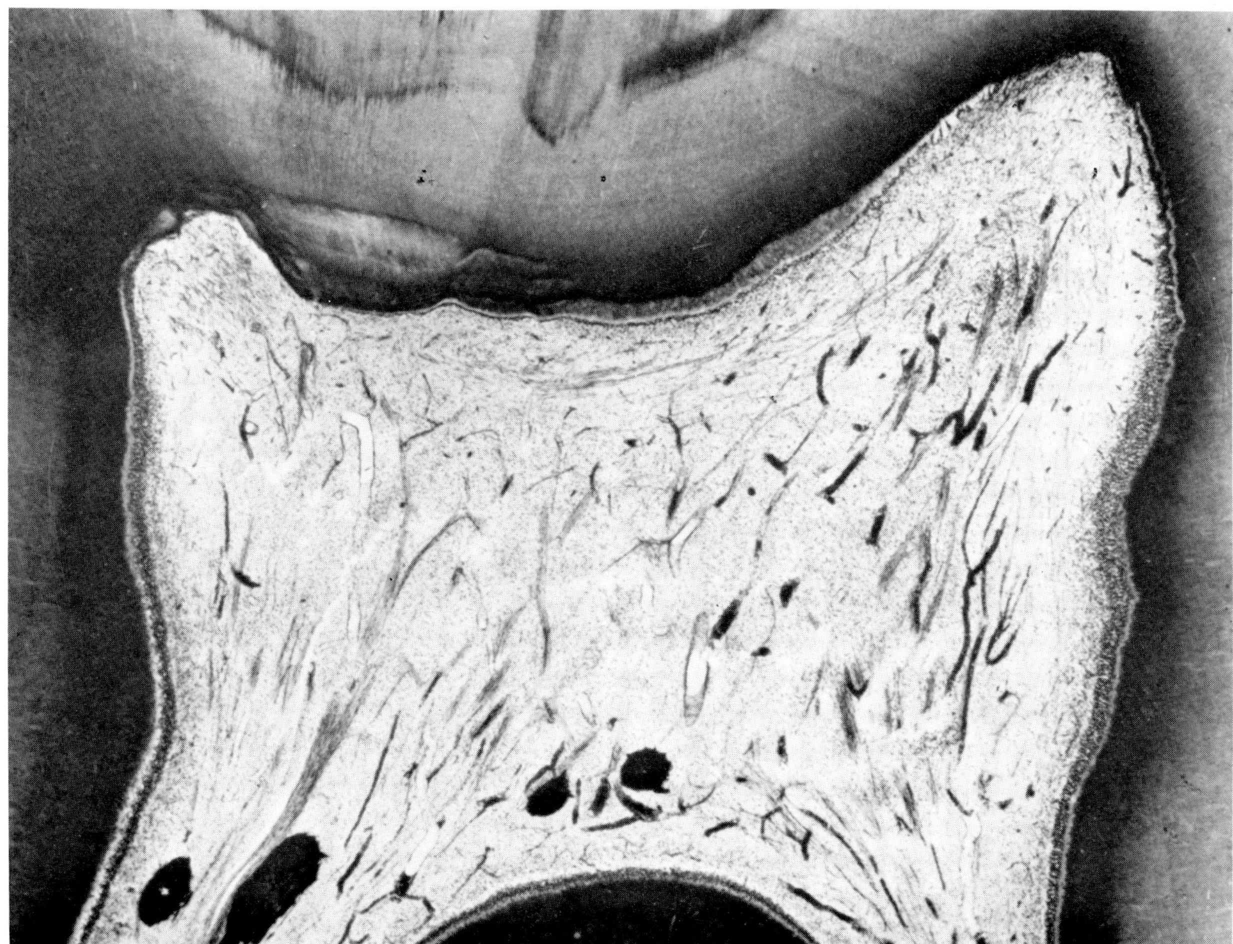

Fig. 8–3. Hyperemia in adult human pulp. Many capillaries and some larger vessels are dilated throughout coronal pulp. Small focus of round cells is evident near right pulp horn. This section, therefore, may represent concurrent hyperemia and localized pulpitis, or transition from hyperemia to localized pulpitis. (From Matsumiya, S.: *Atlas of Oral Pathology*. Tokyo Dental College Press, 1955.)

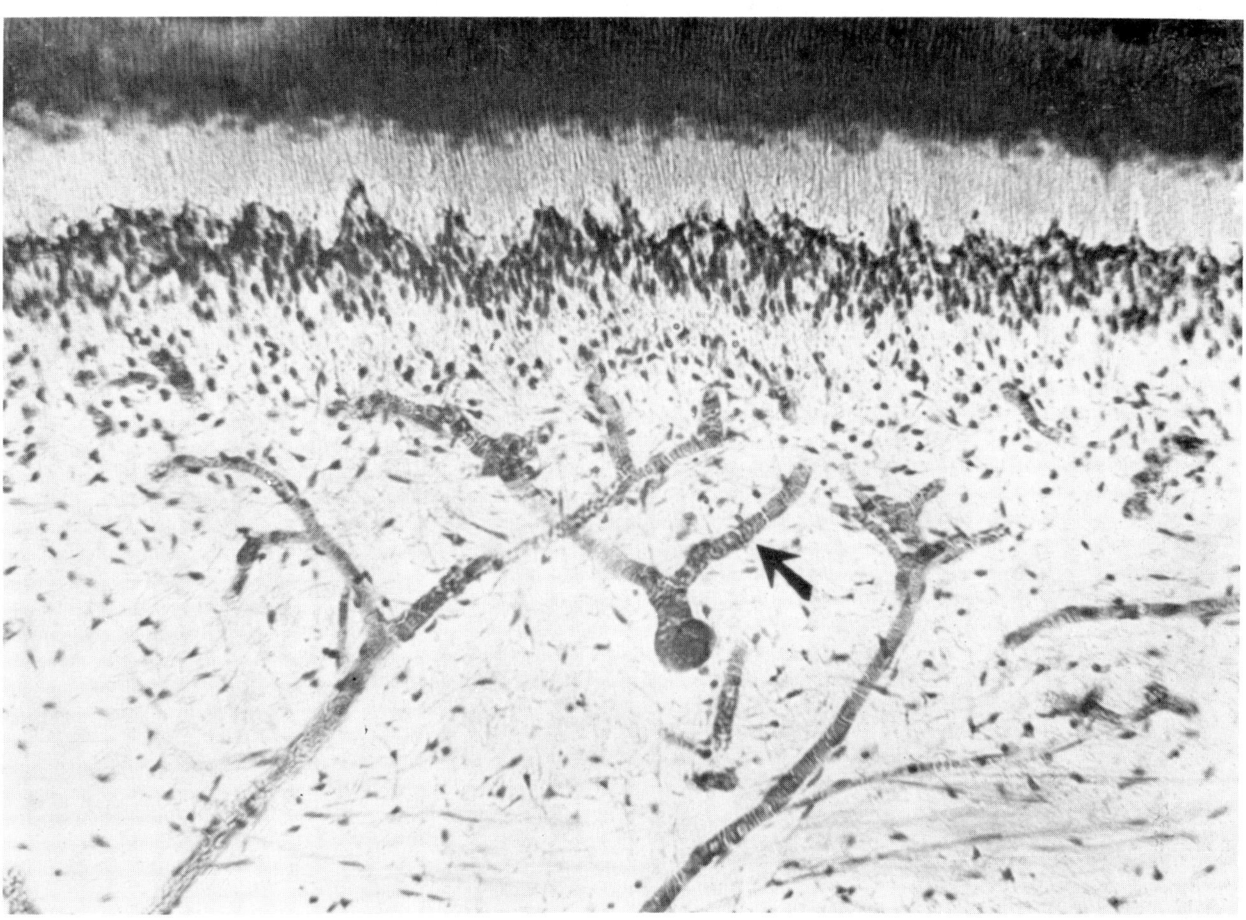

Fig. 8–4. Hyperemia of coronal pulp of adult human tooth. Dilatation of capillaries *(arrow)* of subodontoblastic plexus is dramatically shown. Erythrocytes appear densely packed within these capillaries. In contrast to situation during early pulpitis, odontoblast cell layer here is intact and there has been little or no migration of odontoblast nuclei. (From Matsumiya, S.: *Atlas of Oral Pathology.* Tokyo Dental College Press, 1955.)

deviations from the microscopically normal pulp and is the first to be given histopathologic description. In a pulp so involved, much or all of the capillary bed in the "cell-free" zone, and elsewhere, is brought into active function (Figs. 8–3 and 8–4). Many capillaries undergo a dilatation that is clearly evident. The endothelial cell nuclei become more widely separated. Masses of erythrocytes are seen in close aggregations as they move through the hyperemic capillaries (Fig. 8–5). Actual extravasation of cells beyond the capillary wall, however, does not appear to be a feature of the transitory hyperemia.

PULPITIS

Once these phenomena associated with the hyperreactive pulp are left behind, the microscopic aspects of pulp disease assume the nature of a spectrum. Soon it becomes evident to the observer that disease of the pulp usually implies involvement by ***inflamma-***

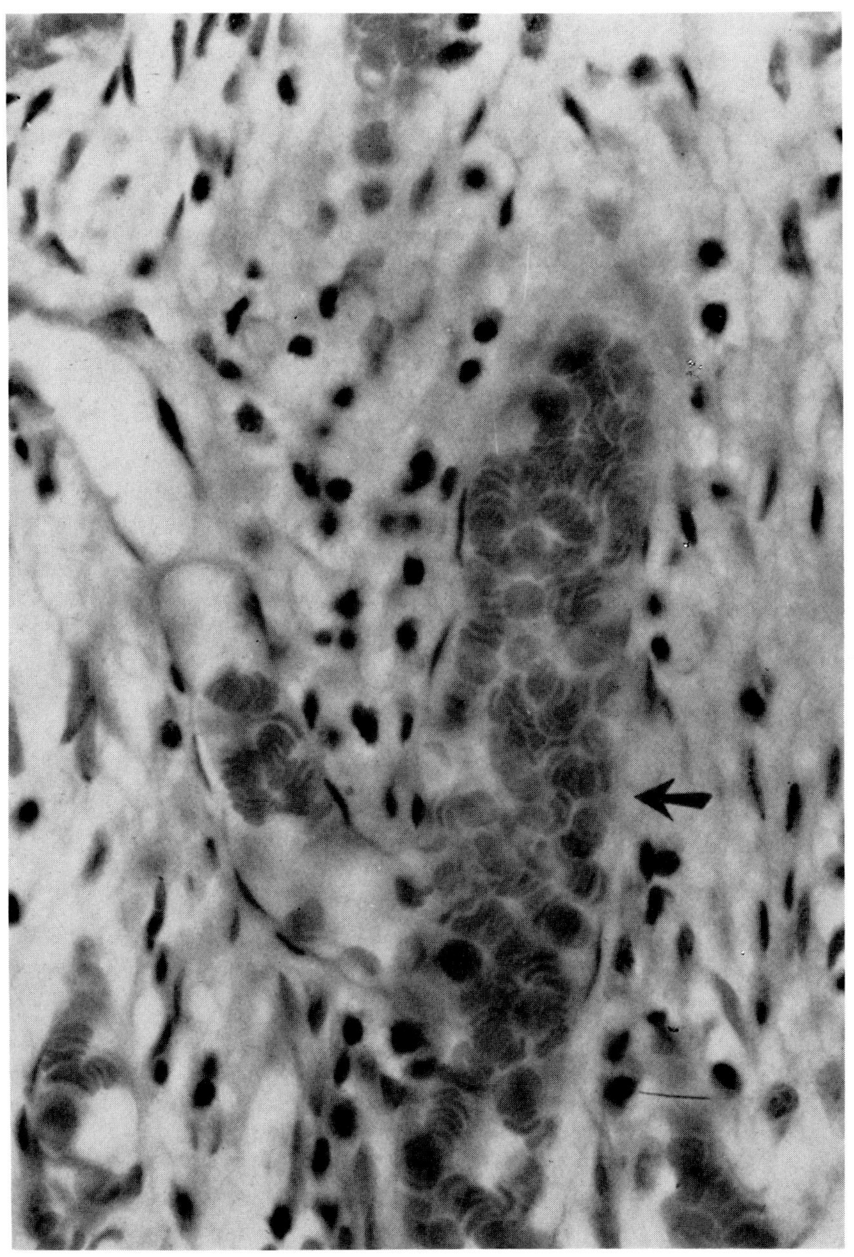

Fig. 8–5. Vascular response characteristic of hyperemia of pulp. Marked dilatation of capillary *(arrow)* is apparent. Many erythrocytes remain within vessel walls. Adult human pulp. (Orban collection.)

tion to a greater or lesser degree. It proves difficult, often impossible, to establish with the microscope that the inflammatory response in one pulp differs qualitatively from that in another. This being the case, the delineation of clinical pulpalgias (pulp pains) from one another on a microscopic basis is bound to prove inadequate. For example, the tooth that is clinically involved by an undeniably ***acute pulpalgia*** is usually found to contain the microscopic evidence of a ***chronic pulp inflammation.*** Even more confounding, the pulp may be almost totally necrotic.

A number of well-qualified authors have attempted to effect a clinical-histopathologic correlation.[6–9] Too often, unfortunately, the student reacts to the contradictions involved by performing a short-lived feat of memory.

In this text we will emphasize that clinical pulpalgia and histopathologic change within the pulp defy accurate correlation. Pulp reaction to a stimulus is far from being synonymous with the production of pulp pain. For example, a certain microscopic reaction follows the mere passage of a rotating dental stone across the external surface of enamel.[1] Seldom is such a stimulus productive of pain. A microscopic response

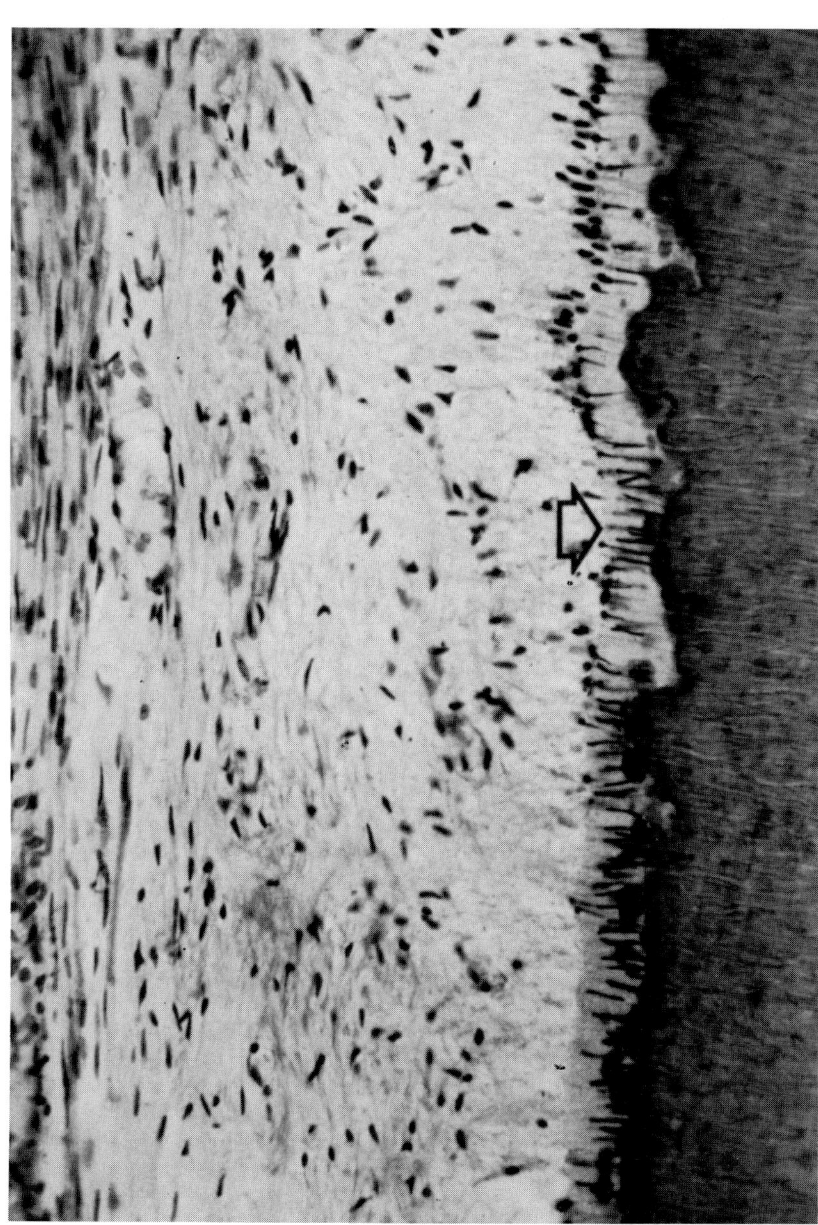

Fig. 8–6. Displacement or migration of odontoblast cell nuclei. Many nuclei *(arrow)* have left pulp and are within dentinal tubules. This has been described as initial pulp reaction to injury of tooth. It is first response to injury which is routinely seen in microsections. Apart from this change, pulp appears intact. (Orban collection.)

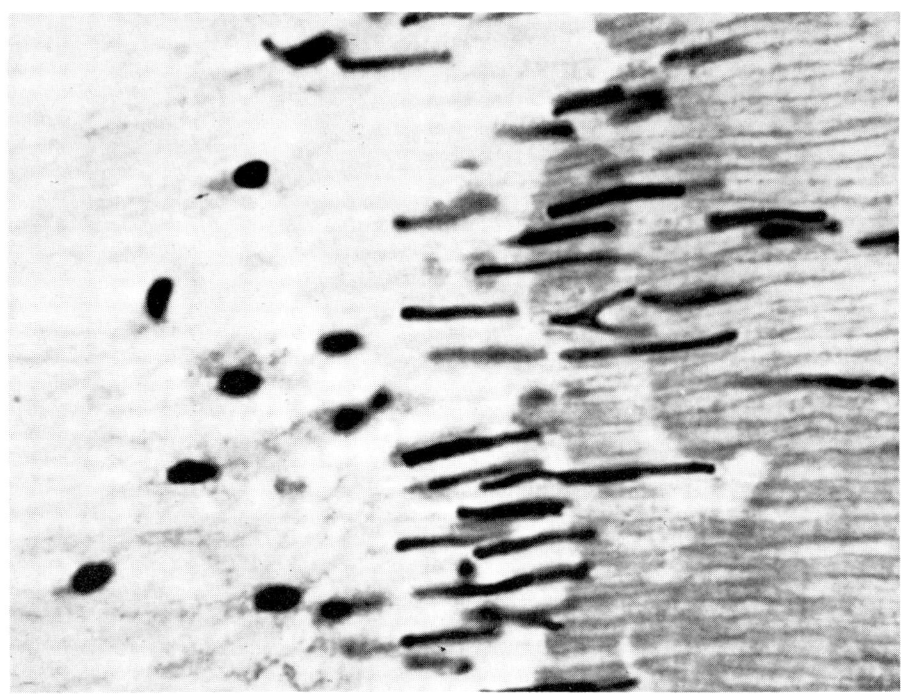

Fig. 8–7. Displacement of odontoblast cell nuclei, as seen at higher magnification. Several degrees of displacement are illustrated, from first stage of migration to advance of nucleus well into tubule proper. Following displacement of its nucleus, entire odontoblast cell is believed to degenerate within tubule. (Orban collection.)

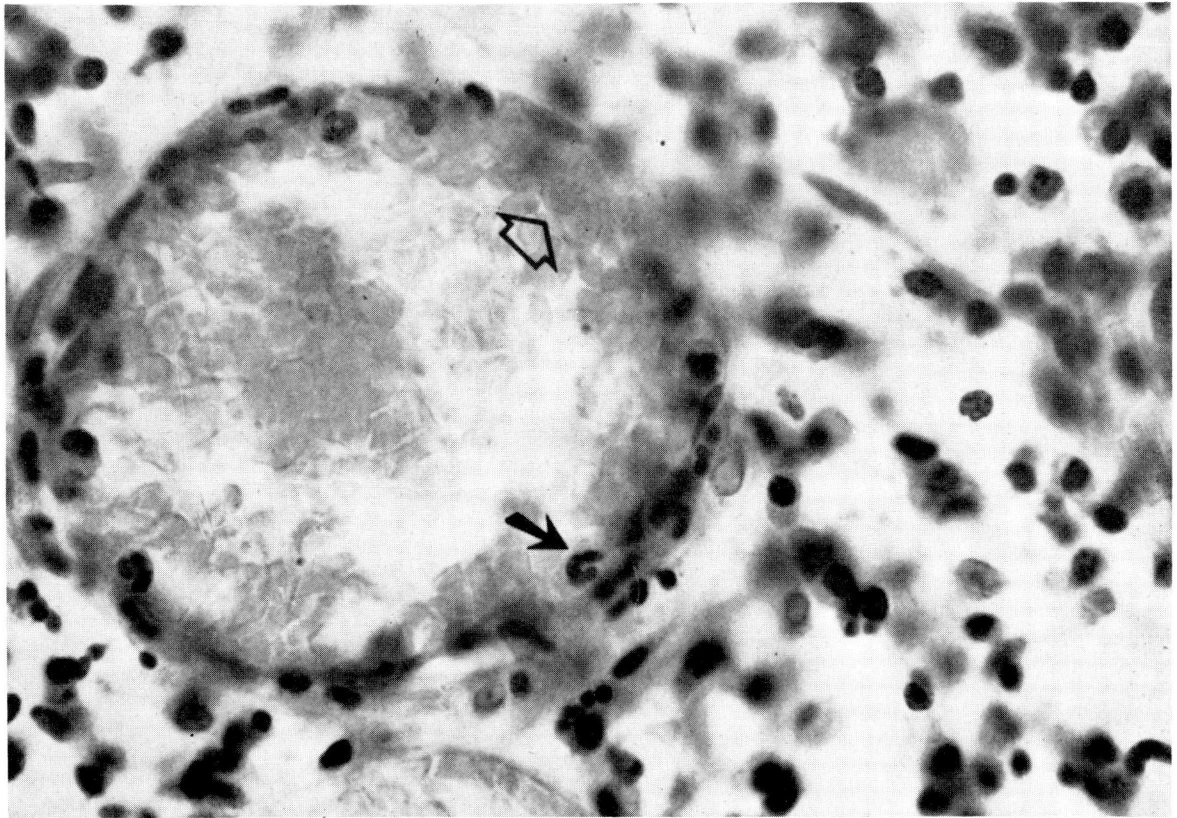

Fig. 8–8. Initial vascular changes associated with inflammation in pulp. Sludging of erythrocytes *(open arrow)* and pavementing of leukocytes *(black arrow)* are evident on perimeter of this capillary. Margination or pavementing of leukocytes develops when speed of blood passing through vessel is slowed and when, at same time, vessel is dilated. (From Matsumiya, S.: *Atlas of Oral Pathology,* Tokyo Dental College Press, 1955.)

also follows fluctuation in the temperature of the air, food or drink that comes in contact with the teeth.[3] The latter stimulus, by contrast, is often productive of pain, albeit mild and fleeting. Most would agree that the application of a revolving bur to dentin, without adequate coolant, is a relatively severe stimulus which both heats and desiccates the dentin. Pulp reaction is even more pronounced in this situation[10] and pain almost certain. In summary, then, (1) the pulp demonstrates a cellular response to almost all stimuli, (2) the extent of the cellular response depends in part on the severity of the insult to the tooth, (3) pulp pain is not evoked by all stimuli, although the likelihood of pain grows with the severity of the stimulus.

It is worthwhile to survey the pulp response to injury from start to finish. The features of inflammation in the pulp are those of inflammation in any connective tissue. There is an increase in the permeability of vessels nearest the site of injury and an extravasation of fluid from these vessels into the connective tissue spaces (edema). The intrapulp pressure rises.[4] At this stage a "side-effect" of inflammation occurs, directly attributable to the unique environment of the pulp and thought to be the result of the increased pulp pressure. The phenomenon is the displacement or migration of odontoblast nuclei into dentinal tubules (less accurately referred to as the "aspiration of odontoblasts"). It has been described as the initial pulp reaction to injury of the dental structures.[11,12] Certainly it is a readily observable change and the first response to injury to be routinely seen in microscopic sections (Figs. 8–6 and 8–7). As far as can be observed, the odontoblast nuclei do not return to their original locale. Instead, the entire odontoblast cells degenerate, and their breakdown products contribute, as additional irritants, to the inflammatory process.[11]

More classic inflammatory changes soon occur deep to the affected odontoblast cell layer. There is a chemical modification of the ground substance, often evidenced by an increased eosinophilia (eosinophilic staining) of the connective tissue.[13,14] Marked dilatation of blood vessels is accompanied by the "sludging" of erythrocytes[5] and the pavementing of leukocytes along the vessel walls[3,15] (Fig. 8–8). Diapedesis of leukocytes occurs through the same walls[15,16] (Fig. 8–9).

Around the dilated vessels a rich "infiltrate" of leukocytes is soon noticeable (Fig. 8–10). Before long the cells of this inflammatory infiltrate come to dominate the scene at the expense of the original connective tissue cell population. More often than not, so-called "chronic" inflammatory cells dominate in turn the influx of leukocytes (Fig. 8–11). In fact, the presence of the distinctive round cells in a microsection is often used to establish the pulp as inflamed.

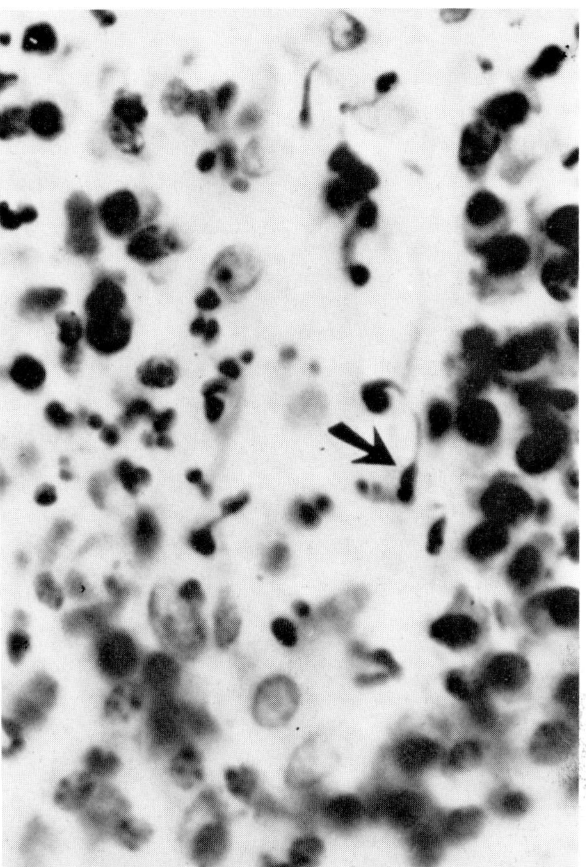

Fig. 8–9. Diapedesis of polymorphonuclear leukocytes during pulpitis. Neutrophil *(arrow)* has made partial transition through capillary wall. Other leukocytes also can be seen leaving vessel. There is edema in connective tissue, and inflammatory cells are numerous. Human pulp. (Orban collection.)

What particular cells comprise the "infiltrate" in pulp sections? The variety in the types of cells and their proportionment is considerable. Leukocytes, yes, but what particular ones? As has been stated, the "chronic" forms usually dominate the scene. Small leukocytes, macrophages, and plasma cells are therefore abundant. Neutrophils are also commonplace when the inflammation is a localized process and presumably of short duration. Seldom, however, is there a predominance of neutrophils or even of the

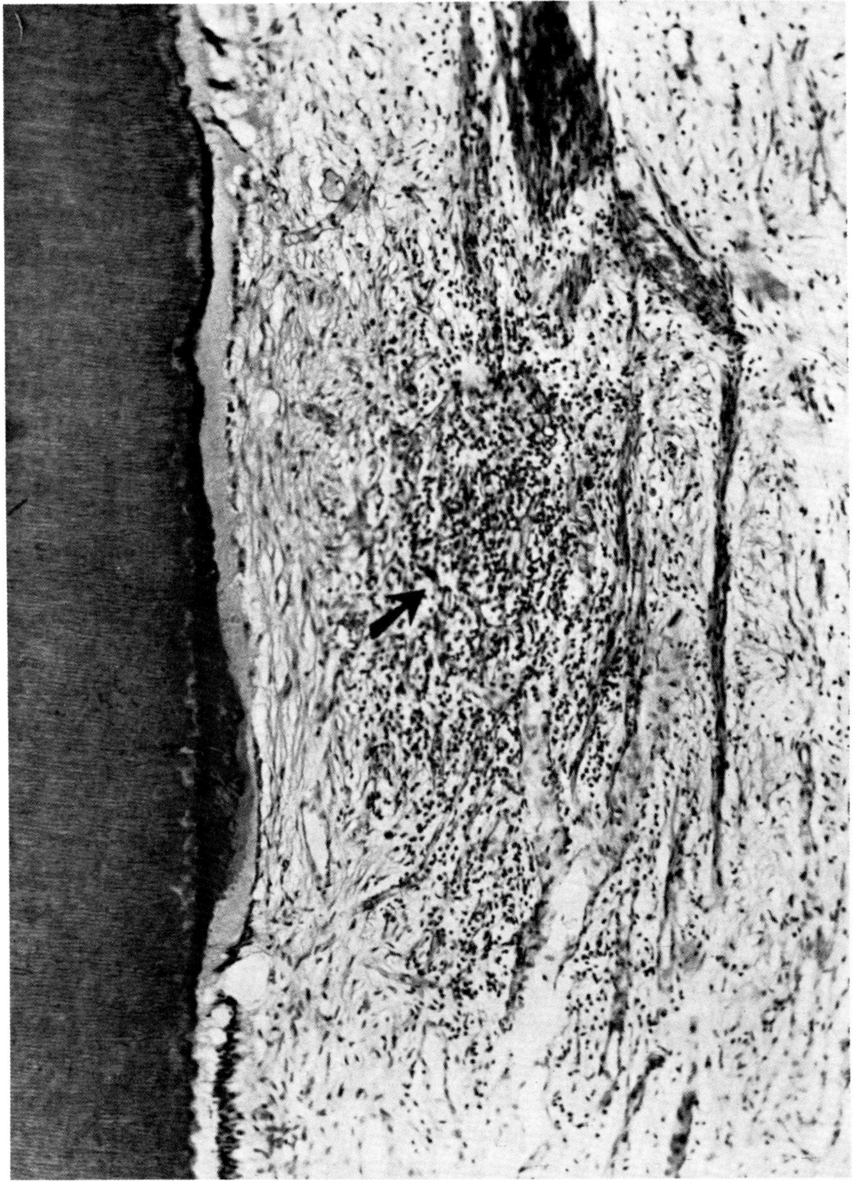

Fig. 8–10. Incipient pulpitis showing circumscribed area of inflammation near pulp wall. Blood vessels in area are enlarged. Many connective tissue elements within pulp at this site have been displaced or eliminated. Adjacent odontoblasts have been either destroyed or greatly modified. (Orban collection.)

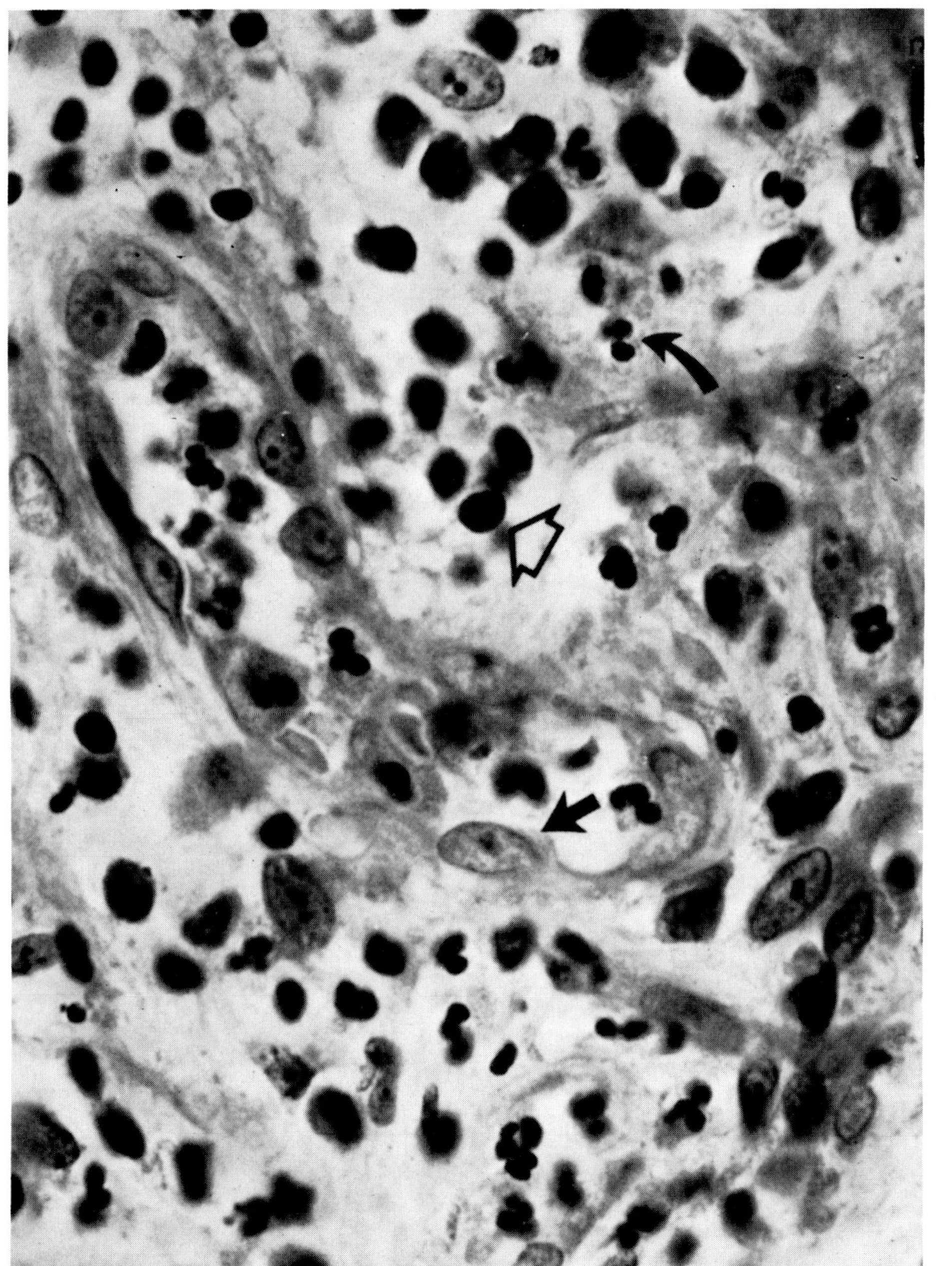

Fig. 8–11. Inflammatory cell infiltrate of pulpitis. Capillary with swollen endothelial cell nuclei *(black arrow)* is prominent in center of field. Leukocytes lie within vessels and in even greater abundance beyond them. White-cell population includes neutrophil *(curved arrow)* and plasma cells *(open arrow)*. (Orban collection.)

polymorphs as a group. It is for this reason that the true "acute" inflammation of microscopic definition is said to be absent in pulp sections.

The process of pulp inflammation is often reversed, and effective connective tissue ***repair*** is then the end result. This resolution occurs where there has been localized rather than a generalized pulpitis. The tooth concerned has experienced, say, a single relatively minor insult, or a gradually approaching threat to the pulp, such as caries, has been removed. Irritation has not been severe, certainly.

A consistent feature of pulp repair is the re-establishment of odontoblast cells lost in the course of inflammation. Apparently the cells that are lost are not replaced through the mitosis of adjacent odontoblasts.[17] Rather, underlying mesenchymal cells provide the reservoir. In one sense, the source of new odontoblasts depends on the extent of the damage to the original odontoblast layer and the adjacent connective tissue. If the injury has been minor and only scattered odontoblasts have died, the undifferentiated mesenchymal cells of the "cell-rich" zone are the replacement source. Regeneration is then comparatively rapid. If, on the other hand, all the odontoblasts in an area are destroyed, and with them the elements of the "cell-free" and "cell-rich" zones, then regeneration takes longer. In the latter instance, the new odontoblasts must come from mesenchymal cells even deeper within the pulp.[18,19] However, this is not simply a matter of undifferentiated cells moving out to the dentin and there being transformed directly into odontoblasts. Instead, through a series of mitotic divisions, cells derived from the stimulated

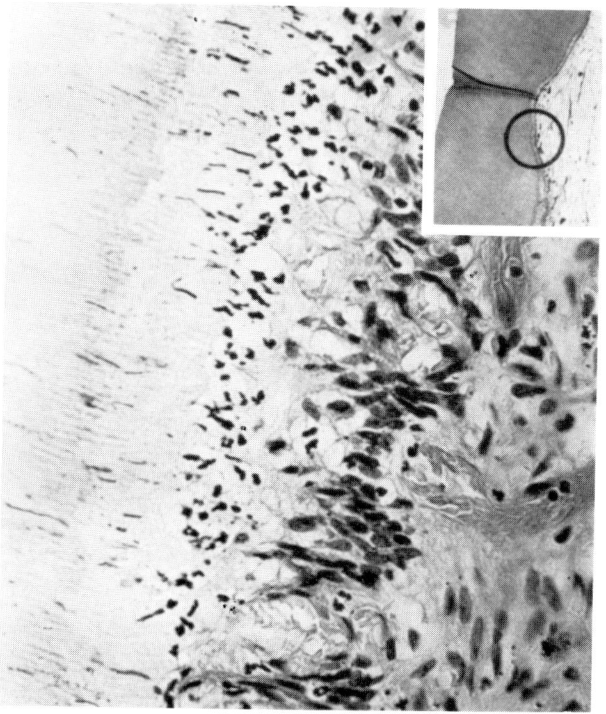

Fig. 8–12. Fibroblast cell proliferation in human pulp in response to mild stimulus. New fibroblasts are evident in cell-rich zone with orientation of their nuclei toward odontoblastic layer. Displacement of some odontoblast nuclei is noticeable to left. New odontoblast cells will appear later. Section of pulp six days after experimental cavity preparation. (From Swerdlow, H. and Stanley, H. R.: J.A.D.A., *56*:317, Mar., 1958.)

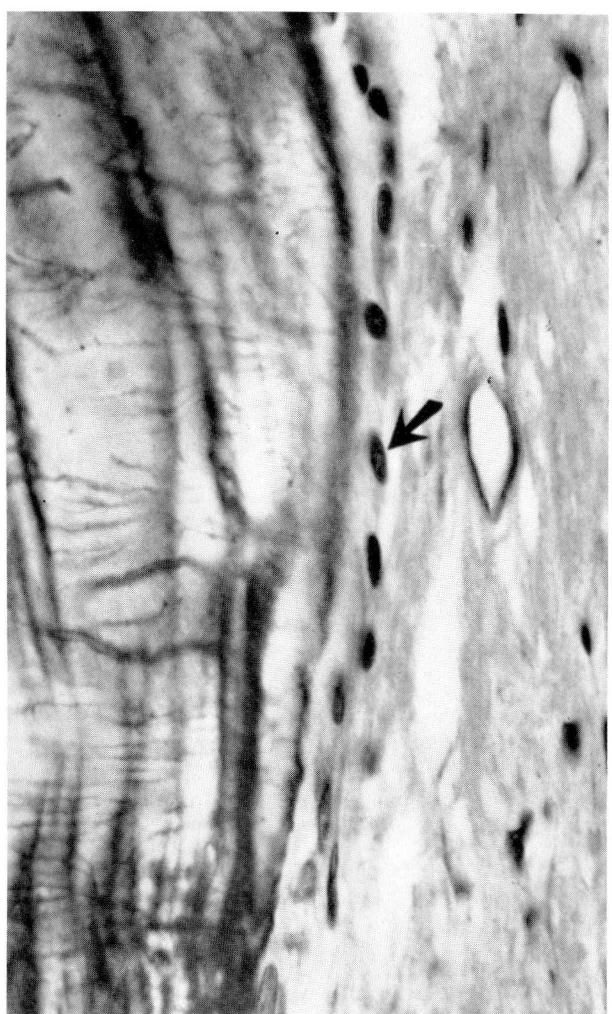

Fig. 8–13. Replacement odontoblast *(arrow)* on surface of new zone of predentin. Cell bodies of these odontoblasts are cuboidal to low columnar in form. Reparative dentin produced by preexisting odontoblasts is to the left. (Orban collection.)

mesenchymal cells move wave-like toward the pulp periphery. On the advancing front, these successive generations of daughter cells increasingly assume the potentialities of odontoblasts. The cells of the sequence which finally contact dentin are the ones that make up the new odontoblast layer.[19]

The stimulus of a mild irritant does more to the "cell-rich" zone than provoke a differentiation of odontoblasts. To an even greater extent it encourages the growth of new fibroblasts, also from the mesenchymal elements of the zone. Swerdlow and Stanley noted a massing of fibroblasts within six days of experimental cavity preparation[20] (Fig. 8–12). Unquestionably, this concentration of cells is a prelude to the new connective tissue which must "back-stop" the regenerating odontoblasts. Meanwhile, any normal delineation of the "cell-free" zone is quite lost in this ferment of inflammation, necrosis, and repair.

A limited inflammatory reaction is often followed by, and may even be accompanied by, the laying down of reparative dentin. The stimulus to this localized dentin production is the external irritant. If the inflammation is restricted and does not completely destroy the odontoblasts at the site, the odontoblasts may form reparative dentin in coexistence with the nearby round cell infiltrate. Otherwise, the new dentin will appear when replacement odontoblasts reach the dentin wall (Fig. 8–13).

When one considers how many insults can produce pulp inflammation, the need for care in ascribing a particular inflammatory reaction to a particular irritant becomes obvious. For example, the question facing the student who examines a pulp section may boil down to this: Does the observed round cell infiltrate represent the response to the small carious lesion which was noted in the enamel of the tooth before sectioning? To establish such a connection with reasonable certainty, the following would need to prevail: (1) the pulp lesion would be a localized one; (2) the pulp lesion would either emanate from the dentin-pulp junction or be near the dentin, even though separated from it by a zone of normal pulp tissue[21] (Fig. 8–14); (3) the dentinal tubules leading peripherally from this site would end in the caries lesion or be continuous with enamel rods that did.[1,22]

We have just alluded to the development of a center of pulp inflammation at a distance removed from the dentin wall (Fig. 8–14). This situation appears to exist much more often than it actually does. Serial sections of the entire pulp are required to

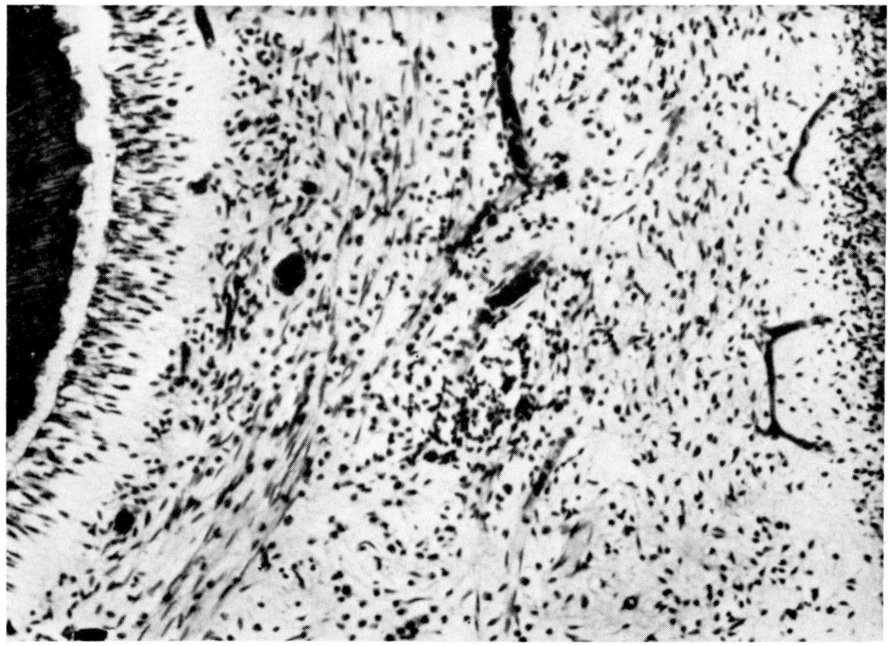

Fig. 8–14. Isolated zone of incipient pulpitis at distance removed from dentin wall. Concentration of inflammatory cells can be seen in center of field. Odontoblast layer *(left)* and subjacent connective tissue are normal. This pulp inflammation is response to caries in outer part of dentin. (From Langeland, K.: *Tissue Changes in the Dental Pulp.* Oslo University Press, 1957.)

demonstrate that the seemingly isolated zone is in truth a lateral section of a more extensive inflammatory process extending centrally from the dentin. The establishment of such an inflammatory zone, when it does exist, apparently follows the initial reactions of odontoblast nuclei displacement and the creation of new odontoblasts from mesenchymal cells. Thus, localized central inflammation is long term in nature, a response to a mild irritant.

When a single irritant applied to a pulp has been too massive, or cumulative small insults have proved too numerous, then what began as a localized process of inflammation spreads to involve more and more of the coronal pulp. Usually this extension is a slow

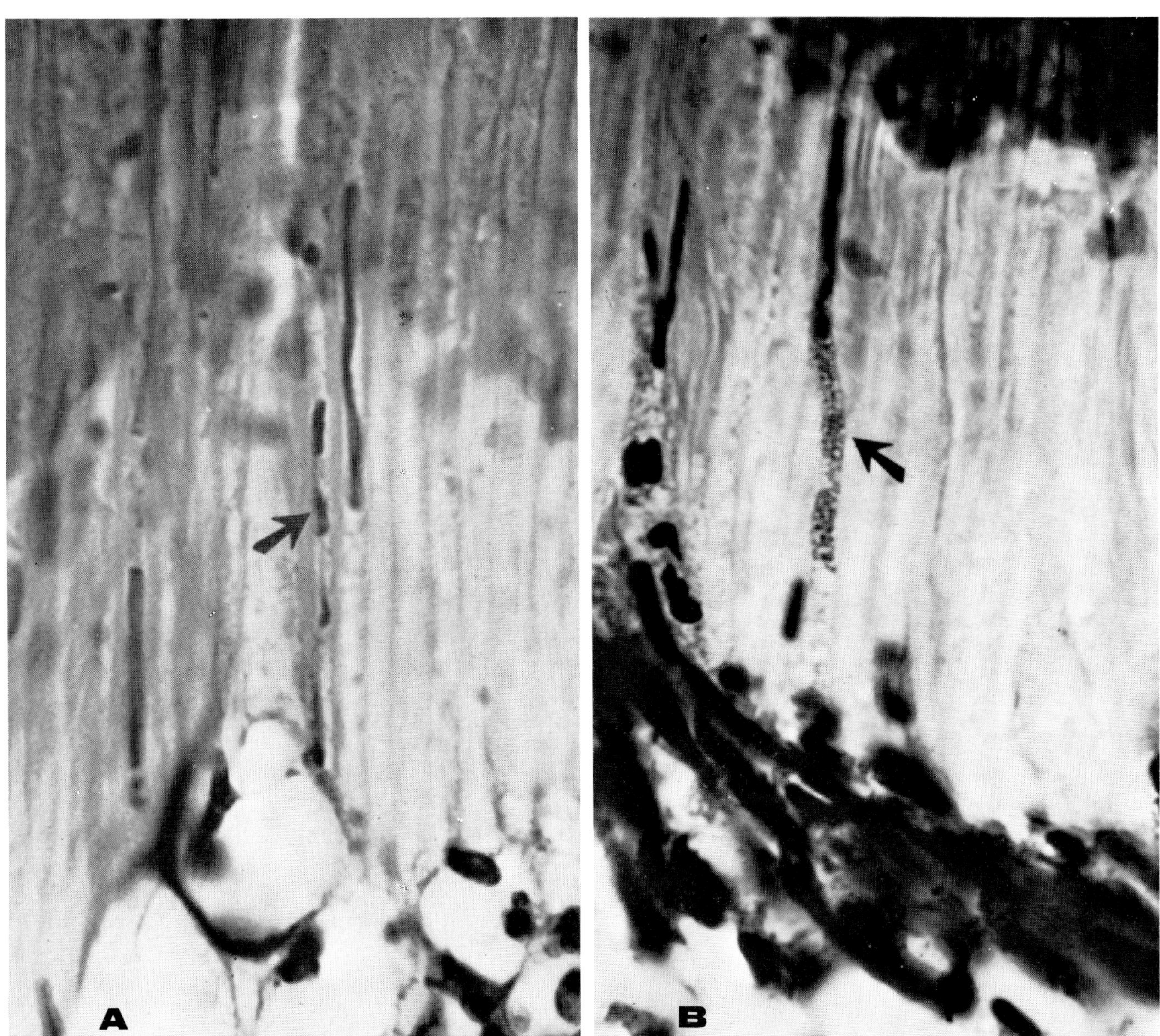

Fig. 8–15 *A*, Neutrophil *(arrow)* which has migrated from pulp into dentinal tubule. Each lobule of three-lobed nucleus is linked to next by chromatin thread. Elongation of leukocyte was necessary before it could migrate. Cell is thought to migrate in order to phagocytose remnants of odontoblast, which originally occupied tubule. Human tooth. *B*, Eosinophil within dentinal tubule. Most eosinophilic granules *(arrow)* have remained on pulp side of cell nucleus. This particular leukocyte is entirely within uncalcified predentin zone. Human tooth. (Orban collection.)

process, but occasionally it will display great speed. The end result, once a large segment of a coronal pulp has become inflamed, is total necrosis of that pulp. Hyperplastic pulpitis is the single exception.

The advance of inflammation within the pulp can be effectively studied with reference to a series of photomicrographs. The first phases of the progression have been noted. Vascular dilatation, localized edema, and displacement of odontoblast cell nuclei are followed by the establishment of the inflammatory infiltrate (Figs. 8–7, 8–8 and 8–10). The infiltrate actually represents cell ***and*** fluid inflow, the fluid being the "edema fluid" and a highly significant part of the connective tissue change. The cellular portion, or "round cell" part of the infiltrate, is composed of the various leukocytes. The phenomena of margination and diapedesis have enabled white cells by now to escape the vessels and become part of this infiltrate. Orban photographed many of the polymorphonuclear group (both neutrophils and eosinophils) within the actual dentinal tubules (Fig. 8–15). Presumably the polymorphonuclear cell that moves into a tubule disintegrates there as did the odontoblast cell before it.[23]

Localized vascular disturbance, destruction of odontoblasts, and round cell infiltrate may be all the reaction that can be associated with an initial carious lesion in dentin. Furthermore, as a rule, only the pulp immediately adjacent to the invaded tubules will show microscopic disturbance (Fig. 8–16*B*).

Vascular change continues as inflammation becomes more solidly entrenched in a particular part of

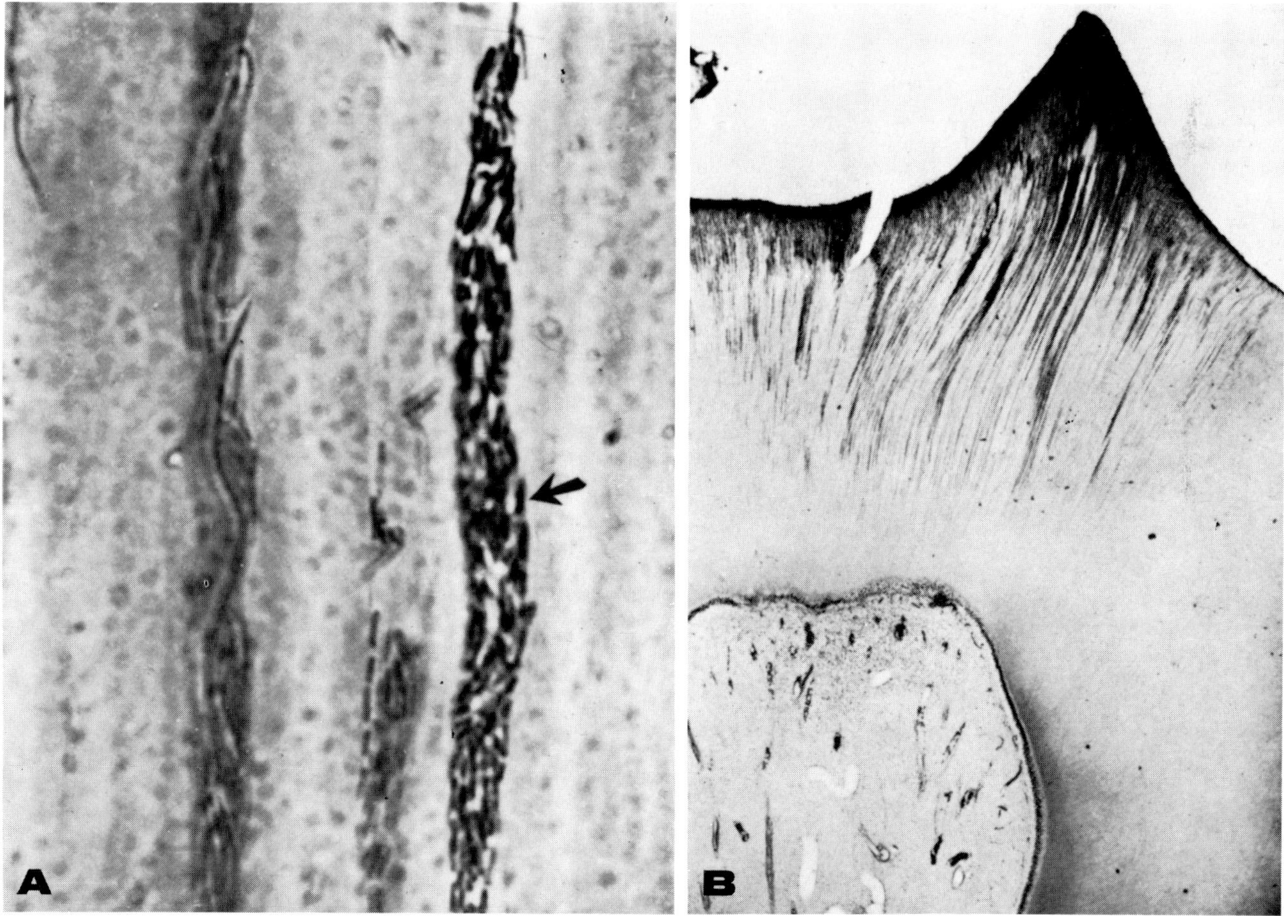

Fig. 8–16. *A,* Bacilli *(arrow)* within tubules of human carious dentin. Decalcified section. Gram-Weigert stain for bacteria. (From Matsumiya, S.: *Atlas of Oral Pathology.* Tokyo Dental College Press, 1955.) *B,* Pulp reaction to bacterial invasion of dentinal tubules prior to existence of gross carious lesion in dentin. Only pulp adjacent to invaded tubules shows evidence of inflammation. Odontoblasts are disrupted, pulp vessels are enlarged, and there is massing of round cells. Human tooth. (Orban collection.)

the pulp. The endothelial cell nuclei become swollen. Each endothelial cell appears to encroach upon the lumen far more than it would in the normally functioning vessel. Leukocytes fill the lumen to the exclusion of most erythrocytes. An obvious slowing of the flow within the vessel takes place[3] (Fig. 8–11).

Throughout the stroma around the vessel, fiber and fibril have given way to fluid and cell. The small lymphocyte abounds. Fibroblasts persist, but like the endothelial cell, these appear large and atypical. Histiocytes of the once-normal pulp can be seen in the process of change to the macrophage form (Fig. 8–17). Eosinophils are surprisingly numerous (Fig. 8–18). Where bacteria are free within the pulp in small numbers, they undergo phagocytosis. The macrophages perform this work, as clearly demonstrated by Orban (Fig. 8–19).

Frank infection of the pulp or, in other words, the actual entry of bacteria into the pulp tissue, often leads to the development of the microabscess. An abscess of the pulp, of course, may be sterile. Progression of the inflammatory process to the stage of abscess, however, is most significant, and infection is often a forerunner of it.

The microabscess of the pulp begins as a tiny zone of necrosis within a dense round-cell infiltrate (see Fig. 7–19). When this lesion exists, as it often does, on the actual dentin wall, it is frequently found in connection with a carious exposure (Fig. 8–20; see also Fig. 8–21*A*). On those occasions when the abscess develops away from the dentin wall, the classic abscess structure is evident, *i.e.*, the central suppurative core, the zone of the cellular infiltrate and dying fibroblasts, and the peripheral fibrous capsule (Figs. 8–21*A* and *B*). The fibrous capsule of the pulp abscess, to be sure, often lacks continuity and clarity (Fig. 8–21*C*). Were the host tissue more dense, more fibrous, this would hardly be the case.

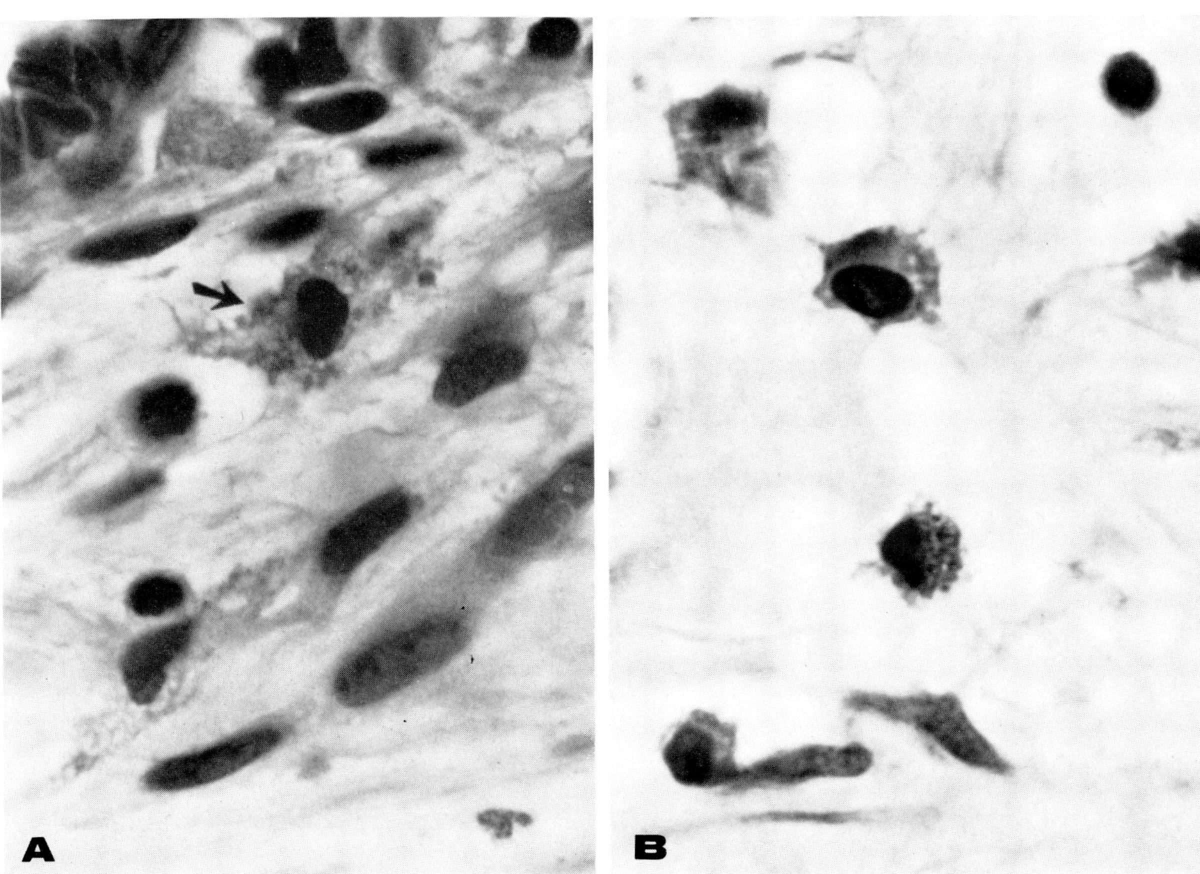

Fig. 8–17. *A*, Histiocyte of human pulp which is changing into macrophage *(arrow)*. Stimulus for change is inflammation in pulp. (Orban collection.) *B*, Completion of transformation of histiocyte into macrophage *(top center)*. Eosinophil with its granules lies below macrophage, and small lymphocyte is visible in top right. Human pulp. (Orban collection.)

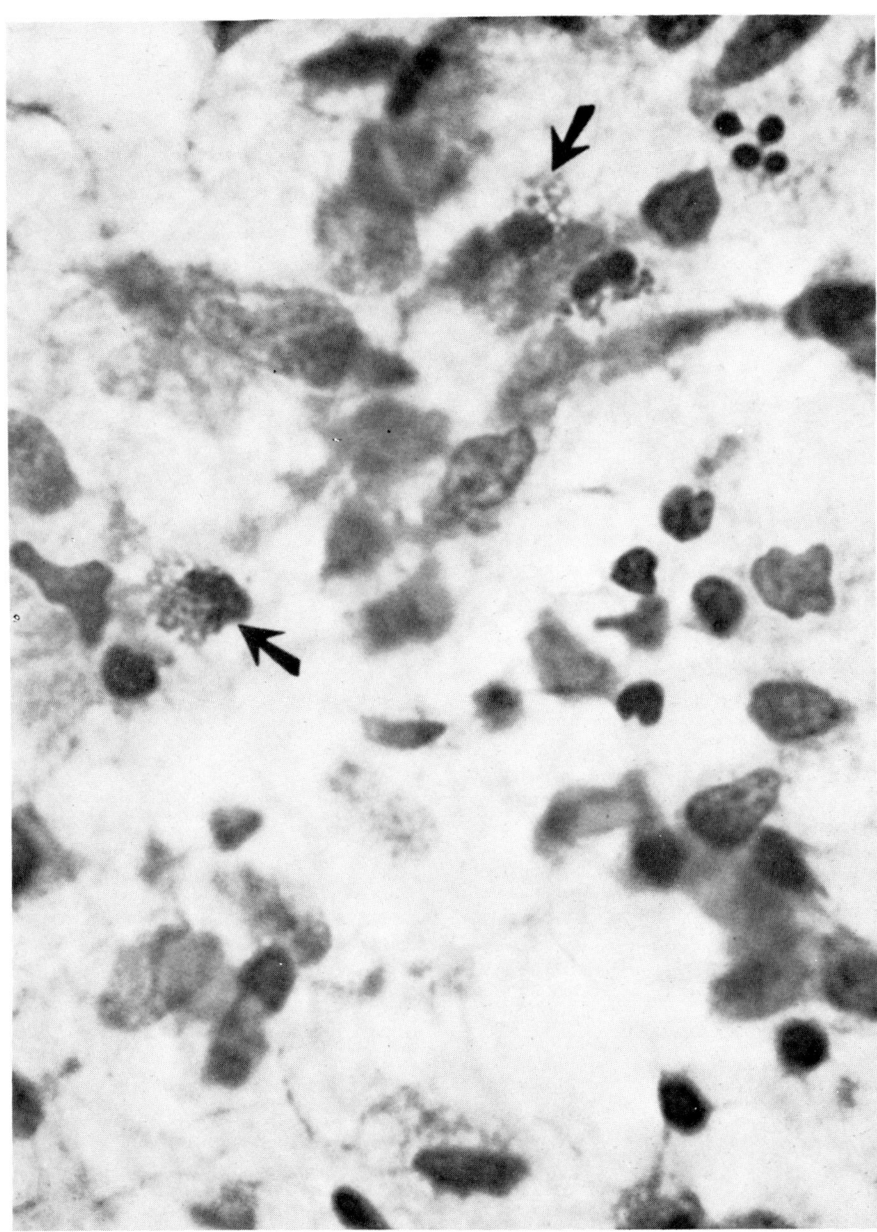

Fig. 8–18. Eosinophils *(arrows)* within inflamed human pulp. Fibroblast nuclei are evident as pale elliptical structures in background. (Orban collection.)

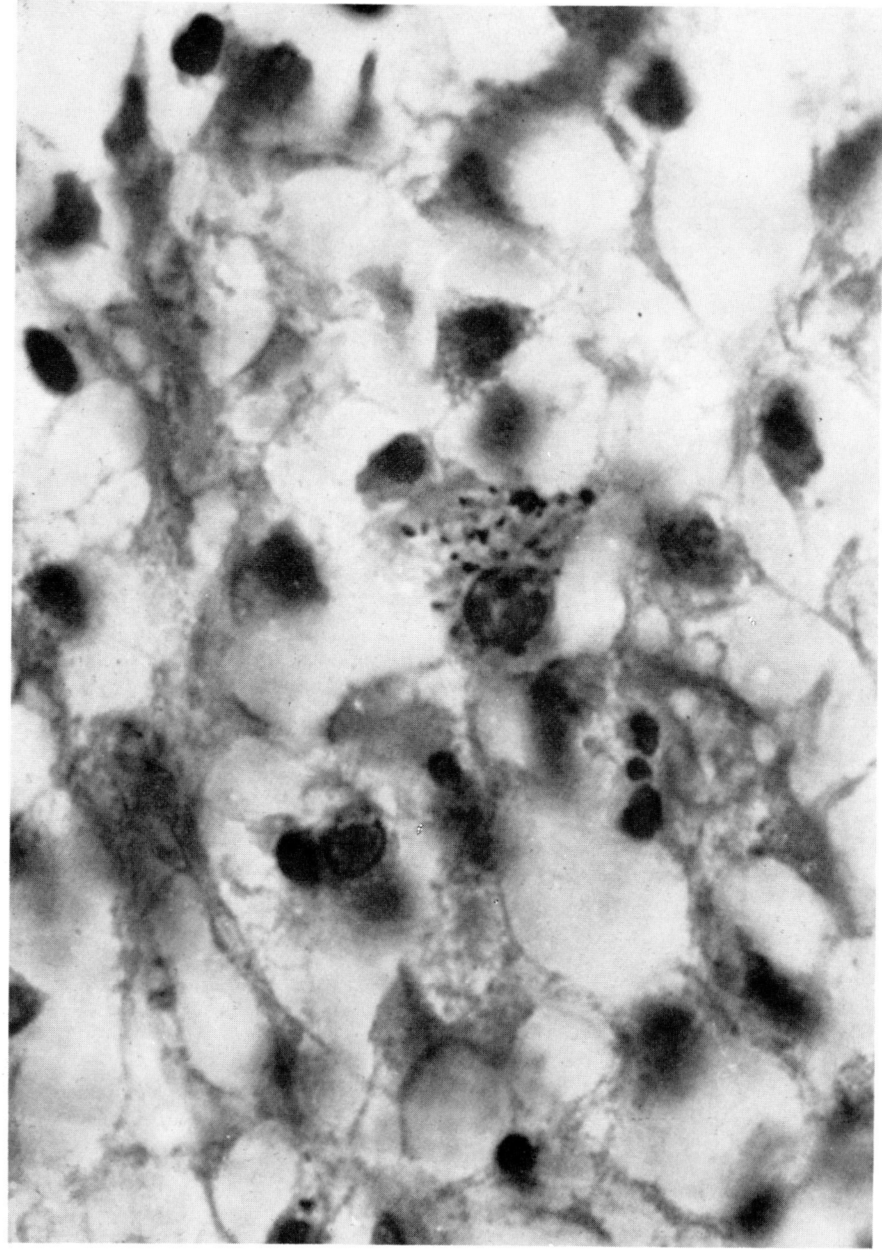

Fig. 8–19. Pulp macrophage loaded with phagocytosed bacteria. Phagocytosis of bacteria is effective part of inflammatory response in pulp when number of bacteria involved is not great. Human pulp. (Orban collection.)

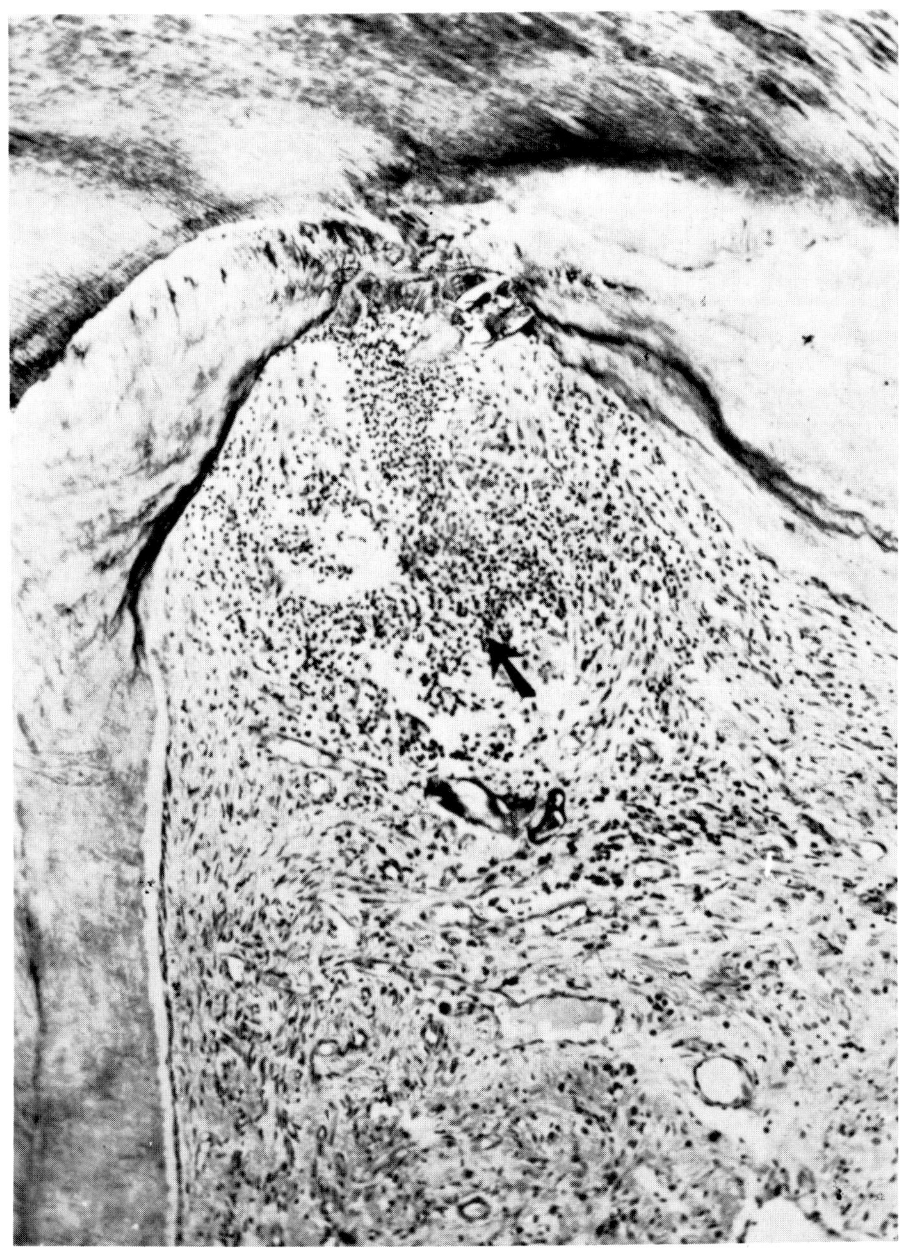

Fig. 8–20. Microabscess of human pulp at area of carious exposure extended through reparative dentin. Zone of necrosis *(arrow)* is continuous with area of exposure. (Orban collection.)

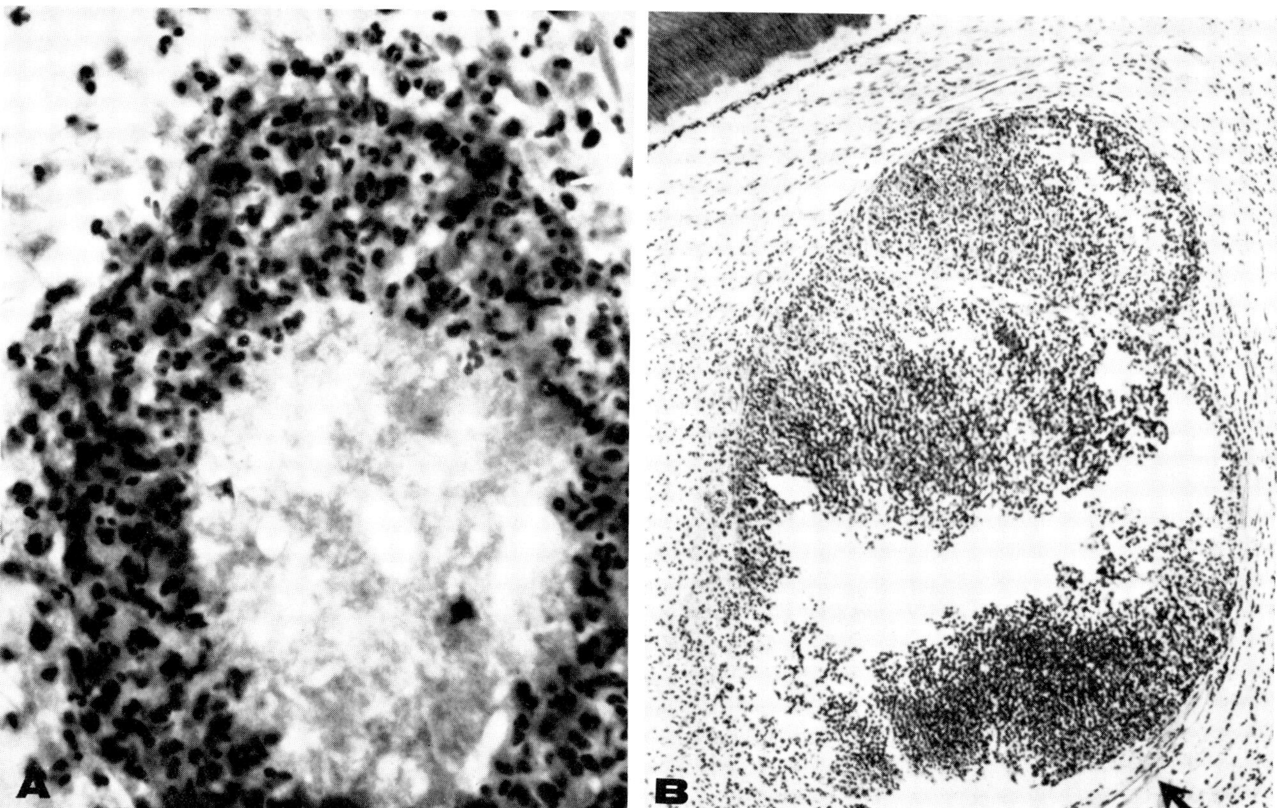

Fig. 8–21. *A,* Microabscess in pulp which has developed in classic form away from dentin wall. This photomicrograph portrays only central suppurative core, and zone of cellular infiltrate and dying fibroblasts. Peripheral fibrous capsule is not visible. Human pulp. (Orban collection.) *B,* Fibrous capsule *(arrow)* on periphery of microabscess. There has been compaction of pulp tissue on periphery of this rapidly expanding abscess, and localized destruction only. Human pulp. (Orban collection.) *C, Above:* Absence of fibrous capsule around pulp abscess. Pulpitis (p) is evident with liquefaction necrosis (ln) in central zone. Many pulp abscesses, like this one, do not have capsule. Asymptomatic mandibular third molar; 19-year-old male. *Below:* Pulp inflammation *(above)* has extended to periapex. (*d*—dentin, *p*—pulp, *inf*—inflammation of the periapical tissue.) (From Seltzer, S., Bender, I. B., and Ziontz, M.: Oral Surg., *16*:846, July, 1963.)

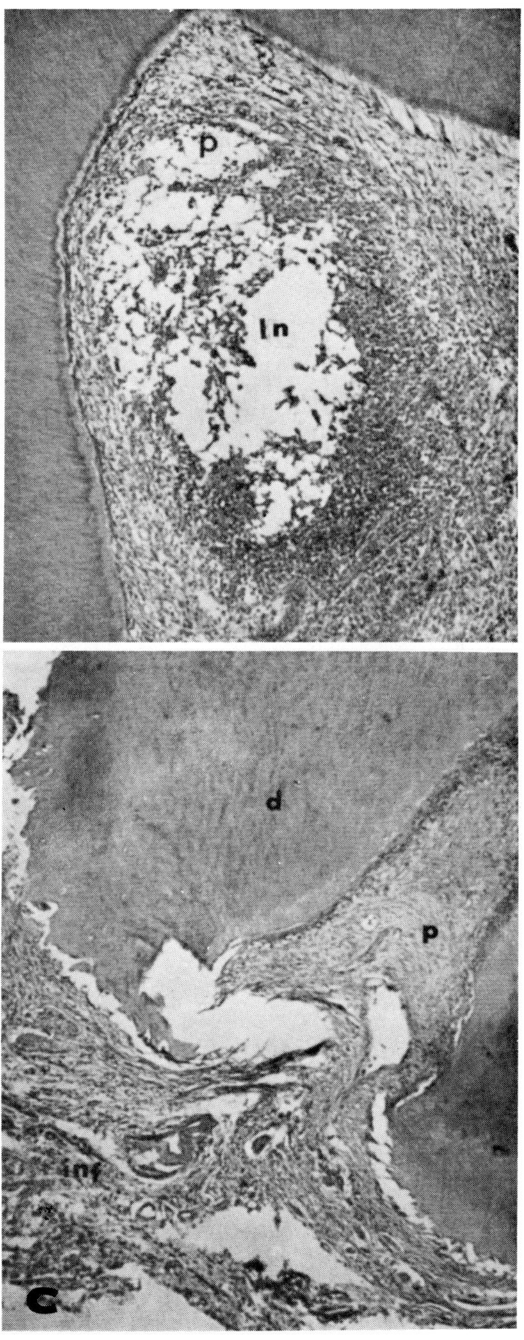

Fig. 8–21*C*.

In histopathologic terms the nature of pulp response to caries attack is more variable. When the caries process advances unchecked, eventually to penetrate the zone of reparative dentin, it is not enough to say that a chronic pulp inflammation is established, or that this inflammation terminates in a suppurative microabscess. The duration of involvement and the resistance of the pulp are obviously of significance. In the isolated microsection that is studied without a clinical history, these factors always remain unknown. Despite such limitations, the histologic nature of the various responses is worth studying. One pulp may be involved with a carious exposure and contain a single abscess. Another, with approximately the same observable caries lesion, may contain not one but numerous tiny abscesses (Fig. 8–22). Still another pulp may give evidence of having undergone a rapid transition from localized abscess to widespread necrosis. This latter response can be accompanied by bacterial growth within the pulp chamber (Fig. 8–23). If the organisms are saprophytic in nature, then what is known clinically as the "gangrenous pulp" will be created in the process.

Many pulps, on the other hand, respond to carious exposure by surface ulceration. In this way it appears that they are able to offer long-term resistance and to delay extensive breakdown of their soft tissue mass. Even though the entire occlusal surface of the coronal pulp is ulcerated, the deeper connective tissue may be normal (Fig. 8–24). Beneath the necrotic surface of the ulcer lies a zone of dense leukocytic infiltration (Fig. 8–25). Beyond this, a zone of proliferating

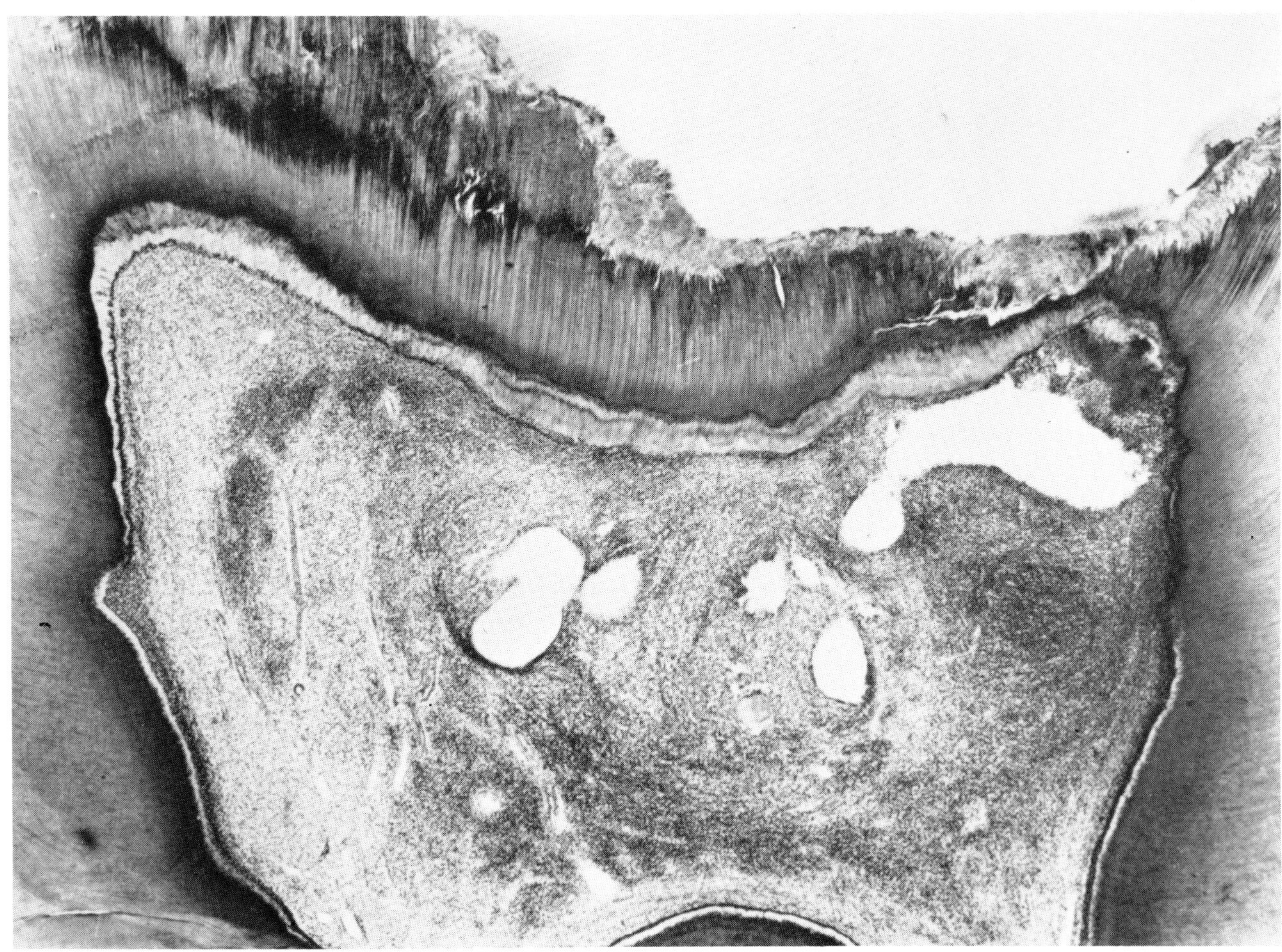

Fig. 8–22. Multiple abscesses in human molar pulp. Caries penetration has been extensive and inflammatory change in pulp connective tissue is far advanced. Round cells are everywhere. Space in center of each abscess represents lysed and necrotic material, which was lost in preparation of section. (From Matsumiya, S.: *Atlas of Oral Pathology.* Tokyo Dental College Press, 1955.)

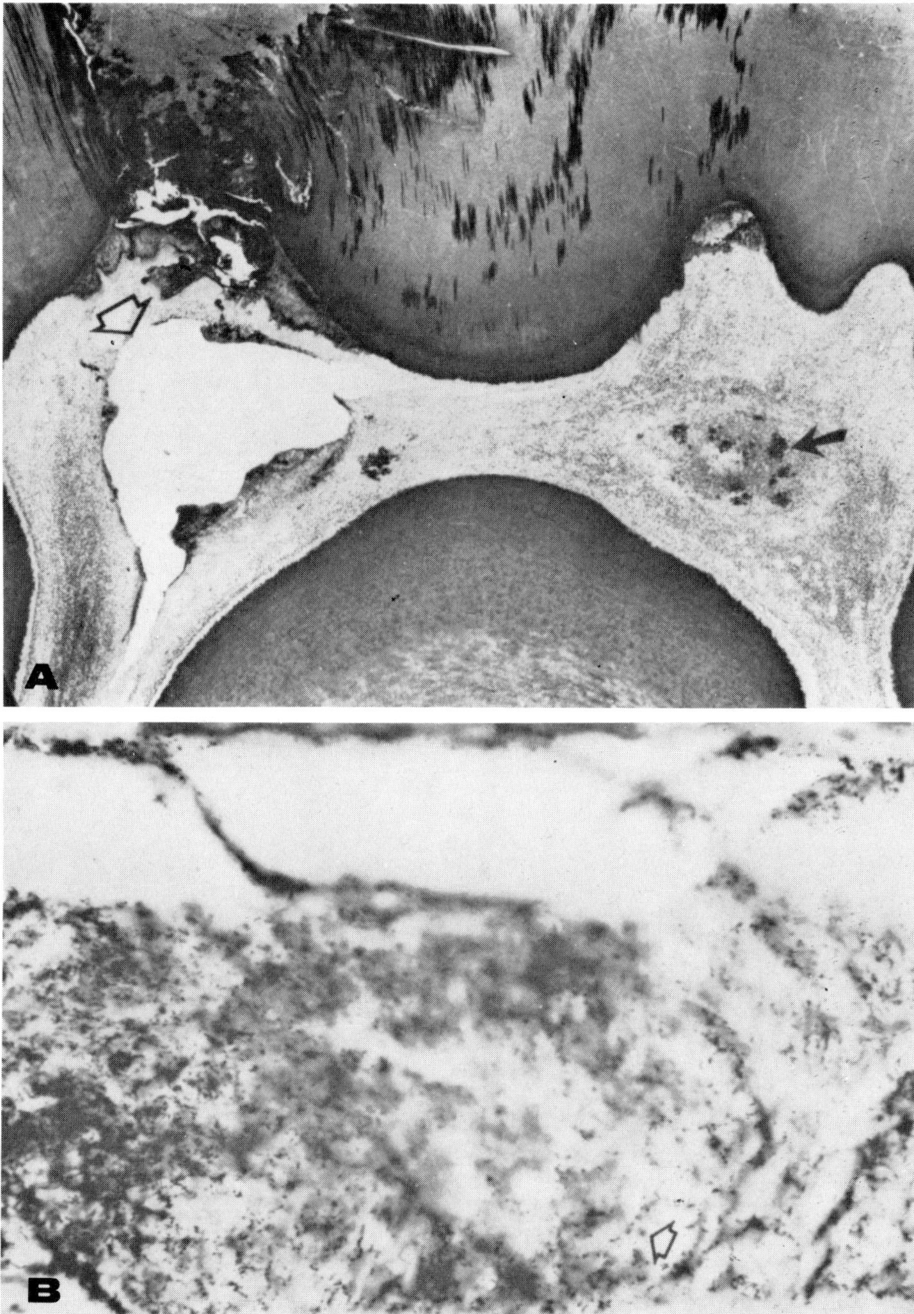

Fig. 8–23. *A,* Massive and rapidly advancing pulp necrosis accompanied by bacterial growth. Bacterial penetration resulted in development of abscess *(open arrow).* Bacteria were not contained by defenses and spread rapidly through coronal pulp. Much pulp became necrotic without undergoing typical liquefaction. Dots *(black arrow)* are bacterial masses. When resident bacteria such as these are saprophytic, pulp is putrescent and is known as "gangrenous pulp." Human molar tooth. (From Matsumiya, S.: *Atlas of Oral Pathology.* Tokyo Dental College Press, 1955.) *B,* Bacteria in necrotic tissue of gangrenous pulp. Cocci predominate. Some are clumped. Other cocci *(arrow)* are individually distinct. Spaces above are artifacts. (Orban collection.)

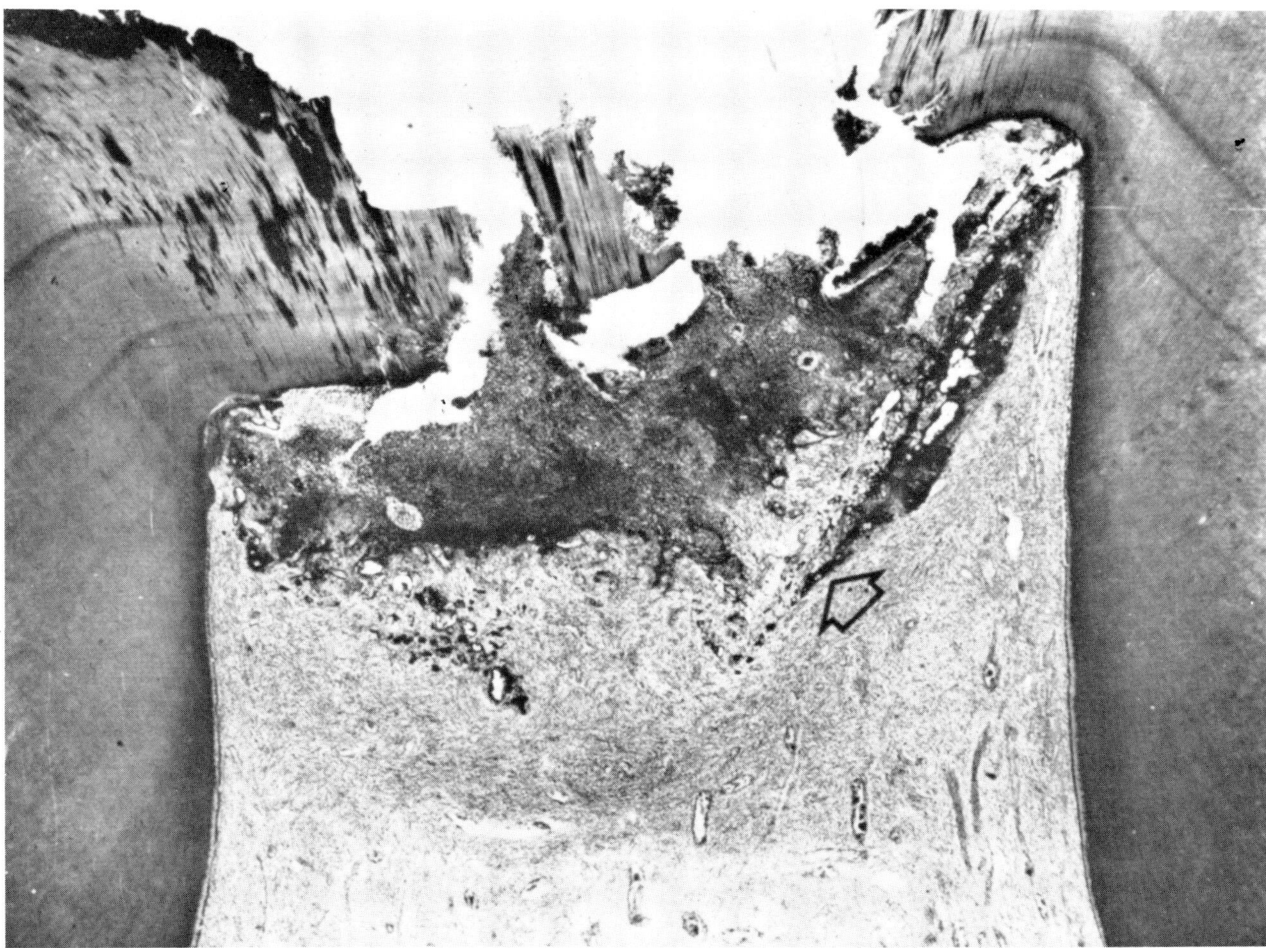

Fig. 8–24. Ulceration of entire surface of human pulp, in response to carious exposure. Beneath necrotic surface of ulcer is zone of dense leukocytic infiltration. Below this is zone of proliferating fibroblast cells and collagenous fibers, *i.e.*, "collagenous zone" or fibrous zone. Irregular calcifying masses *(arrow)* are sometimes found in this area. Toward floor of pulp chamber connective tissue is relatively normal. (From Matsumiya, S.: *Atlas of Oral Pathology.* Tokyo Dental College Press, 1955.)

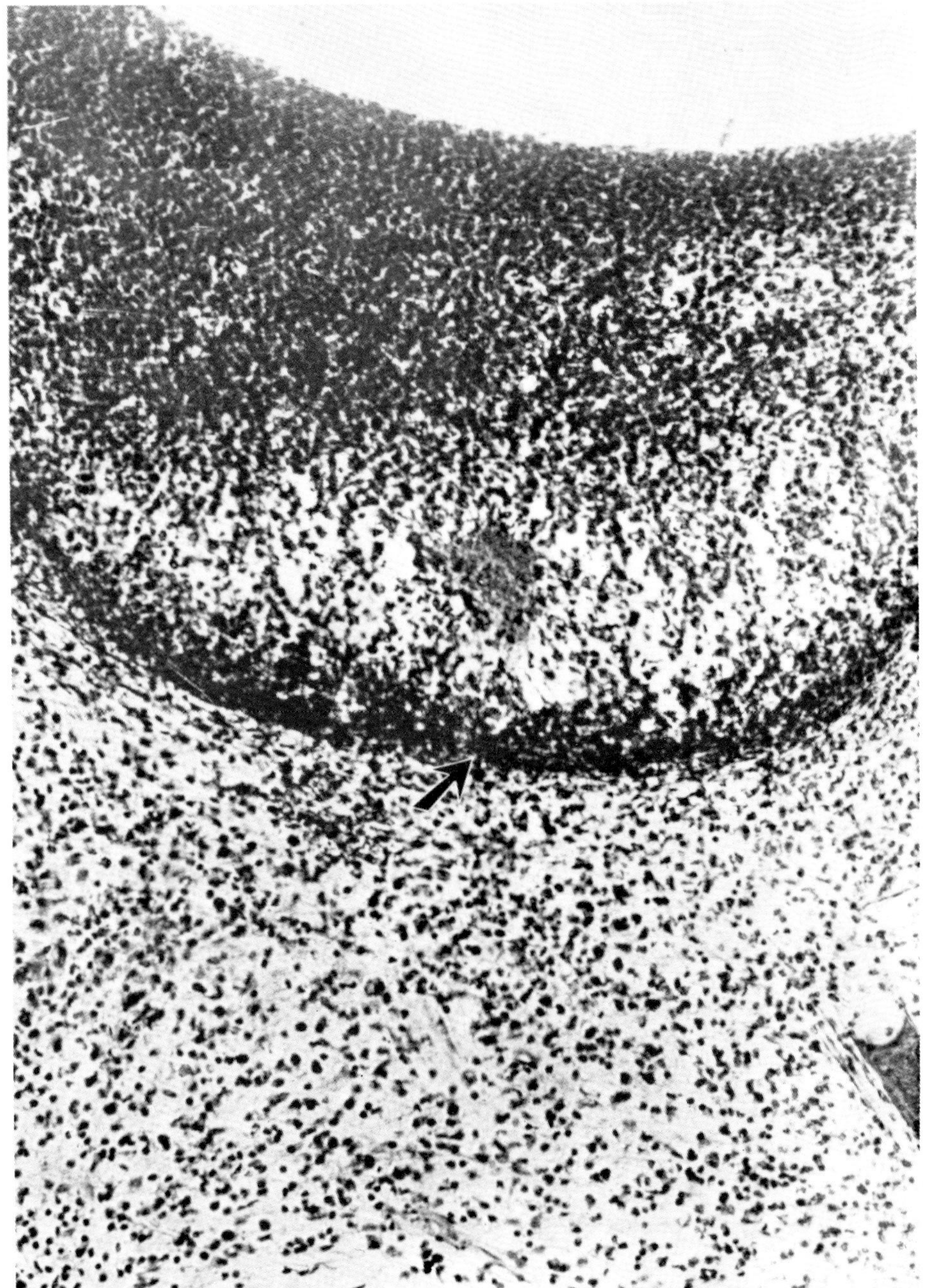

Fig. 8–25. Surface of ulcerated human pulp. True surface of ulcer is distinct *(arrow)*. Zone of dense leukocytic infiltration, which is part of ulcer, lies beneath. Above actual ulcer is wide layer of necrotic "pus" cells. (From Matsumiya, S.: *Atlas of Oral Pathology*. Tokyo Dental College Press, 1955.)

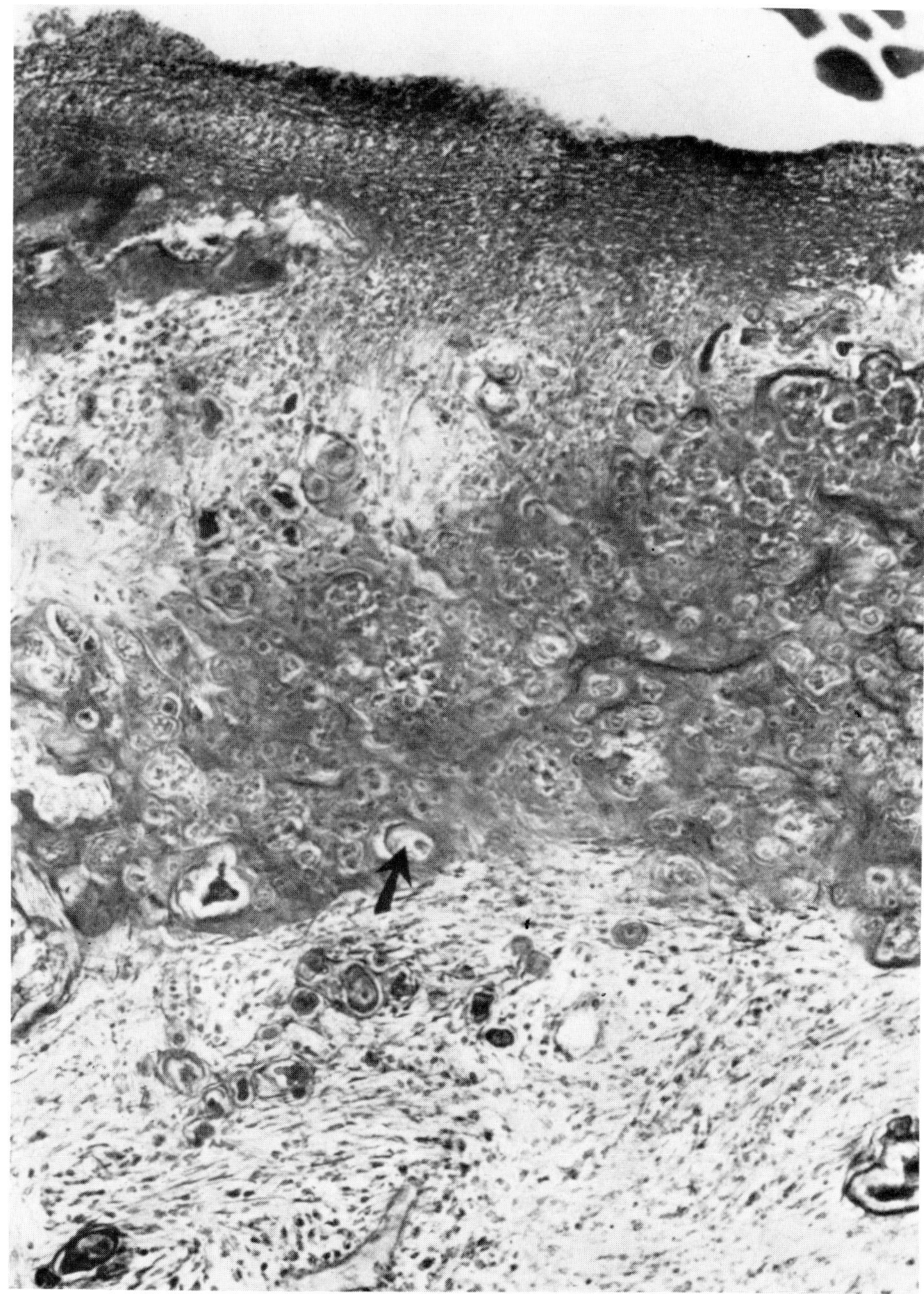

Fig. 8–26. Irregular calcific masses within collagenous zone, deep to ulcer of human pulp. Center of each mass *(arrow)* is uncalcified or incompletely calcified. Necrotic cells may serve as foci for inorganic salt deposition. These calcifications are described by Matsumiya as part of defensive process. (From Matsumiya, S.: *Atlas of Oral Pathology.* Tokyo Dental College Press, 1955.)

fibroblast cells and collagenous fibers serves to limit the process. It is within this "collagenous zone" that one finds the irregular calcific masses described by Matsumiya and considered to be a part of the defensive process. Necrotic cells may serve as nuclei for the inorganic salt deposition. Many such nuclei adhere and coalesce. In their center the masses are considered to be either uncalcified or incompletely calcified[24] (Fig. 8–26). At one stage or another such barriers as are provided by the ulcer no longer prove adequate. The fibrous zone is breached and inflammatory change permeates the entire pulp (Fig. 8–27).

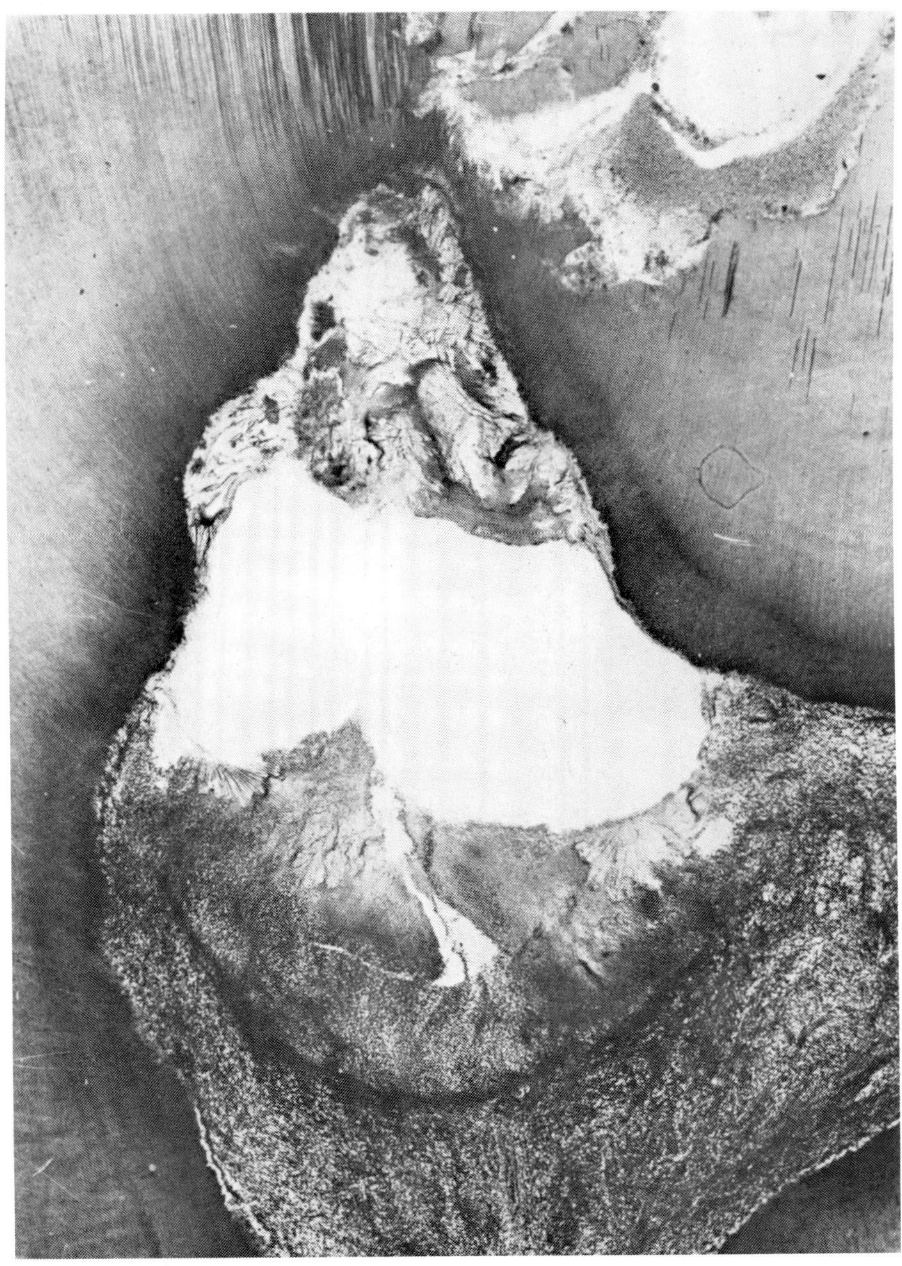

Fig. 8–27. Transformation of pulp ulcer into generalized chronic inflammation of entire pulp. Barrier provided by collagenous zone has been breached. Inflammatory round cells now permeate entire pulp. Carious exposure. Human tooth. (From Matsumiya, S.: *Atlas of Oral Pathology*. Tokyo Dental College Press, 1955.)

NECROSIS

Necrosis is the constant companion of inflammatory change within the pulp. It precedes the regeneration of odontoblasts in pulp repair. It is present, at least locally, within most zones of round-cell infiltration. We have observed it as a constant feature of the pulp abscess and of the ulcerated pulp (Figs. 8–20 and 8–25). It forms an integral part of the thrombus which is produced in many a pulp vessel (Fig. 8–28). Necrosis within an arteriole of the pulp is of unusual significance. Because the pulp lacks significant collateral circulation, the tissue breakdown is not localized as it would be in most connective tissues. Instead, an extravascular necrosis of unusual size may be the outcome.

We have seen that inflammatory change may envelop a pulp slowly or swiftly. The conversion of an inflamed pulp into a necrotic one likewise may occur

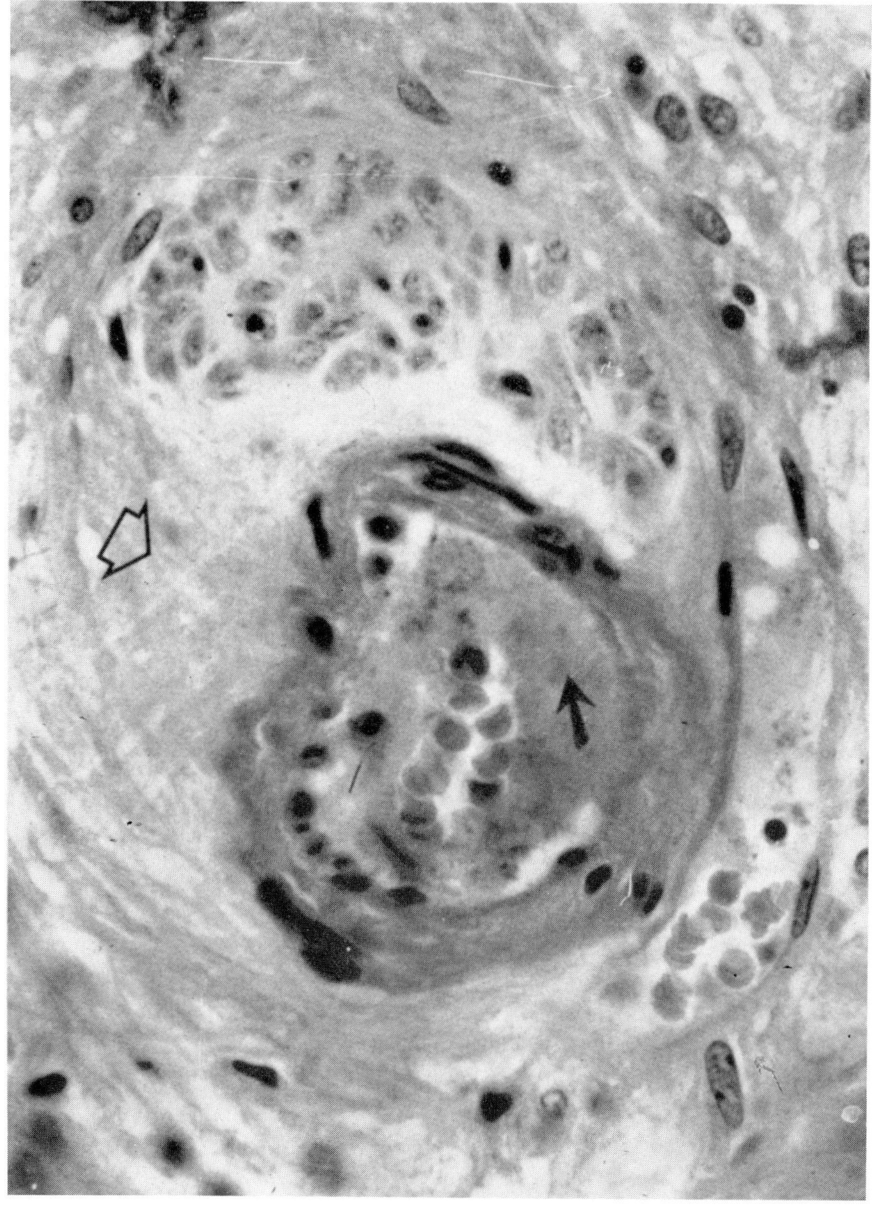

Fig. 8–28. Thrombus *(black arrow)* in arteriole of human pulp. Extravascular necrosis *(open arrow)* has already begun. There is also thrombus within capillary to right of arteriole. (Orban collection.)

in a matter of hours or may require years of time. Certain elements of the original pulp, such as the nerve fibrils, may linger beyond the rest, but in the end destruction is complete (Fig. 8–29).

PULPOSIS

Pulposis is a term used to designate a dystrophic pulp condition, a degenerative change of unknown cause. It implies a type of change distinct from the hyperreactive state, pulpitis, and necrosis. Within the designation "pulposis" are included at least four departures from normal: atrophic pulposis (atrophy of the pulp), calcific pulposis (calcific degeneration of the pulp), hyperplastic pulposis (hyperplasia of the pulp), and the idiopathic resorptions (internal and external).

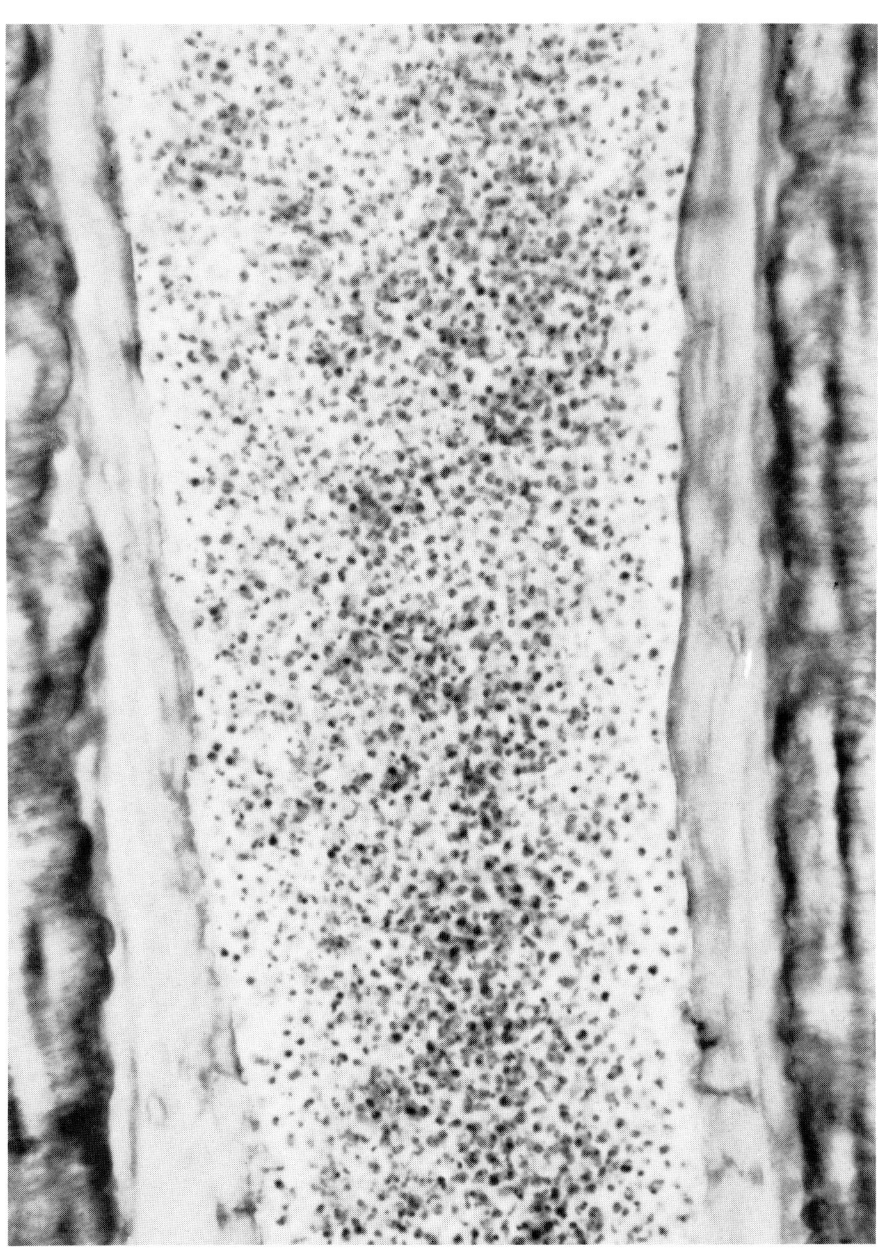

Fig. 8–29. Total necrosis of pulp tissue within root canal. All normal elements of pulp have been eliminated. Root canal is filled with dead leukocytes (pus). Human pulp. (Orban collection.)

Atrophic Pulposis

Atrophic change in the pulp is increasingly open to question. Recent studies of the artifacts produced by delayed fixation and by acid decalcification have demonstrated that these artifacts and "atrophic change" have much in common. Whenever an intact tooth is placed in fixative without prior removal of the root end, a significant delay occurs in the penetration of fixative through the narrow foramen and root canal to all the reaches of the pulp.[25] The delay permits postextraction autolysis to proceed before the fixative can complete its work.[26] "Reticular atrophy," with its typical "fish-net" mosaic, can, in fact, be

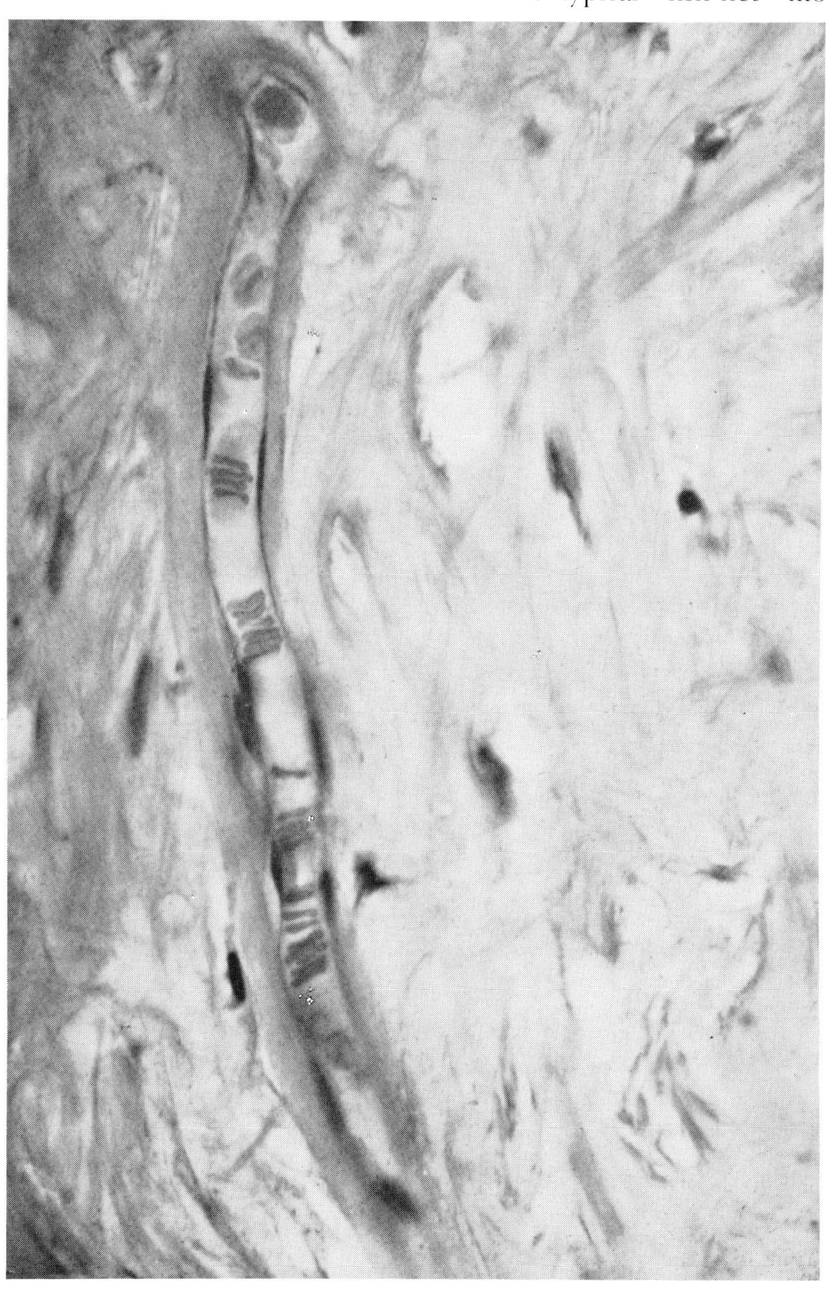

Fig. 8–30. Physiologic atrophy of pulp associated with aging. Three characteristic features are evident: reduction in total cell count; reduction in size of fibroblast cells that do remain; and dominance of fibrous elements. Human pulp. (Orban collection.)

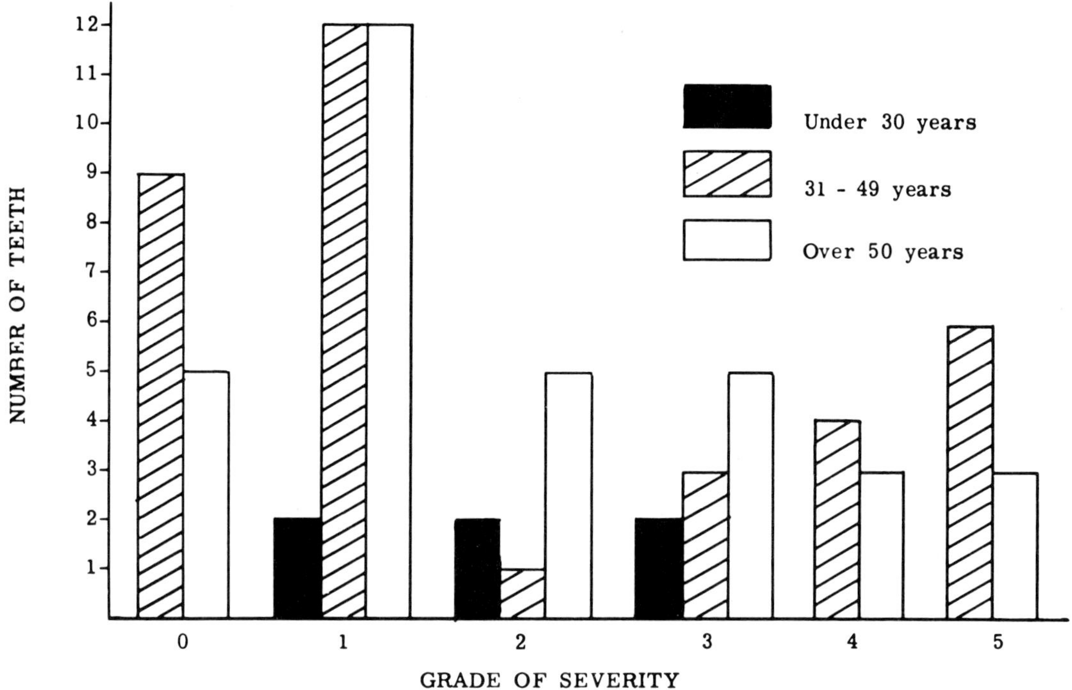

Table 8–1. Random distribution of stones and diffuse calcification of the pulp in 3 age groups. The direct correlation between age and pulp calcification is apparent. (From Rubach, W., and Mitchell, D. F.: Oral Surg., *19*:482, Apr., 1965.)

induced by merely delaying the fixation of extracted normal young teeth.[27]

To a lesser extent the use of strong acids and the failure to change acid solutions during decalcification also create artifact. Here the changes involve loss of cellular detail rather than the sweeping erasure seen in reticular atrophy.[26]

A sensible approach is needed in the matter of atrophic pulposis versus artifact. It would seem wise to question any histopathologic diagnosis of atrophy when the techniques employed in fixation and decalcification are not known. Atrophy in the tooth of a young person is also improbable.

On the other hand, atrophic change is a valid consideration when we are dealing with an adult tooth. Seltzer, Bender, and Ziontz emphasize that numerous changes occur in any pulp as a feature of advancing age.[7] They point out that dental caries and operative procedures appear to accelerate the change. Fibrosis of the pulp, for instance, is thought to be more prevalent in teeth that have received one or more restorations.[7] Certainly the frequent observance of a reduction in cell size and in the total number of cells within the aging pulp is undeniable. Most observers consider these changes to be a part of the ***physiologic atrophy*** of aging[7,28] (Fig. 8–30).

Calcific Pulposis

Pulp calcifications and atrophic changes in the pulp are closely associated. Both are commonplace. Certain forms of both are considered to be part of the normal aging process (Table 8–1). In pulposis we are concerned, of course, with calcific changes other than those that produce reparative dentin and the pulp stone. ***Calcific pulposis,*** therefore, encompasses the vascular wall calcifications seen in atherosclerosis[29] (Fig. 8–31), and the so-called linear calcifications (Fig. 8–32).

Contrasted to atrophy, calcific pulposis stands on a firmer base because it is an undeniable entity. It cannot be simulated by tardy or incomplete fixation

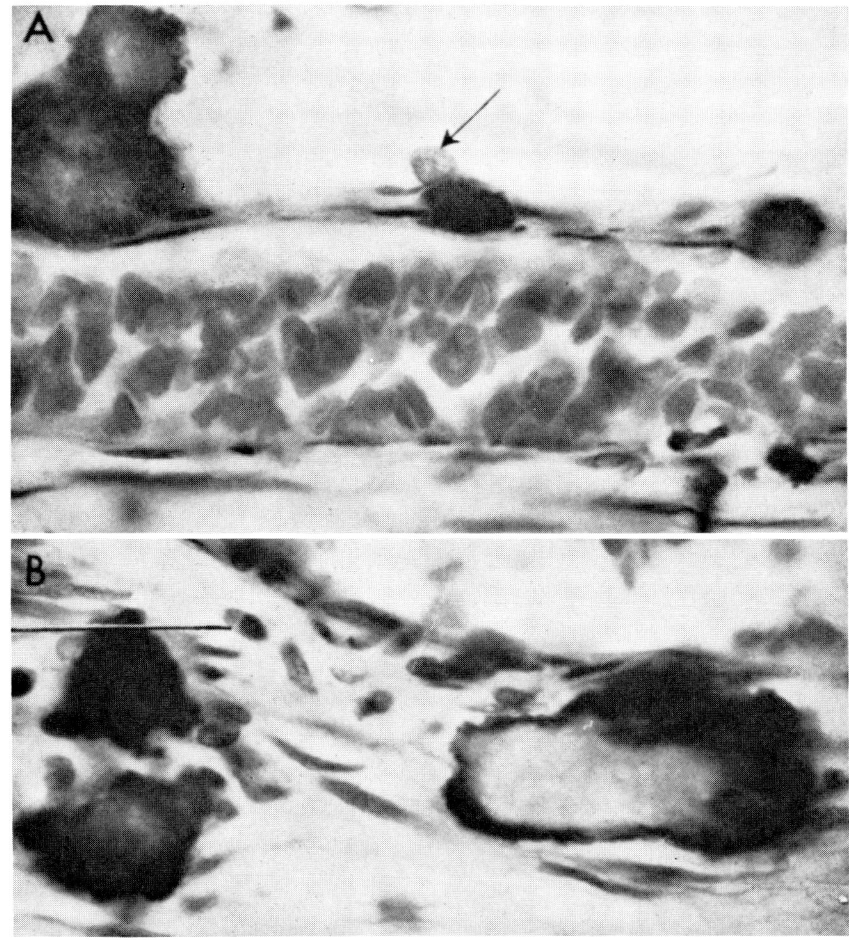

Fig. 8–31. *A,* Calcifications along walls of pulp vessel. Large mass can be seen in upper left, adhering to connective tissue of vessel wall itself. Arrow (center) indicates cell adjacent to smaller calcification. Human pulp. (From Langeland, K.: *Tissue Changes in the Dental Pulp.* Oslo University Press, 1957.) *B,* Calcific bodies adjacent to wall of pulp vessel. Large mass to right shows calcification on its perimeter, but has uncalcified central area. Human pulp. (From Langeland, K.: *Tissue Changes in the Dental Pulp.* Oslo University Press, 1957.)

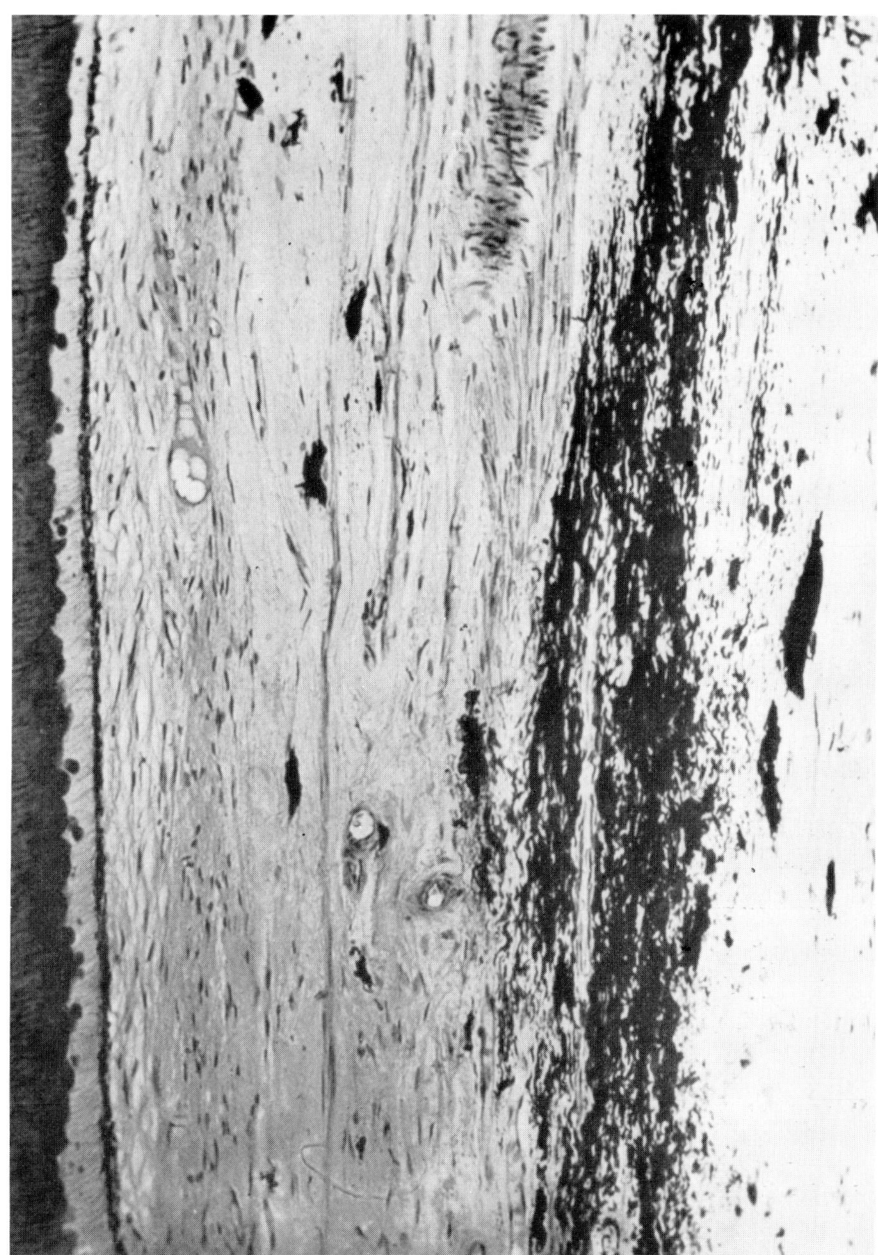

Fig. 8–32. "Linear calcification" within root canal of human tooth. Calcifications follow direction of nerves and connective tissue fibers. Many individual centers of calcification tend to fuse. No inflammatory reaction is evident. Pulps with linear calcification are difficult to anesthetize. (Orban collection.)

or by the action of too vigorous an acid for too long a time. Atrophy is a condition demonstrable only with the microscope. Areas of calcification, on the other hand (provided they exist in sufficient mass and density), are demonstrable clinically with both the radiograph and the root canal instrument.

Calcific pulposis is a widespread phenomenon. It is seen in the pulp at an early age. Schroff has commented on the higher frequency and more widespread distribution in root canals.[30] Seltzer, Bender, and Ziontz found dystrophic calcification to a varying degree in most pulps. "In some pulps where there had been no caries or operative interventions, the coronal portions were relatively free of calcifications. Even in those teeth, however, the apical portion of the pulp, especially in regions of collagen fibers, contained scattered calcifications. In teeth with periodontal disease, dystrophic calcifications increased tremendously in both coronal and radicular portions of the pulp. In teeth whose pulps were chronically inflamed, dystrophic calcifications were found in regions of previous liquefaction necrosis and, in varying amounts, in the remaining pulp tissue."[7]

Unquestionably, calcification tends to localize at sites of necrosis within a pulp. Since minute foci of necrosis are often widespread, the calcified deposits may be extensive. The calcific pulposis that develops on this basis is often termed "diffuse calcific degeneration" or "diffuse calcification."[31,32] Calcified bodies may even form around the nuclei of individual necrotic cells in the inflamed pulp (Fig. 8–33). By the same token, a larger zone of tissue, orginally cellular, may show amorphous deposit (Fig. 8–34).

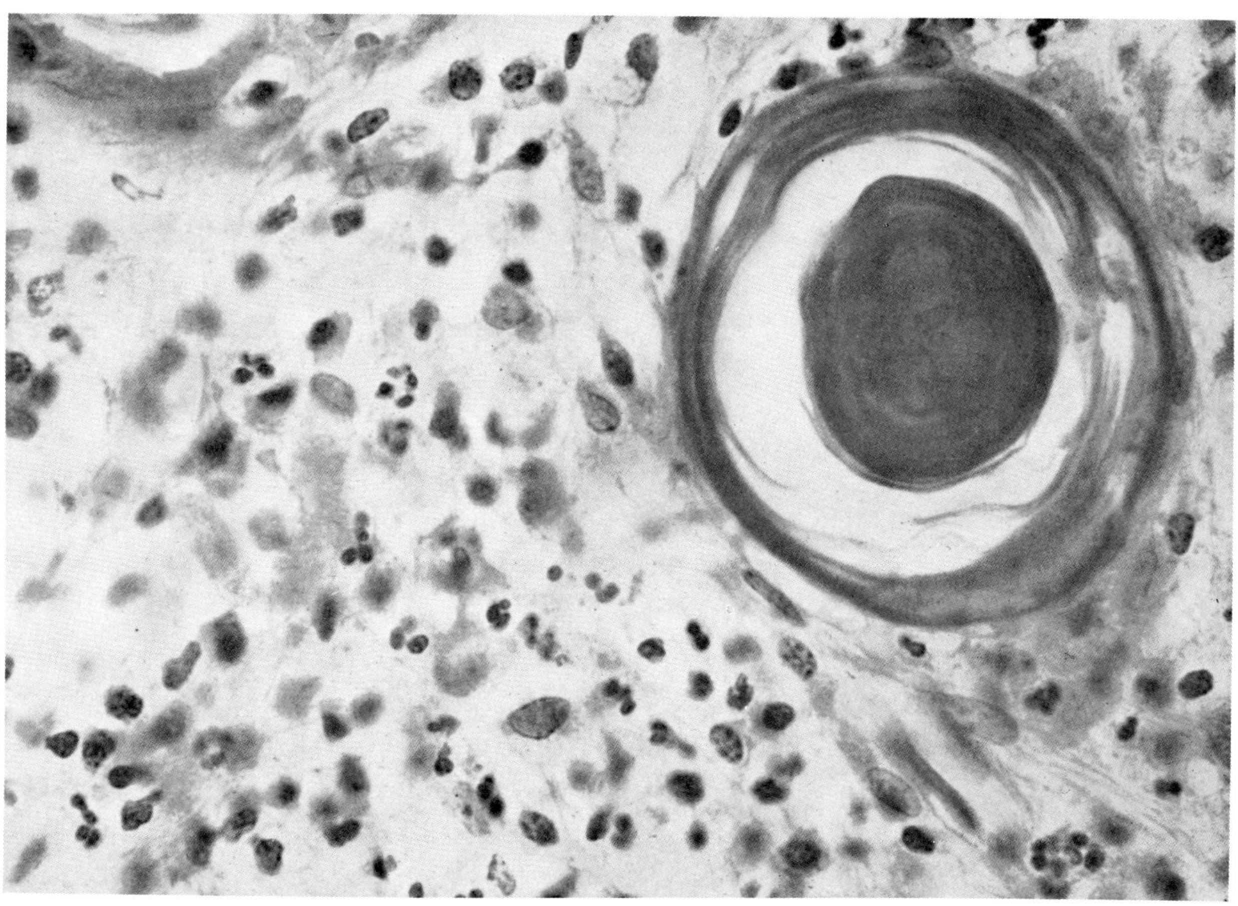

Fig. 8–33. Calcification of necrotic cells in inflamed pulp. Shadow of necrotic cells can still be seen at center of this calcified body (upper right). There are numerous plasma cells and several neutrophils in surrounding tissue. Human tooth. (Orban collection.)

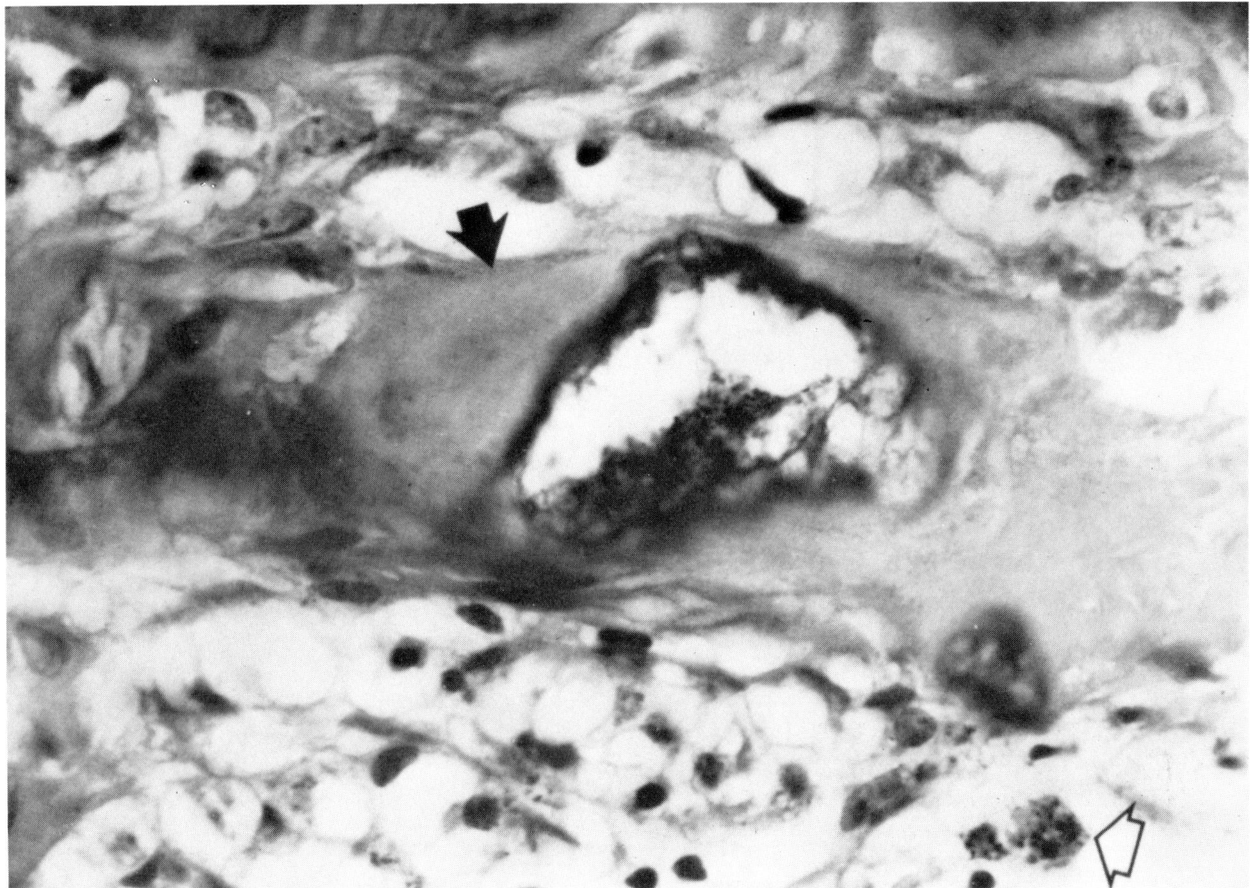

Fig. 8–34. Calcific pulposis *(black arrow)* involving larger mass of tissue. Bacteria are present in center of calcific area. Phagocytes *(open arrow)* containing bacteria are also visible beyond calcified tissue. Human pulp. Bacterial stain. (Orban collection.)

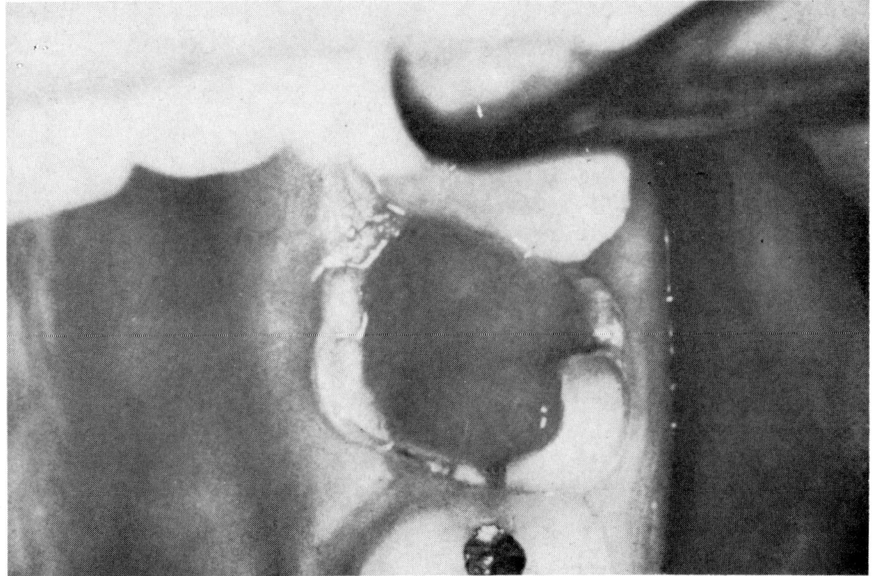

Fig. 8–35. Hyperplastic pulposis in molar tooth. Roof of pulp chamber has long since been eliminated by caries. Rising out of shell of crown is mushroom of living pulp tissue, firm and indifferent to touch. Pulp and nearby gingiva have fused.

Hyperplastic Pulposis
(Hyperplastic Pulpitis) (Pulp Polyp)

Hyperplastic pulposis, which begins as pulpitis, is the most visually dramatic of all the pulp responses. When it is present in a mouth, we are drawn to it at first glance. The occlusal surface of the afflicted tooth has disappeared, having long since been removed by caries. Rising out of the shell of the crown is a mushroom of living pulp tissue, firm and indifferent to the touch (Fig. 8–35).

The chronically inflamed young pulp, widely exposed by caries on its occlusal aspect, is the forerunner of this unique growth. What amounts to a successful delaying action is fought against the inevitable total necrosis. Proliferative growth of inflammatory connective tissue is the weapon employed. Such vigorous counteraction would be impossible for most adult pulps. But the capacity of the young pulp to resist necrosis is often great. For one thing, blood supply is ample because of the wide apical foramen. It is as though the destruction of the pulp is resisted by the creation of a buffer zone of new tissue, within which most of the inflammatory battle is concentrated.

Microscopically, the hyperplastic pulposis is a complex of new capillaries, proliferating fibroblasts, and all-pervasive inflammatory cells. As a rule, that part of the pulp from which it develops is usually composed of the same elements (Figs. 8–36 and 8–37). More distant areas of the pulp tend to be

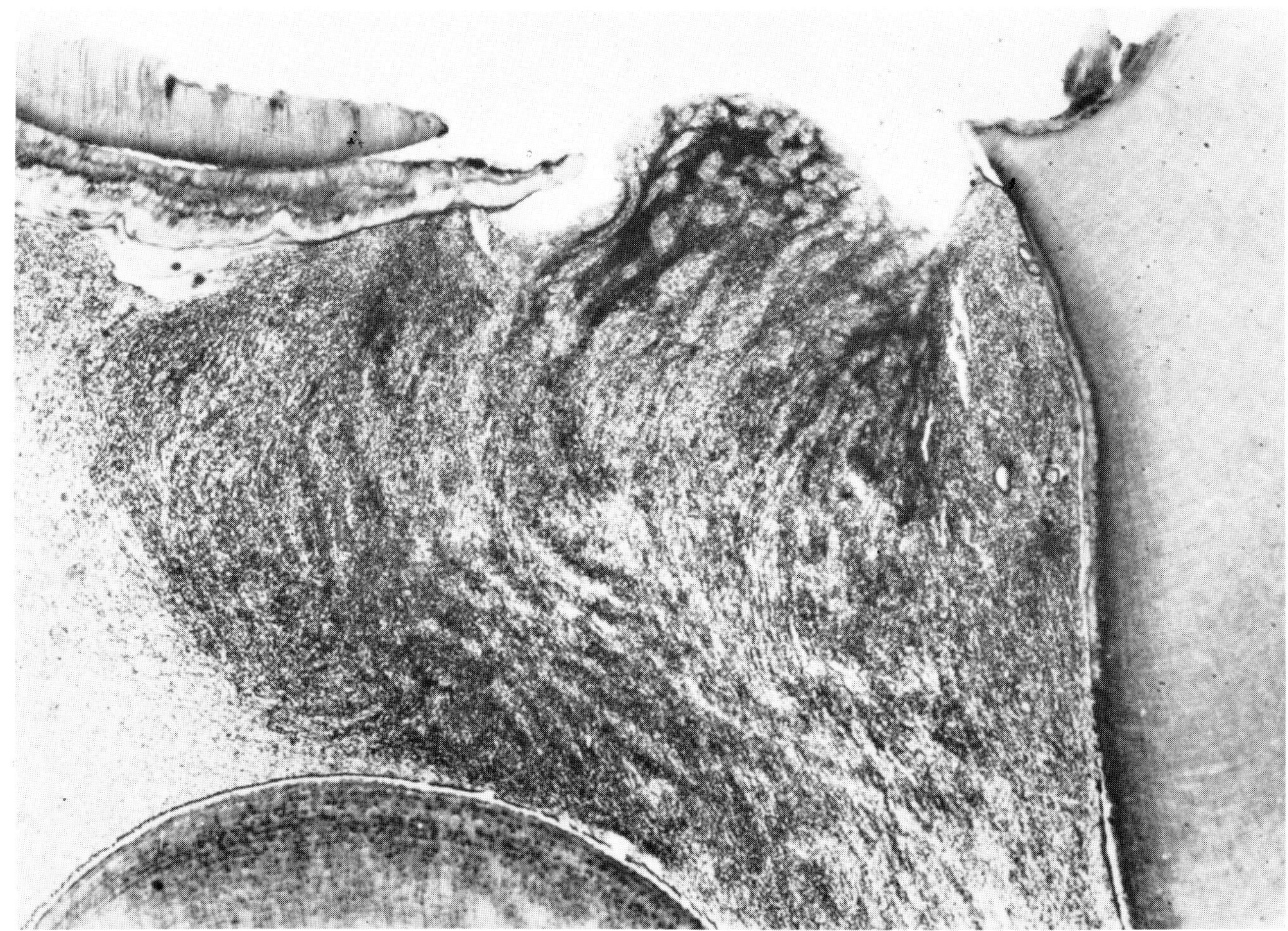

Fig. 8–36. Hyperplastic pulposis in its early stage of development. Surface of outgrowth consists of necrotic cells and leukocytes and is not epithelialized. Hyperplastic tissue below is complex of fibrils, proliferating fibroblasts, and new capillaries. It is pervaded by inflammatory cells. More distant areas of pulp are gradually being transformed into similar chronic inflammatory tissue. Human pulp. (From Matsumiya, S.: *Atlas of Oral Pathology.* Tokyo Dental College Press, 1955.)

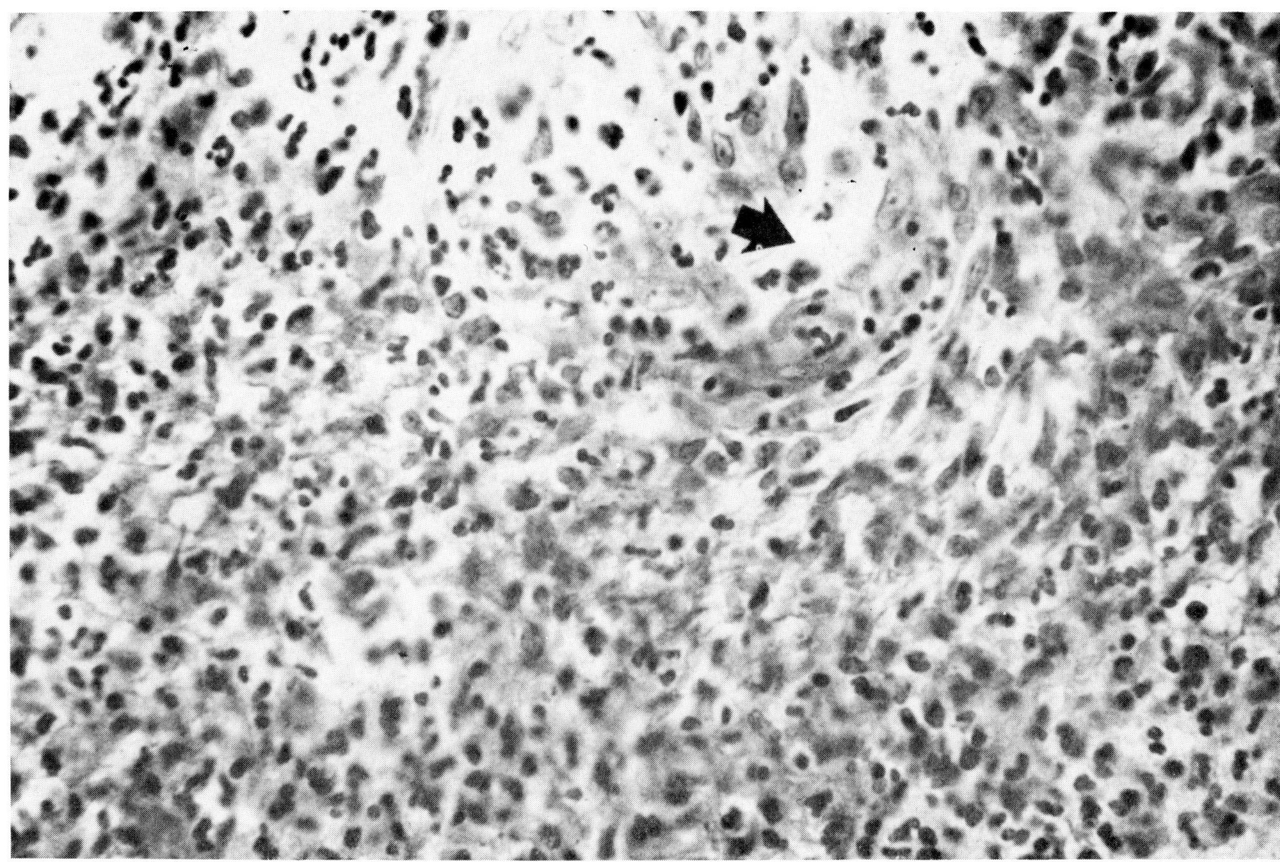

Fig. 8–37. Chronic inflammatory tissue of hyperplastic pulp (pulp polyp). Inflammatory cells are so numerous that they obscure most other elements. Capillaries *(arrow)* are abundant. Note leukocytes within lumen of this vessel and enlarged endothelial cell nuclei. Human pulp. (Orban collection.)

transformed eventually into the same type of inflammatory tissue. Support for the protruding mass is supplied by collagenous fibers that are rooted in the deeper pulp tissue of the chamber (Fig. 8–38). Sensory nerve elements are almost totally absent, a contrast to the rich innervation and exquisite sensitivity of an exposed pulp which is ***not*** hyperplastic.

Before the lesion has grown to any extent, its surface layer consists of massed necrotic cells and leukocytes (Fig. 8–36). Beneath lies inflammatory tissue in a wide zone of variable width. As the mass expands, it either retains the surface layer of necrotic connective tissue or it acquires an epithelial "cap" (Fig. 8–39). Epithelium on the surface assumes stratified squamous form without delay. Linear ridges of epithelium interdigitate with the connective tissue below. Despite all this, the epithelial cover of the polyp seldom provides protection comparable, say, to that seen in the attached gingiva. The epithelium is invariably riddled with round cells from the continuous inflammatory process in the underlying connective tissue. Ulceration is commonplace. For these reasons alone the ready hemorrhage of even the epithelialized polyp should come as no surprise (Fig. 8–40).

To encounter a hyperplastic pulp that is isolated within tooth structure and yet epithelialized is to ask the question, "Just where does the surface epithelium originate?" Most probably a true epithelial cell graft occurs. Cells of the oral mucosa floating free in the saliva effect a "take" upon the highly vascularized young connective tissue of the exposed pulp. This done, they grow freely in all directions to clothe the surface.

On other occasions a pulp polyp will be observed which has made contact with the gingiva and is no longer an island (Fig. 8–35). Continued expansion of the once isolated mass, or a breaking down of the

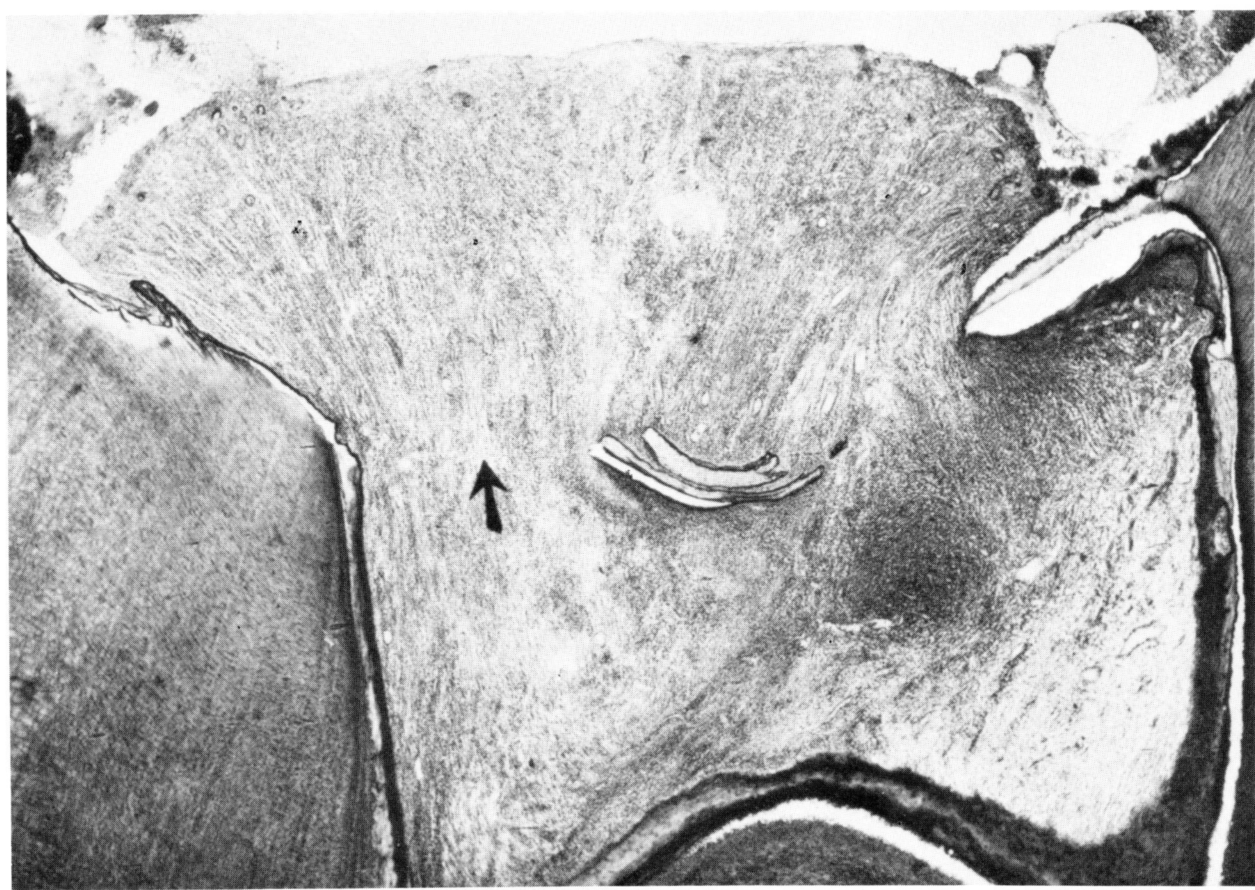

Fig. 8–38. Collagenous fiber matrix which is present within pulp polyp (hyperplastic pulposis). Collagenous fibers *(arrow)* radiate, fan-like, from depth of pulp to surface of enlarged mass. These fibers support and strengthen polyp, permitting it to withstand considerable surface pressure. Fragments of dentin are visible within. Some original pulp of crown remains *(lower right)*. (Orban collection.)

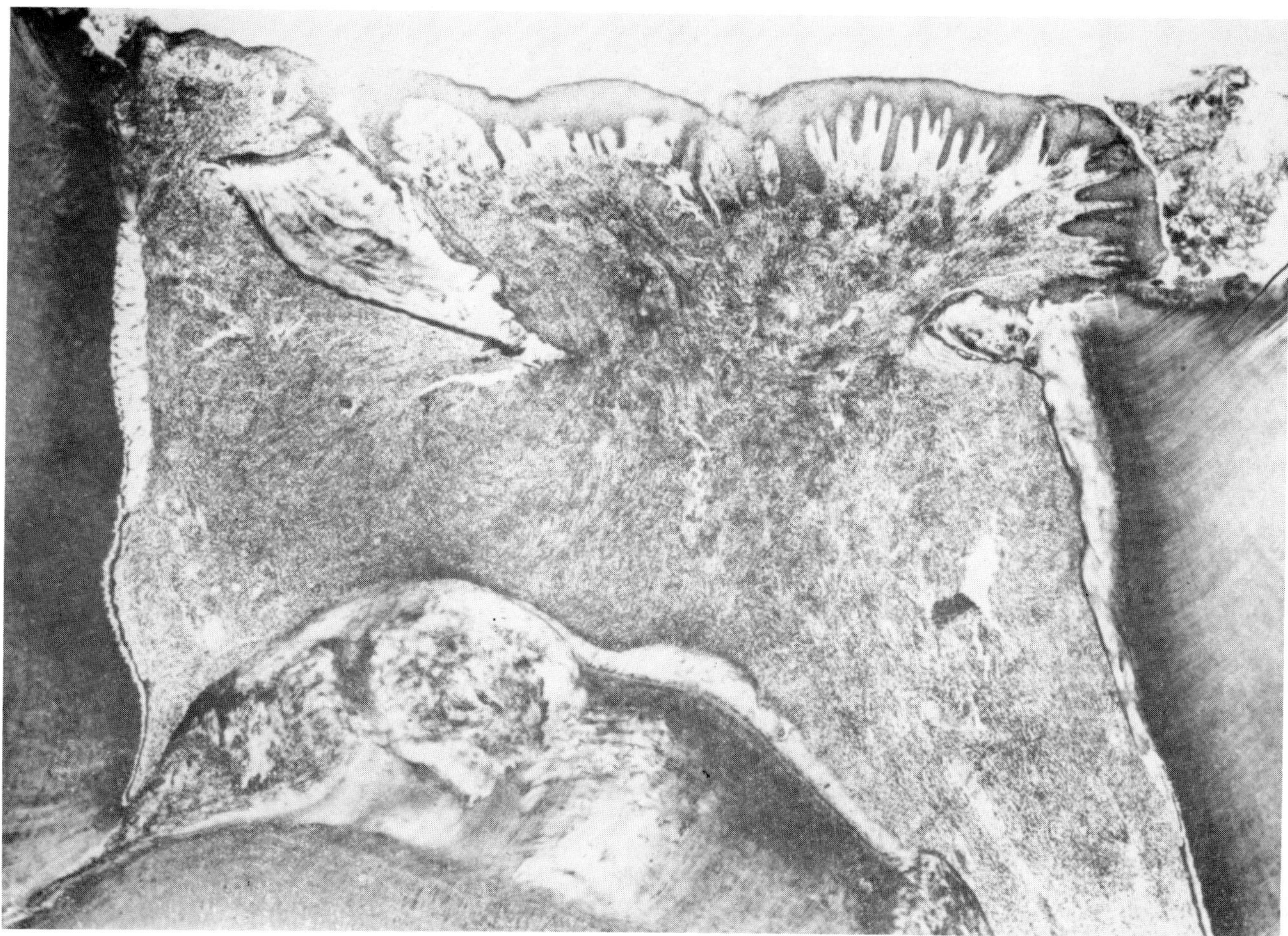

Fig. 8–39. Completely epithelialized pulp polyp. Stratified squamous epithelium covers entire surface. (Fig. 8–38, by contrast, shows polyp with surface layer of necrotic connective tissue.) Mass beneath epithelium in upper left is large fragment of dentin. Human pulp. (From Matsumiya, S.: *Atlas of Oral Pathology.* Tokyo Dental College Press, 1955.)

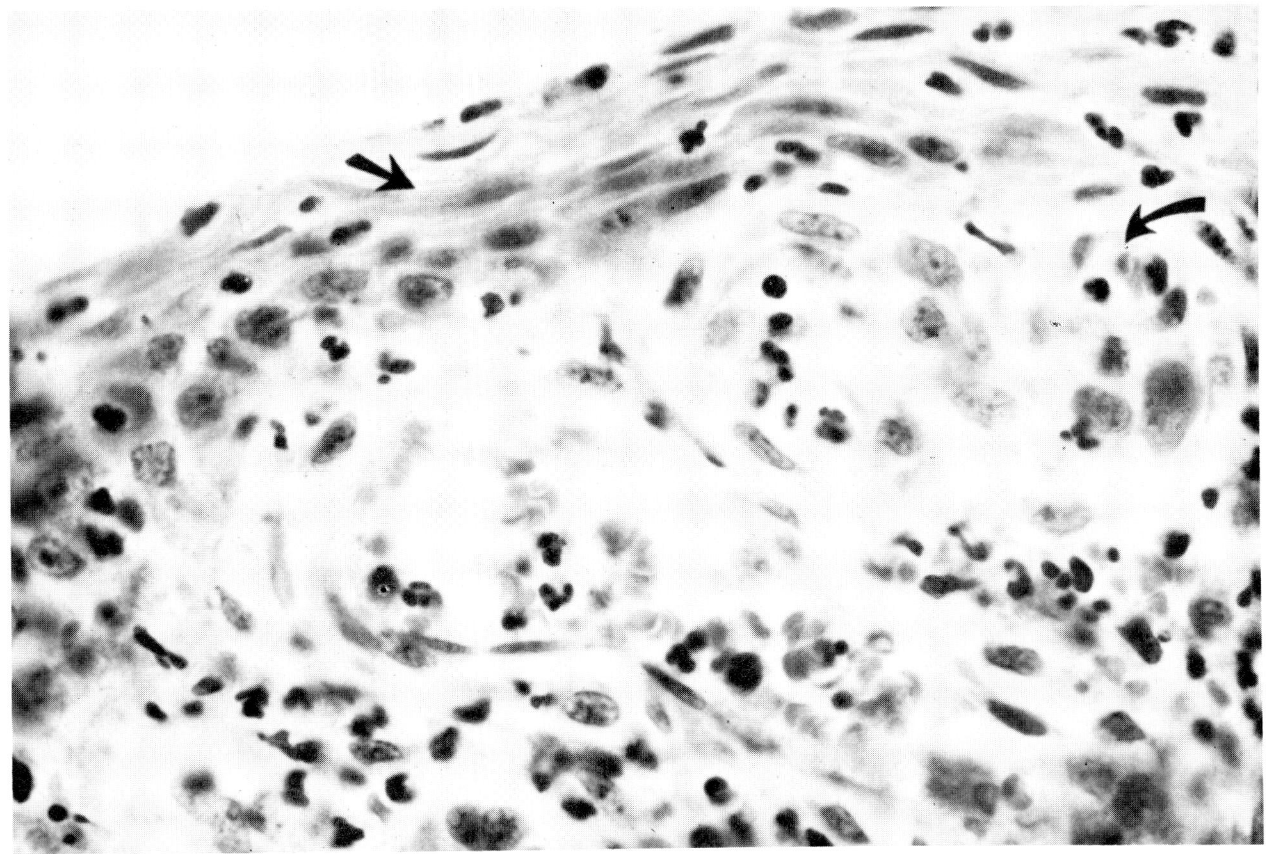

Fig. 8–40. Stratified squamous epithelium *(straight arrow)* of hyperplastic pulp. Epithelium is often thin, and capillaries *(curved arrow)* are always close to it. Leukocytes *(left of straight arrow)* from connective tissue can be seen passing through epithelium to surface. Human pulp. (Orban collection.)

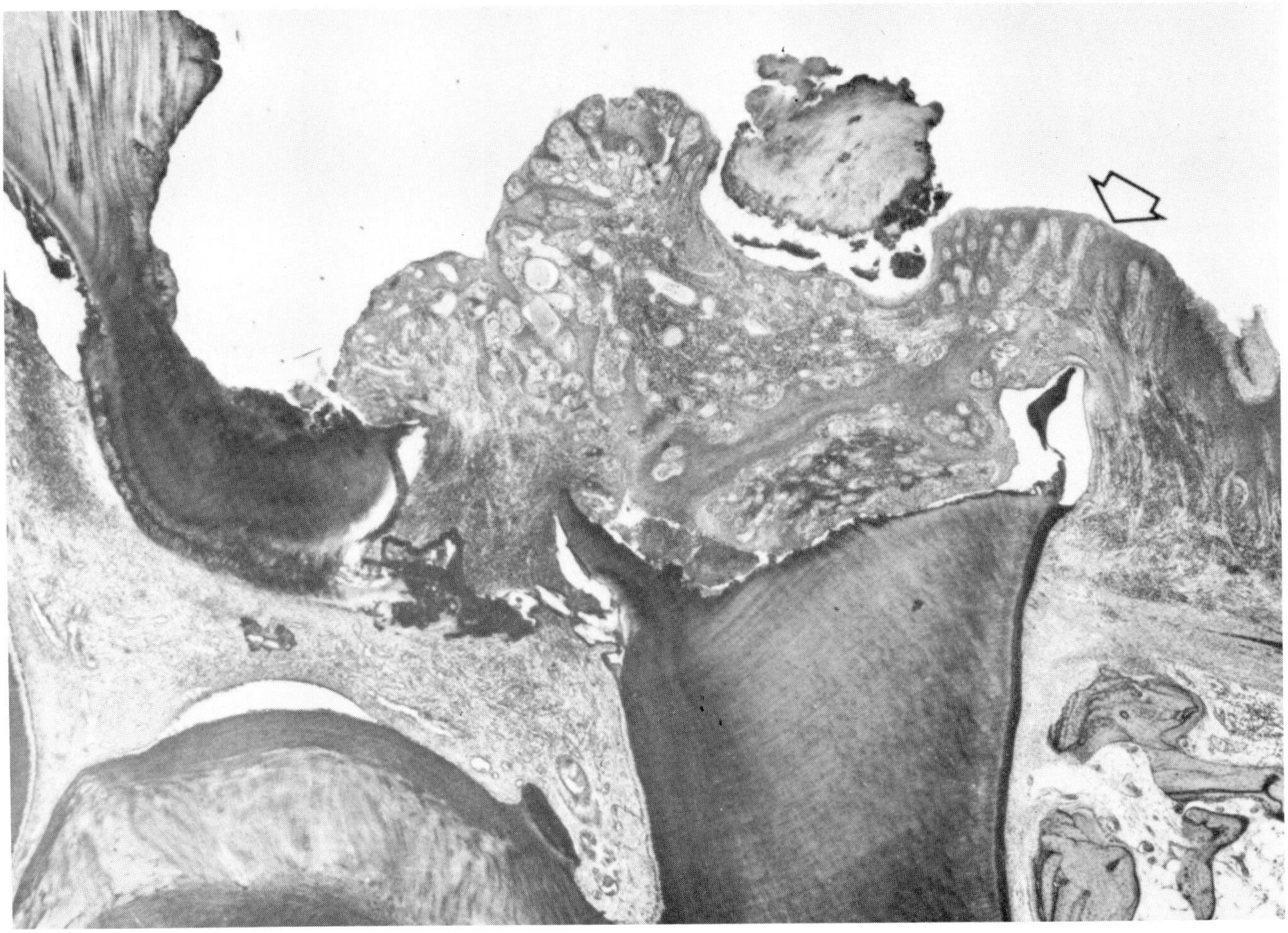

Fig. 8–41. Continuity of pulp polyp and gingiva *(arrow)*. Crown of tooth was destroyed by caries. Pulp tissue grew out of pulp chamber and merged with gingiva. In this case it is probable that direct migration of epithelial cells occurred from gingiva across entire surface of proliferating pulp. Human tooth. (From Matsumiya, S.: *Atlas of Oral Pathology*. Tokyo Dental College Press, 1955.)

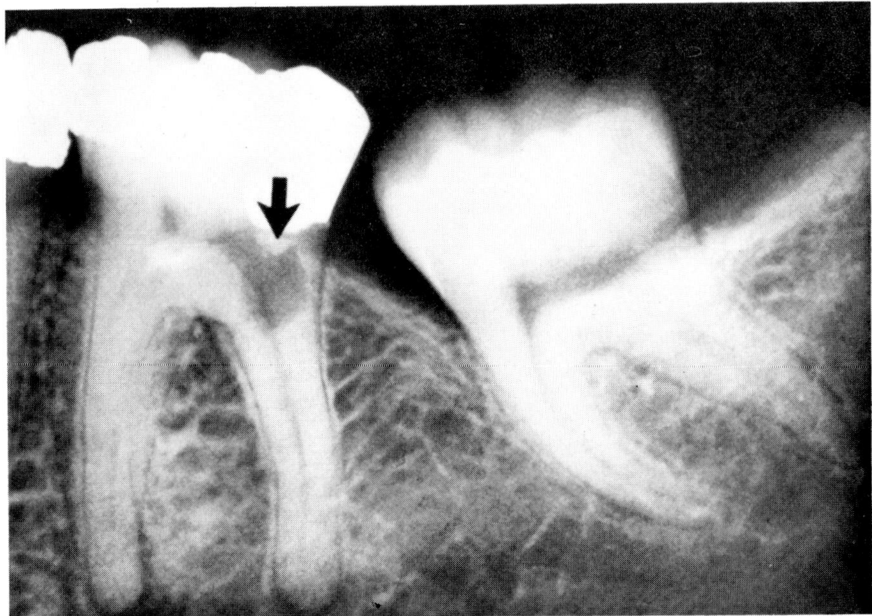

Fig. 8–42. Advanced internal resorption of mandibular first molar. Process of resorption has spread distally from pulp to undermine restoration and has perforated to external surface of tooth. Note evidence of calcific repair *(arrow)* within area of resorption, and extension of pulp inflammation to periapex.

carious walls of the pulp chamber, has brought about this contact and the eventual fusion of pulp and gingiva. Knowing the nature of epithelium, we can be sure that often in these circumstances a direct migration of epithelial cells occurs, from the gingiva across the entire surface of the pulp connective tissue[33,34] (Fig. 8–41).

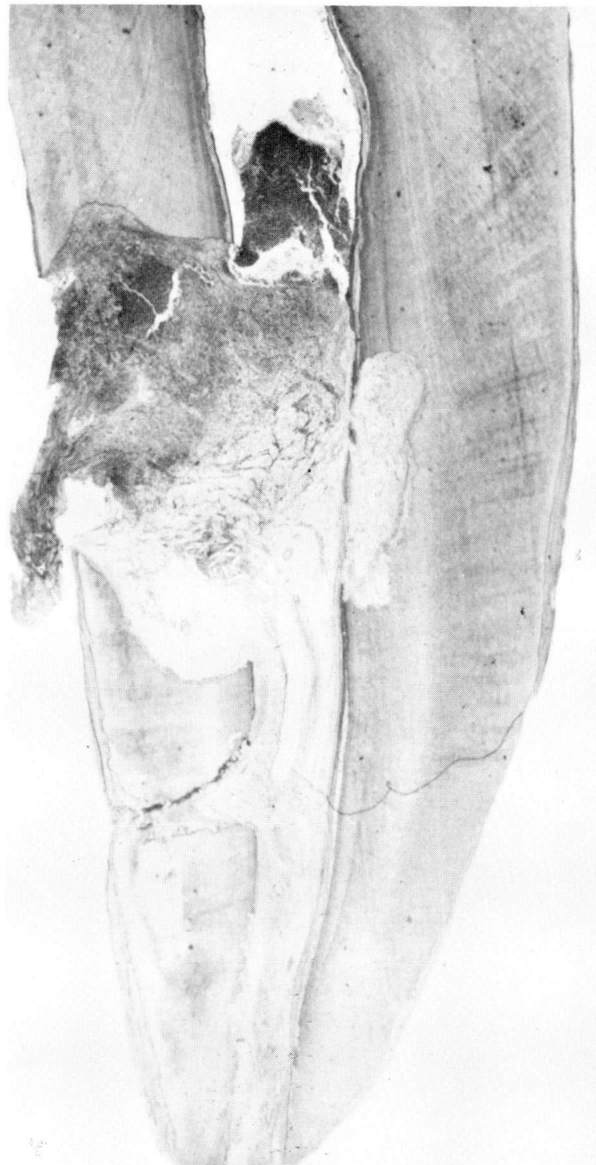

Fig. 8–43. Idiopathic resorption of root dentin. Without clinical history it is impossible to say from this section that resorptive process represents internal resorption rather than external resorption. Dense basophilic staining of connective tissue within resorbed area points to presence of marked inflammatory infiltrate. Note also accessory canal. (Orban collection.)

Idiopathic Resorptions

Internal Resorption. Internal resorption is the term applied to a peculiar dystrophy of the pulp which results in destruction of the dental hard tissues. The process begins in the pulp and spreads laterally through the dentin. Hitherto a definite example of the process was identifiable only on rare occasions. The resorptive lesion, when detected, had often perforated to the external surface of the tooth (Fig. 8–42). Once this situation prevailed it was impossible to say with accuracy that the resorption was not an example of ***external*** resportion (Fig. 8–43).

Recent years have seen an increased emphasis on pulp disease and the serial sectioning of many teeth in the early stages of pulp disease. As a result, true ***internal*** resorption is being detected more often. It is now appreciated that resorption of dentin on the

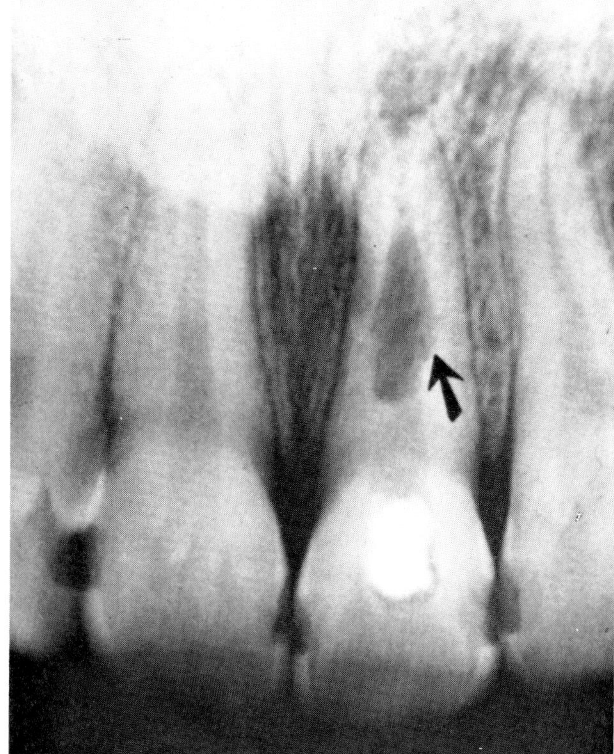

Fig. 8–44. Internal resorption of upper central incisor, clearly associated with pulpitis. Partial pulpectomy had been carried out some time before as treatment for pulpitis in tooth. Marked internal resorption of root dentin *(arrow)* was later noted in this post-treatment film. Involved tooth also demonstrates periapical pathosis and resorption of dentin at apex, a fairly common occurrence.

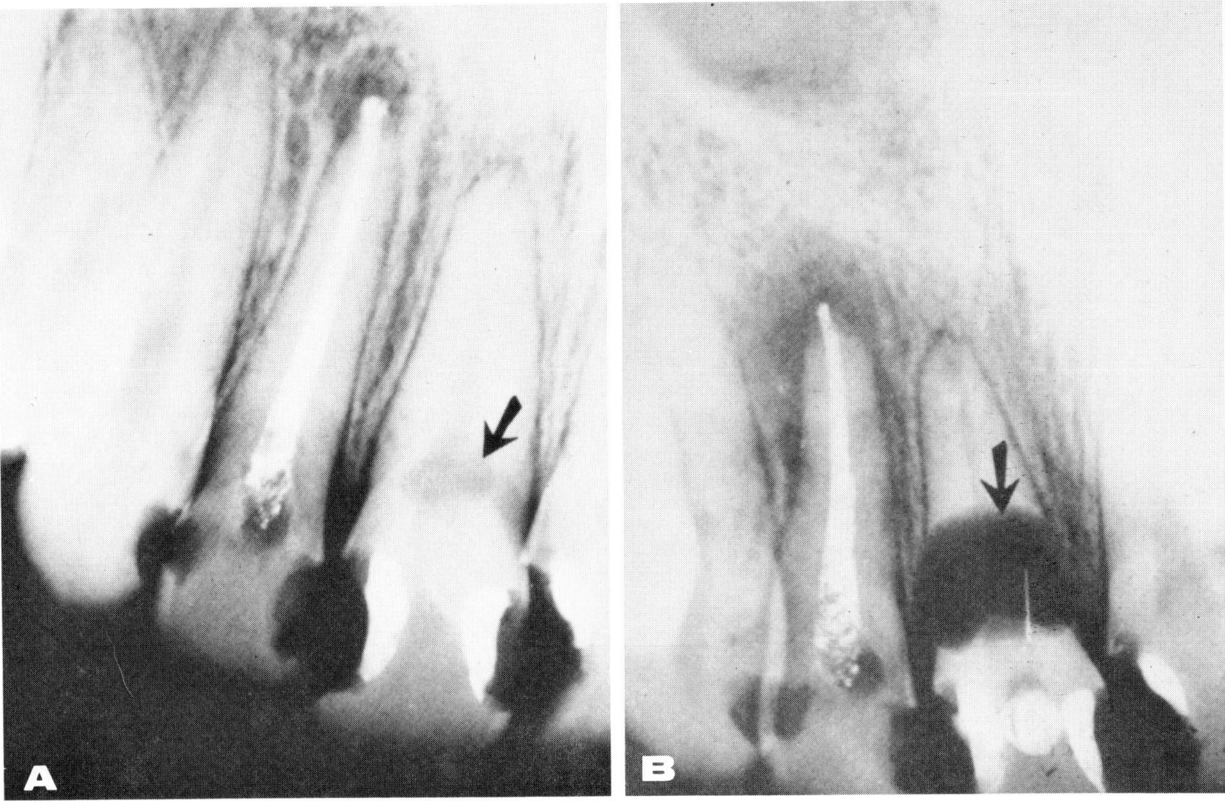

Fig. 8–45. *A,* Early internal resorption *(arrow)* of upper central incisor. In all likelihood, pulpitis preceded resorption. *B,* Destruction in six months of upper central incisor by internal resorption. Limited area of resorption noted in A, changed to this massive lesion *(arrow),* which virtually severed crown of tooth from root.

pulp wall is often related to existent pulpitis[30,35,36] (Fig. 8–44). Whether all internal resorption begins as an unpredictable accompaniment of pulp inflammation is not known. A history of trauma to the involved tooth can sometimes be brought forth, but the precise cause of the pulp derangement that leads to internal resorption has never been clarified.[35,37] The resorptions often move swiftly.[36] Some obviously progress to the point of destroying the usefulness of the tooth (Fig. 8–45). Others wane after a time and are then repaired.[36]

In all probability internal resorption, like other hard tissue resorptions, is the work of macrophages and multinucleated giant cells.[36,38,39] The latter are found in close apposition to the dentin surface, often within "bays" of their own creation. They are indistinguishable from the osteoclast cells which resorb bone. The dentin that is lost is replaced by a chronic inflammatory tissue (Fig. 8–46).

Since the process of internal resorption is intermittent, repair often follows resorption in a given area. During the lull in resorption, cells akin to either odontoblasts or osteoblasts differentiate from the mesenchymal cells of the pulp. Tissue resembling both dentin and bone is deposited (Fig. 8–47). When the process of resorption leads to massive destruction of dentin, the incomplete hard tissue repair consists of bone or a bone-like tissue arranged in random trabeculae (Fig. 8–48). On the other hand, if the internal resorption comes to an end after a comparatively small amount of dentin has been removed, the repair is usually accomplished with dentin, at first atypical and irregular. This first deposit is shortly overlaid by dentin, characteristically tubular (Fig. 8–49). In the repair of cementum resorption, and in the establishment of reparative dentin after the localized death of odontoblasts, a similar two-stage deposit of hard tissue is often noted. The first layer is amorphous. Typical cementum or dentin comes later, after the environment has become more "stable."[40]

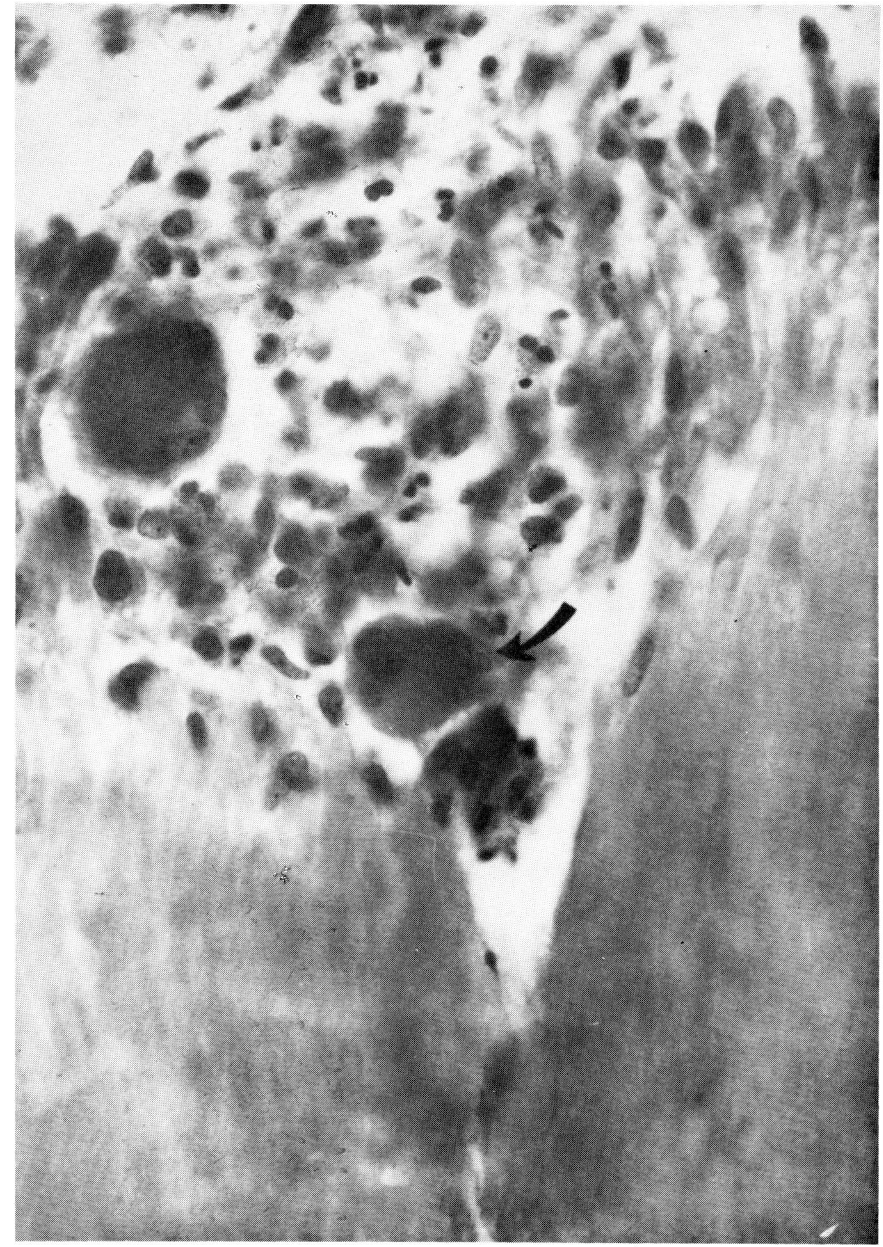

Fig. 8–46. Internal resorption on pulp wall of human tooth. Bay-like defect has been created. Dentin lost through resorption is being replaced by chronic inflammatory tissue. Multinucleated giant cells *(arrow)* are prominent at dentin surface. (Orban collection.)

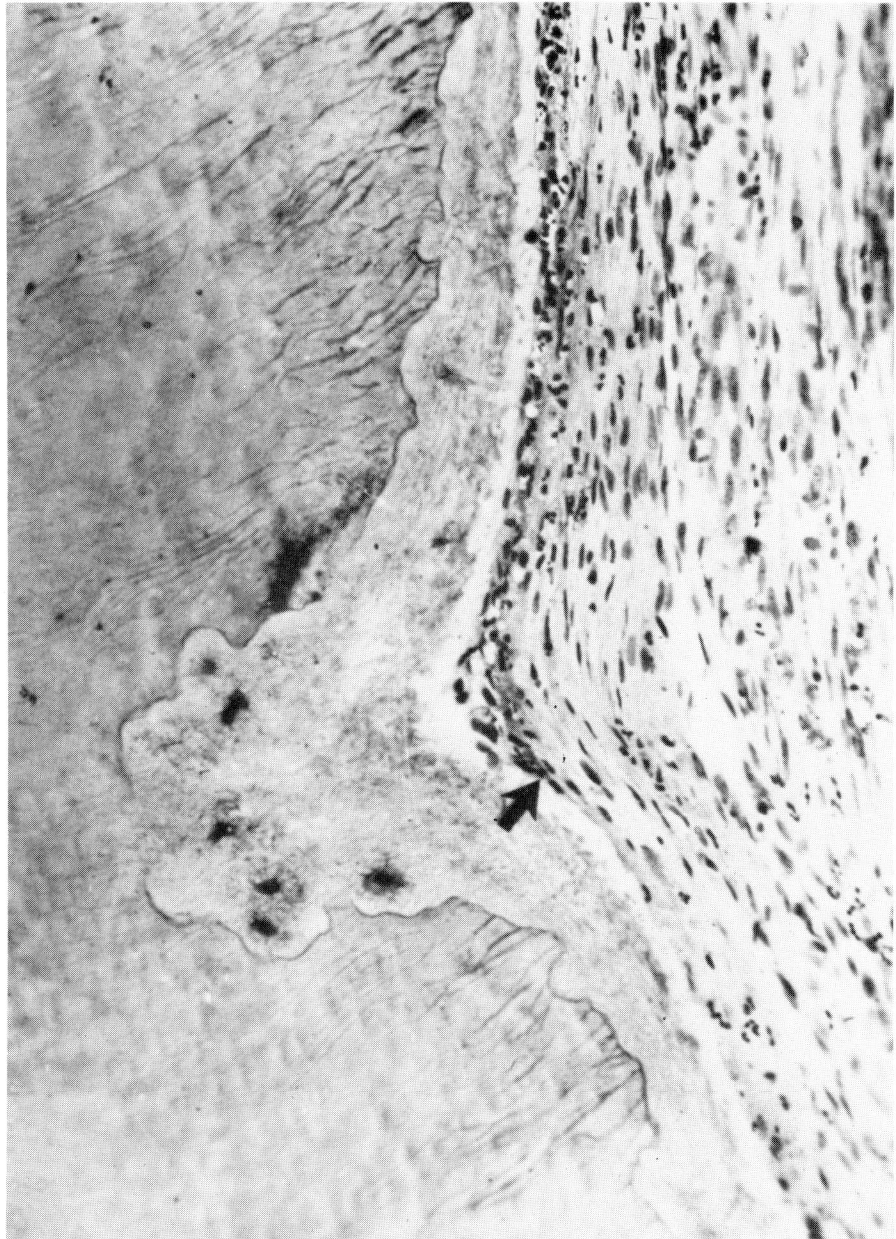

Fig. 8–47. One form of repair associated with minor internal resorption. Tissue similar in some respects to both reparative dentin and bone has filled in resorption area. It contains cells resembling osteocytes within lacunae. Formative cells are present against predentin-like zone *(arrow).* Pulp appears comparatively normal. (Orban collection.)

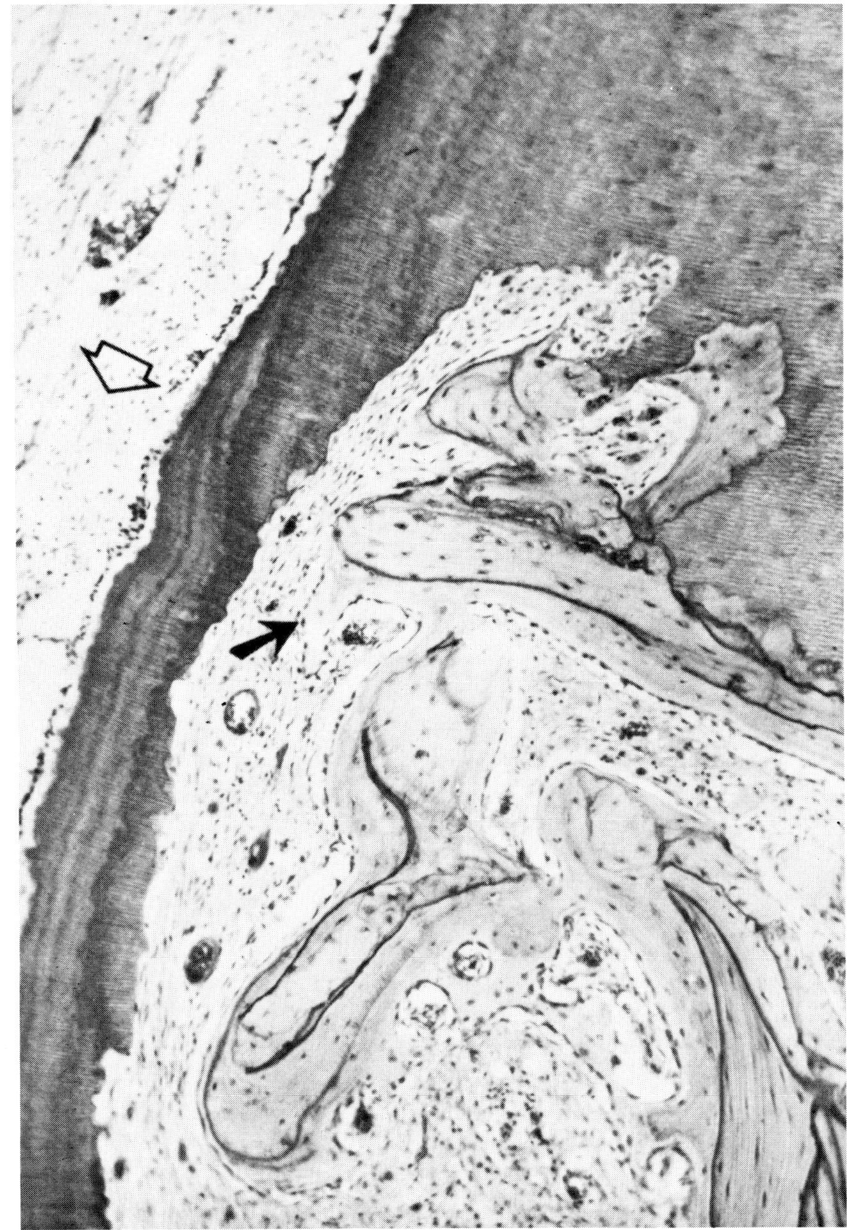

Fig. 8–48. Partial repair of massive internal resorption by osseous tissue. Continuation of repair is evidenced by osteoblasts *(black arrow)* on surface of bone-like trabeculae. Resorption area was found in other sections to be continuous with pulp *(open arrow)*. (From Hine, M. K., and Ritchey, B. D.: J.A.D.A., *34*:468, Apr., 1947.)

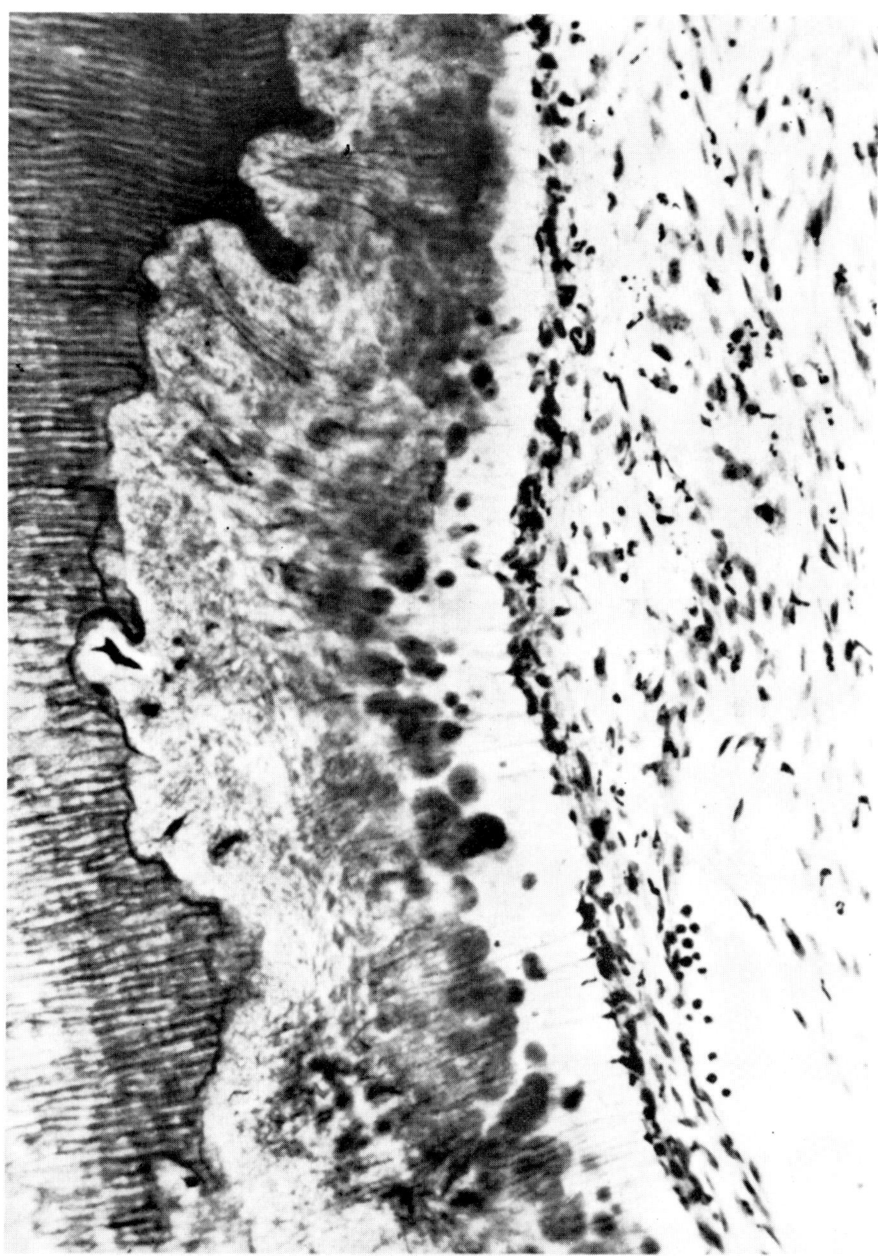

Fig. 8–49. Repair of internal resorption by dentin. Line of furthest advance of resorption is clearly seen to left. Repair may be complete, but deposit of reparative dentin continues. (From Hine, M. K., and Ritchey, B. D.: J.A.D.A., *34*:468, Apr., 1947.)

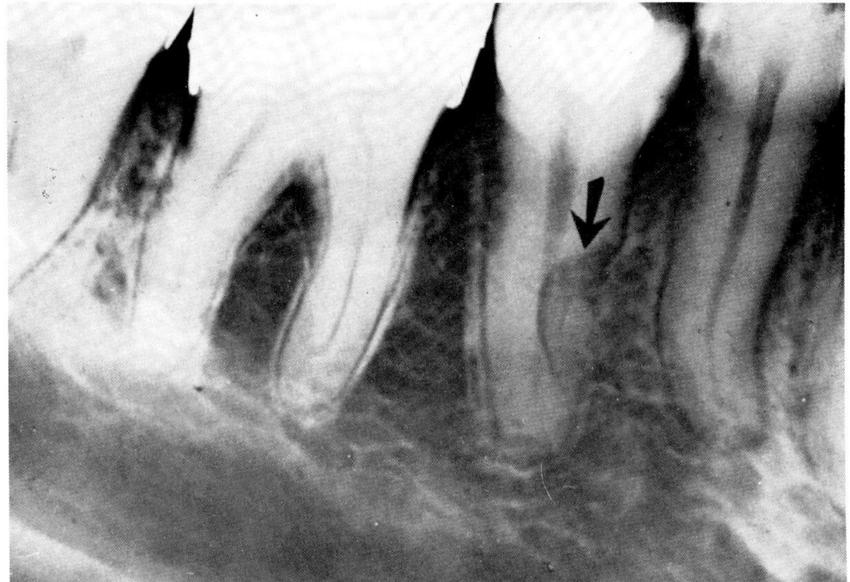

Fig. 8–50. External resorption *(arrow)* on massive scale. Actual penetration to pulp has occurred. In this case lesion was known to have begun in cementum on mesial root surface.

External Resorption. There is a form of root resorption that begins in the periodontal connective tissue rather than in the pulp. The innumerable resorptions encountered in root cementum testify to the frequency of the process in its usual limited form. In other words, minute external resorptions of cementum are commonplace. Occasionally the lesion is progressive to the point where there is massive destruction of dentin and an actual penetration to the pulp[41] (Fig. 8–50). Once the pulp is entered, a pulp pathosis is established which is often indistinguishable from that of internal resorption. Metamorphosis of the pulp and the further destruction of original dentin proceed as we have already observed.

REFERENCES

1. Stanley, H. R.: The Cells of the Dental Pulp. Part of a Symposium, *Biology of the Pulp.* American Association of Endodontists, Chicago, Illinois, Feb. 2, 1961.
2. Langeland, K.: Graduate Lecture. University of Washington, Nov. 15, 1962.
3. Scheinin, A.: Flow characteristics of the pulpal vessels. J. Dent. Res., *42*:438, Jan.-Feb., 1963.
4. Beveridge, E. E., and Brown, A. C.: The measurement of human intrapulpal pressure and its response to clinical variables. Oral Surg., *19*:655, May, 1965.
5. Pohto, M., and Scheinin, A.: Microcinematography of the Living Dental Pulp. University of Helsinki, Finland, 1957, 16 mm., sound, color, 38 min. Bureau of Audio-Visual Service, American Dental Association, DT 178.
6. Coolidge, E. D., and Kesel, R. G.: *A Textbook of Endodontology.* 2nd Ed., Philadelphia, Lea & Febiger, 1956, Chapt. 8, pp. 141–154.
7. Seltzer, S., Bender, I. B., and Ziontz, M.: The dynamics of pulp inflammation: correlations between diagnostic data and actual histologic findings in the pulp. Oral Surg., *16*:846, July, 1963.
8. Grossman, L. I.: *Endodontic Practice.* 8th Ed., Philadelphia, Lea & Febiger, 1974, Chap. 2, pp. 48–64.
9. Seltzer, S., Bender, I. B., and Nazimov, H.: Differential diagnosis of pulp conditions. Oral Surg., *19*:383, Mar., 1965.
10. Swerdlow, H., and Stanley, H. R.: Reaction of human pulp to cavity preparations: results produced by eight different operative grinding technics. J.A.D.A., *58*:49, May, 1959.
11. Langeland, K.: *Tissue Changes in the Dental Pulp.* Norwegian Institute of Dental Research, Oslo, Oslo University Press, 1957, p. 134.
12. Ostrom, C. A.: Pulp damage by induced inflammation. Dent. Prog., *3*:207, July, 1963.
13. Ibid, p. 56.
14. Swerdlow, H., and Stanley, H. R.: Reaction of the human dental pulp to cavity preparation. II. At 150,000 r.p.m. with an air-water spray. J. Prosth. Dent., *9*:112, Jan.-Feb., 1959.
15. Matsumiya, S., Kondo, S., Takuma, S., Suzuki, A., and Osawa, Y.: *Atlas of Oral Pathology.* Tokyo, The Tokyo Dental College Press, 1955, p. 165.
16. Orban, B.: Unpublished data.
17. Langeland, K.: Op. cit., p. 135.
18. Sicher, H.: *Orban's Oral Histology and Embryology.* 5th Ed., St. Louis, The C. V. Mosby Co., 1962, p. 152.
19. Stanley, H. R.: The cells of the dental pulp. Oral Surg., *15*:849, July, 1962.

20. Swerdlow, H., and Stanley, H. R.: Reaction of the human dental pulp to cavity preparation. I. Effect of water spray at 20,000 r.p.m. J.A.D.A., *56*:317, Mar., 1958.
21. Langeland, K.: Op. cit., p., 69.
22. Ibid., p. 73.
23. Orban, B.: Migration of leukocytes into the dentinal tubules. J.A.D.A., *27*:239, Feb., 1940.
24. Matsumiya, S., *et al.:* Op. cit., p. 439.
25. Langeland, K.: Op. cit., p. 14.
26. Stanley, H. R.: Op. cit., p. 850.
27. Ibid, p. 851.
28. Sicher, H.: Op. cit., p. 160.
29. Langeland, K.: Op. cit., p. 49.
30. Schroff, F. R.: Pathology of the dental pulp. Austral. Dent. J., *59*:95, Apr., 1955.
31. Gardner, A. F.: *Pathoogy of the Dental Pulp with Clinical Correlations.* Practical Dental Monographs. Chicago, Year Book Publishers, Inc., May, 1963, p. 30.
32. Boyle, P. E.: *Kronfeld's Histopathology of the Teeth and Their Surrounding Structures.* 4th Ed., Philadelphia, Lea & Febiger, 1955, p. 105.
33. Hartwell, S. W.: Surgical wounds in human beings. I. Epithelial healing. Arch. Surg., *19*:835, Nov., 1929.
34. Matsumiya, S., *et al.:* Op. cit., p. 197.
35. Simpson, H. E.: Internal resorption. J. Canad. Assoc., *30*: 355, June, 1964.
36. Warner, G. R., Orban, B., Hine, M. K., and Ritchey, B. T.: Internal resorption of teeth: interpretation of histologic findings. J.A.D.A., *34*:468, Apr., 1947.
37. Boyle, P. E.: Op. cit., p. 290.
38. Goldhaber, P.: Behaviour of bone in tissue culture. From Calcification in Biological Systems, Washington, D.C., American Association for the Advancement of Science, 1960, p. 370.
39. Sullivan, H. R., and Jolly, M.: Idiopathic resorption. Austral. Dent. J., *61*:193, Aug., 1957.
40. Henry, J. L., and Weinmann, J. P.: The pattern of resorption and repair of human cementum. J.A.D.A., *42*:270, Mar., 1951.
41. Thoma, K., and Goldman, H. M.: *Oral Pathology.* 5th Ed., St. Louis, The C. V. Mosby Co., 1960, p. 248.

Chapter 9

Periapical Pathosis

ALFRED L. OGILVIE

The study of periapical disease is in some respects a more satisfying experience than the venture into pulp disease. The size and locale of the pulp tend to frustrate the dentist in his effort to base treatment on accurate diagnosis. Beyond the tooth, however, the scene changes. For one thing the periodontium is a larger canvas than the pulp. We are concerned there with a more varied complex of tissues. Lesions assume a greater size. Alveolar bone is involved sooner or later with accompanying roentgenographic change. What is more, we know that periapical disease as a rule meets a more effective resistance within the periodontium than does pulp disease within the pulp. Battle is joined outside the tooth where the full resources of the body can be utilized. Resistance and containment take forms similar to those seen in other bone and soft tissue complexes of the body. The dentist's understanding of periapical lesions, therefore, is reinforced by his past learning. It is also sustained by his success in correlating the diagnosis of these lesions with their effective treatment in day-to-day practice.

The relationship between pulp and periapical disease is a close one. Pulp involvement is almost always the forerunner. Our examination of periapical pathosis, therefore, follows logically upon the survey of pulp pathosis. Inflammation and its sequelae are shared by both (Fig. 9–1). Certain developments, however, are more commonplace in the periapex. The cyst is almost unknown in the pulp, but is a frequent periapical lesion. Repair is far more often achieved periapically than intrapulpally.

We have previously traced (Chapter 6) the inseparable connective tissues of pulp chamber, root canal, foramens, and periapical zone. Given the existence of this continuum, the spread of disease beyond the tooth apex is most understandable. Certain structures of the apical periodontium exert a strong influence on the nature of the lesions that arise. Most apparent is the continuous periodontal ligament, its rich collateral blood supply, and its epithelial network. Beyond is the cribriform plate of the alveolar bone proper, through which, at many points, the interstitial connective tissue of the ligament merges with the marrow of the alveolar supporting bone.

The net result of these features of the periapical zone is that a more adequate cellular defense can be mounted around the tooth apex than within the pulp. And it is well that this is so. To have the pulp succumb to bacterial invasion, and to have pulp chamber and root canal then become a nidus for bacteria and organic toxins, is one thing. Within the tooth these agents are to a great extent "outside" the body. It is quite a different matter when bacteria and/or toxins escape the root canal into the connective tissue at the root apex. Now the rich collateral circulation of the periodontal ligament becomes both a blessing and a curse. In the pulp a dual resistance is provided by (1) the physical barrier of the dentin, and (2) the connective tissue response. At the periapex, defense rests more heavily upon the cellular and vascular reactions to the external threat. Here, even more than in the pulp, defense hinges upon inflammation.

The histopathologic aspects of periapical disease fall better into place after a brief preview of the reactions that are possible in the apical area. The

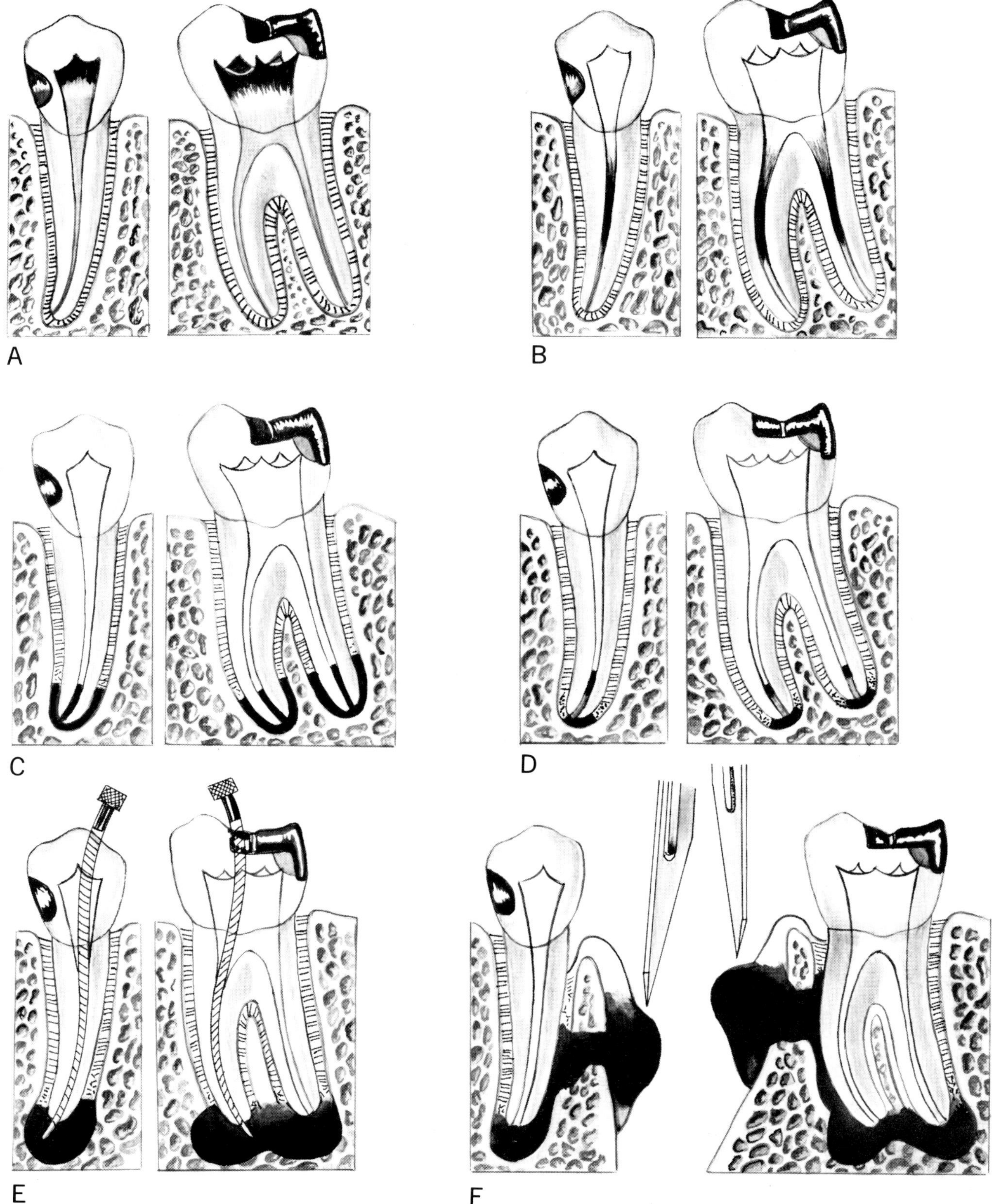

Fig. 9–1. Continuum of pulpal-periapical inflammation and infection. *A,* Early pulpitis triggered by bacteria from deep caries and placement of restoration. *B,* Inflammation spreads down canal as coronal pulp becomes necrotic. *C,* Inflammation reaches apex and spreads into tissue of periodontal ligament—beginning acute apical periodontitis. *D,* Necrosis of PDL along with inflammation is earliest sign of chronic apical periodontitis. *E,* Chronic, suppurative apical periodontitis has developed. Pulp is totally necrotic. Drainage through canal may be gained by trephining apical foramen. *F,* If infected with virulent bacteria, acute apical abscess or phoenix abscess may develop. Incision and drainage may be necessary. (Courtesy Dr. James D. Zidell.)

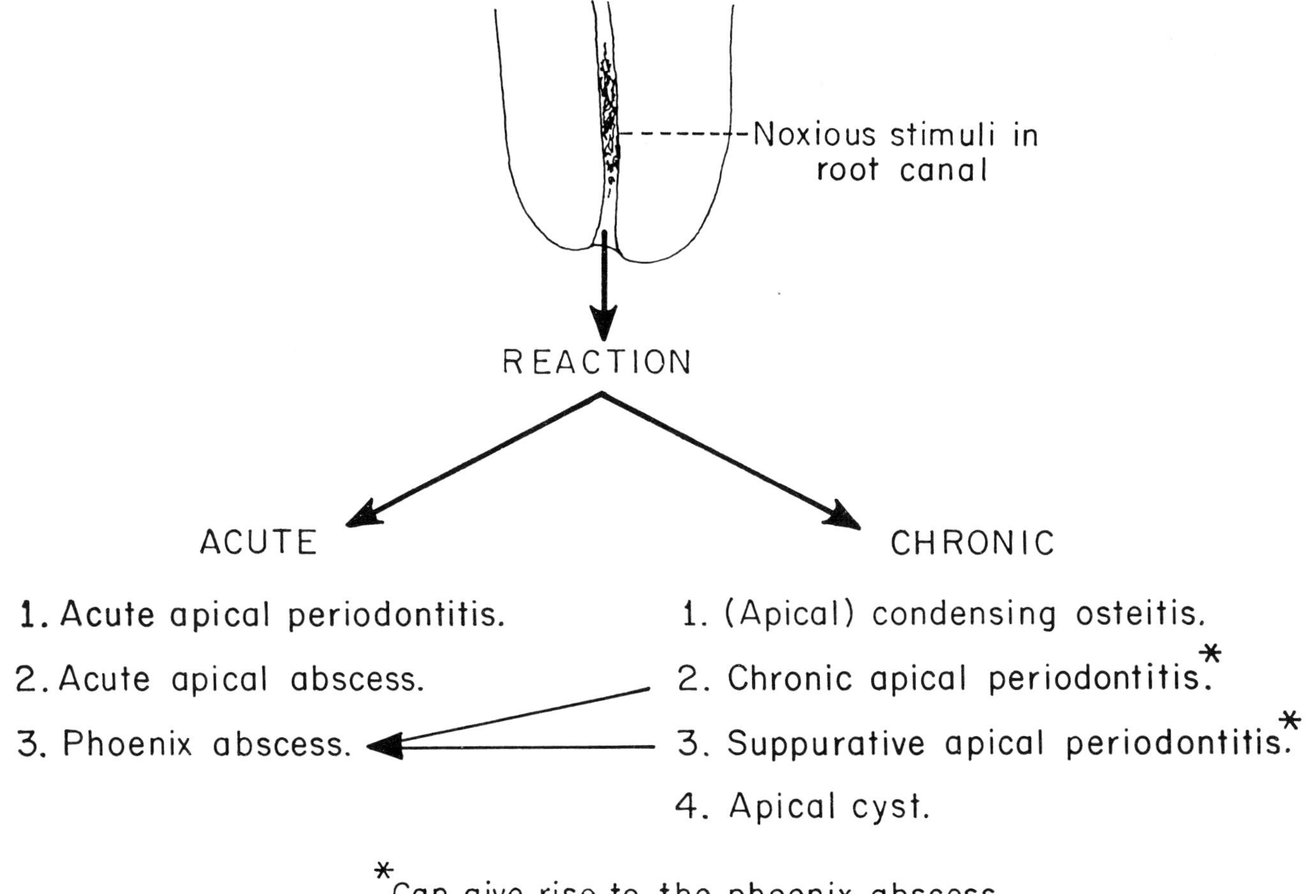

Fig. 9–2. Patterns of reaction to noxious stimuli which pass from root canal into tissues beyond apex. Either acute reaction or chronic reaction appears. Two forms of chronic reaction (chronic apical periodontitis and suppurative apical periodontitis) can change abruptly into an acute condition, namely, phoenix abscess.

response to noxious stimuli, which pass from the root canal into the tissues beyond the root apex, assumes one or the other of two patterns (Fig. 9–2). An ***acute*** reaction may develop and take the form of an ***apical periodontitis.*** Such is often found to be the response to mechanical instrumentation accidentally carried beyond the canal. The acute response is also illustrated by the ***apical abscess.*** In contrast, the periapical response to noxious stimuli from the root canal may be ***chronic*** in nature. Periapical change then follows in one of three ways. (1) Most commonly, a stand-off or balance between local (body) resistance and the noxious agent develops. We are then dealing with the ***chronic apical periodontitis*** (granuloma). (2) On other occasions the noxious stimuli increase in number or degree, as, for example, when the number and/or virulence of bacteria within the root canal rises or the bodily resistance falls. This signals a transition from chronic apical periodontitis to ***suppurative apical periodontitis*** with characteristic suppuration and drainage by way of the fistula and stoma. (3) A third chronic lesion may develop in either of the first two ways when epithelial rest cells are stimulated to proliferate and produce an ***apical cyst.*** In this periapical lesion, epithelial cells line a cavity in a continuous sheet and may promote growth of this cavity (cyst) through their secretion of fluid into the space.

The understanding of periapical disease is accelerated when mnemonics* is employed on the basis of a simple descriptive vocabulary. Thus, for any inflammatory state of the periodontal complex, only one

*Mnemonics—a technique of improving the efficiency of the memory.[1]

word, "periodontitis," need be learned. By prefacing with the term "apical," the location of the inflammation is suggested. Similarly, the term "apical" repeated with each periapical lesion will bring to mind the accompanying term as an endodontic one. Other terms, denoting pathologic change in the apical region, but not of pulp origin, are used without the "apical" prefix. By way of illustration, "ankylosis" should not, or need not, be preceded by the term "apical."[2]

APICAL PERIODONTITIS

Acute Apical Periodontitis (AAP)

Acute apical periodontitis arises most frequently as a sequel to pulp disease and endodontic treatment. The tenderness that is felt at the root apex after even the most straightforward vital pulpectomy is a case in point. On other occasions, the acute reaction is set off by the accidental passage of an instrument beyond the canal. Or, the instrument may remain within the canal and yet may push into the periodontal ligament such irritants as necrotic pulp tissue, bacteria, or dentin fragments. Inflammation is then a certainty. Overmedication or overextended root canal filling material can set up the same acute response and the same almost diagnostic apical tenderness.

Acute apical periodontitis should be recognized for what it is, namely, an inflammation around the apex of a tooth. The distinctive features are microscopic rather than roentgenographic, symptomatic rather than visible. From a necrotic pulp, for example, toxic elements or bacteria may advance beyond the foramen. A localized inflammatory infiltrate then develops in the periodontal ligament (Fig. 9–3). The cellular part of the infiltrate includes many "round cells" as well as neutrophils. The accompanying

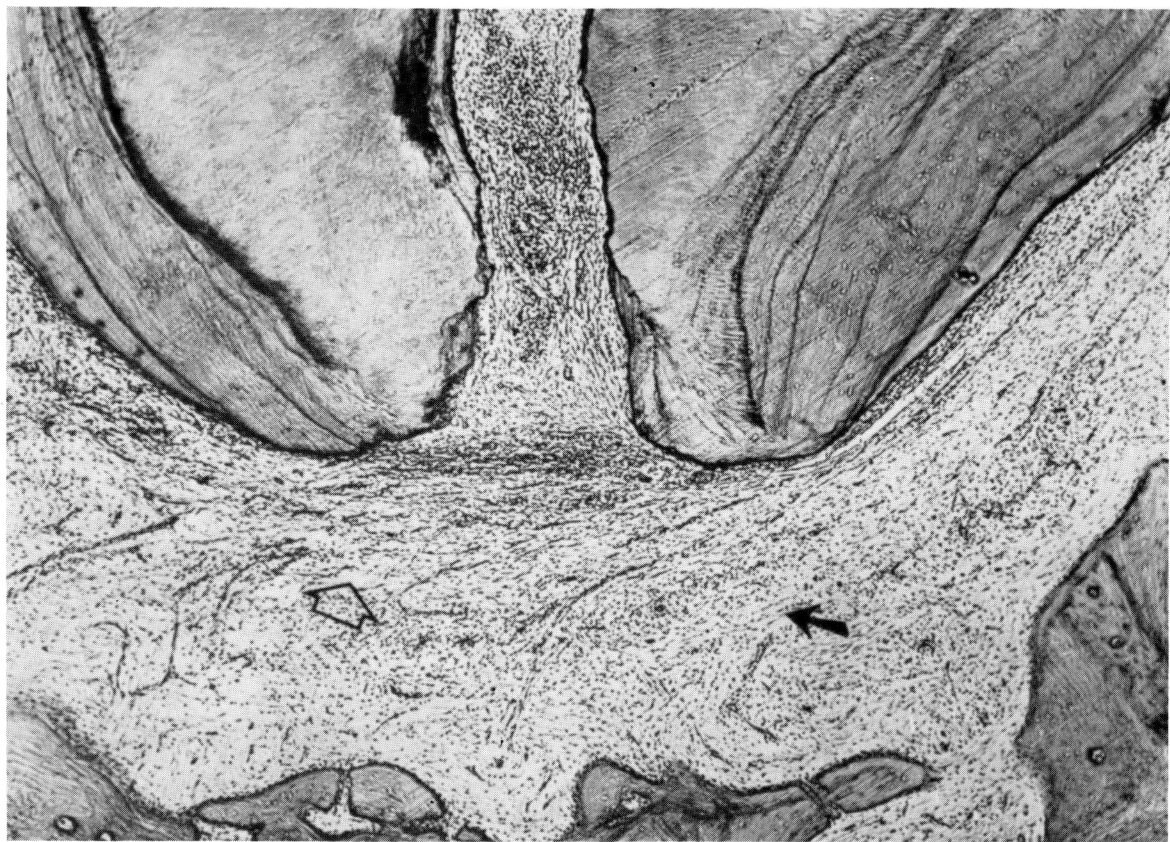

Fig. 9–3. Microscopic features of acute apical periodontitis. From necrotic pulp, toxic elements and/or bacteria have penetrated periodontal ligament at apex of tooth. There is localized inflammatory infiltrate, including edema *(open arrow)*, with ligament. Beginnings of fibrous capsule *(black arrow)* can be detected between cellular infiltrate and alveolar bone. Human tooth. (From Matsumiya, S.: *Atlas of Oral Pathology.* Tokyo Dental College Press, 1955.)

vascular changes and the edema create pressure on the sensory nerve endings in the area. Elevation of the tooth, as a result of the increase in intercellular fluid, adds to the tenderness. Where the reaction is of some duration (as may be presumed in Fig. 9–3), the beginnings of a fibrous capsule can be detected between the cellular infiltrate and the alveolar bone.

An acute lesion anywhere either heals or becomes a chronic one: so with the acute apical periodontitis. The outcome depends primarily on the duration of the inciting irritant and the severity of the irritant. The insult of pulpectomy, for instance, is quickly past and the acute apical periodontitis that is produced by this trauma is rapidly repaired. On the other hand, the continued presence of a necrotic pulp in an untreated tooth prohibits repair. Nature then does the next best thing. Following the principle of encapsulation, the irritant is "walled off" at the apex of the tooth by connective tissue (the chronic apical periodontitis).

Of course, when the irritant is massive or extremely virulent, the mild inflammatory process of acute apical periodontitis is bypassed entirely. Containment of the irritant is again achieved, but only at the cost of a much more acute and widespread inflammatory reaction. This we recognize as the acute apical abscess.

Chronic Apical Periodontitis (CAP)

Chronic apical periodontitis (the so-called dental granuloma) represents a "stand-off" between local resistance and the noxious stimuli emerging from the root canal. In the presence of an untreated nonvital tooth it is impossible for the defenses of the body to eliminate the irritants within the root canal. Occasionally endodontic treatment, supposedly adequate, will perpetuate this chronic process or even initiate it. Inflammation can scarcely be avoided when the apical connective tissue is in contact with root canal filling material, which is itself irritating, or when there is gross overextension of even a nonirritating material.[3,4]

The condition has been misnamed "dental granuloma" and even "root abscess" for many years. Essentially, one is concerned here with a mass of chronic inflammatory tissue. The qualities of a tumor are wanting, hence the unsuitability of the suffix "oma." Likewise, the growth is quite removed from the new connective tissue of wound repair, which can properly be termed granulation tissue.[5] The term ***"chronic apical periodontitis"*** suggests the length of time the lesion has been present, the mild state of its symptoms, and the microscopic picture of chronic inflammation.[2]

The diseased area in chronic apical periodontitis tends to grow to a certain size and then to go no further. The expansion occurs first at the cost of the normal periodontal ligament and alveolar bone. This is the usual slow replacement of specialized tissue in the face of chronic inflammation. Cementum and dentin resorption is also commonplace[6] (Fig. 9–4). As the apical lesion grows and ages, its structure tends to change, but our attention should first be directed to features that remain characteristic despite enlargement. Nerve tissue has been demonstrated in a high percentage (80%) of periapical inflammatory lesions.[7] We would expect, and do find, the most intense cellular reaction around the root apex and especially at the foramen. A "round cell" infiltration is often prominent there (Fig. 9–5). Plasma cells and small lymphocytes abound. A variable number of polymorphonuclear leukocytes, including eosinophils, are present. Small capillaries are numerous, their endothelial cell outgrowth keeping pace with the soft tissue expansion (Figs. 9–6 and 9–7). Fibroblasts are also differentiated. They, in their turn, provide the innumerable fibrils that interlace and encapsulate the mass (Figs. 9–5 and 9–7).

Epithelial tissue is a distinctive and surprisingly widespread feature of chronic apical periodontitis. Actually this should come as no surprise. Given the abundance of epithelial cells in the periodontal ligament, it is inevitable that the inflammatory process should encompass and stimulate many of these normally dormant residents. To one degree or another then, the epithelium proliferates within the new inflammatory tissue, tending always to ramify in the direction of the receding bone. The epithelium may also apply itself widely to the root surface (Fig. 9–8). Round cells find the epithelium no barrier. They are everywhere among the squamous layers, demonstrating once again that epithelium and inflammatory connective tissue are compatible.

As we pass from the center of the "granuloma" toward the periphery, the loose complex of cells, ground substance, fibrils, and vessels gives way to a more fibrous capsule (Fig. 9–5). Here it is the fibroblasts that are the more numerous and more active, rather than the round cells. The prominence of the "capsule" is, of course, a variable thing.

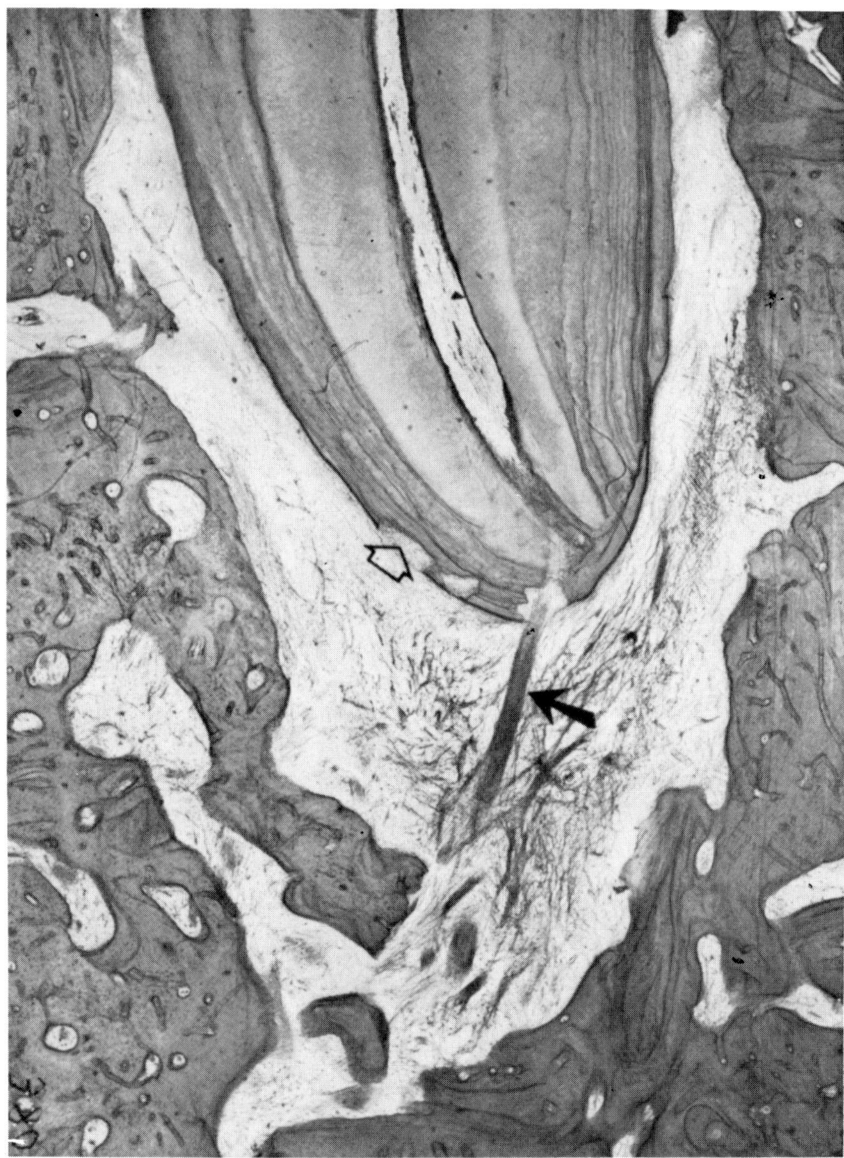

Fig. 9–4. Chronic apical periodontitis of low activity. Area of inflammatory connective tissue has developed around apex of tooth at expense of normal periodontal ligament and alveolar bone proper. Prominent nerve fiber bundle *(arrow)* passes through inflammatory tissue to foramen. Such persistence of vital nerve tissue in face of inflammation is well known. Pulp of tooth is not completely necrotic. Intensity of irritant(s) from this pulp was probably low. Certainly inflammatory reaction is not marked and bone on margin is unusually compact. Cemental resorption *(open arrow)* is apparent, however. Human tooth. (Orban collection.)

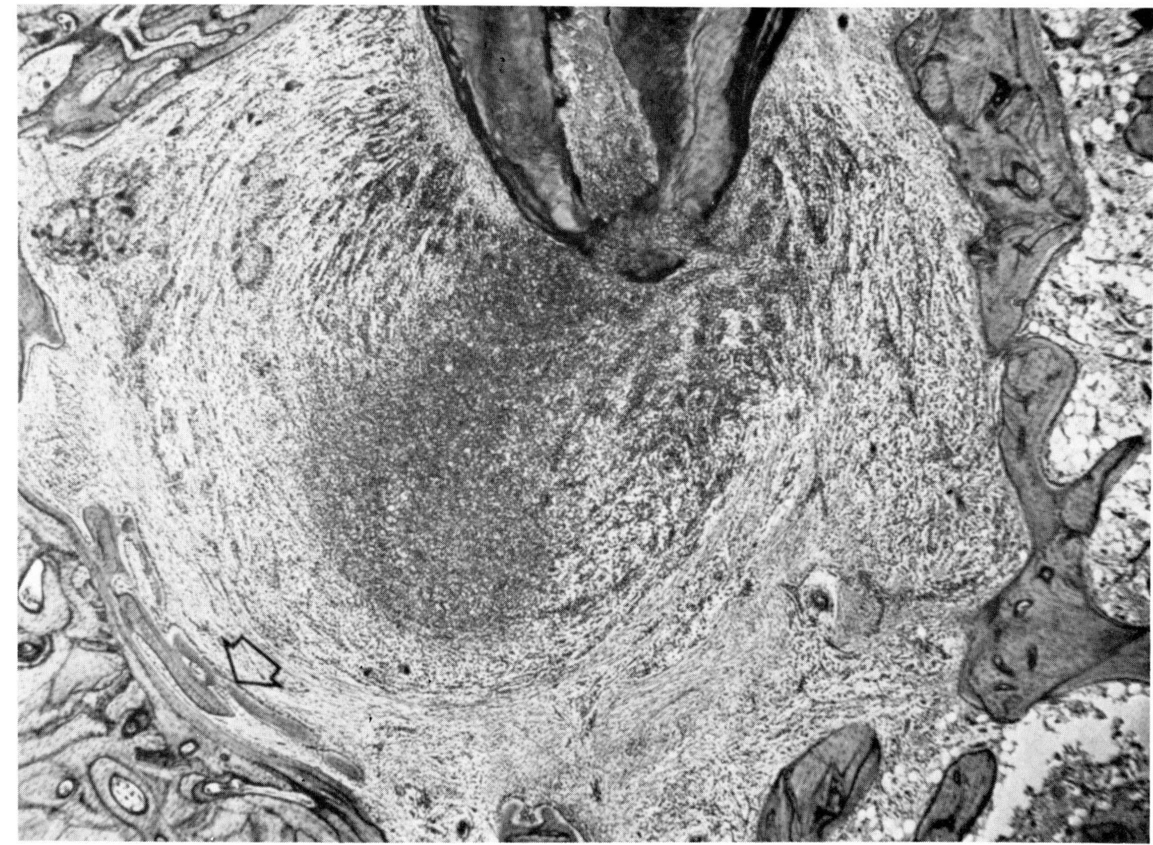

Fig. 9–5. Chronic apical periodontitis in its more classic form. Central zone is dense with round cells (plasma cells and small lymphocytes). Beyond is circular layer of fibrous capsule. Limited bone regeneration *(arrow)* can be clearly seen at outer margin of capsule. Human tooth. (From Matsumiya, S.: *Atlas of Oral Pathology.* Tokyo Dental College Press, 1955.)

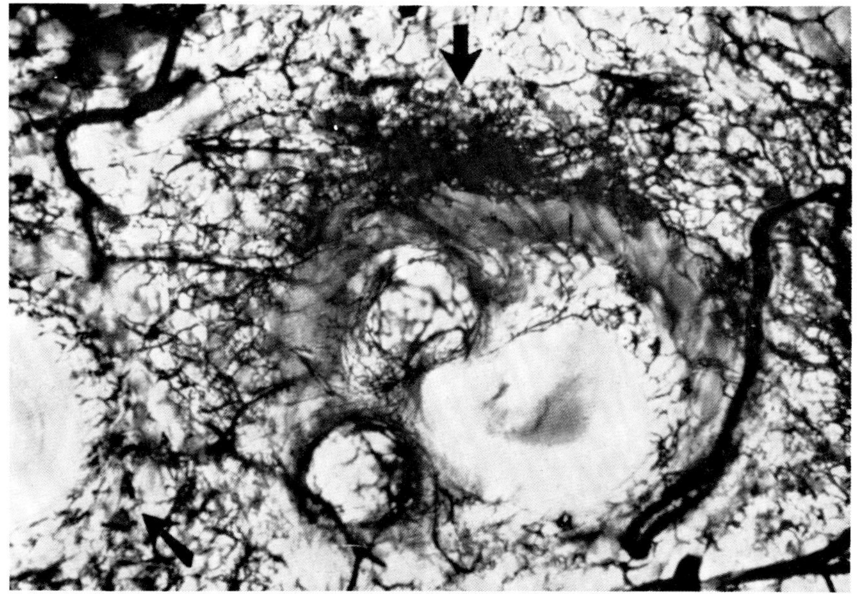

Fig. 9–6. Vascular change at periapex associated with chronic apical periodontitis. Contrast vascularity evident around normal tooth *(lower arrow)* with that seen in pathologic area *(upper arrow).* Lesion has greatly increased vascular supply. Horizontal section through apices of teeth in perfused monkey. (Courtesy Dr. D. Walter Cohen.)

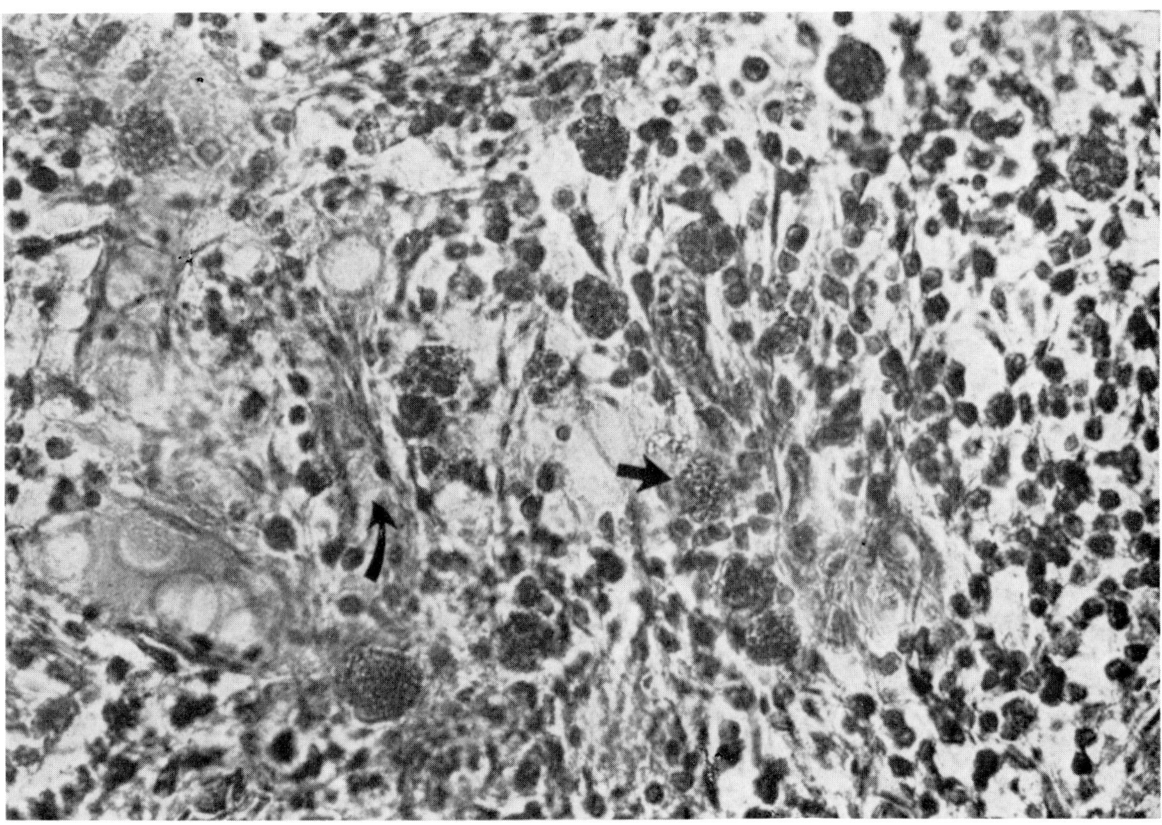

Fig. 9–7. Inflammatory tissue within central zone of chronic apical periodontitis. Tissue consists essentially of semi-fluid ground substance, fibrils, fibroblasts, round cells, and capillaries. Curved, tube-like structures *(left arrow)* are newly-formed capillaries. Eosinophils *(center arrow)* are numerous in this particular section. Human periapex. (From Matsumiya, S.: *Atlas of Oral Pathology.* Tokyo Dental College Press, 1955.)

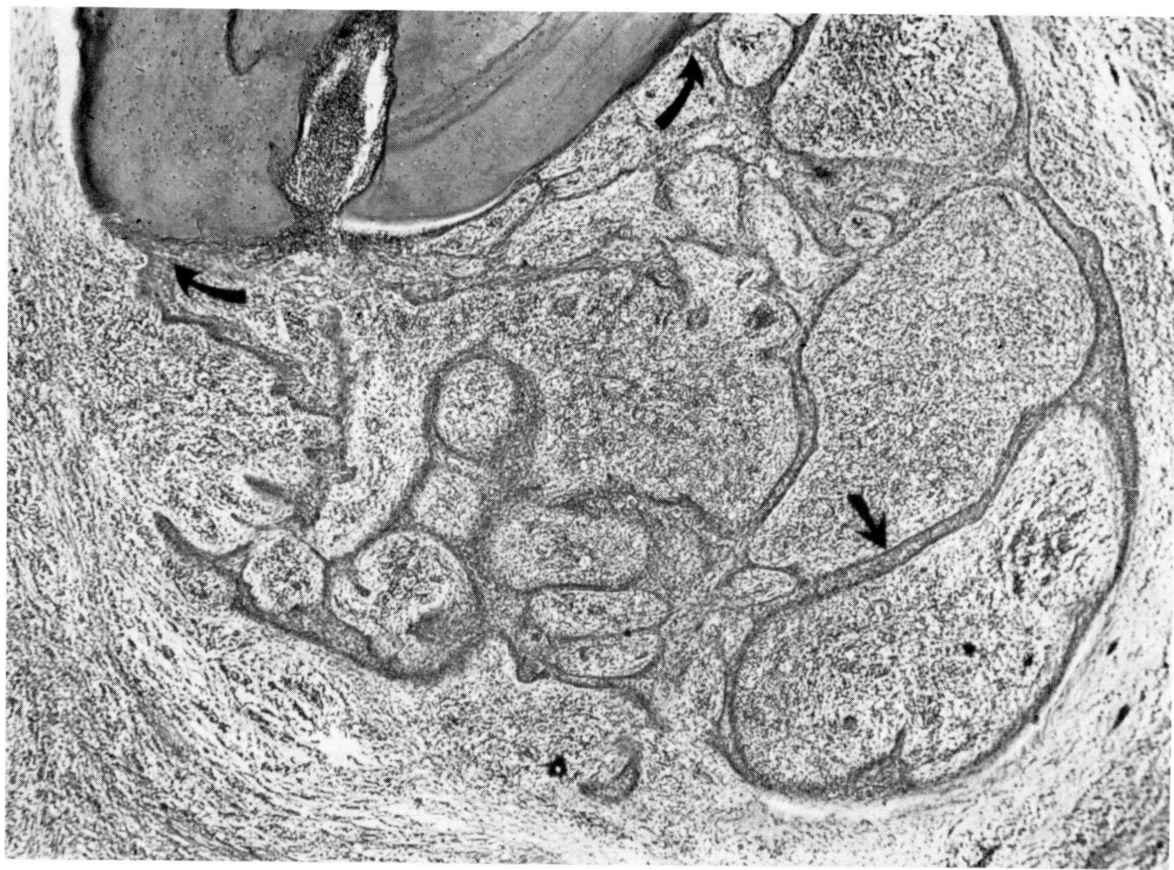

Fig. 9–8. Chronic apical periodontitis with contained epithelium. Epithelial cells of periodontal ligament have proliferated within new inflammatory tissue. Epithelium tends to ramify in reticular pattern *(straight arrow)* toward receding bone. It also may, as in this case, apply itself widely to root surface *(curved arrows)*. Infiltration of epithelium by round cells is everywhere apparent. Human tooth. (From Matsumiya, S.: *Atlas of Oral Pathology*. Tokyo Dental College Press, 1955.)

(Compare Figure 9–4 with Figure 9–5.) Age of the lesion, intensity of the irritant, and intensity of the inflammatory response are all influential.

These same factors determine, to a large extent, the response of the alveolar bone at any given time in the history of the lesion. "Bone regeneration associated with apical inflammatory processes is not uncommon. It is an expression of the fluctuating character of the process; periods of activity, during which bone is resorbed, alternate with periods of inactivity during which the bone is regenerated."[8] In Figure 9–5, for example, bone regeneration can clearly be seen on the periphery of the fibrous capsule.

The clinical and roentgenographic features of chronic apical periodontitis should be well known. The condition may remain asymptomatic for a long time. On other occasions, the tooth involved feels slightly elevated and sensitive to pressure. Loss of vitality of the pulp is an invariable finding. In the dental film, the lesion appears as a radiolucent, circular-to-ovoid area which encloses the root end and extends apically from it. Should the mass be static in size, or only slowly progressive, it is apparently possible for the cancellous supporting (marrow) bone on the margin to become more compact and radiopaque.[9,10] This is the state of affairs suggested in Figure 9–9 and also in Figure 9–4.

Most of the aforementioned features are shared by the apical cyst. Accurate distinction between chronic apical periodontitis and the apical cyst is therefore impossible on the basis of clinical and roentgenographic findings alone.

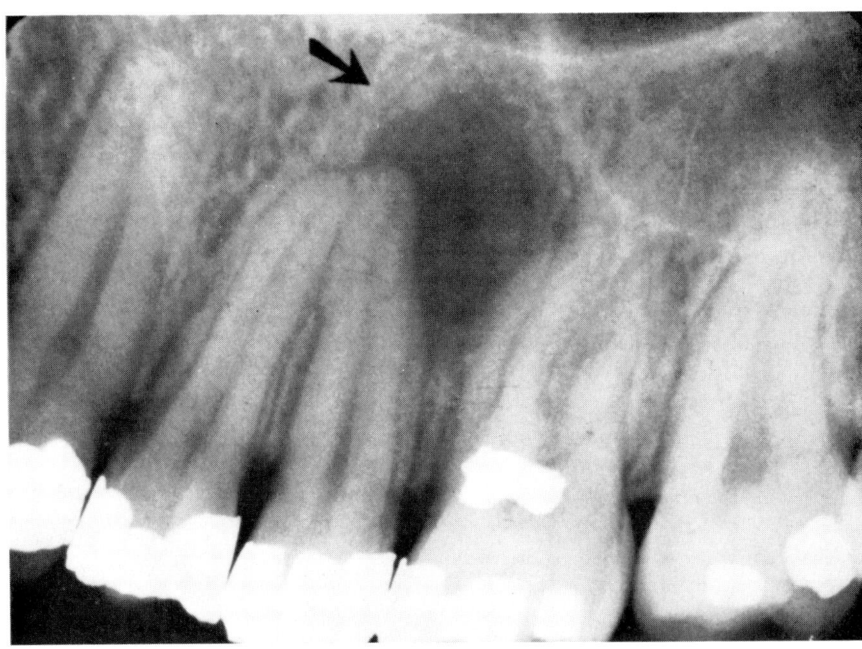

Fig. 9–9. Roentgenographic appearance of chronic apical periodontitis. Lesion is evident as circular-to-ovoid area at apex of maxillary second premolar. Bone on mesial margin *(arrow)* of radiolucency appears more opaque than elsewhere. Chronic apical periodontitis and apical cyst have similar radiographic features. For this reason they cannot be diagnosed on strength of radiograph alone. (Courtesy Dr. Neal Chilton.)

Suppurative Apical Periodontitis (SAP)

When the "stand-off" or balance between local resistance and the noxious stimuli is upset, the low-grade inflammatory lesion changes character abruptly. The balance may be altered by: (1) an increase in the quantity of a given irritant on the scene, (2) an increase in the virulence of bacteria that may be present, or (3) a decrease in the bodily resistance. ***Suppurative apical periodontitis*** ensues, with its accompanying fistula and stoma ("gum boil") (Fig. 9–10). The term "suppurative" before "apical periodontitis" implies the presence of frank pus. This fluid we observe as it emerges from the stoma, or when the apical area is exposed during operation, or in microsection. The term "chronic alveolar abscess" is too frequently understood to mean a chronic continuation of the acute alveolar abscess, which is seldom the case.[2]

There is good reason to stress that the dentist is dealing with an apical periodontitis which has become suppurative. Proteolytic enzymes released by the polymorphonuclear cells of the area have liquefied the collagen, ground substance, tissue cells, and bacteria alike. The outcome is pus.[11]

Active pus formation calls for drainage. Occasionally, the root canal itself will serve this purpose. However, when the root canal is blocked, a new exit must be created. When periapical necrosis (hence pus formation) is extensive, the same holds true. Then even an open root canal cannot remove the volume of exudate with sufficient speed. It is for these reasons that the lateral drainage pathway, or fistula, is such a common finding.

The ***early*** stage of suppurative apical periodontitis is shown in Figures 9–11 and 9–12. Roentgenographic evidence of widening of the periodontal ligament space and a slight radiolucency of the alveolar bone are apparent. A fistula has not had time to form. The production of pus has begun, as evidenced by the empty space and abundant necrotic cells in the microsection (Fig. 9–12). Clinically, there is little or no pain.

This same type of lesion, at a ***later*** stage, demonstrates active suppuration (Fig. 9–13). A well-defined fistula exists. This channel has been created through bone, periosteum, and mucosa in turn, by enzymes such as necrosin, and cells such as the osteoclast and the macrophage. Since the route of the fistula is curved and devious, its lumen is evident in a plane section only at intervals. Ulceration of the tract

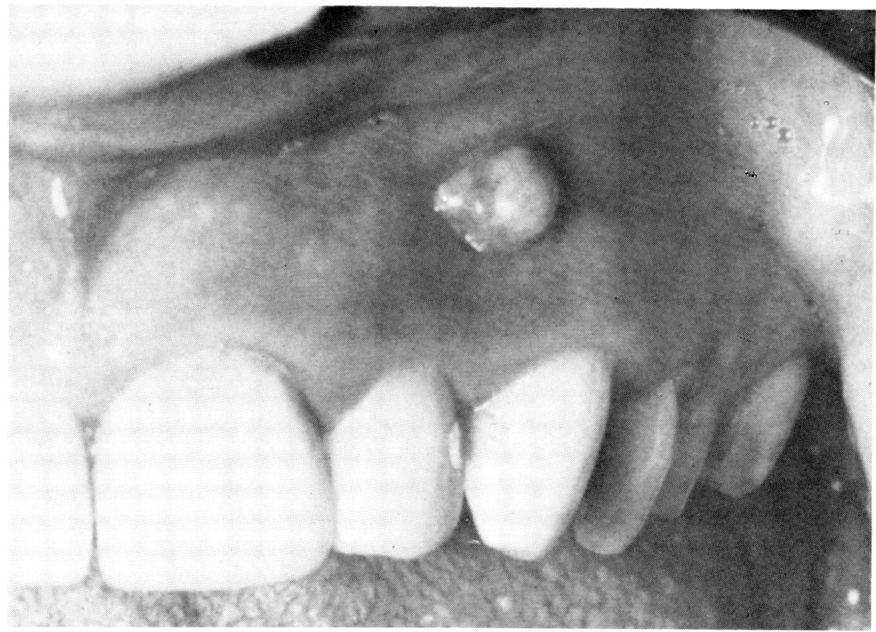

Fig. 9–10. Suppurative apical periodontitis and its stoma ("gum boil"). Drainage is occurring periodically from primary lesion at apex of maxillary lateral incisor (see Fig. 9–14). At the moment stoma is closed and there is no visible pus. Exudate is obviously just below surface, however, and it will soon drain actively.

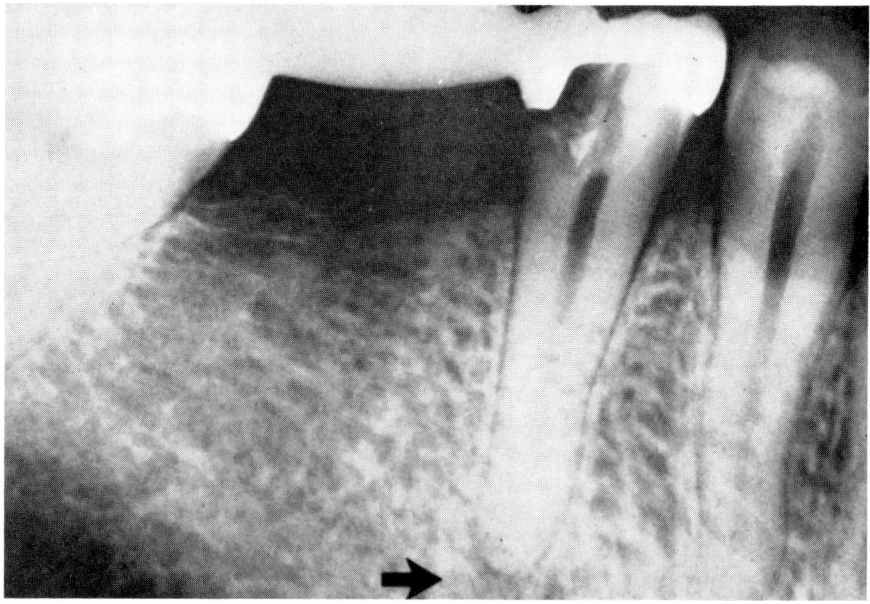

Fig. 9–11. Roentgenographic features of early suppurative apical periodontitis. Mandibular second premolar is involved. Widening of periodontal ligament space has occurred at apex and limited radiolucency *(arrow)* can be seen there. In this case, as in Figure 9–12, fistula has not had time to form.

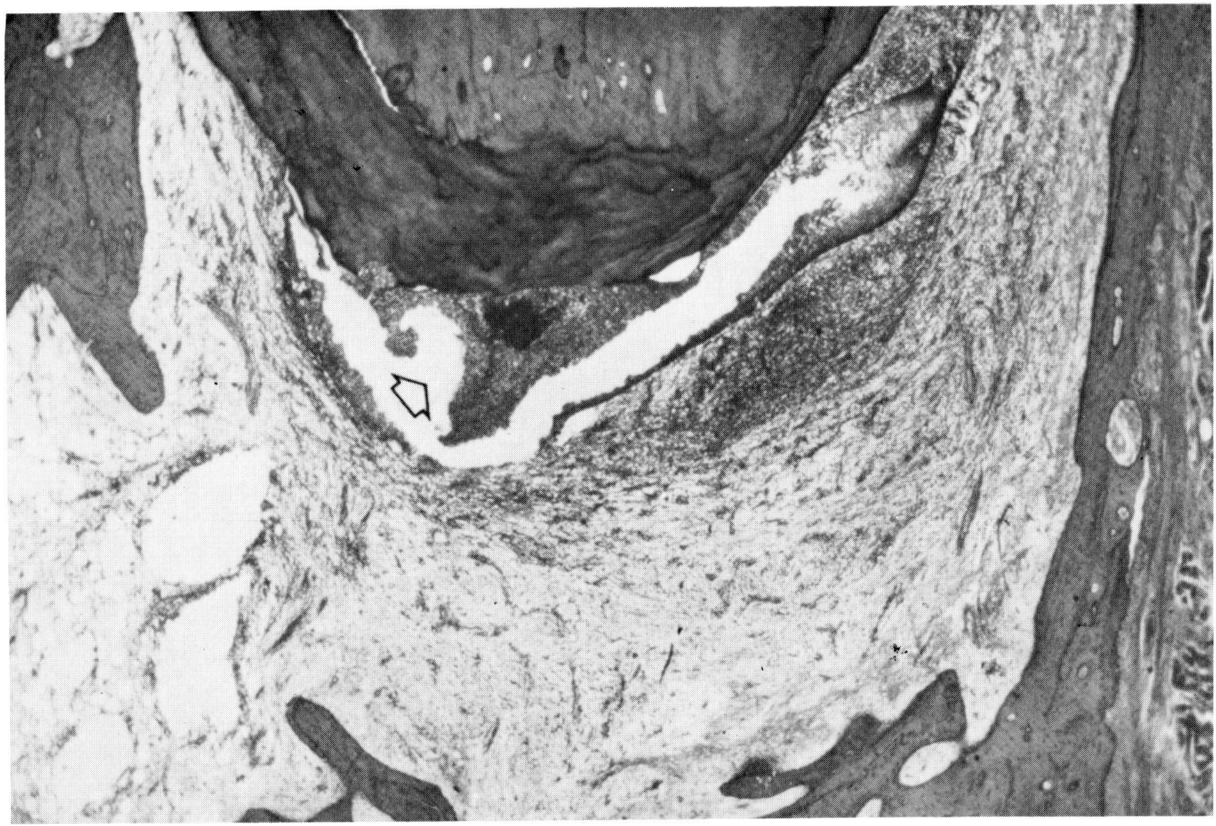

Fig. 9–12. Early stage of suppurative apical periodontitis. Chronic apical periodontitis had existed for some time. Production of pus has begun, as evidenced by empty space and abundant necrotic cells *(arrow)* at immediate apex. Fistula is not yet established. Human tooth. (Orban collection.)

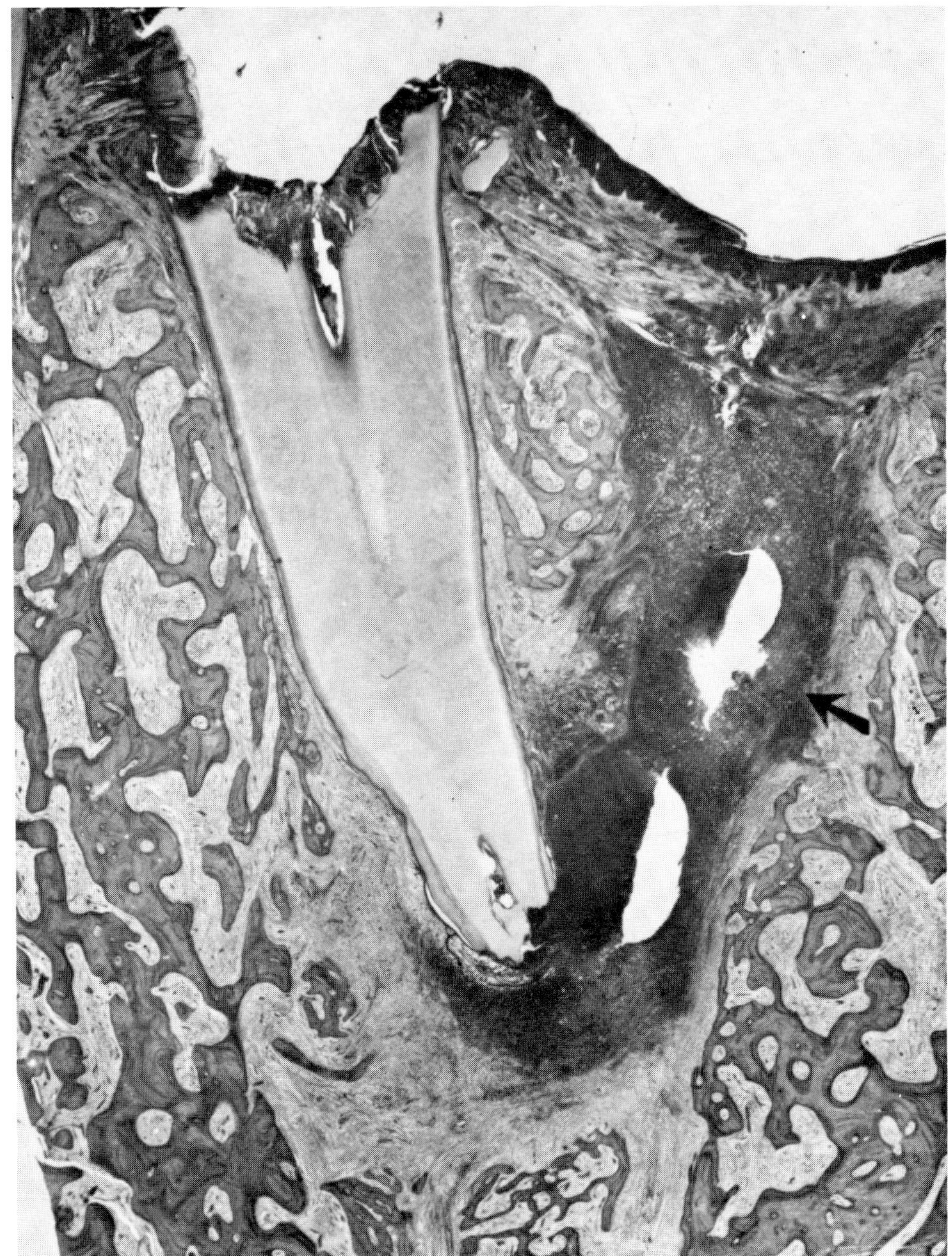

Fig. 9–13. Later stage of suppurative apical periodontitis. By this time well-defined fistula exists. Because fistula has provided adequate drainage, there has been little enlargement of area of bone destruction created earlier by chronic apical periodontitis. Much of fistular tract is lined, not by epithelium but by ulcerated, heavily infiltrated connective tissue *(arrow)*. Human mandibular premolar tooth. (From Matsumiya, S.: *Atlas of Oral Pathology*. Tokyo Dental College Press, 1955.)

wall is shown, together with a dense chronic inflammation of the connective tissue forming the sheath of the tract. It should also be evident that when a suppurative periodontitis can find a path of drainage, it does not usually lead to any marked extension of the apical area of bone loss, beyond that created by the chronic lesion that preceded it.

The roentgenographic picture of this more mature lesion complements the histopathologic. Because of the bone destruction inherent in the creation of the fistula, the area of radiolucency coronal to the apex may be greater than in chronic apical periodontitis (Fig. 9–14). The roentgenogram brings out a further point. Where the anteroposterior width of the alveolar process is minimal (*e.g.*, around the upper lateral incisor), a completely radiolucent zone may be produced adjacent to the root.

Frank pus is being produced in quantity. Either periodically or almost continuously, this is discharged at the stoma. Figure 9–10 shows a case in which, at the time of photography, there was no active drainage. Figure 9–15, on the other hand, illustrates the continuous escape of pus from a fistula reaching to the surface of the chin. Far more often a dental fistula will terminate intraorally. The fistula from a mandibular or maxillary anterior tooth usually penetrates to the adjacent vestibule (Fig. 9–16). Microscopic features of such a lesion are evident in Figure 9–17. This case illustrates a tract fully epithelialized from apical area to mucosal surface. The gingival epithelium has proliferated through the inflammatory tissue around the fistular canal to the periapical area. There it has joined with epithelium present near the apex.

Characteristically, the purulent exudate reaches for the surface along the route offering the least resistance. The encasement of bone and soft tissue will be penetrated at its thinnest point. In the anterior mouth this will be on the labial of the tooth, opposite the apical third of the root length.

The exudate from a maxillary posterior tooth may utilize the maxillary antrum in its escape. Anatomic factors of root position, antrum floor location, and bone thickness overlying the root apex will dictate this outcome. Figure 9–18 shows suppurative apical periodontitis of the distobuccal root of an upper first molar. The inflammatory focus at the root end exhibits a wide abscess cavity which has become lined with epithelium. Pus can be seen within. A fistular canal has broken through the bony overlay onto the

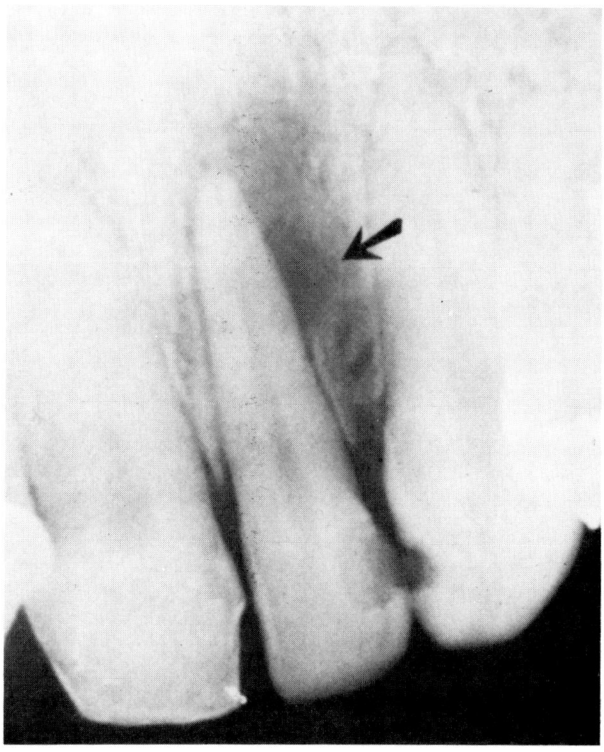

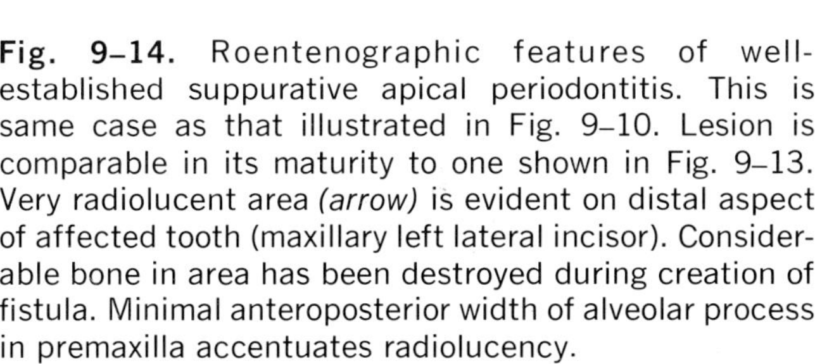

Fig. 9–14. Roentenographic features of well-established suppurative apical periodontitis. This is same case as that illustrated in Fig. 9–10. Lesion is comparable in its maturity to one shown in Fig. 9–13. Very radiolucent area *(arrow)* is evident on distal aspect of affected tooth (maxillary left lateral incisor). Considerable bone in area has been destroyed during creation of fistula. Minimal anteroposterior width of alveolar process in premaxilla accentuates radiolucency.

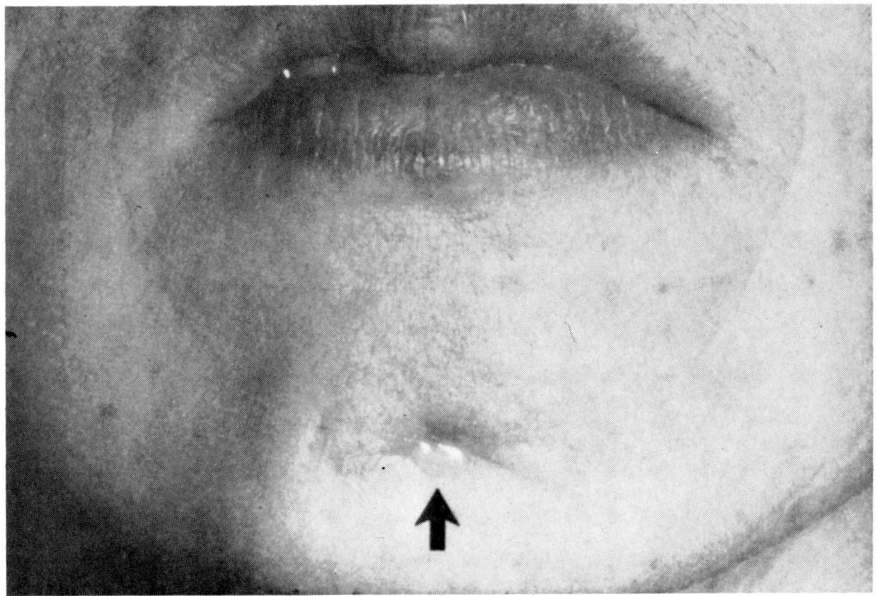

Fig. 9–15. Flow of pus from stoma associated with suppurative apical periodontitis. Drainage to surface of chin is uncommon finding. Far more often fistula of suppurative apical periodontitis in anterior mandible will terminate intraorally. Chin is not enlarged because adequate drainage exists. This is in sharp contrast to swelling seen when acute apical abscess is located in same area (Fig. 9–19).

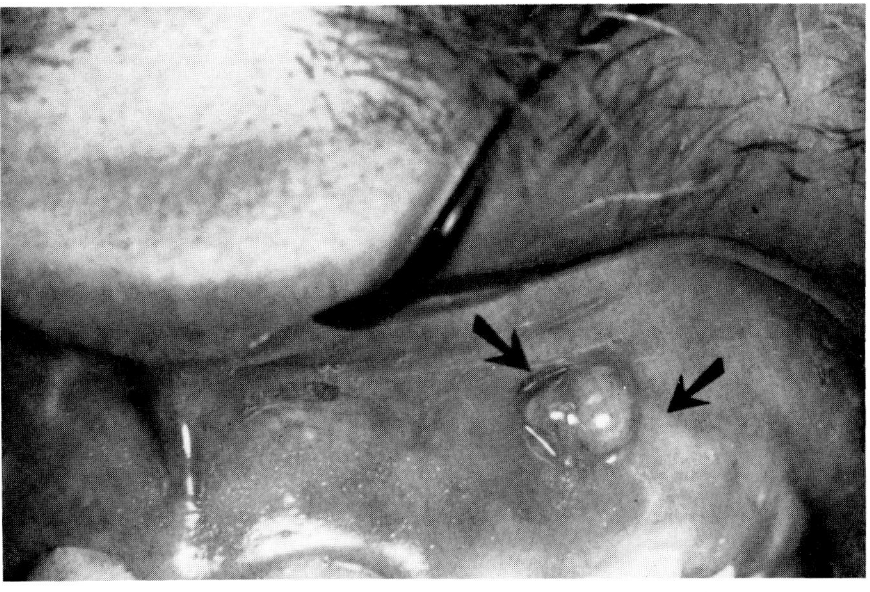

Fig. 9–16. Typical exit of drainage from suppurative apical periodontitis involving anterior tooth. Drainage is intraoral. Stoma *(left arrow)* is on facial aspect of alveolar process, at or near level of mucogingival junction *(right arrow)*.

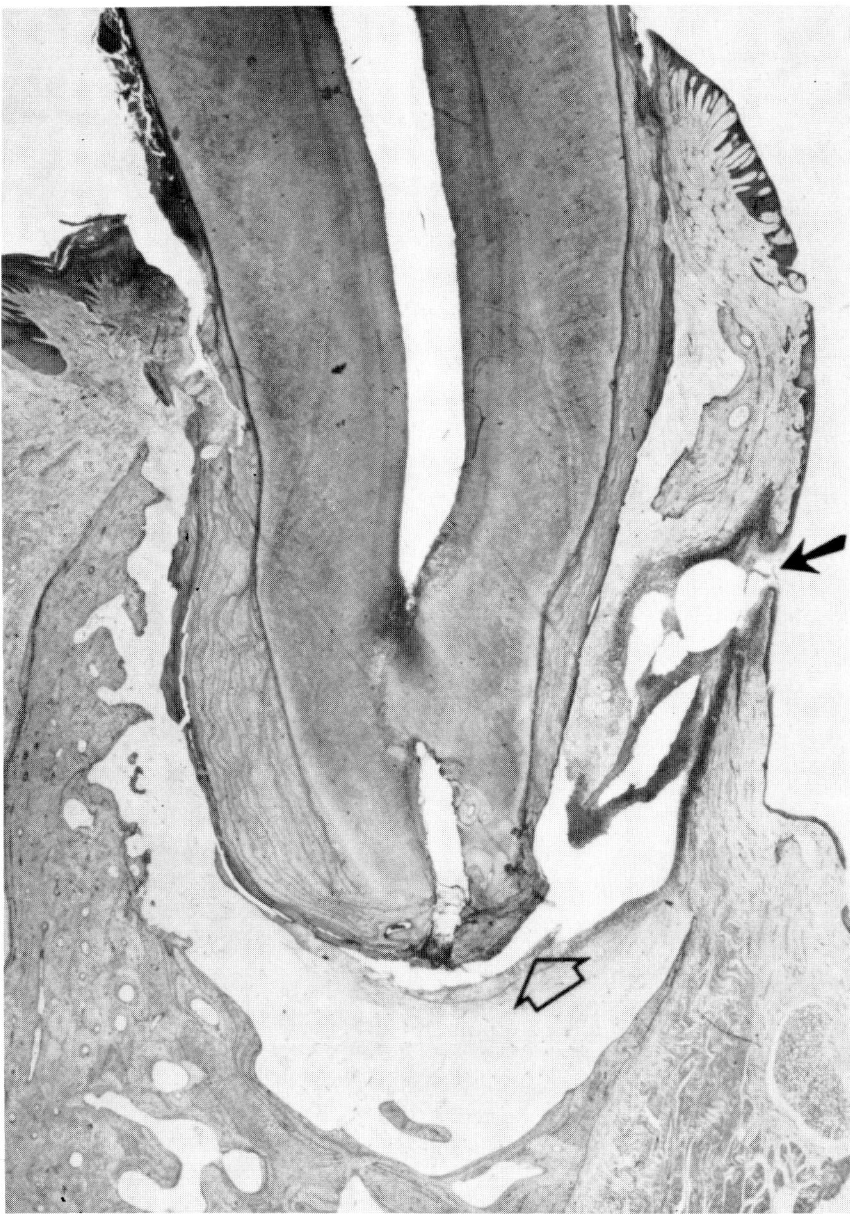

Fig. 9–17. Fistula, completely epithelialized, leading from periapical area to mucosal surface. Oral epithelium has migrated along connective tissue wall of fistula to periapical area and has merged with epithelium *(open arrow)* already present there. Fistula ends in stoma *(black arrow)* which lies just apical to mucogingival junction on facial aspect. Human mandibular incisor tooth. (Orban collection.)

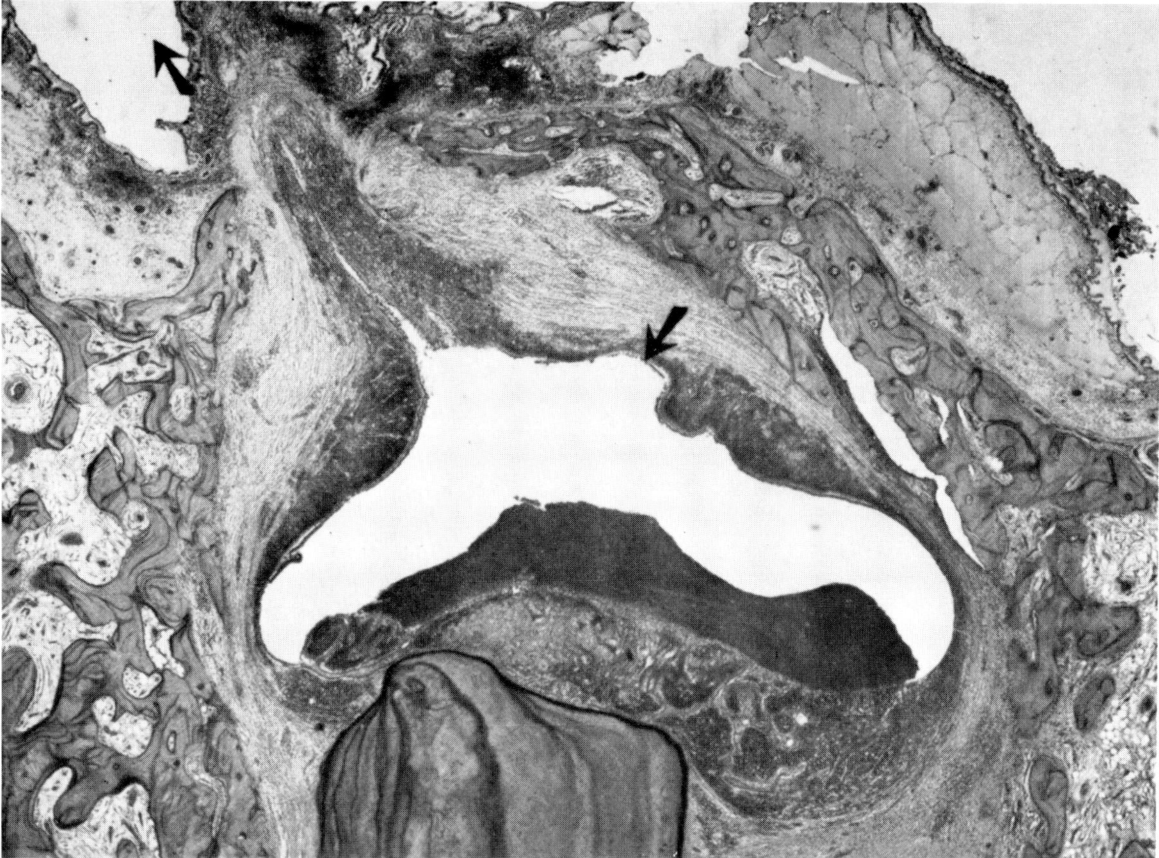

Fig. 9–18. Suppurative apical periodontitis of maxillary molar, with drainage to maxillary sinus. Large abscess cavity can be seen at end of distobuccal root of this first molar. Fistular canal has broken through bony overlay onto floor of sinus above. Inflamed, polyp-like tissue rings orifice of fistula and protrudes into antrum *(upper arrow)*. Ciliated epithelium from sinus has proliferated down fistula and onto abscess wall *(lower arrow)* to join epithelium in periapical area. Human tooth. (From Matsumiya, S.: *Atlas of Oral Pathology*. Tokyo Dental College Press, 1955.)

floor of the antrum. The mucosa around the mouth of the canal has become inflamed. Polyp-like tissue rings the orifice and protrudes into the antrum.[12]

APICAL ABSCESS

Apical abscess is a term chosen to designate an abscess related to the root apex. Learning is aided by this choice of "apical abscess" over the term "acute alveolar abscess," even though the latter term has been employed for a long time. A periodontal abscess is also, strictly speaking, an alveolar abscess. In fact, the periodontal abscess is confined to the true alveolar process of the mandible or maxilla more frequently than is the apical abscess, which may extend well beyond the alveolar process into the body of the bone. Diagnosis is thus clarified: the "apical abscess" has its origin through the root canal, the "periodontal abscess" has its origin through the periodontium.[2]

Acute Apical Abscess (AAA)

The ***acute apical abscess*** is an acute inflammation of the apical tissues. Rapid onset, acute pain, extreme sensitivity of the tooth to touch, and massive swelling are its clinical features (Fig. 9–19). Obviously, it represents a major effort on the part of the body to first localize and then destroy an invasive agent. As a rule, it stems from an infection. Virulent bacteria moving from the root canal into the apical periodontal ligament provide the immediate threat. Occasionally, the toxins of a sterile pulp necrosis may be indicted.

Histopathologic illustrations of this acute process,

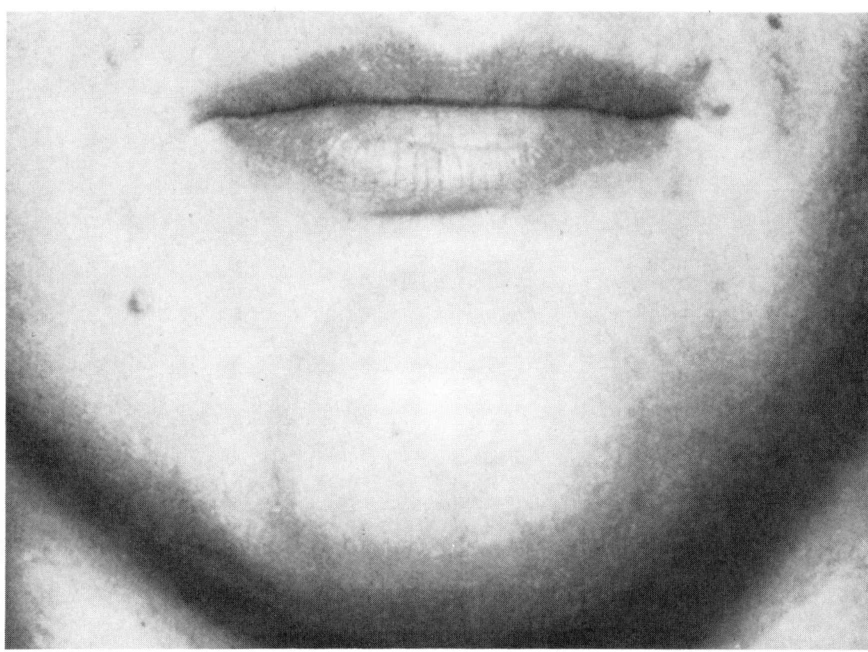

Fig. 9–19. Acute apical abscess involving mandibular incisor tooth. There is massive swelling of chin, produced by intense leukotaxis, vascular engorgement, and edema within. Lesion represents major effort on part of body, first to localize and then to destroy invasive agent.

when it is fully developed, are just not available. Biopsy is ruled out because of the impossibility of obtaining a specimen from a patient with this massive swelling. The brief life of the abscess before it is resolved by spontaneous or therapeutic drainage, or is transformed into a different lesion, has also precluded the finding of an example at autopsy. Nonetheless, we can assume that the changes that occur at the genesis of the abscess bear some resemblance to those already seen in acute apical periodontitis (Fig. 9–3). Quickly, of course, the reaction intensifies and, while still in its early development, resembles what we see in Figure 9–20. There are now many polymorphonuclear leukocytes and round cells on the scene. Enlargement of the apical blood vessels is obvious. As for the intense leukotaxis, the vascular engorgement and the edema, which together comprise the acute apical abscess as the dentist observes it (Fig. 9–19), these come later.

Roentgenographic confirmation of the acute apical abscess is also impossible. An abscess modifies bone greatly, it is true. Decalcification, however, such as is necessary for roentgenographically visible change, is a delayed process seen only after the acute inflammation has persisted in the area for several days.[13] All that is usually observed is a slight widening of the periodontal ligament space. In sum, positive diagnosis rests on the clinical findings.

Phoenix Abscess (PA)

We have just been dealing with the acute inflammation that attacks normal tissues. Chronic apical inflammation can also burst into flame. Thus, the term applied to this very situation—the ***phoenix* abscess***—is the apical lesion that develops as an acute exacerbation of a chronic or suppurative apical periodontitis.

Clinically, the phoenix abscess is often indistinguishable from the acute apical abscess. In the roentgenogram, fortunately, there is a difference. A large area of radiolucency can be seen in the film (Fig. 15–35*B*), and this eliminates any speculation in diagnosis. The radiolucency is created by inflammatory connective tissue, which has long since replaced alveolar bone at the tooth apex. Now, for the first or just another time, the dormant lesion has become the seat of an acute inflammation.

*Phoenix—one that experiences a renewal or seeming rebirth.[1]

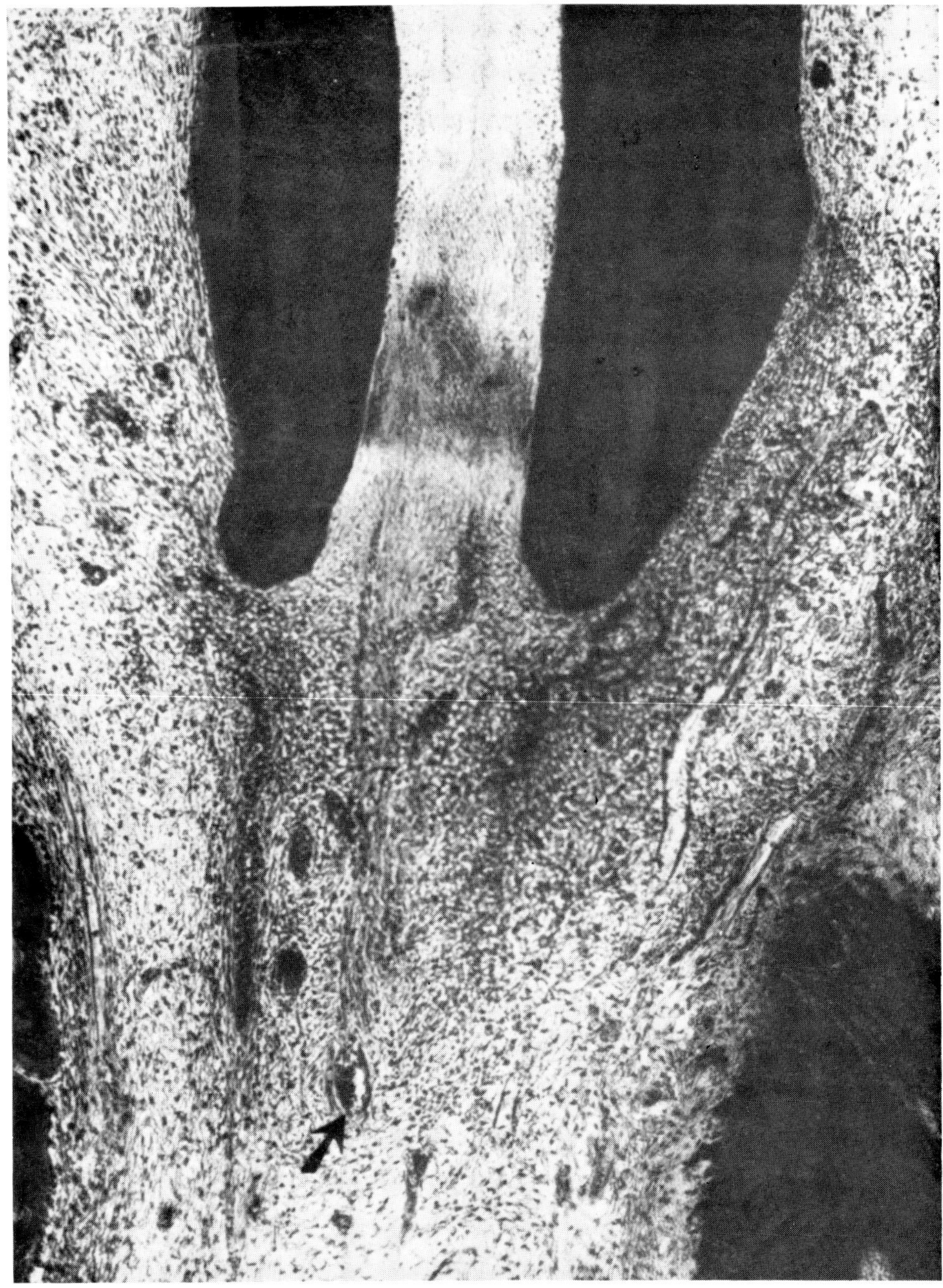

Fig. 9–20. Acute apical abscess in early stage of development before it would be observable clinically. Many polymorphonuclear leukocytes and round cells have been drawn to periapex through leukotaxis. Apical blood vessels *(arrow)* are enlarged. (From Matsumiya, S.: *Atlas of Oral Pathology.* Tokyo Dental College Press, 1955.)

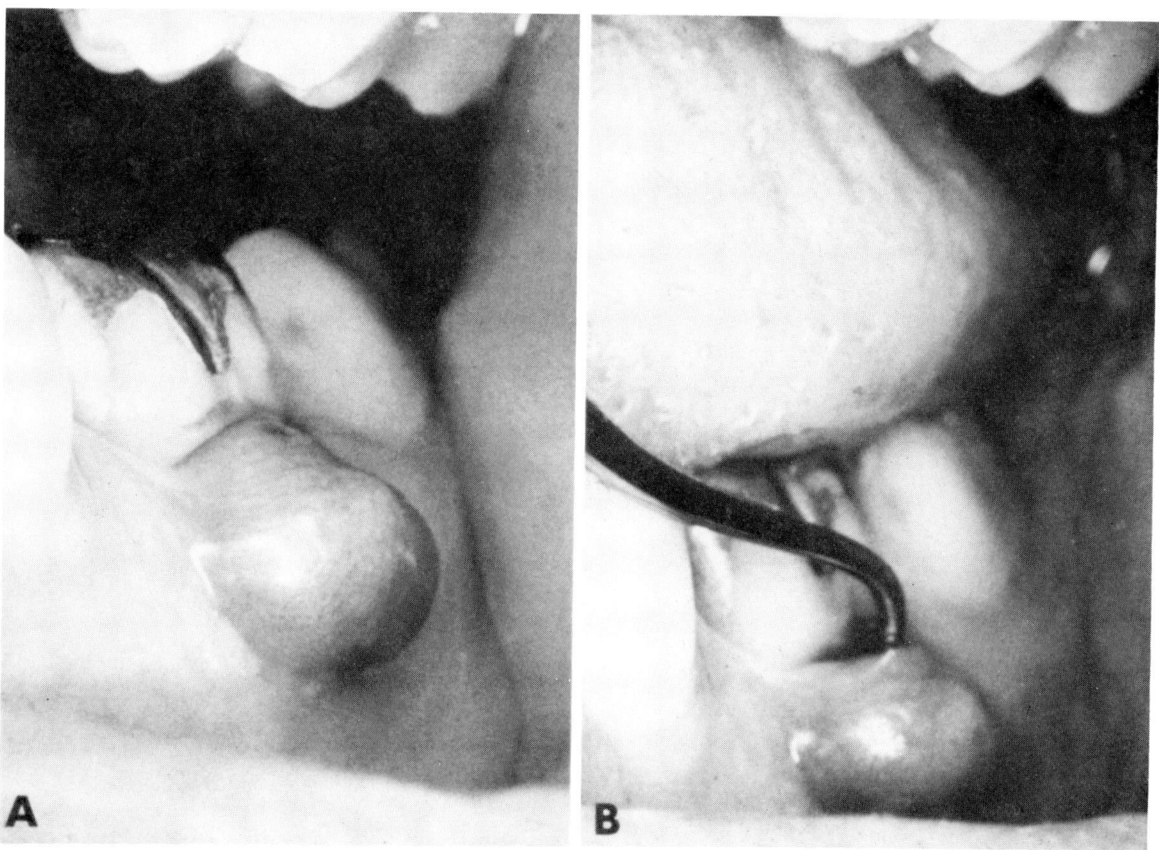

Fig. 9–21. *A,* Phoenix abscess which has pointed to oral cavity by way of buccal periodontal pocket, rather than through alveolar bone. At first glance this lesion might appear to be simply periodontal abscess. Mandibular first molar tooth. *B,* Same phoenix abscess shown in *A*. Periodontal probe has been passed far down buccal surface of tooth. Probe demonstrates continuity between apical area, furca of tooth, and gingival sulcus.

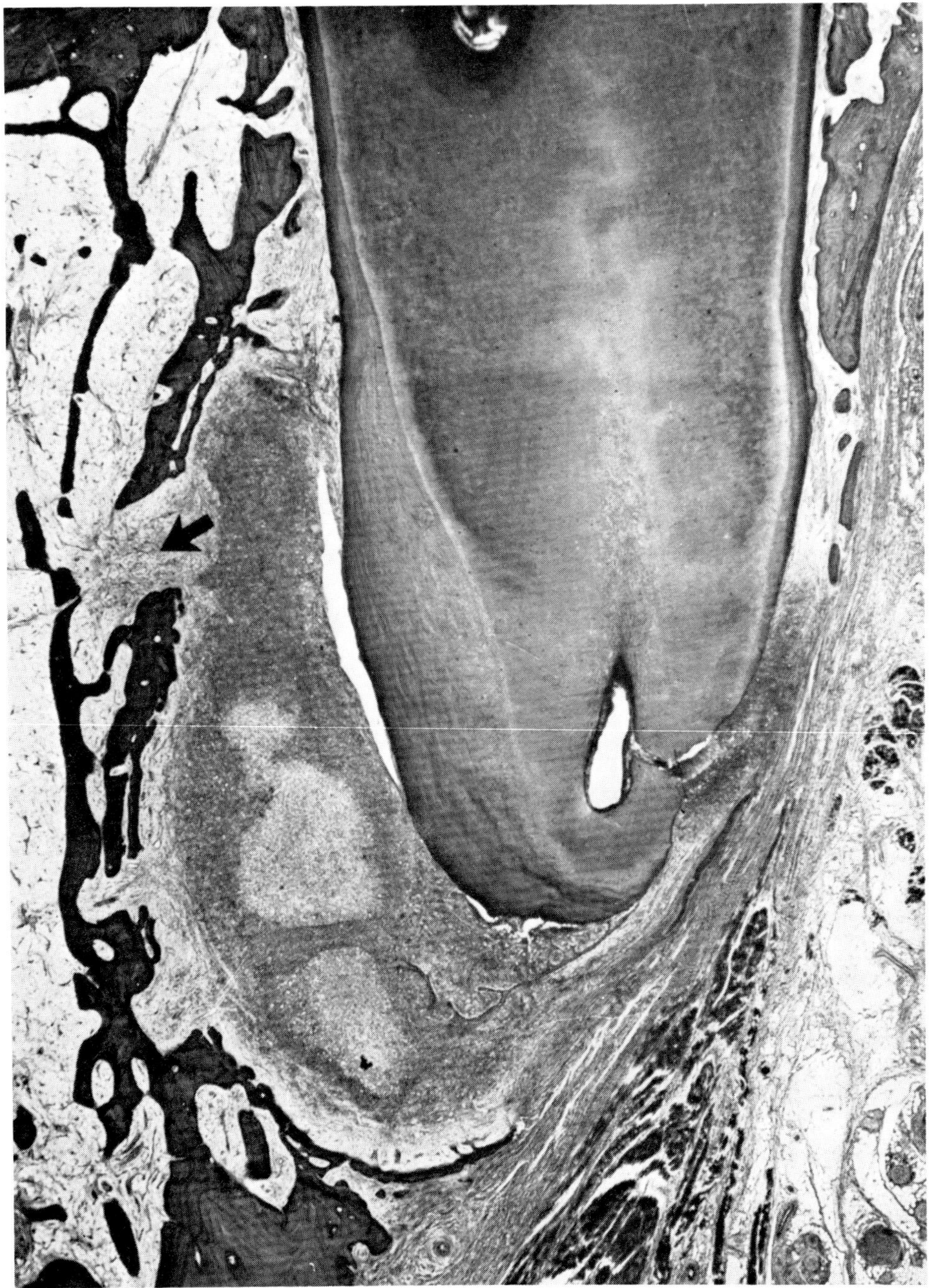

Fig. 9–22. Histopathologic features of phoenix abscess. Active abscess has developed within longstanding chronic apical periodontitis. Central zone of abscess is filled with necrotic elements. Neutrophils and round cells *(arrow)* are spreading through fibrous capsule into surrounding bone marrow spaces. (From Matsumiya, S.: *Atlas of Oral Pathology.* Tokyo Dental College Press, 1955.)

The first of the two clinical views (Fig. 9–21*A*) is that of a phoenix abscess which has "pointed" to the oral cavity, not through the alveolar housing, but instead by way of a buccal periodontal pocket. What appears to be a periodontal abscess actually is not. The companion photograph (Fig. 9–21*B*) demonstrates the continuity that did exist between the apical area, the furca, and the gingival sulcus in this patient.

Matsumiya provides an excellent photomicrograph of the phoenix abscess (Fig. 9–22). Reconstructing the clinical background he notes that an earlier abscess had breached the buccal wall of the alveolar bone. The inflammation subsided, however, and a chronic apical periodontitis remained. Later, a strong bacterial infection recurred within the focus and the present condition resulted. A large number of cells, chiefly neutrophils, have infiltrated the chronic inflammatory tissue on the abscess wall and are spreading into the surrounding bone marrow spaces. The abscess is filled with "pus cells" and other necrotic elements. An active inflammation exists.[14]

APICAL CYST

The ***apical cyst*** is a significant dental lesion. Among the periapical disorders, only the acute apical periodontitis and the chronic apical periodontitis occur more frequently. Most agree that the apical cyst is a true cyst, *i.e.*, a pathologic cavity that is lined with epithelium and often fluid-filled.

The term apical cyst is substituted (again for mnemonic reasons) in place of the time-honored "radicular cyst." The prefix "apical" directs attention to the location of the cyst and also suggests the etiology as endodontic in nature. The adjective "radicular," while it implies root, also signifies that the cyst may be at any location along the root. Thus a "lateral cyst" and the "apical cyst" are both "radicular cysts," even though the lateral cyst is found on the lateral surface of the root and is not necessarily associated with a pulpless tooth.[2]

The presence of epithelium within apical inflammatory lesions has been repeatedly confirmed.[15–17] This epithelium, with few exceptions, is derived from the epithelial rests of Malassez. The apical cyst develops within such apical lesions and from this epithelium. Actually a lined cystic cavity can develop at the site of either the chronic or the suppurative form of periodontitis. The latter metamorphosis (suppurative periodontitis to apical cyst) is, of course, less often seen.

Why and how does the cystic cavity form? The

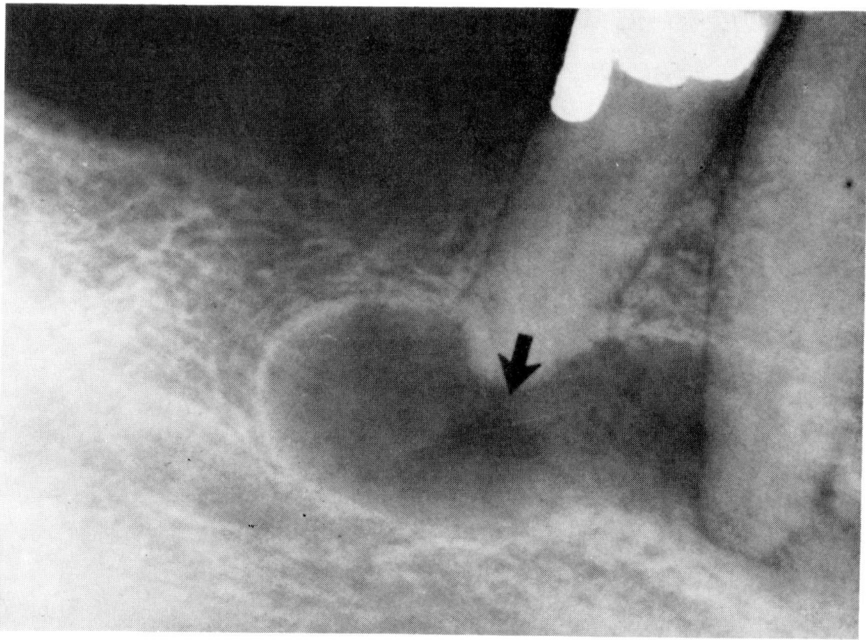

Fig. 9–23. Apical cyst of large size. Ovoid radiolucent area is very distinct. Originating within chronic apical periodontitis at apex of mandibular first premolar *(arrow)*, cyst has expanded to occupy considerable portion of mandible. Cuspid tooth remains vital. (Courtesy Dr. Clifford Ames.)

consensus views inflammation as the primary stimulus. Excited by inflammation, the epithelial cells in the apical area proliferate widely. The reticular pattern of their growth at this stage is quite dramatic (Fig. 9–8). Mitosis occurs in the basal layer of cells along the periphery of the epithelial cords and clusters. More and more layers of squamous cells are produced. Eventually, the central cells of this epithelial mass die, because they have become too far removed from the connective tissue, which is their source of nourishment. The common death of central epithelial cells leads to necrosis, necrosis to liquefaction, and liquefaction to the apical cyst—a fluid-filled cavity within epithelium. There remains unanswered, of course, an important question. Why do only some lesions of chronic apical periodontitis become apical cysts when epithelium and inflammation are present in all?

Growth of the apical cyst is a slow process. At the outset the cyst can be likened to an epithelial parasite within the apical "granuloma." Once established, the apical cyst will ***occasionally*** press on its own into new territory far beyond the CAP, into the cavity of the maxillary sinus, for example. In such an instance the original connective tissue lesion and additional alveolar bone give way before the cyst. Most apical cysts remain small. Many, in fact, stay within the limits of the inflammatory lesion which preceded them. For others, the process of local expansion continues, but at an extremely slow rate. Figures 9–23 and 9–24 provide a contrast between a larger expansive apical cyst and the common localized lesion.

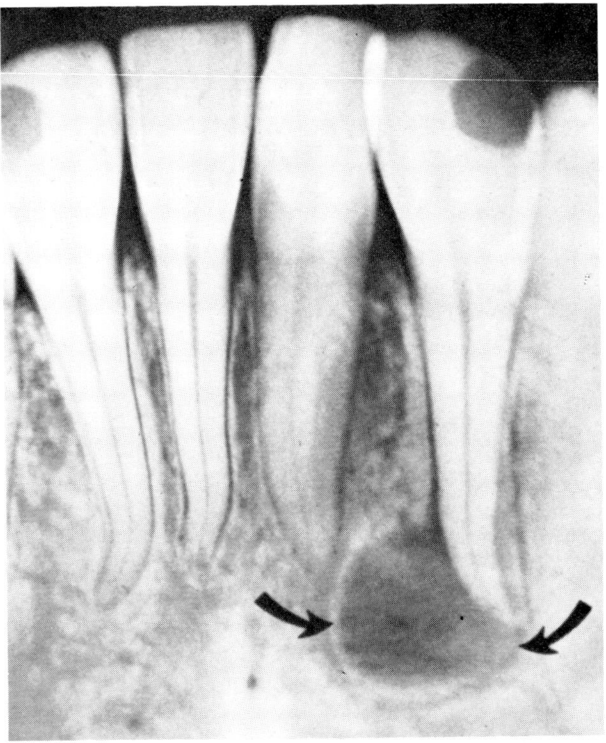

Fig. 9–24. Apical cyst of more common localized type. Boundary of cyst *(arrows)* is well demarcated in this case. However, "condensation" of peripheral bone can be feature of both apical cyst and chronic apical periodontitis (see Fig. 9–9).

How does the minute cyst become a larger one? A continued apical inflammation, the unending mitosis of epithelial cells of the cyst wall, the necrosis and liquefaction of cells, epithelial and other, which are desquamated into the cyst cavity, the resultant increase in cyst content, and finally, the resorption of bone in response to pressure from this growing volume of cyst fluid—all contribute to the expansion.

Apical cysts have in common: (1) epithelium, (2) a central lumen lined by the epithelial sheet, (3) a fluid or semi-fluid substance within the lumen, and (4) an outer capsule of connective tissue. When the cyst is young, its epithelium is continuous with the network of epithelium which has already ramified at the apex of the tooth (Fig. 9–25). Later the accessory fingers and cords seem to "retract," leaving a consolidated cyst wall (Fig. 9–26). It is impossible to ignore the inflammatory overlay in many apical cysts. Round cells often permeate both the epithelium and the immediate connective tissue (Fig. 9–27). They also enter the cyst fluid in quantity. Should inflammation dominate, the epithelial lining may be thinned or interrupted (Fig. 9–28).

A curious fluid fills the cavity of the cyst. Its slippery yet crystalline feel, and the often amber tint, render this fluid unique. Erythrocytes are rarely found when the fluid is aspirated from a cyst *in situ*. Free-floating epithelial cells and leukocytes, however, are often detected (Fig. 9–28). Cholesterol is sometimes abundant and always unmistakable when encountered. The elliptical spaces and "slits" seen in microsections are indicative of places where this crystalline substance had been before tissue preparation dissolved it away (Fig. 9–27).

The connective tissue wall of the cyst is usually composed of an inner and an outer layer. The inner zone, made up of inflammatory connective tissue, underlies the epithelium in all its ramifications. The outer peripheral layer is the true "capsule" of the cyst. Collagenous fibers here are often densely arranged. Their connections with the alveolar bone are com-

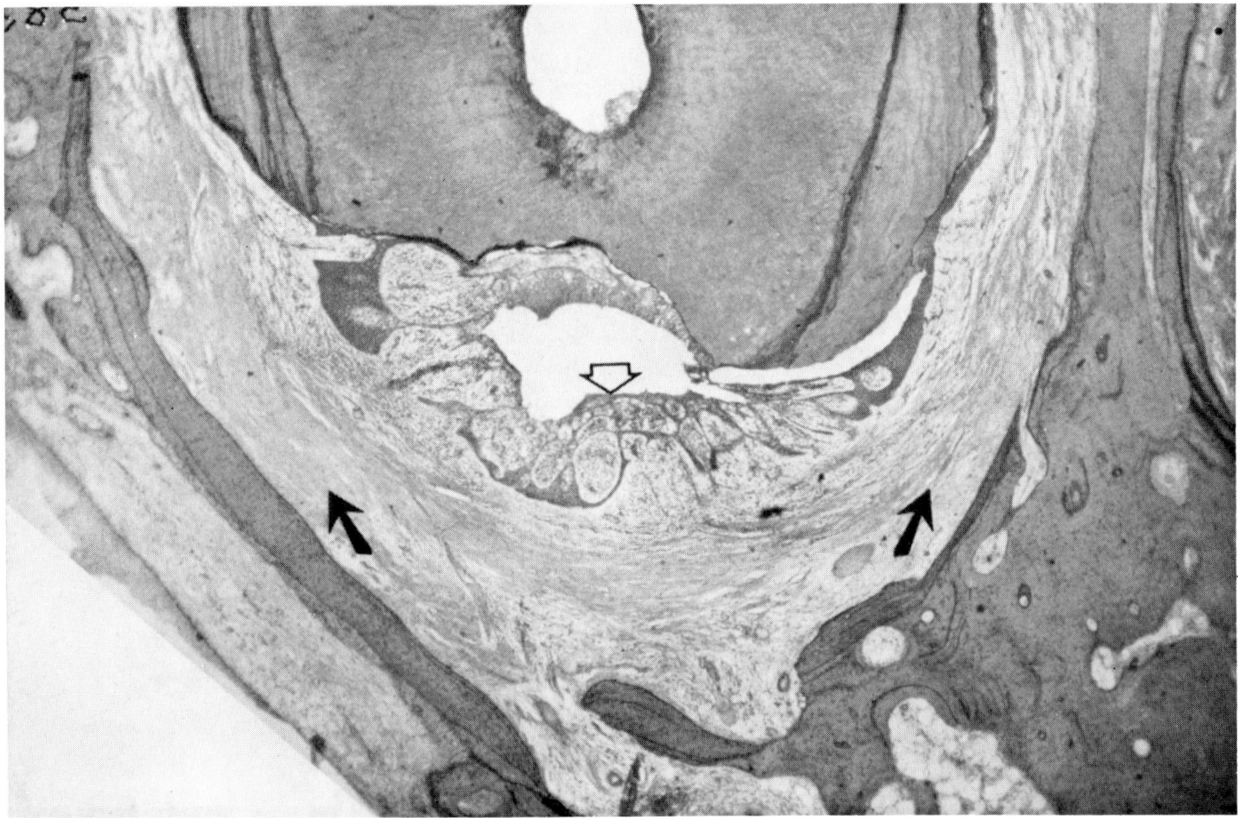

Fig. 9–25. Apical cyst, early in its development. Cyst is already characteristic. Lumen is lined by epithelium *(open arrow)* and there is distinct outer capsule *(black arrows)* of fibrous connective tissue. Preexisting epithelium merges with that of new cyst. Human tooth. (Orban collection.)

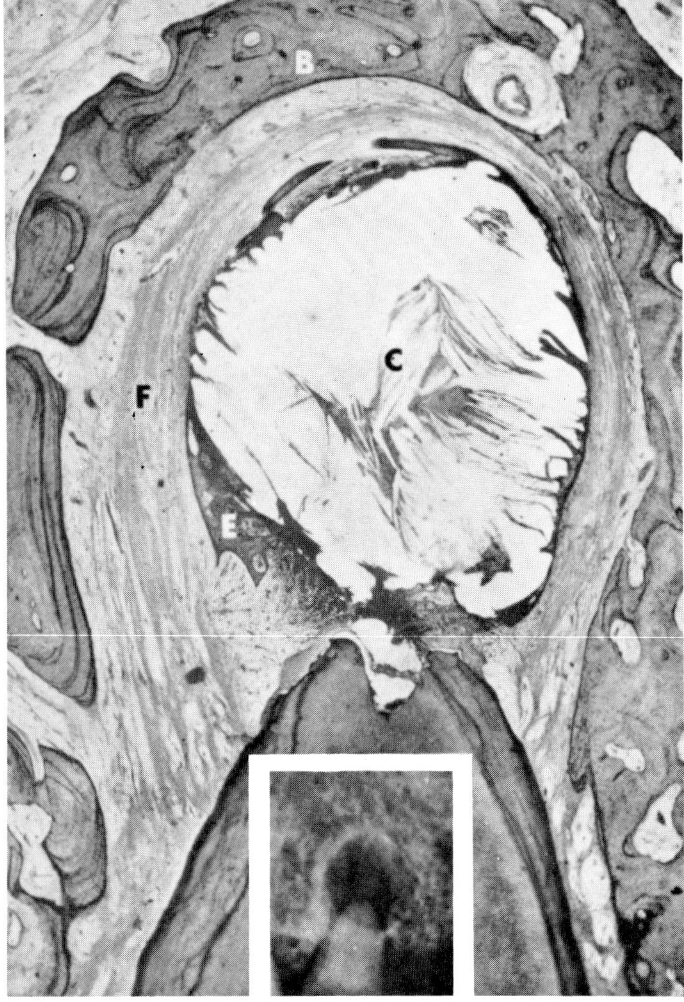

Fig. 9–26. Correlation of radiograph and biopsy of apical cyst. In this more mature cyst *(C)* accessory fingers of epithelium have "retracted," leaving consolidated cyst wall. Alveolar bone *(B)* on perimeter of cyst capsule *(F)* is also noticeably compact. This bone resembles bone of tooth socket, *i.e.*, alveolar bone proper. Human maxillary central incisor tooth. (Orban collection.)

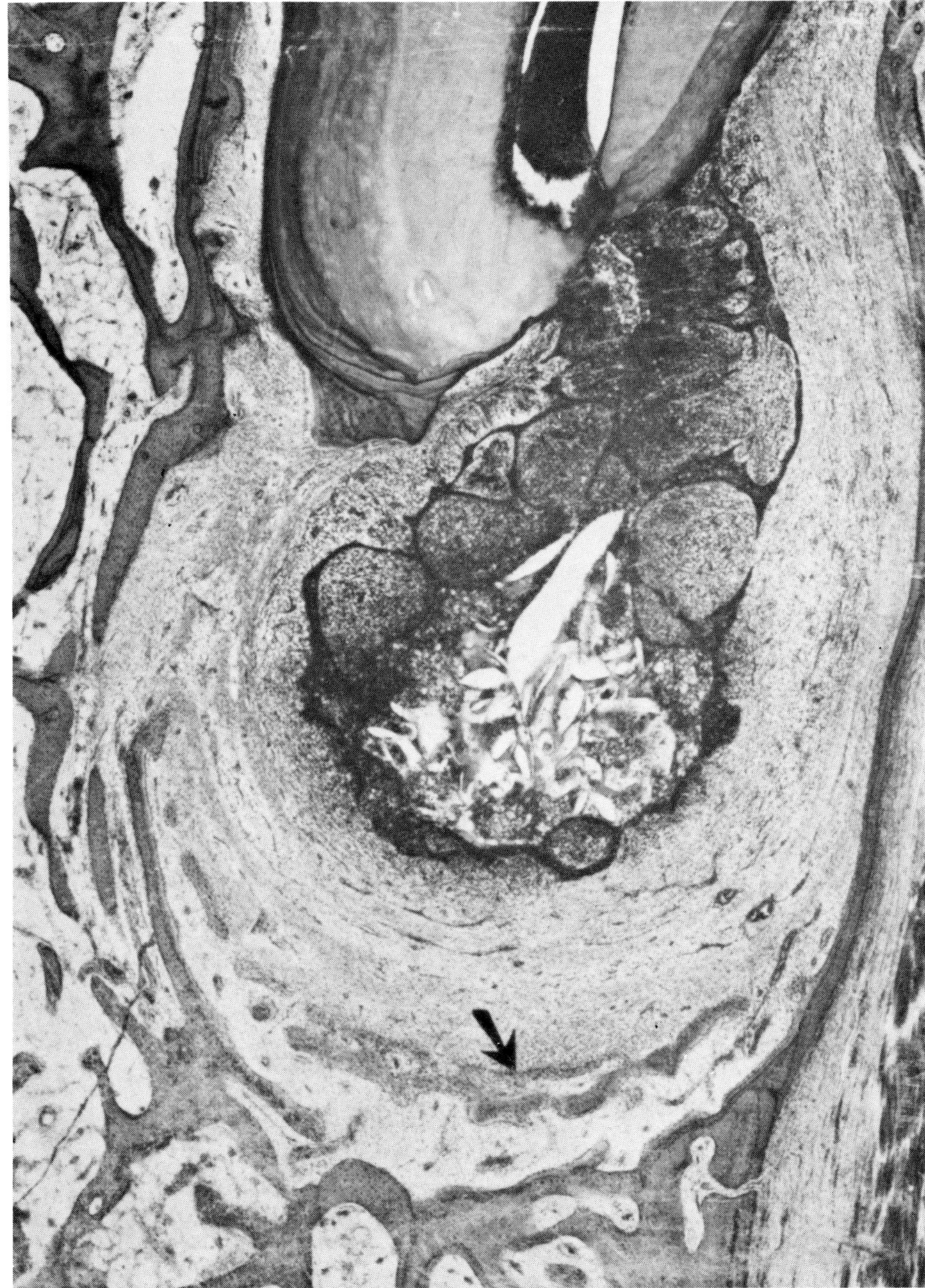

Fig. 9–27. Apical cyst with marked inflammatory overlay. Round cells permeate both epithelium and connective tissue immediately deep to it. Spaces indicate where crystalline cholesterol has formed within cyst. Bone formation is evident *(arrow)*. This may reflect narrowing of width of connective tissue zone, as occurs in some apical cysts. Human tooth. (From Matsumiya, S.: *Atlas of Oral Pathology*. Tokyo Dental College Press, 1955.)

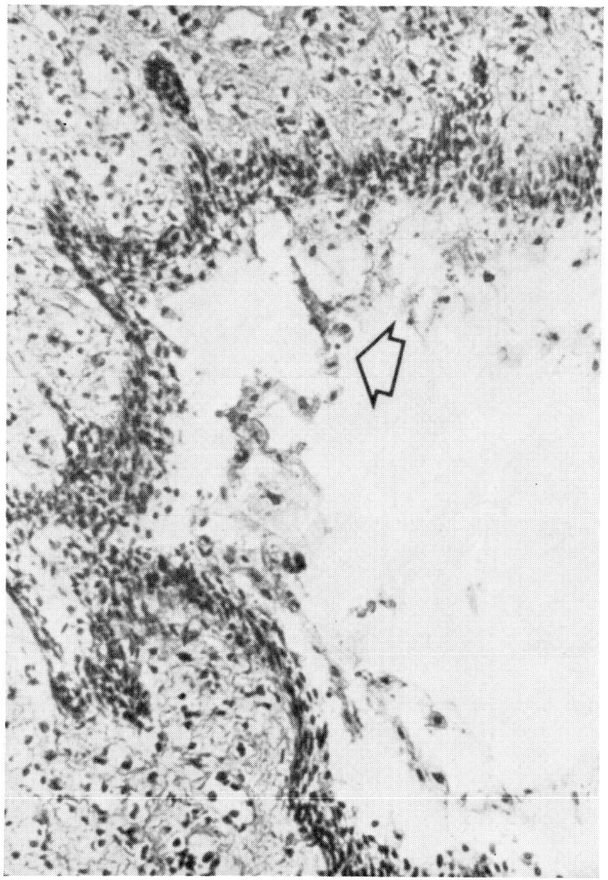

Fig. 9–28. Central cavity, epithelial lining and some of the connective tissue wall of human apical cysts. Both epithelial cells and leukocytes are floating free within cyst cavity *(arrow)*. Epithelial lining is thin and penetrated by many round cells. Connective tissue shows moderate chronic inflammation.

paratively loose, however. For this reason, it is often possible to enucleate an apical cyst intact. Occasionally, tooth and cyst are removed as one (Fig. 9–29).

The outermost boundary, of course, is the alveolar bone. Always responsive, the bone tells its own story of growth or *status quo* in the life of the cyst. Evidences of new peripheral bone are often seen (Fig. 9–27). These may reflect a narrowing of the connective tissue zone as the inflammatory process diminishes. The majority of jaw sections available to us show trabeculae of compact bone on the margins of the apical cysts. In fact, the bone that forms the cystic enclosure and the bone of the alveolar tooth socket (alveolar bone proper) present a similar appearance (Fig. 9–26).

The apical cyst has many of the clinical and roentgenographic features of chronic apical periodontitis. This is to be expected. After all, the cyst arises as a rule within an existing apical CAP and often remains a minor feature of that inflammatory tissue mass. Both grow slowly. Both are asymptomatic. Seldom does either expand to a size greater than that of a large pea. On a roentgenographic basis alone, distinction between the two is usually impossible. To merely state the obvious, the roentgenogram can reveal neither the epithelial lining nor the fluid content of a cyst. The observation of a fine radiopaque line on the circumference of the area (Fig. 9–24) cannot be considered diagnostic. Several studies have made clear that this "condensation" of peripheral bone is not limited to the apical cyst, but occurs in the case of chronic apical periodontitis as well.[18–20] It is interesting to note that both CAP and cyst may be invisible in the roentgenogram. Should either lesion grow entirely within cancellous bone, the intact outer cortical plate of the alveolar process can impart a normal image despite the presence of the lesion inside.[21]

Direct observation of apical lesions during treatment reveals much to the dentist. But many a small cyst, we may be sure, passes unnoticed during the clinical inspection. Only serial microscopic sections, carefully studied, reveal the epithelium-lined cavity of the early cyst. Bhaskar recently completed an analysis of 2,348 radiolucencies (Table 9–1). The incidence of apical cysts was found to be high (42.7%) and only a little below that of chronic and suppurative apical periodontitis combined (48.1%).[22]

Table 9–1. Analysis of 2,348 Apical Radiolucencies

Type of Periapical Lesion	*Incidence (%)*
Chronic and suppurative apical periodontitis	48.1
Apical cyst	42.7
Residual cyst	3.6
Apical scar	2.7
Cementoma (periapical osteofibrosis—stage 1)	1.3
Apical abscess	1.1
Cholestotoma	0.4
Giant cell lesion	0.1
	100.0

From Bhaskar, S. N.: Personal communication, 1964.

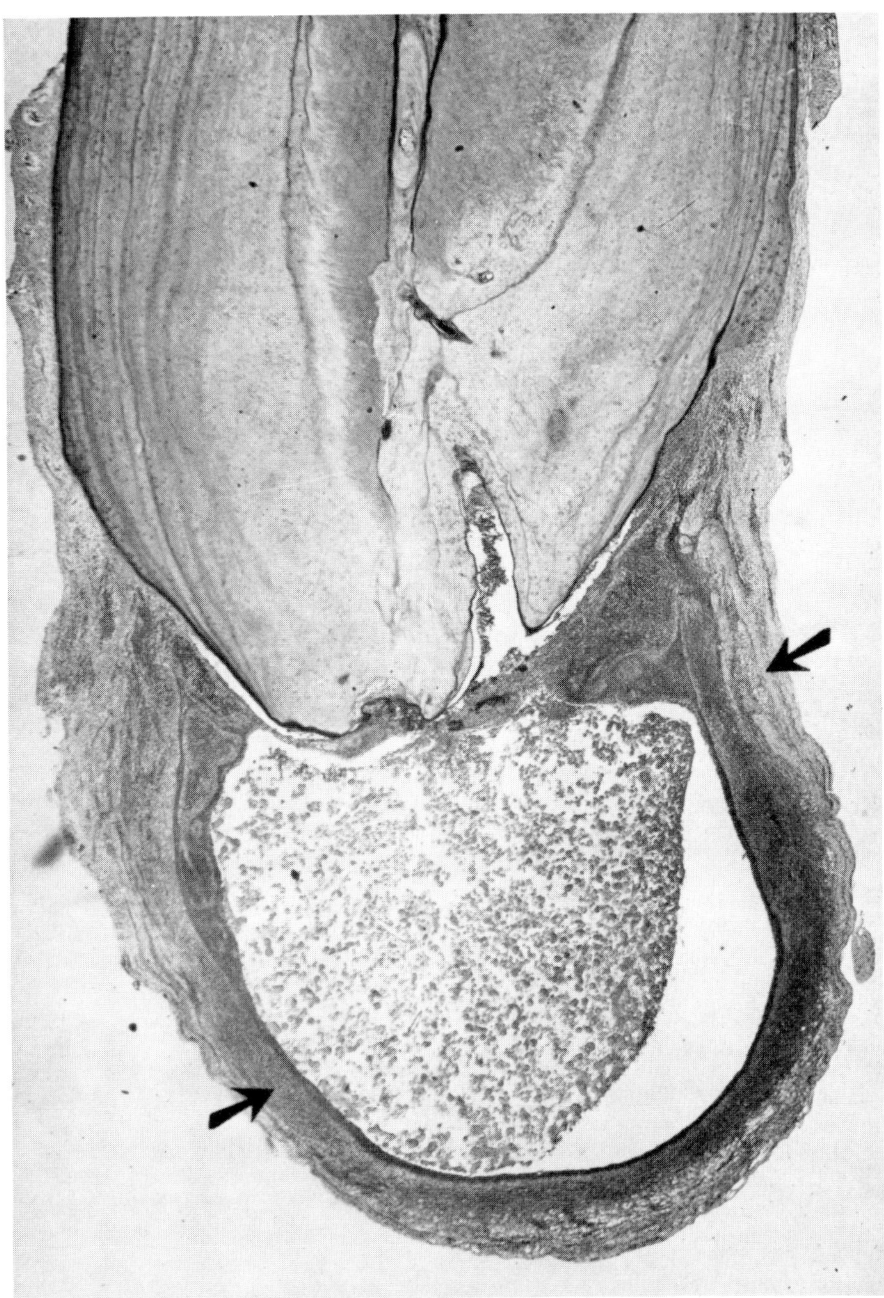

Fig. 9–29. Intact apical cyst with its associated tooth. Inner layer *(right arrow),* made up of inflammatory connective tissue, underlies epithelium. Outer layer *(left arrow)* is true "capsule" of cyst. Collagenous fibers within "capsule" are often densely arranged. Their connections with alveolar bone are comparatively loose, however, and for this reason it is often possible to enucleate apical cyst intact. Human tooth. (From Matsumiya, S.: *Atlas of Oral Pathology.* Tokyo Dental College Press, 1955.)

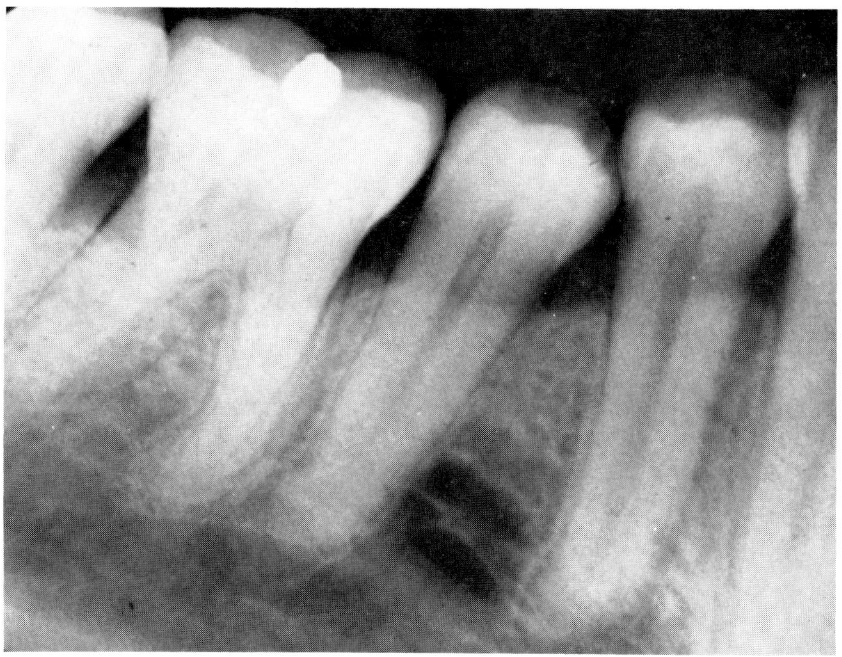

Fig. 9–30. Residual cyst in alveolar bone of mandible. Radiolucent area between roots of two premolar teeth was found during course of routine roentgenographic survey. Both premolars have vital pulps and area is completely asymptomatic.

RESIDUAL CYST

Occasionally the dentist sees an isolated radiolucent area in the alveolar bone that proves to be a ***residual cyst*** (Fig. 9–30). Theoretically these should be more prevalent than is the case. After all, many an apical cyst lining is incompletely removed or is left behind following tooth extraction. Evidently a certain stimulus must be provided the residual epithelium before it will develop into a new cyst. The same holds true, of course, in chronic apical periodontitis.

Only a few specimens of residual cyst have been closely described. Kronfeld noted the basic epithelium, cavity, and capsule.[16] He stressed the absence of inflammatory cells, both in the epithelial lining and in the connective tissue zone. Uncommon and uncomplicated, the lesion offers few problems.

GLOBULOMAXILLARY CYST

When a distinct radiolucency is noted in the maxillary anterior, the ***globulomaxillary cyst*** must be kept in mind. This is a nondental cyst arising from epithelial remnants along the fusion line of the median nasal and maxillary processes. Accordingly, while it may envelop the root ends of the lateral incisor and/or the cuspid, these teeth remain vital. If

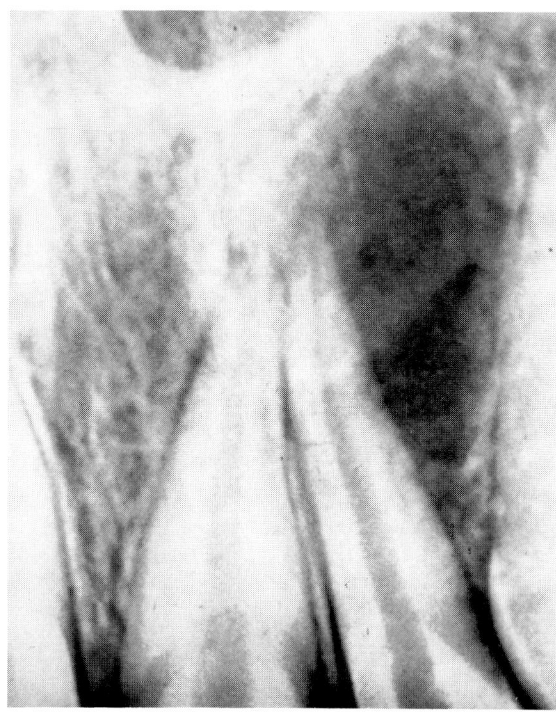

Fig. 9–31. Almond-shaped globulomaxillary cyst which has developed from epithelial remnants in suture line of premaxilla, *i.e.*, fusion line of median nasal and maxillary processes. (Courtesy Dr. S. N. Bhaskar and Walter Reed Army Institute of Research.)

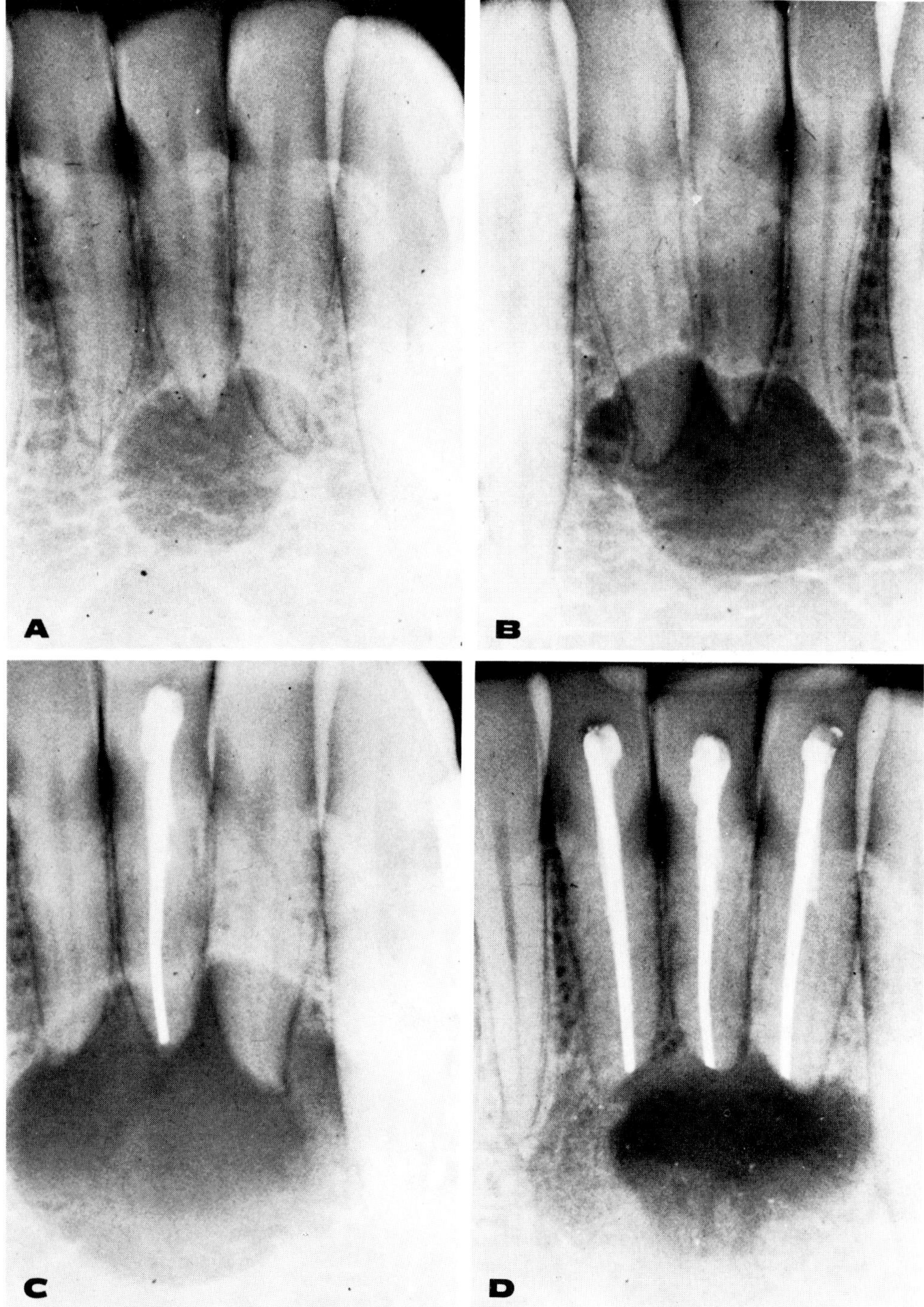

Fig. 9–32. Recurrence of a keratinizing follicular cyst. *A,* Initial radiograph of lesion at apex of pulpless left central incisor. *B*, Obvious increase in size within five months. Root canal therapy was done at this time—no sugery. *C*, Four months later lesion has greatly increased in size. *D,* Enucleation and biopsy proved lesion to be keratinizing follicular cyst. Root canal therapy was done on two adjacent incisors. Six months postoperative film shows some improvement.

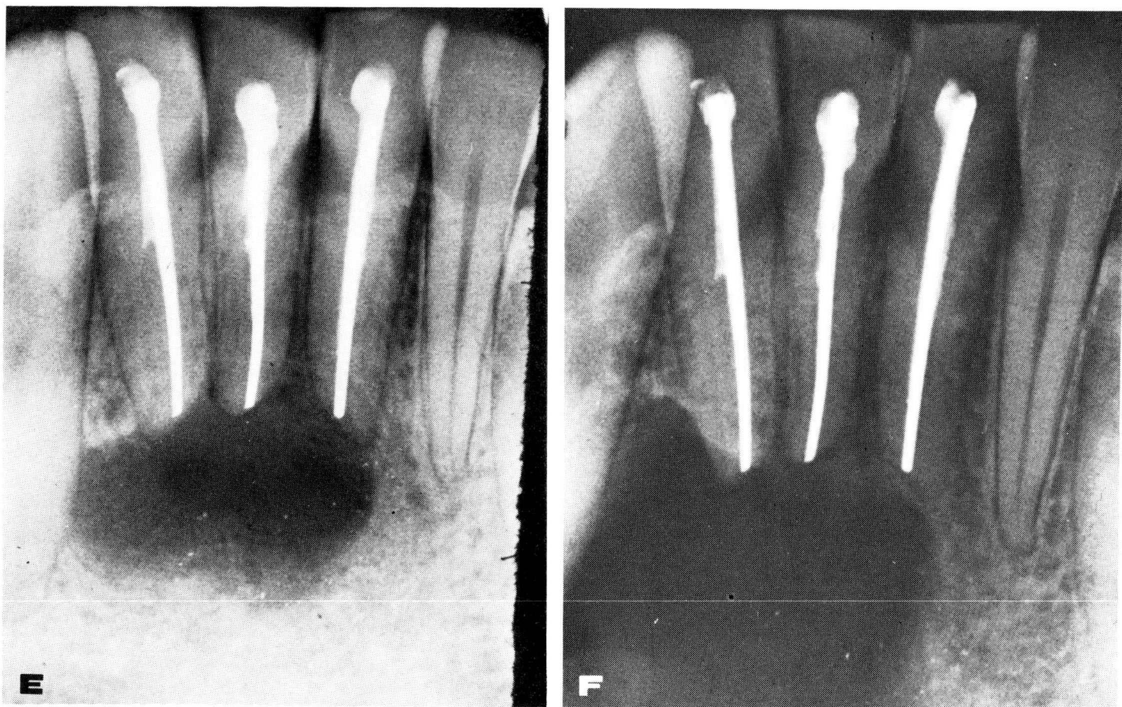

Fig. 9–32 continued. *E,* At 22 months lesion is again increasing in size. *F,* One year later lesion is 2 × 2 cm., swollen and painful. Biopsy following surgery proved lesion to be a recurrent keratinizing follicular cyst. (From Melrose, R. J., Cooperman, H. H., and Abrams, A. M.: J. South. Cal. Dent. Assoc., *37*:186, Apr., 1969.)

it were an apical cyst, at least one of these teeth would be nonvital. Histopathologic features are those of a noninflamed cyst. Diagnosis of the globulomaxillary cyst, therefore, means the placing of emphasis on roentgenographic evidence (Fig. 9–31) and the use of the biopsy more as a confirmation.

KERATINIZING FOLLICULAR CYST

The keratinizing follicular cyst has an unusual biologic potential—it has a marked propensity for recurrence. In a series of 250 consecutive cases of keratinizing cysts, Crawford found approximately a 10% recurrence rate.[24]

Melrose, Cooperman, and Abrams have pointed out the primordial origin of these cysts—follicular rather than dentigerous as is the more common apical cyst.[25] Keratinizing cysts arise from either the enamel organ epithelium or remnants of the dental lamina. They "are considered to be the most aggressive of the jaw cysts in terms of their ability to destroy bone and attain considerable size before discovery" (Fig. 9–32).

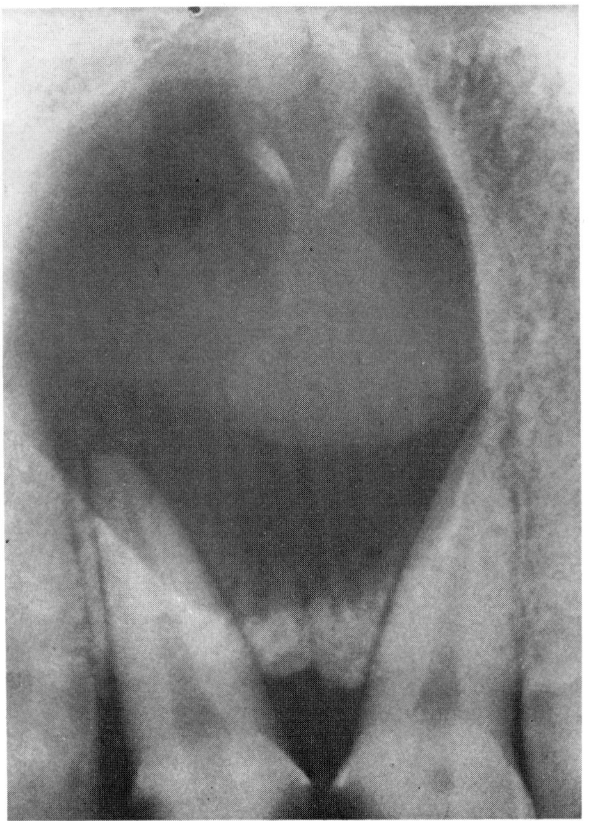

Fig. 9–33. Divergent roots of central incisors is pathognomonic of cyst. Biopsy proved this to be median palatine cyst. (From Courage, G. R., North, A. F., and Hansen, L. S.: Oral Surg., *37*:745, May, 1974.)

MEDIAN PALATINE CYST

"The median palatine cyst is defined as a fissural cyst located in the midline of the hard palate, posterior to the anterior palatine papilla. Pathogenesis of this cyst has been ascribed to proliferation of epithelial remnants entrapped within the palatal suture."[26] It is often confused with the nasopalatine duct cyst or other cysts in the area including apical cysts of the central incisors.

Courage, North, and Hansen reviewed 12 cases reported since 1957, a fact that makes this a rare cyst.[26] It has the pathognomonic propensity of all cysts to move teeth, in this case widely diverging the roots (Fig. 9–33).

PERIAPICAL OSTEOFIBROSIS

What is commonly termed the cementoma is more accurately a ***periapical osteofibrosis.***[27] The true cementoma, on the other hand, is a rare neoplasm of cementum which is attached to the tooth root.[28,29]

Periapical osteofibrosis has an interesting evolution. The trend is from normal alveolar bone, to fibrosis, to a dense, atypical reossification. The initial stage (fibrosis stage or osteolytic stage) is characterized by a proliferation of fibroblasts and collagenous fibers in the apical periodontal ligament. The resultant mass induces resorption of the lamina dura and its surrounding medullary bone (Fig. 9–34). Unlike the tissue of apical periodontitis or apical cyst, this new growth is free of inflammation. Furthermore, nerves and vessels "ignore" it as they make their passage to and from the root canal.

In time, cementoblasts or osteoblasts differentiate within the soft tissue and a central focus of calcification appears (the intermediate stage) (Fig. 9–35). A deposit of bone-like tissue may be continued over years of time until nearly all the fibrotic tissue is reossified (Fig. 9–36). When this occurs the evolution has reached its third and final stage[30] (Fig. 9–37*A*, *B*, and *C*).

Problems of diagnosis arise in conjunction with the initial radiolucent stage of periapical osteofibrosis (Fig. 9–38). These are reviewed in Chapter 10.

The true cementoma is a neoplasm of calcified tissue resembling both bone and cementum. As a rule it takes the form of a growing mass confluent with the root of the tooth (Fig. 9–37*D*). The student of endodontics should keep in mind that the tumor does on occasion advance up the root canal.[31,32] A column of pulp tissue remains in the root canal. Thus the

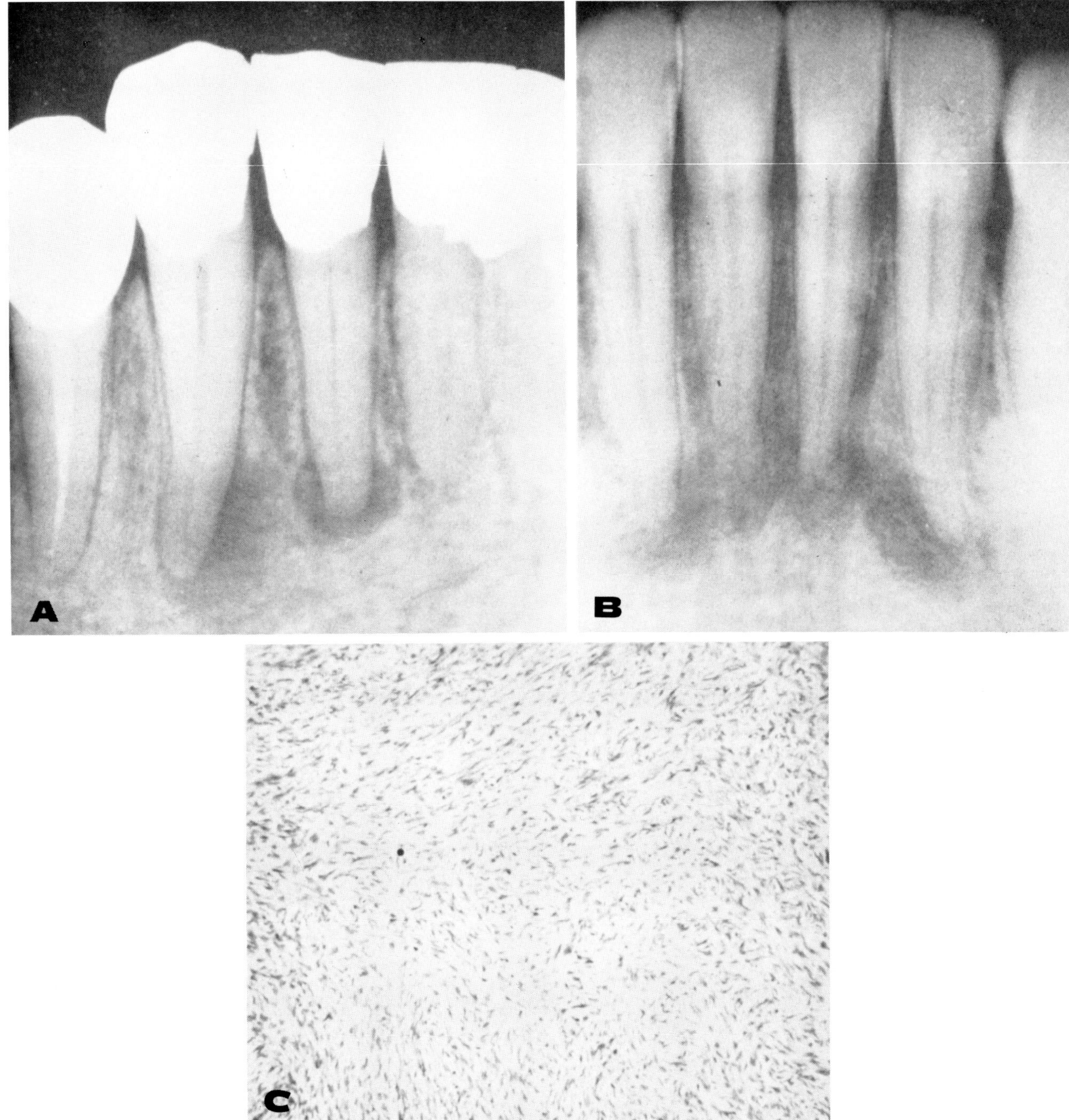

Fig. 9–34. *A,* Periapical osteofibrosis, stage one. Pulps in both teeth are vital. Transition to stage two is developing in roentgenogram, *B.* *C,* Biopsy of periapical osteofibrosis, stage one. Fibrous connective tissue lesion has replaced cancellous bone. (Photomicrograph courtesy Dr. S. N. Bhaskar and the Walter Reed Army Institute of Research. U.S. Army Photograph.)

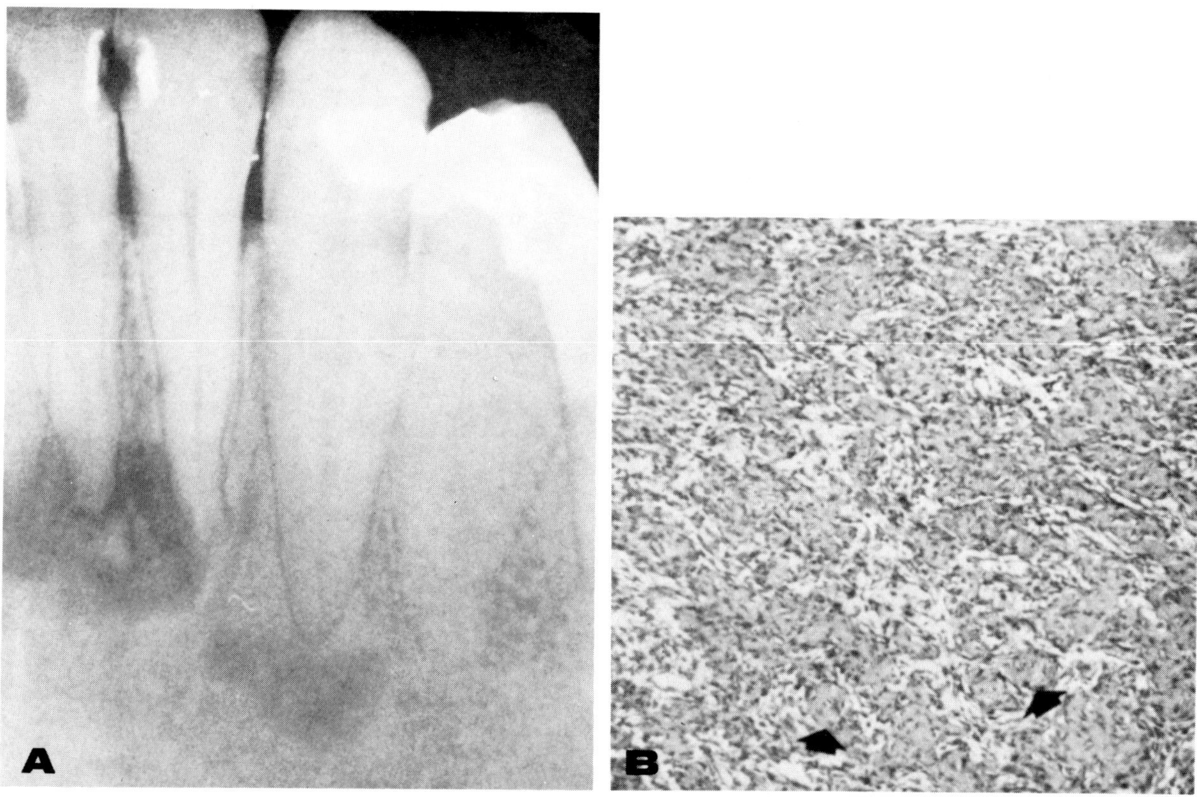

Fig. 9–35. *A,* Periapical osteofibrosis, stage two. Slight calcification of fibrotic lesion is now developing. Pulps are vital. *B,* Biopsy of stage two with foci *(arrows)* of calcification appearing throughout lesion. (Photomicrograph courtesy Dr. S. N. Bhaskar and the Walter Reed Army Institute of Research. U.S. Army Photograph.)

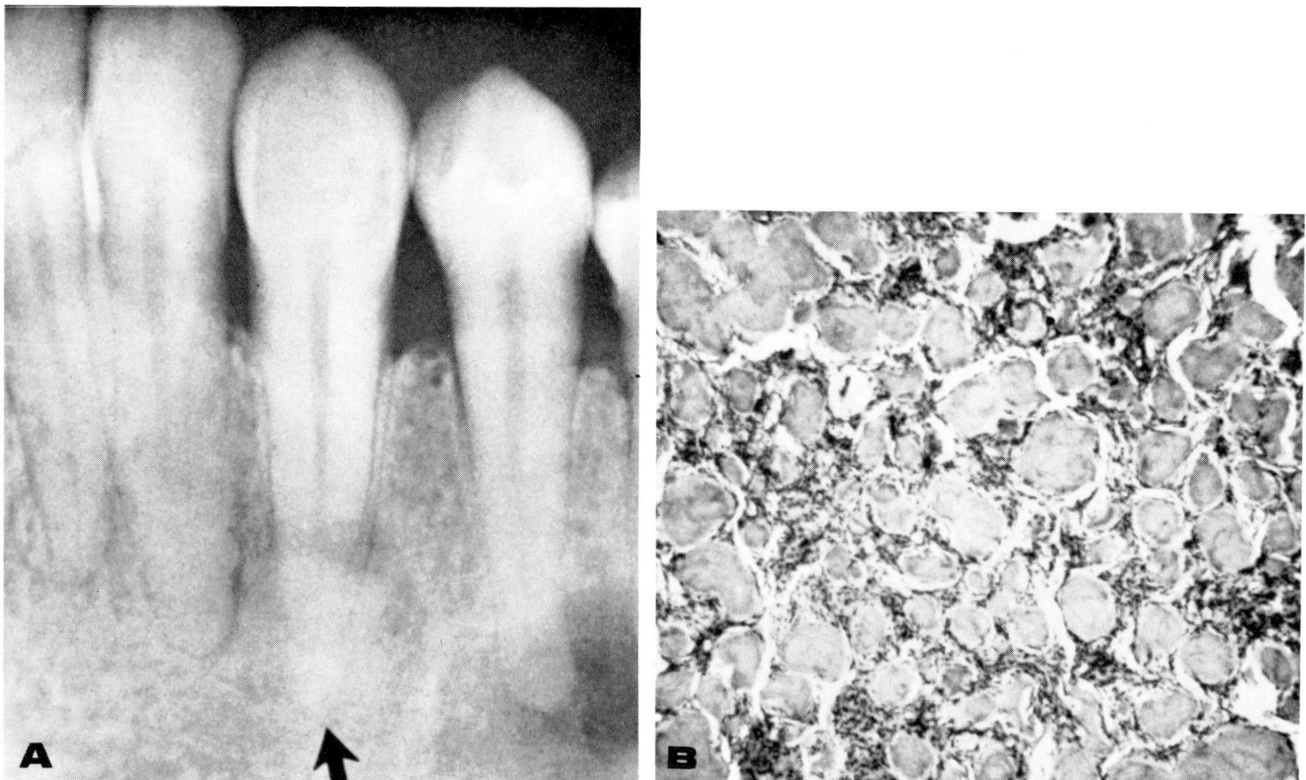

Fig. 9–36. *A,* Periapical osteofibrosis, stage three. Osseous calcification *(arrow)* associated with vital pulp. Fibrotic stage one is seen at periapex of first premolar. *B,* Biopsy of stage three with advanced, dense calcification. (Photomicrograph courtesy Dr. S. N. Bhaskar and the Walter Reed Army Institute of Research. U.S. Army Photograph.)

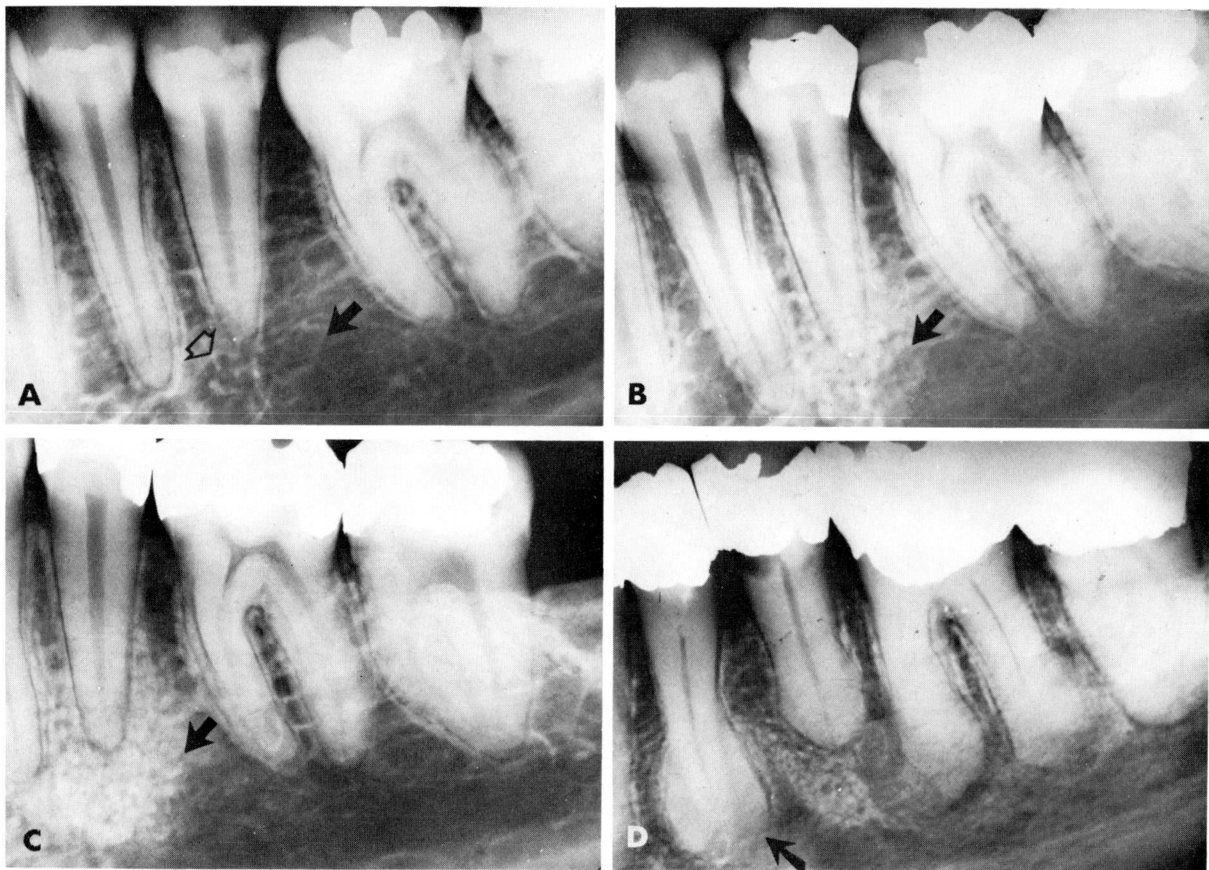

Fig. 9–37. Five year, chronologic development of periapical osteofibrosis in young female patient. *A,* Stage one. Lesion *(black arrow)* is hardly discernible from surrounding radiolucency. Slightly lobulated appearance *(open arrow)* is only discernible feature.

B, Stage two. Osteofibrosis two years later.

C, Stage three. Osteofibrosis five years following initial roentgenogram. Mandibular lesions are bilateral.

D, Roentgenogram of ***mother*** of patient shown in *A, B,* and *C.* The cementoma *(arrow)* and periapical osteofibrosis in daughter bring out possible familial background. (Courtesy Dr. Clifford Ames.)

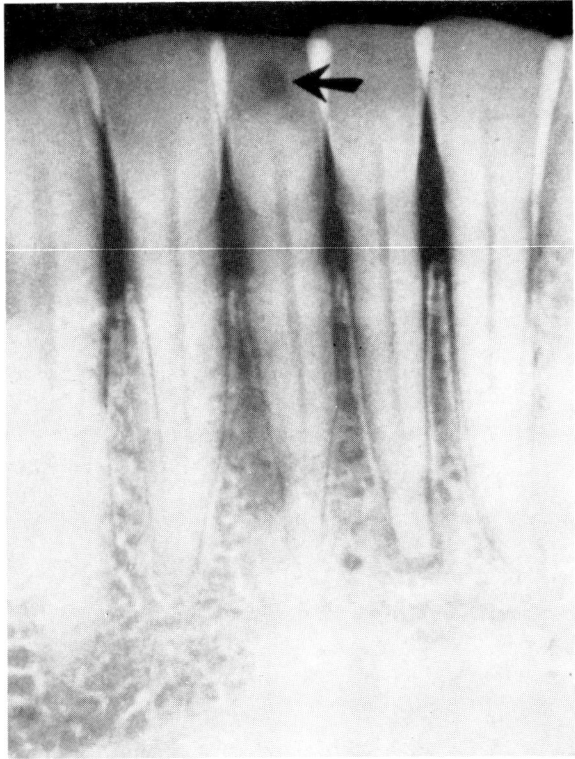

Fig. 9–38. Error in diagnosis of periapical osteofibrosis. Referring dentist has started to open into vital pulp *(arrow)* on roentgenographic evidence alone when lesion was in radiolucent fibrotic stage one. Lesion is now calcified to stage three. Adjacent incisor exhibits stage one fibrosis.

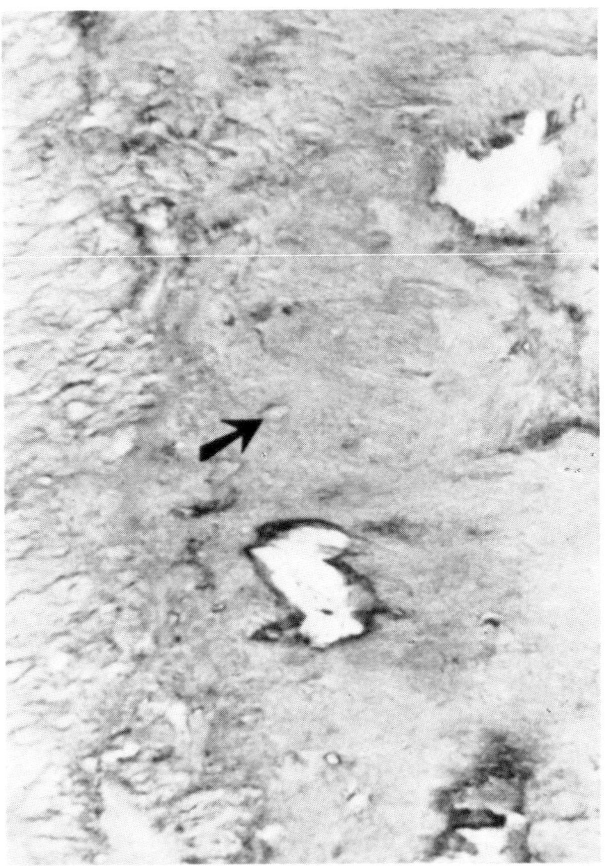

Fig. 9–39. Biopsy features of either "true" cementoma or third stage ("mature") periapical osteofibrosis. Tissue resembles compact bone more than cellular cementum. Minute spaces *(arrow)* closely resemble lacunae of bone. Several large clear areas are reminiscent of nutrient canals. Fibers similar to Sharpey's fibers or periodontal ligament fibers can be seen entering left margin. Biopsy of calcified mass which was attached to root of human tooth.

tumor as well as the pulp of the coronal chamber are sustained.

There is little if any microscopic distinction to be made between the "true" cementoma and the "mature" periapical osteofibrosis. The tissue in its bulk and morphology resembles compact bone much more than even cellular cementum (Fig. 9–39).

(APICAL) CONDENSING OSTEITIS

Increased calcification of bone at the apex of teeth is a common finding in dental practice. An example has already been noted during the third stage of periapical osteofibrosis. More often than not, though, the circumscribed radiopaque area at a root apex represents a response of alveolar bone to pulp inflammation or to pulp necrosis. Instead of the customary removal of apical bone in the face of inflammation, there is a stimulation of the osseous tissue. Osteoblasts form more bony trabeculae, the trabeculae merge, and marrow spaces are reduced to a minimum (Fig. 9–40). All this implies strong resistance to irritants released at the apical foramen. The lesion is noted most often, therefore, around the apices of young permanent teeth involved in chronic pulpitis. Endodontic treatment can bring about a reversal of the process and the disappearance of the radiopaque area (Fig. 9–41).

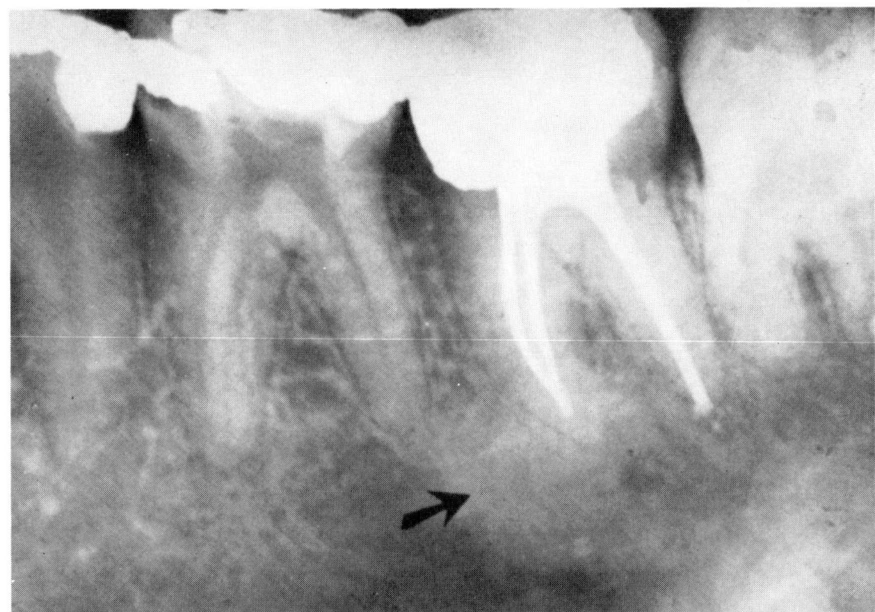

Fig. 9–40. Apical condensing osteitis which developed in response to chronic pulpitis. Radiopaque area *(arrow)* can be observed in alveolar bone at apex of mesial root of second molar. Additional bony trabeculae have been formed and marrow spaces have been reduced to minimum. Periodontal ligament space is visible, despite increased radiopacity of nearby bone. Endodontic treatment of tooth has only recently been completed. Condensing osteitis predated this treatment.

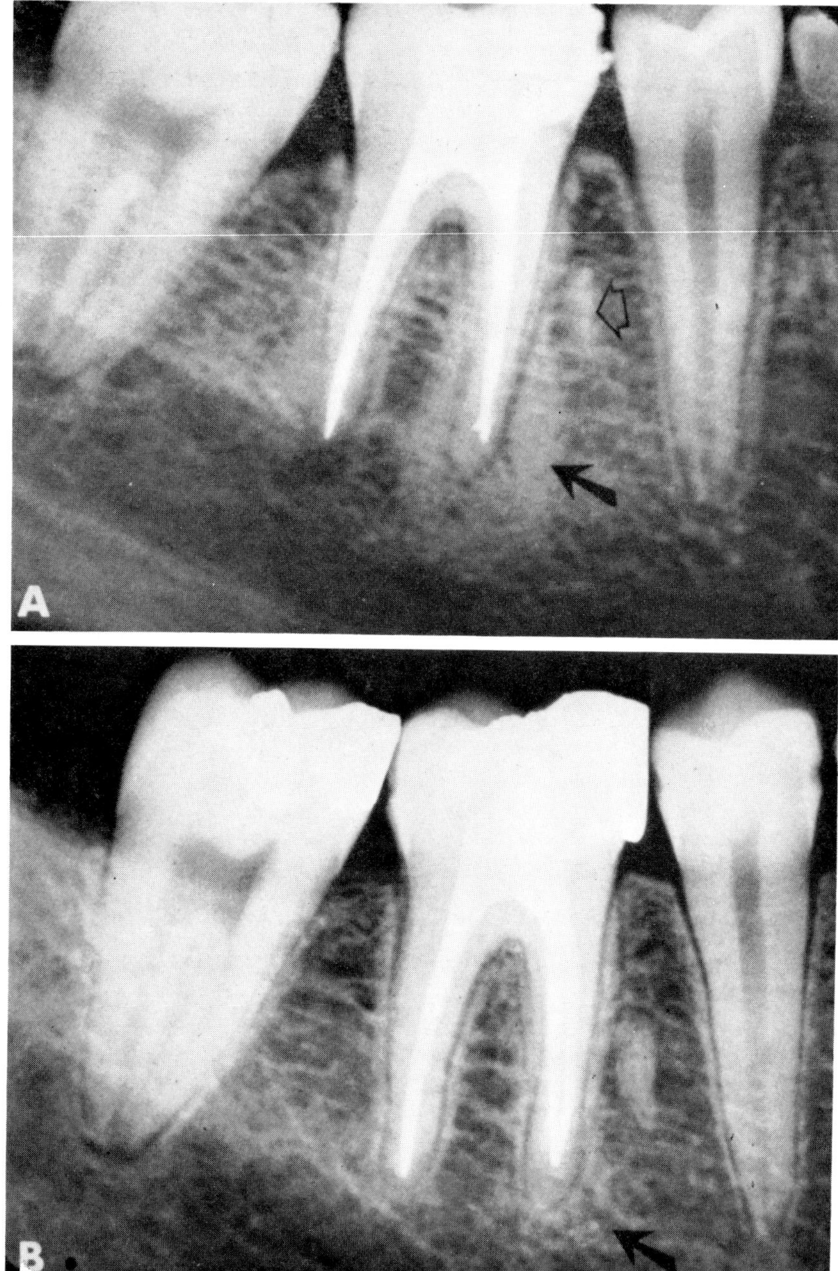

Fig. 9–41. *A,* Apical condensing osteitis associated with chronic pulpitis. Endodontic treatment has just been completed. Obvious condensation of alveolar bone *(black arrow)* is noticeable around mesial root of first molar. Radiolucent area is evident at apex of distal root of same tooth. Retained primary molar root tip *(open arrow)* lies within alveolar septum mesial to molar. *B,* Resolution *(arrow)* of apical condensing osteitis shown in *A* one year following endodontic treatment. From radiographic standpoint complete repair of both periapical lesions has been obtained. Reversal of apical condensing osteitis and disappearance of radiopaque area is possible.

TUMORS

Both benign and malignant tumors occur in the oral cavity—some primary in origin, others metastatic. Often the radiographic evidence of their existence mimics bone lesions associated with endodontic periapical disease. In addition, pulps may be devitalized by the invasive malignant disease to complicate and confuse accurate diagnosis.

Carcinoma of primary oral origin, beginning on oral mucous membranes and invading the bone (Fig. 9–42), is, of course, more easily diagnosed than primary sarcoma or metastatic tumors. Bone-invasive oral carcinoma may be ***seen*** on physical examination as well as radiographically. However, primary sarcoma or adenocarcinoma of the salivary glands that invades the jaws may be more difficult to differentiate.

Unquestionably the most difficult to diagnose is metastatic disease. Abrams and Melrose have reported such a case from the Oral Tumor Board at the University of Southern California.[33] A 50-year-old woman was initially seen with a swelling in the lower right jaw (Fig. 9–43). She complained of a numbness and a lump in her jaw of two weeks duration. She also claimed the teeth felt "a little loose." Past history revealed the patient had been treated for carcinoma of the left breast six months previously by radical mastectomy and postoperative cobalt 60.

Oral examination revealed buccal swelling in the right mandible, which was slightly painful to palpation. The premolar teeth were quite loose and the canine was moderately mobile. No periodontal pockets were probed.

Electric pulp testing revealed that the canine, both premolars, and the second molar (the first molar was missing) all tested nonvital.

In the roentgenogram (Fig. 9–44), the unusual vague outline of the bony lesion is apparent as well as the external resorption of the three teeth directly involved. The "moth-eaten" root resorption, as well as the sharp chisel-shaped apical resorption, is not at all typical of the usual periapical lesion.

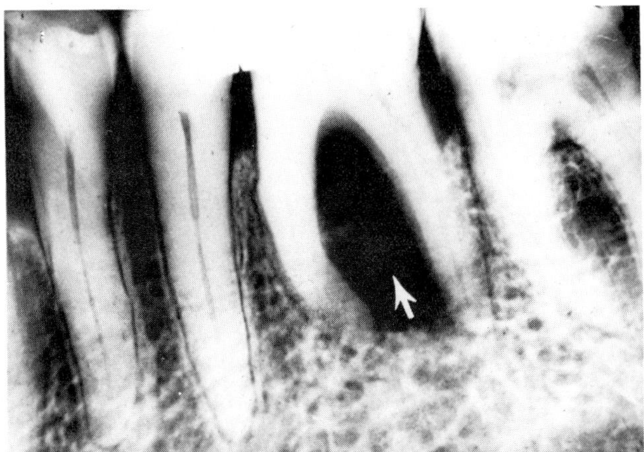

Fig. 9–42. Squamous carcinoma of gingiva invasive of underlying bone. Carcinoma was readily visible on gingiva. However, image in radiograph *per se* resembles pulp-periodontal disease. (Courtesy Dr. Albert Abrams and Dr. Raymond Melrose.)

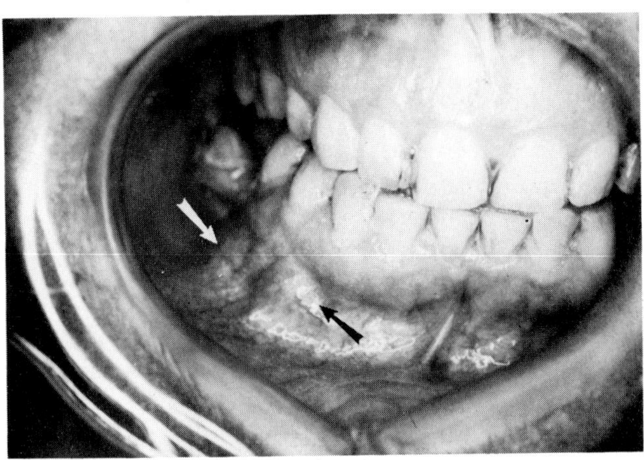

Fig. 9–43. Vestibular-buccal swelling from metastatic breast cancer. Appearance and symptoms can be confused with apical cyst or acute abscess. (Courtesy Dr. Raymond Melrose and Dr. Albert Abrams.)

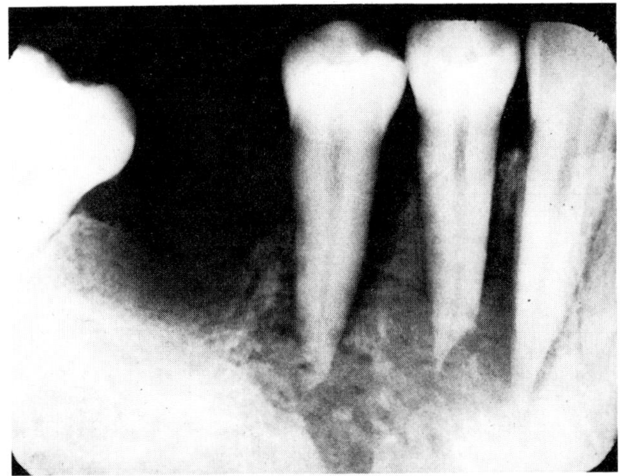

Fig. 9–44. Radiograph of metastatic cancer of breast. All three teeth test nonvital. Unusual chisel edge and moth-eaten resorption are not typical of inflammatory osseous lesion. Biopsy proved lesion malignant. (Courtesy Dr. Raymond Melrose and Dr. Albert Abrams.)

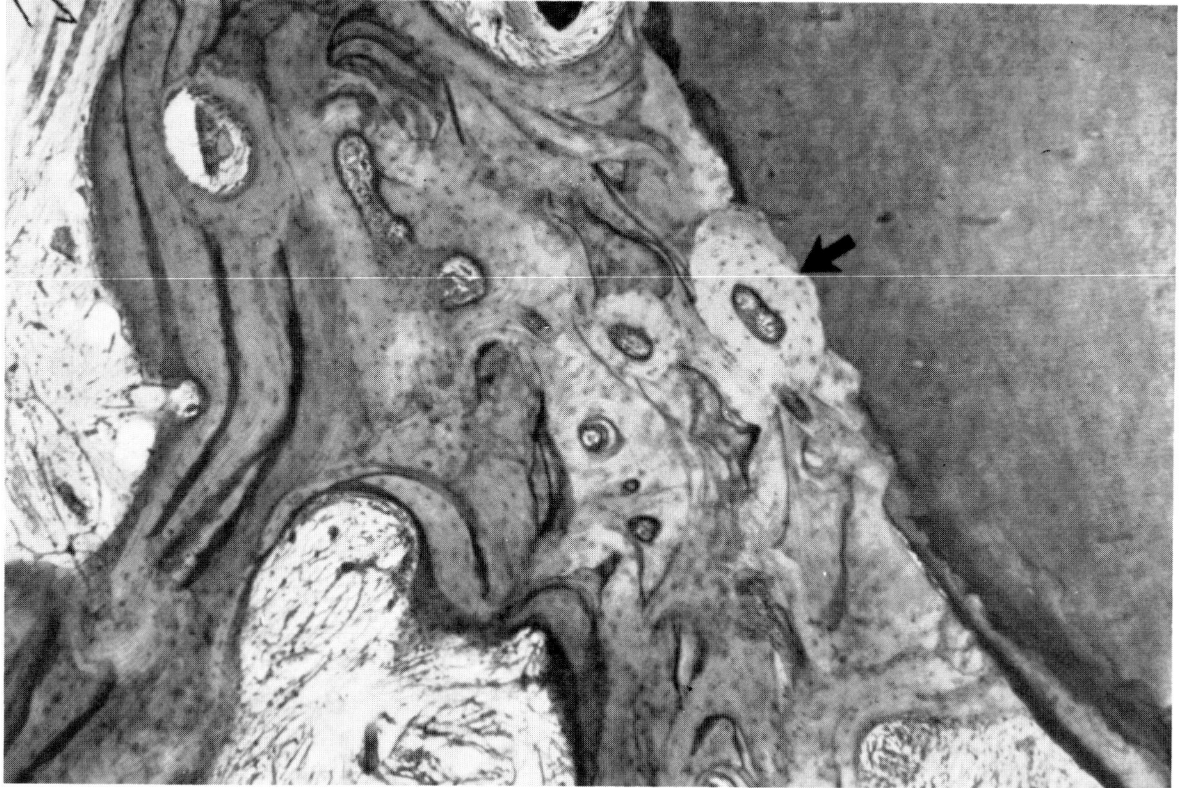

Fig. 9–45. Ankylosis of alveolar bone proper with dentin and cementum. Bridge of bone extends from alveolar process to tooth. At one point haversian system of bone *(arrow)* has fused with dentin of root. This particular ankylosis occurred in connection with chronic apical periodontitis and followed resorption of dentin and cementum in area *(arrow)*. Kronfeld has emphasized that ankylosis usually occurs during attempted repair of root resorption. (From Kronfeld, R.: J.A.D.A., *25*:1457, Sept. 1938.)

Biopsy proved the metastatic spread of the breast cancer to the mandible. A hemimandibulectomy was performed, but the patient died of further metastasis.

ANKYLOSIS

Once in a long while the alveolar bone may fuse with cementum and/or dentin of the root surface after root canal therapy.[34] A permanent union or ***ankylosis*** of tooth and bone results[35] (Fig. 9–45). The existence of such a bond can seldom be suspected, far less confirmed, in the roentgenogram.[36] Detection is a clinical matter, with percussion and tooth rigidity the key factors.

PERIAPICAL REPAIR

Periapical repair in the sense of healing is usually achieved only after endodontic treatment. The reason for the paucity of spontaneous healing should be evident. Most apical lesions are inflammatory responses to an irritant or irritants emanating from the root canal. They signify containment. At the same time they are testimony to the fact that the source of the irritant, the root canal, is beyond the reach of the body defenses. Until treatment removes the irritant, the lesion is bound to persist.

All chronic disease, of course, represents a form of balance between repair and destruction. Throughout the history of any chronic periapical lesion, a measure of repair is taking place. New bone may form on the periphery of an apical area, for example, even though the lesion remains (Fig. 9–27).

Fortunately, true healing is now commonplace in endodontic practice. One of a variety of treatment procedures may be used. These include: (1) root canal treatment without surgical entry to the periapex, (2) root canal treatment, then surgical entry with removal of the periapical lesion and curettement of the exposed apex, (3) root canal treatment, then

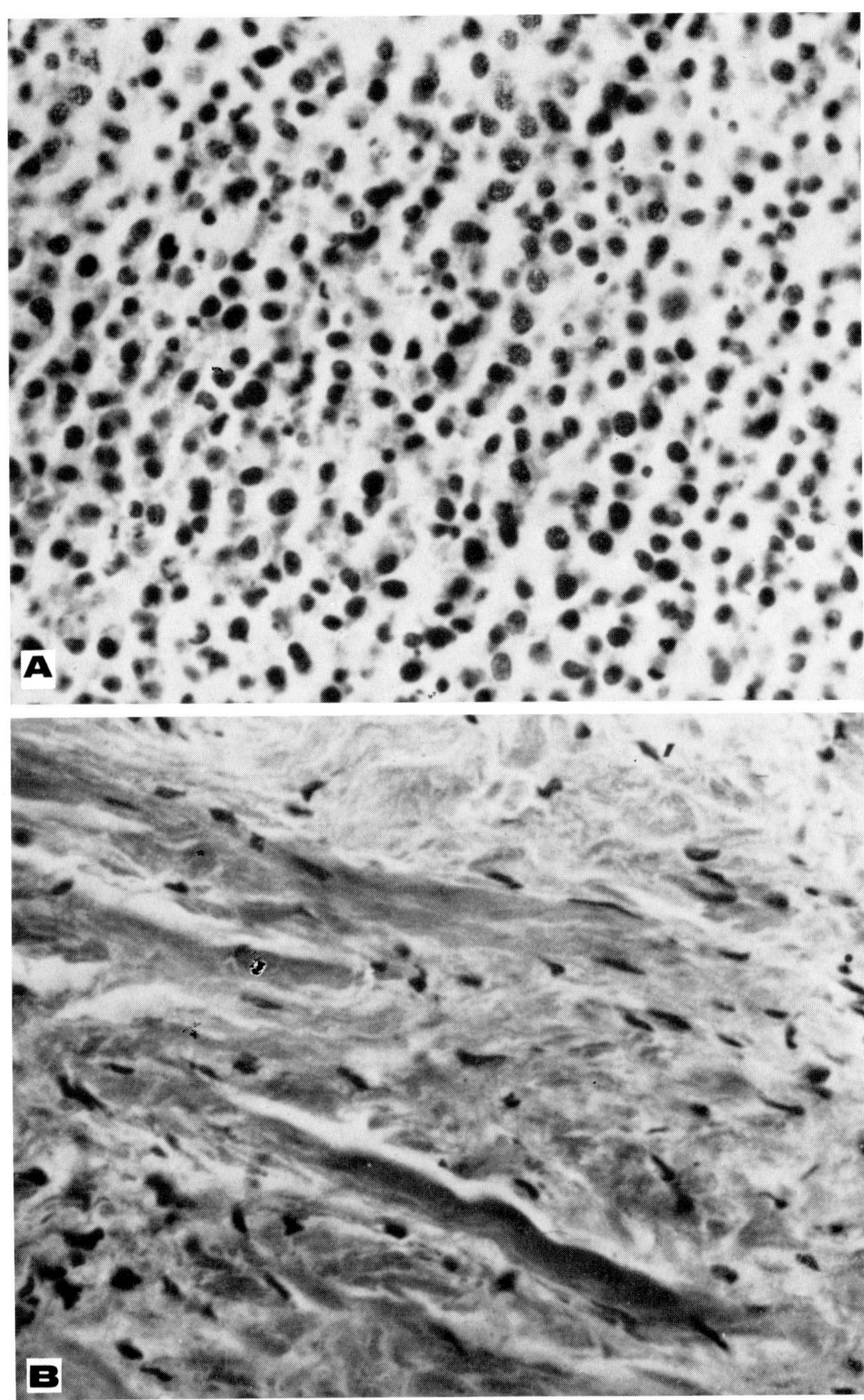

Fig. 9–46. *A,* Periapical tissue obtained from case of suppurative apical periodontitis. Cells and extracellular elements are those of chronic inflammatory tissue. There is little in way of organized fiber pattern. (From Ingle, J. I., and Ogilvie, A.L.: J. Canad. Dent. Assoc., *18*:565, Oct. 1952.) *B,* Repeat biopsy of same periapical area dealt with in *A,* ***one week*** after completion of initial periapical surgery. This section demonstrates cell-fiber pattern of young connective tissue which has filled the surgical defect. Alveolar bone, cementum, and periodontal ligament will later emerge from this vigorous new tissue to repair defect. (From Ingle, J. I., and Ogilvie, A. L.: J. Canad. Dent. Assoc., *18,* 565, Oct., 1952.)

surgical entry with amputation of the root end and removal of the periapical lesion, (4) combined endodontic-periodontic therapy, in which a periapical area and a confluent periodontal pocket are entered surgically and thoroughly curetted.

The nature of periapical repair varies with the procedure used for treatment. When chronic apical periodontitis is resolved by procedure 1, obviously the reparative sequence will differ from that prevailing when procedure 2 is carried out. In the first instance, inflammatory tissue is left at the apex to be converted into new connective tissue reasonably free of inflammation. In the second an apical void is created, which must be filled by young connective tissue. The extent of the cellular transformation that occurs within one week of treatment is illustrated in Figure 9–46. A biopsy section of suppurative apical periodontitis is contrasted to another biopsy section of the same area obtained during the repair that followed. An entirely different potential is evident following treatment.

Once new connective tissue has replaced the lesion, the process of repair is similar regardless of the lesion and the type of treatment. In due course, trabeculae of bone extend through the young connective tissue from the periphery of the defect toward the center (Fig. 9–47). These trabeculae thicken, rearrange themselves, and gradually assume the pattern of alveolar supporting bone. (Comparable bone activity is evident during the filling-in of an extraction socket.)[37,38] With young connective tissue now adjacent to the root itself, cementoblasts differentiate and cementum is deposited. In fact, new lamellae of cementum may progressively seal over the entire root end, including the filling material present there.[39] Repair can also take the form of an apical scar of dense collagenous connective tissue (see Fig. 15–32). The bone defect in such cases seldom fills in.[40]

Usually, however, regeneration is complete. After preliminary attachment and organization, a new periodontal fiber complex again links bone and tooth.[39,41] It is interesting to note that the periodontal ligament, first of the apical structures to make way for disease, is the last to resume normal form.

Periapical repair is routinely assessed on the basis of the disappearance of symptoms and the return of normal landmarks in the post-treatment roentgenogram. The time required for the elimination of the radiolucent area is quite variable. Twelve months after the treatment of chronic or suppurative apical periodontitis, osseous healing usually appears complete (Figs. 9–48 and 9–49).

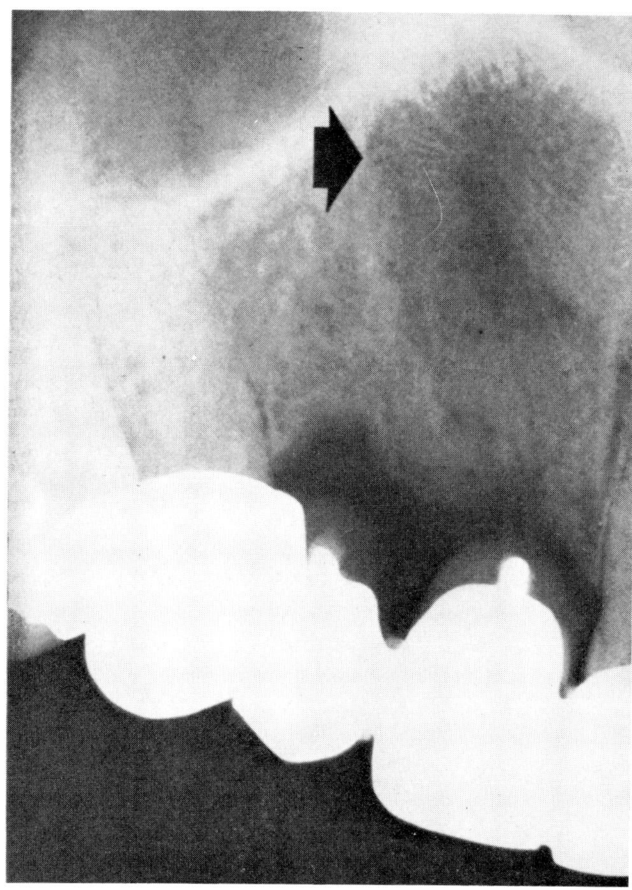

Fig. 9–47. "Sun-burst" effect seen during periapical repair. In this case tooth concerned has been removed. Trabeculae of new bone *(arrow)* are extending from periphery of former apical defect toward its center. Later these same trabeculae will assume pattern of alveolar supporting bone. (Courtesy Dr. Jerome Zech.)

Radiolucency may persist despite treatment. Most frequently this is attributable to inadequate filling of the canal.[42] There is always the possibility that an apical cyst was present originally, and persists while the inflammatory reaction fades. A mild inflammation may also be sustained in response to overfilling of the canal.[43] As we have mentioned, persistent radiolucency occasionally indicates repair in the form of the apical "scar."

Endodontic treatment paves the way for healing under a variety of conditions. In the past the repair of large cystic defects seemed the ultimate in complexity. Actually, though, repair of the closed bony defect is reasonably straightforward, whatever the size of the defect. Combined endodontic-periodontic therapy has shown that more involved forms of repair can be

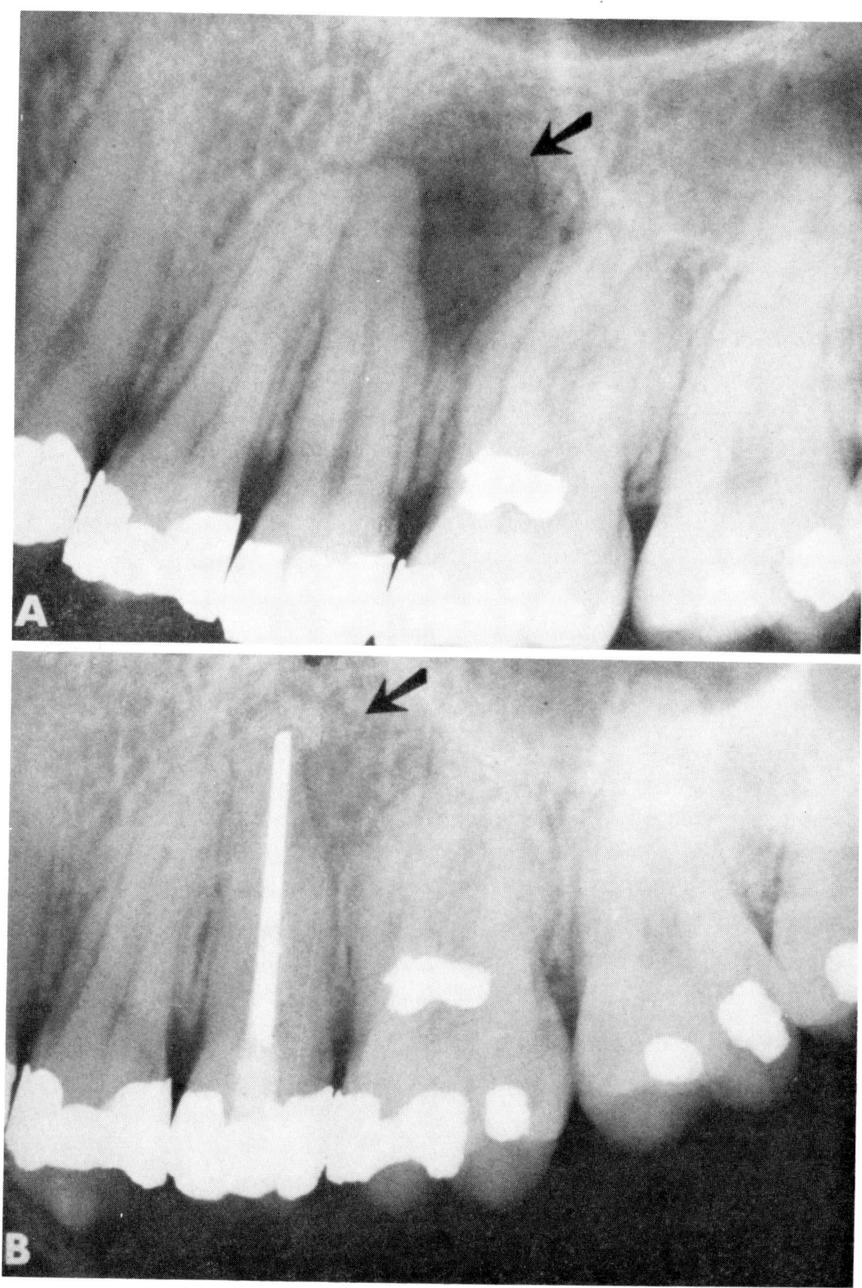

Fig. 9–48. *A,* Pretreatment roentgenogram of chronic apical periodontitis *(arrow)* related to maxillary second premolar. This is same lesion illustrated in Figure 9–9. (Courtesy Dr. Neal Chilton.) *B,* Repair *(arrow)* of chronic apical periodontitis illustrated in *A*. This roentgenogram was taken 12 months after successful endodontic treatment. It shows almost complete regeneration of tissues around second premolar. Trabeculation of bone is normal for individual, and much of periodontal ligament space is again visible. Endodontic treatment was completed without periapical surgery. (Courtesy Dr. Neal Chilton.)

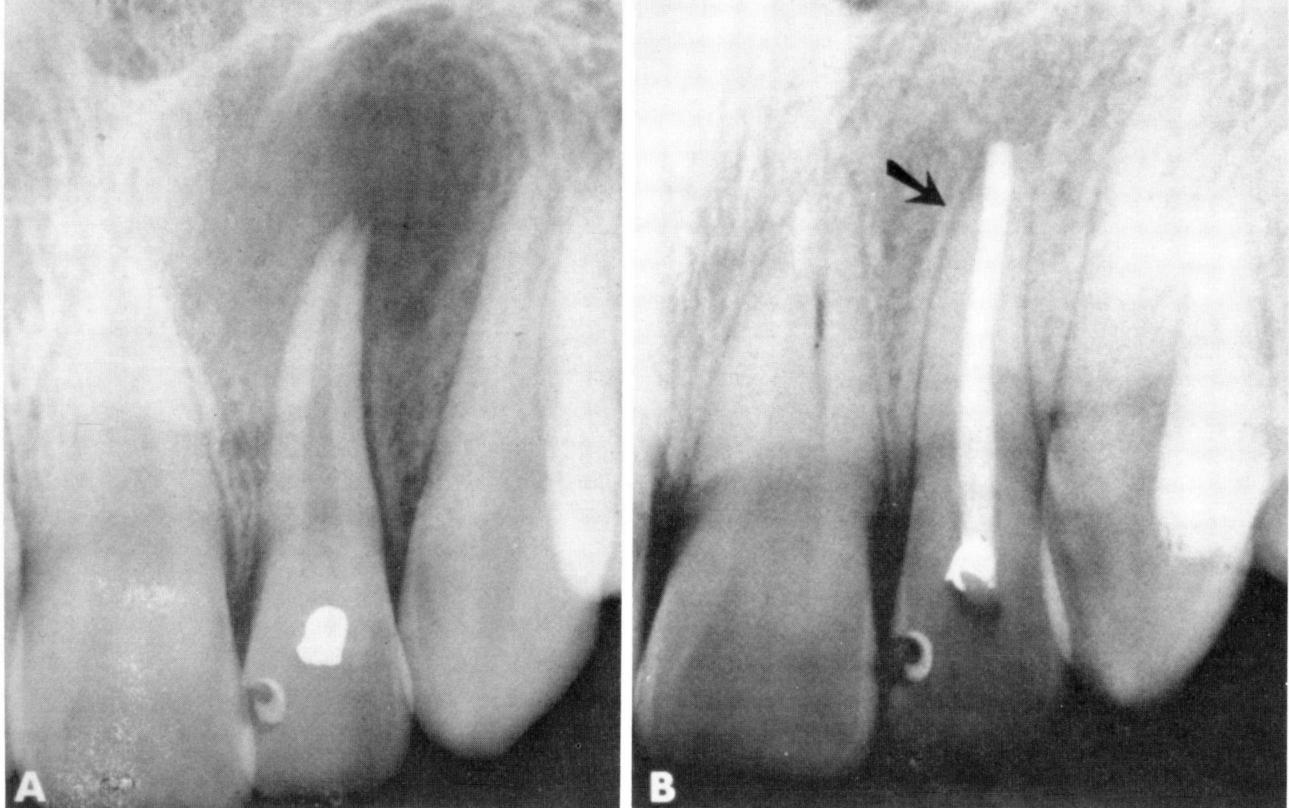

Fig. 9–49. *A,* Suppurative apical periodontitis as viewed in pre-treatment film. Disappearance of normal periapical landmarks is evident. Lesion is large and has spread from apex of lateral incisor to involve much of mesial surface of adjacent cuspid. (Courtesy Dr. Neal Chilton.) *B,* Adequate repair of suppurative apical periodontitis. This is 12-month post-treatment roentgenogram of case shown in *A*. Normal osseous landmarks, such as lamina dura *(arrow),* have returned. Endodontic treatment was completed without periapical surgery. (Courtesy Dr. Neal Chilton.)

induced.[44,45] It is now evident that under certain conditions both the apical periodontium and the marginal periodontium can be reestablished at the same time (see Fig. 15–59).

REFERENCES

1. *Webster's Third New International Dictionary,* Springfield, Mass., G. & C. Merriam, 1961.
2. Ingle, J. I.: A suggested nomenclature for pulpal and periapical pathosis. J. Seattle Distr. Dent. Soc., *1*:11, Apr., 1963.
3. Schilder, H., and Amsterdam, M.: Inflammatory potential of root canal medicaments. Oral Surg., *12*:211, Feb., 1959.
4. Rappaport, H. M., Lilly, G. E., and Kapsimalis, P.: Toxicity of endodontic filling materials. Oral Surg., *18*:785, Dec., 1964.
5. Florey, H.: *General Pathology.* 3rd Ed. Philadelphia, W. B. Saunders Co., 1962, p. 473.
6. Boyle, P. E.: *Kronfeld's Histopathology of the Teeth and Their Surrounding Structures.* 4th Ed. Philadelphia, Lea & Febiger, 1955, p. 198.
7. Bynum, J. W., and Flieder, D. E.: Demonstration of nerve tissue in periapical inflammatory lesions. J. Dent. Res., *39*:737, July-Aug., 1960 (Abstract).
8. Boyle, P. E.: op. cit., p. 199.
9. Worth, H. M.: *Principles and Practice of Oral Radiologic Interpretation.* Chicago, Year Book Medical Publishers, Inc., 1963, p. 257.
10. Shafer, W. G., Hine, M. K., and Levy, B. M.: *A Textbook of Oral Pathology.* 2nd Ed. Philadelphia, W. B. Saunders Co., 1963, p. 387.
11. Colby, R. A., Kerr, D. A., and Robinson, H. B. G.: *Color Atlas of Oral Pathology.* 2nd Ed., Philadelphia, J. B. Lippincott Co., 1961, p. 74.
12. Matsumiya, S., Kondo, S., Takuma, S., Suzuki, A., and Osawa, Y.: *Atlas of Oral Pathology.* Tokyo, The Tokyo Dental College Press, 1955, p. 241.

13. Worth, H. M.: op. cit., p. 253.
14. Matsumiya, S., *et. al.*: op. cit., p. 27.
15. Hill, T. J.: Epithelium in dental granulomata. J. Dent. Res., *10*:323, June, 1930.
16. Kronfeld, R.: The epithelium in chronic apical periodontitis. Proc. Ninth Austral. Dental Congress, 1937, p. 578.
17. Shafer, W. G., Hine, M. K., and Levy, B. M.: op. cit., p. 389.
18. Linenberg, W. B., Waldron, C. A., and De Laune, G. F.: A clinical, roentgenographic and histopathologic evaluation of periapical lesions. Oral Surg., *17*:457, Apr., 1964.
19. Priebe, W. A., Lazansky, J. P., and Wuehrmann, A. H.: The value of the roentgenographic film in the differential diagnosis of periapical lesions. Oral Surg., 7:979, Sept., 1954.
20. Stafne, E. C.: *Oral Roentgenographic Diagnosis*. 2nd Ed. Philadelphia, W. B. Saunders Co., 1963, p. 88.
21. Bender, I. B., and Seltzer, S.: Roentgenographic and direct observation of experimental lesions in bone. J.A.D.A., *62*:152, Feb., 1961.
22. Bhaskar, S. N.: Personal communication, 1964.
23. Boyle, P. E.: op. cit., p. 217.
24. Crawford, W. H.: Personal communication (unpublished data).
25. Melrose, R. J., Cooperman, H. H., and Abrams, A. J.: Clinical pathologic conference. J. South. Cal. Dent. Assoc., *37*:186, Apr., 1969.
26. Courage, G. R., North, A. F., and Hansen, L. S.: Median palatine cysts. Oral Surg., *37*:745, May, 1974.
27. Worth, H. M.: op. cit., p. 596.
28. Shafer, W. G., Hine, M. K., and Levy, B. M.: op. cit., p. 226.
29. Gorlin, R. J., Meskin, L. H., and Bradey, R.: Odontogenic tumors in man and animals: pathologic classification and clinical behaviour—a review. Ann. N.Y. Acad. Sci., *108*:722, Nov. 4, 1963.
30. Zegarelli, E. V., and Kutscher, A. H.: The cementoma. Dental Radiog. and Photog., *34*:4, 1961.
31. Blum, T.: Clinical oral surgery, with special emphasis on its related pathology. III. J. Dent. Res., *10*:377, June, 1930.
32. Wertheimer, F. W., Driscoll, E. J., and Stanley, H. R.: "True" (attached) cementoma with root canal involvement. Oral Surg., *14*:630, May, 1961.
33. Abrams, A. M., and Melrose, R. J.: Clinical Pathologic Conference, Univ. So. Calif., 1970.
34. Shafer, W. G., Hine, M. K., and Levy, B. M.: op. cit., p. 438.
35. Kronfeld, R.: The biology of the cementum. J.A.D.A., *25*:1451, Sept., 1938.
36. Worth, H. M.: op. cit., p. 207.
37. Weinmann, P., and Sicher, H.: *Bone and Bones*. 2nd Ed. St. Louis, C. V. Mosby Co., 1955, p. 333.
38. Matsumiya, S., Suzuki, I., and Takuma, S.: *Atlas of Clinical Oral Pathology*. Vol. II, Tokyo, The Tokyo Dental College Press, 1963, p. 85.
39. Coolidge, E. D.: The status of pulpless teeth as interpreted by tissue tolerance and repair following root canal filling. J.A.D.A., *20*:2216, Dec., 1933.
40. Penick, E. C.: Periapical repair by dense fibrous connective tissue following conservative endodontic therapy. Oral Surg., *14*:239, Feb., 1961.
41. Matsumiya, S., Suzuki, I. and Takuma, S.: op. cit., p. 80.
42. Ingle, J. I.: Existos y Francasos en Endodoncia. Revista de la Assoc. Odonto. Argentina, *50*:67, Feb., 1962.
43. Seltzer, S., Turkenkopf, S., Vito, A., Green, D., and Bender, I. B.: A histologic evaluation of periapical repair following positive and negative root canal cultures. Oral Surg., *17*:507, Apr., 1964.
44. Prichard, J.: The infrabony technique as a predictable procedure. J. Periodont., *28*:202, July, 1957.
45. Hiatt, W. H.: Periodontal pocket elimination by combined endodontic-periodontic therapy. J. Am. Soc. Periodont., *1*:152, July-Aug., 1963.

Chapter 10

Diagnostic Procedures

JOHN I. INGLE, EDWARD E. BEVERIDGE, CYRIL GAUM, and RONALD R. SLOWEY

What is Diagnosis? Proper diagnosis is a continuing process. Data, based on a complete history and examination, must be gathered, sorted and analyzed, and then a conclusion drawn. From this a plan of treatment is developed. It is important to remember that one of the limiting factors in diagnosis is the dentist himself; proper diagnosis coming only when the dentist strives for the highest possible accuracy in recognition and analysis of ***all*** criteria. In view of these assumptions, diagnosis may be defined as obtaining answers to clinical questions which determine the course of preventive, educational, and therapeutic services to be rendered the patient. This definition suggests that diagnosis must be described not only in terms of pathologic conditions present, but in terms of patient- and dentist-related complications as well. Only when diagnosis considers ***all*** factors can it be termed "proper."

Diagnosis of pulp disease and of the sequelae of pulp disease ranges from the obvious to the obscure. Differential diagnosis of an obscure facial pain or a vague yet referring pulpalgia can be most complex. On the other hand, the obvious fracture or obvious carious lesion immediately directs attention to the involved tooth. Many diagnostic problems will try the patience and test the skill of the most sophisticated diagnostician. To become sophisticated, however, the dentist must discipline himself to a repeatable routine. Diagnostic procedures should become as orderly as the preparation of, say, a class II amalgam filling.

The examination-diagnosis appointment is often the first doctor-patient encounter and should be conducted under optimal conditions. The dentist should be fresh and relaxed and have adequate time scheduled. His demeanor must be one of kindliness and attentiveness, for the patient may consider this appointment a confrontation and be filled with anxiety and apprehension. He may have experienced pain for many days.

Before embarking on a detailed discussion of history and examination, a word must be said about record keeping. Dentists are notorious for not keeping proper records. Surely every normal finding in the mouth need not be recorded, but certainly the pathologic or potentially pathologic conditions, and the date of their discovery, should be recorded. It is particularly important to record the findings on examination following an accident.

As dentists become more and more involved with evaluation by their own Professional Standards Review Organizations, perfect records emerge as increasingly important. The whole problem of "paper work" may be lightened if the dentist dictates his findings at the chair to an assistant. A kind of verbal "shorthand" can be developed, later to be translated to the patient during the informed consent procedure. In any case, it must all be written down.

HISTORY AND HISTORY-TAKING (ANAMNESIS)

Anamnesis is the first step in developing a diagnosis; a history of the patient's immediate problem, of his past related problems, and, finally, of his general health. This is best developed by following the time-honored formula of establishing the ***chief complaint,*** enlarging upon this complaint by questioning about the ***present illness,*** and, finally, determining the advisability of the treatment approach by establishing the facts related to ***past illness*** of both the chief complaint and general health.

The extent of the dental-medical history varies with each case. The patient who presents himself with a new complaint, but who has previously been under the care of the same dentist, will undoubtedly have a well-established history on record. Questioning in this case may not go beyond the ***chief complaint*** and a discussion of the ***present illness.*** In marked contrast, hours may be spent in taking the history of a patient who is in pain, but is being seen for the first time.

The chief complaint may not be a verbal "complaint" by the patient, but rather an observation by the dentist of a condition unknown to the patient. Many asymptomatic pulpless teeth, for example, are discovered in a routine roentgenographic survey.

Chief Complaint

The ***chief complaint*** of the new or referred patient is most easily established by asking "what is your problem?" The patient with a problem related to a pulpless tooth will have had pain or swelling or a traumatic accident, or he will have noted something different, such as a draining fistula or a darkened tooth, or he may have been referred by another dentist and told what his problem is.

In any case his answer will usually be quite definite; "This tooth (pointing) is painful; or is discolored; or is draining." The chief complant should be written in the patient's own words; "I have a gum-boil," for example.

As soon as the chief complaint is established and recorded, the examiner proceeds to questions regarding the patient's present illness.

Present Illness

"How long have you had this condition (or problem or pain)?" is a logical question to follow the ***chief complaint.*** The duration of the complaint is also pertinent. If the patient has pain, it is necessary to know how long the discomfort has been present and how long each episode of pain exists. Such questions as "How long ago did the accident happen? When did you first notice the swelling? How long has the tooth been painful to bite on?" often bring answers necessary to determine the chronicity of the lesion.

When the duration of the problem has been established, it is then necessary to discover the precipitating factors. The quickest way to get at the problem of pulpalgia is to enquire of the effect of thermal extremes. "Does the tooth ache when you eat or drink something hot or cold?" Answers in the affirmative suggest pulp vitality with pulpitis, whereas negative answers usually signify nonvital pulp with a beginning apical periodontitis, particularly if the tooth is painful on mastication.

The question, "When does the tooth ache?" often elicits an answer that establishes the diagnosis. Such answers as, "When I lie down in the evening" (moderate acute pulpalgia); "When I go out in the cold air" (moderate acute pulpalgia); "Only when I scratch the tooth at the gum line" (hypersensitivity); "It began aching violently when I drank hot coffee" (advanced acute pulpalgia); or "Each time I even touch the tooth with my tongue" (acute apical periodontitis).

Logical questions such as, "Is the tooth painful to bite on?" or "Do you feel the area is swollen?" could provide the lead to a beginning acute abscess. Early swelling may be felt by the patient, but not observed on casual examination.

The emergent nature of the patient's discomfort, determined by the questioning or by his demeanor, will determine the ***next step in examination.*** If the patient is obviously suffering, the history-taking of present illness should be put aside and a cursory examination begun to determine which tooth is involved. From this history and short examination, the exact diagnosis may be made and immediate relief extended to the patient with a local anesthetic. Time is gained by dealing with a pain-free and more rational patient. Under no circumstances should an injection be made unless the examiner is sure of his diagnosis, for further examination will be greatly limited under block anesthesia.

If the patient is not in severe pain during questioning, the history-taking should be continued to establish facts about ***past illness.*** By these questions two areas of past history may be explored; a specific past history about the present complaint and related oral conditions, and a past history of the patient's physical status.

Past Illness

The question, "Did you ever have this problem (or pain) before?" occasionally brings to light the fact that the chief complaint is a recurrent one, *e.g.*, a fistula that has drained for years. A history of long-standing severe pain should make one suspicious of a condition other than pulpalgia, possibly a neurogenic or psychogenic pain. Questions regarding past illness of the chief complaint will logically follow answers derived from the first question about chronicity.

Developing a history of ***past illnesses*** to determine the patient's state of health should follow. Typical questions to be asked are:

How is your health?
Has there been any change in your health in the last year?
Has your weight changed?
Are you presently under the care of a physician?
If so, for what condition?
When was your last medical examination?
Have you ever been hospitalized?
Have you ever had any operations? Serious accidents?
Are you wearing a heart pacemaker?
Have you had (or do you have) diabetes, rheumatic fever, rheumatoid arthritis, infectious or serum hepatitis, kidney trouble, sinusitis, headaches, heart condition, a blood pressure problem, a heart murmur, asthma, allergic conditions, or hay fever?
Have you ever had penicillin or other antibiotics?
If so, are you allergic to any of these?
Are you taking any medications (anticoagulants, antidepressants, tranquilizers, corticosteroids, Dilantin)?
Do any medications make you ill?
Have you ever had any adverse reaction to injected dental anesthetics?
Do you clot quickly after a cut or injury?
Do you heal quickly?
Do you have trouble sleeping?
Do you often have to urinate?
Are you occasionally nervous or tense?
How does this tension show itself? In what part of your body do you feel the tension?
Women should be asked questions about child-bearing, menstrual, or menopausal problems.

Positive answers to these questions must be weighed and evaluated to determine the risk of treatment against the risk of nontreatment. Positive answers of a serious nature should be followed by a review of the system involved: cardiac, respiratory, and so on. The patient's physician should also be consulted if any history of a serious nature is uncovered.

During the interview the dentist-patient relationship tends to crystallize. Rapport is established, and this is relevant to all future relationships. This is a period when the terrified patient is reassured. Many patients are so frightened, however, they are not at ease until an uneventful first treatment is completed. Kindliness and attention to the patient's concern will do much to ease emotional trauma, particularly if a thorough and painless examination follows.

EXAMINATION

Blood Pressure and Pulse Rate

Before undertaking a direct examination of the face, neck, and oral cavity, the patient's blood pressure and pulse rate should be taken and recorded. Routine use of the sphygmomanometer occasionally brings to light unsuspected cases of hypertension in patients who are going to the dentist but not seeing a physician regularly. Halpern found that only about 18% of the dental clinic patients at Temple University "were seeing their physicians."[1] Not only will information about hypertension materially affect considerations for treatment in the dental office, but the dentist is legally bound to inform the patient of the level of his blood pressure when seeking consent to proceed with treatment. A blood pressure reading of 140/90 might arbitrarily be considered a level for referral to a physician. Elevated pressures should be re-checked before each treatment. Recording the patient's temperature could also be a good habit to establish.

Extraoral Examination

A common fault among practitioners is to begin the examination intraorally. One must discipline oneself to initiate the examination ***extraorally,*** thereby observing extraoral fistulas, swellings, or asymmetries. Facial or neck ecchymosis, abrasions, or scars should be noted as they relate to traumatic accidents that may have injured the teeth or jaws. During digital examination, one should palpate for lymphadenopathy of the submaxillary, submental, and anterior and posterior jugular lymph nodes. At this time, the patient should be instructed to report areas of tenderness.

Intraoral Examination

Visual Examination

The presence of a pulpless tooth often is established during conversation with a patient. Discolored teeth or fractured teeth are readily apparent. Teeth with obvious caries or large restorations are also suspect, including those teeth restored by full coverage. It is when the examiner sees a mouth in which every tooth has been fully covered that the true "puzzlement" begins.

It is a cardinal rule that visual examination of the mouth should always begin in the oral vestibule. It is a good idea to examine the lips first—visually and by palpation. The examiner should then stand in front of the patient, and using both hands, he should widely separate the lips and cheeks down to the depth of the fornix. He then asks the patient to close. This act exposes all the buccolabial tissue from molar to molar. If a fistula is present, draining into the vestibule, it will be easily seen. The patient's head should be turned from side to side to facilitate examination of the buccal vestibule. Buccal caries and restorations are noted at this time, as are discolored pulpless teeth. Findings are dictated to the assistant and lips and cheeks are then released. The examiner steps to the side or behind the patient, and the visual examination continues with an explorer, a periodontal probe, and a mouth mirror.

For psychologic reasons the most obvious tooth is examined first, particularly if the patient, the history, the symptoms, or the signs call attention to a certain tooth. Is there a large restoration or caries? Is the tooth discolored? Is there a fistula? When an explorer is used, does the tooth become painful if caries is probed? Does the periodontal probe reveal a periodontal pocket?

What is the condition of the teeth in the immediate vicinity? What is the general state of oral care and repair for the whole mouth? Does the involved tooth have an opponent? Is the involved tooth salvageable or necessary? These are some of the questions the examiner must ask himself during the visual examination.

Strong light may be shone through anterior teeth for ***transillumination.*** If a pulpless tooth is only slightly discolored, the color change may show only by this method. The mouth mirror is held in shadow in the palate, and variance in color from tooth to tooth is noted in reflection.

If the exact involved tooth is not known, but a region or half arch is suspected, then all the teeth in the area must be carefully examined until the most likely candidate is found. Again, the size of a carious lesion or a restoration often points to the involved tooth. Remember, a full crown is often a prime suspect. Periodontal probing throughout the area is also indicated.

After the dentist has completed the local examination dealing with the chief complaint, he should then complete the oral examination both for the patient's protection and (in today's world) for his own as well. First, the tongue should be grasped with a 2 × 2 gauze square and extended to permit examination of its ventral surface, first on one side and then on the other and, with a pre-warmed mouth mirror, examination of the superior, lateral, and posterior portions of the tongue, the fauces, and the nasopharynx. Once the tongue and throat have been examined, the floor of the mouth should be palpated with the index finger of one hand intraorally and the index finger of the other hand extraorally, and the tissue in between carefully assessed.

Next, the hard and soft palate should be examined for fistulas, tori, and fluctuant swellings from periapical lesions. One's attention should now be directed to the alveolar processes and gingival tissues. With the aid of a mouth mirror and a periodontal probe, all pocket depths are measured, and areas of suppuration, bleeding upon touch, and sensitivity are noted. Where periodontal disease is moderate or advanced, particular attention should be devoted to the extent of involvement of bi- or trifurcations.

At this point, and only at this point, should the examiner check the remaining teeth with a mouth mirror and explorer, looking and feeling for caries, defective margins, loose restorations, discolorations, vertical fractures, and enamel invaginations, erosion, and abrasion. The handle of the mouth mirror should also be used for percussion, testing any tooth of questionable periapical health. Finally, occlusal relationships should be carefully examined. It is most important that the patient be informed of any unusual or pathologic change that is present. To remain silent, even for referred patients, is to later stand accused and indicted.

Percussion and Palpation

Percussion and palpation logically follow or literally become a part of the ***visual examination.*** If a tooth is extremely painful to movement, it should only be touched, gently, and not percussed. Another degree of discomfort calls for ***gentle*** percussion of suspected teeth with the fingernail, tapping the incisal edge or cuspal tip.

True percussion of asymptomatic teeth is done with

the mirror handle, but this should never be used if the patient has an acute apical abscess or acute apical periodontitis. Mirror handle percussion against morsal surfaces may bring out minor differences in sensation between teeth. The patient can only say that one tooth "feels" different when it is tapped. This minor difference may prove to be a major clue.

The sophisticated examiner may be able to detect differences in sound elicited by percussion. The tooth involved with an apical cyst or suppurative apical periodontitis often sounds "mushy" when percussed. Normal, vital teeth give off a sharper "twang" sound. Maxillary teeth whose roots are involved in maxillary sinusitis also give a "mushy" sound. The special examination for suspected ***undisclosed fracture*** is discussed under that section in Chapter 11.

Palpation is performed simultaneously with percussion. The region apical to suspected teeth is firmly palpated with the fingertips, unless, of course, an acute abscess is present. Remember to palpate to the lingual as well as the buccal, especially in the mandible. The teeth themselves should also be palpated, for occasionally a tooth reacts painfully to horizontal pressure but not to vertical percussion. Mobile teeth, associated with acute inflammation or advanced alveolar bone loss, can be detected by palpation.

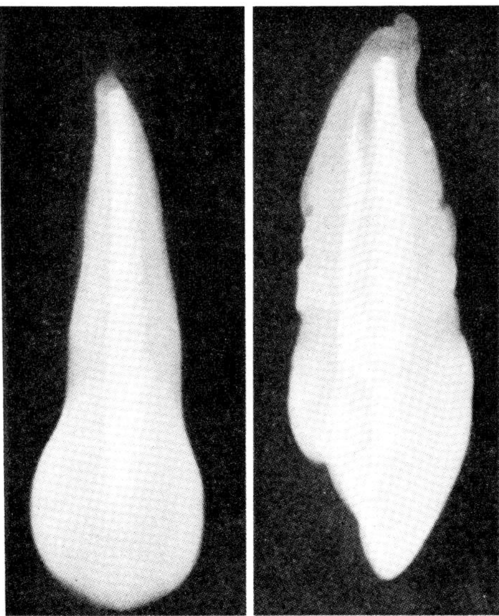

Fig. 10–1. Deceptive quality of roentgenogram. *Left,* Apparently well-obliterated laboratory exercise shown in standard labial-lingual projection. *Right,* Buccal-lingual projection provides third dimension unavailable in *oral* roentgenology. Failure to obliterate canal is apparent here, but was obscured in labial-lingual projection.

Palpation of the temporomandibular joint and muscles of mastication is discussed separately in the chapter on pain, Chapter 11.

All findings from examination by percussion and palpation should be recorded in the patient's record. By this time, certain clues to the nature of the problem and which tooth is involved should begin to materialize. Confirmatory evidence is needed, and the roentgenographic examination is the next logical step. While the film is being processed, the examination may be continued.

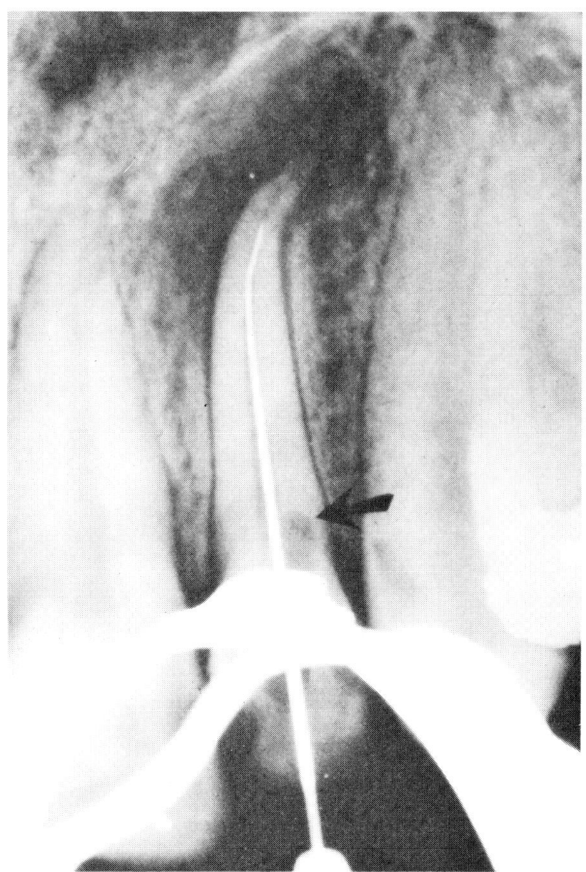

Fig. 10–2. Importance of adequate roentgenogram. Number of important details may be learned from this film: (1) size and character of periapical lesion, (2) curvature of root end, (3) relationship of root to adjacent roots, (4) mesial or distal inclination of root, (5) approximate length of tooth, (6) relationship of exploring instrument to root curve, (7) size of canal, and (8) divergence of coronal cavity *(arrow).* Periodontal lesions could also be apparent. Central beam, directed through periapical region, gives clarity to this important area.

Roentgenographic Examination

No single phase of the endodontic examination will be so rewarding as the roentgenographic examination—or so misleading. The dentist must constantly bear in mind that the roentgen image is a shadow, and has the elusive qualities of all shadows. First and foremost, it is a two-dimensional representation of a three-dimensional problem (Fig. 10–1). Also, like any shadow, it may be too light or too dark, too short or too long. The central beam must be carefully oriented to give detail where detail is required (Fig. 10–2). This will usually require that the central beam be aimed directly through the periapex rather than through the compromise position at the crest of the alveolar process. In addition, two or more exposures are frequently necessary to check out detail from more than one horizontal angle (Fig. 10–3). This is especially true in the case of the normal bony foramens. The mental foramen may be directly superimposed over the apex of the mandibular premolars (Fig. 10–4). The nasopalatine foramen also may be superimposed on the apex of the maxillary central incisors. Because these foramens are actually some distance from the apices of these teeth, their shadows may be shifted far to the mesial or the distal merely by shifting the horizontal angle of the cone of the x-ray machine to the mesial or distal during separate exposures (Fig. 10–5). On the other hand, if the radiolucent area seen in the roentgenogram is actually from a lesion truly associated with the periapex of the involved tooth, its shadow will remain "attached" to the root end and will remain so in spite of a mesial or distal shift in separate films. For details regarding the "horizontal shift," the reader is referred to Chapter 2.

Interpretation. The finest radiologist will be severely handicapped in securing valuable information from a film that has not been properly placed, exposed, and processed. Conversely, the finest film is of limited value if the interpreter is inadequate. Alas, it is a discredit to the profession and a disservice to the public that many practitioners gain little information from roentgenograms because they lack disciplined interpretation.

An organized method of evaluating and interpreting radiographs, from a single film to a full mouth set or a panographic plate, has been suggested by Wuehrmann.[2] By this technique, the dentist reviews

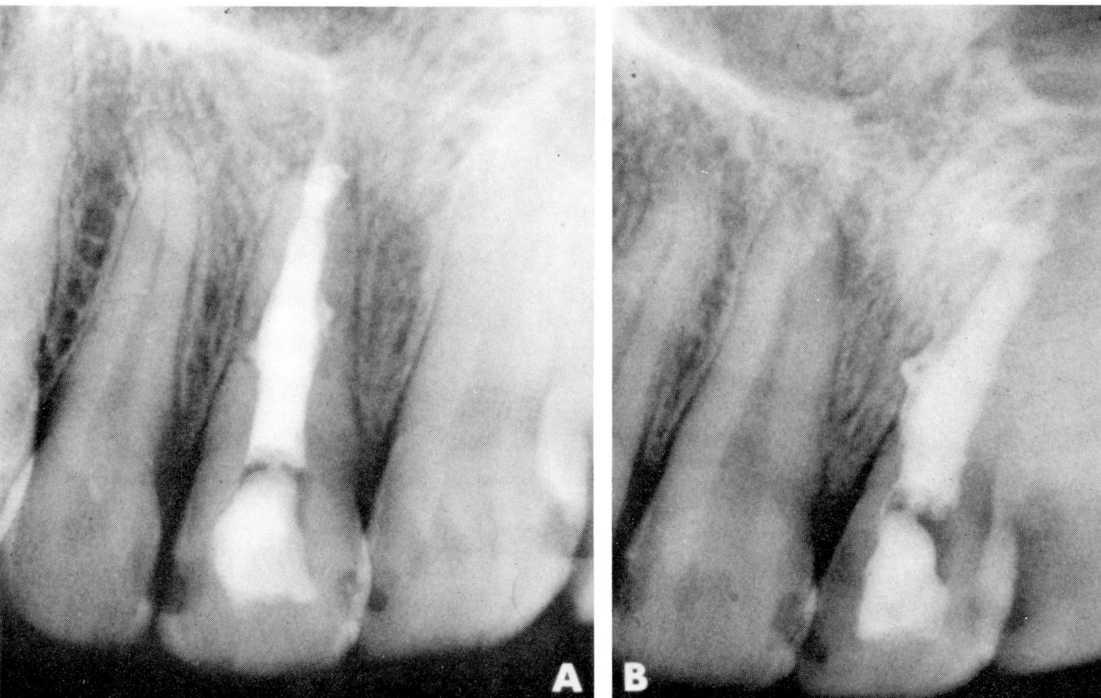

Fig. 10–3. Variations in horizontal angle improve roentgenographic interpretation. *A,* In this straight-on, labial-lingual projection, internal resorption defect is seen. *B,* In mesially directed projection, extension of resorptive defect to mesial-lingual is apparent.

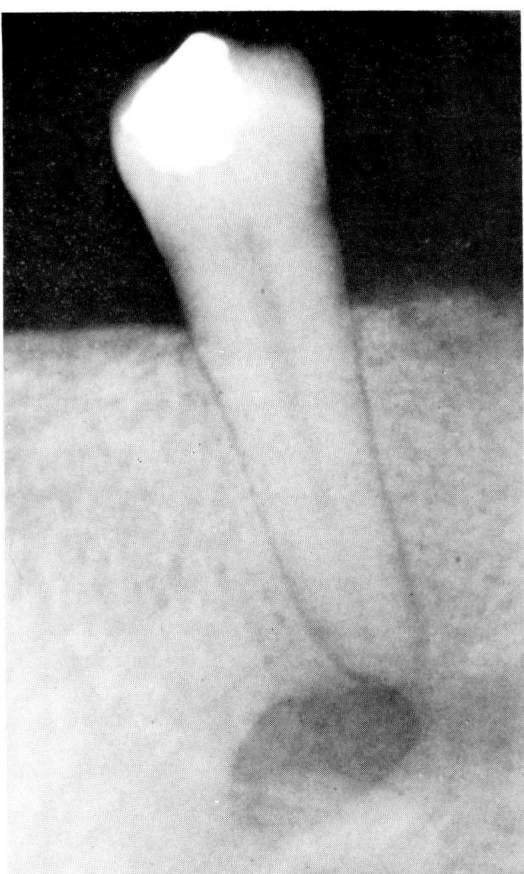

Fig. 10–4. Mental foramen is superimposed exactly at apex of vital mandibular premolar and may easily be mistaken for periapical lesion.

one particular structure at a time, say, the lamina dura. This structure is followed all the way around the first tooth on the left and then around the next tooth and the next until the full film or full mouth survey is scanned. Observations are called out to the assistant who is recording.

Attention is then turned to the next structure, the crowns of the teeth, for example, and again each crown is evaluated independently. The crest of the alveolar process should then be followed from left to right, upper to lower, and all the structures outside the alveolar process should be evaluated as well—the sinuses, floor of the nose, foramens, and so on. In short, radiographic interpretation should be done in an organized habitual way so that nothing is overlooked.

Tracing of the black periodontal membrane space will reveal the number, size, and shape of the roots and their juxtaposition. While observing the roots, one should look for periapical lesions and such root defects as anomalies, fractures, and external resorption. The number, curvature, size, and shape of all the canals and chambers should be noted along with internal resorption, pulp stones, linear calcification, and open apices.

In the crowns the dentist should search for the depth of caries and restorations that reach or nearly reach the pulp, as well as evidence of pulp cappings or pulpotomy, *dens invaginatus* or *dens evaginatus,* and the size of preparations under porcelain or acrylic jacket crowns. Radiographic interpretation is no better than the motivation, systematic evaluation, and skill of the dentist.

Evaluation does come down to a matter of personal interpretation, however, as demonstrated by Goldman and his colleagues.[3] The radiographs of 253 cases, originally examined by three faculty members at Tufts University, were re-examined by them six to eight months later. These endodontists agreed with ***themselves*** from 72 to 88% of the time. In a previous study on the same 253 cases, six of the faculty all agreed with each other only 47% of the time and five of six agreed ***with each other*** only 67% of the time.[4]

One of the reasons for these discrepancies, of course, deals with how we interpret bony lesions. Shoha, Dowson, and Richards were able to demonstrate the variables in this interpretation.[5] They found that lesions were always larger than their radiographic image, especially in the mandibular molar region. Lesions in the premolar area were only slightly larger than their radiographic image and, unlike others, could be seen on the film before cortical bone was lost. Lesions found by hindsight are often difficult to detect initially because of their vague outline.

Root Anatomy. The roentgenographic examination provides essential information relative to normal and abnormal root formation. The dentist preparing to do root canal therapy on the ***mandibular*** anterior teeth, particularly to the incisors, is well advised to move the tube horizontally and to take the roentgenograms from a proximal direction as well as from the standard anterior-posterior position. Mandibular incisors with two roots, or two canals within the tooth, are more apt to be found through this lateral exposure (Fig. 10–6).

Every tooth in the mandible is subject to extra roots and hence root canals. The premolars and molars are no exception (Fig. 10–7). By both radiographic

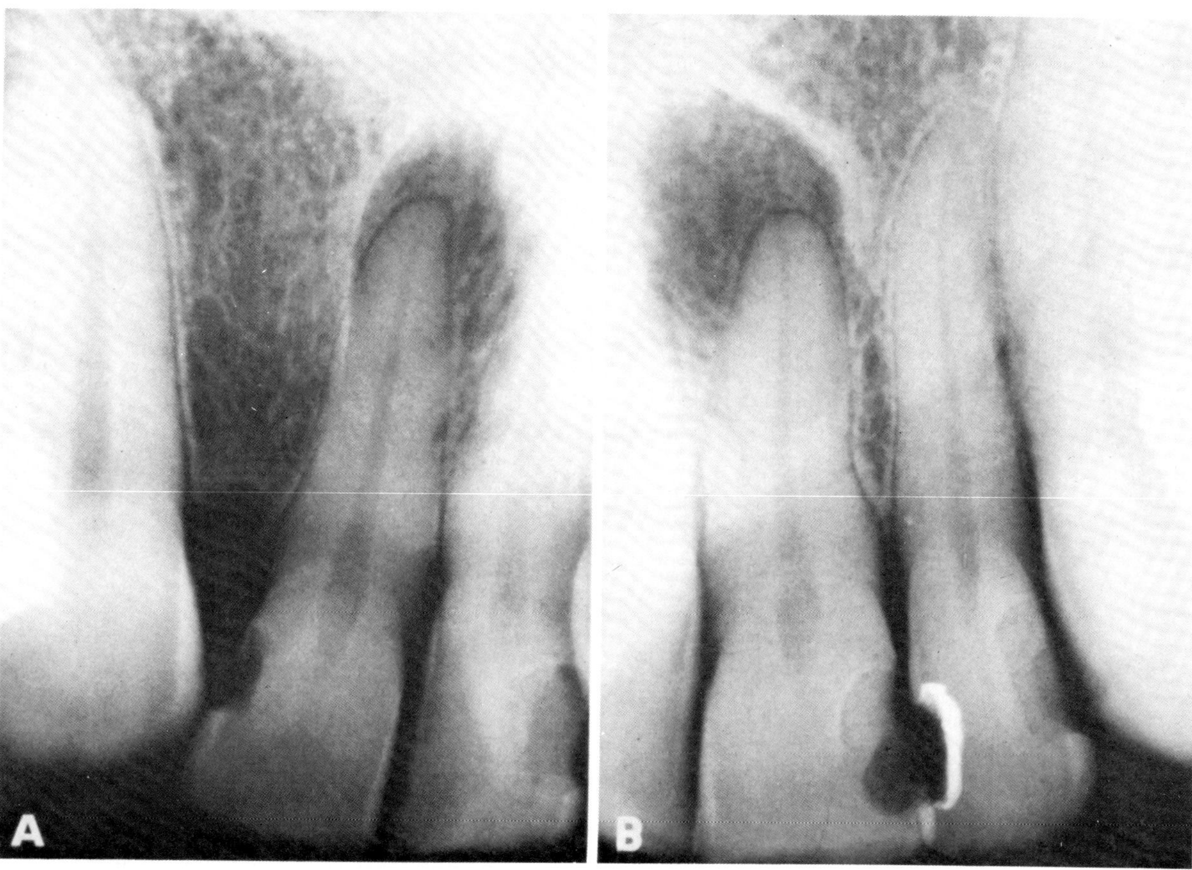

Fig. 10–5. Example of method used to determine relationship of radiolucency to periapex of tooth. *A,* Nasopalatine foramen is superimposed over periapex of *right* central incisor. Right lateral incisor is missing. *B,* By changing horizontal projection, shadow of nasopalatine foramen may also be superimposed over periapex of *left* central incisor, proving that radiolucent area is some distance lingual to apex of both teeth.

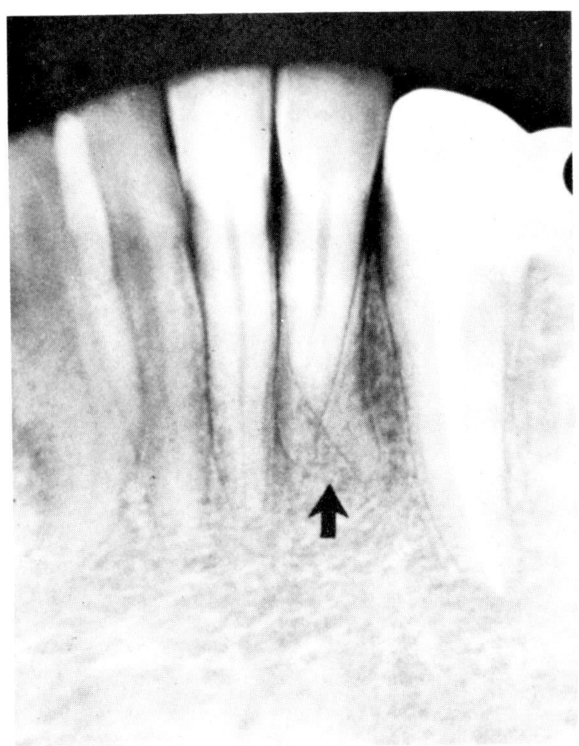

Fig. 10–6. Multiple roots and multiple canals in mandibular incisors may be demonstrated by varied horizontal exposures. Two roots of lateral incisor *(arrow)* are "separated" in this exposure.

and mechanical means (Fig. 10–8), the number of canals and foramens should be determined before enlargement is undertaken. In any case, the dentist should carefully obtain roentgenograms on every candidate for endodontic therapy, and should then exercise the utmost care in evaluating these films, even to examining them with a powerful magnifying glass.

Three-root or three-canal maxillary first premolars are seen more clearly if the projected horizontal direction of the central beam is slightly from the mesial (Fig. 10–9). The normal two roots or two canals of the maxillary first premolar also are easier to find ***if the beam is directed from the mesial.*** In this case the buccal canal or root ***always*** appears to the distal on the film. ("Shoot" from the ***mesial*** and the ***buccal*** root will always be to the ***distal.***)

Slowey has demonstrated how difficult it is to detect extra roots, let alone extra canals.[6] One particularly baffling case involved a maxillary lateral incisor with an unusual extra root. In the post-treatment radiograph, a bony lesion could be seen to the distal (Fig. 10–10*A*), but it was assumed related to invagination from the cingulum. Because the lesion would never heal, the tooth was extracted, and only then was the extra root revealed (Fig. 10–10*B*,*C*). A radiograph of the contralateral incisor reveals what must be a bilateral anomaly (Fig. 10–10*D*). As Slowey points out, "whenever the outline of the root is unclear, has an unusual contour, or strays in any way from the

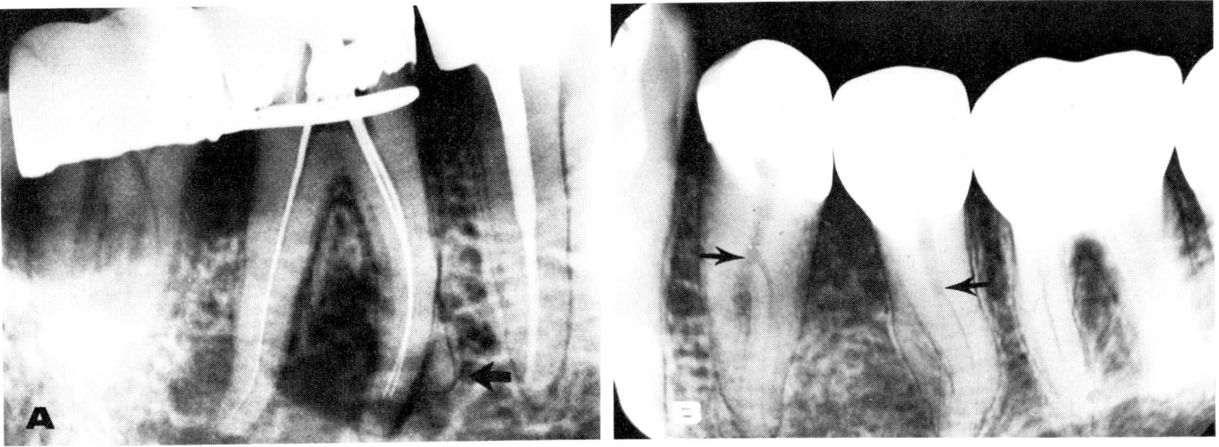

Fig. 10–7. *A,* Mesial root of first molar has not only two separate canals, but additional root as well *(arrow)*. *B,* Two premolars with unusual root and canal formation. "Fast-break" in canal density *(arrows)* indicates canal bifurcation. Both teeth have 3 and possibly 4 canals, but number of apical foramens can only be determined by instrument placement (see Fig. 10–8). (From Slowey, R. R.: Oral Surg., *37*:762, May, 1974.)

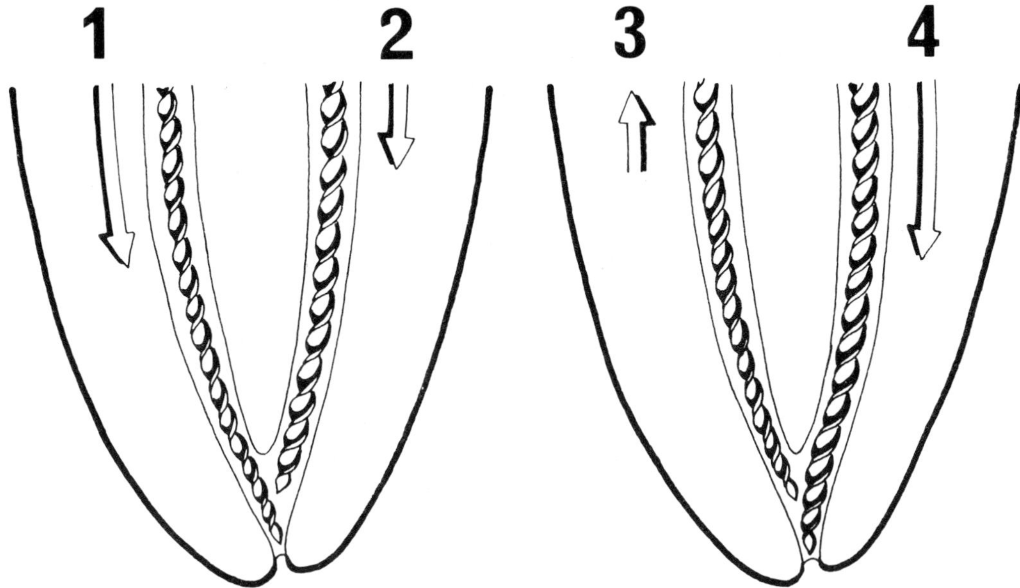

Fig. 10–8. Mechanical means of determining separate or common foramens for two canals. Instrument is placed to full depth in either canal (1) and instrument in second canal (2) is prevented from going fully to place. Single foramens can then be confirmed by raising first instrument (3), allowing second instrument to go fully to place (4). If turned, instruments can be felt to grate against each other. (From Serene, T. P., Krasny, R. M., Zeigler, P. E., Higginbotham, T. L., Longhurst, G. E.: *Principles of Preclinical Endodontics.* Dubuque, Iowa. Kendall/Hunt Publishing Co., 1974.)

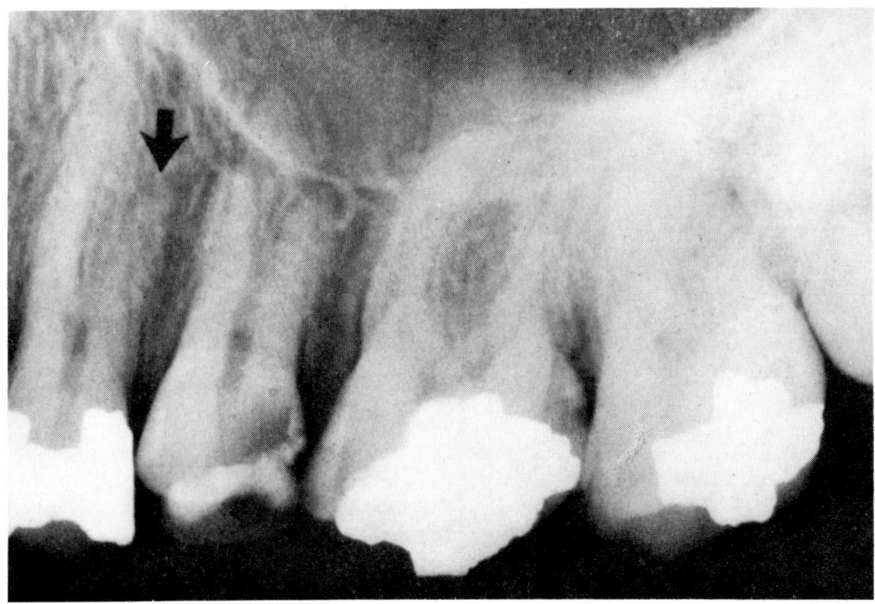

Fig. 10–9. Three rooted maxillary first premolar *(arrow)* and second premolar are readily discerned in this roentgenogram. Clarity of root structure can be improved by "aiming" central beam directly through ***apical*** region.

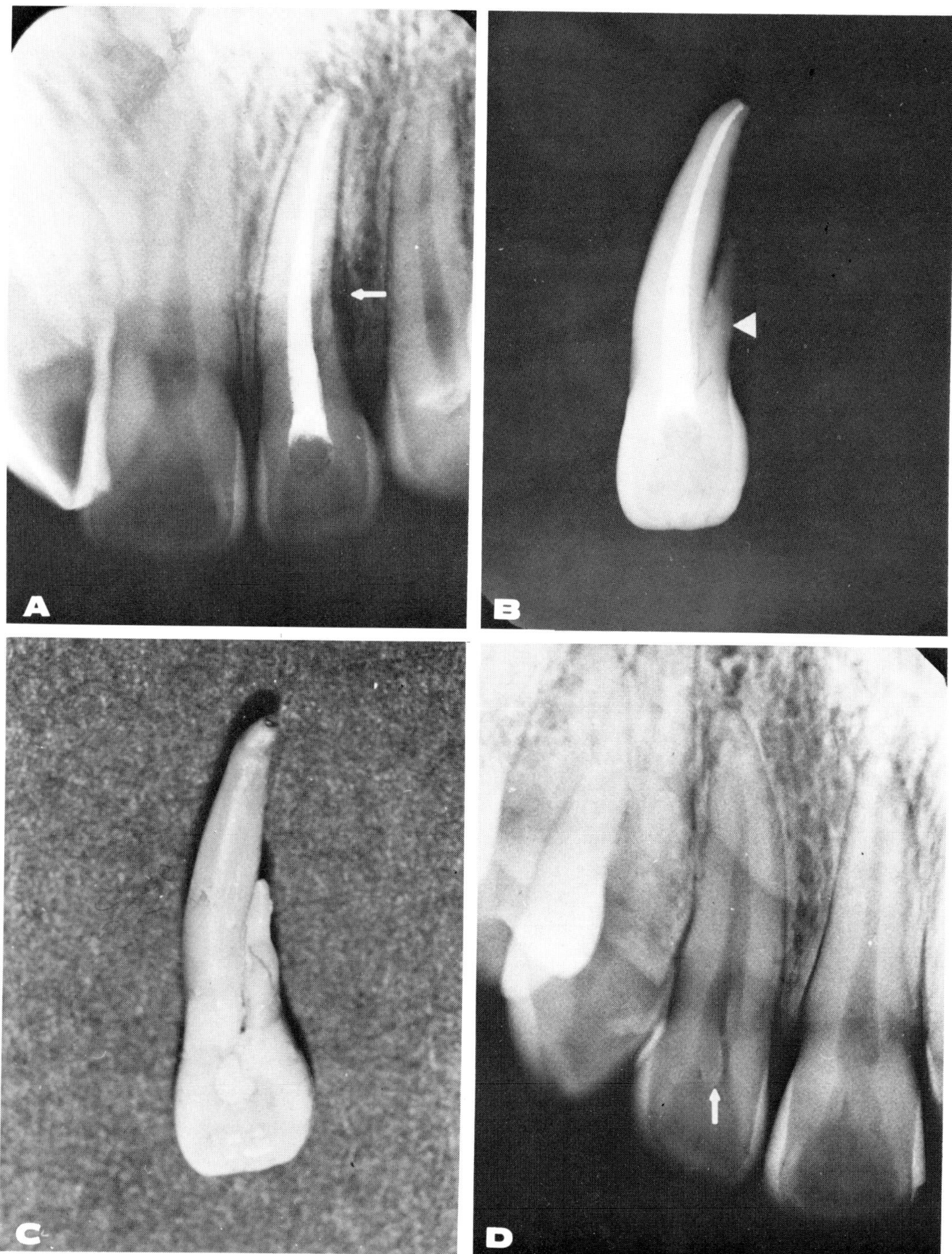

Fig. 10–10. *A,* Continuing lateral lesion (mesial) and acute abscess. Tooth is finally extracted. *B,* Benchtop radiographic view reveals second root and unfilled canal, which was not seen in original films. *C,* Lingual view of second root and invagination from cingulum. *D,* On contralateral side, similar anomaly exists. (From Slowey, R. R.: Oral Surg., *37*:762, May, 1974.)

expected radiographic appearance, one should suspect an additional root canal . . ."[6] He quotes Worth who said "Look at the corners of the radiograph and the center will take care of itself."

The mystery of extra canals within the normal number of roots is more perplexing than the extra root problem itself. Slowey has again given us some tips in how to detect the undetected.[6] One method is to observe carefully in the length-of-tooth film the appearance of the canal, high in the root, just as it breaks out of the chamber. If an ***extra dark line*** is seen in the coronal third of the root, running parallel to the instrument (Fig. 10–11), one should suspect a second canal. This is especially true in the mesiobuccal of upper first molars, where a fourth canal is found 50% of the time, or in the distal of lower first molars (Fig. 10–12).

Slowey also points out another clever diagnostic aid.[6] It could be called "the fast-break." In viewing a radiograph, if one detects a ***sudden change*** in the radiolucency within a canal, this change in density probably signals the beginning of an additional canal (Fig. 10–13), a frequent occurrence in maxillary first premolars. When seen in such teeth as a mandibular canine (Fig. 10–14*A*), however, it requires that the dentist obtain roentgenograms from a different horizontal angle (Fig. 10–14*B*), and that he search out the extra canals with the length-of-tooth instruments (Fig. 10–14*C*).

A frequently overlooked vagary in root formation

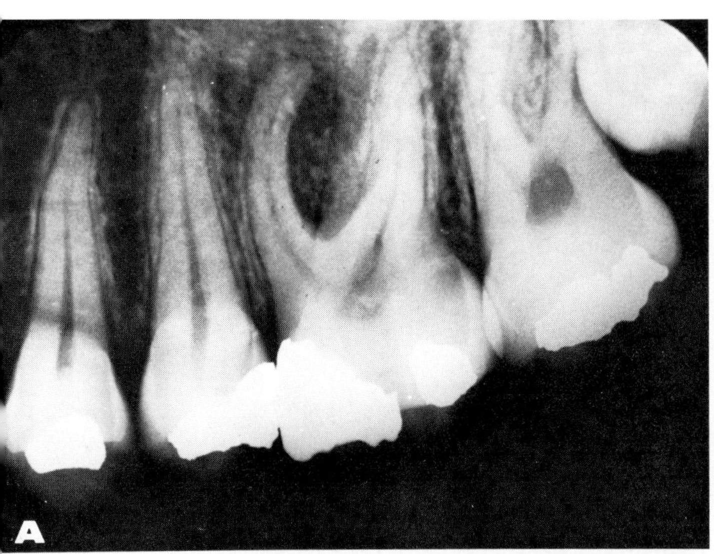

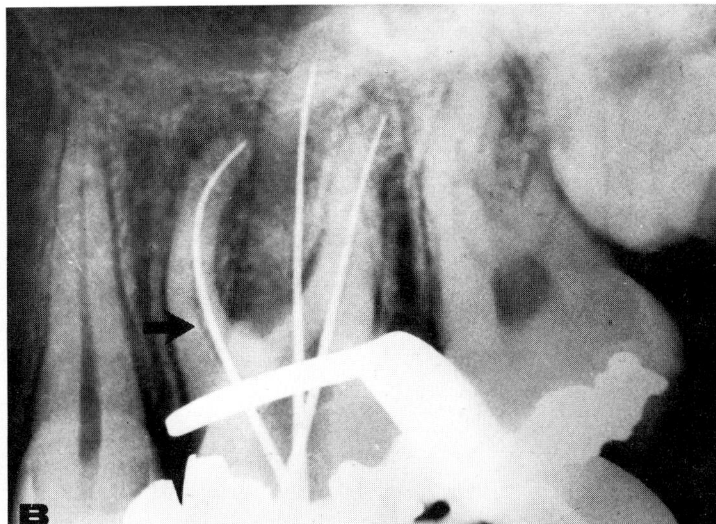

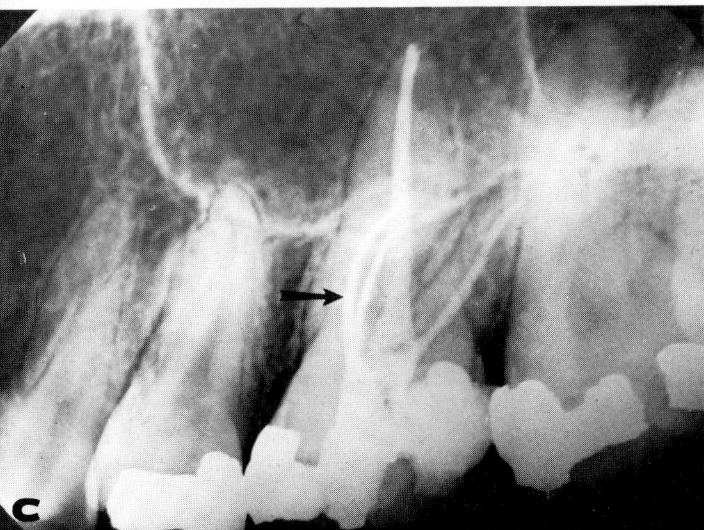

Fig. 10–11. *A,* From viewing initial film, one would not suspect 2 canals in mesiobuccal root of the first molar. *B,* Extra dark line alongside exploring instrument *(arrow)* signals possibility of second canal. *C,* Final film showing 2 separate mesiobuccal canals apparently arising from common orifice. (From Slowey, R. R.: Oral Surg., *37*:762, May, 1974.)

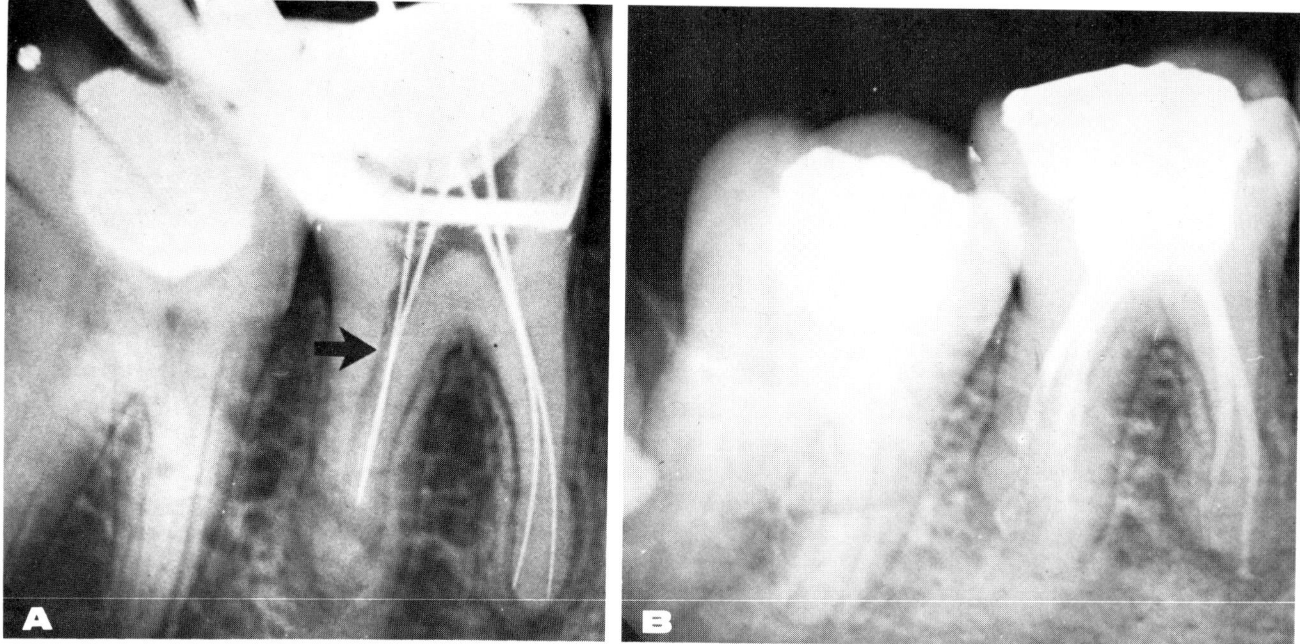

Fig. 10–12. *A,* Two instruments in single canal, but wide extra dark line *(arrow)* indicates additional canal. *B,* Final filling proves 4 canals. (From Slowey, R. R.: Oral Surg., *37*:762, May, 1974.)

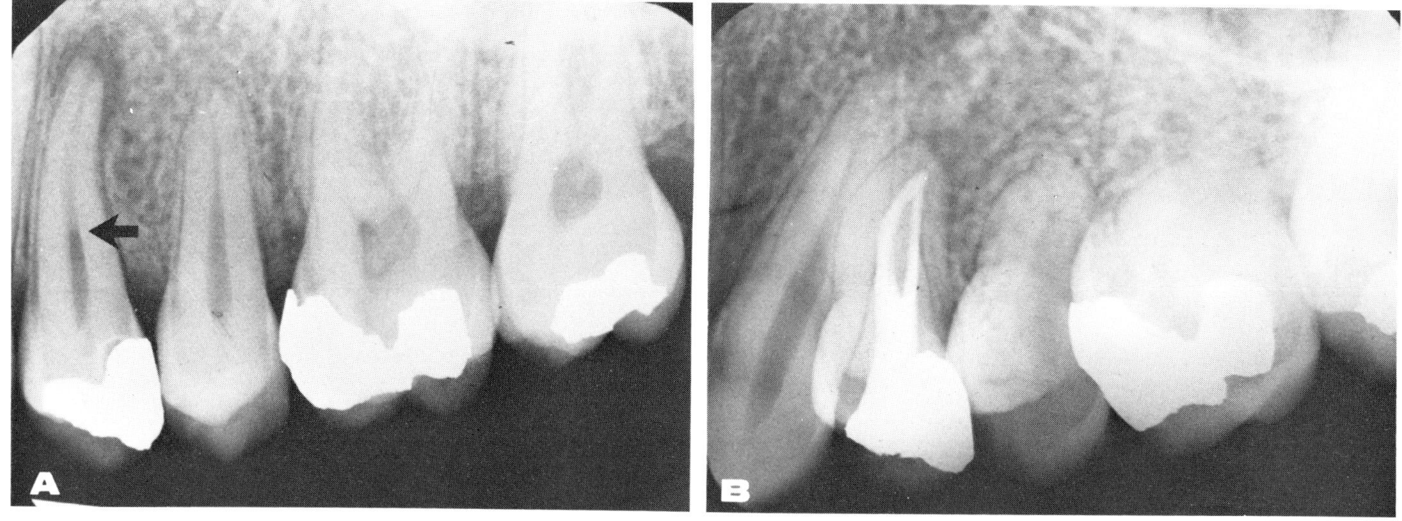

Fig. 10–13. *A,* Sudden change in radiographic density *(arrow)* signals probable canal bifurcation at that point. *B,* Change from right-angle horizontal projection *(A)* to 20-degree projection from distal clearly reveals two canals but single foramen. (From Slowey, R. R.: Oral Surg., *37*:762, May, 1974.)

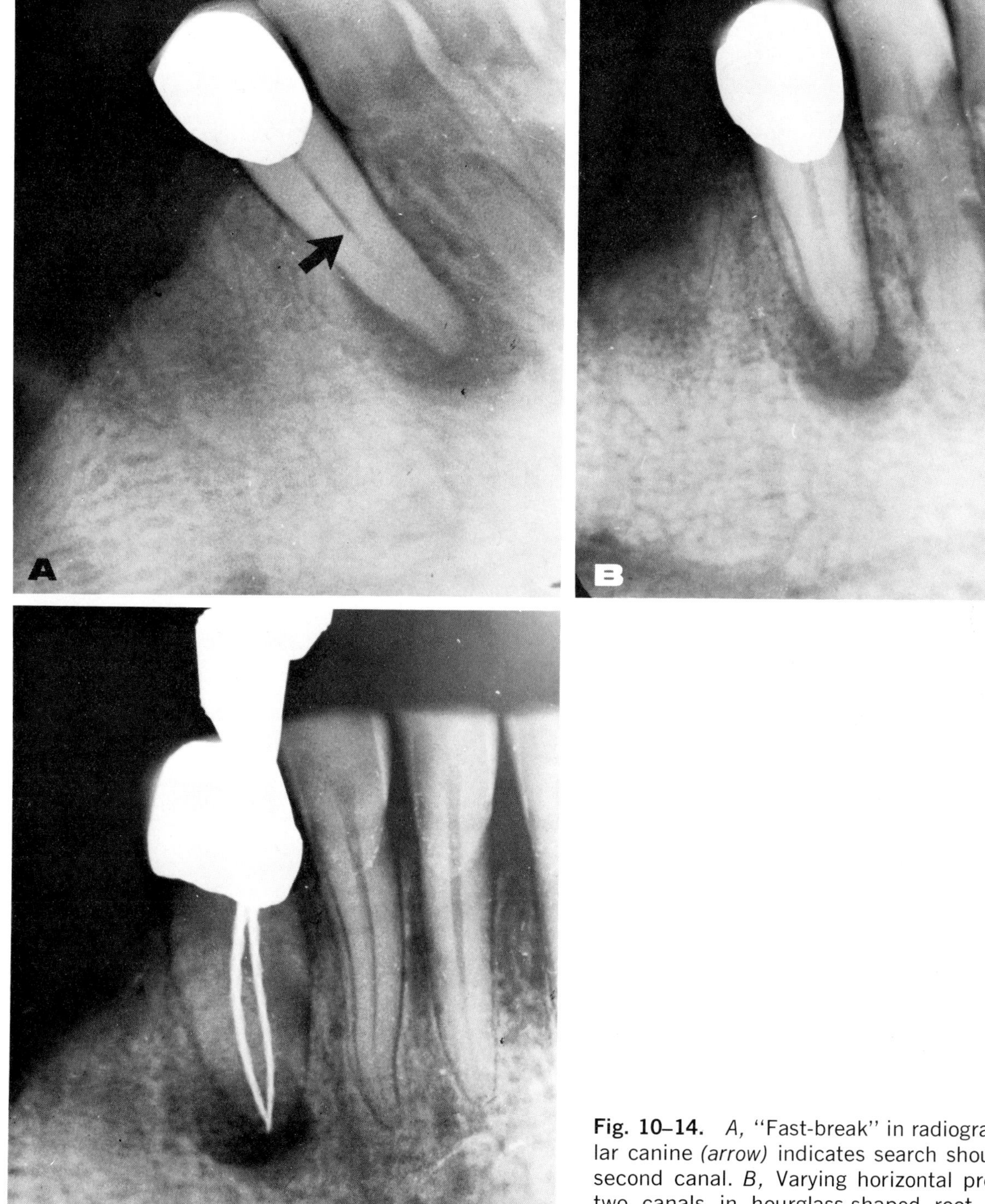

Fig. 10–14. *A,* "Fast-break" in radiograph of mandibular canine *(arrow)* indicates search should be made for second canal. *B,* Varying horizontal projection reveals two canals in hourglass-shaped root. *C,* "Length of tooth" instruments in place reveal single foramen. (From Slowey, R. R.: Oral Surg., *37*:762, May, 1974.)

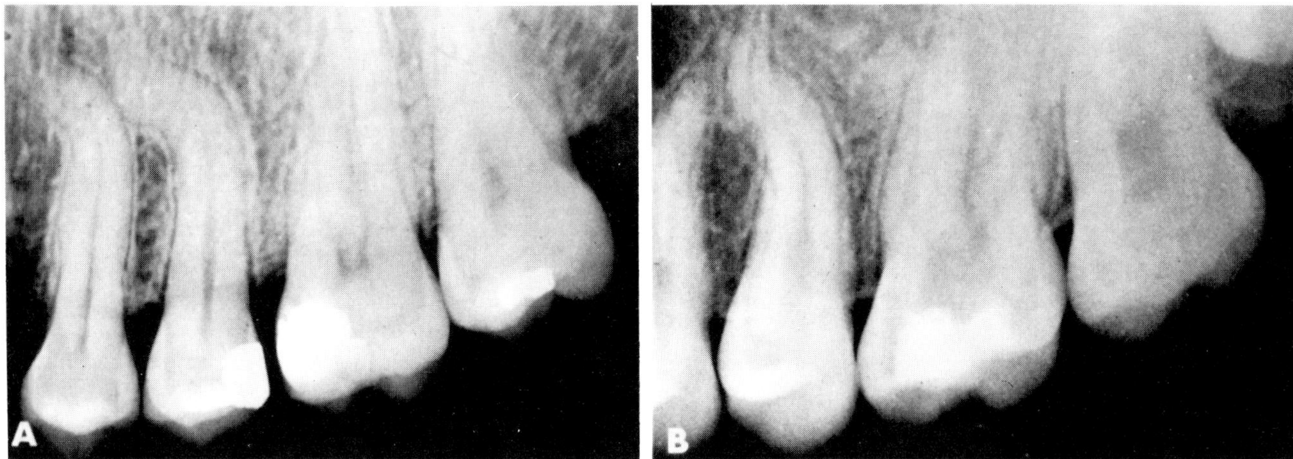

Fig. 10–15. Unusual *mesial* and bayonet curvature seen in three maxillary premolars.

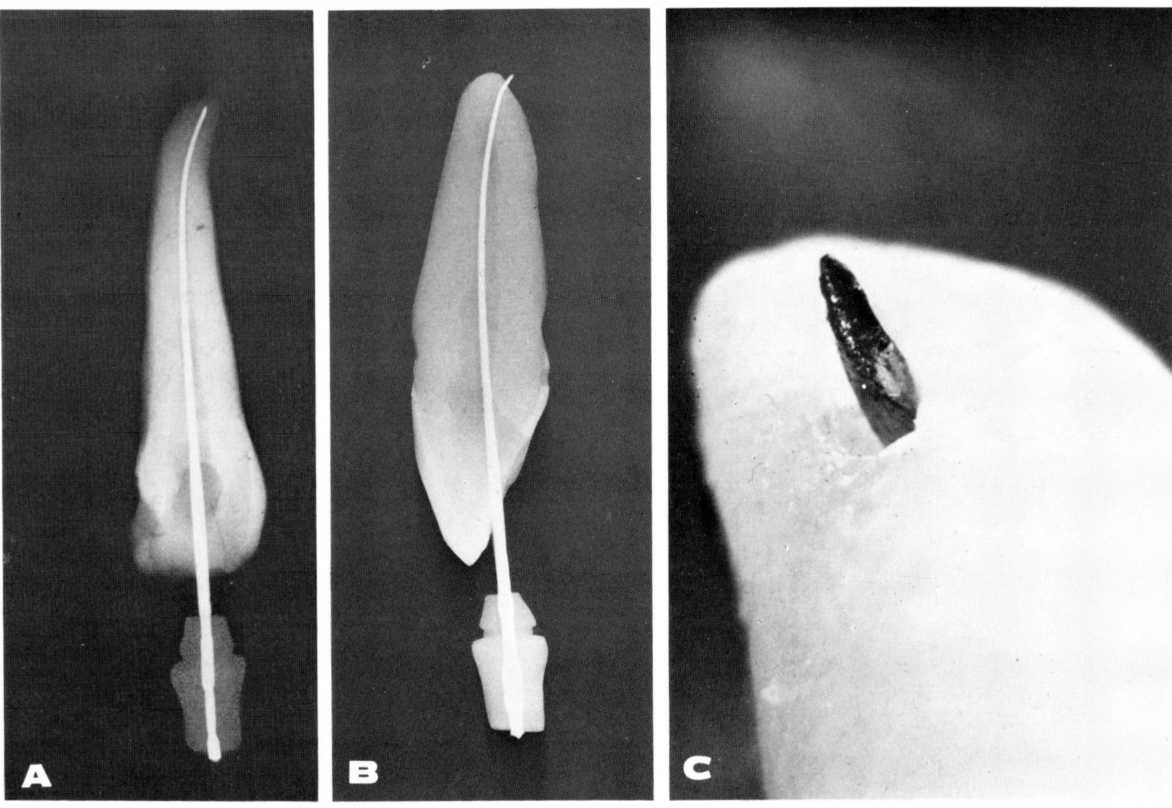

Fig. 10–16. Double root curvature in maxillary lateral incisor. *A,* Radiograph with instrument proves canal exits to distal. *B,* Mesiodistal view of same tooth shows canal also exits to lingual. *C,* Apical photograph of same tooth which demonstrates instrument perforating lingual far short of apex. (Courtesy Dr. Howard Clausen and Dr. John R. Grady.)

is severe curvature. When curvature is to the mesial or distal, so frequently seen in the maxillary lateral incisors (50% of the time) or occasionally seen in premolars (Fig. 10–15), no problem in detection of the curvature exists. When the curvature is to the ***buccal*** or ***lingual,*** however, in the same plane as the central x-ray beam, curvature is difficult to detect (Fig. 10–16). Careful examination may reveal increased radiopacity at the root end, as the root doubles back on itself and is literally "x-rayed" twice. In its extreme, a peculiar "target" or "bullseye" appearance will show in the film (Fig. 10–17).

In addition to "normal" variances in tooth form, certain anomalies that could well affect the vitality of the pulp may appear in the roentgenogram. Invagination and dens in dente are two conditions that frequently have anomalous tracts leading from the enamel surface directly to the pulp (Fig. 10–18). These defects may also extend well up the root, even to the apex. They are accompanied by a deep, bacterial invasion of the pulp, which leads to pulp necrosis and its periapical sequelae (p. 316).

Lesions Within the Tooth Observable by Roentgenogram. Before discussing those lesions within the tooth observable by roentgenogram, a word must

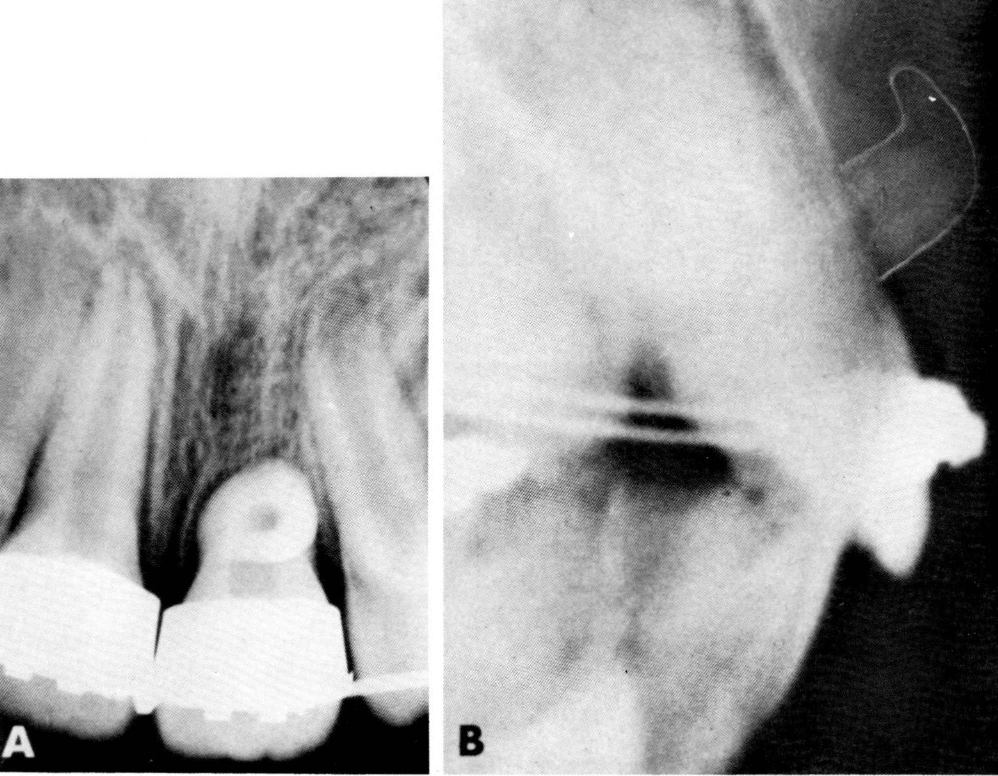

Fig. 10–17. "Target" or "bullseye" phenomena seen in roots that severely curve to buccal or lingual, *i.e.,* in direction of central beam. *A,* Central incisor with dilacerated root under orthodontic realignment. *B,* Lateral head film in which labially dilacerated root is apparent. Photo retouched for clarity. (Courtesy Dr. Alfred T. Baum.)

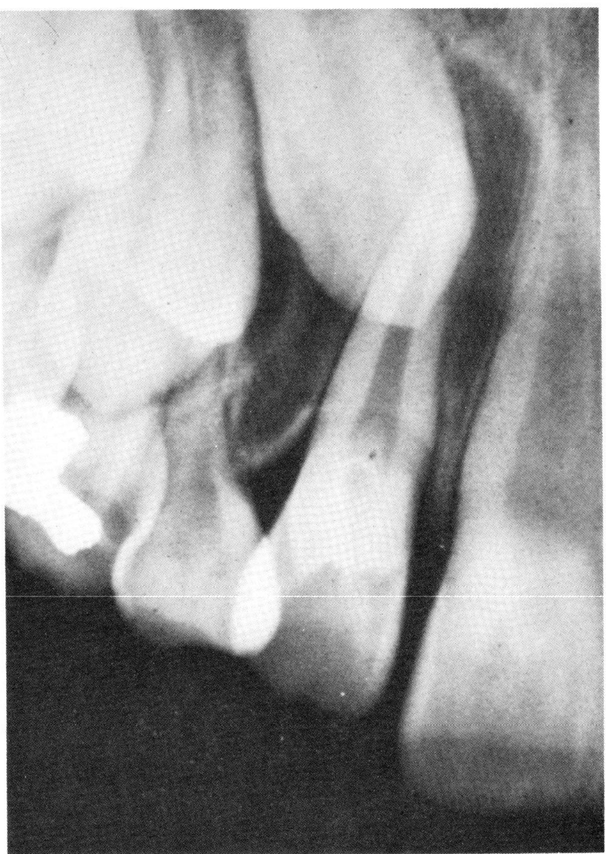

Fig. 10–18. *Dens invaginatus* in cingulum area of maxillary lateral incisor. Anomalous tract seen in this roentgenogram has led to pulp infection and periapical pathosis.

be said about those lesions ***not*** observable in a diagnostic film, for herein lies a common error in diagnosis. The dentist should not expect to see roentgenographic changes within the tooth when examining a patient with hypersensitivity or acute pulpalgia. The roentgenogram shows changes in calcifications; therefore the soft tissue lesion of acute pulpalgia cannot be seen in a film. Necrosis of the pulp also cannot be seen ***within*** the tooth, although ***periapical*** changes usually accompany necrosis. Pulp death in the ***developing tooth,*** in which the pulp is destroyed by traumatic accident, is readily apparent because the root ceases to develop.

In contrast to acute pulpalgia or necrosis, ***chronic*** pulp inflammation may frequently be diagnosed from the roentgenographic changes seen within the tooth. Pulp stones and pulp "gravel" are often associated with chronic pulp disease (Fig. 10–19). This most certainly does not mean that all teeth with pulp stones are involved in chronic pulpitis, for pulp stones are a frequent finding in apparently normal, virgin teeth (Fig. 10–20). The chronically inflamed pulp, however, often produces not only pulp calcifications, but also areas of internal resorption.

Internal resorption often is seen following traumatic injury (Fig. 10–21). Idiopathic internal resorption also may be "picked-up" on roentgenogram. Differentiation between internal resorption and external resorption is quite simple by radiograph.[7] First of all, the lesion of internal resorption has sharp smooth margins that can be clearly defined (Fig. 10–22*A*). It need not be symmetrical, however. Another diagnostic sign is the manner in which the pulp "disappears" into the lesion—not extending ***through*** the lesion in its regular shape (Fig. 10–22*B*).

Initially, the resorbed defect may be confused with dental caries in the roentgenogram (Fig. 10–23). On the other hand, dental caries is a less sharply defined

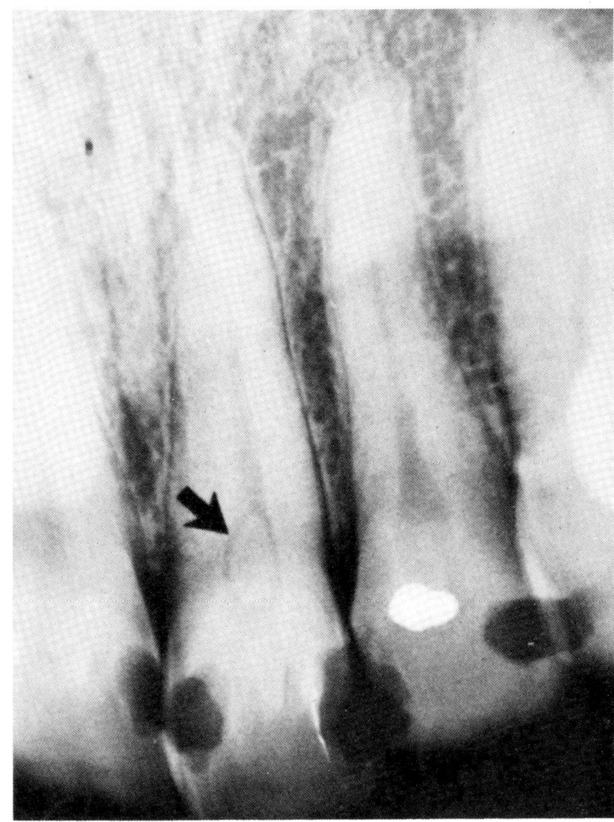

Fig. 10–19. Huge pulp stone *(arrow)* which has developed in association with chronic pulpitis. This "ball and socket" type stone must be fragmented to be removed.

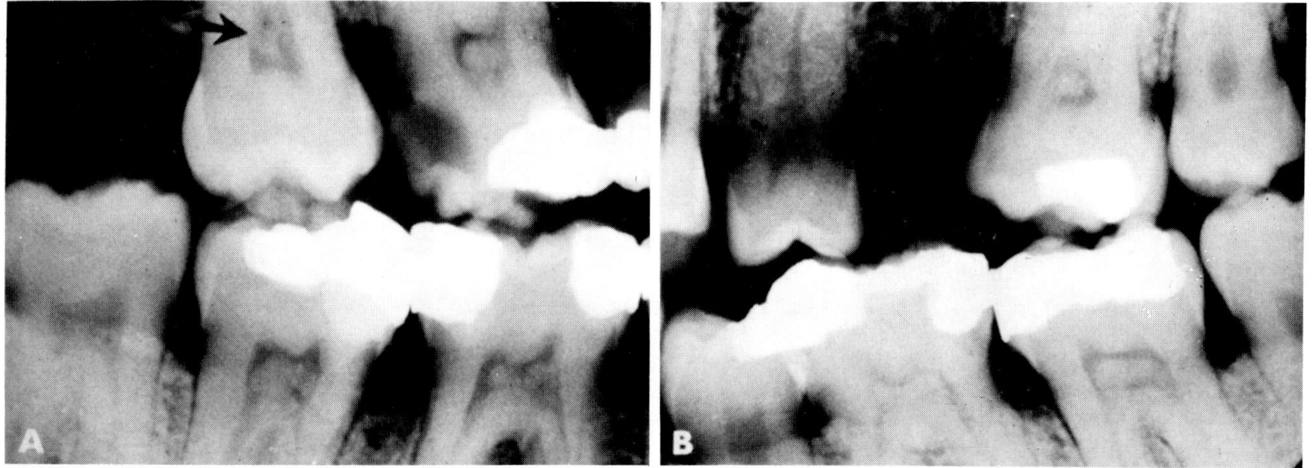

Fig. 10–20. Multiple pulp stones that have developed in molar teeth of one patient. Many stones are related to advanced carious lesions and large restorations. One stone, *left (arrow),* has developed in virgin tooth.

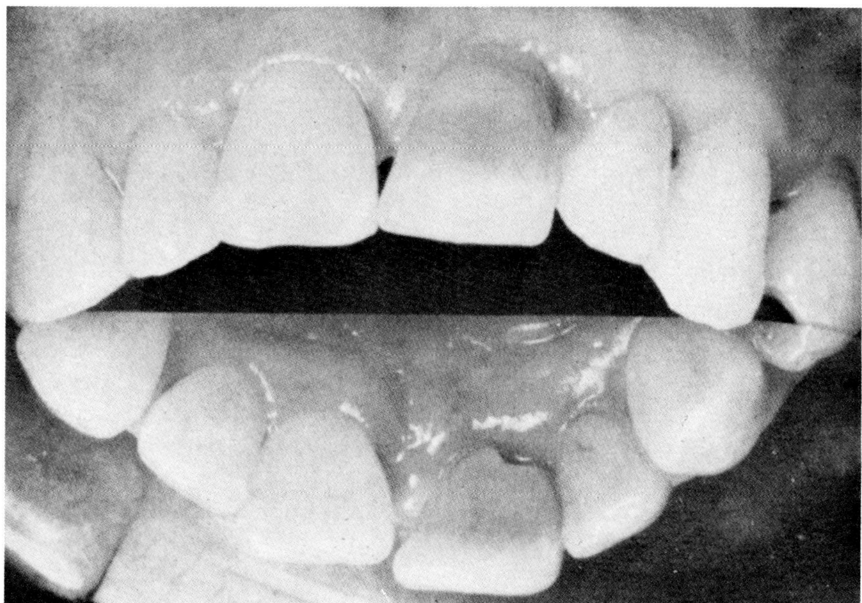

Fig. 10–21. Frontal and mirror views of "pink tooth." Crown is badly involved with internal resorption following impact trauma.

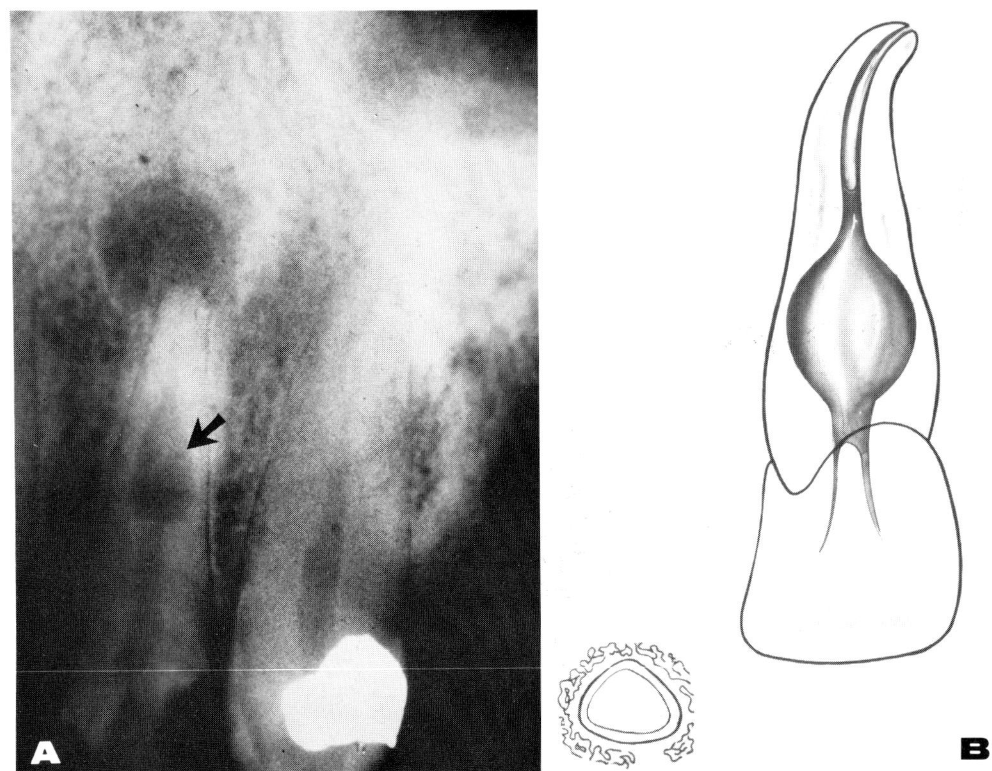

Fig. 10–22. *A,* Radiograph of lesion of ***internal*** resorption. Note sharp smooth margins. *B,* Drawing of internal resorption shows how shadow of pulp "disappears" into lesion. (Courtesy Drs. A. H. Gartner, T. Mack, R. Somerlott, and L. Walsh. Drawing modified from Dr. F. H. Lepp, Caracas, Venezuela, Oral Surg. *27*:185, Feb., 1969.)

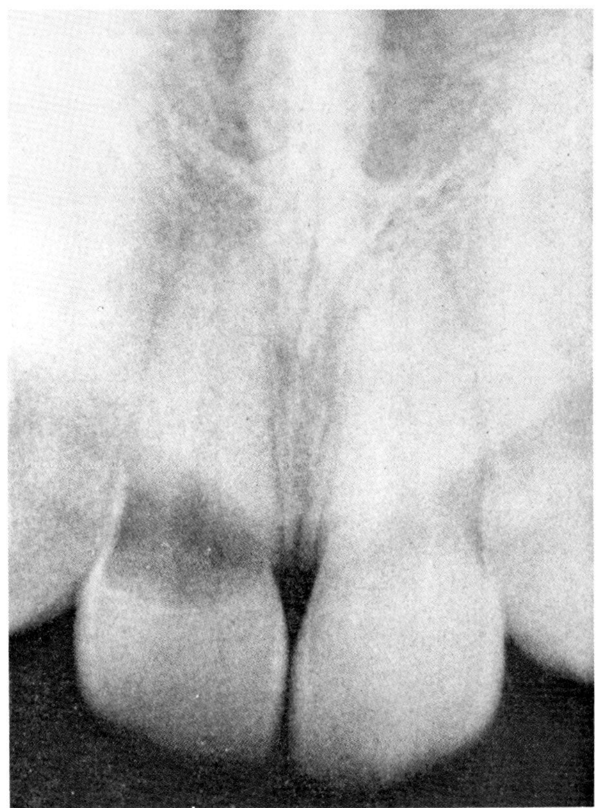

Fig. 10–23. Internal resorption (Fig. 10–21) may easily be confused with dental caries in roentgenogram.

shadow on the radiograph than is internal resorption. A careful visual examination should prove that the carious lesion does not exist. To ignore the resorptive lesion could be fatal to the future of the tooth, as the internal resorption relentlessly progresses to a hopeless state (Fig. 10–24).

Other effects of impact trauma besides internal resorption may be observed by roentgenogram within the tooth. A root fracture, of course, may be seen, but in addition to this, pulp stones, calcifications, or early pulp death may show in diagnostic films (Fig. 10–25).

Roentgenograms may be valuable diagnostic aids in determining which teeth could possibly be involved in pulpalgia. Deep caries and deep restorations, as well as recurrent caries, may have suggested the diagnosis.

Lesions Outside the Tooth Observable by Roentgenogram. Once again, attention must be di-

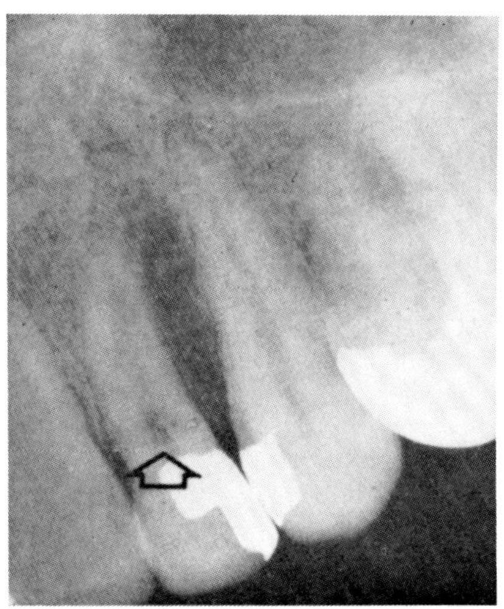

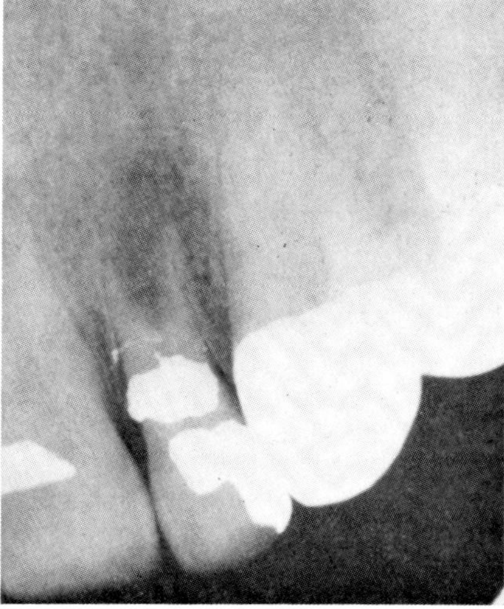

Fig. 10–24. Initial lesions of internal resorption *(left—arrow)* is mistaken for dental caries. Operative intervention *(right)* has stimulated internal resorptive process.

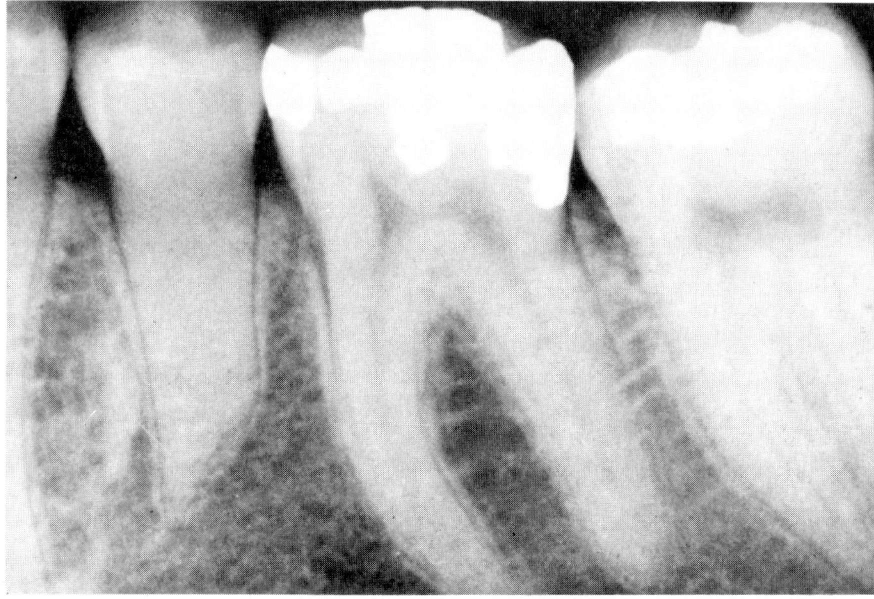

Fig. 10–25. Total pulp calcification and external resorption following injury of mandibular second premolar.

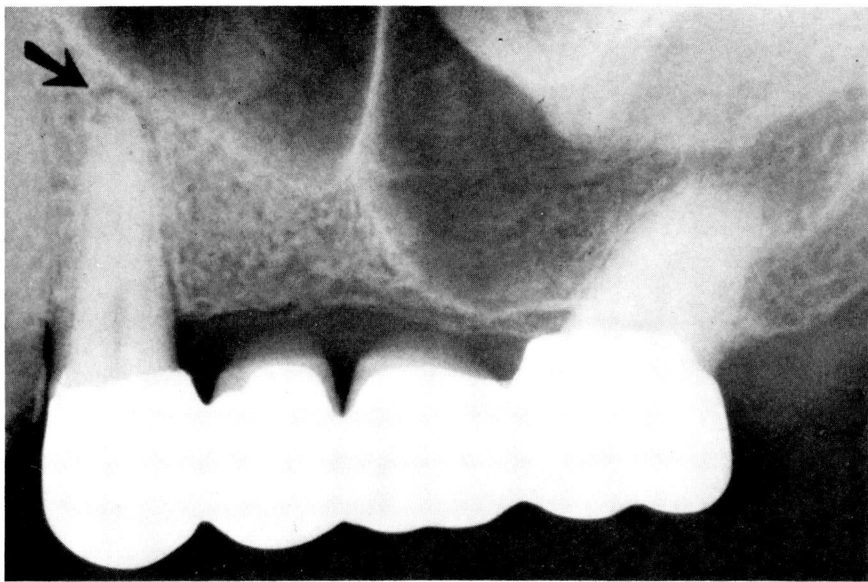

Fig. 10–26. Periapical changes associated with traumatism *(arrow)* are often mistaken for lesions of pulp origin. First premolar is vital but highly mobile.

rected to pulp and periapical conditions in which roentgenographic changes are ***not readily*** observable. No periapical lesions should be expected during ***incipient*** or ***moderate*** pulpalgia; however, a widening of the periodontal space at the apex may be expected along with ***advanced*** pulpalgia. This space develops as inflammation extends from the pulp into the periapical tissues, and the tooth is lifted in its socket by the inflammatory swelling (see Fig. 8–21*C*).

The periapical lesion associated with occlusal traumatism may be mistaken for a lesion of pulp origin. The widened periodontal space and external root resorption can be confused with the changes from advanced pulpitis (Fig. 10–26). History of pulpalgia, and reaction to hot and cold, will aid in differential diagnosis.

The same widened periodontal space should be expected with two other acute conditions; acute apical periodontitis and acute apical abscess. All too frequently dentists expect to see major decalcific changes associated with these violent acute conditions. They overlook, of course, that the decalcification seen on a roentgenogram takes days to develop, and should not be expected to appear with a condition of short duration.

The periapical osseous changes associated with ***chronic pulp disease*** are a paradox. Rather than a decalcifying lesion, as one might expect, the ***radiopaque*** lesion of condensing osteitis often is related to the root end of the tooth involved in chronic pulpitis. In addition to the condensing osteitis, external root resorption also may take place. In this case, the missing tooth structure is replaced by the condensing osteitis (osteosclerosis) (Fig. 10–27). When the chronically inflamed pulp is removed by pulpectomy, and root canal therapy is completed, the condensing bony lesion gradually disappears (see Fig. 9–41).

Differentiating external resorption from internal resorption is remarkably simple.[7] First of all, the walls of the lesion are ragged and irregular (Fig. 10–28*A*). It might appear on the side of the tooth or centered. The pulp always appears to "pass through" the lesion unaltered, maintaining its shape and size to the apex. The lesion appears to be superimposed over the canal (Fig. 10–28*B*).

If the resorption is at the apex, the tooth may appear shortened, blunted, or square, rather than conical, as in teeth moved orthodontically (Fig. 10–29*A*), or it may be obliquely resorbed or have a cupped-out appearance (Fig. 10–29*B*). Another may have the chewed appearance of a tree felled by a beaver (Fig. 10–29*C*). In any event, if apical resorption has taken place, the apical foramen will be in the center of the end of the root. The apical opening can be seen. If the root resorption has a moth-eaten appearance, it is possible that the tooth was traumatically ripped loose from its ligaments and/or was

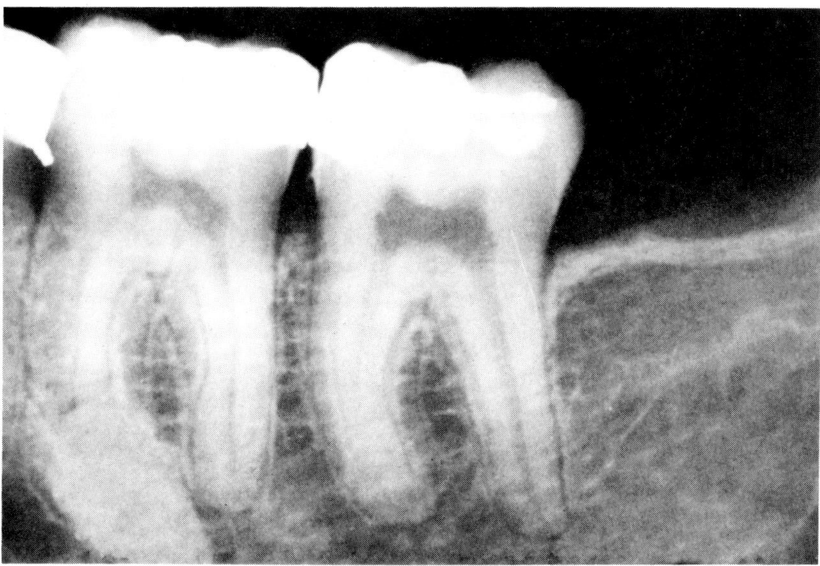

Fig. 10–27. Condensing osteitis, external resorption, and pulp stones associated with chronic pulpitis of first molar. Condensing osteitis will disappear following successful endodontic therapy.

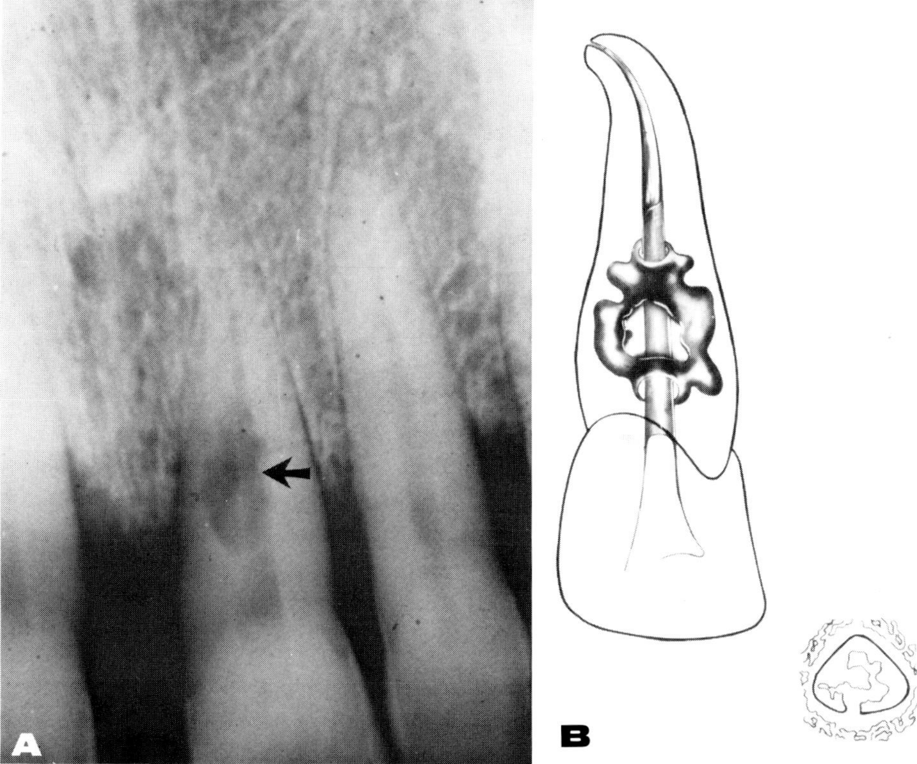

Fig. 10–28. *A,* Radiograph of lesion of ***external*** resorption. Note ragged margins of lesion. *B,* Drawing of external resorption shows how shadow of pulp "passes through" lesion unaltered. (Courtesy Drs. A. H. Gartner, T. Mack, R. Somerlott, and L. Walsh. Drawing modified from Dr. L. H. Lepp, Caracas, Venezuela, Oral Surg. *27*:185, Feb., 1969.)

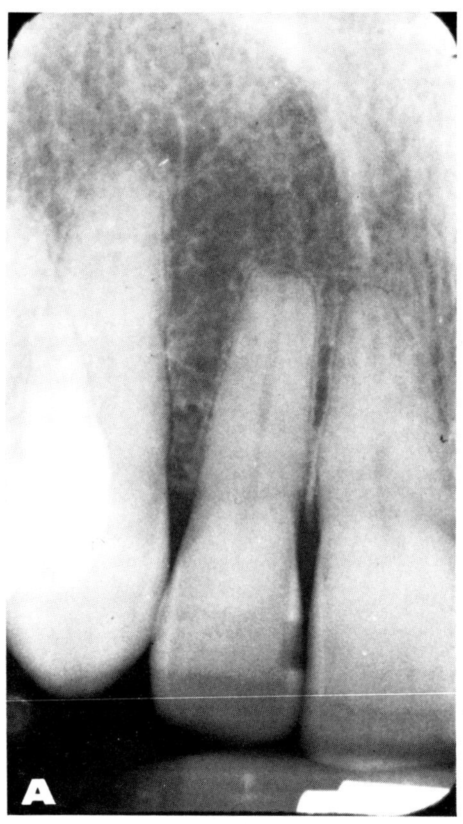

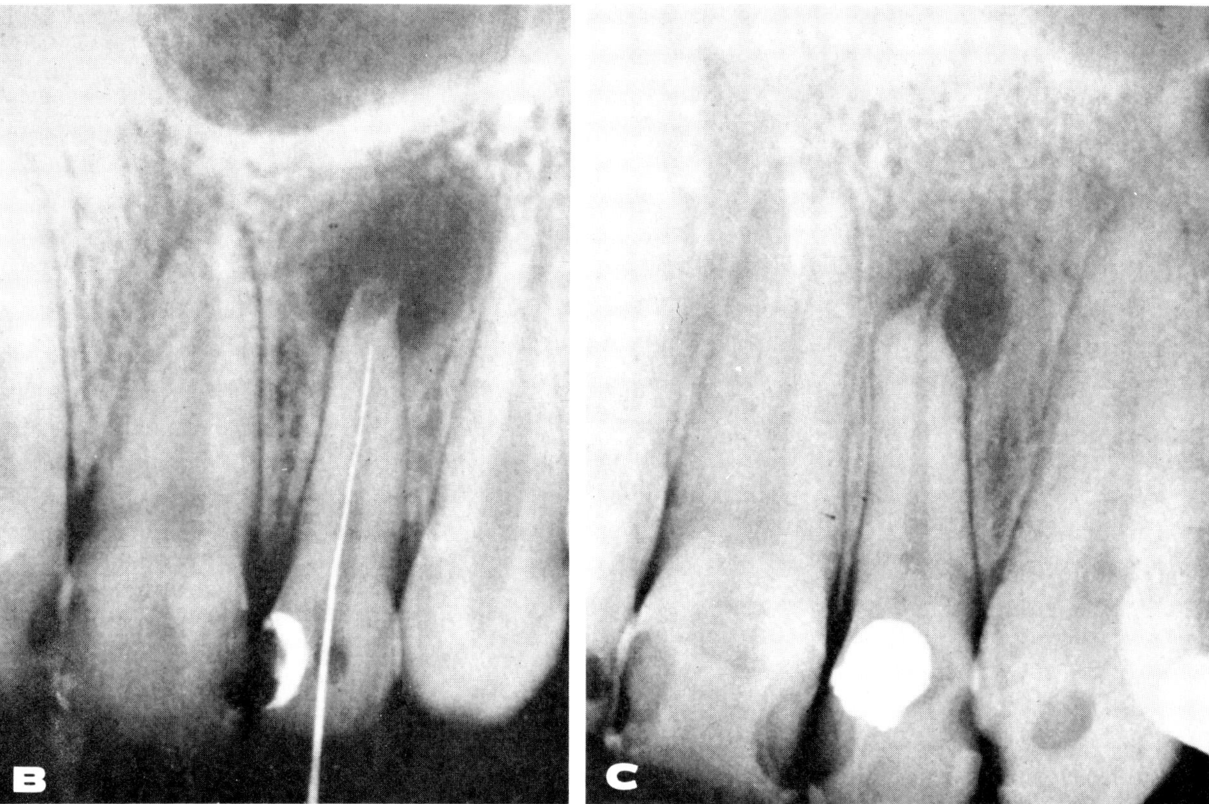

Fig. 10–29. *A,* Blunted apices of teeth moved orthodontically more than 40 years ago. *B* and *C,* Two forms of apical external resorption. *B,* Resorptive defect leaves flaring apical foramen which could not be adequately obturated by conventional methods. *C,* Advanced external resorption of apex makes conventional instrumentation hazardous. (*B* and *C* from Luebke, R. G., Glick, D. H. and Ingle, J. I.: Oral Surg., *18*:97, July, 1964.)

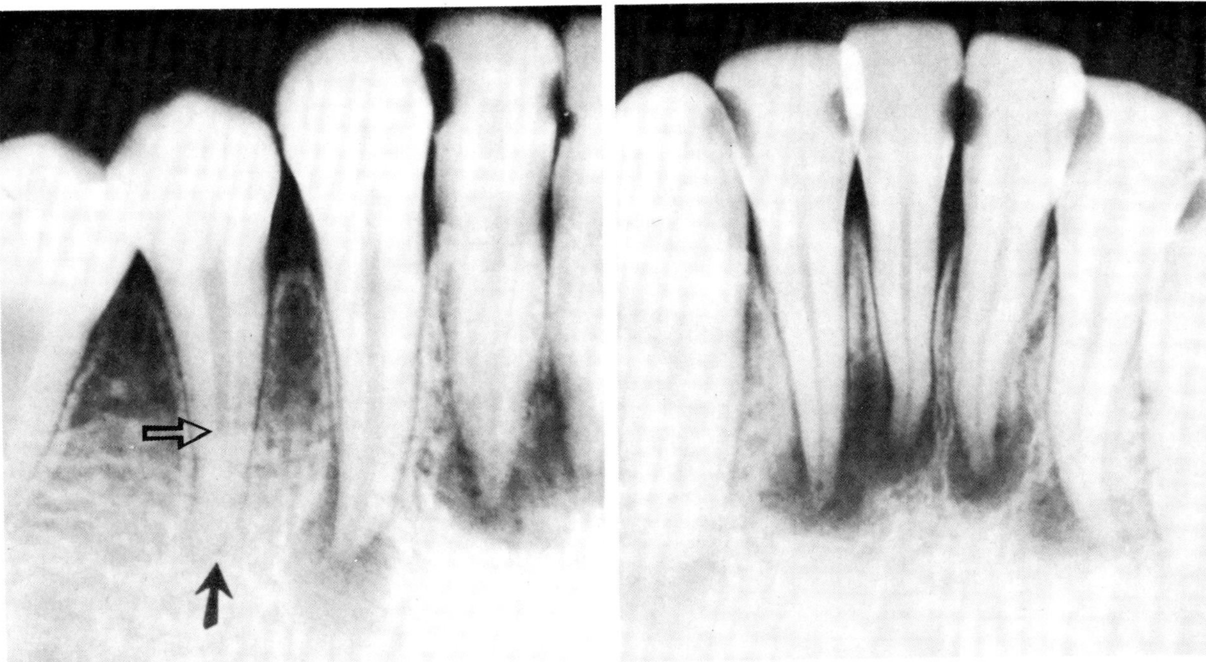

Fig. 10–30. *Chronic* apical periodontitis involving five mandibular anterior teeth. Pulp death from impact trauma. Well-circumscribed lesions and pear-shaped configuration periapical to canine are typical of chronic apical periodontitis. These may be confused with apical cyst. Bifurcated canal *(left, arrow)* is also apparent. Sudden change in radiolucency in canal *(open arrow)* denotes point of separation of canals.

replanted. Sometimes an unexplained lesion in the region strongly suggests malignant disease (see Fig. 9–44).

Roentgenographic Changes as the Sequelae of Pulp Necrosis. The periapical osseous lesions that develop as sequelae of pulp necrosis are by far the most frequently observed regional changes.

Associated with ***chronic apical periodontitis*** is a well-circumscribed osseous lesion. Roentgenographically, it appears as a radiolucent area, varying in size from a few millimeters to a circle the size of a filbert. The bony perimeter of the lesion may appear radiopaque (Fig. 10–30).

It is virtually impossible to differentiate by roentgenogram the lesion of chronic apical periodontitis from that of ***apical cyst.*** On occasion, the cyst may be more circumscribed and have a denser bony perimeter. It also moves roots around (Fig. 10–31).

The roentgenographic appearance of ***suppurative apical periodontitis*** is that of a larger, more diffuse, and irregular lesion (Fig. 10–32). This lesion may also drain into the mouth through a fistula or extraorally onto the neck or chin (Fig. 10–33).

In the event that one of these inflammatory lesions is in contact with the floor of the maxillary sinus, chronic sinusitis may result (Fig. 10–34).

Differential Diagnosis. A number of pathologic changes in and near the alveolar process may be mistaken for true periapical lesions. First to consider would be the nonodontogenic cysts—the globulomaxillary cyst, the midline palatal cyst, and cyst of the nasopalatine canal or foramen. Because these cysts are not associated with the exact root end, they may be roentgenographically "moved" around and away from the root ends if the horizontal direction of the central x-ray beam is varied from side to side (Fig. 10–35). Residual cysts, as well as globulomaxillary cysts, may be found along the lateral surface of the root (see Figs. 9–30 and 9–31). To be further considered in the differential diagnosis of cysts is the vitality of the pulps of associated teeth. The pulp of a tooth with an ***apical*** cyst will test nonvital. This may not be true of the teeth near nonodontogenic cysts, unless traumatic injury caused pulp death and also triggered sutural cyst formation.

Periodontal lesions may easily be mistaken for

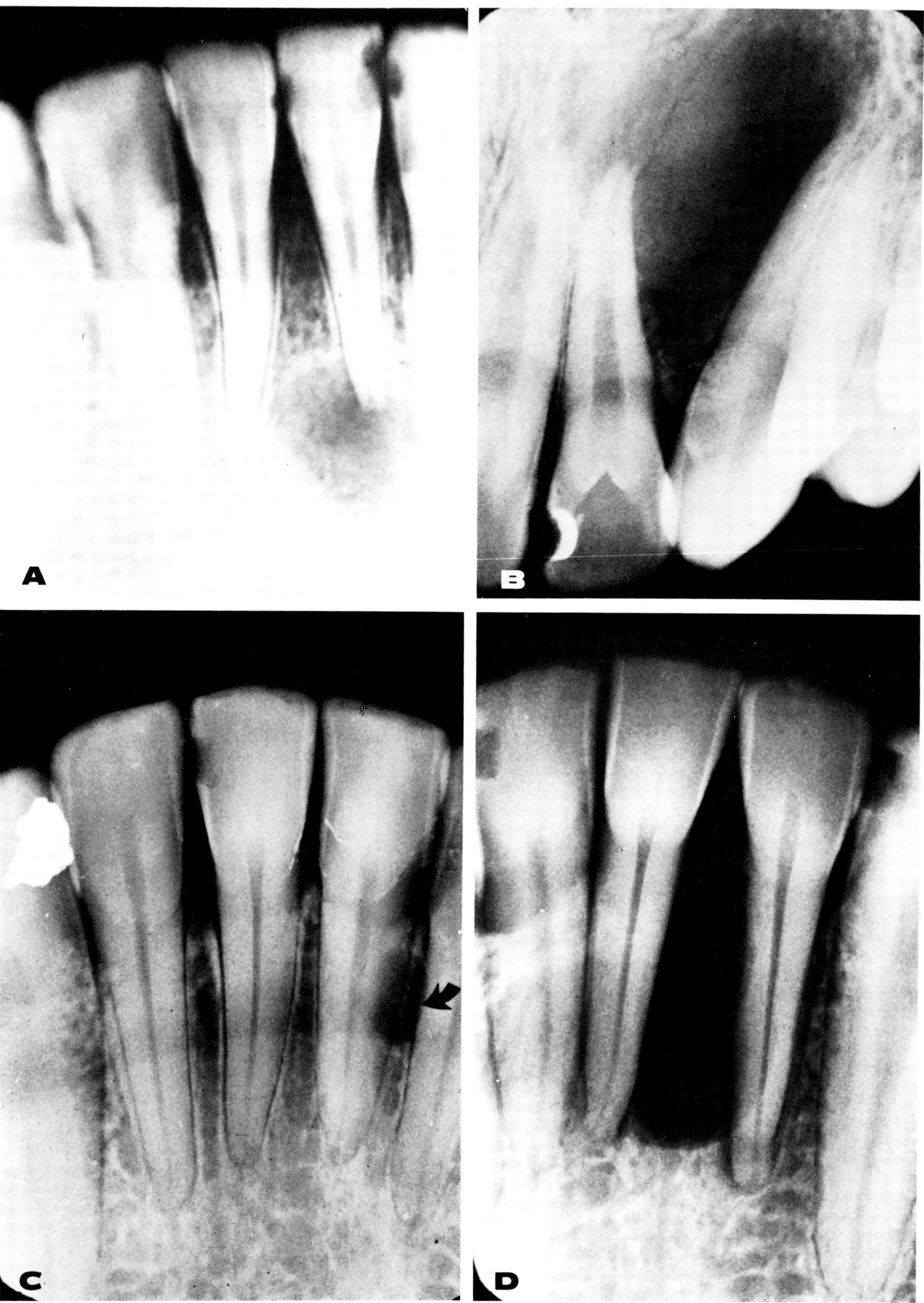

Fig. 10–31. Movement of teeth pathognomonic of cyst. *A,* Root separation beginning from modest cyst development. Typical circumscribed radiopaque perimeter may be confused with chronic apical periodontitis. *B,* Pulpless lateral incisor with infected apical cyst. Canine has been particularly displaced. *C,* Lateral cyst *(arrow)* not involved with pulpless tooth. *D,* Same case, 14 months later. Teeth remain vital. Biopsy, lateral periodontal cyst. (C and D from Degering, C. I.: Oral Surg., *32*:498, Sept. 1971.)

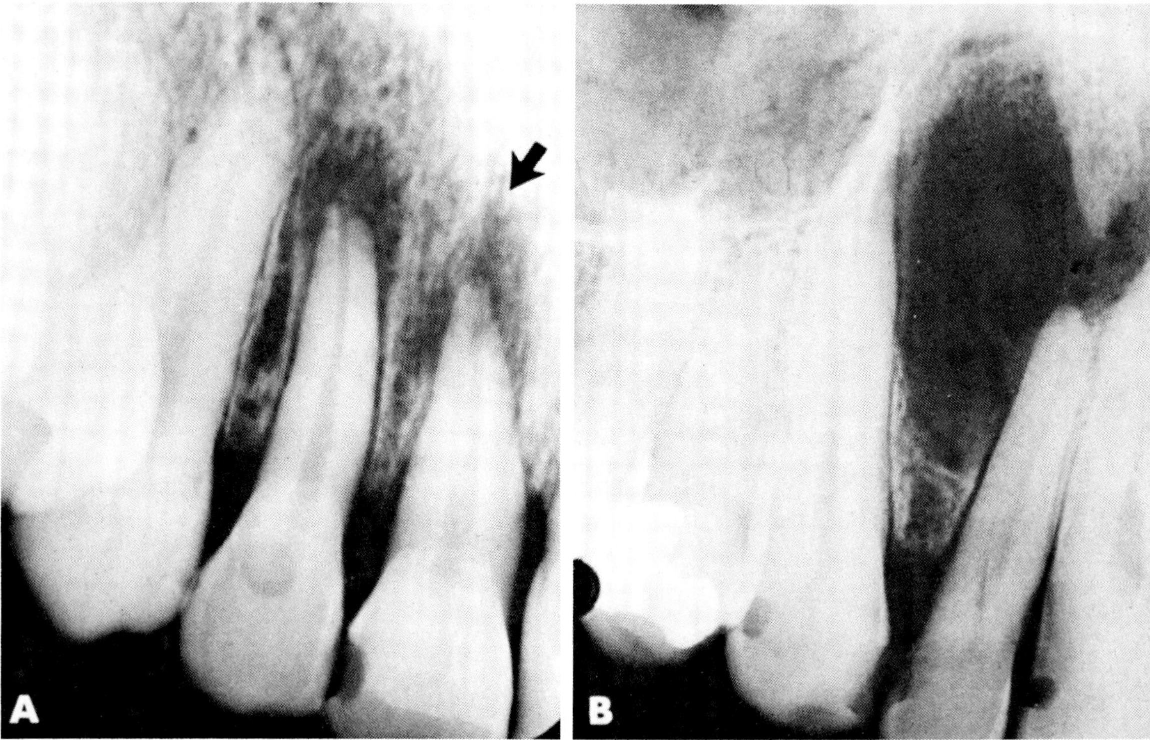

Fig. 10–32. *A,* Diffuse radiolucent appearance *(arrow)* of ***suppurative*** apical periodontitis (with fistula) is here contrasted with circumscribed radiolucency of chronic apical periodontitis associated with lateral incisor. *B,* ***Suppurative*** apical periodontitis with draining fistula following chronic infection of apical cyst. Huge, diffuse radiolucency is typical of suppurative apical periodontitis. Root of tooth was displaced by original apical cyst.

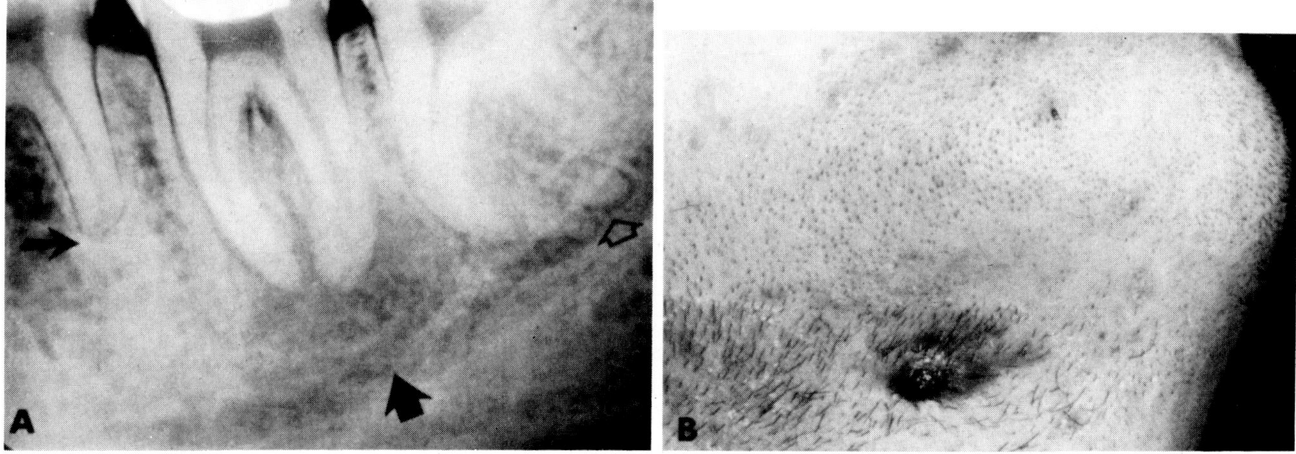

Fig. 10–33. *A,* Diffuse, roentgenographic appearance *(large arrow)* of suppurative apical periodontitis in posterior of mandible may be overlooked, owing to radiopacity of heavy cortical bone. Also noted are condensing osteitis and external resorption from chronic pulpitis *(arrow—left),* and anomalous third root of third molar *(open arrow—right). B,* Extraoral fistula (neck) draining from suppurative apical periodontitis seen in *A* has persisted for eight years. Immediately following root canal therapy, discharge ceased and stoma healed to "navel" of scar tissue.

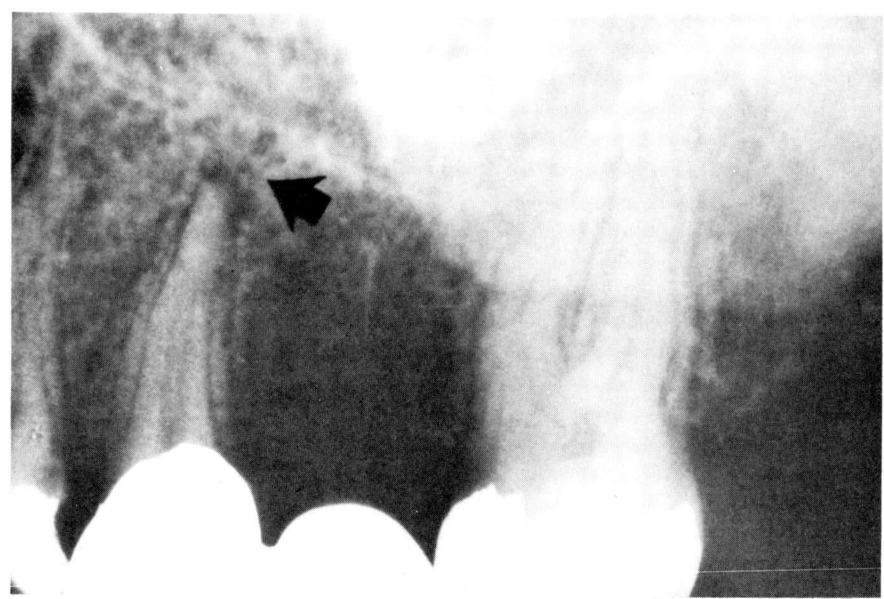

Fig. 10–34. Suppurative apical periodontitis *(arrow)* which has perforated floor of antrum. Patient is suffering from unilateral maxillary sinusitis, which healed following endodontic therapy.

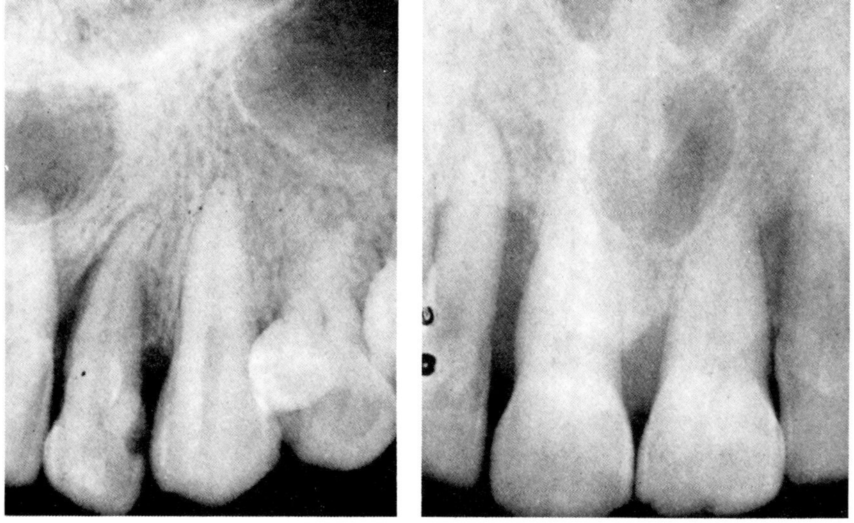

Fig. 10–35. Cyst of nasopalatine canal which may be "moved" from side to side by varying horizontal angle of exposure. Lesion appears to be directly over apex of central incisor *(left)* but has "moved" to middle-line position in direct labio-lingual projection *(right)*. Periodontal disease complicates case.

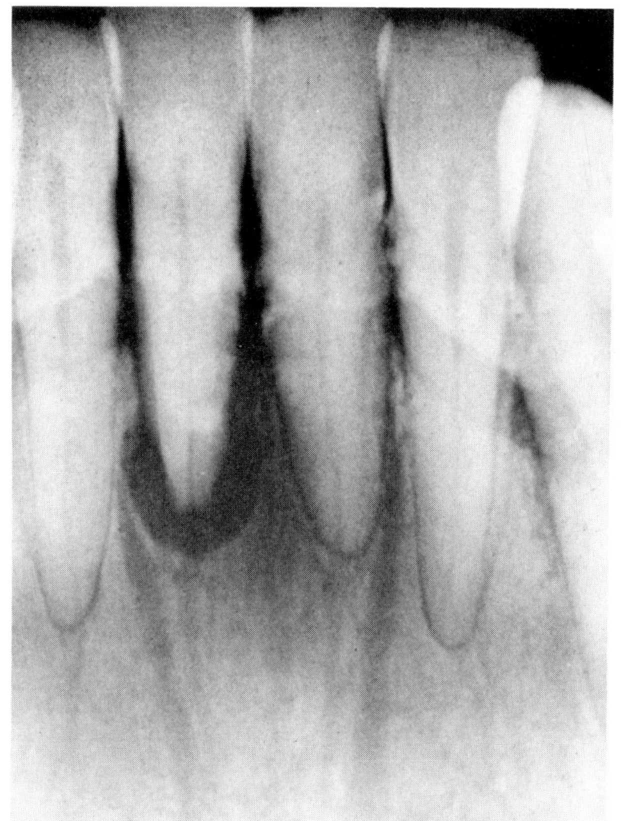

Fig. 10–36. Periodontal lesion which appears as periapical lesion. Involved central incisor is vital. Peculiar radiolucent, horizontal band lies between heavy supragingival calculus and crest of alveolar process. (Courtesy Dr. Jerome Zech.)

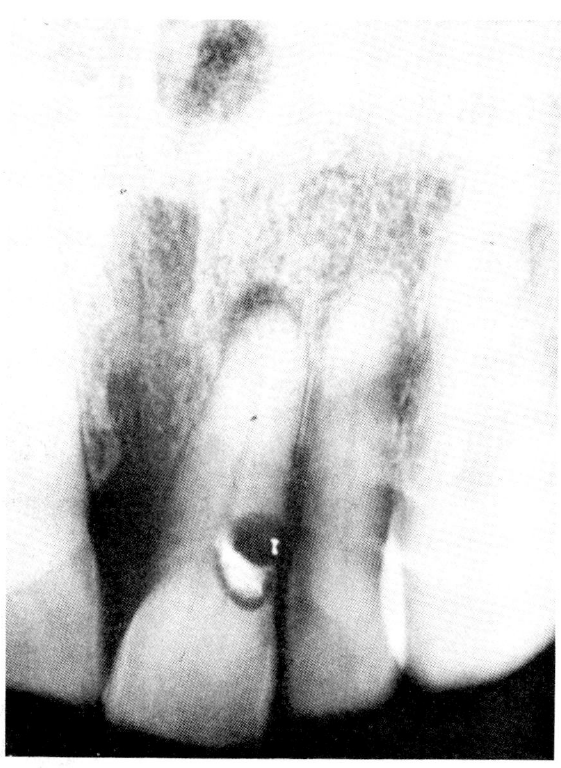

Fig. 10–38. Resorptive lesion following impact injury to tooth. Initially resorption could have been external, but now involves pulp, which has become necrotic.

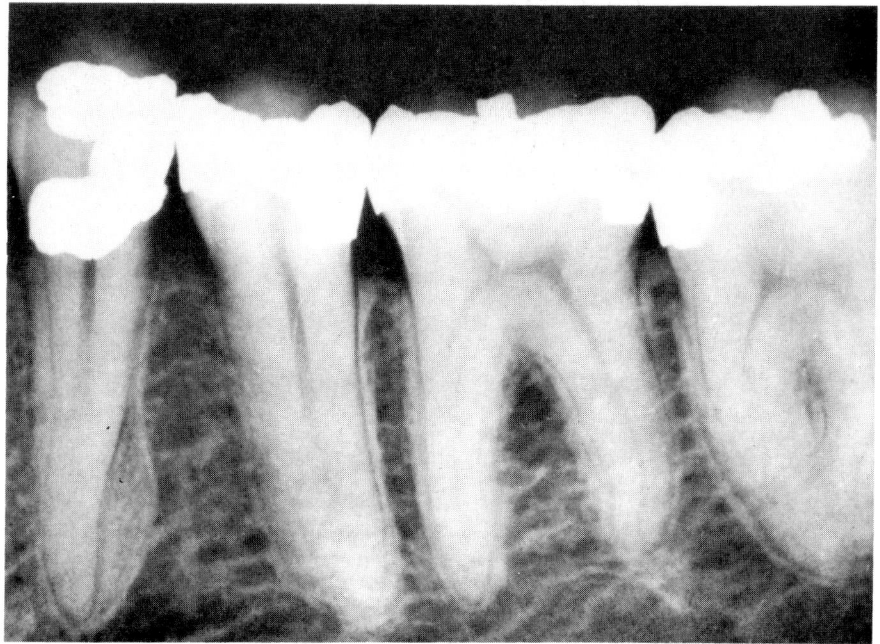

Fig. 10–37. Osteosclerosis distal to first premolar. Lamina dura and periodontal ligament may be traced in area of lesion, indicating that it is not attached cementoma.

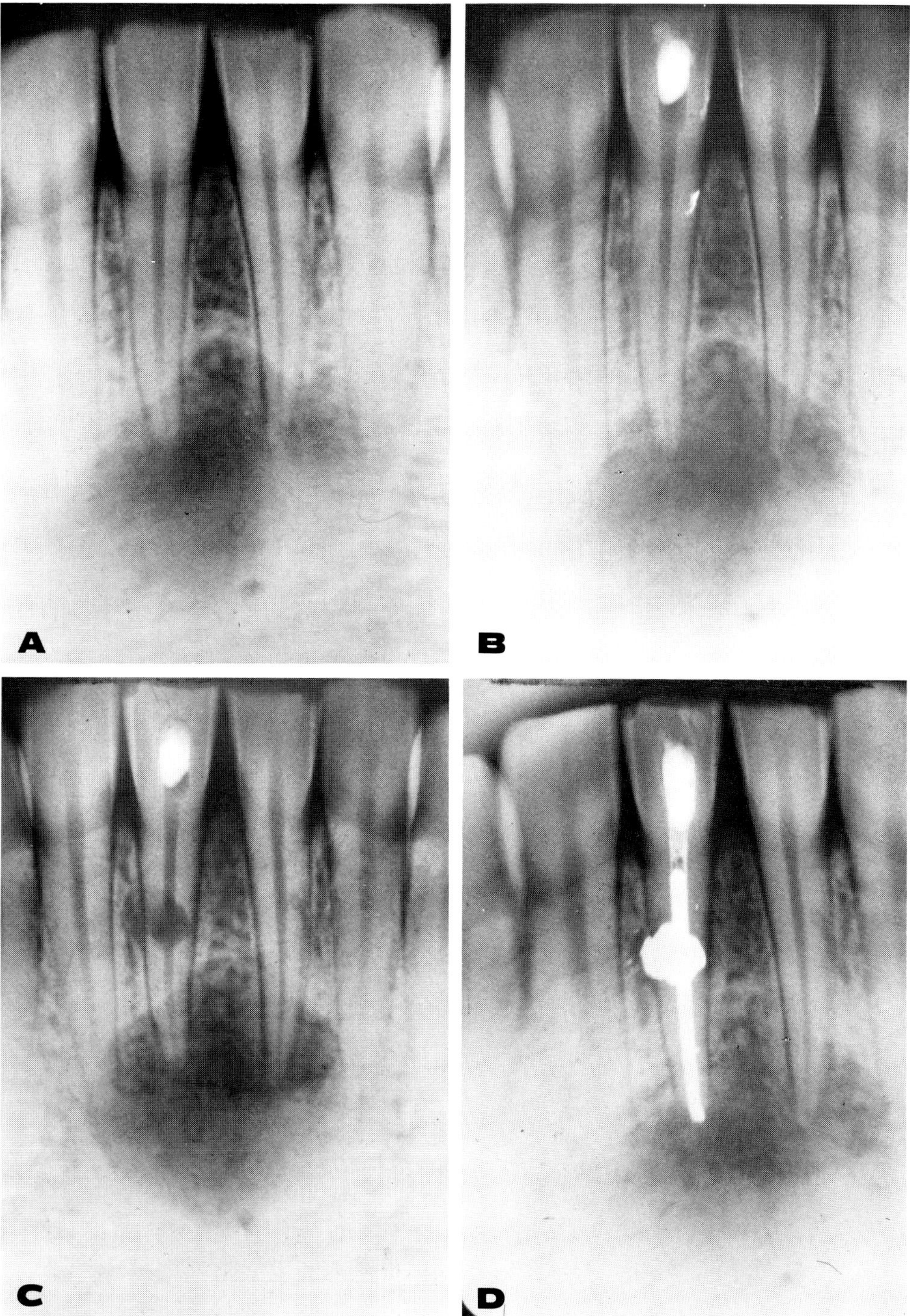

Fig. 10–39. Chronologic development of internal resorptive defect which has become external as well. Patient is adolescent female with bruxism. (See Chapter 7 and Fig. 7–10.) *A*, Mandibular incisors apparently involved with chronic apical periodontitis. Pulps of both teeth are vital. *B*, Referring dentist mistakenly opens into vital pulp of right central incisor. Detecting his error he places a temporary filling and dismisses patient. *C*, Six months later internal resorption from stimulated pulp has perforated root, and external resorption has also begun. *D*, Total pulpectomy, root canal therapy, and amalgam repair of resorptive lesion saves incisor. Left central incisor remains vital. Alleviation of trauma from bruxism will allow healing.

periapical lesions (Fig. 10–36). Here again, the periodontal probe and pulp tester are invaluable in determining the origin of the lesion seen in the roentgenogram. Silver or gutta percha points, placed in the periodontal pocket and examined radiographically in position, will serve as confirmatory evidence to the patient and referring dentist alike.

Common errors in diagnosis center around the lesion of ***periapical osteofibrosis,*** particularly during stage one when radiolucency is so apparent (see Fig. 9–34). By the time the lesion begins to calcify into an osteosclerotic lesion (Fig. 10–37), little doubt should exist about the nature of the lesion (see Fig. 9–35). Errors will still be made, however, in spite of all evidence to the contrary. The pulp tester will invariably reveal teeth with vital pulps, and the dentist must display the good sense to believe the authority of the pulp tester, not just the illusion of disease presented in the roentgenogram (see Fig. 9–36).

Areas of external resorption may also be confused with lesions of pulp origin. A thorough examination will probably reveal a pulp vital to all testing. If it is believed that the area of external resorption has developed from a continuing lesion of internal resorption, endodontic intervention is in order (Fig. 10–38). External resorption may be the result of a traumatic injury to the attachment apparatus, a blow that may have also devitalized the pulp. In this event, endodontic therapy is in order, although the two conditions are not directly associated. Surgical intervention into the external resorptive defect and repair with amalgam will frequently stop the process (Fig. 10–39).

The roentgenogram may prove an invaluable aid in determining which tooth has an associated periapical lesion. At the same time, the roentgenogram may be misleading (Fig. 10–40). This fact emphasizes again the necessity of using multiple tests for pulp disease.

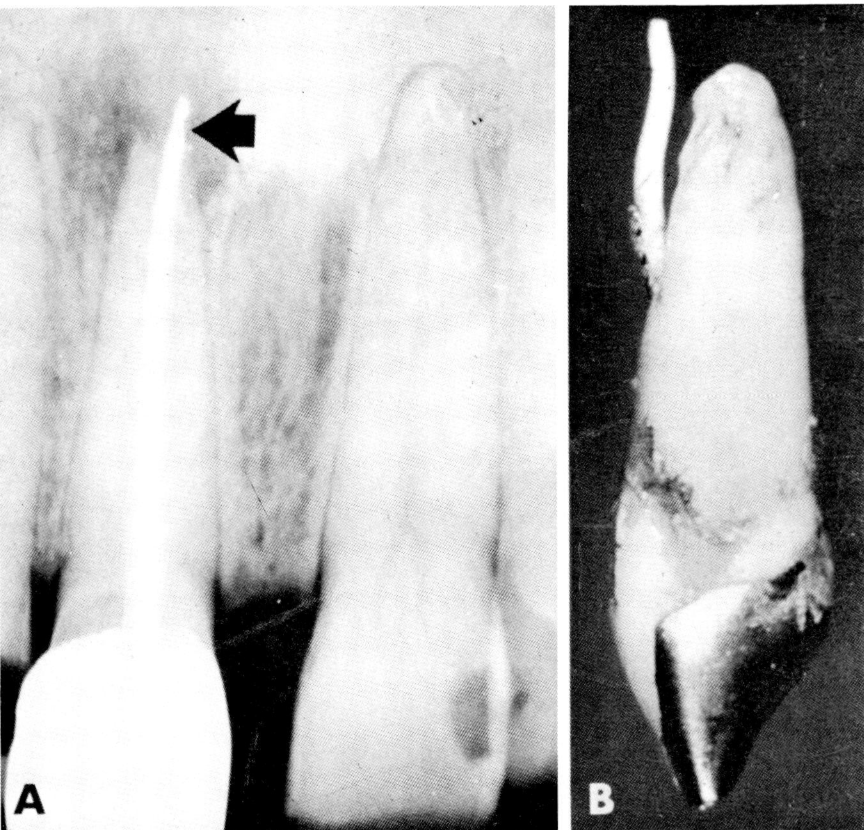

Fig. 10–40. Misleading roentgenogram related to lack of third dimension. *A,* Failing root canal therapy in maxillary central incisor appears to be grossly overfilled. *B,* Extracted tooth seen in roentgenogram proves that case is not overfilled. Perforation was by huge enlarging instruments used through restricted access cavity. (Courtesy Dr. Eugene Meyer.) (Luebke, R. G., Glick, D. H., and Ingle, J. I.: Oral Surg., *18*:97, July, 1964.)

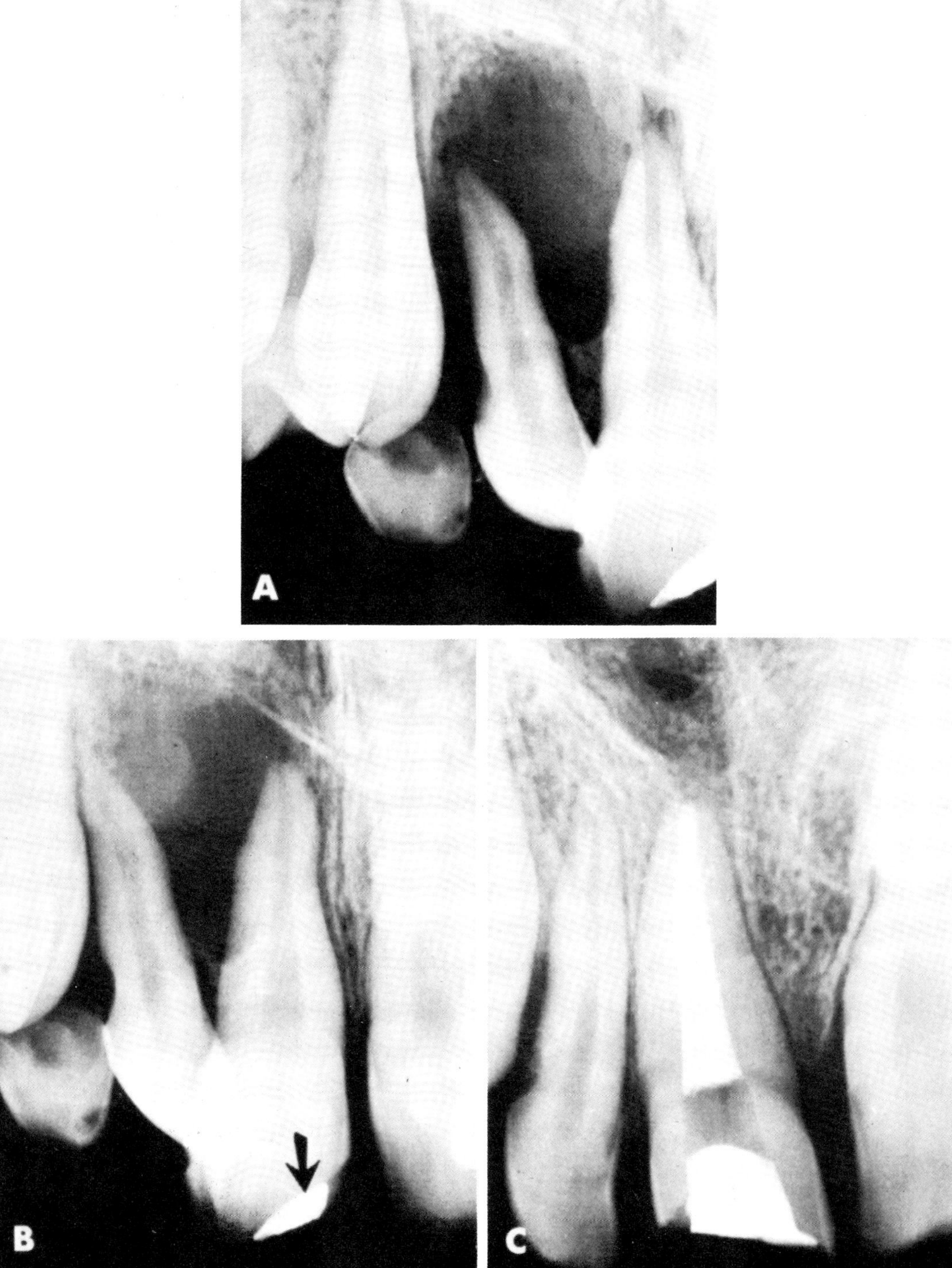

Fig. 10–41. Importance of multiple roentgenographic exposures. *A,* Lateral incisor appears to be principally involved tooth in this direct buccal-lingual projection. *B,* Projection through central incisor shows it is involved in lesion as well. Lateral incisor is vital and central incisor is nonvital, pulp death having developed from trauma *(arrow)*. *C,* Following therapy, new bone develops throughout area and both teeth reattach. (Courtesy Dr. Pierre R. Dow.)

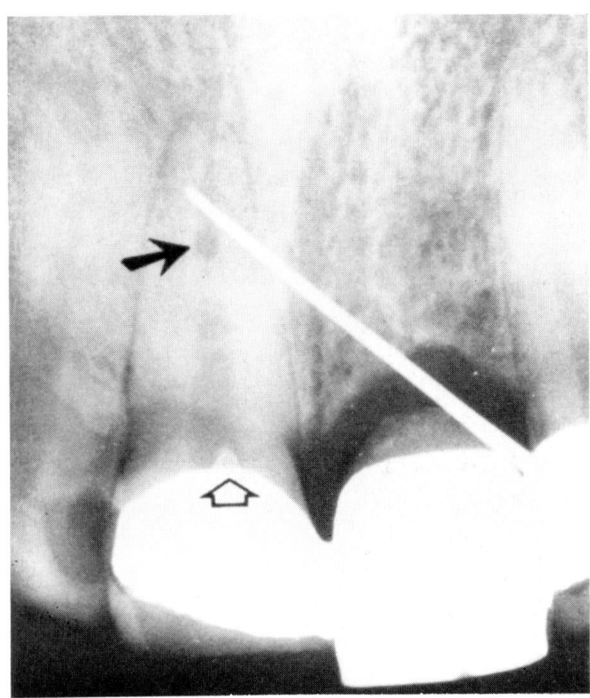

Fig. 10–42. Distant draining fistula is explored with silver point, which directs attention to tiny area of internal resorption *(arrow)* in adjacent incisor. Pulp breakdown probably began when fixed retainer was "anchored" *(open arrow)* in pulp. (Courtesy of Dr. Pierre R. Dow.)

It also points up the necessity of exposing roentgenograms from more than one horizontal angle (Fig. 10–41). In the last analysis, the pulp tester is the final authority and must be believed in spite of the roentgenographic evidence. Roots of teeth may be nearly denuded of bone by lesions not of their own origin, and still the pulp of the "innocent" tooth will remain completely vital (Fig. 10–41).

Occasionally a fistula is noted opposite a tooth that pulp-tests perfectly vital. In this event, a gutta percha or silver point should be passed down the sinus tract, to direct attention in the roentgenogram to the troublemaker (Fig. 10–42).

Finally, something must be said in favor of the occasional use of occlusal films or lateral head films when it is necessary to "reach" beyond the limits of the periapical film. Teeth "lost" by intrusion, or "lost" filling materials or root tips may be shown with these films, but would be missed with a standard periapical film (Fig. 10–43).

Importance of the Initial Roentgenogram. The initial diagnostic roentgenogram must be carefully studied, not only as an aid in diagnosis, but as a "blueprint" of what is ahead during treatment. A number of things should be looked for, and the film should be consulted frequently during treatment, not immediately set aside in the patient's record.

First of all, the size and shape of the pulp chamber and the direction and angulation of the canals as they leave the chamber is most important at the outset, when coronal preparation is begun. Obstructions such as pulp stones are also seen. One realizes how much the initial roentgenogram is depended upon each time a tooth with a full crown is treated. In this film the radiopaque metal crown eliminates a preview of coronal pulp anatomy.

Once the crown is entered, the curvature of the roots and the approximate length of the tooth must be known. Again, the film supplies most of the necessary information, although information about root curvatures to the buccal or lingual is rather sparse.

The inclination of the roots of the teeth to the mesial and the distal is revealed by the roentgenogram and must be cautiously heeded if gouging and perforation are not to result (Fig. 10–44*A*).

The relationship of the roots of the teeth to associated periapical lesions is seen in the initial roentgenogram and such information is invaluable if surgery is planned. Also, the degree of proximity of the involved root to neighboring roots is most important to know before treatment.

Finally, the initial film provides information about previous treatment, including evidence of broken instruments as well as desperate attempts and failure of treatment of which the patient may not be fully aware (Fig. 10–44*B,C,D*). Again the dentist may be completely fooled by the roentgenogram and needs other confirmatory evidence of the true situation. Sometimes raising a surgical flap can provide the only answer.

Importance of Confirmatory Roentgenograms During Treatment. The x-ray is not only a valuable diagnostic tool; it is an indispensable working tool. Only through the use of working roentgenograms can the operator keep abreast of his advances in the tooth during endodontic treatment.

Upon first entering the tooth, if a suspicion exists that the direction of the coronal preparation is going astray, a ***confirmatory film*** should be taken to evaluate

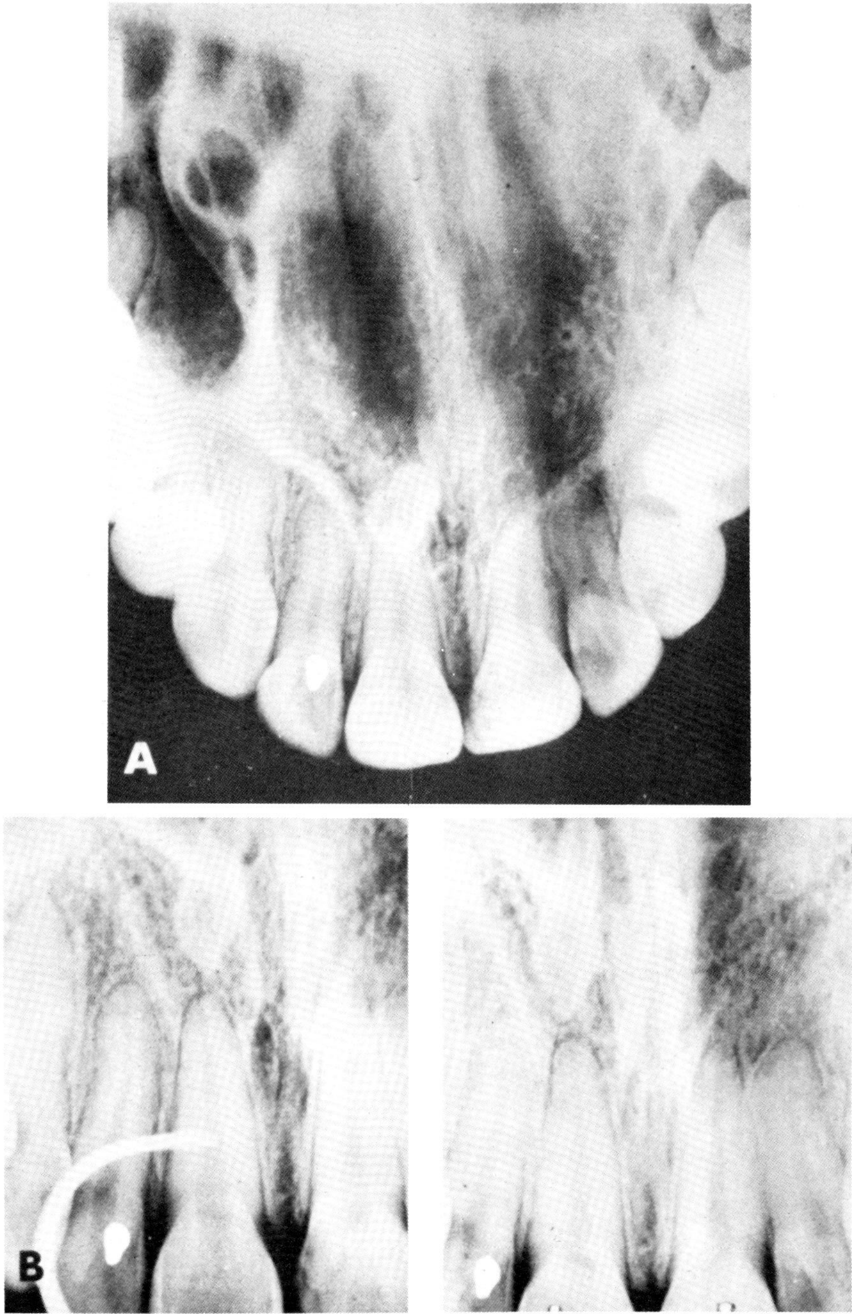

Fig. 10–43. Use of occlusal film to detect and locate structures or lesions beyond "reach" of standard periapical exposure. *A,* Radiopaque object associated with labial fistula appears in occlusal film to be superior to right central incisor. *B, (Left)* Shepherd-hook explorer marks fistula in follow-up roentgenogram. *(Right)* Resorbing deciduous incisor is revealed in very high periapical exposure. At age four, primary tooth was driven into floor of nose. Parents thought tooth had been avulsed. (Courtesy Dr. John Ganzner.)

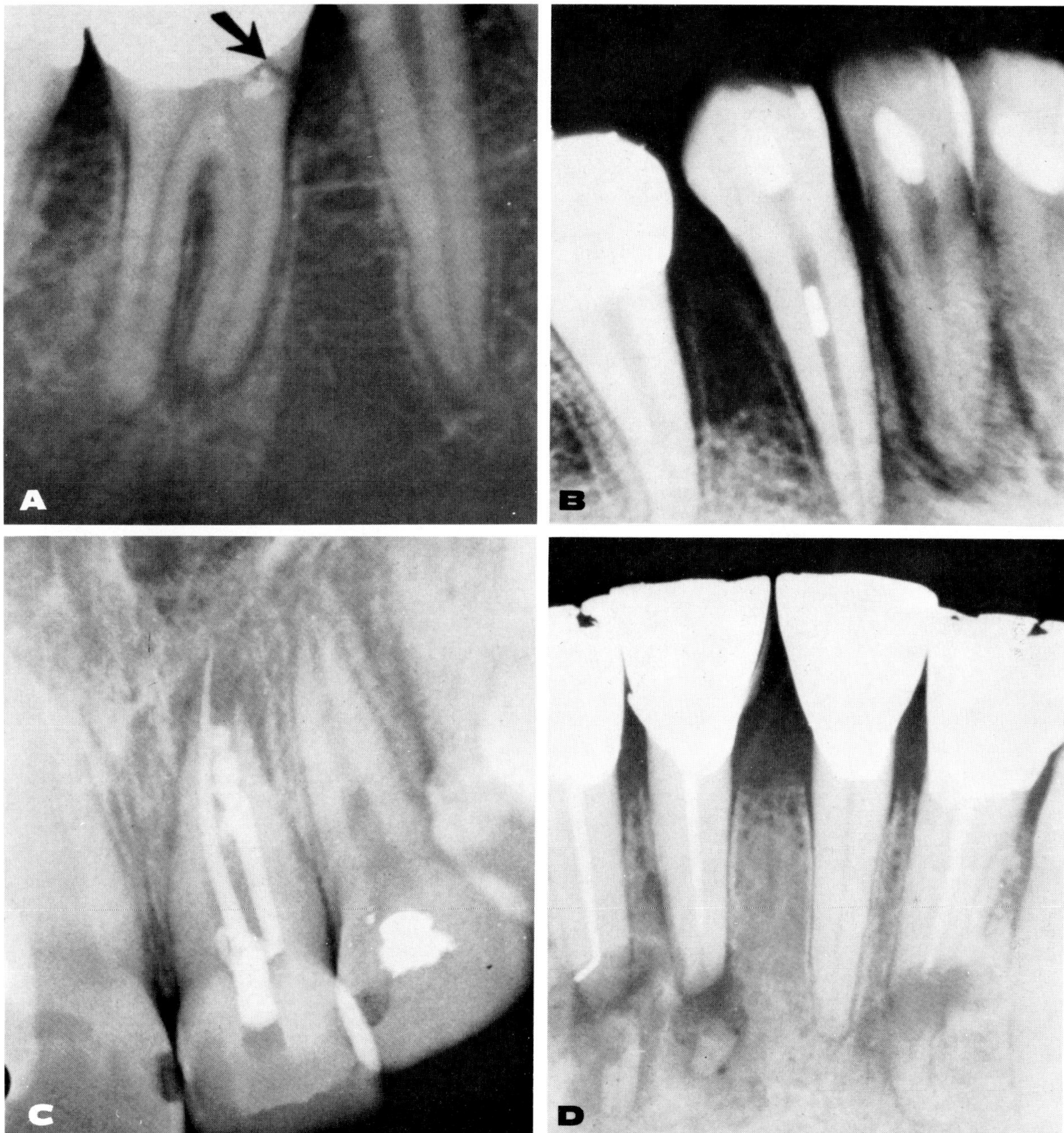

Fig. 10–44. *A,* Root perforation *(arrow)* and associated periodontal lesion is revealed by roentgenogram. Condensing osteitis and external root resorption are related to chronic pulpitis, which was initial complaint.
B, C, and *D,* Treatment errors and failures revealed by roentgenogram.
B, Fissure bur broken in canal.
C, Totally ineffective canal obliteration. Inadequate coronal access cavity is smaller than canal and apex to be debrided and obliterated. *D,* Complete "butchery" and total failure in attempted multiple apicoectomies. Canals are inadequately filled and amputated root tips have been left in place.

alignment (see Fig. 10–2). If the pulp chamber has calcified and the pulp receded, ***confirmatory progress*** films of the operating bur in place will indicate progress toward the distant orifice of the pulp canal. In an attempt to save time, these roentgenograms are often not taken. Actually, hours of time and possible tragedy may be averted by their use. A one-minute developing routine in the darkroom will stimulate the use of multiple treatment exposures.

The ***confirmatory length-of-tooth*** film is undoubtedly the second most valuable film to be taken after the initial diagnostic roentgenogram (Fig. 10–45). After length of tooth is established and canal instrumentation is begun, the dentist should never hesitate to expose confirmatory roentgenograms if he is ever in doubt about the progress of his instrument. Many perforations have been avoided and unusual canal anatomy discovered by the confirmatory roentgenogram. The few minutes spent in exposing and developing the film may save hours of valuable time and ensure success.

The ***confirmatory trial point*** roentgenogram serves two important purposes. First, it confirms the visual and "tug back" judgment of the fit of the initial filling point. Second, it provides the final opportunity to judge the advance of instrumentation. If an error in length of tooth has been made, and the canal has been instrumented short or long, this is the final opportunity to correct the error. Invariably, when the trial point confirmatory film is ignored, trouble ensues.

The ***confirmatory final film*** follows completion of the root canal filling. It should be made before a coronal restoration is placed, for some correction in the canal filling may have to be made. Ideally, the final film for the record, and the duplicate film to be returned if a referring dentist is involved, should be taken with the rubber dam clamp removed (Fig. 10–46).

Confirmatory progress films of work being done outside the tooth may also be necessary. Searching for root tips, lost filling material, the exact apex of a root during trephination or surgery—these are only a few of the uses made of confirmatory roentgenograms.

Importance of Confirmatory Recall Roentgenogram. The importance of the ***recall*** roentgenogram

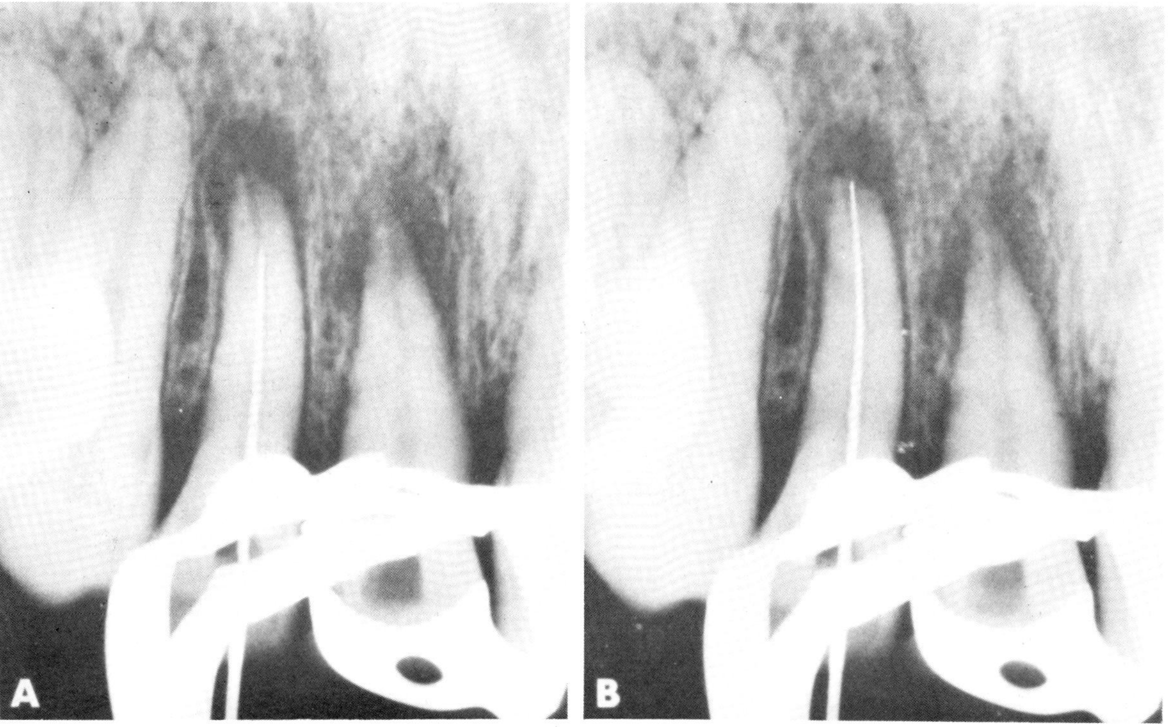

Fig. 10–45. Importance of confirmatory length of tooth roentgenogram. *A*, Length of tooth is established by determining distance from tip of instrument to apex. *B*, After working length of tooth is established, instrument may be placed to this depth and confirmatory roentgenogram taken.

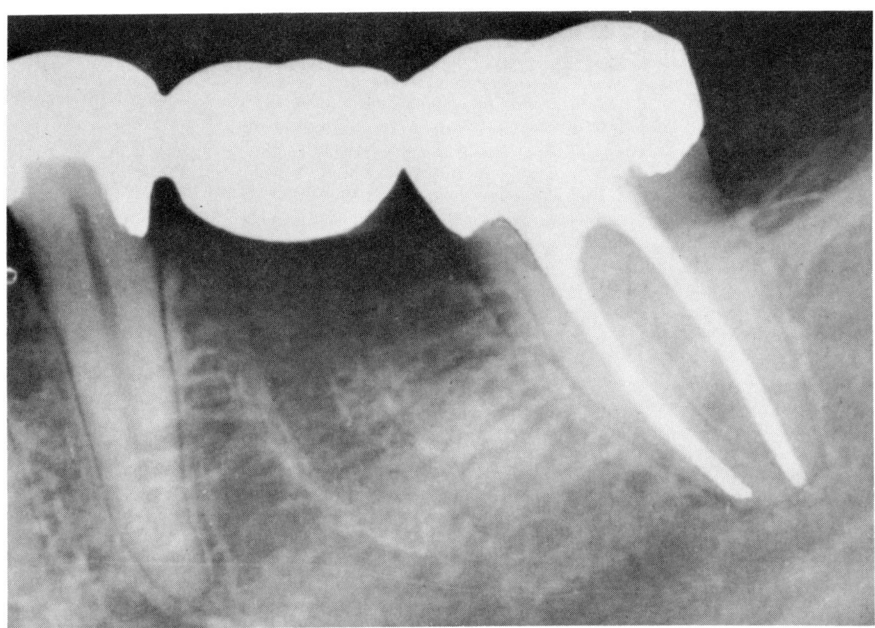

Fig. 10–46. Confirmatory roentgenogram of completed therapy. Quality of canal obliteration, relationship of final root canal filling to apex, and status of periapical region at completion of treatment are all established in final film. First recall roentgenogram should be taken in six months.

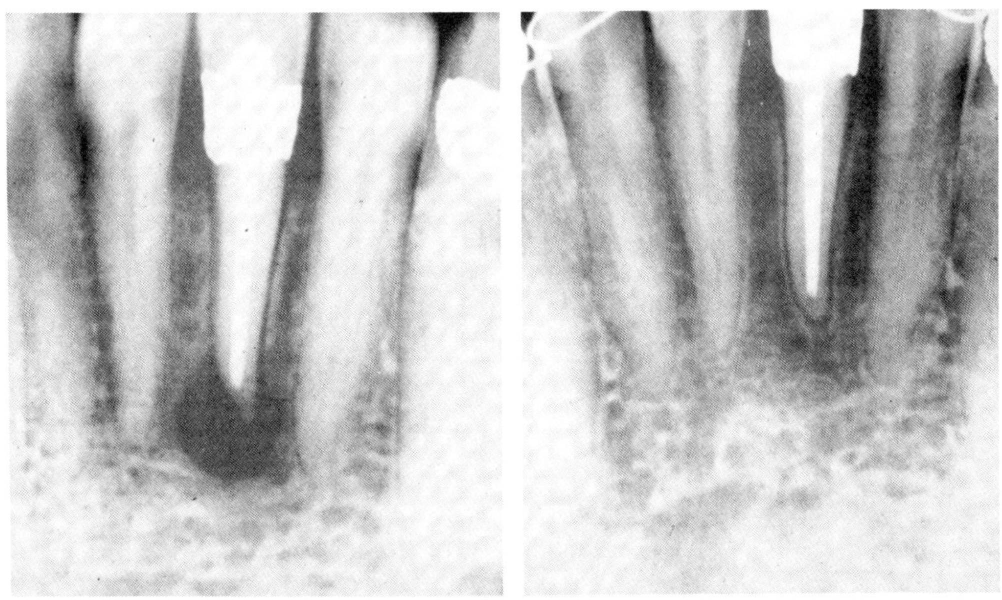

Fig. 10–47. Importance of confirmatory recall roentgenogram. *Left,* Treatment film completed at time of apicoectomy. *Right,* Roentgenogram taken six months later. Complete recalcification is apparent. Lamina dura and periodontal ligament space indicate that new cementum, periodontal ligament, and alveolar bone have developed. Note multiple canals in adjacent teeth.

cannot be emphasized enough. These recall films are best taken over a one-year period at least; in the case of the elderly patient, over a two-year period (Fig. 10–47). If any abnormal or unusual findings are noted, they should be watched carefully, and the recall interval should be stepped-up and possibly extended in time. Unfortunately, not all patients return for their recall radiographs, particularly if they are symptom-free. Riley surveyed 159 Diplomates of the American Board of Endodontics who reported that fewer than half of their patients returned on recall.[8]

It is certainly the dentist's responsibility to act on the findings of the recall roentgenogram. If endodontic failure becomes apparent, the patient should be recalled, the cause of failure should be determined, and if correction of the failure is possible, it should immediately be undertaken.

On the other hand, the forest should not be lost in the trees so that only the endodontically treated tooth is examined in the film. To permit dental caries or another pulpless tooth to develop alongside a treated tooth is inexcusable (Fig. 10–48).

Testing for Pulp Vitality

Granted that the radiograph is an excellent diagnostic tool, one must concede it can be misleading. So can the history derived from the patient. Cross-checking these findings by further testing procedures is a must.

The results of the interview and history are ***subjective findings,*** whereas the patient's response to testing procedures may be considered ***objective***—less open to bias and subjective interpretation. To a certain extent, moreover, it is possible to quantify the responses to testing, and these figures may be consulted in follow-up examinations. This is especially true of the electric pulp tester. In a double-blind situation, Van Hassel and Harrington ran a total of 1,267 test stimuli on matched pairs of normal teeth.[9] They found patients to be remarkably perceptive in determining which tooth was tested—78% accuracy between two teeth in the same quadrant, 95% accuracy between two teeth in opposite arches, and up to 100% accuracy between corresponding teeth across the midline. The foregoing attests to the validity of quantified results.

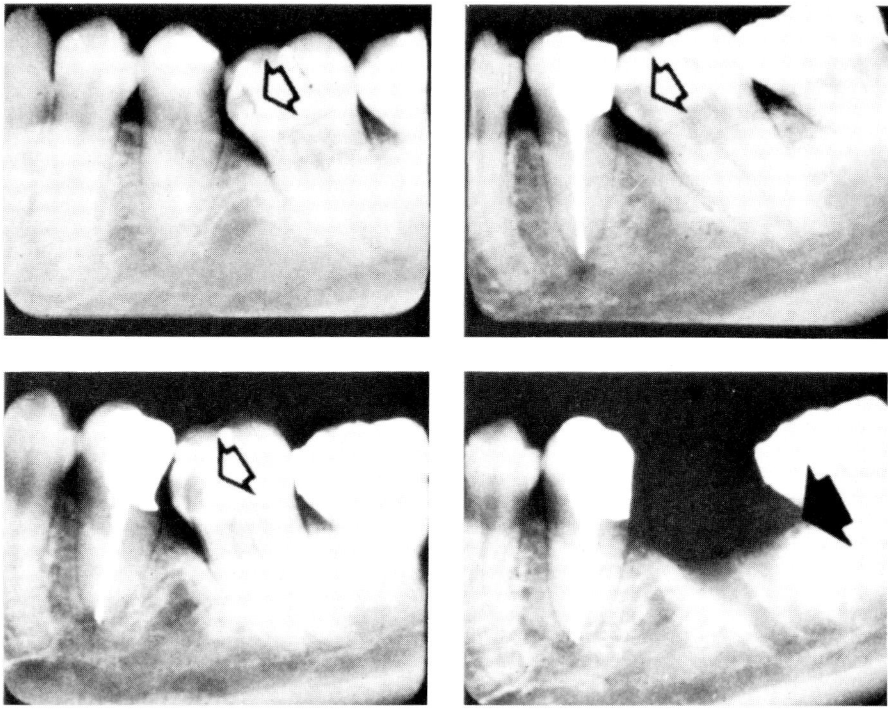

Fig. 10–48. Importance of observing and acting upon other lesions that appear in recall roentgenograms. Increase in carious lesion in molar tooth is visible at six months and one year *(open arrows)*. In two years pulp was involved and tooth was extracted during acute pulpitis. Dentist is condemned for not informing patient of encroaching caries.

A qualifying caveat must be added, however, and that is the modification of any testing procedures (or history for that matter) imposed by the patient's emotional or physical state. This is particularly true of patients suffering prolonged and/or excruciating pain.

Requisites of Testing. In any testing procedure, adequate controls are necessary. If one is questioning the vitality of the maxillary canine, for example, the best control tooth would be a normal, uninvolved canine on the opposite side. Because of the differences in bulk, thickness of the enamel, and size of the pulp, a maxillary lateral incisor certainly would not be a good control tooth for a maxillary canine. Nor is a premolar a good control for a molar. In all instances, the best control tooth is the normal contralateral tooth. Lacking this, a comparable tooth in the opposite arch is a reasonable control. It is necessary, however, to test teeth adjacent or near to the suspected tooth, especially if trauma is an etiologic factor. This applies to thermal tests, but particularly to electric vitality testing. The minimum number of teeth acceptable for interpreting response to testing should be: (1) the tooth in question, (2) the normal contralateral or opposing tooth, and (3) the two adjacent teeth. Any test stimulation should be standardized in terms of quantity of stimulus, length of time it is applied, and quality of stimulus.

Electric Vitality Testing. Degering tested the various methods of determining pulp vitality—air and explorer, application of cold and heat, and the electric pulp tester.[10] Of these methods, he found the electric apparatus to be the most effective. By testing teeth with nonvital pulps and observing no change in the ***galvanic skin response*** of his subjects, he concluded that the pulp tester stimulated only the vital pulp tissue and not the supporting tissue through the sensory nerves of the periodontal ligament space. Paradoxically, he also found that some patients volunteered that they felt a reaction, while the sensitive GSR did not record a measurable physiologic reaction.

The basic premise is wrong, however, in determining vitality by testing the sensory nerve response of the pulp. The vitality of the pulp is not dependent on its ***nerve*** supply, but rather on its vascular supply. The two may not be compatible.

A ***recently erupted tooth*** frequently tests nonvital, yet never in its lifetime will it be more vital. A young tooth traumatized by impact may test nonvital, yet when the pulp is opened, the rush of blood illustrates the error of the test. Three-canal molars often give bizarre pulp test readings when one canal is normal, one canal necrotic, and the third canal acutely inflamed. Again, it is experience gained in using the pulp tester that gives the practitioner confidence. Electric pulp testers measure sensory nerve response to a current of electricity which first must pass through a resistant layer of enamel. Hence, the thicker the enamel on the tooth, the greater the amount of current required to induce a response. The rheostat readings on molar teeth and maxillary canine teeth, therefore, will be much higher than the readings on incisors, particularly the mandibular incisors. The premolars fall somewhere between. Secondary and reparative dentin development also increases the amount of resistant tooth structure between the electrode and pulp. Therefore, calcified teeth in elderly patients or teeth with receded pulps under extensive restorations require a much higher rheostat reading than do young vital teeth. The diagnostic radiograph again is evaluated, this time in light of the varied results of pulp testing.

The degree of pulp inflammation or degeneration causes the greatest variance in pulp response. The hypersensitive-hyperemic pulp reacts in a hypersensitive manner, that is, very low on the rheostat. A pulp involved in advanced acute inflammation requires more current to react than a normal pulp requires. The pulp involved in chronic, long-standing inflammation does not respond on the rheostat until the higher numbers are reached. In fact, current discharged at the top number can usually be tolerated. The necrotic pulp gives a completely negative response to electric testing, that is, the full discharge of current elicits no response by the patient. In this use the pulp tester demonstrates its greatest value—determining the presence or absence of pulp death.

The research area of pulp physiology is moving rapidly, and before long a testing device has to be developed which measures blood flow rather than sensory excitation. For the present, the Burton Vitalometer has long been the standard against which other devices have been measured. This is a high-frequency instrument that plugs into the alternating current. It has the advantage of delivering a repeatable performance, and thus can be used to recheck vitality in the future against a present level. There are presently five or six commercial electric pulp testers on the market, including two portable devices powered by mercury batteries. The others plug into the

110-volt line. Aduddell and Reynolds found reliability and consistency in both types of devices with respect to voltage output at various settings on the same tester, but they found variation between different pulp testers made by the same manufacturer.[11] They did not check battery testers, however, while the batteries were failing.

Precautions in Pulp Tester Use. It has been suggested that employment of electric pulp testers on patients who have an indwelling cardiac pacemaker is contraindicated. After testing the effects of electric pulp testers on dogs with artificial pacemakers, Woodley and his associates concluded that currents of the magnitude of 5 milliamps to 20 milliamps are sufficient to modify normal pacemaker function.[12] After testing one battery-powered device and three using line current, they found that the S. S. White Pulp Tester Model 2A was the only one to cause interference with pacemaker action. They further warned against such devices as desensitizers or electrosurgical units, which could produce unknown current leaks, as one of the pulp testers did.

The question is often asked whether repeated or prolonged use of an electric pulp tester on a single tooth can be damaging to the pulp. McDaniel and his coworkers were unable to demonstrate any pulp changes in teeth of experimental animals after prolonged application of maximum stimulus with a Burton Vitalometer.[13]

Technique of Electric Vitality Testing. To achieve accurate results with an electric pulp tester, a procedure must be carefully followed. The teeth to be tested must be thoroughly air-dried and isolated with cotton rolls. The tip of the tooth electrode of the pulp tester must be covered with toothpaste in order to make good electrical contact. The examiner should place a bit of the toothpaste on the back of his left hand where it is readily available.

The tooth electrode is placed against the dried enamel surface in the gingival third area, with care to avoid contact of electrode or paste with any restorations or gingival tissue. This would cause a false reading. The patient's cheek must be grasped to complete the circuit. The rheostat on the tester is ***slowly and continuously*** advanced, and the patient is instructed to indicate when the sensation is first experienced. Raising the hand or making a sound are good warning signals. The findings should then be recorded for each tooth tested. In order to compare accurately a possible changing vitality, the same pulp tester should always be used on the same patient.

The occasional molar tooth which responds with bizarre symptoms should be tested in a number of areas. It may happen that two areas on a molar will test negative, but a positive test within normal range may be gained in another area. This indicates that the pulp in two canals is necrotic or badly degenerated, whereas the pulp in the third canal is still vital, even though inflamed.

If it is absolutely essential that a tooth fully covered by gold or porcelain be electrically pulp tested, the following method may be used: The cavity is prepared through the restorative material until the dentin is reached. Care must be taken, in penetrating a porcelain crown with a diamond point, not to fracture the crown. Sometimes the action of the bur excites a positive response, and pulp testing is not necessary. If testing is necessary a small metal instrument with a thin coat of toothpaste is placed in the cavity against the dentin. Care is taken not to contact the metal restoration. The instrument is held with a nonconducting piece of rubber dam. The contacting instrument is then touched by the tooth electrode, and the rheostat is carefully advanced. Response of a ***vital*** pulp appears almost immediately for the dentin is contacted, not the usual enamel surface.

Thermal Tests. As Degering has pointed out, thermal stimuli such as ice and heated gutta percha have far more value as testing methods when "the teeth in general were sensitive to temperature changes."[10] It must not be assumed that normal vital pulps will not respond to thermal tests, for they will, particularly to cold. Thermal stimuli, on the other hand, will not give a graded, repeatable performance—only positive or negative replies. When the test is applied, however, the dentist might try counting to himself until a reaction is forthcoming.

Cold is used by spraying ethyl chloride on a large cotton pellet, which is then applied to the buccal surface of the tooth with cotton pliers; cold is more reputable than heat. Cold applied with sticks of ice made by freezing water in discarded anesthetic Carpules is an even better method than the ethyl chloride pellet. The time-honored method of spraying ethyl chloride, a general anesthetic, on the tooth can be dangerous, frightening, and painful, even though a rubber dam protects other teeth. For this technique, a substitute for ethyl chloride is recommended—Fluori-Methane Spray, which comes in the same spray bottle container as ethyl chloride, but is not dangerous.

Heat, applied by heating base plate gutta percha and applying it "smoking" hot to the moistened buccal surface, also raises a positive reply, particularly if the pulp is hypersensitive or inflamed.

Both hot and cold stimuli bring about a reaction from a pulp that is hypersensitive or hyperemic. However, cold is more apt to elicit a response than is heat. A stick of ice or ethyl chloride applied to the buccal surface usually causes a response that lasts only as long as contact is made. Occasionally a stream of ice water can be a better stimulus. Hot gutta percha should be removed as soon as discomfort is noted, so that pulp damage cannot occur. Again, with true hypersensitivity or hyperemia, the sensation fades away upon removal of the stimuli. This is ***not*** true when pulpalgia is present, for with this condition the pain continues after the stimulus is removed.

Thermal stimuli are especially effective in testing for pulp inflammation—to determine which tooth is involved in acute pulpalgia. The pulp afflicted with ***moderate*** pulpalgia is oversensitive to cold, that is, cold actually starts the pulp aching. A lukewarm rinse often alleviates the pain. This same pulp may overreact to the heat test, but it is not as likely to start the discomfort.

Heat applied to the tooth with ***advanced*** acute pulpalgia brings on an instantaneous excruciating pain. Conversely, cold alleviates this pain, and the dentist examining the patient with advanced pulpalgia is well advised to have cold water "at the ready" to stop the exquisite pain brought on by the heat.

Cold as a stimulus is completely negative in chronic pulpalgia or necrosis. Heat rarely elicits a response from the necrotic pulp, but may bring about a slight sensation from the chronically involved pulp.

Percussion. Percussion should be performed with a relatively heavy instrument with a blunt end. Many mouth mirror handles fulfill these two requirements. One should attempt to standardize the amount of force used in percussion. The testing should be started on what is thought to be a normal healthy tooth. Two criteria are used to measure the result of percussion: (1) the ***patient's*** report of pain or its absence, and (2) the sound the ***dentist*** hears as a tooth is percussed. Normal healthy teeth in proper occlusion should not elicit pain on moderate percussion. And they produce a rather clear, sharp sound. Teeth whose apical periodontal membranes are inflamed usually respond with pain and may well produce a dull thud. Inflamed areas of the ***lateral*** portions of the periodontal membrane may ***not*** elicit pain when the tooth is tapped in the vertical direction, but do so upon laterally directed forces. Therefore, percussion should be directed not only in the long axis of the tooth, but against the buccal surface and, when possible, against the lingual surfaces as well.

Test Cavity. As a last resort, a test cavity may have to be prepared to determine the presence or absence of pulp vitality. This is especially true of teeth with advanced pulp recession, which do not respond to any other method of testing. Anesthesia must not be previously administered. When the dentin is entered, the patient experiences the typical sensation that "his tooth is being worked on." Because of the universal use of local anesthesia, many patients have never experienced the sensation of a bur cutting across dentin, and they will be at a loss to know of what the dentist speaks. As the bur (usually a No. 2 round bur) penetrates into the dentin, the patient should feel pain. Few vital pulps can be entered without some warning from the approaching bur.

Another use of the test cavity applies to fully crowned teeth that cannot be electrically pulp-tested and do not respond to thermal stimuli. Careful preparation through the crown, to the dentin, will reveal the state of pulp viability. Gold foil, amalgam, or silicate is used to restore the tiny test cavity if the pulp is found to be vital and healthy.

Anesthetic Test. Another testing method of "last resort" is the anesthetic test. This approach serves to delineate the tooth containing the aching, inflamed pulp, which acts as the primary source of pain being referred to the opposite arch or nearby tooth.

After all testing procedures have been exhausted, the examiner may still be at a loss to determine which tooth is actually aching, for the pain may be referred into a widespread area. In this case, the most logical tooth is first anesthetized. If the assumption proves correct, all the pain, primary and referred, will be alleviated. If the ***referred*** area is anesthetized first, only this area will be relieved, and the primary pain continues or can be stimulated.

The most common use of the anesthetic test involves the pain reference between maxillary and mandibular molars, or between a mandibular molar and pain referred to the ear. Often the patient is not convinced that he does not have a true earache until a mandibular block is given and the earache stops. The same is true of the patient who is absolutely convinced that a maxillary molar is aching when results of other tests point to a mandibular molar.

Bite Test. The bite test is used when a fracture is suspected. A soft lead shot held in a fold of scotch tape (or an orangewood stick or pencil) is placed between the cusps of the suspected tooth while the patient applies moderate pressure. This item can also be placed entirely on one cusp. Two criteria are evaulated: the visual separation of cusps and/or the elicitation of pain.

Transillumination. Transillumination has been suggested since the 1920s, and interest has recently been rekindled by the utilization of fiber optics. However, Reynolds and Aduddell concluded, "The use of fiber optics as a transilluminator for diagnostic purposes is of little value except in the detection of fractures in the crowns of teeth. It should not be considered a substitute for radiographic survey in any instance."[14]

Neurologic Tests. A simple measure of neurologic function is the use of both a cotton wisp and a pinprick with a sterile hypodermic needle. This would be employed when permanent anesthesia, paresthesia, or neurologic disorders affecting the sensory distribution of the trigeminal nerve are suspected.

Biopsy. Indications for biopsy are discussed in greater detail in Chapter 15, which deals with periapical surgery. Certainly, the biopsy must be considered the first line of diagnosis when the differential diagnosis includes a neoplasm.

Laboratory Tests. A number of laboratory tests are needed at times and should be conducted by competent personnel in medical laboratories. These tests might include an anesthetic sensitivity skin test when the patient gives a history of reaction to local anesthetics. Similarly, a history of allergic reaction to antibiotics would necessitate an antibiotic sensitivity skin test if antibiotic therapy is being considered.

Bacterial antibiotic sensitivity tests initiated by culture from either the root canal or the exudate from a fistula or incision and drainage may be necessary when the usual operative treatment and medication have not controlled intracanal and periapical infection (see Chapter 13).

Although the dentist rarely would unilaterally assume the responsibility, he may find it necessary to order a variety of blood tests and have the resources to call upon for their interpretation.

DIAGNOSTIC PERPLEXITIES*

Even after a careful history and examination, some cases still defy immediate diagnosis. The most frequent among these have been cataloged as diagnostic perplexities. Generally they fall into the following categories: (1) fistula, (2) numbness, (3) persistent discomfort, (4) cracked tooth syndrome, (5) bizarre radiographic appearance, and (6) idiopathic root resorption.

1. A ***fistula*** does not always exit in a stoma exactly opposite the seat of the problem. Witness the case of

*Abstracted from a manuscript to be published by Dr. Cyril Gaum, with credit to his associates, Joel Dunsky, Alvin A. Krakow, and Vangel Zissi.

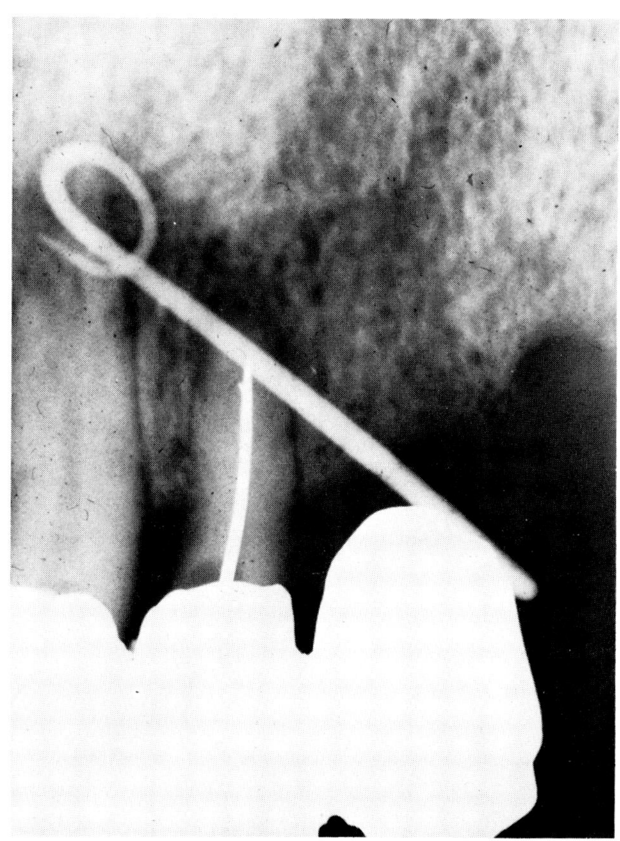

Fig. 10–49. Although stoma of draining sinus track was over canine and treated lateral incisor was suspected as origin, it was actually the more distant central incisor causing problem. (Courtesy Dr. Cyril Gaum.)

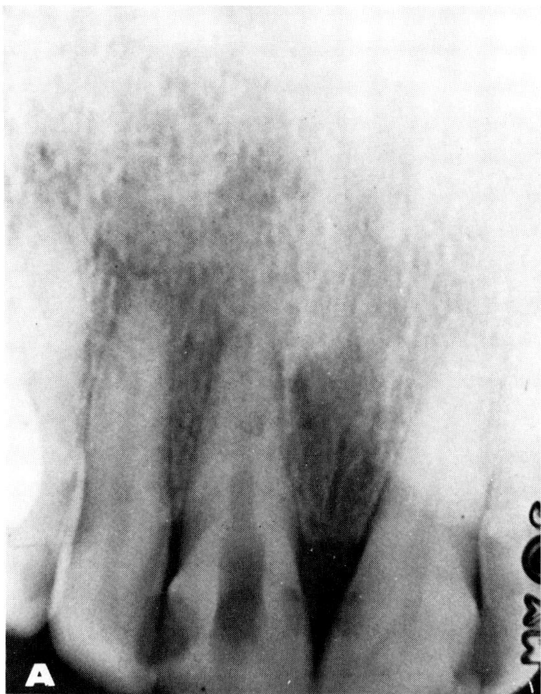

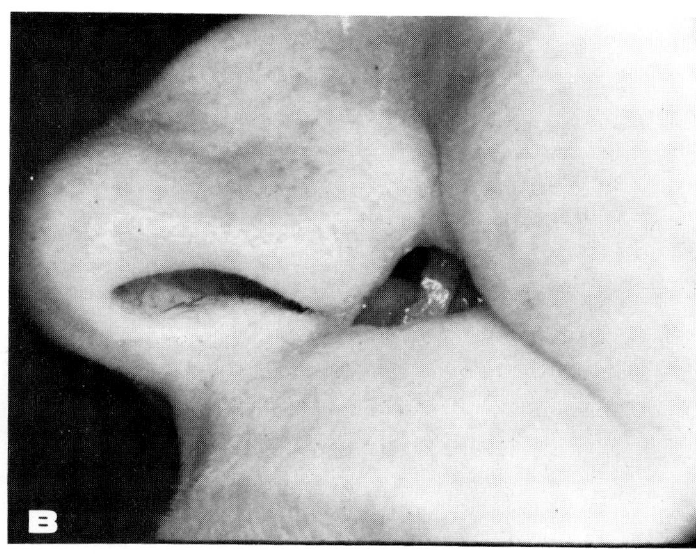

Fig. 10–50. *A*, Pulpless central incisor with vague periapical osseous changes. *B*, Draining fistula associated with infected pulpless incisor in *A*. (From Harris, W. E.: J.A.D.A., *83*:358, Aug. 7, 1971.)

drainage in the area of an extracted canine (Fig. 10–49). Logically, the adjacent pulpless lateral incisor must be suspected. However, a tracer gutta percha point, inserted through the stoma to the depth of the sinus tract, pointed to the pulpless central incisor as the culprit. Harris has revealed a pulpless maxillary central incisor that was draining extraorally through a stoma as far as the angle of the *ala nasi* (Fig. 10–50).[15]

Fistulas related to cracked teeth are most perplexing, and often can be diagnosed only by the laying of a surgical flap. A fistula located midroot on a tooth often indicates a fracture or perforation. In one particular case, the fracture was not discernible in the initial radiograph, but following obturation of the root canal, the horizontal fracture became readily apparent (Fig. 10–51).

2. ***Numbness*** has been encountered in a number of perplexing cases. When numbness is a symptom, one should be concerned with trigeminal neuropathies, tumors, or cysts that involve the innervation. In one particular case, the numbness seemed to be related to a large periapical lesion encroaching on the mandibular canal (Fig. 10–52*A*). Once root canal therapy was completed, the numbness started to leave, and within 14 months the lesion had healed and normal sensation was restored (Fig. 10–52*B*). Numbness associated with an acute alveolar abscess is often noted, but in such cases the diagnosis should be quite obvious.

Sixty-one cases of facial numbness were reviewed by a Mayo Clinic group,[16] who found that 83% of the cases had a definite cause, including 48% in which the numbness was of dental origin. Thrush and Small reported on seven cases of facial numbness, only one case of which was dental—typical mandibular numbness following a most profound local anesthesia and molar extraction.[17] The remaining cases of numbness were caused by carcinoma of the nasopharynx, tumor invasion of the gasserian ganglion, adenocarcinoma of the brain stem, and cerebrovascular accident. All these patients exhibited numbness of the jaws, lips, tongue, or palate. They summarized their report by saying, "The most important task is to exclude neoplasia." They recommended basal views of the skull and examination of the nasopharynx.

3. ***Persistent discomfort*** may continue after obturation or radicular surgery, or it may develop some time later. In a case in the latter category, the patient was

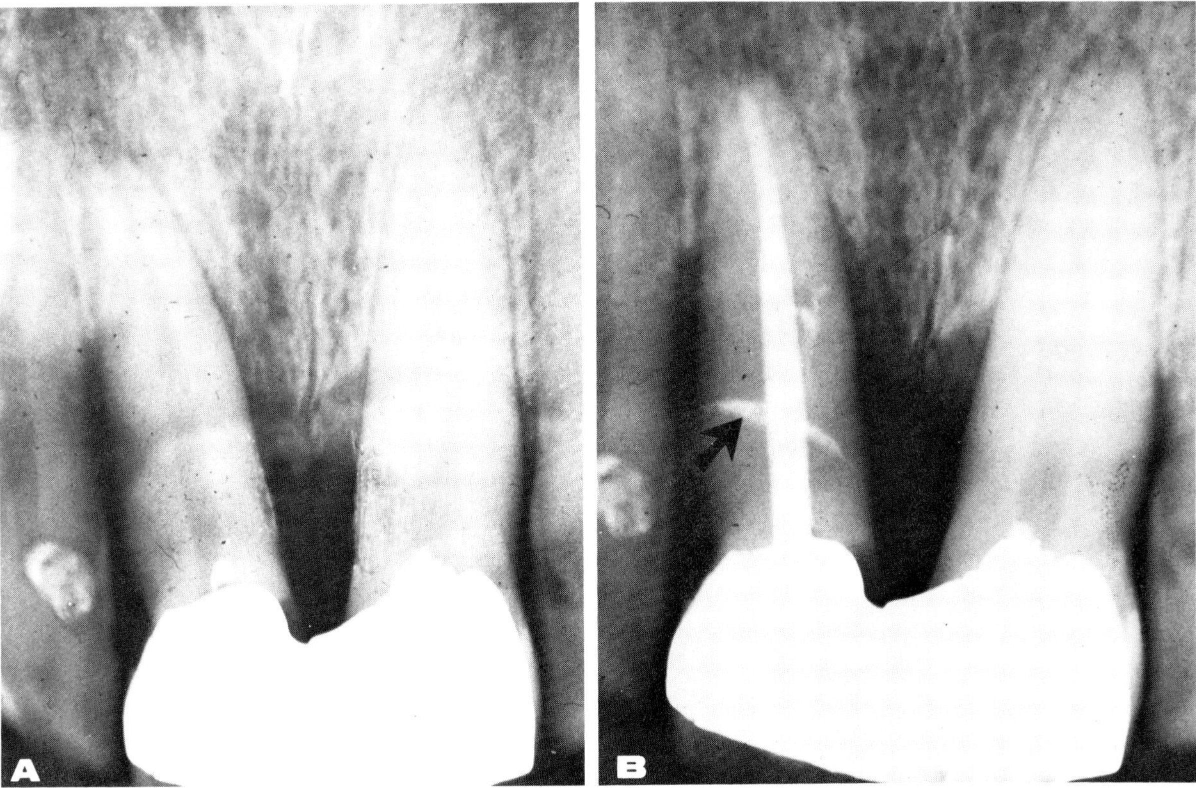

Fig. 10–51. *A,* Preoperative film reveals no fracture line associated with chronic fistula. *B,* Cement is extruded into fracture line. (Courtesy Dr. Cyril Gaum.)

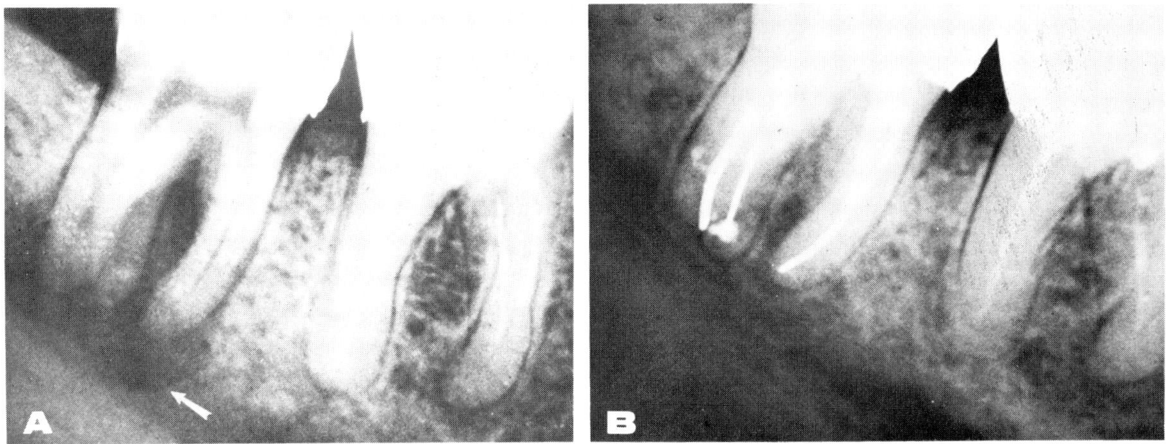

Fig. 10–52. *A,* Extensive periapical lesion encroaching upon mandibular canal *(arrow).* Numbness results. *B,* Successful endodontic result, 14 months later. Numbness disappeared as healing advanced. Note 2 distal canals and lateral canal as well. (Courtesy Dr. Cyril Gaum.)

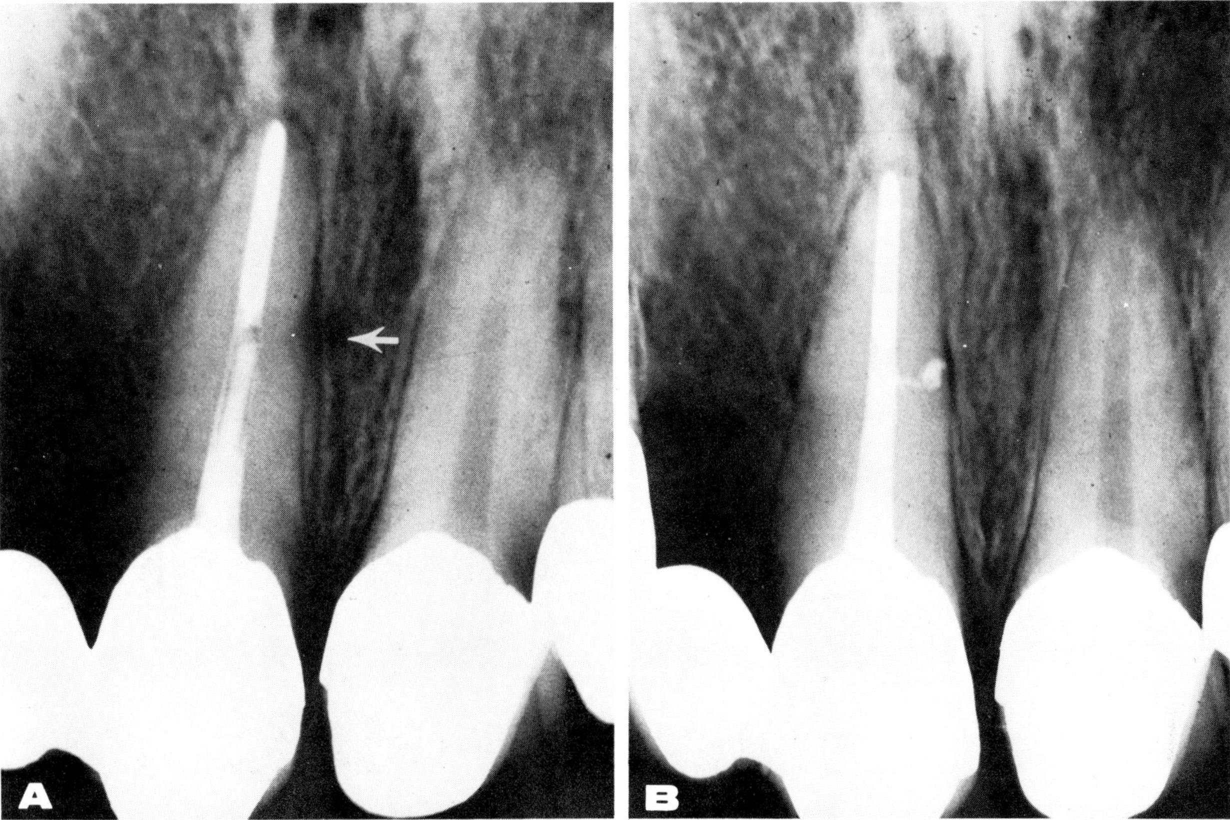

Fig. 10–53. *A,* Persistent discomfort after endodontic treatment and bridge placement. Lesion *(arrow)* midroot with some resorption, indicates patent accessory canal. *B,* Retreatment obturates accessory lateral canal, healing occurs, and discomfort is alleviated. (Courtesy Dr. Joel L. Dunsky.)

examined radiographically months after root canal therapy and placement of a bridge abutment. The discomfort was "mid tooth" and the radiograph revealed a bony lesion in that area along with external root resorption and a poorly obturated mid canal (Fig. 10–53*A*). Because a lateral canal was suspected, the main canal was re-obturated from the crown, and immediately the discomfort disappeared (Fig. 10–53*B*). This case well demonstrates the necessity to obturate all of the canal, not just the apical third.

Another case of persistent discomfort came from a maxillary molar where cotton had been left in the pulp chamber under the cement base and a class I amalgam filling. Merely removing the cotton and placing a solid base "cured" the discomfort. Conjecture about the cause of the pain includes the presence of a hairline fracture or an accessory canal in the floor of the chamber.

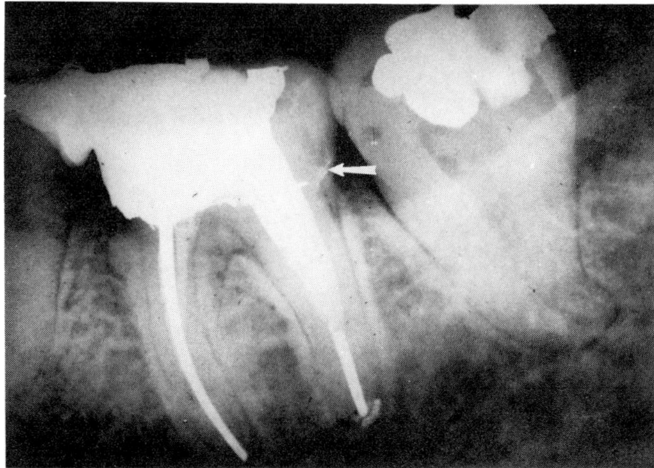

Fig. 10–54. Cement extruded through undisclosed hairline fracture *(arrow)* reveals source of persistent discomfort. (Courtesy Dr. Cyril Gaum.)

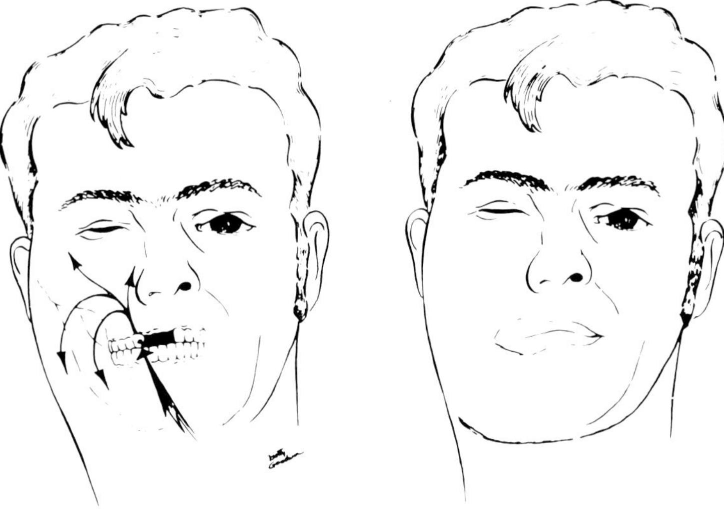

Fig. 10–55. During transient periods of increased pressure in deeply submerged submarine, extracorporeal air entered facial interstitial spaces through empty root canal. (From Verunac, J. J.: J.A.D.A., *87*:1192, Nov., 1973.)

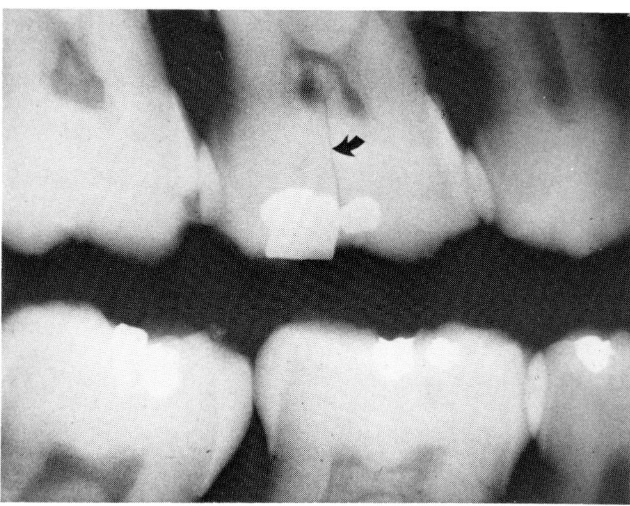

Fig. 10–56. Vertical fracture of the crown revealed in bitewing film not apparent in periapical film. (Courtesy Dr. Cyril Gaum.)

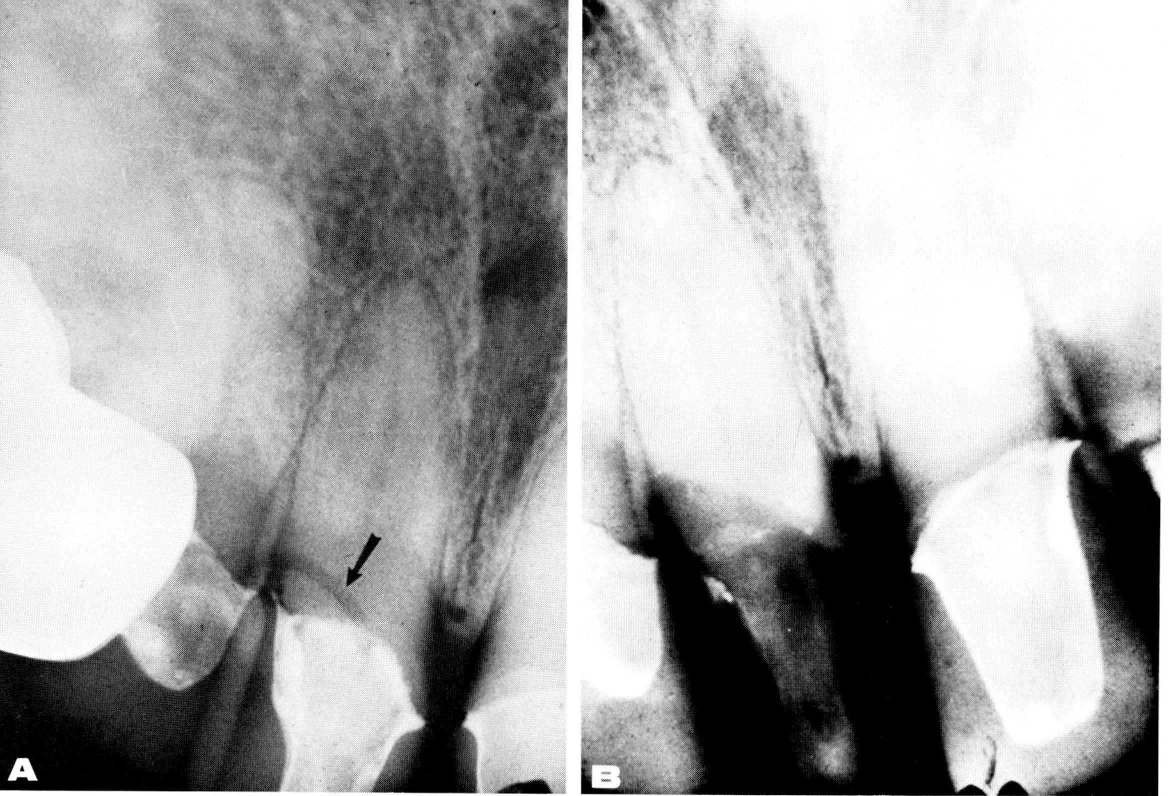

Fig. 10–57. *A,* Radiolucent line *(arrow)* is suspected of being fracture under jacket crown. *B,* Jacket crown is removed and "fracture" becomes high chamfer preparation. (Courtesy Dr. Cyril Gaum.)

In a similar case, cotton and Cavit were sealed in a postpreparation in the distal canal of a lower molar, and this resulted in continuous pain. Because the dentist did not utilize the retentive cavity, the patient was recalled and the preparation was filled permanently. The cause of discomfort immediately became apparent when cement was forced out of a minute fracture line (Fig. 10–54).

A most perplexing and life-threatening case, reported by Verunac,[18] was that of the young submariner who consistently developed massive facial emphysema each time the submarine dived. The swelling would become pronounced after the submarine was deeply submerged for 15 hours (Fig. 10–55). Within four or five days after surfacing, the swelling would disappear. Navy physicians had given him antibiotics to no avail and had recommended his discharge from the service.

Examination by a dentist revealed a lingual cusp fractured away from a maxillary first premolar and exposing the lingual canal which was patent through the foramen. The air under submerged pressure was being forced through this tiny hole into the entire side of the face and neck (Fig. 10–55).

4. ***The cracked tooth syndrome*** accounts for many perplexing diagnostic problems. A typical case is that of the patient who experienced intermittent episodes of acute pain radiating over the entire side of the head. The periapical radiograph revealed a periapical lesion, and vitality testing proved the pulp to be nonvital. Just before endodontic therapy was started, a bitewing radiograph was taken which revealed a

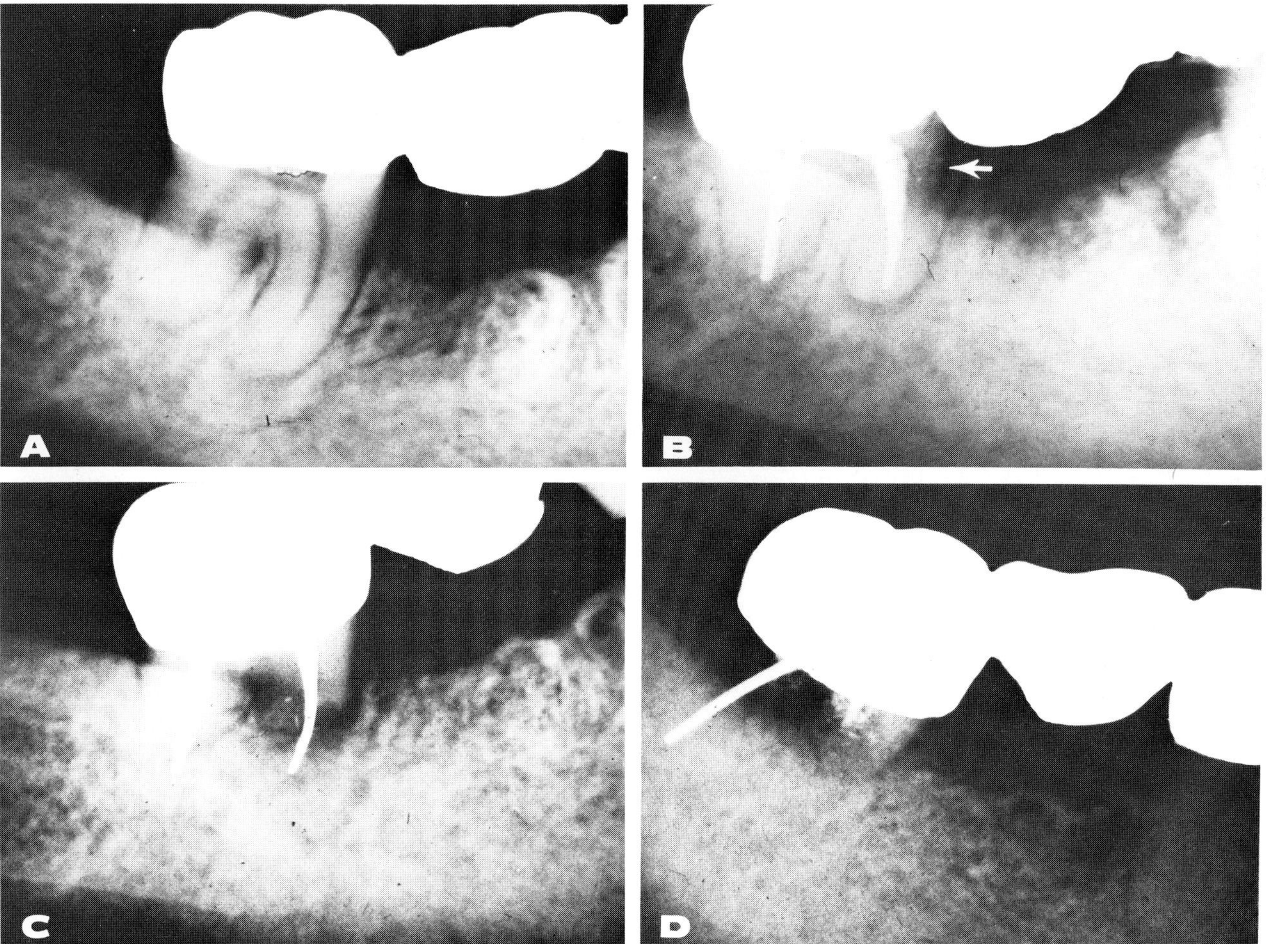

Fig. 10–58. Unexplained root resorption of bridge abutment in patient with breast cancer. *A*, Initial film. *B*, One month later. *C*, Seven months later. *D*, Two and one-half years later. (Courtesy Dr. Cyril Gaum.)

vertical fracture into the pulp (Fig. 10–56). It is interesting that the crack could not be seen in the periapical film, but did show in the bitewing. Crown fractures may be more easily detected by bitewing radiographs.

5. ***Radiographic appearances*** are not all they appear to be. Just such a case is illustrated in a film of a maxillary incisor. The tooth was exquisitely tender to percussion and was mobile. In the radiograph a horizontal radiolucency appears above the margin of the porcelain jacket crown (Fig. 10–57*A*), which was diagnosed as a fracture with pulp involvement. The crown was removed, and what appeared to be a fracture turned out to be a high chamfer crown preparation. This was verified with a second radiograph (Fig. 10–57*B*). The pulp was necrotic.

6. ***Idiopathic Root Resorption.*** Although one expects occasionally to see root resorption in a maxillary lateral incisor, or in severely traumatized or replanted teeth, one is perplexed indeed by cases of root resorption for which no logical explanation exists.

One such case involved the roots of a mandibular molar bridge abutment, where resorption began shortly after root canal therapy (Fig. 10–58*A*). Within two and a half years the roots had completely resorbed away.

One might speculate that this resorption could have been related to the patient's breast cancer. It has been postulated that a parathyroidlike hormone is secreted by tumor cells and there is a high incidence of hypercalcemia in patients with breast cancer.

Breast cancer could not have been an etiologic factor in a similar case reported by Poliak.[19] His patient was a middle-aged male motion picture producer who developed an unexplained resorption five years following therapy of an endodontically treated mandibular second molar. Within two years the entire root structure had essentially resorbed away (Fig. 10–59).

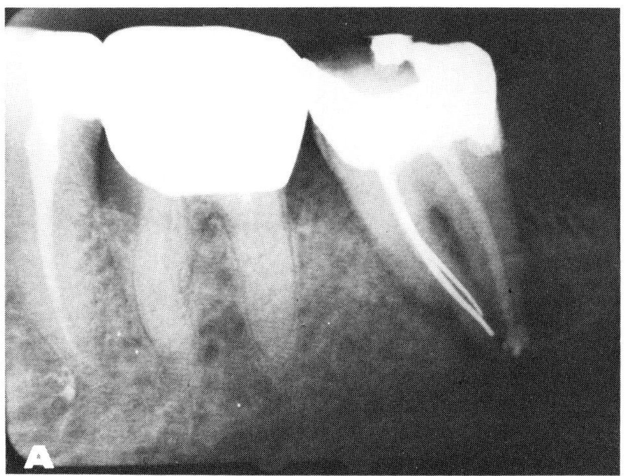

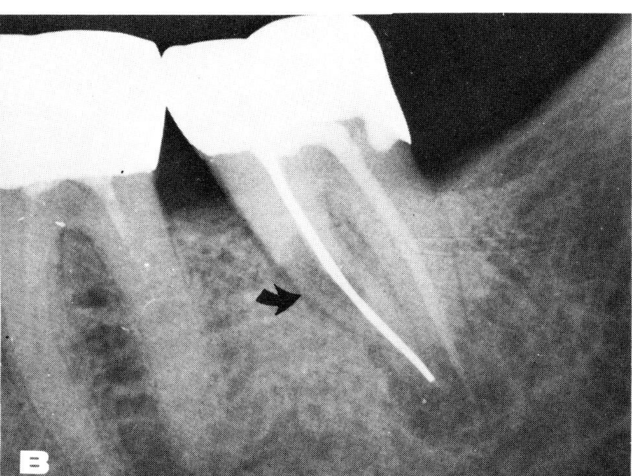

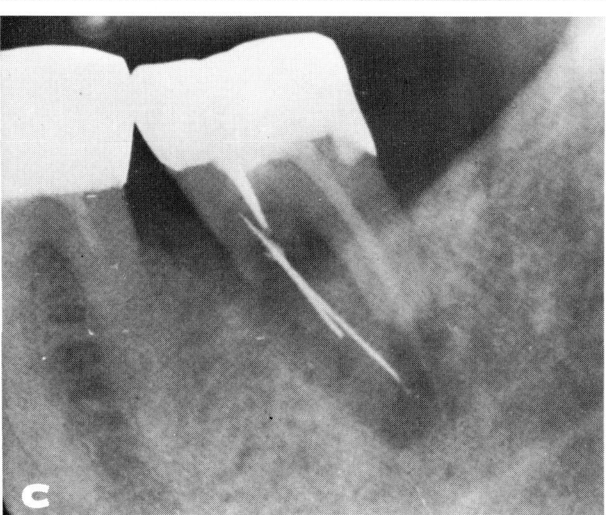

Fig. 10–59. Unexplained root resorption in middle-aged male in good health. *A,* Final treatment film. *B,* Five-year recall radiograph, first time external resorption appeared *(arrow)*. *C,* Two years later (seven-year recall) tooth is hopelessly resorbed and must be extracted. (Courtesy Dr. Bernard Poliak.)

REFERENCES

1. Halpern, I. L.: Patient's medical status—a factor in dental treatment. Oral Surg., *39*:216, Feb., 1975.
2. Wuehrmann, A. H.: Radiation hygiene and its practice in dentistry are related to film viewing procedures and radiographic interpretation. J.A.D.A., *80*:346, Feb., 1970.
3. Goldman, M., Pearson, A. H., and Darzenta, N.: Reliability of radiographic interpretations. Oral Surg., *38*:287, Aug., 1974.
4. Goldman, M., Pearson, A. H., and Darzenta, N.: Endodontic success—who's reading the radiograph? Oral Surg., *33*:432, 1972.
5. Shoha, R. R., Dowson, J., and Richards, A. G.: Radiographic interpretation of experimentally produced bony lesion. Oral Surg., *38*:294, Aug., 1974.
6. Slowey, R. R.: Radiographic aids in the detection of extra root canals. Oral Surg., *37*:762, May, 1974.
7. Gartner, A. H., Somerlott, R., and Walsh, L.: Differential diagnosis of internal and external resorption. Paper presented at Meeting of Am. Assoc. Endodont., April 25, 1975.
8. Riley, R. R.: Endodontic recall procedures. Oral Surg., *37*:118, Jan., 1974.
9. Van Hassel, H. J., and Harrington, G.: Localization of pulpal sensation. Oral Surg., *28*:753, Nov., 1969.
10. Degering, C. I.: Physiologic evaluation of dental pulp testing methods. J. Dent. Res., *41*:695, May-June, 1962.
11. Aduddell, A. C., and Reynolds, R.: Pulp testers. Oral Surg. To be published.
12. Woodley, L, Woodworth, J., and Dobbs, J. L.: A preliminary evaluation of the effect of electric pulp testers on dogs with artificial pacemakers. J.A.D.A., *89*:1099, Nov., 1974.
13. McDaniel, K. F., Rowe, N. H., and Charbeneau, G. I.: Tissue response to an electric pulp tester. J. Prosthet. Dent., *29*:84, Jan., 1973.
14. Reynolds, R. L., and Aduddell, A. C.: A clinical evaluation of fiber optics and transillumination in diagnosis. J. South. Cal. Dent. Assoc., *39*:896, Nov., 1971.
15. Harris, W. E.: Unusual endodontic complication: report of a case. J.A.D.A., *83*:358, Aug., 1971.
16. Goldstein, N., Gibilisco, J., and Rushton, J.: Trigeminal neuropathy and neuritis. J.A.M.A., *184*:458, May, 1963.
17. Thrush, D. C., and Small, M.: How benign a symptom is facial numbness? Lancet, *2*:851, Oct. 24, 1970.
18. Verunac, J. J.: Recurrent severe facial emphysema in a submariner. J.A.D.A., *87*:1192, Nov., 1973.
19. Poliak, B. H.: Personal communication, 1975.

Chapter 11

Differential Diagnosis and Treatment of Oral and Perioral Pain

JOHN I. INGLE, DUDLEY H. GLICK, and L. DANIEL SCHAEFFER

"Pain is perfect misery, the worst of all evils; and, excessive over-turns all patience."
John Milton—*Paradise Lost*[1]

A well-trained dentist may render a patient many services, services which gain him a deep personal satisfaction. Foremost among these is the diagnosis and relief of excruciating or long-lasting pain. These are the occasions patients remember most vividly: "the night you came back at midnight and relieved my terrible toothache," or ". . . you diagnosed the constant pain I had for two years, Doctor, and after everyone else had given up."

These problem cases are rarely rewarding financially, but are those few moments we as a profession enjoy, setting us apart from the lay public. These are the problems that try one's patience and ingenuity. Only the skilled will be successful in diagnosing the really difficult cases.

Pity the dentist who pursues his professional career with a nagging uncertainty about any but the most obvious pain problems. Disdain accrues as well for the dentist whose only solution to problems of pain lies with extraction forceps. The patients who have suffered this mistreatment stand as a pitiful indictment of a poorly-trained, insecure, and disinterested segment of our profession.

Dental diagnosis is a personal experience; therefore, many of the qualities of a good diagnostician are of a personal nature. In this regard, dental diagnosis today is to be compared with medical diagnosis of the past. We still diagnose " by the seat of our pants," so to say. Medicine, on the other hand, is slowly moving from the "art" of personal diagnosis to the so-called "science" of diagnosis. Rightly or wrongly, the electrocardiograph and electroencephalograph, liver and kidney function tests, complete blood count, 17-ketosteroid determination, echocardiography, and a host of roentgenograms are only a few of the tools which have changed the character of medical diagnosis.

REQUIREMENTS OF A DIAGNOSTICIAN

There are a number of assets a dentist must have to be a successful diagnostician. Most important would be: knowledge, interest, intuition, curiosity and patience. He must also have an acuity of senses and the necessary tools for diagnosis.

Knowledge. Primarily, the dentist must depend upon himself, not the laboratory; therefore, ***knowledge*** is the most important single asset the dentist must possess. This includes familiarity with all local oral causes of pain as well as the numerous systemic, neurogenic, and psychogenic causes. Conversely, the dentist must also be aware of the many physical and mental effects brought about by protracted severe pain. He must know that constant overwhelming pain can effect dysfunction of every organ of the body. Bonica, in discussing the pain victim, emphasizes these facts: that the pulse rate slows while the blood pressure and respiratory rate increases. The pupils dilate. The patient is affected by nausea, slow digestion, and a diminution of renal function. Moreover, many patients become hysterical, with reaction ranging from docile to unmanageable.[2]

Under ***knowledge*** must also be listed the important asset of ***knowing when and where to refer the patient*** for additional consultation. This comes with experience and the slow careful development over the years of a group of physicians and fellow dentists who may be depended upon to assist in diagnosis. Often the patient is referred because examination reveals a problem clearly in the province of the neurologist or otolaryngologist. Sometimes the patient is referred because the examiner has exhausted his knowledge and frankly needs help in diagnosis—the recognition of fallibility and limitation (when to yell for help).

Interest. ***Interest*** is the second important asset possessed by a good diagnostician. The dentist must have a keen interest in the patient and his problem, and must evidence this interest in handling the patient. If this attitude is not natural to the dentist, he will render the patient and the profession a service by referring all diagnostic problems to an interested and competent fellow practitioner.

Intuition. In addition to ***interest*** and ***knowledge,*** the good diagnostician requires ***intuition*** or "sixth sense." There must be developed within the best examiner a psychic perception of the true basis of a problem, or the presence of the unusual. This is the ability, possessed by so few, which sometimes allows for instant and unusual diagnosis. Sir William Osler must have been one of these people.

It is ***intuition*** that tells the dentist the patient is holding back information or is not telling the complete truth. Moreover, intuition immediately puts the examiner on guard with the patient who "knows too much," *i.e.,* all the words and symptoms related to a certain condition. Intuition allows one to suspect the unusual, but it also goes hand-in-hand with still another prime asset of the good diagnostician . . . ***curiosity.***

Curiosity. One must pursue or develop a natural ***curiosity*** about the patient and his disease, if perseverance is to be maintained in arriving at a diagnosis. Dr. Harry Sicher has likened dental diagnosis to the actions of a good detective, and curiosity is a detective's greatest asset. Medawar describes diagnosis as the "use of the hypothetico-deductive system."[3] Again, ***curiosity*** goes with ***interest,*** and the dentist who is bored by the painstaking methods of diagnosis will never have the ***curiosity*** to delve a little deeper, probe a little further, ask the unusual. All this takes time and thus requires ***patience.***

Patience. Oftentimes, diagnosis of unusual pain may take hours to develop. This time may be expended in one or two sittings or spread over many weeks. Remember, some patients who complain of unusual pain have suffered this pain for years, and so one cannot expect to make a snap diagnosis in a matter of minutes. This is the reason, as we stated earlier, that difficult diagnosis may be unrewarding financially but very rewarding emotionally. Again, if the dentist is not willing to sacrifice the time to attempt to help these individuals, he is urged to refer the patient for diagnosis, rather than make an incorrect, quick diagnosis which usually results in his reaching for the forceps.

The dentist obviously cannot abandon his other patients to see one person repeatedly. Too frequently the problem patient is asked to return at the end of the day when both dentist and patient are tired and irritable. A better solution is to see the patient in the morning, before office hours. This is an imposition many dentists are not willing to assume, so again they are urged to refer the patient to their more altruistic colleagues.

Senses. The good diagnostician must have the astuteness to grasp what his senses reveal to him.

First, he has a voice to ask questions and ears to hear the answers; he has eyes to see and hands to probe and palpate. In short, he has senses with which he communicates with the sick patient. But as Friedman has pointed out,[4] "one must learn to listen with the third ear and see with the third eye."

Controlling these senses, however, is the ***mind,*** and if the mind does not inquire and then reason, or has not accumulated the knowledge necessary to inquire and finally to analyze, then the senses are useless. His mind must list all the possible causes of the pain and then, more often than not, eliminate them one by one until the correct diagnosis is made.

There is a "language of pain" which must be comprehended by the examiner—language the patient uses to describe symptoms that should signify something to the astute. Melzack and Torgerson have categorized the words describing pain into classes and subclasses—words that describe the ***sensory*** qualities as well as the pain-***affective*** qualities of fear and tension, and the ***evaluative*** words describing the overall intensity of the experience.[5]

"Clinical investigators have long recognized the varieties of pain—the burning qualities of causalgia, the stabbing, cramping qualities of visceral pains, the splitting, pounding qualities of headaches, the nagging pain of rheumatism, the cramping heavy qualities of menstrual pain, the smarting, itching qualities apparently well known to sufferers of piles."[5] These valid descriptors are vividly played each evening on the television.

Melzack and Torgerson give the patient a vast choice of descriptive words that often provide the clues to diagnosis in response to the question, "What does your pain feel like?"[5]

Terms Describing Pain

Sensory

Temporal: Beating, flickering, pounding, pulsing, quivering, throbbing, thumping.
Spatial: Darting, flashing, jumping, radiating, shooting, spreading.
Punctate Pressure: Boring, drilling, lancinating, penetrating, piercing, pricking, stabbing.
Incisive Pressure: Cutting, lacerating, sharp.
Constrictive Pressure: Binding, biting, cramping, crushing, gnawing, gripping, nipping, pinching, pressing, squeezing, tight.
Traction Pressure: Grinding, pulling, tugging, wrenching.
Thermal: Burning, hot, scalding, searing, cool, cold.
Brightness: Itchy, smarting, stinging, tickling, tingling.
Dullness: Aching, blurred, drawing, dull, heavy, hurting, numbing, sore, splitting, steady, tender.

Affective

Tension: Dragging, exhausting, fatiguing, nagging, tiring.
Autonomic: Choking, nauseating, sickening, suffocating, wretched.
Fear: Awful, dreadful, fearful, frightful, terrifying.
Punishment: Cruel, gruelling, killing, punishing, racking, torturing, vicious, wicked.

Evaluative

Agonizing, annoying, bearable, discomforting, distracting, distressing, excruciating, horrible, intense, intolerable, mild, miserable, savage, troublesome, ugly, unbearable, violent.

The terms "cold and cool" were only used by patients to described dental pain.

By focusing on 20 key words from this master list, Dr. Melzack can derive a pain-rating index which enables him to correct inaccurate estimates of pain that patients from different cultural backgrounds tend to make. Patients are usually delighted with the pain-describing adjectives—"Now I can tell exactly how it feels. Before, I couldn't think of just the right words."

Anchor words for intensity are particularly helpful, ranging from mild (1) to excruciating (5), with discomforting (2), distressing (3), and horrible (4) in between. The patient may be given a 10-inch ruler and asked "how many inches of pain do you have?"

Melzack concluded that pains described as "flickering, jumping, and pinching" are less severe than those termed "pounding, shooting, or cramping."[6] Patients are suspect who describe pain with low-rank value words, *i.e.,* pinching and tender, and then insist their pain is "excruciating."

Equipment. The examiner must also have some basic instruments available. The electric pulp tester, the x-ray machine, materials for thermal tests, the mirror, explorer and probe are all vital to the examination, and are thoroughly discussed in Chapter 10, Methods of Diagnosis.

If the altruistic dentist is armed with the knowledge and interest, the curiosity and patience, and finally, the instruments of diagnosis, he is prepared for a most rewarding experience: identifying the source of pain and relieving the suffering of a fellow human being.

The modern dentist, who is oriented to the value of retaining the pulpless tooth, will think of endodontic problems when a patient complains of pain. This has not always been so. In the past the oral surgeon was the diagnostician most frequently consulted. Today, however, the endodontist and the periodontist are often called upon to make the decisions in "oral medicine" and regarding pain.

If the foregoing paragraphs sound like a sermon, they were meant to be. One cannot emphasize too strongly the personal nature of good diagnosis. If the dentist is ever to deserve the title "oral physician," it will be earned in the field of diagnosis. This is also the area in which the dentist is most apt, on a professional basis, to earn the respect and friendship of his medical colleagues.

The personal nature of diagnosis was emphasized by Dr. Arthur B. Hertzler, who states, "My patients have told me what to write and I have put it down to the best of my ability, slowly and painfully. . . . I have always found it impossible to write of things I have not seen."[7]

And so it is with this discussion of pain. These are the things we have seen. This is what our patients—by their words, actions, signs, and symptoms—have led us to write. These are the results of knowledge and experience, not just a review of the literature.

One final comment. Students frequently ask why they should spend time learning the shades of difference in the pain of pulpalgia. "What's the difference?" they will ask, "You always remove the pulp anyway—one disease, one treatment."

"What is the difference?" one might ask. The answer lies in the necessity of knowledge. One must know the normal before recognizing the abnormal; the commonplace before the unusual. For this reason we study histology before pathology. For this reason we must know intimately all the signs and symptoms of the most obvious and frequent syndromes before we undertake studying the complex and rare syndrome. The importance of this basic knowledge is rudely brought home when one becomes aware that the patient sitting across from you is not really suffering true dental pain, but is actually psychotic.

THE PHENOMENON OF PAIN*

Before facial or oral pain can be explained or understood, a knowledge of pain in general must exist. What actually is pain? What are its components? Do all people "suffer" to the same intensity? Can some people ignore pain, or as Milton said, "Does excessive pain overturn all patience?" Before we discuss specific pain, a brief explanation of the phenomenon of pain is necessary: the anatomic, physiologic, and psychologic substrata of pain.

*Abstracted from a manuscript to be published by L. Daniel Schaeffer.

The deceptively simple question, "What is pain?" is not simple to answer. Aristotle described it as a "quale; a passion of the soul," rather than an ordinary sensory experience. Erasmus Darwin anticipated the "intensive" theory of pain when he stated that pain resulted from the overstimulation of any of the other senses, as by extremes of temperature. Later research has shown that pain is mediated by end organs and neural pathways separated from those of other senses. Monheim has said: "Pain may be defined as an unpleasant sensation created by a noxious stimulus which is mediated along specific nerve pathways into the central nervous system, where it is interpreted as such."[8]

Because of the psychic content of pain, however, the words of Sir Thomas Lewis are equally appropriate: "Pain, like similar subjective things, is known to us by experience and described by illustration."[9]

Physical Substratum of Pain. A simple, yet important, concept to be kept in mind throughout this discussion is illustrated by the chain of events diagrammed in Figure 11–1, stages 1 through 6.

Noxious stimuli causing tissue damage impinge on a widely distributed system of afferent fibers, the pain receptors. Any energy of sufficient intensity to cause tissue damage elicits action potentials (impulses) in these fibers as a linear function of the log of the

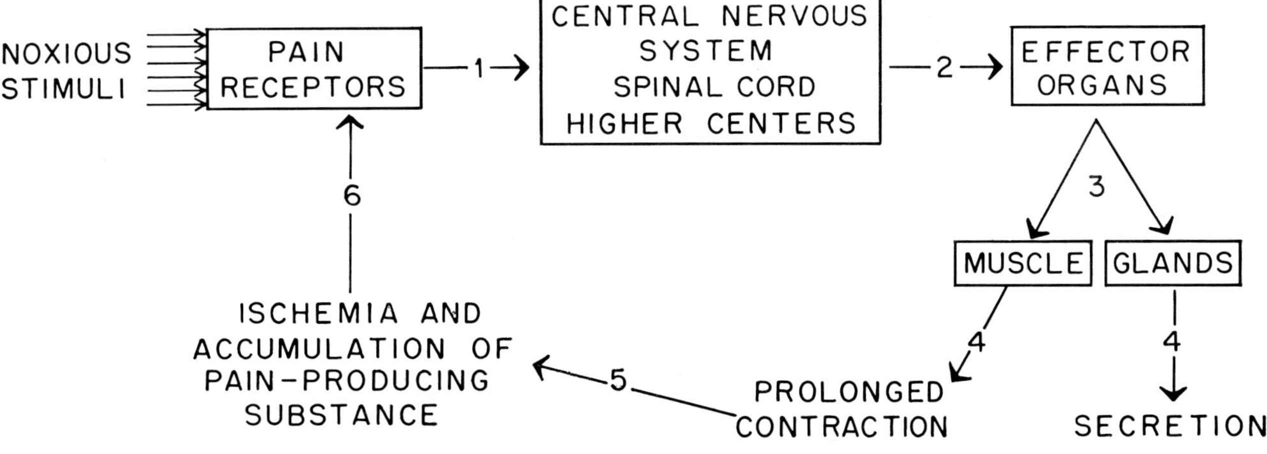

Fig. 11–1.

intensity of the stimulus (Weber-Fechner law).[10] Pain produced by muscle spasm can be used as an example of noxious stimuli, which could even be emotional, setting off a cycle of muscle contraction leading to pain. These impulses pass (1) to the central nervous system where the information is processed and sent (2) to various effector organs such as muscle and gland tissue (3), which respond by contracting or secreting (4). Long-standing noxious stimuli may result in prolonged muscular contraction (4), which produces, in turn, the accumulation of potassium ions (5), which act again as noxious stimuli (6) for pain receptors in the muscle itself. Thus the pain-spasm-pain-spasm cycle is perpetuated. This cycle may ***persist*** even after the primary noxious stimulus is eliminated.[11]

Psychic Substratum of Pain. The "higher centers" illustrated in Figure 11–1 stress the importance of the psyche in the overall pain experience. Monheim has pointed out that pain has two aspects: pain ***perception*** and pain ***reaction.***[12] Pain ***perception*** is relatively constant from person to person, whereas pain ***reaction*** is quite variable in different individuals and in the same individual at different times. The variability is an expression of one's past experience: how he has been taught to react to pain and conceive of pain; in short, the total of his learning experiences.

In addition to the psychic overlay, a number of studies have shown differing cultural and racial reactions to pain. This difference is important because the diagnostician routinely depends on a patient's spoken response to determine the degree of pain, its location, and its localization or diffuseness. Zola has shown that these responses may not be reliable.[13] He contrasted two patients of different ethnic origins who came to an eye, ear, nose, and throat clinic. One confined his complaint to the eye, ear, nose, or throat, whereas the other chose another part of his body. One would deny the presence of pain, calling it instead a "throbbing" or "congestion or pressure—not really pain." The other could make the pain "go away" by rubbing a remote site.

Pain is communicated in many different ways, and so knowledge of a patient's social and cultural background can help one to understand the communication. People learn to express their reactions to stimuli by observing the reactions of those who are similar to oneself. The first important source of comparison is the family transmitting cultural norms to its children. In a study of dental fears,[14] children whose mothers had high anxiety scores showed more negative behavior during an extraction than children of mothers with low anxiety scores. As we have already illustrated, behavior may well be related to one's cultural or ethnic origins.[15] Using electric shock as a noxious stimulus, Yankee, Irish, Jewish and Italian women were asked to respond to two levels of discomfort—where they first experienced the shock and where they could no longer "stand the pain." Although all the ethnic groups first discerned the shock at the same level, a good deal of difference was apparent in accepting the pain. The Italians tolerated the least amount of shock and were ***considerably*** less tolerant than the Yankees and the Jews. The Irish were also on the low end of the tolerance scale somewhere between the Italians and the Jews.[15] It has also been shown that the stronger the identification one has with his ethnic group, the more willing he is to tolerate pain, to conform to the group norm.[16] No difference in pain reactions of White or Black women obstetrical patients has been found, however.[17]

Neurons and Synapses. The basic element of the nervous system is the neuron. Typically, the neuron consists of a cell body and its threadlike processes, the axon and the dendrites (Fig. 11–2). Within the cell body of the neuron are located the nucleus and numerous cytoplasmic structures, *e.g.*, neuroplasm, Nissl bodies, mitochondria, neurofibrils, Golgi apparatus, endoplasmic reticulum, lysosomes, and pigmental inclusions.

There is not a single type of neuron, the nervous system being composed of a wide variety of shapes and sizes. Despite their tremendous diversity, however, all neurons exhibit three fundamental characteristic properties: (1) they have a specialized capacity to respond to stimuli; (2) they are able to transmit their "excitations" (action potentials) to all portions of the cell; and (3) they have the unique ability to "excite" receptor cells whether they be other neurons or muscle or glandular cells.

When a nerve cell is "fired," the action potential (excitation) traverses the length of the threadlike axon and terminates at the point where the terminal fibers of the axon contact another nerve cell. This junction between two neurons is called a synapse. The synapse is of prime significance, since it is an integrative connector of the neurons. An impulse, for instance, can be transmitted ***within*** the neuron, either toward or away from the cell body. However, ***conduction*** of an impulse from one neuron to the next can only be in one direction.

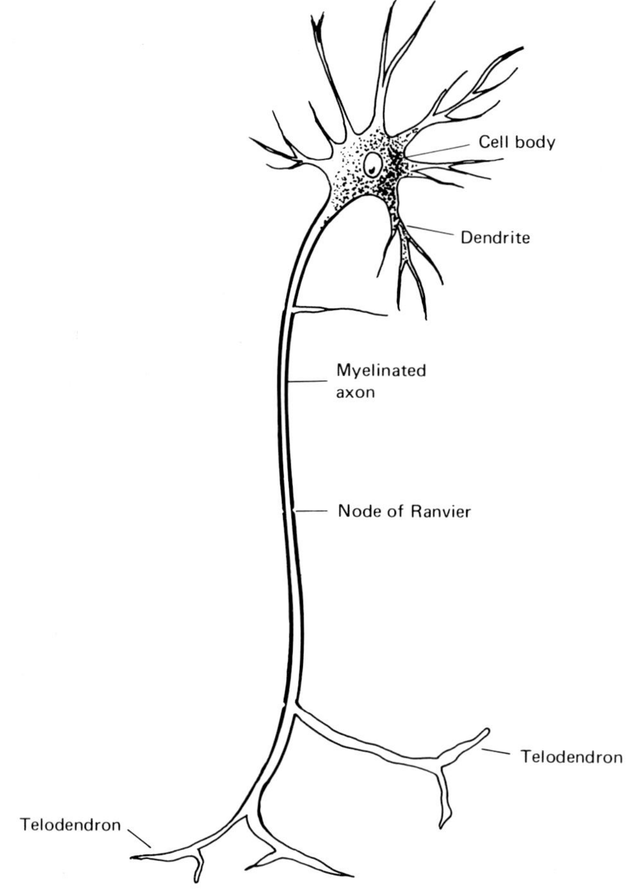

Fig. 11–2. Neuron with dendrites and axon extending out of cell body.

Unidirectional conduction is dependent on the chemical "one-way" transmission of action potentials from one neuron to the next. Thus, the synapse permits the ***pre***synaptic action potential of an axon to exert its influence across the synaptic cleft to the dendrite or cell body of an adjacent neuron. The ***pre***synaptic neuron "generates" an action potential in the ***post***synaptic neuron by releasing synaptic vesicles containing the neurochemical transmitter, acetylcholine, which then diffuses across the synaptic cleft and attaches to its specific receptor sites located on the postsynaptic cell membrane.* Only after a finite number of these neurotransmitter molecules have become "bound" to the receptor sites of the postsynaptic membrane will the following neuron generate an action potential. Presumably this is brought about by the postsynaptic membrane becoming momentarily sieve-like and more permeable to sodium and potassium ions. It is this flux of ions that changes the electrical potential across the postsynaptic membrane and thus elicits an action potential in the postsynaptic cell. The transmission across the synapse usually requires from 0.3 to 1.0 millisecond.

*The exact mechanism of action of acetylcholine on the postsynaptic membrane remains elusive.

Unlike the axon, which is essentially not fatigable, the synapse is fatigable. Also, synaptic transmission succumbs much more readily to such conditions as anoxia and ischemia caused by anesthetic agents than does axonal transmission. This fatigability of the synapse probably results from depletion of stored synaptic vesicles containing the neurochemical transmitter, acetylcholine. The rapid recovery of the postsynaptic membrane is related to the hydrolytic splitting of acetylcholine by the enzyme acetylcholine-esterase to acetate and choline.

Basic Neuron Physiology. A nerve fiber conducts nerve impulses, *viz.,* action potentials. This readily observable phenomenon is intimately related to the physicochemical properties of the neuron's cellular membrane (neurilemma). Although difficult to define, an impulse may be considered "a physicochemical charge transmitted by the nerve fiber."

The first essential for the conduction of a nerve impulse is the establishment of a potential across the selectively permeable cellular membrane, utilizing a metabolic process known as the "sodium pump." This mechanism sets up concentration differences of certain positive and negative ions between the two sides of the membrane. It is this selective separation of ionic charges that constitutes the ***resting*** potential.

An ***action*** potential may be generated by a variety of external stimuli—pressure, heat, light, mechanical force, or electrical stimuli. The nerve impulse is generated by the entry of sodium ions into the axon. The voltage change associated with this transient reversal of potential (from approximately −70 mVolts to +30 mVolts) is known as the "spike" or "action potential."

Pain Receptors and Afferent Nerve Fiber Pathways. Before one can understand the neural structure and functions of the pain process, the anatomic features of the various components must be discussed. Facial and oropharyngeal pain results from appropriate stimulation of receptors or free nerve endings, which are acknowledged to be naked (nonencapsulated) endings found in virtually every structure of the body. They are located in superficial layers of the skin or mucous membrane of the maxillofacial areas, adventitia of blood vessels, aponeurotic sheaths, periosteum, dental pulp, and predentin areas of the tooth. The parent primary neurons sub-branch to form finely divided nets. These networks of receptors may overlap and interdigitate, although they do not establish direct connections with one another.

Pain is elicited from pain receptors by any nonspecific noxious agent that causes destructive injuries of cells or tissues surrounding the receptors. Thus, pain is not produced by direct stimulation of a nerve fiber, but by some disturbance of tissues which leads to generation of an action potential in the general vicinity of the terminal ending of the fiber. Lim has presented evidence that the nerve endings mediating pain are specialized chemoreceptors that are sensitive to chemicals released by tissues in response to noxious stimuli.[18,19]

Once the ***pain*** impulse is generated in the peripheral afferent pain receptors, it is transmitted to the sensory modalities of the postcentral gyrus of the cerebral cortex by two neuronal fiber systems. The first system is composed of small myelinated fibers designated as "A delta" fibers, whose sizes range from 2 to 5μ in diameter. These fibers exhibit conduction velocities from 12 to 30 meters per second. The second neuronal system is composed of yet smaller unmyelinated fibers, designated "dorsal C" fibers, whose diameters range from 0.4 to 1.2 microns. As the name implies, these fibers are located in the lateral divisions of the dorsal roots of the spinal cord. Their conduction velocities are significantly slower than A delta fibers, ranging from 0.5 to 2.0 meters per second. Both the dorsal root C and A delta fiber systems terminate on the lateral spinal thalamic tract neurons of the spinal cord.

Pain impulses emanating from the face and mouth

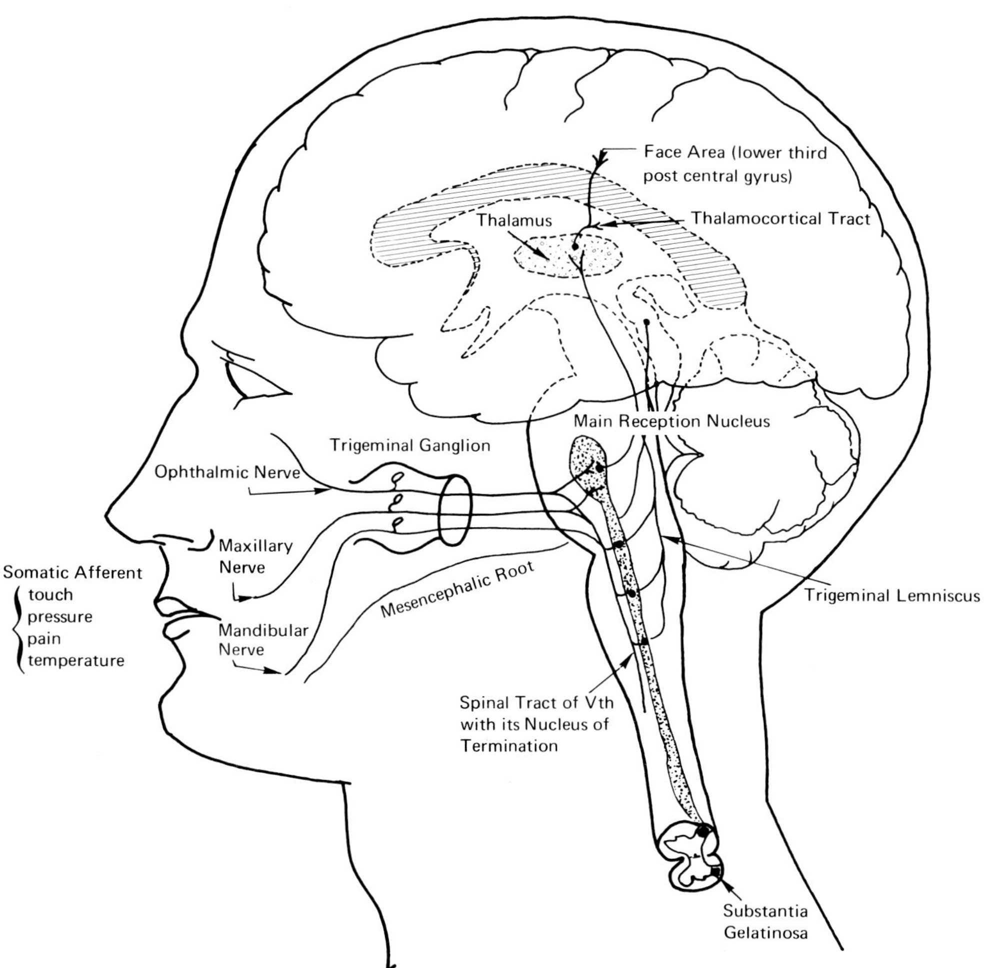

Fig. 11–3. Trigeminal (V) nerve relaying pain impulses to postcentral gyrus of cerebral cortex for recognition as pain.

regions are mediated centrally by way of afferent fibers that travel through the posterior roots of the trigeminal (V), facial (VII), glossopharyngeal (IX), and vagus (X) cranial nerves; and the first, second, and third cervical spinal nerves; and, also, by way of sympathetic afferent fibers descending through the posterior roots of the upper thoracic spinal nerves. The nerve cell bodies of the primary sensory neurons are located in the posterior root ganglion of the nerve through which they pass. Pain impulses are transmitted to the cognitive areas of the cerebral cortex by three orders of afferent neurons. The first-order neurons that transmit pain impulses from the maxillofacial areas terminate in the nucleus caudalis of the brain stem. For example, each branch of the trigeminal nerve has its cell body in the trigeminal ganglion, and pseudounipolar fibers continue through the sensory root to enter the pons. These fibers constitute the descending tract of the trigeminal nucleus. The nucleus caudalis is the lower caudal portion of the trigeminal spinal tract nucleus. The second-order trigeminal neurons begin where the initial synapse occurs within the substantia (pars) gelatinosa of the nucleus caudalis. These second-order trigeminal neurons are transmitted to the ventral posteromedial and posterolateral nuclei of the thalamus, where they terminate in several nuclei. The final synapse occurs there with the third-order trigeminal neurons. Considerable convergence takes place at each synapse as the pain impulse is projected to the cerebral cortex from these nuclei. The pain impulses are then relayed to the postcentral gyri of the cerebral cortex, where they become "recognized" as sensory pain (Fig. 11–3).

Hypotheses of Central Nervous System Modulation of Pain. The physiology of pain involves complex mechanisms and is not entirely understood. Collins et al. have reported the relationship between sensation and fiber size in human beings.[20,21] Historically, two concepts of pain impulse have prevailed. In the "specificity theory" concept, the pain impulse is thought to be simply conducted by A delta and small C fibers to a pain center in the brain. The second historical theory is the "pattern theory," which states that all fiber endings, except those that innervate hair cells, are alike and that the pattern for pain is produced by ***intense*** stimulation of nonspecific receptors which undergo central summation. Neither of these theories satisfactorily explains the many known facts about pain, including input control and central summation, and both have been challenged. More recently, Melzack and Wall have proposed a "gate-control" theory, which appears to be comprehensive and plausible.[22]

Gate-Control Theory of Pain. Once the peripheral nerves have been activated, impulses are transmitted over fibers that vary greatly in speed of transmission and diameter. It is also believed that different kinds of nerve fibers carry different kinds of sensory information, *viz.*, noxious versus mechanical information,[23] and that a physiologic balance between these kinds of impulse information determines whether pain will be consciously perceived. It is generally felt that A alpha neurons carry impulses that are non-noxious in character (*e.g.*, mechanical stimuli such as touch and pressure); whereas, A delta and dorsal C nerve fibers carry noxious pain stimuli.[23] Activation of these nerve fibers does not always produce pain, however, and so it is believed that several important interactions must occur between the input information from the various fiber groups in specific synaptic regions of the spinal cord and brain stem. This inhibitory-excitatory interaction of afferent fiber synapses is proposed to occur within the spinal cord and has been proposed by Melzack and Wall as the "gate-control" theory of pain.[22]

In this theory, when skin is noxiously stimulated, many different afferent impulses are transmitted to the central nervous system via both the large A alpha fibers and the smaller A delta fibers and C fibers. Since the large A alpha fibers have higher conduction velocities than the smaller pain fibers, the volleys of large fiber impulses reach the substantia gelatinosa faster than those transmitted by the small pain-carrying fibers. The overall effect of large-fiber activity is to "close the gate" for the passage of pain impulses to the transmission cells. The "gate" represents the initial synapse between the peripheral neurons and the secondary medullary neurons located in the substantia gelatinosa of the central nervous system. In other words, when the telephone line is busy, the next signal cannot be heard.

In this proposed "spinal-gate" theory of pain, the effects of small-fiber transmission may be further influenced by fibers that descend from higher centers of the central nervous system (*viz.*, somesthetic centers of the cortex and possibly the reticular formation). If the inhibitory effects of the large afferent fibers and those descending from the brain predominate, a response to pain stimulus will not occur. Instead, a variety of nonspecific sensations may occur, *viz.*, either stretching, pressure, touch, or thermal sensations. On the other hand, if impulses from the smaller afferent pain fibers predominate at the gate, they will overcome the nonspecific inhibitory effects, the gate will be opened, and the appropriate CNS pain reflexive actions will occur.

The gate-control theory is used to explain how Chinese acupuncture works. The twirling acupuncture needles constantly stimulate all of the peripheral nerves, but because the A alpha (proprioceptive) nerves are larger and therefore faster, they continue to "keep the gate closed" at the synapse in the substantia gelatinosa, thus effectively blocking the ***pain*** message from the slower, smaller fibers from getting through to the higher centers where it can be perceived. It is the repetitive stimulation by the needles that keeps the gate closed. The Chinese have shown that if procaine is injected into the spot where the needle is to be placed, acupuncture will not produce analgesia at some remote site as it usually does.

The neuroanatomic basis for applying the gate control of pain effects, in the maxillofacial area of the body, can be explained. The first, second, and third branches of the trigeminal cranial nerve, which contain both sensory and motor fibers, enter the cranium in the middle cranial fossa and join with ventral portions of the Gasserian ganglion where cell bodies of various sizes are located. No synapses occur at this point. Central fibers of pseudounipolar trigeminal cells continue in the sensory root and enter the pons, where the fibers constitute the nucleus of the descending tract of the trigeminal nerve. Many of the larger A alpha fibers bifurcate and turn medially to terminate in synapses in the chief sensory nucleus in the midbrain. Fibers projecting from the chief sensory nucleus to the thalamus and cortex are known to be largely involved with the transmission of fine ***tactile*** functions of the maxillofacial areas. The remaining descending tract fibers turn caudally and terminate medially by synapsing at all levels from the medulla to the third or fourth cervical spinal cord levels (Fig. 11–3).

It is in the caudal portions of the trigeminal nuclear descending tract that an important gate-control interaction appears to occur in an interneuronal region called the pars gelatinosa.[24] If the reflexive pain mechanisms proposed by Melzack and Wall for the spinal cord were transposed to the activated reflexive pathways that emanate from the nucleus caudalis of the descending tract of the trigeminal nerve, the pain "gate" would be opened and the neurophysiologic components of pain would begin.[22]

The most basic pain activities are due to localized reflex areas between the various nuclei of the trigeminal descending tract and the somatic and visceral motor nuclei of the lower brain stem as shown in Figure 11–3. For example, a noxious stimulus (trigeminal pain) localized in the maxillofacial area may cause reflexive parasympathetic responses, *viz.*, increased salivation and tearing, through altered activity of the appropriate nuclei within the brain stem.

Generally, this discriminative-perceptive aspect of pain is attributable to the lemniscal pathways, which may reach the somesthetic regions of the sensory cortex via a double synaptic neuronal pathway. Thus, in the CNS (central nervous system) the larger fiber tract begins in the chief sensory and descending tract nuclei and ascends to the posteroventrolateral thalamus, where synapse occurs, before projecting directly to the somatosensory cerebral cortex for the area of the face. Since these impulses are transmitted rapidly through this system, with little divergence, it is well suited for rapid and precise transmission of spatial and temporal pain information.[25]

In summary, the gate-control theory remains the best model system for studying pain mechanisms encountered throughout the entire body. In all probability, as more and more basic experimental and clinical research is applied to this hypothesis, some details may have to be modified to become more applicable to the exact mechanisms of the action of pain.

Projection. If a pain fiber is stimulated artificially at a point central to its terminus, the sensation is also felt as having come from the periphery. For example, part of the pain felt when one strikes the ulnar nerve ***seems*** to come from the fingers. The explanation of this phenomenon is that the central nervous system has ***learned*** that impulses generally originate in the end organs (fingers) themselves, rather than along the nerve trunk, and so interprets any impulses as such.

Referred Pain. In referred pain, the sensation is interpreted as coming from one area, although it actually originates elsewhere; thus, the pain of angina pectoris is often felt in the left arm.

A convenient rule to explain or trace the source of referred pain is the ***dermatome rule.*** In essence, it states that pain in a viscus is often felt in a somatic area of the body that developed from the same embryonic segment as the structure in which the pain originates. The brain, having more awareness of somatic than of visceral structures through past experience, interprets the pain coming from the regions subserved by the somatic afferent fibers. In certain cases, however, pain arising in a visceral organ may be felt in that organ alone and not referred.

For example, pain fibers from the central portion of the diaphragmatic pleura travel in the phrenic nerve and synapse at the level of C3 and C4. Thus, pain arising in this region of the diaphragm is referred to the neck.[26]

The somatic area is more likely to be an area of referral if it is already the source of ***subliminal*** afferent pain inputs. The concomitant feature of muscle tenderness in an area of referral is due to the overflow of excitation into efferent neurons which go to the muscles. This outflow causes prolonged muscular contraction, which results in ischemia and pain from the accumulation of K ions in the muscle tissue. Long-standing conditions of this sort may result in the establishment of a vicious pain cycle.

Central Pain. We should realize, although its treatment is certainly not within our province, that there can be lesions of the thalamus or spinothalamic tract which result in so-called "central pain." In this condition there is complaint of constant discomfort. The mechanism of the phenomenon is not well understood, and little investigation has been done.[27]

Psychologic Factors Modifying Pain. ***Eliciting Pain.*** As mentioned before, the highest centers of the central nervous system play a great role in the individual's assessment and reaction to pain. It is there that past conscious and unconscious experiences are integrated with present situations.

Although most pain is elicited by noxious stimulation of peripheral receptors, it may also be a purely psychic experience. Pain plays a great role in the individual's psychic development. Engel[28] lists five aspects of its role:

1. "Pain . . . contributes to the . . . concept of body image . . . That which hurts belongs to one's own body."[28] "It is significant that phantoms (limbs) have ***not*** been noted in those with absence of a limb resulting from a congenital defect or from infantile amputations."[29]
2. "Pain is much involved in the development of object relationships." An infant learns that his cries of pain will bring comfort from his mother. He learns to associate the unpleasantness of pain with the pleasure of relief.
3. "Early in childhood, pain and punishment become linked." Thus, one comes to expect punishment and, by association, pain when he is 'bad.' "Guilt, conscious or unconscious, is an invariable factor in choice of pain as the symptom . . ."
4. "Pain also early becomes very closely associated with aggression and power." A child discovers that he can impose his will on others by threatening or actually inflicting pain, and can also control his own aggressions by realizing that the outcome may be painful to himself.
5. "Pain may also be associated with sexual development." There are some persons who prefer pain to sexual experience.

Thus we see that pain plays a great role in the individual's psychic development; that it becomes associated early in one's life with punishment; and that pain can be experienced as an expiation for feelings of guilt. Persons in whom these associations are found are said to be pain-prone. They seem to have more than their share of suffering, illnesses, operations, and the like, and are "unusually tolerant of pain inflicted upon them by nature. . . ."[30] An overabundance of suffering, aggression, violence, and a lack of human warmth are conditions most often found in the early life history of such persons. Pain episodes may be precipitated in these individuals when certain circumstances arise—strangely enough, when things are going too well and when the environment is causing no suffering to expiate their guilt feelings.

One must also realize that pain may be used as an escape mechanism by some patients. Sternbach et al. have described a constellation of characteristics in patients with chronic low-back pain—"low-back losers."[31] In "Pain As an Old Friend," Penman suggests that pain may become a sufferer's major preoccupation or defense, and that not all patients who are relieved of their pain are uniformly grateful.[32]

The role of anxiety in the production and control of pain is also important. The greater the patient's anxiety, the less his or her tolerance for pain.[33] The reduction of anxiety is indeed one of the common techniques employed by dentists to alleviate pain.

Relieving Pain. If psychologic factors can produce or intensify pain, so too can they be used to modify and reduce the perception of and reaction to pain. Baldwin and Weisenberg recently reviewed the modalities for mitigating pain.[34] Baldwin cleverly demonstrated the reduction of anxiety to forthcoming tooth extraction in children by properly informing them and preparing them for exactly what they should expect.[35] Egbert's approach to psychologic preparation also has direct application for the terrified endodontic patient, particularly the one facing surgery.[36] It includes several variables: (1) ***information*** about what to expect before, during, and after the operation; (2) ***reassurance*** from an authoritative figure (in this case the dentist); (3) specific ***instructions*** on how to relieve pain, and (4) frequent ***interpersonal contact*** to reinforce motivation and support. An inquiring or comforting phone call the evening before and following treatment is a good example of such interpersonal contact.

Opton has detailed a number of ***coping mechanisms*** for pain control.[37] They include: (1) distraction or displacement of attention away from the threat, often done by talking to the patient during a distressful moment, (2) verbalization by the patient to relieve his tension by expressing his true feelings, (3) relinquishing control to an authority figure or (4) affiliation behavior—that is, ***affiliation*** with an authority figure—a close or trusting relationship with the doctor, assistant, friend, parent, or even fellow patient enables one to feel he or she is not facing the ordeal alone,[38] (5) telling oneself to relax—the heart of the "natural childbirth" approach, and (6) mental rehearsal—the "work of worrying"—going over in one's mind the sequence of anticipated events, appraising and reappraising the threats involved.

Each person has his own repertoire of such coping mechanisms. "The larger the repertoire, the more effective is the patient's ability to successfully cope with the situation."[39] Many dentists quite naturally employ many of these techniques to dispel fear, anxiety, and pain—the warm friendly "chairside manner," the explanation and preparation to aid "mental rehearsal," the encouragement of patients to speak out, to verbalize, giving patients some control of the situation.

Other techniques used to reduce anxiety and fear, hence pain, are: relaxation training, hypnosis, placebos, psychologic desensitization, biofeedback, audioanalgesia, and acupuncture.

CLASSIFICATION OF ORAL AND FACIAL PAIN

The origin of oral and facial pain may be classified as follows: regional pain, neurologic pain, atypical facial pain, and referred pain.

Regional Pain

The most frequently encountered cephalic pains are ***regional*** in location. The various origins of regional pain are: pulp pain, periapical pain, periodontal pain, and myofascial pain–dysfunction syndrome.

Pulp Pain

Pulp pain, or ***pulpalgia,*** is by far the most commonly experienced pain in and near the oral cavity, and may be classified according to the degree of severity as well as the pathologic process present:

1. Hyperreactive pulpalgia
   a. Hypersensitivity
   b. Hyperemia
2. Acute pulpalgia
   a. Incipient
   b. Moderate
   c. Advanced
3. Chronic pulpalgia
4. Hyperplastic pulposis
5. Necrotic pulp
6. Internal resorption (pulposis)
7. Traumatic occlusion
8. Incomplete fracture

The mildest pulp discomfort is that experienced when no inflammation is present, ***hyperreactive pulpalgia.***

Hyperreactive Pulpalgia. Hyperreactive pulpalgia is characterized by a ***short, sharp shock;*** that is, the "pain" is best described as a sensation of sudden ***shock.*** The sensation is as ***sharp*** as it is sudden and ***must be elicited*** by some exciting factor. ***It is never spontaneous.*** The pain is of ***short*** duration, lasting only slightly longer than the time the irritating element is in contact with the tooth. In some manner the odontoblastic cellular body within the dentin must be excited by a noxious stimulus, be it hot or cold, sweet or sour, or touch. Excitation of the odontoblast conducts the excitation to the pulp nerves. These "dentinal receptors have the characteristics of slow adaptation."[40]

It is difficult to explain to a patient that the severe pain he experiences when eating ice cream—a blinding pain that extends upward through the eye and into the forehead—is really normal and not pathologic. We can only tell him that the cold excites the nerve in the tooth, and the pain is so severe that it is referred upward through the eye.

The dentist, however, requires a more sophisticated explanation. Although this is hard to come by, the best explanation revolves around our thinking of the fluid in the dentinal tubules, along with the odontoblast cells, as a "pump"—a hydrodynamic theory, if you will, the fluid moving back and forth to excite the pulp nerves.

Brannstrom has pointed out that "the displacement of tubule contents, if the movement occurs rapidly enough, may produce deformation of nerve fibers in the pulp or predentin or damage to the cells; both these effects may be capable of producing pain. Such a mechanical transmission of the stimulus would account for the hitherto inexplicably great sensitivity of the dentin to pain, in spite of the apparent absence of nerve fibers in this tissue."[41]

Brannstrom goes on to say, "Sensation due to cold stimulation of human dentin does not seem to depend upon the simple physical conduction of the cold stimulus through the dentin to excite the nervous elements at the pulpal-dentinal junction directly, but upon a faster and more peripherally placed receptor and propagating mechanism in the dentin, the physiology of which is not understood."

Scott has pointed out "the probability that 'cold' excitation takes place, not at the receptor terminals but on the terminal axons, which may be in the predentin and odontoblast layer, since the observed potentials have the same properties as conducted potentials in other peripheral axons."[41a]

Beveridge demonstrated that the application of cold to a tooth caused a fall in intrapulp pressure (Fig. 11–4).[42] Measuring pulp blood flow by photoplethysmography, an Israeli group confirmed the fall in "interstitial" pressure, but measured an increase in "arterial transmural pressure." One could speculate that the sudden filling of the pulp capillaries from the increase in arterial pressure brought on by the cold could cause the shooting pain of cold hypersensitivity.[43]

Hyperreactive pulpalgia due to the application of heat is more easily explained. Again, Beveridge easily demonstrated a true increase in intrapulp pressure when heat was applied to the tooth (Fig. 11–5). An increase of pressure within the pulp serves to excite the sensory pulp nerves.[42]

Three different types of response to heat have also been recorded from pulp nerve fibers: (1) a transient type of response when pulp nerve fiber was excited by heat over 43°C; the response ceased as soon as the temperature fell below the firing points; (2) a long-lasting type of response which started at over 45°C and continued even after the temperature had returned to the initial level for a few minutes; (3) a

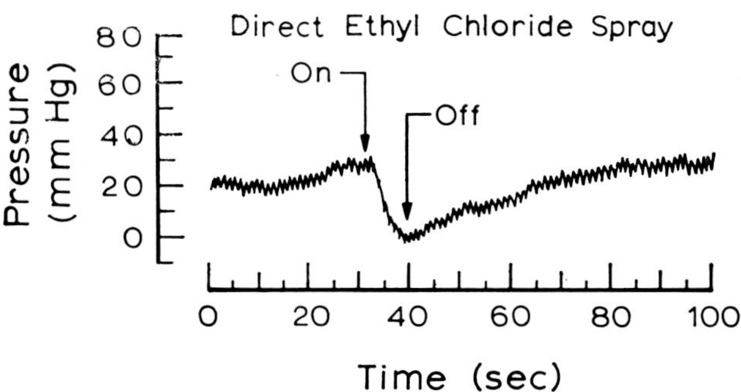

Fig. 11–4. Effect on intrapulp pressure by application of cold ethyl chloride spray to anesthetized mandibular premolar in 13-year-old male. Within eight seconds, intrapulp pressure had dropped 30 mm. Hg to nearly zero. After irritant was removed, pressure returned to initial base line within one minute. (From Beveridge, E. E., and Brown, A. C.: Oral Surg., *19*:655, May, 1965).

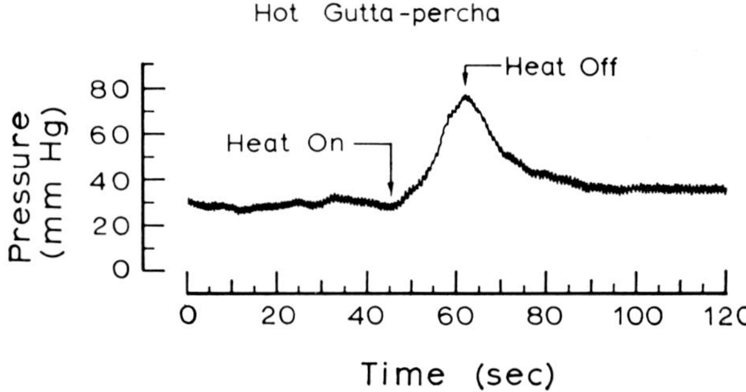

Fig. 11–5. Effect on intrapulp pressure by application of hot gutta percha to anesthetized maxillary premolar in 12-year-old female. Within fifteen seconds, intrapulp pressure had more than doubled. After heat was removed, intrapulp pressure dropped precipitously, but not to original base line. (From Beveridge, E. E., and Brown, A. C.: Oral Surg., 19:655, May, 1965).

pulsating type of response in which the discharge of the fiber was synchronized with the heart beat.[44]

Brannstrom added to the understanding of the "pumping" excitation by dentinal fluid when he pointed out, "Fluids have a considerably greater coefficient of expansion than solids—a sudden rise in temperature of 20°C at the outer one-third of the closed tubule might result in an immediate pulpward movement of about 5 micra of the content of the tubules."[45]

Hyperreactive pulpalgia is common following the placement of a new restoration. Patients also complain after root planing and curettage, or following periodontal surgery, which exposes the root surface. Hyperreactive pulpalgia also may be present in the tooth with a carious lesion. Teeth being traumatized by bruxism or teeth incompletely fractured are generally more hyperreactive, as are the maxillary teeth involved in maxillary sinusitis.

It is possible, with our present level of knowledge, to divide the sensations of hyperreactive pulpalgia into hypersensitivity and hyperemia.

Hypersensitivity. The exciting factors of a hypersensitive pulp are usually cold food or drink or cold air, contact of two dissimilar metals which will yield a galvanic shock, or stimulation of the exposed dentin on the root surface by cold, sweet or sour substances, vegetable or fruit acid, salt, glycerine, or often by just touching the surface with a fingernail, a toothbrush, an interdental stimulator, or an explorer. One should not be surprised at this latter reaction when the microanatomy of the dentin and pulp is reviewed. The cementum covering the gingival root dentin frequently is missing or has been removed by curettage or brushing, exposing the dentin and thereby exposing the long branching processes of the odontoblast within the dentinal tubules. To irritate these extensions of the odontoblast is likely to be as painful as to stimulate the entire cell.

The sensation derived from a physical irritation of the odontoblastic processes in the dentin might best be explained as follows: The odontoblast cell bodies in the pulp are supplied by afferent sensory nerve endings. Scratching across the exposed dentin and thus across the odontoblasts themselves stimulates the cell, producing stimuli that are received by the odontoblastic and interodontoblastic nerve endings. "The stimulus produced by the damaged odontoblast may be envisioned as either a change in the chemism or in the electrical surface potential of the odontoblast."[46] This is the major sensation experienced when a bur cuts across the dentin.

Explaining hypersensitivity from cold is more difficult. As previously explained, it is possible that the physical presence of the cold itself stimulates a fall in the interstitial fluid pressure but an increase in the arterial transmural pressure. The sudden filling of the pulp capillaries may trigger the pain everyone has experienced when eating ice cream.

One is led to conjecture about the pulp sensation stimulated by sour substances, fruit juices, sugar, salt, and dissimilar metals, which may be described as an electric current flowing between the oral cavity and the pulp. Sicher postulated that the oral cavity is positively charged and the pulp is negatively charged.[47] Any electrolyte, such as salt or fruit acid, upsets this ionic balance and the resultant current stimulates the nerve endings to the odontoblasts. The sensation disappears as soon as the electrolyte is diluted away, or metal (such as aluminum foil) is removed. In addition to the current flow theory, Anderson believes that "pain can be evoked from dentin by applying to it solutions which exert high osmotic pressure."[48] Brannstrom pursues this idea further with the following hypothesis:[45]

"The application of sugar solution or short air blast to the exposed dentin may remove small amounts of the tubule content by dehydration or evaporation respectively. A 30-second blast has been found to result in a distal movement of the content of about 100 μ, a 2-second air blast would presumably cause a movement of about 5 to 10 μ."

Hyperemia. All minor pulp sensations were at one time thought to be associated with hyperemia—an increased blood flow in the pulp. The investigations of Beveridge and Brown demonstrated, however, that an increase in intrapulp tissue pressure is produced only when heat is applied to the tooth, not cold.[42,49] The increased pressure against the sensory nerve endings in the pulp might well produce the sensation associated with hyperemia. Quite possibly this will explain why the pain appears to be of a different intensity and character with applications of cold or heat, the cold producing a hypersensitivity response and the heat producing true transient hyperemia.

The converse of "pain from pressure" also appears to be true. Beveridge and Brown have shown the ***effect of pain*** on intrapulp pressure.[49] Paradoxically, pulp pain causes first a fall and then, when removed,

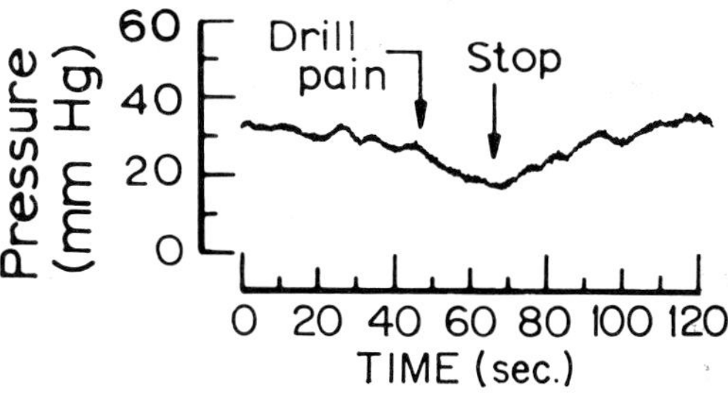

Fig. 11–6. Effect on partially anesthetized pulp from pain elicited by cavity preparation on maxillary premolar of 11-year-old female. Intrapulp pressure dropped about 10 mm. Hg within twenty-five seconds during which patient experienced pain. When drilling ceased, intrapulp pressure climbed slowly to level slightly higher than original base line. (From Beveridge, E. E., and Brown, A. C.: Oral Surg., *19*:655, May, 1965.)

a rise in intrapulp tissue pressure (Fig. 11–6). "This again raises the question of the role of neural control in the regulation of intrapulp pressure."[49] It was also discovered that intrapulp pressure decreased when the patient fell asleep and increased when he awakened.

Examination. Examining to determine which tooth is hyperreactive is not always as simple a step as it might seem. A patient may complain of the symptoms of hypersensitivity on taking cold water into the mouth. On the other hand, ice on the suspected tooth during examination may not elicit an unusual reaction. In this case the entire tooth must be surrounded by cold for the pulp to react. This particular condition is best checked by isolating the teeth adjacent to the suspected tooth behind a heavy rubber dam, and then playing a stream of ice water onto the tooth being examined.

If the tooth has had a recent restoration, it usually responds to applications of ice or of Fluori-Methane* or ethyl chloride sprayed on a large cotton pellet. Scratching exposed cervical dentin may also elicit a pain response. Hyperreactive teeth are said to be more sensitive to the pulp tester, but this is not always true.

Treatment. Grossman has stated, "The best treatment for hyperemia lies in its prevention." This is sound advice.[50] The insulating base under metallic restorations materially reduces most hypersensitivity. Moreover, this sensation usually diminishes gradually as reparative dentin builds to protect the dental pulp.

Since a true hyperreactive pulp is not a pathologic condition, it may go on for years, acting as a distress signal, warning against insult to a particular tooth. The patient learns to avoid the involved tooth and often becomes a unilateral masticator in the process. The pulp seems well able to accept constant insult, and the statement that long-standing "hyperemia" eventually terminates in pulp inflammation and death is patently false. Apparently something more than hypersensitivity or hyperemia must be present to lead to necrosis. One would suspect inflammation.

There is no one good treatment to prevent hypersensitivity associated with root surfaces. The most consistently successful treatment, however, has been the use of the 3M Ionator (F-19), an ionophoretic device reported to deposit phosphate fluoride on the root surface. Using this technique, Simmons has reported 94 to 99% reduction in hypersensitivity.[51] According to a recent report from India,[52] a comparative evaluation of the desensitizing effects of the topical application of 33.3% sodium fluoride paste, of iontophoresis with a 1% solution of sodium fluoride, and of iontophoresis with the patient's own saliva was made. All the teeth treated by iontophoresis with 1% sodium fluoride solution showed either good (55.55%) or moderate (44.45%) relief immediately after one application. Following two to three applications of 33.3% sodium fluoride paste, only 33.33% of the teeth had obtained good relief, 52.94% had moderate relief, and 13.73% had no relief after two and four weeks of observation. Iontophoresis with the patient's own saliva did not produce good relief in any of the patients treated. However, 35.13% of the teeth had moderate relief in two- and four-week observation periods.

Iontophoresis with sodium fluoride produced immediate relief after one application, whereas topical application required two to three applications (Table 11–1).

The study shows that both deposition of fluoride ions into the dentin and formation of secondary dentin are possible mechanisms by which iontophoresis causes desensitization. The author concluded, "Iontophoresis with 1% sodium fluoride is the method of choice for the treatment of hypersensitive dentin, as it meets all the requirements of an ideal desensitizing agent except permanency of effect, which requires further investigation."

Hodosh also recently reported the topical application of saturated solutions of potassium nitrate as well as pastes for home use containing 10% potassium nitrate.[53] "Relief of hypersensitivity was notable and rapid in most instances," he reported. "Potassium nitrate is also an extremely safe chemical."

*Gebauer Chemical Co., 9410 St. Catherine Ave., Cleveland, Ohio 44104. Fluori-Methane has proved as effective as and less dangerous than ethyl chloride spray.

Table 11-1. Comparison of Desensitizing Methods

	Group		
Degree of relief	*I** (%)	*II*† (%)	*III*‡ (%)
Good	33.33	55.55	—
Moderate	52.94	44.45	35.13
None	13.73	—	64.87

*Treatment by topical application using a 33.3% solution of sodium fluoride.
†Treatment by ionophoresis using a 1% solution of sodium fluoride.
‡Treatment by ionophoresis with patient's own saliva.

Commercial toothpastes are available which the manufacturers claim reduce sensitivity. These contain either a formalin or a strontium chloride preparation. In a double-blind study, however, Smith and Ash demonstrated the ineffectiveness of both products in reducing sensitivity.[54,55]

Acute Pulpalgia. True pulpalgia begins with the development of pulp inflammation or pulpitis. Beveridge and Brown have shown that an increased intrapulp tissue pressure is possible.[49] It may be postulated that this pressure might well be the stimulus applied to the sensory nerves of the pulp which leads to severe toothache.

Incipient Acute Pulpalgia. The mild discomfort experienced as the anesthetic wears off following cavity preparation is a good example of ***incipient pulpalgia.*** The patient may be vaguely aware that the tooth feels different, "as though it has been worked on," but the sensation disappears by the next morning.

Stanley and Swerdlow have shown extravascular migration of inflammatory cells following even the modest irritation of a controlled and cooled cavity preparation.[56] It is most fortunate that from the incipient stage, pulpitis is reversible and the discomfort vanishes. One would suspect that incipient pulpalgia is so mild that the pulpitis it predicts is often ignored by the patient until it is too late. This could well be true of the initial sensation developing with a new carious lesion—the slight ache in response to cold or sweets (see Figs. 8–10 and 8–14).

Excitation. Incipient acute pulpalgia must be stimulated by an irritant such as cavity preparation, cold, sugar or traumatic occlusion.

Examination. If the pulpalgia follows cavity preparation, the involved tooth is obvious. If dental caries is the noxious stimulus, the cavity is found by explorer and roentgenograms. The lesion may be quite small, just into the dentin. The patient can usually tell which quadrant is involved and may even point out the involved tooth. Cold is the best stimulus to initiate ***incipient acute pulpalgia.*** The pulp tester is of questionable value in these cases.

When traumatic occlusion is causing the pain, the diagnosis becomes more difficult. (See Traumatic Occlusion, p. 507.)

Treatment. Removal of the carious lesion followed by a sedative cement for a few days may be all that is required to arrest ***incipient acute pulpalgia.*** Watchful waiting following cavity preparation should not extend to procrastination leading to moderate or advanced acute pulpalgia. Corticosteroids placed in the cavity following preparation or used on the dentin surface prior to cementation of extensive restorations, has proved effective for reducing postoperative pain.[57]

Moderate Acute Pulpalgia. The pain of ***moderate acute pulpalgia*** is a true toothache, but one which the patient can usually tolerate. Many patients report for dental attention after hours, or sometimes days, of discomfort from the developing pulpitis. The pain is frequently described as a "nagging" or a "boring" pain, which may at first be localized, but finally becomes diffuse or referred to another area. The pain differs from that of a hyperreactive pulp in that it is not just a short uncomfortable sensation, but an extended pain. Moreover, the pain does not necessarily resolve when the irritant is removed, but may go on aching for minutes or hours, or days for that matter.

Excitation. ***Moderate pulpalgia*** may start spontaneously from such a simple act as lying down. This alone accounts for the seeming prevalence of toothache at night. Some patients report that the pulp aches each evening, "when I'm tired." Others say that "leaning over to tie a shoe," or "going up or down stairs," will start the pain—any act that raises the cephalic blood pressure. The list of inciting irritants would not be complete without mentioning hot food or drink, "sucking on the cavity," and "biting food into the cavity." Most pain of ***moderate pulpalgia,*** however, is started by eating, usually something cold. A warm water rinse does not usually relieve the pain, and cold water makes it worse. The patient may find, however, that two or three aspirin or APC tablets bring relief. He may continue to take analgesics for days, while wishfully thinking that the pulp will recover. Too many dentists also practice this same game of self-deception.

Examination. Attempting to determine which tooth is involved with ***moderate acute pulpalgia*** is often a difficult experience. The patient may report after days of discomfort, and by this time the pain, though still present, may be widespread and vague. The patient believes he can pinpoint the exact tooth, but then he becomes confused. The typical statement, "the tooth stopped aching as soon as I entered the office," is commonly heard. No amount of irritation will start it again. If the patient is on heavy analgesics or mild narcotics, it is best to postpone examination until responses will not be clouded by drugs.

If the pain has been constant for some time, all the

pulps on the affected side seem to ache, and frequently two or three give approximately the same response to the pulp tester or thermal testing. This is where intuition comes into play. The examiner gets a "feeling" about one particular tooth. It might respond a shade sooner to the pulp tester, or it may ache just a bit longer after cold is applied. The restoration seen in the roentgenogram may be just a little deeper. All too frequently, in this day of "full coverage," a number of teeth may be restored with full crowns—a situation which manifestly compounds the problem.

If the pain is only vague when the patient is first seen, the dentist should attempt, by careful questioning, to obtain a general idea of the area of the pain. Usually the patient can tell which side is involved and frequently whether the pain is in the maxilla or the mandible. This may not be absolute, however, for the pain may be referred from one arch to the other. The patient may remember where the pain started initially, hours or days before. Examination of the suspected area may immediately reveal the involved tooth, obvious by a large carious lesion or huge restoration. Then again, nothing unusual may be present.

Roentgenograms may give an immediate clue in the form of a huge interproximal cavity or a restoration impinging upon the pulp chamber. If nothing is learned from roentgenographic examination, the electric pulp tester is then employed, but generally without great success.

A tooth involved in ***moderate acute pulpalgia*** is hypersensitive and will respond sooner, or lower, on the scale of the pulp tester. Then again, all the teeth in the area may be hypersensitive and respond the same to pulp testing, so that no definite conclusions may be drawn from this test.

This leaves the thermal test as the final arbiter, since percussion and palpation rarely reveal any response, although the tooth may be slightly sensitive to percussion.

The first thermal evaluation to use is the cold test, for the pulp is more likely to respond to this stimulus. The tooth that is under the greatest suspicion should be tested first. The examiner should block the adjacent teeth with his fingers, being careful that the melting ice does not run onto these teeth. The immediate response to cold may be quite sudden, violent, and lasting. On the other hand, the initial pain may go away immediately when the ice is removed. ***This is the time to stop!*** Do not test any more teeth for about five minutes. The reason for this is quite obvious. The pain in the tested tooth which stops aching may rebound within a few minutes, and if the dentist has proceeded to test other teeth, neither he nor the patient will be able to differentiate the aching tooth. If the pulp starts to ache, however, reapplying the cold should increase and prolong the pain.

Infrequently, heat is the stimulus that starts the symptoms. Sometimes, however, nothing will start the ache, and the patient must be dismissed and asked to return when the tooth is again painful.

Occasionally the search is narrowed down to a maxillary ***and*** a mandibular tooth, both prime suspects because both are aching. One molar is the problem tooth and the other the "referred" tooth. If an anesthetic is injected into the suspected arch, and the hunch was correct, the pain should stop. If the pain doesn't stop, the offending tooth is in the opposite arch. Again, by means of the anesthetic test, aching mandibular ***premolars*** may be differentiated from molars by the use of a mental injection that will anesthetize from the second premolar toward the midline. A zygomatic injection in the maxillary arch for the maxillary molars, or a careful slow infiltration for the maxillary premolars injected well forward toward the canine, may differentiate between these confusingly similar pains. The anesthetic test is a last resort and should be used after all other means have been exhausted.

In diagnosing ***moderate acute pulpalgia,*** above all, the examiner must ***think;*** he must be shrewd; he must not panic. If in doubt, hesitate! Often, one more day may make a real difference. The patient should be warned to return to the office without having taken any analgesics.

Treatment. The treatment for ***moderate pulpalgia*** is quite simple; pulpectomy and endodontic therapy if the tooth can and should be saved, or extraction if the tooth should be sacrificed. If endodontic therapy is indicated, it may be completed in one appointment (Chap. 5, p. 278).

Advanced Acute Pulpalgia. There is never any question about the patient suffering the pain of ***advanced acute pulpalgia.*** He is experiencing one of the most excruciating acute pains known to man, comparable to otic abscess, renal colic, and childbirth. If every dentist personally experienced the pain of ***advanced acute pulpalgia,*** he would be a more sympathetic practitioner for the experience.

This patient is in exquisite agony, and sometimes

becomes hysterical from the pain. The patient often is seen crying and virtually unmanageable. One patient who had to drive forty miles to a dentist reported he could stand the pain no longer, so he stopped the car, took out a pair of pliers, and pulled his own tooth. Patients have confessed contemplating suicide to escape the pain.

The relief for this pain is embarrassingly simple—***cold water,*** preferably iced. Cold water rinsed over the tooth is all that is usually needed to temporarily arrest the pain. The patient might discover this fact while taking aspirin, and in so doing receive immediate relief. He then reports to the dentist with a thermos or jar of ice water in hand, stopping only to sip as the pain gradually returns. Frequently, he times the periods of relief much as the expectant mother times her labor pains. The relief often lasts 30 to 45 seconds.

When a patient telephones, reporting a toothache, and especially late at night, the dentist should always inquire, "Have you tried ***rinsing*** cold water on the tooth?" If the answer is negative, request that the patient do so and return to the phone to report results. If the cold gives relief, the compassionate professional man meets the patient as soon as possible to give permanent relief. If the cold aggravates the pain, the patient has moderate pulpalgia, which might well become ***advanced pulpalgia*** by morning. The patient with ***advanced pulpalgia*** would have to continue rinsing with cold water throughout the night, and even then, the cold may no longer give relief. Thus a tired and "frazzled" patient becomes a hysterical one.

Examination. The examination for advanced acute pulpalgia, in comparison to that for moderate pulpalgia, is relatively simple, even if the tooth is not aching when the patient presents himself. The involved tooth always has a closed pulp chamber as revealed by the roentgenogram. Otherwise the tremendous intrapulp pressure could not develop.

The history is self-incriminating. Symptoms are violent! The involved tooth usually can be pointed out by the patient, and is sometimes tender to percussion as well. These teeth are said to be less sensitive to the pulp tester (requiring a higher reading), but the performance of this test is merely "gilding the lily."

Because the inflamed pulp reacts so violently to heat, the most decisive test is the heat test, although one must have a cold water syringe in the other hand, ready to give immediate relief. As soon as the hot gutta percha touches the involved tooth, the patient develops what Sicher has called ***the subgluteal vacuum;*** he suddenly rises up in the chair as if stabbed. Cold water is instantly applied and the pain subsides.

The thermal test is conclusive! When the patient is again comfortable, however, the adjacent teeth should also be tested to ascertain that not more than one tooth is involved, or that the suspected tooth gives the most violent reaction. The patient should be assured that the involved tooth will not again be warmed.

Local anesthesia gives blessed relief, and the dentist has from that moment made a friend for life. The friendship will be the more lasting if the tooth is saved by endodontic therapy rather than extracted.

Treatment. The treatment for ***advanced pulpalgia*** is the same as for moderate pulpalgia: pulpectomy and endodontic therapy for the salvageable tooth, and extraction for the hopeless one.

Complete anesthesia of an inflamed pulp may be difficult even though all outward signs would indicate the conduction or infiltration injection to be successful. In this case, an intrapulp injection of lidocaine or pressure anesthesia with lidocaine or cocaine may be necessary (pp. 85–88).

Following pulpectomy, the pulpless tooth should be relieved of occlusal contact by grinding. Endodontic therapy should be completed at a later appointment.

Chronic Pulpalgia. The discomfort from ***chronic pulpalgia*** is best described as a "grumble," which is a term commonly used by patients who often withstand the mild pain for months or years. Often the pain can easily be kept under control with one or two aspirin tablets, two or three times daily. Frequently the patient seeks relief only when the pulp begins to ache every night.

The pain from ***chronic pulpalgia*** is quite diffuse, and the patient may have difficulty locating the source of annoyance. Patients frequently say they have a "vague pain in my lower jaw." ***Chronic pulpalgia*** is likely to cause referred pain, also mild. Other patients may appear with beginning acute apical abscess and confess to knowing something was "wrong" with the tooth for months. Other patients comment on the bad taste or odor constantly noted.

Excitation. The pulp involved in ***chronic pulpalgia*** is not affected by cold, but may ache slightly upon contact with hot liquids. The most common report is, "The tooth is sore to bite on." If meat or bread crust, for example, is crushed into the cavity present, the pain lasts until the irritant is dislodged. The patient may report that the tooth begins to pain late in the day, "when I'm tired," or more frequently, "when I lie down."

One patient confessed to discomfort each Monday morning and Friday evening. These were the times each week when he crossed a 4,000 foot mountain pass in his travel across the State of Washington. Here, the slight difference in barometric pressure was enough to excite the pain response. The same may be true during a plane trip.

Examination. Determining which tooth is involved with ***chronic pulpalgia*** is often ridiculously simple, and on other occasions most difficult. Frequently a large carious lesion is present, or an amalgam restoration is fractured at the isthmus. Another common offender is recurrent caries under a restoration, usually an inlay. These are the lesions that are painful when compressed by food packed into the cavity.

The leathery dentin covering these lesions may be removed with a spoon excavator, often without anesthesia and with no great discomfort. The pulp lies revealed, covered with a gray scum of surface necrosis. Biopsy would show degeneration of the remainder of the pulp, which accounts for the lack of severe pain.

Chronic pulpalgia most difficult to diagnose lies under a full crown, which is impossible to pulp test electrically; or under a three-quarter crown where recurrent caries is not revealed by roentgenogram. The electric pulp tester and the roentgenogram are the best tools for locating the tooth involved with ***chronic pulpalgia.*** The tooth sometimes responds as "necrotic" to electric testing, that is to say, it will take the maximum discharge from the tester. In any case, a high reading on the rheostat should be expected. England et al. demonstrated intact nerve fibers, with some variations from normal, in pulp specimens with "irreversible pulpitis."[58] In the necrotic pulp, dissolution of the fibers was apparent.

The roentgenogram often reveals interproximal or root caries, or recurrent caries under a restoration. In ***chronic pulpalgia,*** the so-called thickened periodontal membrane also may be present, indicating that the inflammatory process is not confined completely to the pulp. These cases may also demonstrate condensing osteitis of the cancellous bone at the apices. Interestingly, this osteosclerosis disappears after successful endodontic therapy (see Fig. 9–41).

The apices of the involved roots also show external resorption, although this condition is more prevalent following pulp necrosis and complete periapical involvement (see Fig. 10–27).

Thermal tests are of little value in a positive sense in diagnosing ***chronic pulpalgia,*** although in some cases slight pain may be experienced in response to extreme heat. This is in accord with the patient's history of no response to iced drinks, but the occasional response to hot coffee.

Percussion has a good deal to offer in many of these cases. Often the patient is vaguely aware that something feels "different" about the involved tooth when it is percussed. Palpation is virtually useless. However, having the patient bite on an applicator stick sometimes reveals soreness of a particular tooth.

Chronic pulpalgia has the aggravating habit of referring its vague pains throughout the region. The patient may insist that a mandibular molar is aching when examination reveals a maxillary molar offender. Often, anesthetizing the involved tooth is the only convincing proof to the patient that he is wrong. Twice patients have reported with aching of a maxillary molar when the maxillary lateral incisor has been found to be the offender. If the tooth suspected by the patient appears normal to all examination and testing, the examiner should be suspicious of ***chronic pulpalgia*** in another tooth on the same side. The mandibular molar involved in ***chronic pulpalgia*** is not so apt to refer pain to the ear as it is in acute pulpalgia.

Treatment. The treatment for ***chronic pulpalgia*** is quite basic; pulp extirpation and endodontic therapy if the tooth is to be saved; otherwise, extraction. Anesthesia is no problem.

Hyperplastic Pulposis. The exposed pulp of ***hyperplastic pulposis*** is practically symptom-free unless stimulated directly.

Excitation. The discomfort of a ***hyperplastic pulp*** results from compressing food against the exposed pulp during mastication. Extremes of heat and cold, such as hot coffee or ice cream, may produce mild discomfort.

Examination. Discovery of the ***hyperplastic pulp*** is quite simple. It "erupts" up out of its open bed of caries for all to see. Differential diagnosis is concerned with only one problem, namely that of discerning whether the polyp is pulp or gingival in origin, for both are covered by epithelium (see Fig. 8–41).

The pulp polyp may be lifted away from the walls with a spoon excavator, and the pedicle of its origin thus revealed. It is remarkably painless to handle and may even be excised with a sharp spoon excavator with no great discomfort.

Treatment. Frequently the teeth involved in ***hyperplastic pulposis*** are so badly decayed that restoration is virtually impossible. Hence, extraction is usually indicated. On the other hand, if the tooth can be restored, pulpectomy and endodontic therapy are recommended prior to restoration.

Glick reports limited success with pulpotomy of these cases.[59] Done originally as an experiment on three cases with good bleeding, he was surprised to see periapical repair take place.

Necrotic Pulp. There are no true symptoms of complete ***pulp necrosis,*** for the simple reason that the pulp with its sensory nerves is totally destroyed. Often, however, only partial necrosis has occurred, and the patient has the same vague, comparatively mild discomfort described for chronic pulpalgia.

The examiner also must bear in mind that the pulp in one or two canals in multi-rooted teeth may be necrotic, and the pulp in a second or third canal may be vital and quite probably involved in acute or chronic pulpitis. The results of examination in these cases are most bizarre, for each level of pulp vitality is represented by a confused response.

Examination. A routine roentgenographic survey or coronal discoloration may present the first indication that something is amiss in the case of the tooth with a necrotic pulp. Upon questioning, the patient may recall an accident of years ago, or a bout of pulpalgia long since forgotten.

Many cases of ***pulp necrosis*** are discovered because of the discoloration of the crown. this applies primarily to the anterior teeth and ranges from a vague discoloration, visible only to the trained eye, to the frank discoloration of the darkened tooth. A discernible difference may sometimes be demonstrated by transillumination.

The roentgenogram may be helpful if a periapical lesion exists, for its presence usually indicates associated pulp death. Roentgenographically, the tooth with the ***necrotic pulp*** may exhibit only slight periapical change; in other words, a radiolucency is usually found by hindsight rather than foresight. Then again, a sizeable periapical bony lesion may accompany the ***necrotic pulp.*** No changes in the canal are noted roentgenographically to indicate necrosis.

One of the first lessons to be learned from the dental roentgenogram, however, is ***never*** to trust a roentgenogram alone in diagnosing ***pulp necrosis.*** A snap judgment of the periapical radiolucency that exists with periapical osteofibrosis associated with perfectly normal, vital pulps will lead to error if the examiner depends upon x-ray evidence alone (Chap. 9, p. 425). It is imperative ***always to pulp test the tooth.***

The electric pulp tester, therefore, is the instrument of choice for determining pulp necrosis. With complete necrosis no response will be given at any level on the tester. With partial necrosis, a vague response that can easily be tolerated may be elicited at the top of the scale.

The tooth with a necrotic pulp may also be slightly painful to percussion.

Treatment. There is no treatment for pulp necrosis *per se,* for the necrotic pulp has long since been destroyed. If the tooth can be saved, endodontic therapy is indicated.

Internal Resorption. ***Internal resorption*** is an insidious process when the afflicted pulp is completely symptom-free. On the other hand, this condition has been known to mimic moderate acute pulpalgia in pain intensity. The usual case, however, closely resembles the chronic pulpalgia syndrome, *i.e.,* mild pain at the tolerable level. When confined to the crown, enough tooth structure may be destroyed for the pulp to show through the enamel. Hence, the synonym for ***internal resorption***—"pink tooth."

Excitation. Symptoms of ***internal resorption*** depend primarily on whether the process has broken through the external tooth surface. If the pulp destroys enough tooth structure finally to erupt into the oral cavity, it responds much as the hyperplastic pulp, painful only to pressures of mastication.

Because the pulp is undergoing dystrophy localized to a single area, it is not as likely to be excited by the drinking of hot or cold fluids. The pulp that erodes through the root surface may give vague symptoms primarily with mastication, but the patient usually remembers these symptoms in retrospect after the condition is pointed out on the roentgenogram.

Examination. Two methods of examination reveal the case of ***internal resorption:*** visual examination if the crown is involved, and roentgenographic for the crown and root. Thermal tests and the electric pulp tester may provide confirming, yet only partially reliable, evidence.

The case of ***internal resorption*** truly difficult to diagnose is the one of coronal involvement often hiding behind the full or three-quarter crown, and thus not revealed in the roentgenogram. The patient complains of vague symptoms and referred pain, but response of the involved pulp to the testing procedures may be similar to that of the other teeth. Percussion may be of slight value. In these cases an intuitive hunch is needed. If one is fortunate, the correct tooth, when tested, may exhibit slight variances from the other teeth in the area. On the basis of these minor variances, the suspected tooth is chosen; however, the presence of ***internal resorption*** is not confirmed until the coronal pulp is entered.

Treatment. Pulpectomy is the only treatment for ***internal resorption.*** As long as the pulp remains it is most likely to continue its destructive process. If the tooth can be saved by endodontic restoration, the reader is referred to the section on ***Internal Resorption,*** Chapter 4, pp. 244–245.

Traumatic Occlusion. A tooth ***traumatized*** by bruxism or ***traumatized*** because a restoration is in hyperocclusion often responds much as the tooth with mild pulpalgia. First of all, the pulp usually is hypersensitive, reacting primarily to cold. In addition, the pain may be vague, reminiscent of chronic pulpalgia.

The patient may complain of being bothered by pulp discomfort upon awakening in the morning or possibly of being awakened by the discomfort. The story of pain at the end of a rather trying day is also characteristic. Pathognomonically, the patient reports relief after only one aspirin. Moreover, he usually says that the tooth is not painful on mastication; at least this is not his chief complaint.

Paradoxically, even a ***well-treated*** pulpless tooth being traumatized by bruxism presents the vague symptoms of pseudopulpalgia. It, of course, does not respond to thermal stimuli but still feels like a mild toothache.

Examination. From the patient's history usually comes the clue to diagnosing the pain from trauma. History of "toothache" upon awakening is an unusual symptom and should direct one's thinking toward bruxism at night. The discussion of a tense daily situation is another clue. The vagueness of the pain is most important, for one expects to be dealing with chronic pulpalgia, and yet the thermal and pulp tester response is often like that of a normal or hyperreactive pulp. The fact that a low dosage of a mild analgesic can control the pain is pathognomonic.

If one suspects pain from trauma, one should look for facets of wear on the tooth. Articulating paper may be helpful; however, the point of contact may not be readily apparent. One patient shifted her mandible forward during sleep and ground the distal of the mandibular second molar against the mesial of the maxillary first molar, a protrusive shift of a full centimeter. One could not believe that the two well-worn facets would match, and yet, when the youngster was teased into protruding her mandible to this extent, causing contact between the two surfaces, her eyes lighted in delight and she sensuously began compulsive bruxism.*

It should be remembered that the mandible also may be retruded in sleep, causing facets distal to masticatory facets to be involved. Examination for these annoying contacts should be carried out with the patient supine in the dental chair.

Too many dentists examine the median occlusion position (centric) and the lateral excursion of ***function*** (working bite) and completely neglect to examine for ***nonfunctional*** (balancing bite) ***traumatic contacts.*** So often the nonfunctional contact is the patient's compulsive position. Some patients even bring diagrams to the office to describe the point of interference, demonstrating an abnormal and exaggerated oral awareness.

Peculiarly enough, the involved tooth or teeth are frequently not sensitive to percussion but are sensitive to mastication. Biting or chewing on a narrow cotton roll or orangewood stick will sometimes elicit discomfort.

The roentgenogram may show no periapical changes, or may exhibit a widened periodontal space and apical external root resorption (see Fig. 10–26).

Treatment. Treatment for these cases obviously involves relieving the point of occlusal trauma by judicious grinding to reshape the involved tooth and its opponent. Actually, the tooth should be completely disoccluded to give the inflamed tissue a chance to recover.

Many times the dentist is unsure of his diagnosis, especially in cases which so closely resemble or actually are pulpitis. The pulp should be given the benefit of the doubt, particularly if a fully restored crown is involved and complete testing is impossible. If symptoms and signs are vague, the case should first be handled as a problem of traumatic occlusion, especially if there is some evidence that this might be true. If, after careful adjustments, the pulp does not respond with almost immediate relief, the possibility

*Contraction or stretch of muscles (as in yawning) is often pleasurable!

of pulpitis should be reconsidered. But only after all the excursions of the mandible and the patient's history are rechecked.

Sometimes the patient will report relief as soon as the occlusion corrections are completed, even before leaving the chair.

Incomplete Fracture or Split Tooth. The tooth that is ***split*** or ***cracked*** but not yet fractured will present some of the most bizarre symptoms encountered in practice. These symptoms will range from those of a constant, unexplained hypersensitive pulp to constant, unexplained toothache.

The tooth may be uncomfortable only occasionally during mastication, and at that time the pain may be one quick unbearable stab. This is when the crack in the dentin suddenly spreads as the cusp is separated from the remainder of the tooth. The pulp may be only hypersensitive, and this for years. In one case, follow-up continued for eight years, and the pulp hypersensitivity immediately ceased when the buccal cusp fractured away.

Many of the cases involve noncarious, unrestored teeth; hence it is hard to believe that anything could be wrong with the tooth. If the ***split*** has extended through the pulp, bacterial invasion occurs and true pulpitis results. These cases are comparatively easy to diagnose because of the obvious symptoms.

The most frequent complaint is that of a tooth painful to bite on, with an occasional mild ache. One case was diagnosed over the telephone on the basis of a report of these classic symptoms by the harassed referring dentist. The patient confirmed the diagnosis by reporting the same day with the buccal cusp of a maxillary premolar in hand.

Excitation. The discomfort of the ***split*** tooth is elicited by biting on the tooth or contacting cold fluids. If the pulp is involved in the fracture, any exciting agent for pulpalgia will bring on discomfort.

Examination. First of all, one thinks of carefully examining the tooth, dried and under good light, to find the crack in the enamel. Usually, the search goes unrewarded, for the examiner sees no cracks at all, or finds similar enamel crazing in every tooth.

The pulp tester customarily gives a normal reading unless the pulp is involved. Thermal tests may be valuable if a cold or hot stream is played on the tooth, or hot or cold fluids are rinsed against the possible culprit. Hot gutta percha or a stick of ice, on the other hand, is usually valueless.

Percussion alone, surprisingly enough, is usually not helpful, yet biting on an applicator stick or cotton roll may give the spreading action needed to elicit pain.

The crown may also be painted with tincture of iodine, which is washed off after two minutes. The crack often appears as a dark line (see Fig. 7–2).

One of the best implements for examining may be made by folding a piece of No. 7 lead shot or the head of a round bur in a handle of cellophane tape (Fig. 11–7). This may be placed in various positions on a suspected tooth, and by having the patient bite around on the shot, one may determine quite accurately which cusp is ***splitting*** away.

The roentgenogram records an obvious split only if it is in correct alignment to the central rays (Fig. 11–8). It will completely fail to reveal the almost microscopic split, which elicits the really bizarre syndrome.

Treatment. If an ***incomplete fracture*** is suspected, but the pulp is not involved, the crown should be prepared for a full crown, which should then be cemented temporarily with zinc oxide and eugenol cement. The full crown binds the remaining tooth structure much as the hoops contain the staves of a barrel.

If the ***incomplete fracture*** has entered the pulp and a true pulpalgia indicates that pulpitis is present, then root canal therapy should first be completed, followed by full coverage to prevent a total fracture. If the fracture has extended completely through, into the periodontal ligament and pulp, the chances of saving the entire tooth are remote indeed. The possibility of saving a portion of the tooth is discussed in Chapter 16, p. 709.

Periapical Pain

Periapical pain may be almost as excruciating as pulp pain and may often continue for a longer period of time. Periapical lesions that may produce discomfort are: (1) acute apical periodontitis (AAP), (2) acute apical abscess (AAA), (3) chronic apical periodontitis (CAP), (4) suppurative apical periodontitis (SAP), and (5) apical cyst. The prefix "acute," used here, refers to the severity as well as the rapidity of the course of the lesion. Acute apical periodontitis is by far the most distressing periapical lesion.

Acute Apical Periodontitis (AAP). Symptoms. This acute form of periapical pain can be most excruciating and sometimes lasts for days. The tooth is

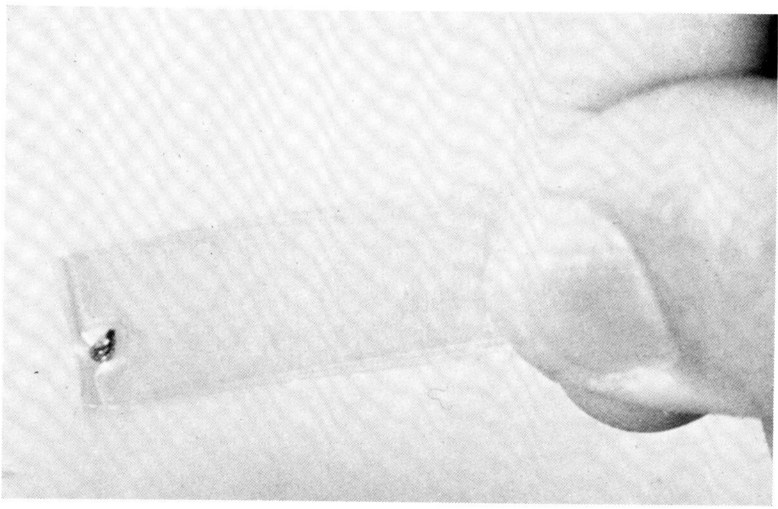

Fig. 11–7. Head of round bur (or No. 7 lead shot) held in "handle" of doubled cellophane tape. Biting on object will determine area of undetected fracture.

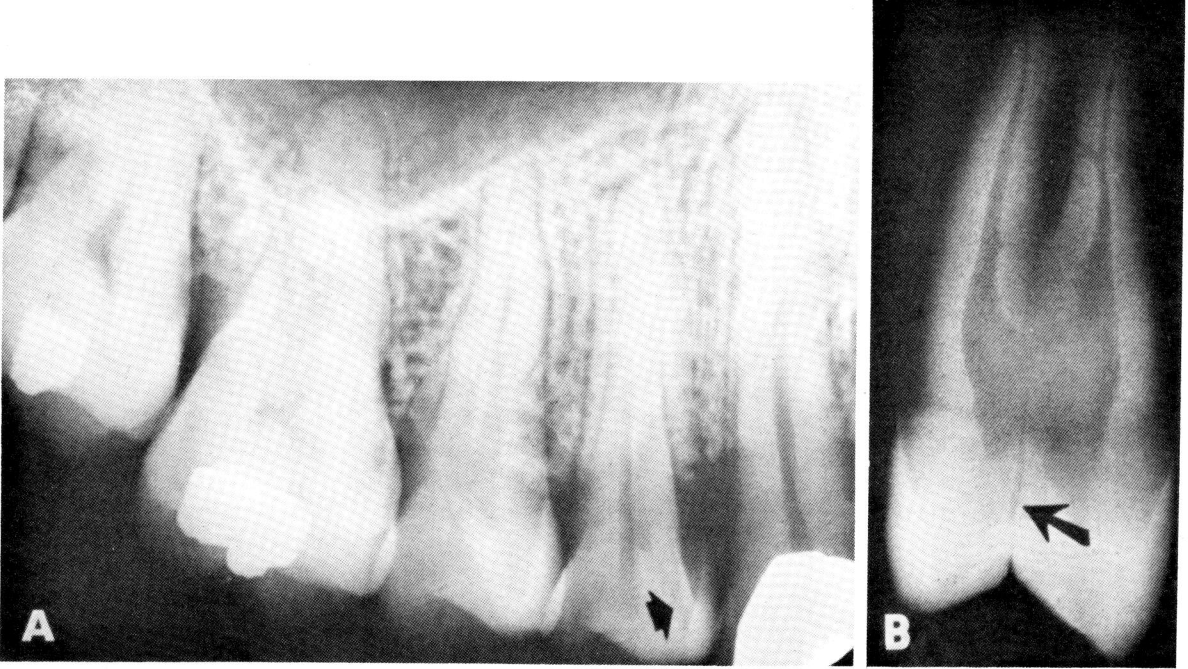

Fig. 11–8. Roentgenograms are usually useless in diagnosing undetected fracture. *A,* Point of fracture *(arrow)* cannot be seen in clinical roentgenogram.
B, After tooth is extracted and radiographed in mesial-distal direction, fracture into pulp becomes apparent. Also note lateral canals. (Courtesy Dr. Dudley H. Glick.)

exquisitely painful to touch, and even contacting the tooth in closure may bring a flood of tears. The pain is most persistent, lasting 24 hours of the day.

The pain has been described as constant, gnawing, throbbing, and pounding. Eventually the patient may gain blessed relief only to bite on the tooth in eating or during sleep, starting the pain cycle once more. Many patients beg to have the tooth extracted. Yielding to their wishes, this has been done, only to have the pain continue for another 48 hours owing to osteitis.

There is no overt swelling involved, just a grossly painful tooth elevated slightly in its socket. One week of discomfort is to be expected if nothing is done! The ***mildly*** uncomfortable case of apical periodontitis associated with ***occlusal trauma*** and bruxism is discussed on pages 507–508.

Etiology. The degree of discomfort described in the preceding paragraphs may be iatrogenic. That is, the clinician perforates the root apex during endodontic therapy, forces caustic medicaments or irritating solutions through the apical foramen, or forcibly deposits necrotic and toxic canal contents into the periapical tissue. These irritants produce a violent inflammatory reaction. If bacteria are present in the canal and are extruded apically, an acute abscess also develops to complicate the picture.

Typically ***acute apical periodontitis*** follows initial endodontic treatment. The mandibular premolars and molars are the teeth most frequently and violently involved, the premolars especially. This fact could be attributed to their invitingly straight, tapered canals, which encourage abuse of the periapex with reamer or file. Furthermore, the thick bony cortex and the small amount of cancellous bone found in this area limit the space allowable for swelling. This limitation greatly increases the pressure in the area, and hence the pain.

Examination. Diagnosis of acute apical periodontitis is relatively easy; the patient is in severe pain and the involved tooth is exquisitely painful to touch. The tooth is in supraclusion and the mandible cannot be closed without initial impact on the involved tooth.

Treatment. The soundest treatment of acute apical periodontitis is its prevention. Care in ***instrumentation*** is the most significant preventive measure. Care in ***medication*** is another precautionary measure. Overmedication and irritating medicaments cause a high percentage of these exasperating cases. Virtually all the intracanal medicaments used today are toxic to periapical tissue. It is essential, therefore, that medicaments be confined to the pulp chamber, that canals ***not*** be "flooded" with medicaments, and that paper points saturated with a drug ***not*** be sealed in canals.

In spite of precautionary measures, acute apical periodontitis may still develop. When it does, the greatest problem involves maintaining the patient in comfort for the entire period of healing and repair. To allow a patient to remain in violent, uncontrolled pain borders on criminal neglect.

When the patient reports with these acute symptoms, the tooth need only be touched to determine the location. To relieve the pain, an immediate injection of a ***long-lasting*** local anesthetic, such as lidocaine with epinephrine 1:50,000, should be given.

As soon as the tooth is comfortable under anesthesia, the occlusion should be adjusted to free the tooth completely from contact in closure or in any excursion. If possible, occlusal ***corrections should be made in the opposite arch*** to prevent more insult to the affected tooth.

A rubber dam should then be placed, and the temporary filling removed very carefully. The tooth must be supported with the fingers to prevent further trauma. A bacteriologic culture should then be taken and the culture sent to the laboratory for an antibiotic sensitivity test (see Chap. 12, p. 574). If the problem is being complicated by infection, it is important to know which antibiotic to use systemically. This is the time to culture the canal contents, before salivary contamination is present.

Using paper points with great care, the ***chamber and canal should be cleared of any liquid contents.*** An instrument is placed in the canal, ***short*** of the registered tooth length, and a roentgenogram taken to check the original tooth length. The present determination of accurate tooth length is most important. Earlier instrumentation at an elongated, inaccurate tooth length may be the basis for the present serious trouble. When the length of tooth is known, a reamer with an instrument stop should be set for this exact length and then employed to ***just barely*** perforate (trephine) through the apical foramen. Sometimes this brings forth a flow of blood and fluid, which materially reduces the periapical pressure. This must be done in a dry, clean canal and with the greatest caution not to further traumatize the periapical tissue.

The advent of the corticosteroids as ***anti-inflammatory*** agents has improved the treatment of acute apical periodontitis. Hydrocortisone, combined with neomycin,* is recommended as an anti-inflammatory-antibacterial medicament. The canal is flooded with this liquid suspension and then, very gently, the fluid is "teased" out the trephined apex with a fresh sterile instrument. A loose cotton pellet is then placed in the chamber and a ***thin*** temporary filling placed without undue pressure. The canal should ***not*** be filled to overflowing with the corticoid solution in order to allow space for inflammatory swelling. There will be some "lag-time" before the antiphlogistic effect of the hydrocortisone takes place.

If the tooth continues to be painful after the analgesia wears off, the patient is instructed to return to the office to have the procedure repeated. Removing the temporary (with a dam in place) once again allows for drainage, and the canal is medicated with Neo-Cortef 1.5%.* The temporary is replaced to prevent secondary contamination. Each time the rubber dam is removed, the occlusion should again be checked. Frequently, further adjustment is necessary because the tooth has again been elevated in the alveolus. The patient is warned not to eat on this side; however, the warning is usually superfluous.

When the patient is leaving the office, he should be instructed that if the pain becomes unbearable at night, he can remove the temporary at home. He should be shown in a mirror how to pick out the thin temporary filling by using a safety pin that has been straightened out. Exposed to the saliva, the canal of course becomes contaminated. This is a modest problem, however, compared to a sleepless night of pain that might be suffered by the patient.

The patient should also be carried on systemic antibiotics and corticosteroids: erythromycin 250 mg., every four hours, for four days, and dexamethasone (Hexadrol) 0.75 mg., 2 tablets a day for four days. By that time, the problem should be resolved.

The patient should also be given a narcotic for analgesia: 30 to 60 mg. (0.5 to 1 gr.) codeine is the initial prescription, taken every three hours with 10 gr. aspirin. If the patient does not obtain relief from codeine or cannot tolerate the drug, 50 to 100 mg. meperidine (Demerol) is prescribed every four hours, depending on the patient's age and weight. A few patients have had such intense prolonged pain they required morphine. Other patients have found it necessary to return every five or six hours for injections of local anesthetic into the affected area.

*Neo-Cortef 1.5%, Eye-Ear Drops, Sterile suspension, Upjohn Co.

Alveolar trephination is another means of relieving the severe pain of acute ***apical periodontitis.*** Trephination, or surgical fistulation, is thoroughly discussed in Chapter 15, pp. 623–624.

In any event, the patient should be seen daily until the symptoms have resolved. Endodontic therapy should not be undertaken until the tooth is comfortable.

Acute Apical Abscess (AAA). The pain of ***acute apical abscess*** is similar to that described for acute apical periodontitis, but is somewhat lower in intensity. After all, necrosis is an extension of the inflammatory cycle, which begins with acute apical periodontitis and continues to the abscess state if not checked.

Necrosis of the ***acute abscess*** usually destroys enough tissue to permit fluid dispersement. The extravasated fluid breaks out into the soft tissue and marrow spaces where swelling is not as confined as it was at the periapex. This is not to say that the ***acute apical abscess*** is not painful. On the contrary, it is quite painful, but in comparison with acute apical periodontitis, the unbearable pain has gone and in its place is a full systolic throbbing pain, particularly on palpation. The involved tooth is also painful to movement or mastication.

Etiology. The discomfort of ***acute apical abscess*** develops gradually as the abscess grows in size. The condition is invariably related to bacterial invasion of the periapical region from a necrotic, infected pulp canal. The ***abscess*** may develop spontaneously from an infected pulpless tooth or may follow initial endodontic treatment if bacteria are forced into the periapical tissue.

In any event, the initial discomfort may be mild, but gradually builds in intensity as the abscess becomes indurated or hardened. When the alveolar plate is "eroded" by the process and the abscess gathers into frank pus, the entire area softens and feels fluctuant to palpation, and the pain is greatly reduced.

Examination. Diagnosis of acute apical abscess is a relatively simple matter. The patient has pain and, invariably, swelling. Although the swelling may not always be observable to the examiner, the patient feels the tenseness of the swollen area. The degree of swelling varies from the initial undetected to gross cellulitis and massive asymmetry. The involved tooth also is extremely painful to percussion or palpation. Roentgenographically, the picture may vary from a widened periodontal space to a large alveolar radiolucency. Actually, the roentgenogram is not the best means of diagnosis, for it frequently reveals nothing of true diagnostic value.

Outside of percussion, electric pulp testing is the best method of diagnosis, for the pulp of the tooth involved in ***acute apical abscess*** is invariably necrotic. The vitality test, moreover, is the best criterion to differentiate an ***acute apical abscess*** from an acute ***periodontal*** abscess. In the case of the periodontal abscess, the pulp of the involved tooth is not likely to be necrotic, although of course it could be. Percussion proves that the periodontal abscess is not so painful as the apical abscess. The reason is quite clear. The periodontal abscess is a "lateral" abscess, found on the lateral aspect of the root, so that percussion causes little increase in pressure. On the other hand, percussion against the inflamed ***periapex*** of the tooth with ***acute apical abscess*** induces a great increase in pressure due to the wedging effect of the tapering root.

The adjacent teeth involved in the swollen area may also be painful to percussion, and they register an increased reading on the pulp tester owing to the collateral edema. The adjacent teeth, however, are not nearly so painful to percussion as the involved tooth and usually register within normal limits in pulp testing. Multiple loss of vitality may follow an accident, so that a number of adjacent teeth could test nonvital, but only one is abscessed.

In contrast to percussion, thermal tests have little value. Extremes of heat may increase gas expansion in the area and thereby increase the pain momentarily. Cold may give slight relief, but usually does nothing at all. Palpation of the area reveals the swelling, and the pressure increases the discomfort.

Treatment. Treatment of the acute apical abscess is discussed in detail under a special section devoted to these problems, Chapter 15, p. 619. Suffice it to say here, drainage is established through the root canal if the abscess is in its initial stage, or by incision if the abscess is fluctuant. Trephination may also be performed to establish drainage and relieve pressure. The occlusion is relieved and the patient is prescribed a regimen of systemic antibiotics and either hot rinses or cold applications, depending on the stage of development of the abscess.

The pain often can be controlled with mild analgesics such as aspirin. However, codeine or meperidine (Demerol) must be prescribed for the severe case.

Endodontic therapy or extraction, whichever is indicated, is completed after the acute symptoms have subsided and while the patient is still receiving antibiotics. Periapical surgery is rarely necessary in treating these cases.

Chronic Apical Periodontitis (CAP). ***Chronic apical periodontitis*** is seldom painful, and is thoroughly discussed in Chapter 9 under Periapical Pathology (p. 398).

Treatment. Endodontic therapy is usually indicated for the tooth involved with ***chronic apical periodontitis.*** This is sometimes followed by periapical surgery, but only where indicated.

Suppurative Apical Periodontitis (SAP). ***Suppurative apical periodontitis*** is generally symptom-free. There may be stages in the long history of such a lesion when a draining fistula closes, and mild swelling and discomfort ensue. The patient reports that the abscess drains daily or that he often opens the abscess with a needle to relieve the discomfort.

Many cases of ***suppurative apical periodontitis*** are so painless that they go undetected for years until revealed by roentgenogram.

Etiology. ***Suppurative apical periodontitis*** is the inflammatory response to an infection by bacteria of low virulence from the root canal. As stated previously, the only discomfort associated with ***suppurative apical periodontitis*** is that related to the occasional closing of the draining fistula with attendant pressure. This chronic lesion, however, may develop an acute exacerbation, the ***phoenix abscess,*** and when this happens, the patient has all the problems of an acute apical abscess. In this event, the pain and swelling are magnified owing to the large pre-existing lesion.

Examination. Upon questioning, the patient with previously undetected ***suppurative apical periodontitis*** may remember a particularly stormy session in the involved area, or perhaps a traumatic incident in which the pulp was devitalized by a blow. He has had no discomfort since, however.

Suppurative apical periodontitis is frequently associated with long-standing dental restorations such as full gold or jacket crowns, large silicates or amalgam, and extensive bridgework. Occasionally a routine roentgenogram reveals ***suppurative apical periodontitis*** associated with a discolored anterior tooth. This may appear as an area of ***diffuse radiolucency*** around the apex of the tooth in question, and may vary from a minor lesion to a massive loss of bone. External resorption of the root end is also a common finding.

The lesion of ***suppurative apical periodontitis,*** easiest to detect, has an associated draining fistula, usually intraoral, seldom cutaneous. This sinus tract, lined with inflammatory tissue, drains the abscess through a stoma into the oral cavity. It is the closing of this tract that causes the patient discomfort.

Treatment. If the tooth involved with ***suppurative apical periodontitis*** can be saved, it may be retained by endodontic therapy. Periapical surgery is sometimes indicated for these pathologic lesions. The chronic lesion that becomes acutely infected must be treated as an acute apical abscess until the symptoms have subsided. The tooth may then be handled as an endodontic case or extracted, as conditions indicate.

Apical Cyst. The ***apical cyst*** *per se* is painless unless it becomes infected. In this event the case should be handled as an acute apical abscess. The apical cyst is discussed in Chapter 9, under Periapical Pathology (p. 415).

Treatment. When treated endodontically, the apical cyst may be enucleated during periapical surgery.

Periodontal Lesion Pain

Few periodontal lesions are severely painful. These lesions are divided into diseases that attack just the gingiva and those that involve the deeper periodontal complex. Two uncomfortable lesions that involve the gingiva and mucosa are ***necrotic ulcerative gingivitis*** and ***herpes simplex.*** These diseases offer no severe problems in the differential diagnosis of pain, because both lesions are diagnosed from their appearance.

Two painful conditions that involve the pericemental structures and must be differentiated are the ***acute gingival*** or ***periodontal abscess and pericoronitis.***

Acute Gingival or Periodontal Abscess. The patient with an ***acute periodontal abscess*** seeks treatment for a tooth that is painful to move or to bite upon. The pain, however, is not so deep-seated or so throbbing as that of an acute apical abscess. Although some localized swelling is present, it is not so extensive as with the acute apical abscess.

Etiology. The ***acute periodontal or gingival abscess*** develops from a virulent infection of an existing periodontal pocket, or as an apical extension of infection from a gingival pocket. Most ***gingival abscesses*** are associated with traumatic injury to the gingiva or periodontium by a mechanical force. Both types of abscess are frequently seen in patients who have compulsive clenching or bruxism.

Examination. Although the involved tooth may be painful to movement, it is not so painful as the tooth involved in an acute apical abscess. Furthermore, the location of the abscess is usually different; the ***periodontal abscess "pointing" opposite*** the ***coronal third*** of the root, whereas the ***apical abscess*** generally ***"points" opposite*** the ***apex.***

The electric pulp tester is the surest method of differentiation. The necrotic, infected pulp causing an apical abscess always gives an essentially negative response to testing, whereas the tooth involved with the ***periodontal abscess*** is generally vital. Use of the periodontal probe often reveals a tract from the gingival sulcus to the abscess.

Treatment. The reader is referred to a periodontic text for information on treatment.

Pericoronitis. The common complaint of the patient with ***pericoronitis*** is severe radiating pain in the posterior mouth and the inability comfortably to open or close the mandible. Not only is it painful to close against the inflamed operculum distal to the erupting mandibular molar, but the pain of muscle trismus limits translation of the mandible as well. The tissue distal to the erupting molar is most painful to touch, especially during eating. The pain radiates through the region, down into the neck, and up into the ear, and can easily be confused with pulp pain. Occasionally an erupting third molar elicits the same, deep spreading pain well before the tooth breaks through the oral epithelium.

Etiology. ***Pericoronitis*** is caused by injury and infection of the pericoronal tissue associated with erupting molars, usually mandibular third molars. The tissue may be injured during eating by trauma from such food as peanuts or bread crust. The infection begins under the operculum and extends with attendant swelling around the entire unerupted crown. This area is frequently a source of primary infection with Borrelia vincentii and Fusiformis dentium.

Examination. The history of trismus and discomfort on opening or closing the mandible is indicative of ***pericoronitis.*** When the operculum is palpated or probed, it is found to be swollen and exquisitely painful. The patient usually assumes it is the tooth that is painful.

Pericoronitis must sometimes be differentiated from a periodontal abscess commonly occurring along the distal aspect of the second molars. Again, the periodontal abscess is not nearly so painful as ***pericoronitis.***

Treatment. The reader is referred to an oral surgery text for information on treatment of ***pericoronitis.***

Myofascial Pain-Dysfunction (MPD) Syndrome

The patient with myofascial discomfort complains of bilateral or unilateral dull pain in the region of the ascending ramus and, almost always, a form of "earache." The ache has been constant, and the patient has usually suffered for a number of days or weeks before reporting for attention. Trismus of the muscles on the same side as the pain limits mandibular opening. Because the pain frequently is referred into the region of the temporomandibular joint, and because of the difficulty in opening the mouth, this condition has often been referred to as ***temporomandibular joint pain-dysfunction syndrome*** (TMJPD). In injury cases, the joint may actually be involved. Arthritis of the TM joint is rare, although Chun has reported acute gouty arthritis as a common yet remedial TMJ affliction in Filipinos, Chinese, and Japanese, particularly after thiazide therapy.[60] Chalmers and Blair, on the other hand, have stated that "involvement of the temporomandibular joint does not appear to be a feature of primary osteoarthritis."[61] Feder has also pointed out that TMJPD syndrome may be secondary to displacement of the condyles by an overextended hearing aid worn in the external auditory meatus.[62]

The typical patient may complain of clicking in the joint during mandibular movement. She also frequently reports the pain as more severe when arising in the morning. Aspirin or codeine may reduce the widespread pain, but the trismus persists. Schwartz has described the pain as "a dull, constant, diffuse, disagreeable ache."[63]

Etiology. Cases of ***myofascial pain-dysfunction*** (MPD) are almost always due to spasm of the muscles of mastication. The usual precipitating cause of the spasm is clenching and grinding or gnashing the teeth due to a stressful life situation. The patients are routinely noted to have a personality defect. Kydd psychologically tested 30 patients with temporomandibular joint complaint, and found 23 of the 30 patients tested to be emotionally unstable.[64] He could also demonstrate by electromyography that in 20 of the 30 subjects, neuron action potentials in the muscles of mastication disappeared when the subjects relaxed, talking about neutral subjects. Weisengreen and Elliot also noted electromyographic abnormalities in a group with so-called temporomandibular joint complaint.[65]

One such emotional woman, as soon as history-taking started, began a tirade about her mother-in-law and broke into tears. When later examined by an associate, she duplicated the performance, and again gave a third and identical performance before a graduate seminar. The patient vehemently protested when the correlation between the tensions of her life situation and her compulsive clenching was pointed out.

Another group of individuals, those suffering from anxiety and frustration, develop muscle spasm through clenching and bruxism. To test the hypothesis that anxiety leads to bruxism and spasm, Thomas, Tiber, and Schireson, of the Myofascial Pain Clinic at the University of Southern California, tested two groups of patients—ten patients with myofascial pain-dysfunction syndrome against a control group of ten matched "normal" patients.[66]

Using electric shock on the forearm to produce ***anxiety,*** and electromyographic (EMG) recordings of the masseter and temporalis muscles to record muscle spasm, the researchers found the "normal" patients demonstrated no muscle clenching in response to anxiety. The stressed MPD patients, on the other hand, showed a significant increase of EMG activity, indicative of bruxism and muscle clenching.

In a second series of tests, ***frustration*** was produced by blindfolding the patients and instructing them to complete a puzzle form board as a "measure of their intelligence." During the test the subjects were constantly harassed by their experimenter to increase their frustration. Although the control and MPD groups both showed increased EMG activity, the reactions of the MPD group "were significantly greater under conditions of frustration than under conditions of anxiety." It is interesting to note that only one female MPD patient showed no tensional increase under conditions of frustration, but at the debriefing session, she slapped the experimenter. "Without knowing it, the patient employed a behavior therapy procedure known as emotive imagery." The conclusion drawn by the USC clinicians was that anxiety, and particularly frustration, led to bruxism and tooth clenching in those patients who had demonstrated the symptoms of myofascial spasm and pain.

The same observations regarding anxiety and frustration were noted by a research group at New York University.[67] Using the Cornell Medical Index and the Rosenzweig Picture Frustration Study, 86 patients—42 with known bruxism and 44 without—were tested for anxiety and frustration. The Cornell Medical Index showed that "bruxistic patients tend to be more anxious than nonbruxistic patients." Furthermore, the Rosenzweig Frustration Study demonstrated that patients with bruxism tend to turn their hostility inward in order to remove frustration, whereas patients who do not have bruxism direct their frustration outward against another person or an object.

The MPD syndrome clinic at the University of Illinois has made similar observations. Lupton classified the MPD syndrome patients with anxiety into two groups.[68] The first group, with suppressed anxiety, was quite unwilling to acknowledge any relationship between their physical symptoms and their mental health. The second group, on the other hand, was characterized by their openly expressed anxiety and a willingness to accept psychotherapy.

To support their contention that ***MPD syndrome is often an emotionally induced psycho-physiologic disorder,*** the Illinois clinicians noted that the usual 30% of the MPD patients given a placebo drug for their "condition" responded favorably.[69] Further, when another placebo drug dubbed "myolax" was dispensed with ***positive verbal clues*** of being "especially helpful for MPD problems," the rate of remission or improvement shot up to 44%, a clear increase of 14% for the placebo effect.[70]

The Illinois clinic also demonstrated remission or noticeable improvement in MPD symptoms for 40% of the patients wearing a ***placebo,*** a nonoccluding palatal appliance (false nightguard) that did not directly modify occlusal contact or alter mandibular placement.[71] Their conclusions were clear—anxiety and frustration lead to muscle spasm and pain, and even placebos give relief.

In England, Rothwell used the Eyesenck Personality Inventory to test 87 MPD patients.[72] He found their neuroticism scores significantly different from those of a normal sample. Rothwell concluded, "It is interesting to note that all the (MPD) patients who did not respond to treatment were married women in the highest socioeconomic groups."

Marback and Dworkin have suggested that the typical MPD patient is passive-aggressive—"wants to remain dependent while struggling with the need to aggressively assert himself."[73] The MPD symptoms provide a secondary gain—attention, sympathy, the opportunity to manipulate others while providing a constant justification for feelings of depression and the desire for isolation. Elimination of the symptoms, the goal of the clinician, seems to run counter to the psychologic needs of the patient. As long as the patient maintains the illusion of seeking a cure, he may avoid a solution of his problems. Dentists become unwilling and unsuspecting victims.

The pioneer in the study of myofascial pain dysfunction syndrome, Dr. Janet Travell, pointed out as early as 1942 the pain-dysfunction cycle related to muscle spasm. By 1952 she had demonstrated the myofascial genesis of facial pain from spasm of the muscles of mastication.[74] In 1960 she published a classic treatise on head and neck myofascial pain-dysfunction in which she discussed the widespread referral of pain arising from spasm of each of the muscles of mastication.[75] For the latest discussion of myofascial pain and dysfunction, the reader is referred to a recent paper by Janet Travell.[75a]

Travell has shown that spasm of the temporalis muscle refers pain into the homolateral maxillary teeth as well as into the maxilla, the frontal region, and the area of the joint (Fig. 11–9 *left*). Spasm of both external pterygoid muscles refers pain directly into the joint region and the area of the maxillary sinus (Fig. 11–9 *right*).

Masseter muscle spasm refers pain into all the homolateral posterior teeth, into the joint, and deep into the ear (Fig. 11–10).

Even the trapezius muscle in spasm refers pain from the posterior neck to the angle of the mandible and to the mandibular posterior teeth, as well as to the temporal region (Fig. 11–11). This widespread reference is not unusual when one considers that the reverse is also true[76]—mandibular jaw pain, in turn, causes spasm of the trapezius muscle (see Fig. 11–27).

Travell discusses occlusal imbalance and emotional stress as two of the precipitating factors in the development of muscle spasm. The patient may realize that the muscles are foreshortening when he notices limitation of his oral opening. She found considerable difference in jaw aperture between a group of "normals" and a matched group suffering from skeletal muscle head pain with limited opening.[75] She has also pointed out the important role played by herpes simplex virus, in and around the

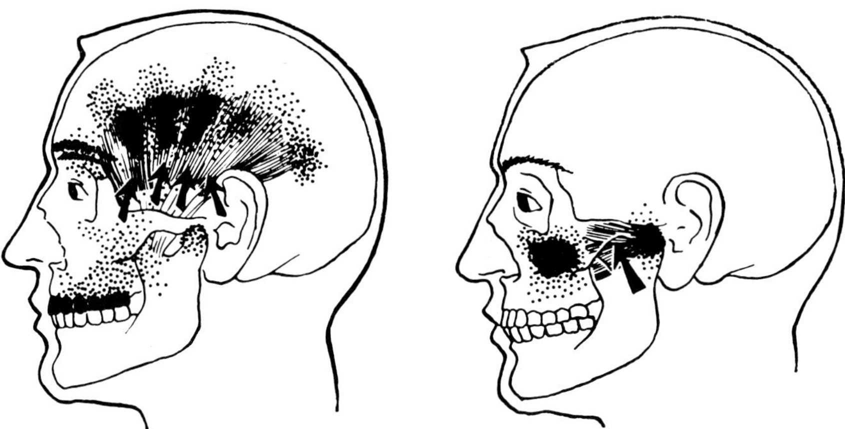

Fig. 11–9. Composite pain reference patterns of two muscles of mastication. Trigger areas are indicated by arrows; zone of referred pain by stippled and black regions. *Left,* Temporalis muscle. Note referred pain into region of temporomandibular joint, supraorbital area and maxillary teeth. *Right,* External pterygoid muscle. Concentrated areas of referred pain are in region of temporomandibular joint and maxillary sinus. (From Travell, J.: J. Prosth. Dent., *10*:745, July-Aug., 1960.)

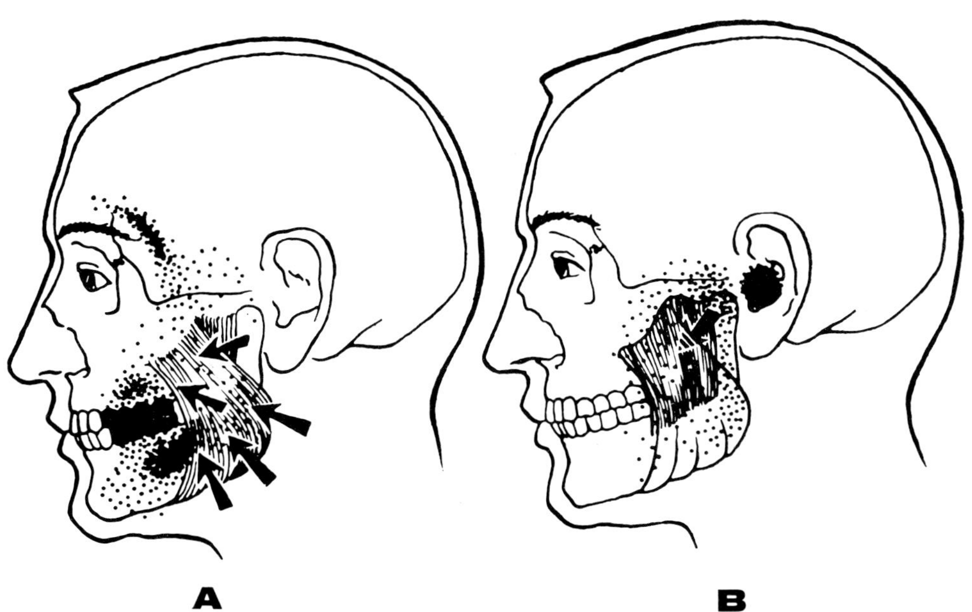

Fig. 11–10. Pain reference patterns of masseter muscle: *A,* Superficial layer. *B,* Deep layer. Trigger areas are indicated by arrows and their pain reference zones by stippled and black regions. (From Travell, J.: J. Prosth. Dent., *10*:745, July-Aug., 1960.)

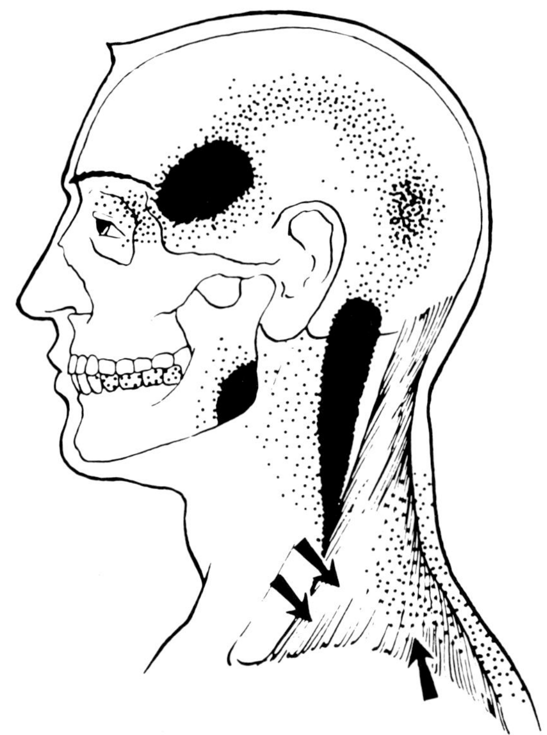

Fig. 11–11. Composite pain reference pattern of trapezius muscle, suprascapular region. Trigger areas are indicated by arrows, and pain reference zones by black and stippled regions. (From Travell, J.: J. Prosth. Dent., *10*:745, July-Aug., 1960.)

mouth and nose, in the development of muscle spasm of the head and neck, believing the herpes virus to have a myotropic affinity for these muscles.[77]

Shanelec conjectured about the role of ischemia of the muscles of mastication as a cause of spasm.[78] He noted that intolerable pain could be produced in the forearm from ischemia caused by repeated clenching of the fist. He also noted the possibility of ischemia and resultant pain developing from repeated clenching of the jaw muscles similar to intermittent claudication caused by the narrowing of the arterial supply to the legs. Claudication of the jaw muscles, produced by chewing and talking as a symptom of ischemia associated with temporal arteritis, was noted by Horton as early as 1944.[79]

Examination. For the extensive examination required for the myofascial pain-dysfunction syndrome, the reader is referred to Schwartz[80] and to Ingle.[81] In brief, however, examination should include a careful history, which covers the patient's relationships with family, friends, associates, and job, as well as a recitation of symptoms and duration of the condition. The iteration of previous dental and medical experiences often is alarming. One may be surprised to learn that pain and dysfunction began with a prolonged dental operation or a traumatic extraction. It might also have begun with an accident, or with yawning, laughing, or shouting.

Special care should be used to elucidate the patient's anxieties and frustrations. Zung has developed a rating instrument for anxiety disorders.[82] Known as the Self-rating Anxiety Scale (SAS), the questionnaire may be used in any office to determine whether a patient is anxious, and if so, to what degree.

The patient is asked to rate each of 20 items as it applied to him within the past week in the following four quantitative terms: none or a little of the time, some of the time, good part of the time, most or all of the time (Table 11–2). The less anxious patient has a low score on the scale and the more anxious patient has a higher score. In scoring the SAS, a value of 1, 2, 3, or 4 is assigned to the response, depending on its positive or negative wording. A key for scoring the scale is shown in Table 11–3.

After testing a group of 209 persons, 100 of whom were normal controls, Zung found an average SAS index of 58.7, plus or minus 13.5, for patients diagnosed as suffering from anxiety disorder, whereas the normal controls' SAS index was 33.8 plus or minus 5.9, a clear difference of 25 points.[82] In between these high and low indices were patients with schizophrenia, depression, and other personality disorders.

It seems reasonable that the Zung Self-rating Anxiety Scale (SAS) could be used in any dental office in rough screening for anxiety and for referral for treatment.

Turning to the oral examination, observation of the midline upon opening frequently gives a clue to muscle trismus or joint dysfunction. The mandible often veers to the affected side. Also, it is important to record the degree of opening.

Palpation of the joints as the patient opens and closes has proved effective in determining whether the joint is the source of pain. Palpation of the muscles of mastication usually reveals a painful "trigger zone" in one or more of the muscles, thought to be the center of the spasm causing the pain and trismus.[75]

Palpating the temporalis muscle is quite simple. As the patient is asked to repeatedly clench his teeth, the

Table 11-2. Zung Self-Rating Anxiety Scale (SAS)

Name ______________________________
Age ______________ Sex ______________
Date ______________________________

	None or a Little of the Time	Some of the Time	Good Part of the Time	Most or All of the Time
1. I feel more nervous and anxious than usual				
2. I feel afraid for no reason at all				
3. I get upset easily or feel panicky				
4. I feel like I'm falling apart and going to pieces				
5. I feel that everything is all right and nothing bad will happen				
6. My arms and legs shake and tremble				
7. I am bothered by headaches, neck and back pains				
8. I feel weak and get tired easily				
9. I feel calm and can sit still easily				
10. I can feel my heart beating fast				
11. I am bothered by dizzy spells				
12. I have fainting spells or feel like it				
13. I can breathe in and out easily				
14. I get feelings of numbness and tingling in my fingers, toes				
15. I am bothered by stomach aches or indigestion				
16. I have to empty my bladder often				
17. My hands are usually dry and warm				
18. My face gets hot and blushes				
19. I fall asleep easily and get a good night's rest				
20. I have nightmares				

Patient is asked to read through items and check to what degree each item applies. SAS is then scored by means of SAS key. (From Zung, W. W. K.: Psychosomatics, *12*:371, Nov.-Dec., 1971. Copyrighted, W. Zung, 1972.)

Table 11-3. SAS Scoring Key

	None or a Little of the Time	*Some of the Time*	*Good Part of the Time*	*Most or All of the Time*
1. I feel more nervous and anxious than usual	1	2	3	4
2. I feel afraid for no reason at all	1	2	3	4
3. I get upset easily or feel panicky	1	2	3	4
4. I feel like I'm falling apart and going to pieces	1	2	3	4
5. I feel that everything is all right and nothing bad will happen	4	3	2	1
6. My arms and legs shake and tremble	1	2	3	4
7. I am bothered by headaches, neck and back pains	1	2	3	4
8. I feel weak and get tired easily	1	2	3	4
9. I feel calm and can sit still easily	4	3	2	1
10. I can feel my heart beating fast	1	2	3	4
11. I am bothered by dizzy spells	1	2	3	4
12. I have fainting spells or feel like it	1	2	3	4
13. I can breathe in and out easily	4	3	2	1
14. I get feelings of numbness and tingling in my fingers, toes	1	2	3	4
15. I am bothered by stomach aches or indigestion	1	2	3	4
16. I have to empty by bladder often	1	2	3	4
17. My hands are usually dry and warm	4	3	2	1
18. My face gets hot and blushes	1	2	3	4
19. I fall asleep easily and get a good night's rest	4	3	2	1
20. I have nightmares	1	2	3	4

Numbers on key are compared with spaces checked by patient after each question on SAS form (Table 11–2). Twenty numbers are then totaled, divided by maximum possible score 80, converted to decimal, and multiplied by 100 to form index. As example, if SAS raw score totals 48, divided by 80 the quotient is 0.6 × 100 equals index of 60, which would indicate patient exhibits slightly more than average (58.7) anxiety. (From Zung, W. W. K.: Psychosomatics, *12*:371, Nov.-Dec.,1971. Copyrighted, W. Zung, 1972.)

examiner's index and middle fingers are pressed with some force against the muscle. After each clenching, the fingers are moved posteriorly and the patient is asked to clench again. If a muscle spasm is present it is very painful and the patient "flinches" away from the palpation. For comparison, the temporalis muscle on the contralateral side should also be palpated.

The external pterygoid muscles are more difficult to palpate (Fig. 11–12) and are best reached with the forefinger or with a large ball burnisher placed high above and distal to the maxillary third molars. The

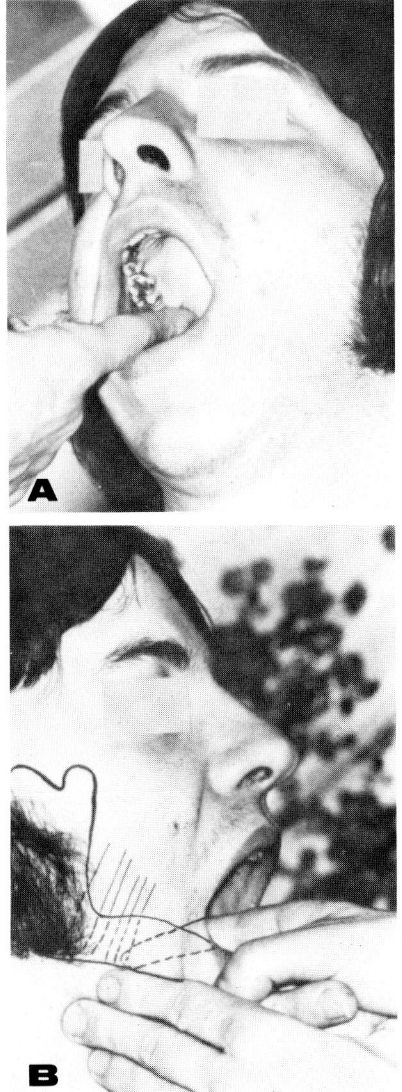

Fig. 11–12. *A,* Palpation of external pterygoid muscle. Lateral distal pressure is applied. *B,* Palpation of internal pterygoid muscle. (From Rosenbaum, M.: Oral Surg., *39*:382, Mar., 1975.)

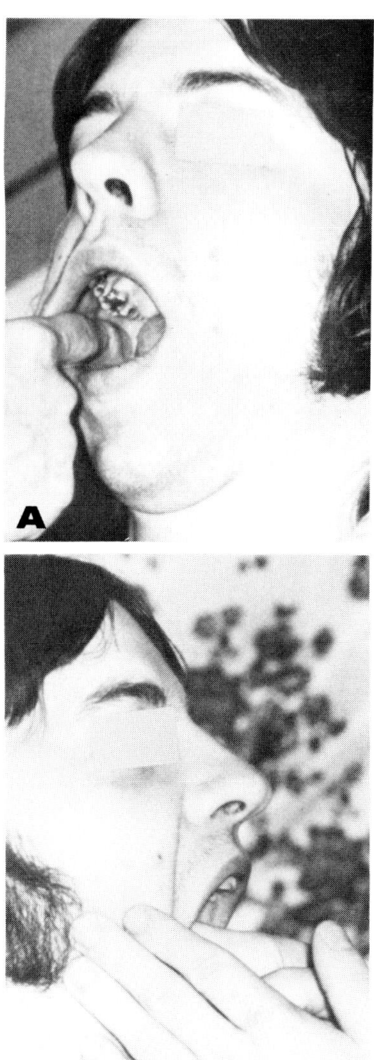

Fig. 11–13. *A,* Intraoral view of palpation of masseter muscle. *B,* Extraoral view of palpation of masseter muscle. (From Rosenbaum, M.: Oral Surg., *39*:382, Mar., 1975.)

masseter and the buccinator muscles are easier to reach (Fig. 11–13). Using two index fingers opposite each other, one inside the cheek and one on the outside, the examiner "traces" along the muscle body as the patient opens and closes. A point of exquisite pain marks the center of the spasm, called the "trigger zone" by Travell.

Sometimes, even the tensor veli palatini muscle is painful as it is palpated around the hamulus in the lateral soft palate. The examiner should also carefully palpate the parotid glands to make sure he is not dealing with infection in the glands or obstruction of the duct. If the parotid is involved, it will be swollen in a very circumscribed pattern due to its capsule. Characteristic is the location below the zygomatic arch.

A stethoscope may be used to listen for clicking or crepitus in the joint, although Schwartz points out that joint sounds usually ***precede*** the spasm and pain.[80] Examination of the teeth both out of contact and in full contact is important, for one invariably finds worn facet pathways, a sure sign of bruxism. In addition, one may also discover a premature contact in the occlusion which appears to divert the mandible in its closing pathway. The examiner must be warned, however, ***that the damaging point of initial contact may have developed because of mandibular shift*** related to the aforementioned muscle spasm, ***rather than vice versa as generally believed.*** Butler et al. found no significant difference between occlusal relationships in MPD symptomatic or asymptomatic patients.[83] They felt the syndrome was sex linked to the female, however.

The examiner must be warned not to confuse toothache with myofascial pain. Just such a confusion has been reported.[84] Vehement denial of the possibility has also been voiced.[85]

Treatment. The variations in treatment of MPD syndrome are as legion as the theories of etiology. A number of modalities have proved effective including occlusal equilibration to eliminate occlusal discrepancies* and bite plates (night guards) to separate the jaws and prevent bruxism. Greene and Laskin found that even a placebo "night guard" worked 40% of the time, whereas wearing a full occlusal splint led to complete or great improvement in two-thirds of the MPD cases.[71] It is conjectured that the muscles cannot be clenched into spasm while a night guard is worn because the interocclusal separation prevents the full muscle contraction necessary for spasm.

Lerman has reported improvement in 84% of previously unsuccessfully treated patients through the use of a "hydrostatic" appliance.[86,87] Taking care that the occlusal vertical dimension did not exceed the freeway space and resting muscle length, Lerman constructed the fluid-bearing appliance for 26 previously unsuccessful MPD patients. The hydrostatic appliance permitted mandibular placement to be self established by the muscles. Twenty-two of the 26 patients improved, but symptoms usually recurred when the appliance was withdrawn and occlusal dysfunctions once again were allowed to guide muscle accommodation.

In addition to the physical treatment that may help the MPD patient, psychologic treatment also may be necessary and effective. If it is concluded that the patient's bruxism is related to frustration or anxiety about his life situation, this correlation should be pointed out to him. He should be told that clenching or grinding his teeth, which leads to painful spasm, is a "safety valve" warning that he is getting "keyed up" over some situation. He should analyze why he is anxious, what it is that is frustrating him, and avoid the cause. The clue to success is the relaxation of the muscle spasm, evidence that the nervous clenching is being eased.

Referring patients with bruxism to a psychiatrist, if this appears to be their only neurotic manifestation, is a form of "overkill." Many dentists have been singularly unimpressed with the results achieved when measured against the duration and cost of psychotherapy.

Pomp, on the other hand, reported good results in treating MPD patients by psychotherapy.[88] Of the 23 MPD patients who completed the 12-week course of therapy, 15 had complete remission of symptoms. Of the eight patients who did not respond to therapy, one improved with the use of a splint and one improved after a change in her living situation. Six patients gained no relief. Thirteen of the patients had constant headache before treatment, and 8 of the 13 became free of their headaches as well as of their muscle spasm.

Pomp concluded, "Clinicians without special psychologic training can still provide proper management for MPD patients if they simply establish an appropriate dentist-patient relationship. They must be prepared to listen sympathetically to complaints, to respond with reassuring explanations, to support the patient emotionally by being strong and confident, and to provide relief from pain and discomfort through therapy.

"It would not be logical to suggest psychotherapy as a ***primary*** treatment for MPD syndrome. Rather, clinicians who deal with these patients should use common-sense psychologic principles of patient management in combination with appropriate pain-

*The MPD clinic at the University of Illinois has shown that "after 2 *mock* equilibrations for treatment of MPD syndrome, 16 out of 25 patients (64%) reported a total or nearly total remission of their symptoms." They further suggested that "occlusal equilibration should not be regarded as either specific or definite therapy for MPD syndrome."[85a]

relieving and muscle-relaxing modalities. Only if a reasonable period of such treatment fails to produce improvement should referral for psychotherapy be considered."

Marback and Dworkin warned against treatment of MPD patients by mechanosurgical procedures, but recommended instead "... supportive palliative and reversible procedures such as exercises, tranquillizers, antidepressants and intramuscular injections of anesthetics and steroids."[73]

Reporting on 100 successfully treated and 35 unsuccessfully treated MPD patients, Greene and Laskin concluded, "In a psychophysiologic disorder such as MPD syndrome the most important factor in successful management does not depend on the specific treatment used, but rather on the general approach to the patient.[89] The establishment of good dentist-patient rapport and an explanation of the nature of the problem appear to be of primary importance." Failure appears to be related to the complex psychologic factors that interfere with the dentist-patient relationship. Greene and Laskin recommended treatment with the most conservative modalities and early avoidance of overtreatment with radical or complex modalities.

Some muscle relaxation has been achieved with tranquilizers. Again, Greene and Laskin reported meprobamate (Equanil) to be 58% effective in treating 90 MPD patients. Of course 31% also responded positively on placebo.[69] Muscle relaxing drugs such as mephanesin (Tolseram) have also been used. Immediate results are not usually achieved, and so the dentist and patient must persist in treatment for a number of days in order to evaluate the drug's effectiveness. Drug dependence should be avoided, however.

It would seem obvious that the best cure for muscle spasm would be muscle relaxation, and any therapy that would break up the spasm would be ideal. As suggested, this might be brought about by physical means (a night guard) or chemical means (meprobamate or mephanesin) or psychotherapy (suggestion). The most direct method, however, is to deal with the muscle in spasm itself.

Again, Travell has provided us with an insight toward breaking the spasm-pain-spasm-pain cycle. "Over 25 years ago she pointed out that 'dry needling' a trigger area is by itself sometimes effective in extinguishing the reverberating pain circuits." She has also proved the efficacy of infiltrating procaine into the trigger point of the spasm. "For procaine infiltration of trigger areas, through a single skin puncture, the needle is moved rapidly in and out to reach all layers of the muscle and to pepper the trigger area thoroughly, while at the same time small amounts of the solution are continuously injected. The total amount used in treating any one trigger area may be only 0.5 to 1.0 ml of procaine."[77]

Travell prefers to use low concentrations of procaine (0.25 to 0.5%) ***without epinephrine.*** These she makes by drawing off 0.5 ml. 1% procaine from a rubber-stoppered bottle and adding 0.5 ml. or 0.75 ml. sterile saline in the syringe for 0.5 or 0.25% solutions respectively.[77] All the while the injection is being made, the patient's mouth is propped wide open to stretch the foreshortened muscle fibers. Travell points out that procaine has a curariform (curare) action on skeletal muscles and that the needling alone "may act by releasing intracellular potassium, which, in turn, blocks nerve conduction temporarily." Dry needling, on the other hand, is more painful and less effective than procaine.

Travell has also introduced passive stretching during vapocooling as a valuable procedure for relieving skeletal muscle spasm, especially in its early stages.[90] To carry out this procedure, the jaw is propped open to place a gentle stretch on the muscles in spasm and

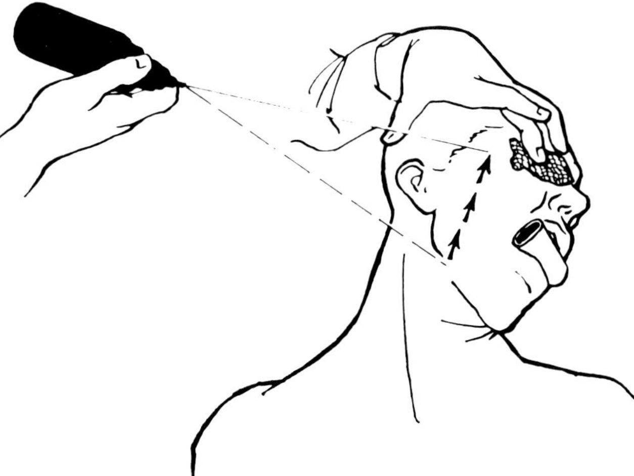

Fig. 11–14. Technique of stretching muscle and applying vapocoolant spray (Fluori-Methane) for relief of masseter muscle spasm. Mouth is propped comfortably at its maximum opening. Each sweep of spray follows muscle lines and travels toward and over related pain reference zones. After prop is removed, hot moist packs are applied for 3 to 4 minutes. Procedure is then repeated. (From Travell, J.: J. Prosth. Dent., *10*:745, July-Aug., 1960.)

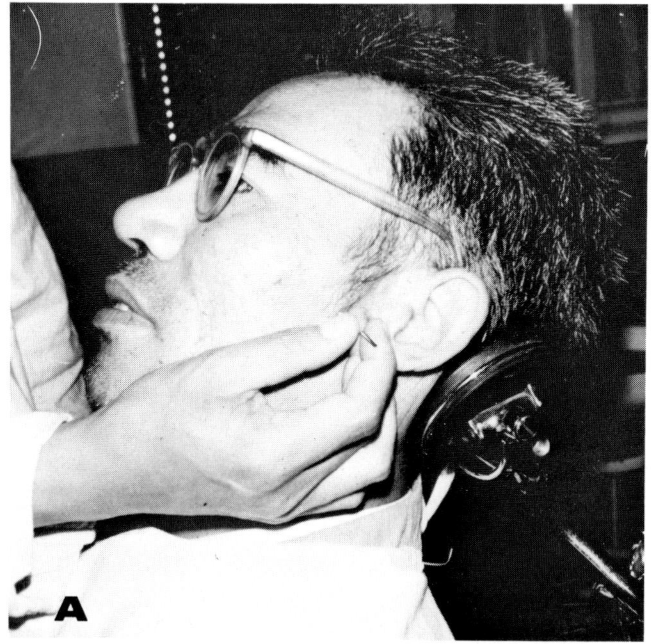

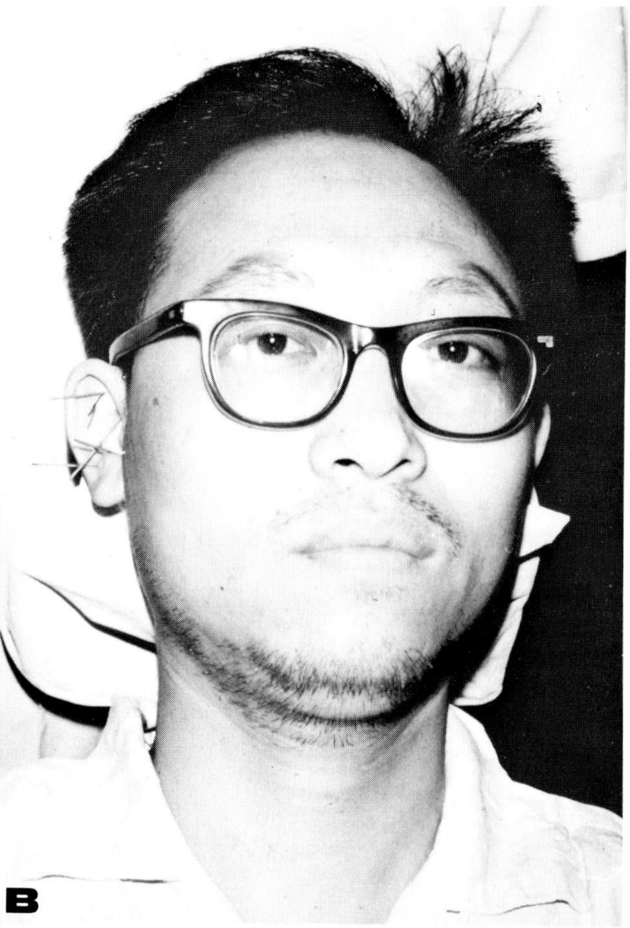

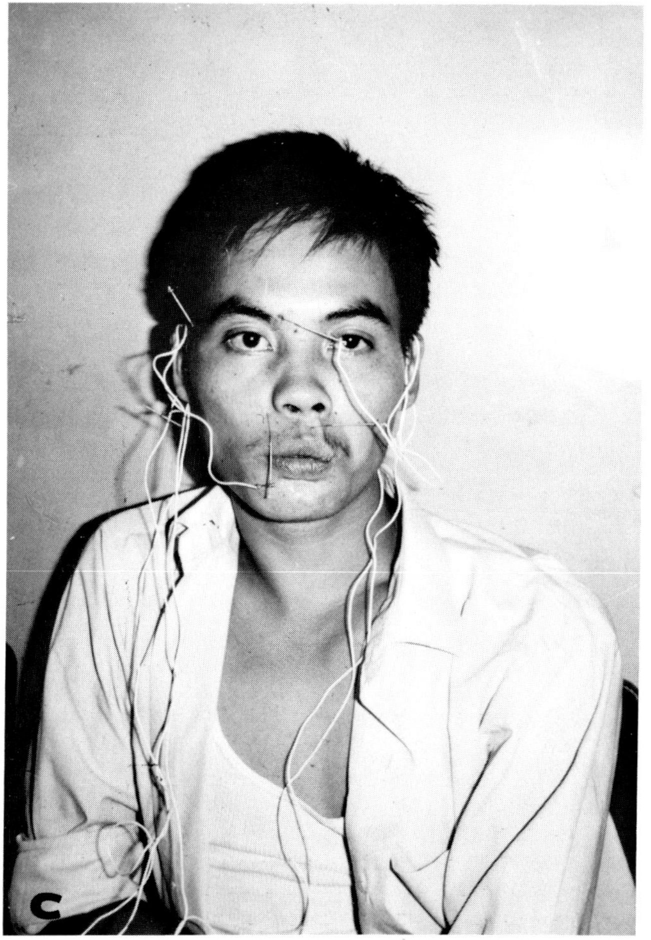

Fig. 11–15. Acupuncture used to treat myofascial pain dysfunction syndrome and seventh nerve palsy in People's Republic of China. *A,* Twirling acupuncture needle to break up spasm of masseter muscle. *B,* Four acupuncture needles placed along meridian in homolateral ear to treat MPD syndrome. *C,* Five needles attached to pulsing stimulator placed homolaterally to treat Bell's Palsy. Partial paralysis is still apparent. (From Ingle, J. I.: CAL, *38*:7, May., 1975.)

a spray of Fluori-Methane is applied in slow, even, interrupted sweeps in one direction only. It is started over the trigger area and travels in the direction of the referred pain (Fig. 11–14).

This process of intermittent spraying takes a minute or two. The prop is then removed, and the patient is instructed to open and close. If jaw aperture has increased, a larger mouth prop is used and spraying is repeated. The cold shock of the spray acts as a surface counterirritant and is thought to block the stream of noxious impulses from the muscle. Pain and cold sensations both travel the spinothalamic tracts and terminate in the same higher centers; thus the "cold impulse" may block the pain impulse interrupting the pain-spasm cycle.

It should be apparent to today's dentist that Chinese acupuncture might be applied as is "dry needling" to break up muscle spasm—and so it is, whether the needles are placed directly into the muscle in spasm or in the region by needling the ear (Fig. 11–15).

In addition to acupuncture, the Chinese use poultices of traditional herbs applied by ionization to the region of the spasm. Concoctions of herbs are also applied to the spasm through the time-honored technique of cupping (Fig. 11–16).

Compared to the ancient art of Chinese traditional medicine, the recent application of analog information feedback to achieve muscle relaxation appears modern indeed. And yet the entire idea is based on the ancient concept of Yoga control of bodily functions.

The idea of muscle relaxation for the reduction of tension and anxiety dates back to Jacobson and is brought up-to-date by his report on the effects of training in ***progressive relaxation.***[91] In this study, patients were able to reduce by 50% action potential levels in the muscles of mastication after one month of daily practice.[92]

Muscle relaxation through meditation became more than a fad in the mid 1970s. Benson, from the Harvard Medical School, demonstrated dramatic reductions in oxygen consumption and blood lactate through a relaxation response modeled after Transcendental Meditation.[92a] Another physician, Bloomfield, chronicled the marked reduction in breathing rate and increase in alpha and theta brain waves characteristic of relaxation.[92b] Using a "technic based on Buddhist meditation," Stone and DeLeo were able to reduce diastolic blood pressure an average of 12 mm. Hg in a group of moderately hypertensive patients. The treated patients also exhibited significant reductions ". . . of plasma dopamine-betahydroxylase activity," thus providing an index of decreased sympathetic nervous system function.[92c] Popular writers, such as Adam Smith, also detailed the relaxing benefits of Transcendental Meditation.[92d]

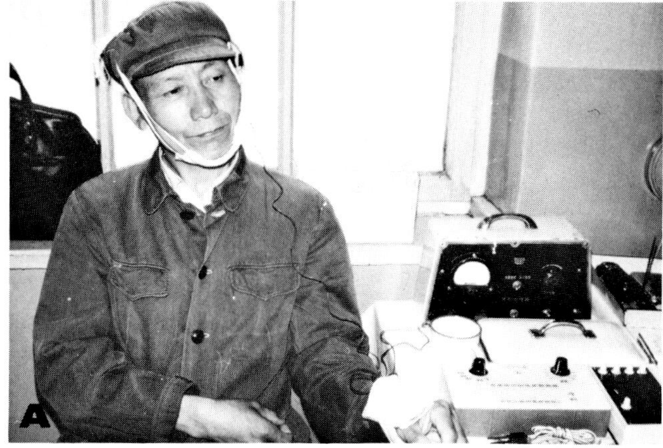

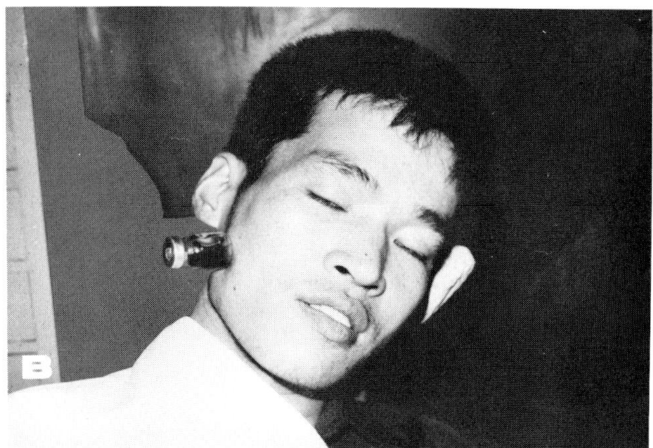

Fig. 11–16. Application of traditional Chinese herbs, by modern and ancient methods, to treat muscle spasm. *A,* Poultice of herbs being ionized into muscles. *B,* "Cupping," an ancient method of counterirritation while herbal concoction is being applied. (From Ingle, J. I.: CAL, *38*:7, May., 1975.)

In order to shorten "practice time" and to reinforce the positive achievements of muscle relaxation, Budzynski and Stoyva devised an analog information feedback system, which attaches to the patient's frontalis muscle in the forehead.[93] The patient was told to lie quietly with his eyes closed and to concentrate on deeply relaxing his frontalis muscle. Electromyographic leads attached to the muscle are passed through Grass amplifiers, so that the EMG output is reproduced as sound—as the muscle activity decreases, the pitch becomes lower. The subject must progressively relax the frontalis muscle to keep the tone at the lower frequencies. Thus, by the continuing feedback the subject's behavior is being shaped, that is, he is taught how to relax muscles in spasm. Adaptation of the biofeedback mechanism to the relaxation of the muscles of mastication has been accomplished in Sweden by monitoring the masseter muscle in patients with MPD.[93a]

For the prevention and treatment of generalized muscle spasm caused by herpes simplex virus as suggested by Travell,[78] she has further recommended the use of idoxuridine (Stoxil) 0.1% ophthalmic solution, swabbed (actually scrubbed) with a cotton applicator into the nostrils, across the lips, and into the oral cavity. Used prophylactically on a regular basis, idoxuridine prevents the proliferation of the herpes simplex virus and its myotropic affinity leading to spasm. It can also be used to treat early herpes lesions. Idoxuridine inhibits the replication of herpes simplex virus by irreversibly inhibiting the incorporation of thymidine into the viral DNA. Gangarosa and his associates have recently confirmed the beneficial effects of Stoxil applied by iontophoresis in the treatment of labial herpes.[93b]

Two approaches to treatment of MPD have been discussed—the direct relaxation of muscle spasm and pain, followed by relief from anxiety and frustration, and conversely, the approach of reducing frustration and anxiety with a concomitant reduction in bruxism and clenching and, hence, myofascial pain and dysfunction.

Neurologic Pain

Neurologic conditions causing pain that frequently is confused with dental pain are: (1) trigeminal neuralgia (tic douloureux), (2) trigeminal neuritis, and (3) herpes zoster neuritis and postherpetic neuralgia.

Other nervous system lesions, even more central, may affect the fifth nerve. The symptoms generated by such a brain lesion are often most confusing and, if paroxysmal in nature, are often misinterpreted as trigeminal neuralgia. Bizarre symptoms accompanied by bizarre behavior (of a truly sick person) may also be judged as psychogenic, and the patient dismissed as a "nut" or a crank. In every case the patient must be given the benefit of the doubt.

The following case histories illustrate the importance of always considering a central nervous system lesion when a diagnosis is being made.

Case History 1: Anderson and Ogle describe a young woman with right hemifacial pain of two years' duration, which began initially as a sharp shooting pain in the lower right face and then localized intraorally and extraorally in the right cheek.[94] Eating and talking increased the pain, and eventually it radiated up the right side of the head. No trigger zone was present. The patient's physician diagnosed the pain as tic douloureux and started drug therapy. When the patient was finally seen by the oral surgeons, the pain had increased in intensity and frequency, lasting in paroxysms between ten minutes and one hour. Results of careful oral examination and of tests of cranial nerves II through XII were essentially normal, except for decreased pulp response of the right mandibular teeth. A central lesion was suspected and a neurologic workup was ordered, including a clivogram, which revealed a right cerebellopontine angle mass. Operation revealed a tumor wrapped around the fifth nerve and displacing it anteriorly against the tentorium. The tumor proved to be an epidermoid cyst, and following operation the patient recovered completely.

Noteworthy in this case are the imitation of the paroxysmal symptoms of trigeminal neuralgia and the bizarre symptoms often exhibited by emotionally disturbed patients. The dentist stands warned that the signs and symptoms from a central lesion may ***cross*** the midline. Bilateral pain is the hallmark of psychogenic pain, hence the confusion.

Case History 2: The case reported by Melrose was equally baffling, but with a poorer prognosis.[95] The patient was a 43-year-old male physician referred for evaluation of paroxysmal attacks of severe pain. He was in good general and oral health until several weeks prior to examination, when he suddenly developed attacks of severe pain in the right mandible, which lasted for several seconds and culminated in numbness and tingling of right upper and lower lips and right tongue. This sensation would gradually disappear over a period of about 20 minutes. The attacks were not predictable, were not associated with any auditory or visual premonitory signs, and had slowly increased in frequency and intensity. The patient did not suffer headaches.

Examination could produce no trigger zone, and the patient could not reproduce the symptoms or relate them to any specific manipulation or episode. "Panorex" and periapical radiographs were not contributory.

Because of the unusual distribution of symptoms and the lack of any obvious dental cause, Melrose suggested that the patient seek neurologic consultation to rule out a more central cause.

About two weeks subsequent to the oral examination, the patient had sudden convulsions and was hospitalized. X-ray examination revealed a large space-occupying mass on the left side. Operation revealed a glioblastoma multiforme apparently involving the trigeminal nucleus.

Following operation, pre-radiation chemotherapy and a course of radiation were administered. Although prognosis is poor with this tumor, the patient survived eleven months.

Granted these are the unusual diagnostic cases, but such conditions must be ruled out in the interest of thoroughness. More frequently, when the pain is other than purely dental, it is neurologic. The most painful and dramatic of the neurologic pains is ***trigeminal neuralgia.***

Trigeminal Neuralgia (Tic Douloureux)

The dental profession probably encounters far less trigeminal neuralgia, a fairly rare condition, than one would suspect from reading the dental literature. Once seen, however, a patient with trigeminal neuralgia is not readily forgotten. The pain, which usually relates to the face and nose, is the symptom that sends the patient to a physician. The disease has three distinct pathognomonic features: (1) intermittent paroxysms of pain along the distribution of one or more divisions of the trigeminal nerve, with complete freedom from the pain between the paroxysms; (2) a unique "trigger mechanism"—stimulation to a particular area of the skin of the face or to the membranes of the mouth, such as washing, shaving, drinking hot or cold liquids, eating rough foods, talking, or even smiling, which sets off paroxysms of pain; and (3) no abnormal neurologic findings except the tic. This unique triad is always produced by true trigeminal neuralgia and never by any other condition.[96]

The first case of tic douloureux seen by me had a trigger zone of dental origin. The patient played first French horn in a symphony orchestra, and complained that whenever he hit a low note on the horn a "tremendous, sharp" pain shot out of a maxillary right canine and up into his eye. Over the telephone this seemed a clear case of pulpitis or incomplete fracture of the tooth. When the patient was examined, however, the canine in question was completely sound, gave a normal pulp tester reading, was normal to hot, cold and percussion, had no restoration, no caries, no apparent fracture, no roentgenographic changes, no severe abrasion or bruxism, no history of trauma, and completely normal responses to all testing.

The patient also complained that occasionally when chewing he would strike the tooth and receive the pain, a symptom reminiscent of an incompletely fractured tooth. A sound canine, however, rarely if ever splits unless involved in an accident.

Examination revealed a shiny facet on a new full crown on the left maxillary first molar, and in closing, the mandible was seen to slide into right eccentric and strike the canine in question. This prematurity in the occlusion was relieved, and the patient was dismissed to observe results.

Two days later the patient called to say he had not had a recurrence of the pain and to express his gratitude. Four other dentists, he stated, had wanted to extract the perfectly sound tooth. He also reported that he had not played his horn.

One month later the patient's wife called to request another appointment. The patient was in such pain he could not even speak over the telephone. The second examination revealed that the pain had begun when he returned to playing his instrument, and now any note, high or low, would excite the pain. The patient's wife, speaking for him, stated that he had seen a number of physicians in the month, and one rhinologist had discovered an obstructed nasal passage on the left side. Believing this condition to be the cause of the trouble, the physician had instructed the patient to place cotton wool in the right nostril to force breathing through the obstructed left nostril. ***And now, each time the wool was placed in the right nostril, the patient was struck with the same vicious pain that originally emanated only from the canine.***

The diagnosis was complete. The trigger zone, formerly in the canine alone, had extended to the right ala of the nose. Two pathognomonic signs of trigeminal neuralgia were present, the paroxysm of pain and the trigger zone to produce the pain. Of course the trigger zone was present previously, but was so similar to referred pain from pulp pathosis that the true state of the disease was masked.*

In some cases of trigeminal neuralgia, suspected teeth have been unadvisedly extracted, only to have the pain continue. In one case ***both*** the second and third branches of the nerve were involved. In another case, ***two trigger zones*** were present, a cutaneous zone along the mandible, which could be triggered only by a wet face cloth, and an intraoral zone, triggered by placing a certain spot on the tongue against a mandibular premolar. Diagnosis in all these peculiar cases was confirmed by a neurologist.

*The patient later had a surgical section of the second division of the trigeminal nerve. Left with parasthesia of the lip, he could no longer play the French horn, and so became a paid official of the musician's union.

In all such cases, the dental examination looms important. If the dentist conducts a thorough and competent examination and every finding is completely normal, the examiner must learn to believe in himself and his abilities and not to panic into extracting or removing a healthy pulp or tooth. Time often solves many problems that would have been treated in error on the basis of a snap diagnosis.

Etiology. Not since the days of Andre in 1756, who coined the phrase "tic douloureux," or Trousseau in 1853, who called the condition "epileptiform neuralgia," has our understanding of the etiology of trigeminal neuralgia improved. It still obtains, however, that the similarities of paroxysmal dysfunction as seen in epilepsy and other pain states, such as trigeminal neuralgia, are most striking. In all honesty, one would have to say that the cause of trigeminal neuralgia is today unknown, in spite of the many and varied theories that have been developed over the past 220 years. Black has postulated, however, that neuronal ***damage*** to the fifth nerve "will result in changes in related areas of the grey matter in the central nervous system. In some susceptible individuals these changes can result in a paroxysmal pain state of central origin."[97] Black has shown in animals that the associated fibers of the fifth nerve, showing degeneration all along the neuron and into the spinal trigeminal nucleus, "prolonged after discharges—very close to stimulation threshold and lasting up to 30 or more seconds," were found on the side of the tooth extraction or pulp extirpation.

Intrigued by Black's apparent implication of dental structures in the etiology of tic douloureux, Ratner, Person, and Kleinman, at the Veterans Administration Hospital in Brooklyn, have approached the diagnosis of trigeminal neuralgia on the assumption that in most instances a distinct pathologic locus (or loci) must exist in the dental or oral structures.[98] They found that such loci do exist, but do not necessarily coincide with sites at which the patient's trigger zone and pain perception are experienced. They further found that the trigger zone and pain perception are referred from the former lesion in reproducible patterns.

Although almost any type of dental and oral lesion capable of producing pain may in certain individuals result in triggering of the trigeminal syndrome, in most instances the location of the pain-related lesion (in 24 of 25 cases) coincided with sites of previous tooth extractions. Such sites may be single or multiple, and are usually present as cavities within the alveolar bone. Dimensions of such cavities may exceed 1 cm. and yet may not be detectable on roentgenograms, because of density of the cortical bony plates. Localization of these cavities is therefore dependent on the empirically derived pain-referral paths aided by a selective local anesthesia procedure devised by the authors.

Following detection and surgical exposure of such sites, curetted material removed from the walls of these cavities contained, in many instances, avascular necrotic bone. Microbiologic sampling of the cavities under maximal aseptic precautions revealed, in many cases, the presence of a wide variety of "non-pathogenic" and pathogenic oral microorganisms.

Treatment consists of combined surgical curettment of the cavities and antibiotic therapy. These authors have found, in a series of 25 cases of idiopathic trigeminal neuralgia, improvements ranging from 70 to 100% as a result of such treatment.

Treatment. Tic douloureux may be self-limiting. The initial treatment recommended today is the use of the drug carbamazepine (Tegretol), which appears to act by depressing synaptic transmission in the spinal trigeminal nucleus. It is also effective in treating some cases of facial migraine, postherpetic neuralgia, or atypical facial pain associated with middle-age depression. Carbamazepine also may be used in combination with diphenylhydantoin (Dilantin). In those infrequent instances when this combination is ineffective, alcohol injection of the sensory root or surgical section or radiofrequency heating to destroy pain fibers of the fifth nerve may be done by a neurosurgeon.[99] The author witnessed tic patients being treated successfully by acupuncture in The People's Republic of China. Although the pain was facial, needles were placed in the soles of the feet.

Trigeminal Neuritis

Whereas trigeminal neuralgia as just described is a paroxysmal sharp pain, ***trigeminal neuritis*** is a constant dull pain involving one or more branches of the fifth nerve. Bonica refers to this condition as secondary (minor) trigeminal neuralgia.[100] Patients with trigeminal neuritis often arrive in a dental office after having seen a number of physicians and dentists. Usually they have had two or three teeth extracted to no avail. The pain is dull enough so that they have been able to live with it by taking copious amounts of aspirin. In one reported case, the patient had widespread pain in the right face, which began anterior to the region of the ear and spread to the temporal scalp. During examination, the painful area was outlined on the face with a pencil. The marked area closely matched the second division innervation of the fifth nerve as well as patches of the region supplied by the auriculotemporal nerve of the third division.

Occasionally, the patient reported, the third division would also be painful, and the cervical muscles would go into painful spasm. The patient had reported to her dentist originally with a toothache in the right maxillary canine, which had been consistently aching for some time. The dentist apparently removed the pulp from the canine, and the patient received temporary relief. Within three days though, the pain recurred and this time over a wider area. The patient then reported to her physician, who treated her for sinusitis, still to no avail.

After three months of pain the patient presented herself for treatment. Examination revealed the pattern of pain previously stated. The maxillary right canine had a temporary filling in place, but a roentgenogram revealed no root canal filling. All the other teeth responded normally.

When the canine was re-entered, about half of a partially vital pulp was found, although pulp testing had been negative. The area was anesthetized, the pulp removed, and an anodyne dressing placed. For two days the generalized neuritis disappeared, only to return after the canal was filled.

The operated tooth was ***not*** painful to percussion. Furthermore, the canal had not been overfilled. After two more weeks of continuous pain (during which time the severity of the pain was increased by a cold breeze blowing across the face), the patient was referred to a neurologist who diagnosed the condition as trigeminal neuritis. The patient remained on codeine and finally aspirin for a full six months before the pain became localized ***lingual*** to the maxillary lateral incisor, on the affected side. The vital teeth on that side all tested normally until finally the maxillary lateral incisor began pulpalgia. When the pulp of the involved incisor was removed, the pain gradually faded from the entire right face.

Another case of trigeminal neuritis followed osteomyelitis of the left mandible, a sequela to periodontal therapy. Pain continued for more than a year.

Etiology. The cause of trigeminal neuritis is unknown. It is suspected, however, that long-standing inflammation and pain along one of the branches of a given division of the nerve gradually leads to "inflammation" of the entire division. When the nerve and its sheath are sectioned and studied histologically, however, no inflammatory changes can be demonstrated along the nerve. Occasionally patients with this condition give a history of having had a virus-like infection in the parotid and joint area, which in turn leads to a long-standing neuritis.

Possibly trigeminal neuritis is similar to Morton's toe syndrome.[101] In this condition a periarteritis develops in the foot, and the sensory nerves that innervate the arteries themselves are apparently responsible for the pain.

Examination. Examination by the dentist consists again of establishing or ruling out any possible oral cause for the widespread pain. Pulpitis of long standing and severity refers pain over the entire involved division of the fifth nerve and even into the other divisions. This is true referred pain, temporary in nature, which disappears when the source of the pain is removed or anesthetized. The chronic pain of trigeminal neuritis, on the other hand, is something else again and usually defies attempts to increase or decrease the intensity of the pain.

If the teeth and the joint appear to be normal, a careful history about past illnesses often reveals a fairly recent illness, which the patient usually describes as a "virus." This resembles an upper respiratory disease, which also involves the region of the temporomandibular joint and the parotid gland. The middle ear might also have been involved. The patient has had swelling in the lateral face and the occlusion disturbed by the shift of the affected condyle. There might also have been decreased salivation. After remission of the acute stage of the disease, the patient may report two or three months of trigeminal neuritis in which the teeth and gingiva, as well as the tissues along the entire facial distribution of the the nerve, may be painful. The pain may be confused with pulpitis or sinusitis or temporomandibular joint pain, but never with trigeminal ***neuralgia.***

Again, care and patience in examination prevent iatrogenic disasters. If the teeth and the joint are found to be normal, the dentist must conclude that something else is causing the trouble. If the distribution of pain accurately follows the divisions of the fifth nerve, one must conclude that ***trigeminal neuritis*** is a strong possibility. The patient should then be referred to a neurologist for complete diagnosis.

Treatment. Any treatment for trigeminal neuritis

should be rendered by a competent physician. Actually the best curative agent is ***time,*** but the patient may be maintained more comfortably during the healing period if analgesics and ataraxic drugs are used. The neurologist should also rule out the possibilities of a neurofibroma or neuroma along the nerve, neoplasia of higher origin, or neoplasia of the maxillary sinus. The dentist should be able to give the patient a "clean bill of health" for the oral cavity.

Herpes Zoster and Postherpetic Neuritis

Patients who develop this syndrome have much the same complaints as patients with trigeminal neuritis. As a matter of fact, Bonica believes that herpes zoster is the most important cause of ***trigeminal neuritis.***[100] The complaint is deep-seated pain, attributable to one division of the fifth nerve. ***The major focus of the pain may be in one tooth.*** Typical herpetic vesiculation may or may not be present and, when present, will follow the course of a nerve.

The pain is constant, quite severe, steady not throbbing, and may be spread over the entire division of the nerve. It may, however, be more severe in some areas than in others. The pain usually does not yield to mild analgesics but necessitates narcotics for relief.

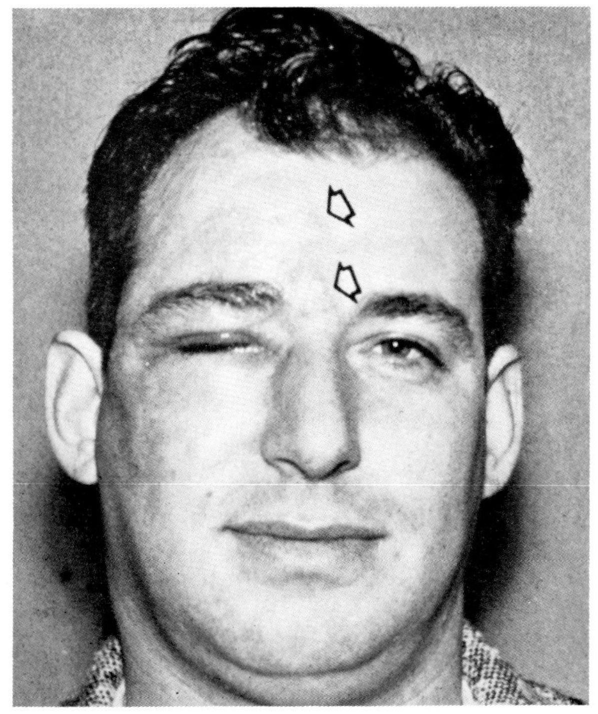

Fig. 11–17. Herpes zoster (shingles) involving first division of trigeminal nerve. Herpetic vesicles *(arrows)* can be seen stopping at midline. Severe pain required morphine potentiated by chlorpromazine for alleviation. Postherpetic neuritis did not develop in this case.

Etiology. The cause of the disease is infection of a sensory ganglion by the herpes zoster virus. The disease continues until the virus is finally controlled by the body defenses.

Examination. If the patient has full-blown herpes zoster and widespread vesiculation, the deep-seated accompanying pain is easy to diagnose (Fig. 11–17). Postherpetic neuritis, on the other hand, may persist or recur some time after the vesicular stage of herpes has healed, often a month or two. If the patient knows he has had severe herpes zoster infection, the diagnosis may well be self-evident. The dentist, however, should carefully check the mouth to ascertain that a severe pulpitis is not superimposed on the condition.

Difficulty in diagnosis arises when the severe vesicular herpetic attack is not manifested, but rather one or two small aphthous ulcers appear in the oral cavity or on the lips or face. The patient with postherpetic neuritis may have difficulty recalling a mild attack one or two months previously.

Patients with this underlying condition may be "certain" that a particular tooth is involved, and that the widespread pain emanates from this tooth. It is up to the dentist to prove to himself and to the patient that this just cannot be true.

Treatment. Postherpetic neuritis is one of the most difficult neurologic conditions to alleviate. The patient with herpes zoster should be under the care of a physician. Nerve block with local anesthetics and stellate ganglion blocks have sometimes proved effective. Although there is no absolute treatment, the disease is self-limiting. Nonetheless the patient may require an extended period of care on analgesics and ataraxics to control the pain.

Atypical Facial Pain

It is often said that the term "atypical facial pain" is a misnomer because the word "atypical" is derived from therapy rather than from pathophysiology. Atypical pain has been named by surgeons who relieve "typical" pain by cutting a nerve. Pain that does not respond to neurectomy, therefore, has become known as "atypical pain." Atypical facial pain does not follow any particular pattern or nerve pathway. "It is a pain that is deep, poorly localized, and vaguely described by the patient. The pain is 'unanatomic' in that it may involve the sensory supply of two or more nerves and may cross the midline. In general this pain is constant and endures for long periods, that is, weeks to years. Trigger zones are lacking." Patients often describe the pain as, "boring, drawing, pressing, pulling, burning, or aching."[102]

Atypical facial pain may be classified under three categories: (1) psychogenic facial pain, (2) dental causalgia and phantom pain, and (3) vasodilating facial pain.

By far the greatest number of these unusual patients are suffering from psychogenic facial pain.

Psychogenic Facial Pain

"Psychogenic pain," according to Bonica, "is pain resulting from the projection of psychic conflicts to some organ without any abnormal activity or tension in the organ to which the pain is referred."[103] The syndrome, states Bonica, is ". . . characterized by the displacement of the pain from the psyche peripherally into the somatic sphere, where it is more tolerable to the ego."

In a study by Rushton, Gibilisco, and Goldstein of 100 patients with ***atypical facial pain*** at the Mayo Clinic, 53% of the patients were classified as suffering from ***psychogenic facial pain.***[104] This group of 53 patients was composed of 46 females and seven males who suffered from depressive reactions, conversion hysteria, or schizophrenia. The ages ranged from 12 years to 70 years with most of the patients in the fourth and fifth decades. The duration of the pain was from one to 36 years.

This interesting study is important to the dental profession for two reasons. First of all, the study brings out the high incidence (53%) of psychotics or psychoneurotics who make up these diagnostic problems, and second, the authors emphasized the unusually high proportion of cases of atypical facial pain that had their ***origin*** in the mouth or followed dental operations.

Rushton, Gibilisco, and Goldstein pointed out that 11 of the 53 psychoneurotic patients in their study ***listed dental operations*** as the beginning of their trouble.[104] The remainder alluded to traumatic blows ("being slapped in the face by my husband") as well as a number of diseases and minor facial operations.

It is frightening to realize that over half the patients with bizarre facial pain syndromes have a functional rather than an organic illness. Fortunately the dental profession sees far fewer patients with functional complaints than does the physician. Because there is no organic reason for the pain does not make the pain any less real to the disturbed patient. It only means that the examiner must be more astute if he is to arrive at a diagnosis, and then recognize that treatment is beyond the usual methods employed in dentistry, or in general medicine for that matter.

The profession must come to realize the psychic importance of the oral cavity, the tremendous value some people place upon their teeth, and the harm that can be done when dental services are forced upon the psychically disturbed patient. The observations of Moulton, a psychiatrist, are succinct in this regard.[105] "Psychiatrists are often shocked at what they consider an appalling lack of psychological insight on the part of the dentist."

"The mouth," says Moulton, "is the earliest area for pleasurable satisfaction, and many adults continue to find their pleasure mainly in its use, as in eating, drinking, smoking, or sexual enjoyment. Pain in this area seems to be especially resented. Often, too, there are specific problems about having the mouth immobilized, because of its use in eating and breathing, and . . . as a primitive weapon of defense . . . used in biting, yelling, and talking back.

"The mouth is also valued highly for its realistic sexual functions and for its use in sexual attraction. It has a special meaning as a sexual symbol, particularly in women, who often fear invasion of the oral cavity, especially by injection needles, and will dramatize this as equivalent to rape. Oral bleeding is frequently used in dreams to refer to rape, menstruation, and abortion. Sexual attraction to the dentist, deep dependency on him, phobic distortions of him, and various other transference problems are about as common as those that develop around the gynecologist and obstetrician . . .

"A tooth may symbolize a person; so its loss means death or abortion. Or again, the loss of a tooth may symbolize some deep anxiety about body injury or loss of power which may or may not be connected with the fear of castration—typical dreams about losing teeth are among the more common anxiety dreams."

Walsh[106] summarizes this approach very well. "It is not sufficiently realized that the mouth is the seat of the most primitive emotions, the first part of the body to win a place in consciousness, and as a result, is often the outlet for the frustrations of adult life. . . . Our mouths are the seat of primitive desires, satisfactions and interests. . . ."

Borland's discussion of these mentally ill people is highly recommended.[107] "Under no circumstances," says Borland, "should a patient ever be told his pains or sensations are imaginary." In addition to Borland, the student is urged to read Engel's outstanding contribution on atypical facial pain.[108] Engel discusses in detail 20 cases (19 female and 1 male) of conversion hysteria with associated facial pain.

Engel found all of the women in the study to be afflicted with dysmenorrhea or sexual problems. This was a similar finding to that of Moulton who states, "These studies seem to point to the mouth as a favorite site for symptoms in women who lack sexual satisfaction. . . ."[105]

Engel's patients described their pain as: "It's like being jabbed with an ice pick," "burning like a red hot coal," "bruised and torn," "like my face is being eaten up."[108] The frequent use of "shooting," "throbbing," "sharp," "nagging," "drawing," "pounding," "aching," "gnawing," "burning," "electricity," "vibration," and "numbness" was also noted.

Engel summarizes, "All the patients were psychologically ill. . . . For the most part, they had all failed to make successful life adjustments. . . . They were a uniformly unhappy and unsatisfied group of people."[108]

In evaluating the patient with psychogenic facial pain, Moulton recognized the striking importance of such precipitating factors as the death of a parent or marital partner upon whom the patient was dependent. She also assigned great importance to exacting perfectionism that covered secret hostility and the inordinate efforts spent by the patient to control and repress strong anger.

More recently mental depression has been suggested as the soil for atypical facial pain. Webb and Lascelles emphasized that people with "depressive illnesses may develop bodily symptoms, and conversely, people with organic diseases tend to become depressed."[109] The authors pointed out that the most common symptoms of depression associated with facial pain are extreme fatigue, lethargy, and irritability. Lascelles stated that these patients are the anxiety depression class, now called unipolar depression, unlike manic depressives, bipolar depression, with a history of at least one episode of mania, loss of appetite, weight and libido along with suicidal behavior.[110] Lascelles, as well as Moulton, was struck with the fact that an unusually high number of the anxiety depressive patients had obsessive, rigid unyielding personality structures ". . . indicated by their overconscientiousness, excessive house-proudness, and a compulsion to check and recheck things they had done." "It may well be," he stated, "that it is this 'obsessive drive' that plays the most prominent part in the persistence of the pain."

Zung described the anxious depressed as "middle-aged and fatigued, with obsessional symptoms and feelings of depersonalization."[111] They are usually hypochondriacs and quite humorless, he said, with "drug dependence, of which alcohol is the most frequent," as well as psychosomatic disorders—headache, asthma, ulcers, muscle pain, and eczema. The most common symptoms, however, are sleep disturbances, a fact also noted by Lascelles.[110]

Gayford, in reviewing atypical facial pain, discusses the obsessional patient and concludes, "The more purely the pain is obsessional, the worse the prognosis."[112] He also makes the rather selfish but realistic observation that the only relief the ***clinician*** "can obtain from such cases, is to hope that the patient will eventually become obsessional about some other region of the body." Gayford noted that some obsessive patients gained relief from their pain by illogical ritual—"two strokes of the buccal mucosa gave considerable relief, but three strokes gave complete relief."

Symptoms. Psychogenic facial pains are mostly deep, constant, and unanatomic pains. Most of the patients are women, and the bizarre symptoms are often matched by the patient's dress or behavior.[113]

Unfortunately, some patients in this group are sincere and well behaved, and they are the ones who lead the dentist on. One patient comes to mind who was addicted to surgery. She was referred for treatment of a pulpless tooth. After an exhaustive and time-consuming examination, done with the patient's complete cooperation, a treatment plan was established and the endodontic procedures were outlined. The patient requested that the work be done "under gas." She was told that no anesthetic of any type would be necessary because the tooth was pulpless. With calm deliberateness the patient outlined the necessity for surgery. Thereupon she proudly described her 11 surgical operations, the last being a tonsillectomy at age 45, which kept her hospitalized for six weeks. She refused endodontic therapy, and her twelfth operation was to have an extraction for the pulpless tooth under gas anesthesia.

Another quite calm patient was referred for the diagnosis of a pain in her palate. Close questioning revealed she had "transferred the pain" to her palate from her tongue, which had previously ached. Finally, amid a flood of tears, the entire story developed.

This 32-year-old woman had had an illegitimate daughter at age sixteen. She, of course, had great feelings of guilt about her daughter's birth, but she assumed a married name and raised her daughter rather than relinquish the child for adoption.

At the age of 12 the daughter developed diabetes mellitus and the mother believed this was a symbol, punishing her through the child. The mother made a martyr of herself caring for the child, and the girl, who had learned of her origins, took unusual delight in taunting the mother. Each day the mother weighed on a gram scale each bite of food the child ate. She also tested the child's urine five or six times each day.

Finally, someone told the mother that if her daughter was "spilling" sugar, her urine would taste sweet. The mother tasted the child's urine and it did taste sweet, but unfortunately the "sweet taste" would not leave her tongue. After a month the "sweet taste" turned into a burning sensation of the tongue and the burning finally became an ache. She "transferred" part of the ache to her palate by pressing her tongue firmly against the palate. At the time this patient came for treatment she had had three maxillary molars extracted to relieve the palatal pain—"surgically destructive treatment" for the patient's neurosis.

Psychiatric consultation revealed the patient's immature personality, deep guilt complex, and obsession.*

Engel had exactly this type of case in mind when he stated, "Aside from the pain in the face and elsewhere, they had long histories of many illnesses, injuries, operations, as well as all sorts of failures, defeats, humiliations, and misfortunes. . . . It became abundantly clear that these patients had a strong unconscious need to suffer. Over and over again they provoked the situations which led to their punishment, failure, or humiliation. . . . In many, a diagnosis of psychic masochism appears justified."[108]

Another woman presented herself for diagnosis and treatment for palatal pain. She had had all of her maxillary teeth extracted except the left canine. For four years she and her husband had been traveling around the nation visiting dentists, physicians, and famous clinics seeking diagnosis. Her pain had started on her face, had spread to her buccal gingiva, into her palate, and across the midline to the other side of her palate.

After a thorough history and examination it was obvious the woman was "psychoneurotic" and she was referred to a psychiatrist in the guise of a neurologist. The psychiatrist confirmed the patient's paranoid state.

When the husband was confronted with the news of his wife's illness he began to weep, and confessed he had been told four years previously his wife was insane. It was the husband who could not face the fact of his wife's illness, and it was he who had been taking her around the nation seeking relief for her functional complaint. The facial pain which initiated the syndrome had originally developed when he slapped his wife's face four years before.*

In relating psychogenic facial pain to unipolar depression, Gayford details a case history in which a 56-year-old housewife developed right maxillary pain following a dental "clearance" (full mouth extractions).[112] "Subsequently she was unable to wear the denture and an alveolectomy was performed on the right maxillary ridge." She was also "seen by a neurosurgeon who avulsed the right infraorbital nerve." The pain persisted. The patient refused psychiatric therapy and became "housebound" because of her pain and her appearance without her dentures.

Boracchia and Boracchia described an interesting case history of a 51-year-old white female who first presented herself to the dentist with pain in the left mandible that had persisted since a bridge was placed six months previously.[114] The pain, described as a burning sensation, began each evening at 6:00 p.m. when the patient was returning home from work. As seen in the roentgenograms (Fig. 11–18*A*), the patient avoided brushing the lower left arch or even eating on that side. Pulp testing with cold proved to be mildly painful on the crowned teeth. Pulp pain could also be started with touch at the gingival and from acidic substances as well.

Finally, the patient became so insistent about the abutment teeth that the dentist (C. B.) devitalized the pulps, performed root canal therapy, and remade the bridge (Fig. 11–18*B*). In spite of the pulp removal, excruciating pain persisted in the teeth. At this point,

*Psychiatric therapy gave the patient an insight into her problem and the pain finally disappeared; however, she reappeared as a patient years later after having married an alcoholic. This time she was suffering from bilateral myofascial pain-dysfunction syndrome.

*Six months of psychiatric therapy relieved the woman of her symptoms and started her toward recovery.

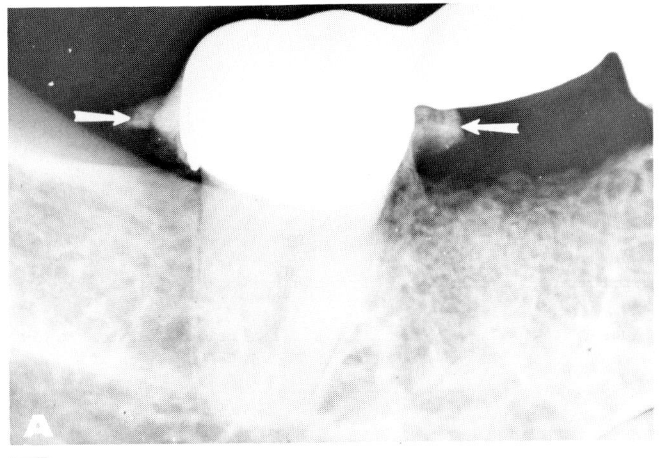

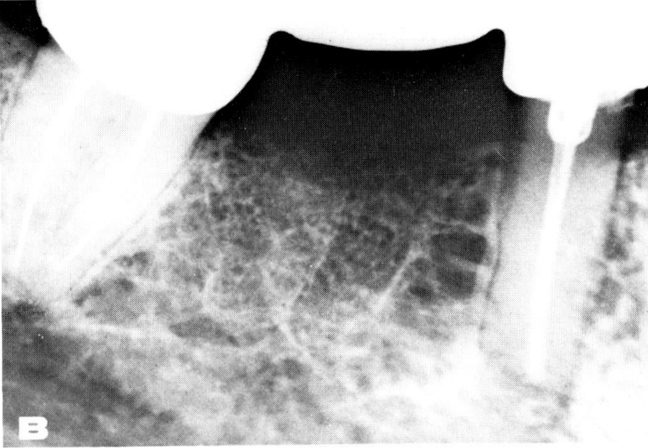

Fig. 11–18. *A,* Left mandible of patient with anxiety depression obsessed of pain in this region. She avoided brushing and eating on this side. *B,* Patient was so insistent about excruciating pain that abutment teeth were endodontically treated. Unfortunately, pain continued. (Courtesy Dr. Carlos Boracchia, Toronto, Ontario.)

the patient was referred to the psychiatrist (M. B. B.) for evaluation and possible treatment.

Examination. The majority of the dentist's time examining the patient suspected of psychogenic pain is spent in history taking, before the oral examination is even approached. The dentist is usually warned well ahead of time that this is a difficult case, either by the referring dentist or by a challenge from the patient.

The questioner should allow the patient to ramble in her responses, and by so doing, reveal a good deal of her personality. Is she too eager? Is she hostile? Does she know all the technical words? Does she sound like a phonograph record having told the story over and over? Can you lead her on to describe pain, sensations, and locations you might suggest? And most important of all, can you, by questioning, "lead" the pain across the midline? ***Anatomically, pain cannot cross the midline.*** If the patient can be led into describing the pain as crossing the midline, the examiner should be suspicious, although Harris has described a case of referred pain from a right mandibular incisor to a left mandibular first molar.[115]

The dental examination should still be most exacting, for the psychoneurotic individual can be suffering from dental as well as mental disease. It is only when the entire dental examination checks out as normal that the dentist has a right to be suspicious of the psychogenic background of the pain.

In order to determine the degree to which a patient is depressed, Boracchia (M. B. B.), a psychiatrist, has suggested that the dentist administer to the patient the Zung Self-Rating Depression Scale (SDS).[114] The SD Scale readily lends itself to use in general practice to uncover the depth of depression in the so-called "hidden depression." Testing and scoring patients usually requires less than five minutes.

The Zung Self-Rating Depression Scale* (Table 11–4) is made up of twenty items—ten worded symptomatically positive and ten symptomatically negative.[116] The diagnostic criteria of the SDS are comprised of the most common characteristics of depression. The patient is asked by the dentist to answer the questions, "In order that I may learn more about you to help me in making a diagnosis." The patient rates the items in quantitative terms—as to how they applied to him at the time of testing—"none or a little of the time, some of the time, a good part of the time, or most or all of the time." Out of sight of the patient, the doctor then scores the replies using a transparent overlay sheet (Table 11–5). From a table attached to the SDS booklet, the "raw score" is converted to the SDS Index which ranges from 25 to 100 (see p. 535). The patient's final SDS Index then serves to determine the state of the patient's mental health—a basis for the decision to refer or not to refer the patient to a psychiatrist or psychologist for a more detailed and professional evaluation.

Using the Self-Rating Depression Scale, Zung demonstrated that 74 was the mean SDS Index for patients diagnosed with depressive disorders (ranging from 63 to 90 on the scale of 25 to 100), whereas

*The Zung Self-Rating Depression Scale, in booklet form with transparent scoring key, may be obtained free of charge by writing Merrell National Laboratories, Cincinnati, Ohio 45215.

Table 11-4. Zung Self-Rating Depression Scale (SDS)

	None or a Little of the Time	*Some of the Time*	*Good Part of the Time*	*Most or All of the Time*
1. I feel down-hearted and blue				
2. Morning is when I feel the best				
3. I have crying spells or feel like it				
4. I have trouble sleeping through the night				
5. I eat as much as I used to				
6. I enjoy looking at, talking to, and being with attractive women/men				
7. I notice that I am losing weight				
8. I have trouble with constipation				
9. My heart beats faster than usual				
10. I get tired for no reason				
11. My mind is as clear as it used to be				
12. I find it easy to do the things I used to				
13. I am restless and can't keep still				
14. I feel hopeful about the future				
15. I am more irritable than usual				
16. I find it easy to make decisions				
17. I feel that I am useful and needed				
18. My life is pretty full				
19. I feel that others would be better off if I were dead				
20. I still enjoy the things I used to do				

Table 11-5. SDS Scoring Key

	None or a Little of the Time	*Some of the Time*	*Good Part of the Time*	*Most or All of the Time*
1. I feel down-hearted and blue	1	2	3	4
2. Morning is when I feel the best	4	3	2	1
3. I have crying spells or feel like it	1	2	3	4
4. I have trouble sleeping through the night	1	2	3	4
5. I eat as much as I used to	4	3	2	1
6. I enjoy looking at, talking to, and being with attractive women/men	4	3	2	1
7. I notice that I am losing weight	1	2	3	4
8. I have trouble with constipation	1	2	3	4
9. My heart beats faster than usual	1	2	3	4
10. I get tired for no reason	1	2	3	4
11. My mind is as clear as it used to be	4	3	2	1
12. I find it easy to do the things I used to	4	3	2	1
13. I am restless and can't keep still	1	2	3	4
14. I feel hopeful about the future	4	3	2	1
15. I am more irritable than usual	1	2	3	4
16. I find it easy to make decisions	4	3	2	1
17. I feel that I am useful and needed	4	3	2	1
18. My life is pretty full	4	3	2	1
19. I feel that others would be better off if I were dead	1	2	3	4
20. I still enjoy the things I used to do	4	3	2	1

Numbers on key are compared with spaces checked by patient on the SDS form. Twenty numbers are then totaled, divided by maximum possible score of 80, converted to decimal, and multiplied by 100 to form index. (Copyrighted, W. Zung, 1974.)

the mean SDS Index for a control group of emotional normals was 33 (range 25 to 43).[116] In between was a group of patients ***initially*** diagnosed as "depressive disorder" who were found to have ***other*** emotional disorders. Their SDS Index was 53 (range 38 to 71) and Zung concluded that symptoms of depression also make up a significant portion of the symptoms of other emotional conditions. He further found the cardinal symptom of depression is sleep disorder, followed by fatigue and decreased appetite. Well down the list were weight loss, decreased libido or suicidal rumination.

In later evaluation of the SD Scale, and using an SDS Index number of 50 as "sick," Zung was able to determine that 360 patients diagnosed as depressed were correctly diagnosed 88% of the time, whereas only 12% were misdiagnosed as "normal."[117] Conversely, he found that 12% of 1108 normal controls would have been diagnosed as "depressed," whereas 88% were found to be emotionally normal. This places the Zung Self-Rating Depression Scale well within the range of acceptance for dentists concerned about their patients' state of mental depression.

In their initial article relating atypical facial pain to depression, Webb and Lascelles described a 60-year-old male kitchen worker with a nine-year history of severe facial pain limited to the second and third divisions of the fifth cranial nerve on the right side.[109] The pain consisted of severe agonizing spasms brought on by chewing and shaving (reminiscent of trigeminal neuralgia), but with an overlay of a ***constant*** burning pain. The patient complained of awakening each day at about 3:00 a.m. and feeling much worse in the mornings than in the evenings (a typical complaint of depression). The patient had had seven teeth removed in unsuccessful attempts to relieve his symptoms.

Another case described by Webb and Lascelles, that of a female with severe pain lasting more than two years, also complained of waking early in the morning, but feeling better in the evening.[109] Her pain was a "severe burning sensation, which started in her left upper lip, spread to involve her nose and the roof of her mouth, and then spread over her head and down her neck."

These cases, along with those previously described by Gayford[112] and the Boracchias[114] hold many clues to the diagnosis of atypical facial pain. Gayford pointed out that the anxiety depression of his patient (three years of pain following a dental "clearance") actually began one year prior to the dental surgery when her husband retired and they moved to a new "area she did not like, away from her friends and relations." The Boracchias' female patient, with the 6:00 p.m. throbbing and burning pain associated with a bridge, had many of the signs of depression—poor sleep and appetite, generalized anxiety and fear, obsession, and constipation.

Boracchia described this patient as extremely anxious, fidgetting and smiling for no reason. She also had an obsessive fear of malignancy and death, while at the same time questioning her own self-worth and "being a female." After two months of psychotherapy, the patient had revealed psychologic material "painful to her." Within the past four years her father had died of cancer of the cecum, her mother of cancer of the stomach, and a brother of leukemia. Although she had guilt feelings for not mourning the loss of her "loved ones," she paradoxically was angry over their loss to her. Her childhood "death wish" for her parents magnified her feelings of guilt and played upon her obsession that punishment, in the form of cancer and death, might be wreaked upon her. Evidently, while working during the day, the patient did not dwell on these thoughts. But after work each evening, returning home, the thoughts and the jaw pain would return.

The cases just described fit very well into the category of the "stressful life events" shown by Holmes and Masuda to play an "important causative role in the natural history of many diseases."[118] Depression and psychogenic facial pain are just such conditions that will follow traumatic life situations. Using some of the stressful or crisis life events denoted by Meyer, Holmes and Rahe developed a questionnaire made up of 43 life events that were empirically derived from clinical experience.[119] This was known as The Social Readjustment Rating Scale (SRRS) (Table 11–6). Using "marriage" as a standard, the patient was asked to rate the series of life events according to their relative degree of necessary readjustment—"Does this event require more or less readjustment than marriage?" From these findings a SRRS profile, measured in Life-Change Units (LCU), was established for each subject.

Plotted against the LCU for a group of 88 subjects, Holmes superimposed a record of health changes experienced by the subjects over the previous ten years. With subjects who had ***major*** life crises, 79% also experienced health changes. Among subjects with ***moderate*** life crises, 51% experienced health changes. Of those with ***mild*** crises, only 37% had

Table 11-6. Social Readjustment Rating Scale

Rank	*Life event*	*Mean value*
1	Death of spouse	100
2	Divorce	73
3	Marital separation	65
4	Jail term	63
5	Death of close family member	63
6	Personal injury or illness	53
7	Marriage	50
8	Fired at work	47
9	Marital reconciliation	45
10	Retirement	45
11	Change in health of family member	44
12	Pregnancy	40
13	Sex difficulties	39
14	Gain of new family member	39
15	Business readjustment	39
16	Change in financial state	38
17	Death of close friend	37
18	Change to different line of work	36
19	Change in number of arguments with spouse	35
20	Mortgage over $10,000	31
21	Foreclosure of mortgage or loan	30
22	Change in responsibilities at work	29
23	Son or daughter leaving home	29
24	Trouble with in-laws	29
25	Outstanding personal achievement	28
26	Wife begin or stop work	26
27	Begin or end school	26
28	Change in living conditions	25
29	Revision of personal habits	24
30	Trouble with boss	23
31	Change in work hours or conditions	20
32	Change in residence	20
33	Change in schools	20
34	Change in recreation	19
35	Change in church activities	19
36	Change in social activities	18
37	Mortgage or loan less than $10,000	17
38	Change in sleeping habits	16
39	Change in number of family get-togethers	15
40	Change in eating habits	15
41	Vacation	13
42	Christmas	12
43	Minor violations of the law	11

Rank order of social readjustment emphasizes *major* life crises and *mild* life crises. Seventy-nine per cent of the former are apt to cause health changes, whereas only 37 per cent of latter experience changes within year. (From Holmes, T. H., and Rahe, R. H.: J. Psychosomat. Res., *11*:213, 1967.)

health changes. On the average, the health changes followed a life crisis by about one year.

In examining Holmes' evidence (Table 11–6), one cannot help but be struck by the impact upon mental or even physical health brought about by the death of a spouse or a close family member or friend, or divorce or separation or even marriages, not to mention being jailed or fired or retired. These could often be the precipitating factors in the latent development of atypical facial pain. The importance of developing this type of information while taking a patient's history cannot be overemphasized.

In discussing history-taking from these patients, Wilson has stated, "It is 'agony' for her to speak, yet she talks with ease almost without ceasing. She is suffering 'death' but she is the picture of health."[120] He goes on to describe a 36-year-old female with the obsession of a "sweet" taste which she felt flowing down the left upper incisors. With this she experienced a deep drawing sensation extending into the palate. Wilson was struck by the fact that this slight complaint had completely upset the patient's life as she searched for a cure. She was agitated and unable to rest.

The patient had graduated from a night law school and entered the bar. "She had immediately been given a case and had been developing it successfully, when this sweet secretion developed, upsetting her to such an extent she was forced to give up not only her case but her practice of law." Only after several weeks in a sanatorium was she persuaded of her obsession, and the "sweet" and the pain disappeared.

Wilson described another woman with severe facial pain that was constant and deep and was intensified by a breeze or by her perspiring. The patient "stated that it caused her the utmost agony" yet she was conducting a big business and was a successful aviatrix. Roentgenograms showed many pulp stones which she had been advised to have removed. It was then discovered that about eight years previously, at the time the pain had started, she and her husband had worked 'the old badger game' on a wealthy and prominent citizen. The remuneration from this had started her business, and although she apparently went about unconcerned, this pain had developed. "The discussion of the episode brought on a severe reaction in the face." After confessing her guilt she "remained free from pain until she had one of her teeth removed."

In taking a case history, if the dentist unfolds the sometimes bizarre but often rather ordinary signs and symptoms discussed here, or determines through the use of a device such as the Zung Self-Rating Depression Scale that the patient is in need of more profound evaluation, then the patient should be referred to a physician or clinical psychologist.

The first medical referral should probably be to a neurologist who can rule out any nerve involvements at a higher level. The neurologist in turn usually is more successful in referring the patient to a psychiatrist. The great American middle class still strongly resists psychiatric care, and dental references frequently are not followed.

Treatment. Patients with psychogenic facial pain need treatment just as much as patients suffering pain from organic sources. Unfortunately, psychic treatment is frequently less successful than the direct surgical or medical therapy used to relieve inflammatory or neurologic pain. For most cases of pain of psychogenic origin, the only course of treatment is psychotherapy. Although it is not within the province of the dentist to institute this therapy, it is his responsibility to know what might be done for his patient and what the prognosis might be.

Fortunately for those cases of psychogenic pain related to depressive illness, great strides have been made with antidepressant drugs, relieving the depression and psychic pain. Lascelles reported on the treatment of 53 patients with psychogenic facial pain, 31 who had previously undergone dental treatment in seeking relief.[110] Thirty-six of the patients were female and 17 male. The most typically descriptive phrase of the patients was, "a deep dull severe ache—unbearable at times." All the patients had depressive symptoms with sleep disturbance (insomnia), general fatigue, irritability, and agitation the most common symptoms—typical of unipolar depression. They also had strong obsessive personalities.

"In the majority of instances," said Lascelles, "the anti-depressant drug phenelzine (Nardil)—together with chlordiazepoxide hydrochloride (Librium) was found adequate for the relief of depression." In some cases imipramine (Tofranil) was substituted for phenelzine. The drug amitryptyline (Elavil) has also been used.

The beneficial effects of the drugs were usually not evident until seven to ten days after the start of treatment. It was also considered essential to give a four-week trial on medication to all patients. If successful, treatment at full dosage was continued for two months and then gradually reduced. The follow-up period lasted seven months. Drug side effects were rare.

Of 53 depressive patients with facial pain, "complete relief" was gained in 55% of the patients, with "significant relief" for an additional 20%. "No relief" or "slight relief" obtained for the remaining 25% of the patients. Those who responded most favorably to the anti-depressant drugs tended to have good previous personalities, the shortest case histories, and to have been "obsessive" in nature. It is interesting to note that four of the patients stopped their therapy when they became symptom-free, and in all four cases, the pain returned within 48 hours.

Lascelles also did a double-blind control study with 40 patients—half on phenelzine and half on placebo.[110] The anti-depressant proved far superior to the placebo in relieving psychogenic facial pain along with depression. He concluded by observing, "The results of treatment for these patients, directed not at their pain but at their underlying depressive illness, show quite clearly the value of taking time to uncover the depressive symptoms by careful inquiry."

The monoamine oxidase (MAO) inhibitors, such as phenelzine (Nardil), exhibit a number of adverse effects and should be used with caution and only under the guidance of an astute and careful physician. The tricyclics, such as imipramine (Tofranil), are recommended by MEDICAL LETTER as the anti-depressants of choice.[121]

Sternbach has pointed out that the anti-depressant drugs have much more value in these cases than the anti-anxiety agents. "Recent biochemical studies," said Sternbach, "suggest that pain and depression may have common metabolic pathways. Supplying a patient with some of the neuroamines that are depleted by serotonin during depression sometimes relieves both his depression and his pain."[6]

Dental Causalgia and Phantom Pain

Causalgia is a rare baffling type of pain seen in approximately 2.5% of peripheral nerve injury cases. ***Dental causalgia,*** though rare, is known to occur as a post-extraction (amputation) phenomenon. Bonica states that causalgia is pre-eminently a result of penetrating wounds, usually due to high velocity missiles.[122] He believes it to be primarily caused by a "stretch" injury of peripheral nerves. It also is frequently an unwelcome sequela of amputation.

Although causalgia is not synonymous with phantom limb, it is frequently associated with this bizarre phenomenon in which the amputee experiences the paradoxical sensation that the amputated member is still in place and is painful.

Elfenbaum postulated an interesting theory for ***dental causalgia*** when he stated "All the patients complain of a peculiar pain pattern in a definite edentulous spot, where a difficult dental extraction has been performed.[123] They tell of the dentist having had an unusual amount of trouble, of lengthy operations, fractured roots that had to be dug out or drilled out, and bone that was hammered or chiseled. Their own apprehension and agonizing experience and, of course, mistrust of the dentist's ability are also part of the history."

Symptoms. The word causalgia means "burning pain" and this is exactly the type of pain experienced by these victims, a "peculiar, nagging, persistent, postextraction pain,"[124] "characterized by constant, spontaneous, often severe burning."[125] Asked to point to the area of the pain, the patient inevitably indicates a ***postextraction area,*** usually a molar, and is adamant in claiming that the pain originates from this region, even though long since healed.

The pain of dental causalgia may begin gradually, often when the patient arises, only to build in intensity as the day with its tensions mounts. One male patient seen by me said the initial morning sensation was that of a piece of chewing gum on the buccal ridge where a maxillary first molar had been extracted two years previously. By the end of the day the pain was of such intensity that it was "beyond the control of codeine." Each night (he admitted sleeping through the night) the severe pain disappeared during sleep, and the next morning the "chewing gum sensation" was again in place. This syndrome had been continuous for two years following extraction. The patient, who was a foreman of an automobile body shop, recognized that the pain increased as his daily tensions increased, while he worked at a job he disliked. The patient was later found to be mildly paranoid.

Etiology. The true etiology of dental causalgia is still unknown. Some theories have arisen, however, concerning the cause of phantom limb pain or causalgia in general. Bonica believes that following amputation of a limb the muscles, bones, and blood vessels in the stump area atrophy, but the nerves continue to grow.[125] These nerves may coil upon themselves, producing a globular mass of nerve tissue called a neuroma. Agnew (Fig. 11–19) has described just such a case, as have Robinson and Slavkin[126,127]—

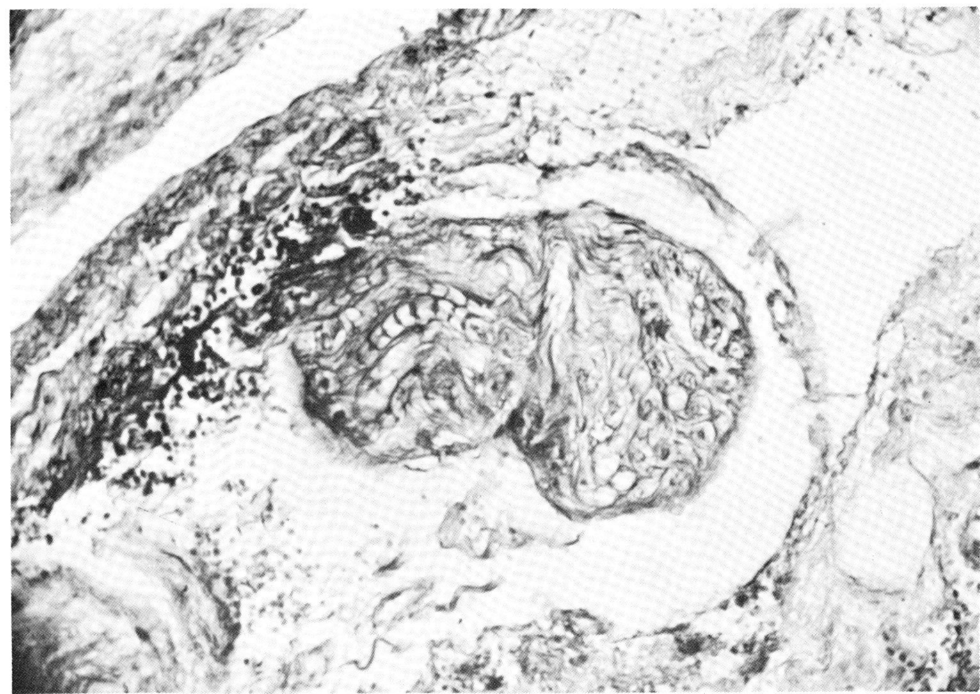

Fig. 11–19. Amputation neuroma revealed by biopsy. Strikingly clearcut, tangled, and well-myelinated fibers, cut at various angles, are massed with irregular sheath and perineural connective tissue into abnormal aggregate of varying size and surrounded by well-vascularized fibrous tissue. Biopsy was occasioned by sharp, intermittent pricking "nerve pain," six months in duration, becoming more diffuse and steady. (Courtesy Dr. R. Gordon Agnew.)

continuous postextraction pain in the anterior palate which, when biopsied, revealed a neuroma.[126] Bonica continues, "The neuroma consists of a branching mass of Schwann cells containing an aggregation of whorled wavy axones embedded in scar tissue."[128] The pressure from the scar might well lead to an anoxic nerve which fires repetitive afferent discharges.

That a neuroma is not always responsible for causalgia is evidenced by the fact that re-operation of the involved area seldom affords relief. Bonica summarizes a discussion on the subject by stating, "Phantom pain epitomized ***Gestalt pain,*** which is the midway point between purely organic and purely psychogenic pain."[129] Psychogenic overlay is also commonplace in causalgic cases.

Elfenbaum, in a succinct review of over 30 cases of dental causalgia (males and females, 36 to 74 years of age) had this to say of his patients: "All patients admit that the syndrome becomes intensified under emotional stress.[123] During the recitation of the symptoms some patients become emotional, and the sharp pain is initiated. Occasionally it is induced when the examiner purposely directs the conversation to some injustice at the person's place of employment or to some disharmony in the family, or when the examiner describes it to someone within the patient's hearing." Elfenbaum went on to say, "Their impatience and irascibility may be among the reasons for their being called crabs and psychopaths by the dentists and physicians who have dismissed them. Medical records of some of the patients show them to be addicts to polysurgery."

Bonica carries this further when he states, "Most of these patients were found to be psychoneurotic. . . . This phenomenon not infrequently occurs following amputation of a breast, an ear, the nose, the penis or a tooth.[130]

"Most . . . patients have fantasied concern over the disposal of the amputated part and cannot bear the idea of their hand or leg or breast being dumped unceremoniously into a garbage can or handled with disrespect."

How frequently the dentist is surprised by the adult patient who demonstrates a morbid interest in his extracted tooth and even asks to take it home with him. One is again reminded of the statement by Moulton, when she writes of the many patients who look upon extraction as a form of amputation or castration.[131]

Facing the act of traumatic extraction in this light, is it any wonder that some patients might well react violently to oral "amputation," possibly magnifying the constant subliminal afferent nerve discharge into a constant, nagging, burning pain?[132] Bonica quotes Cooper and Braceland to the effect that, "The well-integrated adaptive individual can divert his attention from a toothache (or full urinary bladder) if the peripheral stimulus is not physically overpowering."[133] Quite possibly the causalgic victim ***cannot*** divert his attention even from what would be subliminal impulses for most people.

Behrman has also discussed 10 cases of dental causalgia and stated that it occurs only following the extraction of a molar and then only rarely.[134] Elfenbaum has seen the condition occur after the extraction of maxillary first molars as well as maxillary anterior teeth (especially the canines) and mandibular premolars.[135] Rushton, Gibilisco and Goldstein at the Mayo Clinic listed three cases of "postextraction causalgia of the mandibular nerve."[136] We have seen four cases: three males who had maxillary first molars extracted and a very hostile female who had a maxillary first premolar extracted.

Examination. The history and examination leading to a diagnosis of ***dental causalgia*** can be quite frustrating for the dentist. Actually, nothing in a physical sense may be learned by the examination except that the patient has a sensitive area where a tooth was extracted which remains painful. The clue that usually leads to a diagnosis of causalgia or phantom pain lies in the history—the patient's insistence that the primary incident was a traumatic extraction, and his further insistence that the tooth that was extracted still aches.

One should evaluate his patient emotionally. What is the level of his emotional stability? Does he enter into a harangue against the dentist who extracted the tooth? Does he demonstrate a total lack of confidence in this man? How long and varied is his medical-dental history? Has he seen "everyone" about his condition? How does he get along at home, on the job? "The patient who has the pain is to be considered as much as the pain which the patient has."[135]

The examiner would also be advised to question the patient about his concern over losing the tooth. Is his oral image such that he hated losing the tooth and feels as though a beloved part of his body has been "savagely ripped away"?

One must not fall into the trap of immediately suspecting all bizarre pain as causalgic. It is obviously important to rule out all the other more common pain possibilities, such as a tooth in the area with pulpitis, maxillary sinusitis, trigeminal neuritis, postherpetic neuralgia, neuroma, or true neoplasia affecting the fifth nerve. Full-mouth roentgenograms are important, and referral to a rhinologist may be necessary to rule out nasal or paranasal disease. Consultation by a neurologist is inevitable when causalgia is suspected.

Treatment. No true treatment has been suggested for dental causalgia. All the authors are quite pessimistic on the subject. Elfenbaum gave the following excellent advice, however.[137] "Like advising one to lock the barn door after the horse has been stolen, it might appear redundant to say that the best treatment for causalgia is prevention." He went on to say that traumatic exodontia should be widely avoided, especially if the patient's temperament seems to be rooted in "hysterical soil."

For the present sufferer, there is no substitute for teaching the patient how to help himself. Perhaps he can be convinced that the pain is not the only disturbing factor in his life. He should be made aware of the circumstances that trigger and aggravate the pain, and shown how to avoid those situations that are the lifeblood of an anxiety neurosis. Bonica points out psychotherapy, analgesic block (primarily sympathetic block), and surgery as the three possible forms of treatment.[138] The destructive surgical approach is not suggested, but a careful surgical search for neuromas may be indicated.

Hutchins and Reynolds found they could "break up" by analgesic nerve block the hyperirritability of dental innervation produced by a previously painful stimulation.[139] Quite possibly, repeated therapeutic use of this technique might help the victim of causalgia. In any case, the patient probably has to live with the pain the remainder of his life. Analgesics synergistically administered with medium-acting ataraxics might help.

Vasodilating Facial Pain

In the study by Rushton, Gibilisco, and Goldstein referred to previously, *eight* of the 100 patients in the study were suffering from ***vasodilating facial pain.***[136] The tragic aspect of this group lay in misdiagnosis, for six of the patients had arrived at the Mayo Clinic with a misdiagnosis of trigeminal neuralgia. Moreover, six of the eight patients had had various surgical operations to relieve the pain, including tooth extractions, nose and nasal sinus operations, alcohol injections of the fifth nerve, avulsion of the fifth nerve, and decompression of the gasserian ganglion. One patient had undergone ten separate operations to relieve the pain.

Because of the baffling nature and rarity of this syndrome, the dentist may be called upon by a physician to examine these patients. The physician has every right to suspect pulp disease because of the location of the maximal pain in the lower face with pain referred to the molar teeth, and the paroxysmal nature of the attack. The pain quite resembles the far more common pain of advanced acute pulpalgia and, to complicate matters, is frequently nocturnal, as is pulpalgia.

There are a number of similar complex syndromes described over the years that would appear to be much alike in nature. Sphenopalatine neuralgia or Sluder's syndrome, for example, was first discussed in 1908.[140] Conditions since described as histamine headache, cluster headache, and periodic migrainous neuralgia would all seem to be much the same in symptomatology and treatment.[141]

Symptoms. The symptom common to this group of conditions can best be described as a ***unilateral,*** paroxysmal, lower half or lower face headache. The pains are often migrainous in character with flushing and lacrimation of the affected side of the face. Gastrointestinal upset is also a common symptom.

The pain frequently arises at night, an hour or two after retiring. The initial attack may terminate within a 24-hour period. The attacks may last for days or weeks and then mysteriously show remission for weeks or years. Often the initial attack is precipitated by some tensional or emotional disturbance. These conditions are not to be confused with temporal arteritis, which is a higher and more constant pain also due to vasodilation.

Etiology. There is evidence that vasodilating facial pain is a variant of the migraine symptoms complex. Many patients with this facial pain either have migraine or have near relatives with migraine.[141]

Wolff has shown that these headaches or facial pains are due to vasodilation of branches of the external carotid artery, particularly the internal maxillary brach.[142] The pain is produced, says Wolff, not by increased vascular pressure in the area, but rather by increased "traction" or pull on the sensory nerves that ***accompany*** the dilated vessels. Associated spasm of skeletal muscles of the head and neck accounts for the widespread character of the pain into the neck and shoulders. Wolff also points out that the attacks "occur in situations inducing exhaustion, tension, desperation, and frustration. . . ."

This etiology is borne out by a most interesting case, diagnosed by hindsight as vasodilating facial pain. The patient, a colleague, was experiencing repetitive pain, deep in the gingiva, buccal to the mandibular left second molar which was involved with initial periodontal disease. When the pain was present, probing into the involved furca area intensified the pain. At the urging of the patient, periodontal surgery was performed in the area, exposing the furca for better oral hygiene. The operation was minor in nature and uneventful, but when the anesthetic wore off, the patient returned in tears, complaining of the severity of the pain. The intensity and throbbing character of the pain were far out of proportion to the minor surgery. Reinjection of the area afforded some immediate relief, but the patient had to be given morphine for a week to control the severe intermittent pain. After ten days the surgical area was well granulated and the pain could be controlled by codeine.

On the eleventh postoperative day, at 2 a.m., the patient called to say the area was bleeding. Examination revealed hemorrhage from the entire granulation bed and a return of the severe pain. The bleeding was arrested with 2% racemic epinephrine, and the patient was dismissed with some sponges and a bottle of epinephrine. The pain did not subside.

At 4 a.m. the patient called again to say the hemorrhage was greater than ever and the pain was constant. This time the patient was hospitalized. Bleeding and clotting time tests proved to be normal. For three hours, every method to stop the hemorrhage was unsuccessful. Finally at 7 a.m. another colleague was called to assist in suturing the granular bed to the periosteum. This arrested the hemorrhage.

The patient then announced he was violently ill with gastrointestinal cramps. He became ashen in appearance and finally vomited a copious amount of swallowed blood. By this time the chiefs of medicine and anesthesiology had been called in consultation. The severe gastric storm continued for another hour until finally the patient announced, "I'm going to have a migraine. Get my ergotamine." After five

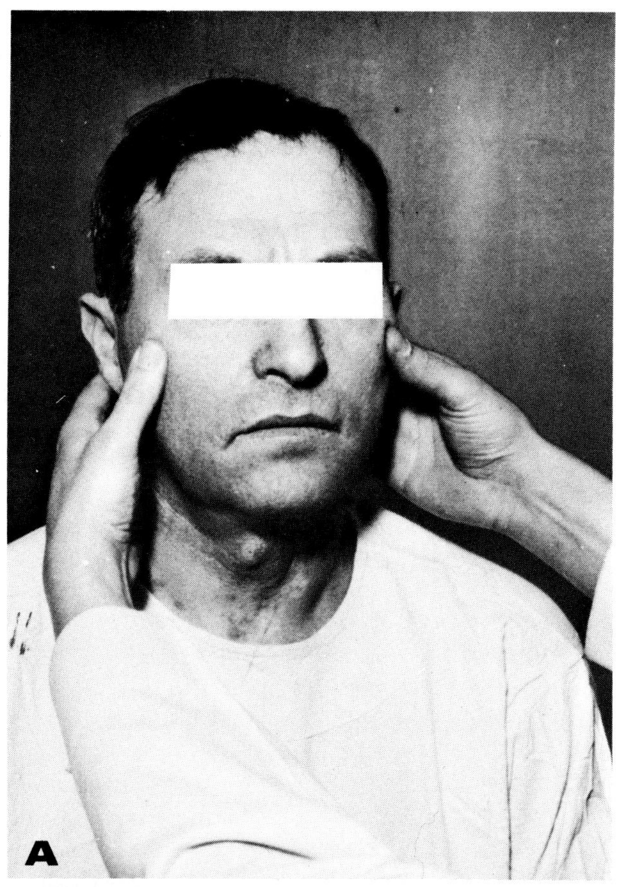

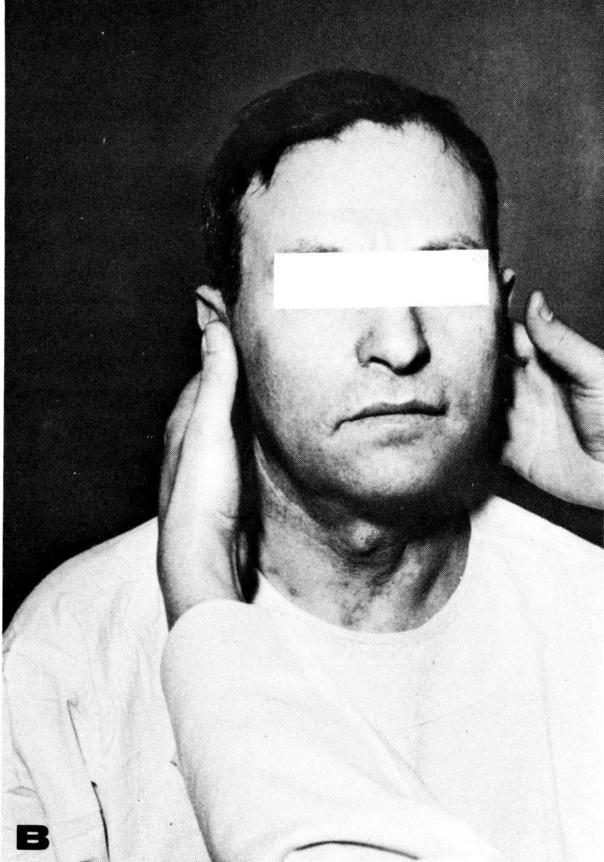

Fig. 11–20. Procedure to differentiate true headache from "functional" type. *A,* Pressure is made with both thumbs against malar area for ten seconds and patient is asked, "Now, what has happened to your pain?" *B,* After patient answers, thumb pressure is suddenly released and question repeated. (From Scott, M.: J.A.M.A., *212*:1214, May 18, 1970.)

hours the severe headache passed and all the oral pain and bleeding ceased as well. Questioning ***after*** the incident revealed that the patient had suffered migraine for years and that he had previously had similar facial pain, but it had not localized in the oral cavity.

In a *post hoc* review of the case, the conclusion was drawn by the principals involved that the intermittent gingival pain was referred vasodilating facial pain, and that the stress of the operation increased the postoperative discomfort. The extensive hemorrhage was due to the vasodilation of the branches of the internal maxillary artery, which grossly increased blood flow to the region, enough so that bleeding developed from the bed of granulation tissue. The final migrainous storm was only the climax of two weeks of suffering the complex syndrome.

Differential diagnosis of vasodilating facial pain may be assisted through the use of a vasoconstrictor. The patient is given a prescription of ergotamine tartrate in sublingual tablet form (Ergomar, 2.0 mg., Cooper) and instructed to place one tablet beneath the tongue as soon as the prodromal symptoms appear. If the usual attack is aborted by the vasoconstrictor, this is good evidence that the condition is caused by vasodilation, and the diagnosis is confirmed. The patient should then be referred to a physician for treatment.

Ergotamine may cause some side effects such as nausea, leg pains, or even precordial distress and pain. Any vasoconstrictor, such as ergotamine, is ***contraindicated*** for any patient with coronary artery disease, suspected arteriosclerosis, hypertension, or pregnancy. Eggleston has also suggested methysergide (Sansert Sandoz), an antiserotonin agent, as synergistic with ergotamine.[143] In addition, inhalation of aerosol epinephrine (3 to 6 inhalations, 10 to 15 minutes apart) has been reported as an effective means of breaking the cyclic pattern of the headache.[144]

Scott has recommended a "simple procedure helpful in differentiating true headache from that of the 'functional' type" or malingering type.[145] "Steady firm pressure is made against both malar bones for ten seconds (Fig. 11–20*A*). The patient is asked during the application, 'What has happened to your pain?' Following the patient's answer, the pressure is suddenly released by dramatically removing the examiner's fingers from the malar area (Fig. 11–20*B*). The patient is again asked, 'Now, what has happened to your pain?' " The emphasis must be placed firmly and dramatically on the NOW.

If the patient has a true headache, he will answer that nothing has happened, or that it "felt better (or worse) when you pressed." However, if the headache is psychogenic or malingering, in most instances, the patient will report complete or marked relief when pressure is applied and sudden return of pain when pressure is released. Repeat trials should give the same results.

Treatment. Treatment of this syndrome is outside the province of dental practice. Satisfactory control may be maintained, however, with self-administered injections of ergotamine tartrate, used whenever the prodromal symptoms appear.

Another form of therapy is desensitization with histamine. A case history best illustrates this method. A patient reported toothache-like pain each time he took a drink of liquor. This connection of vasodilating facial pain with alcohol has been previously noted by Eggleston.[143] The patient exhibited other unilateral symptoms as well—the pain in the lower face and the "runny" nose for example. The diagnosis was confirmed by going to a bar with the patient and having a drink. The vasodilation and the facial pain were immediately apparent. The action of alcohol as a vasodilator and thus the triggering substance for the pain and flushing was explained to the patient. He was referred to a neurologist who confirmed the diagnosis and began a histamine desensitization program by injecting minute but increasingly larger doses of histamine. This treatment is based on the fact that these are "histamine" headaches. Tragically, when the patient was able to resume drinking, he became an alcoholic, losing his family, home, and job.

Another form of therapy that has been applied to vasodilating facial pain was developed by the Menninger Foundation. It is biofeedback. Green and his associates at Menninger's discovered that some patients were relieved of their migraine symptoms, or an attack was aborted, if the patients were taught to raise the temperature of their hands (as much as 10°F) while learning to produce alpha brain waves through electroencephalogram feedback. By watching a dial, the patient could control a transference of vasodilation from the head to the hands. Using a "temperature trainer" that measured the difference between index finger and midforehead temperature, Green was able to show improvement in 74% of the migraine sufferers, including two with "cluster headache."[146]

Referred Pain

One of the difficult problems encountered in oral diagnosis deals with pain referred into, around, and out of the oral cavity. To be sure, the majority of referred oral pain is caused by the various shades of pulpalgia, referring pain to other teeth or to other regions. On the other hand, systemic disease and localized cephalic disease, by referring pain into the jaws, indeed, into individual teeth, calls for acumen on the part of the diagnostician.

The best known example of referred pain encountered by the dentist is that pain originating in the mandibular molars and referring to the homolateral ear. The phenomenon is also seen in reverse, that is, the reference of the pain of otitis media back to the mandibular molars. Common examples of referred pain are: (1) renal colic referring to the groin, (2) acute appendicitis referring to the epigastrium, and (3) angina pectoris referring to the left arm. Equally confusing is the complaint of the acute rheumatic fever victim that all his teeth ache.

Although the mechanism of referred pain is still not clear, it would appear to be related to an "overflow" of painful afferent stimuli entering the sensory neuron pool, and there, where deep and cutaneous neurons overlap, the overflow stimuli from the deep fibers "fire" the cutaneous fibers, thus giving the illusion of pain at the referred site (Fig. 11–21) (see also pp. 496–497).

Sicher summarized this theory by explaining that referred pain is actually a lack of localization of deep pain with concomitant radiation of this deep pain into superficial areas.[147]

The common referred pains with which the dentist must be concerned are those arising from: (1) referred pulp pain, (2) pain referred from the nasal and paranasal tissues, (3) pain referred from myocardial infarction, coronary thrombosis, and angina pectoris.

The broad range of referred oral pain—from the dental pulp, from the ear, or from the thorax—emphasizes the knowledge necessary for complete dental diagnosis. Sicher's comments in this vein are very succinct.[148] "It is redundant to say," he stated,

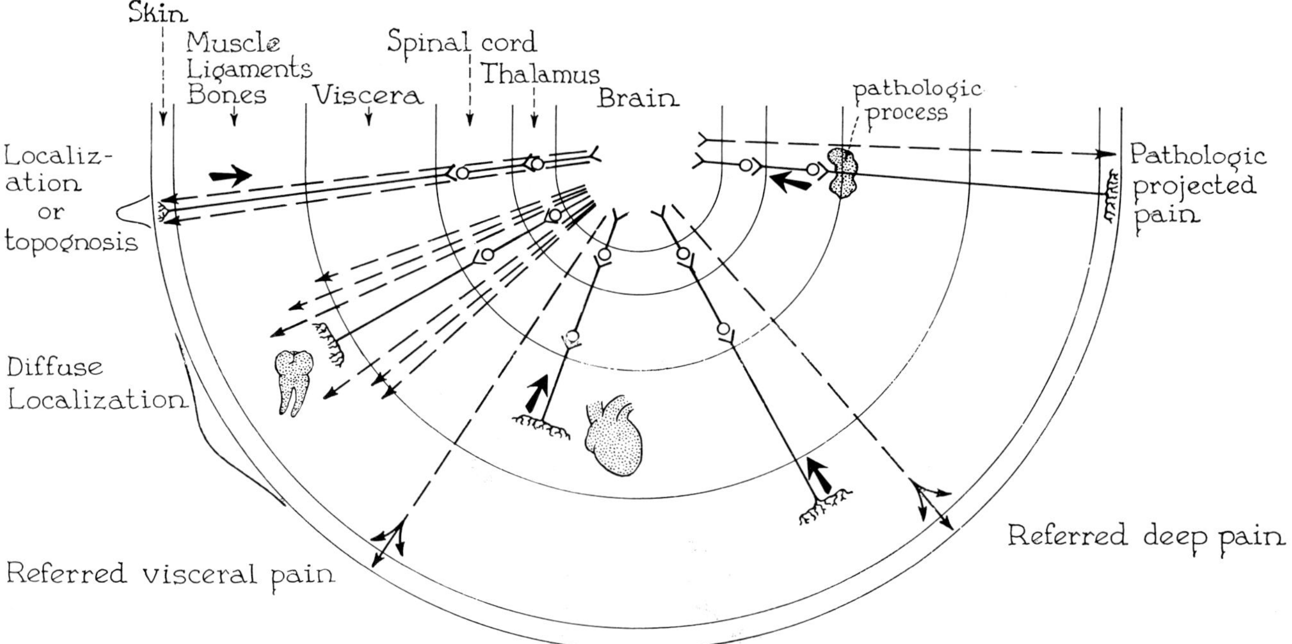

Fig. 11–21. Diagrammatic explanation of referred pain. Solid lines interrupted by synapses represent afferent impulses to brain. Broken lines represent interpretation of pain by brain and efferent impulse back to site of reference. Myocardial pain (heart symbol) is visceral pain referred to muscle, ligaments, and bones (left arm and jaw) as well as skin. Teeth (tooth symbol) within their bony housing present diffused localization of pain, interpreted in brain back to muscles and bones within diffused area. This in contrast to pain originating in skin *(left, top),* which refers back to immediate localized area. (Adapted from Ruch, T. C., and Fulton, J. F.: *Medical Physiology and Biophysics.* 18th Ed., Philadelphia, W. B. Saunders Company, 1960.)

"that the various problems of pain confronting the dentist can be approached and evaluated only if one is thoroughly acquainted with all the known facts and all the unsolved questions. Unfortunately, the tendency to speculate without the indispensable background of facts is a common human frailty. . . ."

Referred Pulp Pain

One of the most frequently encountered and most baffling phenomena with which the dental diagnostician must deal is the problem of referred pulp pain. Texts and articles dealing with this subject frequently give "pat rules" of pain reference with the implication that if pain is to be referred, it is always referred in a particular pattern. This is not so, as anyone active in diagnosis soon discovers. Quite bizarre reference pathways are frequently encountered, and the clinician soon comes to realize that almost any reference, except across the midline, is possible.*

Symptoms. Glick has well illustrated referred pain from pulpalgia—from tooth to tooth and from tooth to nearby cutaneous and deep structures.[149] Figures 11–22 and 11–23 illustrate this information to facilitate diagnosis by visual association.[150]

The leading published scientific study on pulp pain and referred pain is that of Robertson, Wolff, and Goodell.[76] These authors produced toothache by placing stimulating electrodes into defects in the enamel of their own teeth. They found that by delivering up to 10.0 volts to the teeth, severe pain could be induced. Moreover, they discovered that by maintaining the shock for ten minutes the pain would be referred out of the teeth and over the entire distribution of the involved division of the nerve. Wolff described the reference pain from a ***maxillary second premolar*** as follows:[76]

> . . . The voltage was increased gradually to 10 volts. Pain was experienced for the most part locally in the tooth. Occasionally, however, following a momentary break in the stimulating current, the subject experienced a 'jab' of more intense pain, described as a 'narrow column of pain which spread vertically into the eye, the orbital ridge, and the temple.' With extremely intense toothache, pain spread into adjacent teeth and along the maxilla.
>
> The period of toothache was accompanied by intense apprehension, profuse salivation, lacrimation, flushing of the face on the side of the stimulation, and generalized sweating. When the stimulation of the tooth was terminated, the intense pain in the tooth decreased quickly to a pain of less than 1-plus intensity lasting approximately two minutes. This pain was then replaced by a feeling of pressure in and around the tooth that was described as "the sensation of a foreign body lodged between the teeth." Within a few seconds after the termination of the toothache there began a sensation of tightness, slight numbness, and fullness over the cheek, and a tight, stiff sensation in the skin and deep tissues in the temporal region, the forehead, and the scalp on the same side of the head. There was stiffness on motion of the jaw, and occasionally fullness in the ear. Within five to ten minutes after all pain in the tooth was terminated, a steady, aching, diffuse pain of 1-plus intensity was experienced in the homolateral temporal region, along the zygomatic ridge, and for a short distance over the eye. There was no throbbing component to the pain. Bending over and looking into a bright light increased its intensity. It could usually be eliminated by 0.3-Gm. of acetylsalicylic acid.
>
> The headache reached its maximum distribution and intensity of 2 plus within 20 to 30 minutes after termination of the noxious stimulation and cessation of the toothache (Fig. 11–24). The sensation of tightness, fullness, and numbness was comparatively short-lived, whereas the headache persisted for from one to eight hours, and in one instance for 24 hours, gradually diminishing in intensity. During the period of most intense headache there was photophobia and injection of the conjunctiva. In addition the temporal muscle and overlying tissues on the same side as the pain were tender on palpation, and the skin over the painful area was hyperalgesic, *i.e.*, pin prick was sharper.

Wolff also applied the electrical stimulation to teeth in the ***mandible.*** He reported his findings as follows:

> A lower premolar or first molar tooth was stimulated in the manner described above, maintaining a 4- to 8-plus toothache for a period of ten minutes. Throughout the period of stimulation, intense aching pain was experienced locally in the tooth, and there was a less intense aching pain throughout the lower jaw which usually extended into the anterior wall of the ear canal. At the end of the period of stimulation, the pain of high intensity was quickly terminated, but there persisted a sensation of pressure in the tooth. Sometimes together with the pressure there was a dull, diffuse, aching pain of 2- to 3-plus intensity which extended throughout the upper and lower jaws, into the area over the zygoma and the temple to the top of the ear. There was also a sensation of fullness and ache in the ear. This primarily "lower-half" headache was increased in intensity by biting and by bending over. It persisted for periods of one to eight hours.
>
> The effects of noxious stimulation of teeth in the upper and lower jaw were similar (Fig. 11–25), as regards the accompanying apprehension, lacrimation, salivation, flushing of the face, photophobia, and generalized sweating, as well as stiffness of the masseter muscle, and the quality of the pain and response to

*Logan has recently reported (Oral Surg., *18*, 593) pain apparently referred across the midline. The danger of *post hoc ergo propter hoc* diagnosis must be emphasized.

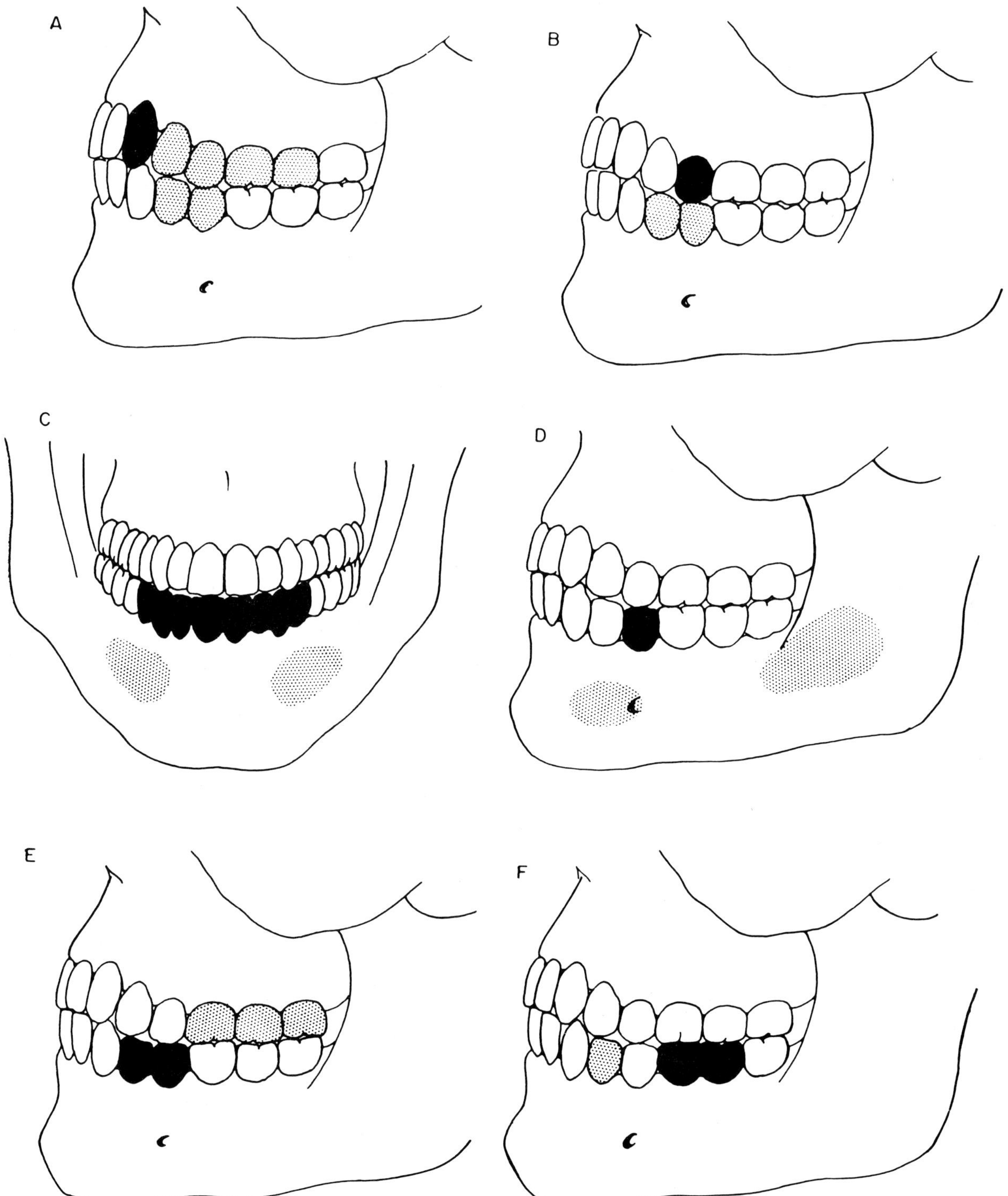

Fig. 11–22. Referred pain pathways from teeth involved with pulpalgia to other teeth as well as to immediate area. *Black* signifies tooth with pulpalgia; *stippled* areas, site of referred pain. *A,* Maxillary canine may refer to maxillary first or second premolars and/or first or second molars; also to mandibular first or second premolars. *B,* Maxillary premolars may refer pain to mandibular premolars. Reverse is also true. *C,* Mandibular incisors, canine, and first premolar may refer pain into mental area. *D,* Mandibular second premolar may refer pain into mental and midramus area. *E,* Mandibular first or second premolars may also refer pain into maxillary molars. *F,* Mandibular molars may refer pain forward to mandibular premolars. (Adapted from Glick, D. H.: Oral Surg., *15*:613, May, 1962.)

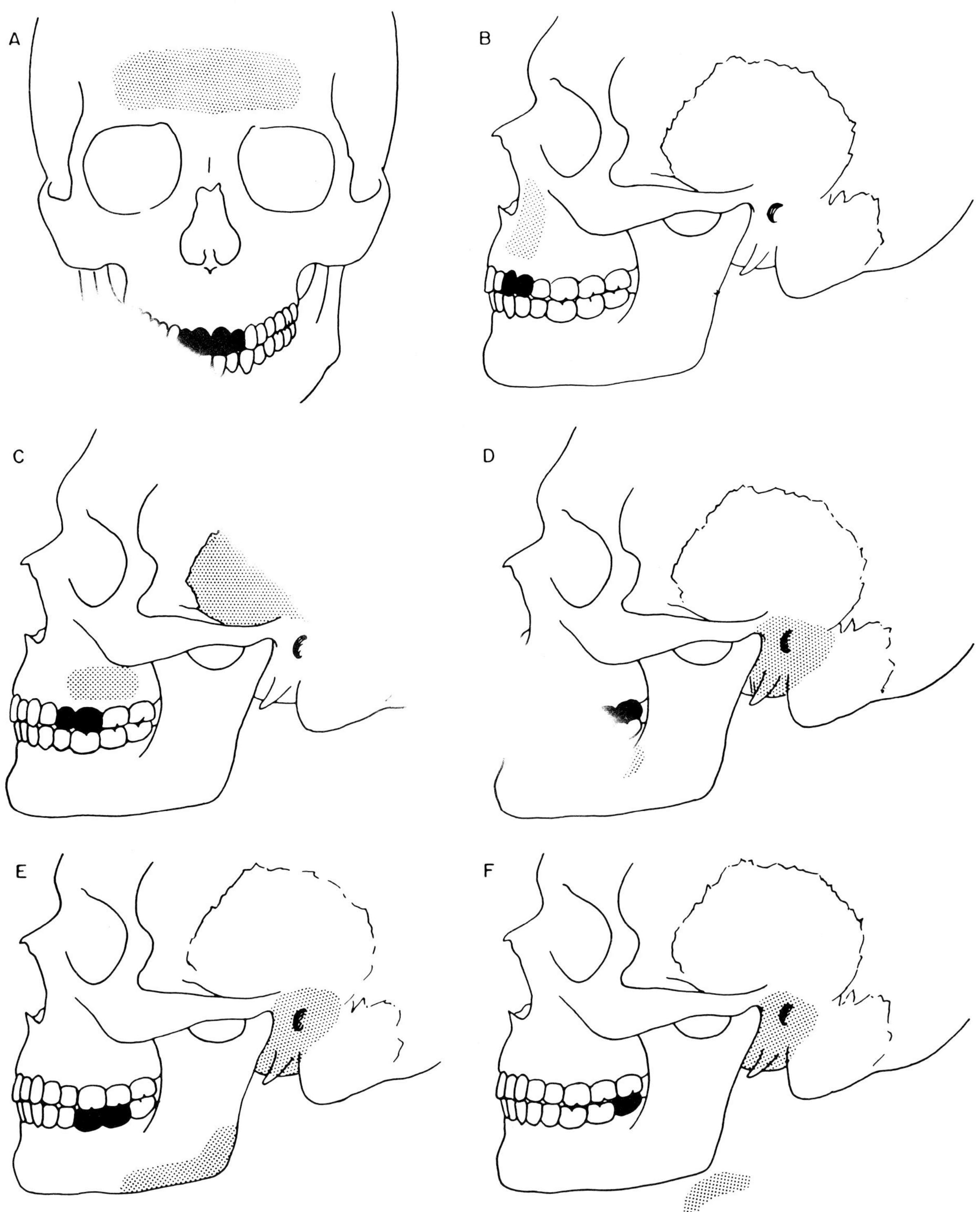

Fig. 11–23. Pain referred from pulpalgia to structures remote from involved tooth. *Black* indicates teeth involved in pulpalgia; *stippled* areas, remote areas of referred pain. *A,* Maxillary incisors may refer pain to frontal area. *B,* Maxillary canine and first premolar may refer pain into nasolabial area and into orbit. *C,* Maxillary second premolar and first molar may refer pain to maxilla and back to temporal region. *D,* Maxillary second and third molars may refer pain to mandibular molar area and occasionally into ear. *E,* Mandibular first and second molars may commonly refer pain to ear and to angle of mandible. *F,* Mandibular third molar may refer pain to ear and occasionally to superior laryngeal area. (Adapted from Glick, D. H.: Oral Surg., *15*:613, May, 1962.)

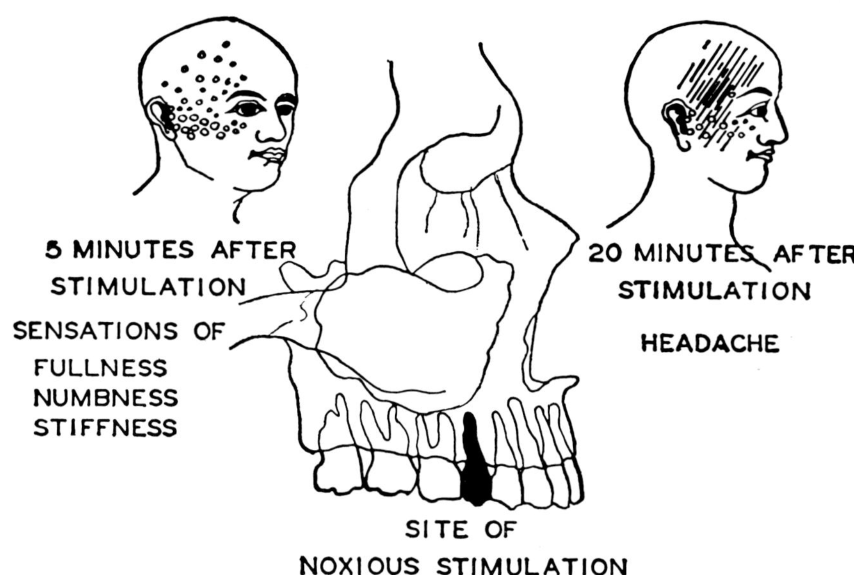

Fig. 11–24. Pain referred from maxillary second premolar. Pain was initially experienced locally in tooth following noxious stimulation by 10 volts of electricity. Within five minutes, numbness, fullness in ear, and muscle stiffness had developed along with steady pain along homolateral temporal, zygomatic, and supraorbital area. Headache reached its maximum distribution and intensity within twenty minutes after cessation of toothache. (From Wolff, H. G.: *Headache and Other Head Pain.* New York, Oxford University Press, 1950.)

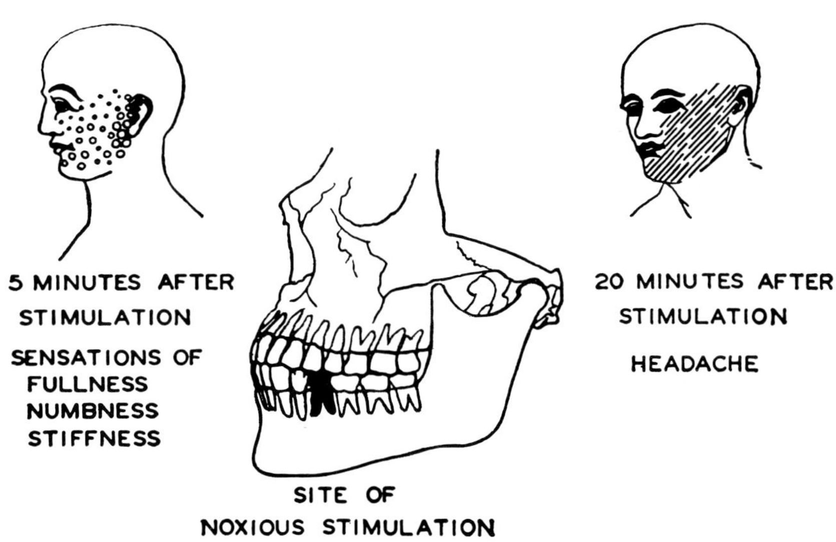

Fig. 11–25. Electrical stimulation of lower first molar maintained severe toothache for period of ten minutes. Pain referred into ear canal and throughout upper and lower jaws, over zygoma and temple, to top of ear; sensation of fullness and ache persisted in ear. Numbness and stiffness of masseter muscle developed. Twenty minutes after stimulation, severe "lower half" headache developed throughout region. (From Wolff, H. G.: *Headache and Other Head Pain.* New York, Oxford University Press, 1950.)

acetylsalicylic acid. Headache did not follow the toothache unless the latter was maintained at 4- to 8-plus intensity for a period of eight to ten minutes. The effects of the noxious stimulation were completely reversible, since no sequelae were noted.

What Wolff has here described from experimentation has been seen countless times by dentists—the patient with advanced acute pulpalgia who is suffering localized and referred pain with all the attendant systemic signs and symptoms.

Wolff further experimented with the reduction of referred pain first by injecting anesthetics into the ***area of referred pain*** on the face and scalp and, second, into the area of the original "noxious stimulation," *i.e.,* the tooth.[76] As Figure 11–26 demonstrates, only ***partial*** relief from pain developed following procaine injection into the ***referred*** area; however, ***complete*** relief from pain was experienced when the region of the ***original*** source of pain was anesthetized.

Wolff also found that protracted pain, as found in osteomyelitis of the mandible, led to sustained contraction and pain of the muscles of the face, head, and neck. In this case (Fig. 11–27), when the source area of pain in the mandible was anesthetized, the referred pain area involved with the third division of the fifth nerve was abolished. On the other hand, the pain areas due to spasm of the muscles of the neck continued. The phenomenon of muscle spasm developing as a result of pulpalgia is exactly the reverse of referred pulp or jaw pain from spasm of the trapezius muscle or the muscles of mastication as described by Travell (see Fig. 11–11).

The interesting research of Wolff and Ray would seem to confirm the reference of deep pulp pain into more superficial and cutaneous associated regions, but could hardly be construed to explain the pain referred from one tooth to another or from the paranasal tissue into the teeth.[151] This type of referred pain has been discussed by Ruch as ***habit reference.***[152]

"Evidence that reference of sensation is a learned phenomenon," states Ruch, "can be found in the clinical observation that a pain may be referred not to its usual point of reference but to the site of a previous surgical operation, trauma, or localized pathological process."

"Habit reference" was verified by Hutchins and Reynolds, who demonstrated that teeth filled ***without*** benefit of local anesthesia could be made to ache when the homolateral nasal wall was stimulated by a needle prick in the vicinity of the maxillary sinus ostium.[153] (See pp. 552–553 for a more complete discussion.)

Ruch, in reviewing the research of Hutchins and Reynolds, looked upon the traumatized sensory nerves of involved dental pulps as a "learned response."[154] Ruch stated further, "The pain impulses from the sinus, conducted in an overlapping path-

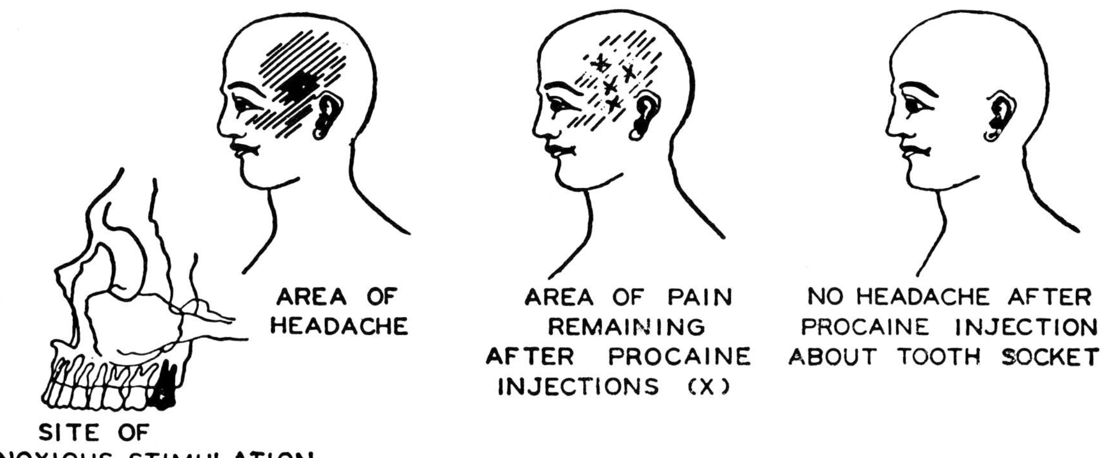

Fig. 11–26. Broad area of referred pain developed from maxillary third molar pulpalgia. Injecting procaine into ***referred area*** alleviated pain only at site of injections. All primary and referred pain was totally eliminated by injecting at site of primary noxious stimuli (third molar). (From Wolff, H. G.: *Headache and Other Head Pain.* New York, Oxford University Press, 1950.)

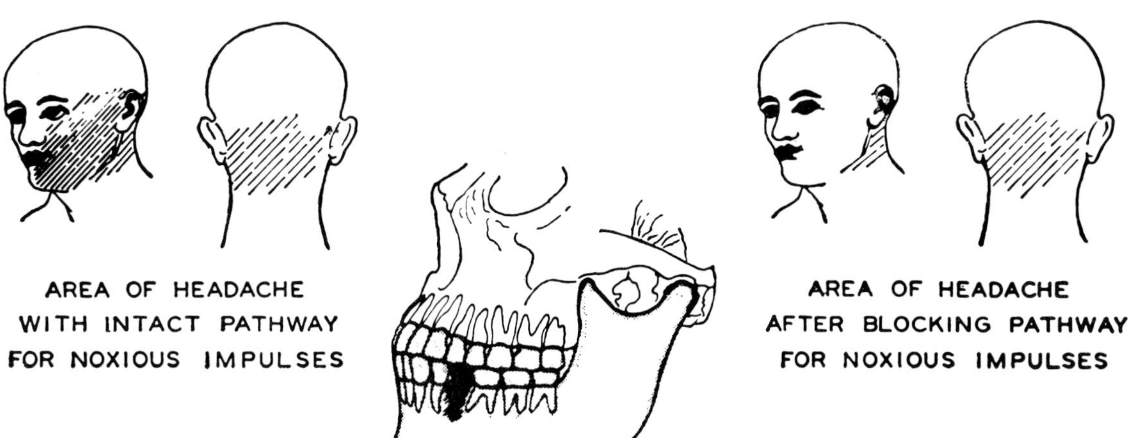

Fig. 11–27. Protracted pain from lower premolar caused not only widespread referred pain (see Fig. 11–25), but pain from spasm of muscles of face, head, and neck. Anesthetizing primary source of pain alleviated pain referred along two divisions of fifth nerve, but did not relieve spasm and pain of muscles of neck. (From Wolff, H. G.: *Headache and Other Head Pain.* New York, Oxford University Press, 1950.)

way, were simply given the previously learned reference for impulses in that path."

This same thought may be projected to explain how pain in one tooth (possibly even in the opposing homolateral arch) could be referred there from pulpitis in another tooth some distance away. The pulp of the referred tooth might well have been previously traumatized by caries, a blow, or dental procedure without anesthesia. This injured pulp then becomes the fertile ground upon which the seeds of referred response could be sown in the future.

This might also explain why pain is referred to teeth when the patient has mumps or inflammation of the temporomandibular joint.

Continuing further with their studies, Reynolds and Hutchins found that they could virtually eliminate referred pulp pain by procaine block anesthesia.[139] This was done by repeating their previous experiment in which they performed traumatic dental work ***without anesthesia*** on both sides of the ***maxillary arch,*** and later demonstrated that ***pain*** was referred to these teeth from a pin prick of the maxillary ostium in the nose. After this fact was well established, the teeth on the ***right*** side were all ***anesthetized.*** Two weeks following these injections, the ***right*** side was again tested with stimulation of the ostium. Amazingly, no referred pain could be elicited on any tooth that had been previously anesthetized. On the ***left*** side, however, which had ***not been anesthetized,*** the teeth still responded with referred pain when the left maxillary ostium was stimulated.

The importance of rendering dental treatment under local anesthesia is emphasized by Reynolds and Hutchins, who found that pain was not referred to teeth that had been treated under local anesthesia.[139]

Maxillary Sinus and Paranasal Pain

The most common ***extraoral*** source of dental pain arises from the maxillary sinus and associated nasal mucosa. Many teeth have been mistakenly extracted because of an incorrect diagnosis of this syndrome. It behooves the dentist to know well the symptoms of these confusing conditions.

Symptoms. The sinusitis patient who reports to the dentist does so with a chief complaint of "toothache." In this case, constant but rather mild pain in a ***number*** of posterior maxillary teeth on one side is almost pathognomonic. All the teeth on this side, whose roots are related to the floor of the sinus, may be aching mildly (see Fig. 10–34).

The teeth feel elongated, as if they "touch first" when the patient closes. The teeth also are tender, and the patient clenches against them saying it "hurts good" to do so. These same maxillary teeth are ***hypersensitive to cold*** fluids as well. Occasionally all the maxillary teeth on the involved side, to the midline, feel uncomfortable and elongated. The pain, mild but deep and nonpulsating, radiates out of this area onto the face, upward toward the temple, and forward toward the nose. A referred frontal headache and cutaneous hyperalgesia along the side of the face and scalp may also be present. The patient frequently reports that the pain began in the early afternoon, or he may give a history of increased pain at altitude when crossing a high mountain pass or when making an air flight.

Etiology. Inflammation with attendant swelling of the mucous membrane of the maxillary sinus is one of the causes of the pain of sinusitis. The most common cause of the discomfort, however, is inflammation and edema of the ***nasal mucosa,*** swelling which in turn blocks off the ostium of the maxillary sinus (Fig. 11–28). An allergy to dust, foods, pollens, feathers, or bacteria usually is responsible for the boggy edematous ***nasal mucosa.*** Anger, fears, tension, and anxiety neuroses also have been shown to be a causative factor of nasal and paranasal inflammation.[155,156] Infection of these nasal tissues and of the sinus mucosa itself also may cause the attack, although infected sinuses are not as common as the public would like to believe.

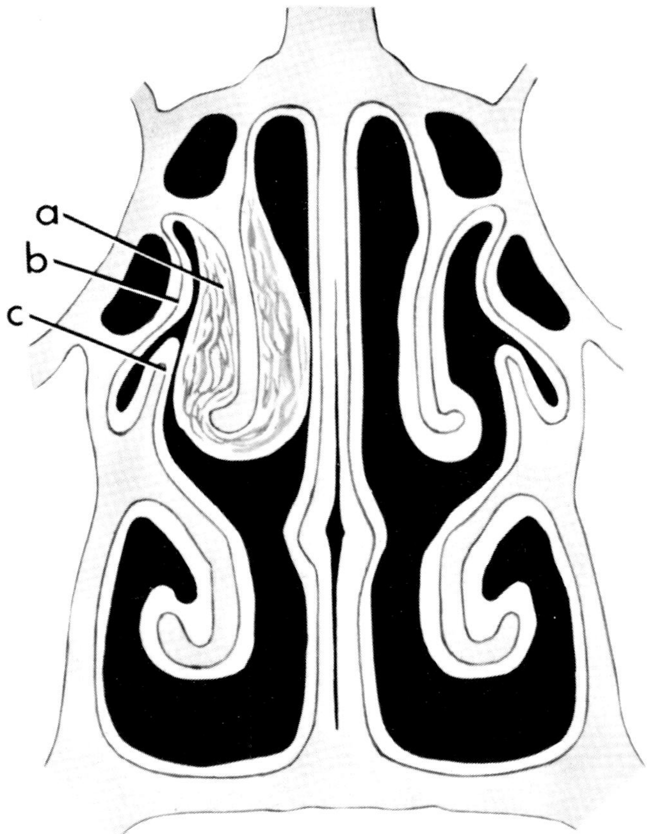

Fig. 11–28. Inflammation of nasal mucosa causes swelling of turbinate and blocks off ostium of maxillary sinus. Pain referred to maxillary teeth may then develop. (From Ballenger, J. J.: *Diseases of the Nose, Throat and Ear.* 11th Ed., Philadelphia, Lea & Febiger, 1969.)

In his excellent book on headache, Wolff ingeniously demonstrates that the majority of so-called sinus pain actually arises from the nasal ***mucosa.***[157] By stimulating with Faradic current the lateral nasal wall in the ***area of the ostium,*** Wolff demonstrated a severe pain sensation ***referred to the maxillary posterior teeth*** on the same side. This pain was of greater intensity than any discomfort that could be elicited by a charged electrode used within the sinus itself. On the other hand, the most sensitive area within the sinus was still in the area of the ostium.

Another interesting experiment was conducted by Wolff through an oral-antral fistula.[158] A balloon was introduced through this opening and inflated. Pressures as great as 100 mm. Hg exerted evenly against all sinus walls were not experienced as sinus pain. However, when a pressure of 80 mm. Hg was exerted for a period of ***two and one-half hours,*** local pain was experienced. The primary reference in this case was still noted ***in the maxillary posterior teeth.*** Wolff concluded that they symptoms usually associated with maxillary sinusitis were primarily related to an ***inflamed nasal mucosa.***

Another interesting study, relating referred tooth pain from the maxillary sinus and associated nasal mucosa, was conducted by Reynolds and Hutchins working with 920 U.S. Marine airmen.[132] These men were repeatedly "ascended" and "descended" in low pressure chambers to "altitudes" of 30,000 feet. Out of the 920 subjects tested, 37 men, representing an incidence of 4.02%, experienced the severe toothache of aerodontalgia. This pain did not appear to be primarily dental pain, but rather a pain referred from the nasal and paranasal region.

Reynolds and Hutchins concluded that the dental pain in each of these cases was related to an occluded maxillary sinus. They arrived at these conclusions after reviewing the following evidence:

1. The aerodontalgia was located in the maxillary posterior teeth in 94.5% of the cases studied. In only 2 cases was pain localized in other teeth.
2. Maxillary sinus pain was concomitant with tooth pain.

3. Pressure equalization methods, such as the Valsalva maneuver (forced expiration, the mouth being closed and the nose held by thumb and forefinger, creating a positive pressure in the oral and nasal pharnyx and middle ear), dramatically relieved the tooth pain in 83.2% of the cases. The remaining 16.8% of cases were relieved spontaneously.

4. The frequent subjective report of the sensation of "breaking loose" indicative of clearing the sinus was associated with relief.

5. Histories of maxillary sinusitis or previous upper respiratory infection were encountered in 78.3% of those individuals reporting aerodontalgia.

6. There was a repeated relationship between aerodontalgia and frontal sinus pain with respect to "altitude" of onset. The frequent finding of concomitant frontal and maxillary sinusitis has been previously noted.

The study also revealed other correlative evidence of dental pain associated with the nasal and paranasal tissue. Individuals previously complaining of aerodontalgia were given repeated "runs" in the low pressure chamber. In this group dental pain recurred 71.4% of the time, showing the consistency of the syndrome.

To evaluate the possible relationship between ***dental disease*** and aerodontalgia, 14 individuals, representing 65 major dental pathologic lesions (including pulp and periapical lesions among others) were repeatedly "ascended" and "descended" in the pressure chamber. In not one instance was aerodontalgia or aerosinusitis experienced in the original or repeated runs. These findings are not in complete agreement with the findings of others, however. Ritchey and Orban, giving contradictory evidence, found aerodontalgia associated with various degrees of pulp inflammation.[159]

Reynolds and Hutchins made the further observation that the majority (90.4%) of the dental pain occurring in the original series of 920 cases occurred in teeth with abnormalities, or in teeth immediately adjacent to those with abnormalities. This phenomenon suggested to the authors the possibility of a "prolonged central excitatory state" in which a "reinforcement of sensory impulses" referred-in by a nearby afferent nerve would trigger sensation in an original excitatory site.

This hypothesis of referred pain, from sinus to tooth or tooth to tooth, they explain as follows.[160]

> The afferent nerve from a tooth, after once being painfully stimulated, as by a blow, deep cavitation, cavity preparation, overfilling resulting in occlusal trauma, pulp exposure, infection, or extraction, continues to react by means of a constant series of excitation waves for a considerable period of time (even years). After the original external stimulus has disappeared, however, ***this excitation subsides to a subliminal level.*** Thus no pain is experienced in the tooth until stimulation of an associated structure (innervated from the same segment) produces a facilitation of the excitation existing in the afferent nerve from the tooth sufficient to carry this excitation to the central nervous system where the subjective sensation of pain arises.

To test this hypothesis, Hutchins and Reynolds tested 14 patients, 10 males and 4 females, whose ages ranged from 14 years to 52 years.[153] On 13 of these patients they bilaterally prepared in posterior teeth shallow class I, II, or V cavities ***without benefit of anesthesia.*** The patients all reported discomfort from the cavity preparations. The cavities (30 in all) were then filled with amalgam without a sedative base. None of the patients reported painful symptoms following the dental procedure. On the fourteenth patient, bilateral maxillary posterior teeth were extracted under nitrous oxide-oxygen anesthesia.

Between nine and 16 days later the patients were recalled, and by means of a needle, the nasal mucosa was stimulated bilaterally at the site of the ostium of the maxillary sinus. The results were very interesting: ***92.8% of the time the patients experienced pain in the tooth*** on which operative dentistry had been completed about two weeks previously. On the other hand, ***only 71.5% of the time did the patients experience pain in the region of the needle prick in the nose.*** In only one case was the stimulation felt exclusively in the nose and not in the tooth; however, ***in 7 cases no sensation was felt in the nose but was experienced exclusively in the teeth.*** In the remaining 22 tests, pain was experienced in both the nose and the tooth. When more than one tooth had been worked on in a quadrant, pain was experienced generally throughout the quadrant.

In summarizing the results of this experiment, Reynolds and Hutchins felt this evidence strengthens the hypothesis that pain referred to the teeth from the maxillary sinus involved ***"spatial summation of the excitation of two separate afferent nerves."***[161]

It is interesting to note that these investigators, as well as Wolff, found the ostium to be the most sensitive area associated with the maxillary sinus, and that its stimulation was most apt to refer pain to the teeth.

Sicher also pointed out that the superior alveolar nerves, supplying the maxillary molar and premolar teeth, pass along the thin wall of the sinuses.[162] The canaliculi are often open toward the sinus; thus the nerves are in direct contact with the inflamed mucoperiosteum of the sinus lining.

The dentist should also remember in making a differential diagnosis that in reverse fashion inflammation or infection ***from*** a root of a ***tooth in contact*** with the sinus floor may be the cause of sinusitis, which in turn will not resolve until the dental trouble is solved.

Examination. The complete diagnosis of maxillary sinusitis must be made by a physician, preferably a rhinologist. The dentist's contribution will be to rule out dental disease as the cause of the pain and correctly refer the patient for complete diagnosis and treatment. In order to do this the dentist must first take a careful history of the pain. Is the pain constant? What kind of pain is it? How severe? Which tooth or teeth are involved? Are the teeth "sore" to bite on? Does hot or cold affect the pain? How long have you noticed the pain? Is it worse now than yesterday?

By asking the same questions that are asked in determining whether pulpitis is present, the dentist elicits, in the case of sinusitis, a number of answers common to sinus pain but not to pulpitis. The pain of sinusitis is not intense; it is in more than one tooth. The teeth in the area are ***all*** hypersensitive to cold. The pain has continued for some time. A ***number*** of posterior teeth are "sore to bite on." The pain is getting worse, for even the upper front teeth are painful now. These answers as they evolve are not typical of dental problems, and the examiner begins to suspect another disease process.

Questions should then be directed toward sinusitis. Have you ever had sinusitis? Do you have a postnasal drip into your throat? Do you have headaches? What part of your head aches? The common referred headache from maxillary sinusitis is a frontal headache. Do not ask the patient whether he has headaches in the front part of his head, but rather let him show you where it aches. He might do so by drawing his hand over his brow. Ask if increasing pressure increases the headache, as when one is leaning over, coughing, straining at stool, or running upstairs.

The extraoral examination should include palpation of the maxillary sinuses under the zygomatic process on each cheek. If maxillary sinusitis is present and is unilateral, the cheek on the involved side, from the canine fossa back to the base of the zygomatic process, will be painful to heavy palpation. The patient may say it feels as if he has been hit in the area, or "frostbitten" is another term used in northern climes. It may also hurt to smile.

If the patient complains of frontal headache, the dentist should check the frontal sinuses by pressing up against the inferior surface of the supraorbital ridge on each side of the nose. If the frontal sinuses are involved, this increased pressure causes pain. All the anterior sinuses may be involved at one time: the maxillaries, the frontals, and the anterior ethmoidal cells. Such pansinusitis is common following an upper respiratory infection.

The intraoral examination should include mobility tests, percussion, electric pulp test, thermal tests, and roentgenograms. The teeth adjacent to the affected maxillary sinus often are mobile when moved between the two index fingers. Furthermore, the are painful to percussion and also sound "mushy" when percussed, if compared to the "twang" sound on percussion of the normal side. The teeth may well prove to be hypersensitive when pulp tested electrically and with ice, and compared to the opposite side.

Roentgenographically, there may be nothing wrong with the involved teeth, and that reconfirms the diagnosis that nothing is wrong orally. The roots of the teeth, however, may be found extending well up into or against the sinus floor, which would account for their involvement. On the other hand, the roentgenogram and pulp test may show a pulpless

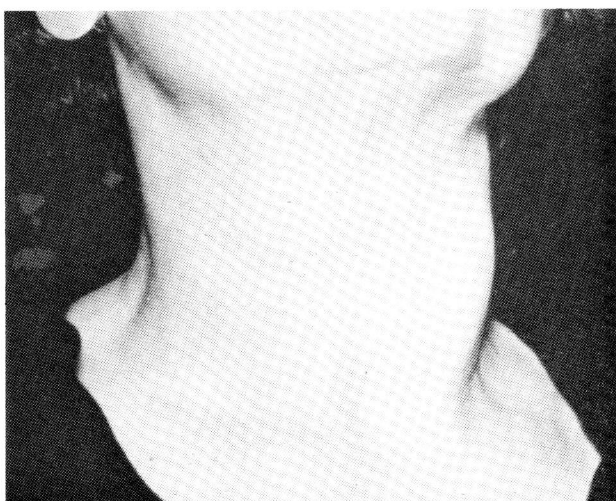

Fig. 11–29. Benign thyroid tumor which recurred following thyroidectomy is referring pain into mandibular first molar on homolateral side.

tooth with a periapical lesion. As stated previously, this could be the cause of a unilateral sinus inflammation. Nenzen and Welander found "local hyperplasia of the maxillary sinus mucosa" in 58% (14 of 24) of the patients who had pulpless teeth with periapical lesions associated with the floor of the sinus.[163]

Persistent pain in this area may be caused by a cyst or neoplasm of the maxillary sinus. In these cases, the pain syndrome is the same as for sinusitis, but of long standing. A roentgenographic study of the area may reveal the lesion.

The differential diagnosis of maxillary sinusitis may be confirmed by spraying 4% lidocaine anesthetic from a spray bottle into the nostril on the affected side. The pain from the congested nasal mucosa and accompanying maxillary sinusitis should be materially reduced within a minute or two.

Treatment. Complete diagnosis and treatment of maxillary sinusitis is left to the rhinologist. Pain may be controlled by aspirin in some cases, but codeine is frequently needed for relief.

Myocardial Infarction, Coronary Thrombosis, and Angina Pectoris

Severe pain referred into the mandible and maxilla from a region outside the head and neck is most commonly referred from the heart. Other sources of referred pain to the jaws are cardiospasm, which is the spasm of the esophageal cardiac sphincter associated with hiatal hernia of the diaphragm, and thyroid disease (Fig. 11–29).

The opposite pain reference has also been seen—pain from pulpalgia referring down the arms. I have dealt with such a case, and Senia has reported an unusual case of pain referred from a mandibular premolar to the homolateral neck, shoulder, arm, and waist in a young physician with chronic pulpitis.[164]

How cardiac pain can be referred as far away as the jaws is difficult to explain; however, an understanding of the sensory dermatomes is helpful in this regard.

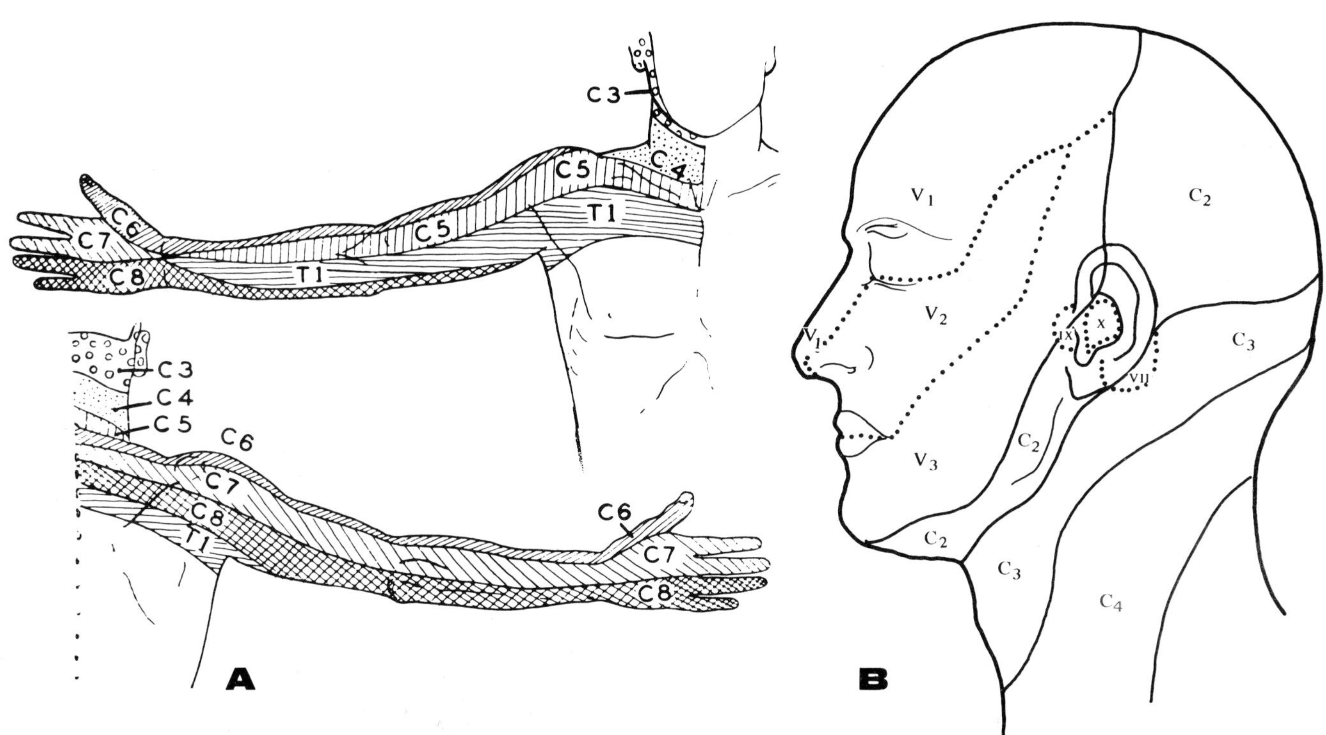

Fig. 11–30. *A*, Dermatome chart of upper extremity of man. Pain referred out of chest from first thoracic dermatome advances by overlapping dermatomes to third cervical dermatome, which in turn overlaps third division of fifth cranial nerve. This has been offered as possible explanation for reference of deep visceral pain from myocardium into jaws and teeth as well as down left arm. (From Keegan, J., and Garrett, F. D.: Anatomical Record, *102*:409, Dec., 1948.) *B*, Detailed map of sensory nerve responsibility. Note how C2 overlaps with V3 (trigeminal-mandibular). (From Clemente, C. D.: *Anatomy: A Regional Atlas of the Human Body.* Philadelphia, Lea & Febiger, 1975.)

Ruch defines a dermatome or sensory root field as "the area of skin supplied with afferent fibers by a single posterior root."[165] He goes on to say, "Dermatomes of adjacent roots overlap greatly so that always two and sometimes three roots supply a single point on the skin." Figure 11–30 demonstrates how the thoracic dermatomes, carrying referred cardiac pain into the chest wall and down the left arm, overlap with the cervical dermatomes which also innervate the arm and shoulder as well as a part of the lower face.[166] The second cervical dermatome in turn slightly overlaps with the fifth cranial nerve which innervates the entire oral complex.

Repetition of a previous paragraph may help to explain this phenomenon: "Referred pain . . . would appear to be related to an 'overflow' of painful afferent stimuli entering the ***sensory neuron pool,*** and there, ***where deep and cutaneous neurons overlap,*** the overflow stimuli from the deep fibers 'fire' the cutaneous fibers, thus giving the illusion of pain at the referred site."

This might well explain the bizarre pain reference from heart to chest wall, to left shoulder and arm, to mandible and maxilla, through the overlapping of the thoracic and cervical dermatomes and the fifth cranial nerve.

Symptoms. I have seen a number of patients with severe pain in the left maxilla and mandible related to coronary occlusion. No other symptoms were present. One patient had the unusual symptoms of referred pain in the ***left*** maxilla and ***right*** arm, but no chest pain. Matson reports a case of coronary thrombosis during which time the patient experienced "pain in ***both*** sides of the ***mandible*** and neck, which radiated to the lateral aspects of the ***zygoma*** and ***temporal*** areas.[167] She specifically denied having chest, shoulder or arm pains . . ."

The ***usual*** symptom complex of myocardial infarction is a sudden but gradually increasing precordial pain, with an overwhelming feeling of suffocation. The squeezing pain radiates upward from the epigastrium, "just under the necktie" to the mandible—the left more frequently than the right. In addition, the inner aspects of the arms ache, again the left more frequently and extensively than the right (Fig. 11–31*A*). Norman discusses four unusual cases of myocardial infarction with pain referred to the right ***and*** left jaws.[168] The left ***maxilla*** is also a common site. Macruz reported that left jaw and arm pain was due to obstruction of the circumflex coronary artery.[169]

Pain directly over the heart, centering around the

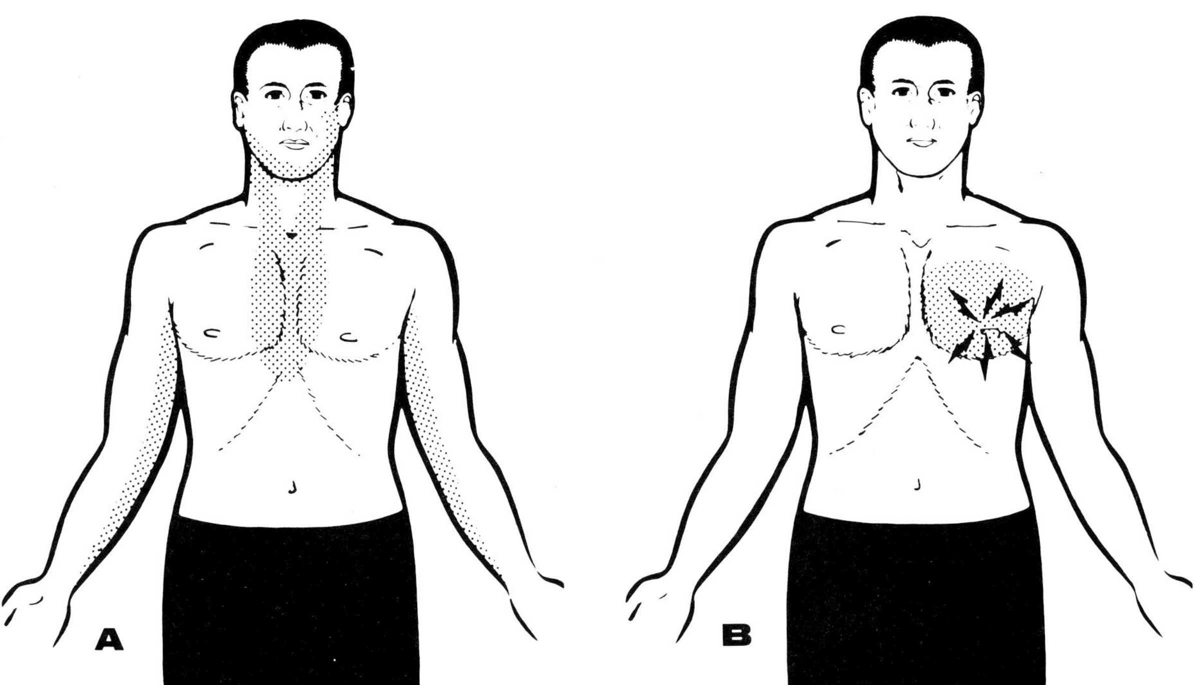

Fig. 11–31. *A,* Pattern of pain and referred pain emanating from myocardial infarction. Central necktie pattern and greater left jaw and arm pain than right side is typical. *B*, Harmless noncardiac pain in left chest. (From Turner, G. O.: Medical World News, April 6, 1973.)

nipple in the left chest (Fig. 11–31*B*), is almost never a sign of heart attack. Left chest direct pain, without the squeezing sensation, may be "confused with paroxysmal tachycardia, pulmonary embolism, hiatus hernia, viral myocarditis, viral pericarditis, gastritis, gallstones, peptic esophagitis, duodenal ulcer, and asthma."[170] "If pain occurs in the arms, raising them above the head will aggravate the pain due to arthritis, bursitis or muscle strain but will not aggravate heart pain."[171]

Such are the common pain symptoms experienced. Accompanying them may be an impending sense of doom or disaster, nausea, and the attendant signs of shock: sweating, cold clammy skin, and a gray complexion. In advanced stages the patient becomes unconscious and cyanotic. If conscious, the patient generally complains of the severe pain and rubs the chest, jaw, and arm. These are the advanced signs and symptoms of a heart attack.

A substantial number of patients with coronary thrombosis do not experience these severe symptoms, but instead experience a reference of pain to the jaws, with none of the chest or arm symptoms. These are the patients who report to the dental office for diagnosis. One such patient reported with pain in the second molar area of the left ***maxilla.*** The pain had suddenly developed the previous day while the patient was working in his garden. He had no chest symptoms, but further questioning revealed he also had pain in his ***right*** arm, an unusual reference point. He had taken an aspirin, had felt nauseated, and vomited. The pain continued. A careful oral examination did not disclose any dental problem that might be responsible for the pain. By elimination, a diagnosis of oral pain referred from a cardiac lesion was made.

The diagnosis of coronary thrombosis was confirmed by a cardiologist who also reported that his more complete history taking had revealed a similar attack two years previously. A glance at the patient's dental chart disclosed that he had reported to the dental clinic with a similar pain two years previously. At that time someone had placed a "bite plate" to correct what was undoubtedly misdiagnosed as "temporomandibular joint pain." During the two-week period the patient had worn the bite plate, his pain had gradually receded, and finally he discarded the plate. Quite probably the original diagnosis was incorrect and the cardiac patient had been treated for the wrong condition. It is possible that he would be alive today if he had not continued heavy labor for two years until his second attack was diagnosed.

Another patient was seen with a history of a severe stabbing pain in the left maxilla which centered in the canine. The patient was in Washington, D.C., undertaking some very trying government business. He had previously had pulpitis, and was certain he again had advanced pulpitis, so severe was the pain. He quite naturally reported to a dentist who examined radiographically and tested the painful canine. The dentist reported he could find absolutely nothing wrong; nevertheless, the recommendation was to extract the tooth. The patient refused treatment, and went to another dentist where the recommendation was repeated. When a third dentist gave him exactly the same diagnosis and treatment plan, he turned his business over to an associate and returned home, tooth intact.

By the time he was seen by the author he was taking Demerol, and so the first examination was rather unsatisfactory. However, it was determined that he did not have any dental problems, but did have two herpetic lesions along the left maxillary buccal gingiva. A tentative diagnosis of herpes zoster was made, and he was referred to a neurologist. He did not go! Gradually, as the herpetic lesions healed, the pain subsided. In a week he replaced the Demerol with 15 gr. aspirin every two hours. In another week he was feeling shaky, but was relatively pain free. He continued under great pressure in his business and six months later suffered a massive myocardial infarction. One year later he died in what might well have been his third attack.

A clinician must review in his mind a case with these symptoms. "Where did I fail?" the conscientious practitioner asks himself over and over. If the patient had not had two herpetic-like lesions in his mouth, more time would have been spent in examination and a proper diagnosis would probably have been made. Again, the fact that the patient refused to go to a physician when a tentative diagnosis of herpes zoster had been rendered may well have contributed to his early death. A clever neurologist would probably have realized he did not have herpes zoster.

In another case a colleague casually discussed the lower left face pain he was experiencing. He had no cavities or restorations on the left, but did have a history suggestive of migraine. A snap diagnosis of vasodilating facial pain was made, and a physician was suggested. The suggestion was ignored and the pain gradually left. Now that the colleague has had two coronary occlusions, hindsight suggests the earlier error in judgment.

It must be emphasized that in each of the several cases described absolutely no heart or chest symptoms were experienced. The usual pain in the left arm was not experienced, the only symptoms being pain in the left mandible and maxilla. One patient, however, did have pain in the right arm.

The importance of being aware of the possibility of referred pain from a myocardial infarction is brought out in a case history related to me by a colleague practicing in a California resort city. The dentist received a telephone call at about 5:30 in the morning from the wife of Moss Hart, the distinguished American playwright. Mrs. Hart stated that her husband had developed a severe toothache during the night and that it had finally become quite unbearable. He was seeking relief at this very early hour.

During the telephone conversation, it was immediately established that the pain was in both the maxilla and mandible on the left side, and that it was not affected by heat or cold. Recalling that Mr. Hart had previously suffered a coronary occlusion, the dentist became suspicious and immediately drove to the Hart residence only a short distance from his own.

He found a distraught patient holding his left jaw and complaining bitterly. Questioning revealed he had no pain except the widespread pain in the left jaws. A hurried examination confirmed the dentist's memory that no grossly suspicious problem existed in the patient's left dentition.

The dentist decided to take Mr. Hart to his nearby office, and if the teeth on the left all responded normally to examination, to take the patient to the hospital. Mrs. Hart was to drive her husband.

Mr. Hart was standing on the lawn as his wife backed their automobile out of the driveway and the dentist was turning his car in the street. In the instant it took to make a U-turn, Mr. Hart had fallen to the ground. The dentist ran to his assistance, but Mr. Hart was dead. Closed-chest cardiopulmonary resuscitation was of no avail.[172]

A number of patients with recurrent angina pectoris have been seen, patients who know they have the disease and who use nitroglycerine to control the attacks. They ***all*** report ***left mandibular*** pain with each spasm. Anginal pain referred to the left posterior teeth was well documented by Natkin, Harrington and Mandel. "In certain instances pain was experienced with concomitant chest pain, and in other instances, pain was confined to the teeth."[172a]

Etiology. Myocardial infarction occurs as the result of the occlusion of one of the coronary arteries. This occlusion may develop from gradual closure of the vessel by atherosclerotic deposits on the vessel wall, or may be due to hemorrhage under an atherosclerotic plaque, raising the plaque to obstruct the vessel lumen.

Recent reports suggest that emotional stress may play an even more important role in the etiology of the disease than do diet, tobacco, heredity, obesity, and lack of physical exercise.[173] Friedman and Rosenman insist that patients with a type A personality (people who walk, speak, drive, eat and work fast even when they don't have to) are much more prone to heart attacks than the more relaxed type B person.[174] "Type A behavior is the No. 1 cause of heart attacks," Rosenman has stated. Others have contended, however, "That the role of personality is at best of the same order as the other factors and is not 'the No. 1 cause of heart disease.'" The "other factors" referred to were smoking, hypertension, and hypercholesterolemia.[175] In this regard, hereditary lipoproteinemia has been described by Fredrickson and Levy as leading to the development of the atherosclerotic plaque and subsequent coronary artery occlusion.[176,177]

Examination. A careful history is important in diagnosing the referred oral pain of myocardial infarction. Usually the patient has a rather unusual story to tell of fairly severe pain which began rather suddenly in the ***left*** jaw, and grew in intensity. It might have moved from mandible to maxilla.

The dentist is anxious to examine and find the tooth involved in pulpitis, for this is exactly what it appears to be. He carefully pulp tests every tooth and finds they all respond normally. He tests with hot and cold and cannot change the character of the constant pain with thermal variation. Roentgenograms of every tooth on the left side are normal.

Then begins the careful questioning. ***Could it be maxillary sinusitis?*** No, it came on too suddenly! Furthermore, his maxilla is not sore to palpation, nor are the left maxillary teeth painful to percussion. ***Then it may be temporomandibular joint or myofascial pain.*** No, it can't be that; no pain can be elicited in the joint upon palpation, and full opening of the mandible elicits no discomfort or dysfunction. ***There may be a periodontal abscess.*** No abscess is visible, and furthermore, the pain is not localized. The examiner realizes he is exhausting the typically oral symptoms, so he returns to the questioning. ***Did the patient have pain anywhere else?*** "No!" ***Are you sure? In your arms?*** "No!" ***How did you feel when you first noticed the pain?*** "I felt like I had indigestion so I took some soda." ***Did it help?*** "No, it made me nauseated and I felt faint. I lay down and broke out in cold sweat." ***And then what happened?*** "The pain in my jaw got worse and moved from the lower jaw to include the upper jaw." ***And then?*** "I took aspirin and tolerated the pain the rest of the night." ***You should have called me last night.*** "I didn't want to disturb you."

This is an actual conversation, and not only reveals the clues to a severe organic disturbance, but also discloses facets of the patient's personality—the self-determination, the concern for others so often expressed by our patients.

Up to this point the diagnosis of coronary artery thrombosis has not definitely been made, but it is suspected. The task that remains is the detective work of eliminating all the other suspects.

Was it trigeminal neuralgia? No, a trigger zone was absent and the pain was constant, not paroxysmal. ***Well, was it trigeminal neuritis then?*** No, it came on too suddenly with no precipitating incident. ***Vasodilating facial pain?*** No, it has lasted too long, and the patient had ***generalized*** sweating and cold clammy skin rather than homolateral facial flushing and lacrimation. ***Could it be psychoneurosis?*** No, obviously not. The patient is too definite, too sensible, and too obviously sick. ***How about herpetic or postherpetic neuritis?*** No, this came on too suddenly and there are no apparent lesions.

Having ruled out such differential diagnoses as localized dental or joint pain, and neurologic or psychogenic pain, one must then consider referred pain from the chest. The pain must, therefore, be cardiac in origin. The patient is referred immediately to a cardiologist, who is then called and will be prepared to receive the patient. The latter is sent in a taxi or taken, but is not frightened by unnecessary concern or dramatic statements.

Treatment. The prompt application of external heart massage—technically, closed-chest cardiopulmonary resuscitation (CPR)—in coronary heart attacks has enabled lives to be saved which would previously have been lost.* A survival rate of 25% has been reported in a series of 1270 patients. The long-term care of the cardiac patient has also greatly changed in the past few years. He should be in the hands of a competent physician, and with good fortune may also be a dental patient for years to come.

*Available from your local Heart Association. Standards for Cardiopulmonary Resuscitation (CPR). Supplement to J.A.M.A., *227*:837–68, Feb. 18, 1974.

REFERENCES

1. Milton, J.: *Paradise Lost.*
2. Bonica, J. J.: *The Management of Pain with Special Emphasis on the Use of Analgesic Block in Diagnosis, Prognosis and Therapy.* Philadelphia, Lea & Febiger, 1953, pp. 154–160.
3. Medawar, P. B.: *The Art of the Soluble.* London, Methuen, 1967.
4. Friedman, N.: Personal communication, 1972.
5. Melzack, R., and Torgerson, W. S.: On the language of pain. Anesthes., *34*:50, Jan., 1971.
6. Pain: usually just a symptom, but it can be a disease state. Dent. Survey, *51*:68, May, 1975.
7. Hertzler, A. B.: *Surgical Pathology of the Mouth and Jaws.* Philadelphia, J. B. Lippincott Co., 1938, p. 5.
8. Monheim, L. M.: *Local Anesthesia and Pain Control in Dental Practice.* St. Louis, C. V. Mosby Co., 1961, p. 21.
9. Lewis, T.: *Pain.* New York, The Macmillan Co., 1942, p. 5.
10. Ruch, T. C., and Fulton, J. F.: Medical Physiology and Biophysics. 18th Ed. Philadelphia, W. B. Saunders Co., 1960, p. 306.
11. Lewis, T.: Op. cit., pp. 29–30.
12. Monheim, L. M.: Op. cit., p. 21.
13. Zola, J. J.: Culture on symptoms: an analysis of patients' presenting complaints. Amer. Sociolog. Rev., *31*:615, 1966.
14. Johnson, R., and Baldwin, D. C., Jr.: Relationship of maternal anxiety to the behavior of young children undergoing dental extraction. J. Dent. Res., *47*:801, 1968.
15. Sternbach, R. A., and Tursky, B.: Ethnic differences among housewives in psychophysical and skin potential responses to electric shock. Psychophysiol., *1*:214, 1965.
16. Buss, A. H., and Portnoy, N. W.: Pain tolerance and group identification. J. Pers. Soc. Psych., *6*:106, 1967.
17. Winsburg, B., and Greenlick, M.: Pain responses in Negro and White obstetrical patients. J. Health and Social Behav., *9*:222, 1968.
18. Lim, R. K. S.: Revised concept of the pain mechanism. In *Pain.* Edited by R. S. Knighton and P. R. Dumke. Boston, Little Brown and Co., 1964.
19. Lim, R. K. S.: Pain. Ann. Rev. Physiolog., *32*:269, 1970.
20. Collins, W. R., and Randt, C. T.: Midbrain evoked responses relating to peripheral unmyelinated or C-fibers in cat. J. Neurophysiol., *23*:47, 1960.
21. Collins, W. R., Nulson, F. E., and Shealy, C. N.: Electrophysiological studies of peripheral and central pathways conducting pain. In *Pain.* Edited by R. S. Knighton and P. R. Dumke. Boston, Little Brown and Co., 1966, pp. 33–46.

22. Melzack, R., and Wall, P. D.: Pain mechanisms: a new theory. Science, *150*:971, 1965.
23. Pearl, E. R.: Is pain a specific sensation? J. Psychiat. Res., *8*:273, 1971.
24. Young, R. F., and King, R. B.: Excitability changes in trigeminal primary afferent fibers in response to noxious and non-noxious stimuli. J. Neurophysiol., *35*:87, 1972.
25. Stewart, W. A., and King, R. B.: Fiber projections from the nucleus caudalis of the spinal trigeminal nucleus. J. Comp. Neurol., *121*:271, 1963.
26. Hardy, J. D., Wolff, H. G., and Goodell, H.: *Pain Sensations and Reactions.* Baltimore, Williams & Wilkins Co., 1952, pp. 40–41.
27. Lewis, T.: Op. cit., pp. 29–30.
28. Engel, G. L.: *Psychological Development in Health and Disease.* Philadelphia, W. B. Saunders Co., 1962, pp. 376–378.
29. Noyes, A. P., and Kolb, L. C.: *Modern Clinical Psychiatry.* 6th Ed., Philadelphia, W. B. Saunders Co., 1963, p. 409.
30. Engel, G. L.: Op. cit., p. 378.
31. Sternbach, R. A., Murphy, R. W., Akeson, W. H., and Wolf, S. R.: Chronic low-back pain. Postgrad. Med., *53*:153, 1973.
32. Penman, J.: Pain as an old friend. Lancet, *1*:633, 1954.
33. Sternbach, R. A.: *Pain: A Psychophysiological Analysis.* New York, Academic Press, 1968.
34. Baldwin, D. C., Jr., and Weisenberg, M.: The role of psychological factors in reducing patient reaction to pain. Paper presented at Am. Assoc. for Advanc. of Sci., 1974.
35. Baldwin, D. C.: An investigation of psychological and behavioral responses to dental extraction in children. J. Dent. Res., *45*:1636, 1966.
36. Egbert, L. D., Battit, G. E., Turndorf, H., and Beecher, H. K.: Value of a preoperative visit by the anesthetist: study of doctor-patient rapport. J.A.M.A., *185*:553, 1963.
37. Opton, E. M.: Psychological stress and coping process in dentistry. Internat. Dent. J., *19*:415, 1969.
38. Helmreich, R. L., and Collins, B. E.: Situational determinants of affiliative preferences under stress. J. Pers. Soc. Psych., *6*:78, 1967.
39. Janis, I.: *Psychological Stress: Psychoanalytic and Behavioral Studies of Surgical Patients.* New York, Wiley, 1958.
40. Yamana, M.: In *Sensory Mechanisms in Dentine.* Edited by D. J. Anderson. New York, The Macmillan Co., 1963, p. 68.
41. Brannstrom, M.: In *Sensory Mechanism in Dentine.* Edited by D. J. Anderson. New York, The Macmillan Co., 1963, p. 78.
41a. Scott, D., Jr.: Personal communication. October 1, 1975.
42. Beveridge, E. E.: Measurement of human dental intrapulpal pressure and its response to clinical variables. Univ. of Washington Master's Thesis, 1964.
43. Shoher, I., Mahler, Y., and Samueloff, S.: Dental pulp photoplethysmography in human beings. Oral Surg., *36*:915, Dec., 1973.
44. Funakoshi, M., and Zotterman, Y.: In *Sensory Mechanisms in Dentine.* Edited by D. J. Anderson. New York, The Macmillan Co., 1963, p. 69.
45. Brannstrom, M.: Op. cit., p. 77.
46. Sicher, H.: The Odontoblast. Private publication.
47. Sicher, H.: Personal communication.
48. Anderson, D. J.: *Sensory Mechanisms in Dentine.* New York, The Macmillan Co., 1963, p. 89.
49. Beveridge, E. E., and Brown, A. C.: The measurement of human dental intrapulpal pressure and its response to clinical variables. Oral Surg., *19*:655, May, 1965.
50. Grossman, L. I.: *Endodontic Practice.* 8th Ed., Philadelphia, Lea & Febiger, 1974, p. 45.
51. Simmons, J. J.: Ionic desensitization of teeth. Texas Dent. J., *79*:11, 1961.
52. Murthy, K. S., Talim, S. T., and Singh, I.: A comparative evaluation of topical application and ionophoresis of sodium fluoride for desensitization of hypersensitive dentin. Oral Surg., *36*:448, Sept., 1973.
53. Hodosh, M.: A superior desensitizer—potassium nitrate. J.A.D.A., *88*:831, Apr., 1974.
54. Smith, B. A., and Ash, M. M.: A study of desensitizing dentifrice and cervical hypersensitivity. J. Perio., *35*:221, May-June, 1964.
55. Smith, B. A., and Ash, M. M.: Evaluation of desensitizing dentifrice. J.A.D.A., *68*:639, May, 1964.
56. Stanley, H. R., and Swerdlow, H.: Reactions of the human pulp to cavity preparation: results produced by eight different operative grinding techniques. J.A.D.A., *58*:49, May, 1959.
57. Stanley, H. R.: Personal communication.
58. England, M. C., Pellis, E. G., and Michanowicz, A. E.: Histopathologic study of the effect of pulpal disease upon the nerve fibers of the human dental pulp. Oral Surg., *38*:783, Nov., 1974.
59. Glick, D. H.: Personal communication.
60. Chun, H. H.: Temporomandibular joint gout. J.A.M.A., *226*:353, Oct. 15, 1973.
61. Chalmers, I. M., and Blair, G. S.: Is the temporomandibular joint involved in primary osteoarthritis? Oral Surg., *38*:74, July, 1974.
62. Feder, M. J., and Stratigos, G. T.: Hearing aids as an etiologic factor in temporomandibular joint pain. Oral Surg., *32*:193, Aug., 1971.
63. Schwartz, L. L.: *Disorders of the Temporomandibular Joint.* Philadelphia, W. B. Saunders Co., 1949, p. 29.
64. Kydd, W. J.: Psychosomatic aspects of temporomandibular joint dysfunction. J.A.D.A., *59*:31, July, 1959.
65. Weisengreen, H., and Elliot, H. W.: Electromyography in patients with orofacial pain. J.A.D.A., *67*:798, Dec., 1963.
66. Thomas, L. J., Tiber, N., and Schireson, S.: The effects of anxiety and tension related to the temporomandibular joint syndrome. Oral Surg., *36*:763, Nov., 1973.
67. Thaller, J. L., Rosen, G., and Saltzman, S.: Study of the relationship of frustration and anxiety to bruxism. J. Perio., *38*:193, 1967.
68. Lupton, D. E.: Differences in developmental background and dynamic psychological patterns of

nonorganic TMJ dysfunction patients. I.A.D.R. Abstr. #240, p. 100, 1969.

69. Greene, C. S., and Laskin, D. M.: Meprobamate therapy for the myofascial pain-dysfunction (MPD) syndrome. J.A.D.A., *82*:587, Mar., 1971.
70. Greene, C. S., and Laskin, D. M.: Correlation of placebo responses and psychological characteristics in myofascial pain-dysfunction (MPD) patients. I.A.D.R. Abstr. #282, p. 119, 1969.
71. Greene, C. S., and Laskin, D. M.: Splint therapy for the myofascial pain dysfunction (MPD) syndrome. J.A.D.A., *84*:624, Mar., 1971.
72. Rothwell, P. S.: Personality and response to treatment of the temporomandibular joint pain-dysfunction syndrome. Oral Surg., *36*:331, Sept., 1973.
73. Marback, J. J., and Dworkin, S. F.: Chronic MPD, group therapy and psychodynamics. J.A.D.A., *90*:827, Apr., 1975.
74. Travell, J., and Rinzler, S. H.: The myofascial genesis of pain. Postgrad. Med., *11*:425, May, 1952.
75. Travell, J.: Temporomandibular joint pain referred from muscles of the head and neck. J. Prosth. Dent., *10*:745, July-Aug., 1960.

75a. Travell, J.: Relief of referred somatic and visceral pain by extinction of myofascial trigger points. Abstracts, First World Congress on Pain, Florence, Italy, International Association for Study of Pain, September, 1975, Abstract No. 129.

76. Robertson, S., Goodell, H., and Wolff, H. G.: The teeth as a source of headache and other pain. Arch. Neurol. Psychiat., *57*:277, 1947.
77. Travell, J.: Personal communication, March, 1974.
78. Shanelec, D. C.: Ischemic Muscle Pain. USC Graduate Student Thesis, Apr. 16, 1971.
79. Horton, B. T.: Transactions of Am. Acad. Ophthal. Otolaryngol. 49th Ann. Meet., pp. 26–27, 1944.
80. Schwartz, L. L.: Op. cit., Chap. 2.
81. Ingle, J. I.: Determination of occlusal discrepancies. J.A.D.A., *59*:6, Jan., 1957.
82. Zung, W. W. K.: A rating instrument for anxiety disorders. Psychosomatics, *12*:371, Nov.-Dec., 1971.
83. Butler, J. H., Folke, L. E. A., and Bandt, C. L.: A descriptive survey of signs and symptoms associated with MPD syndrome. J.A.D.A., *90*:635, Mar., 1975.
84. Duquette, P., and Geobel, W. M.: Pulpitis simulating MPD syndrome: report of three cases. J.A.D.A., *87*:1237, Nov., 1973.
85. Letters to the editor. J.A.D.A., *88*:467, Mar., 1974.

85a. Goodman, P., Greene, C. S., and Laskin, D. M.: Response of patients with myofascial pain-dysfunction syndrome to mock equilibration. J.A.D.A., *92*:755, April, 1976.

86. Lerman, M. D.: The hydrostatic appliance: a new approach to treatment of the TMJ pain-dysfunction syndrome. J.A.D.A., *89*:1343, Dec., 1974.
87. Lerman, M. D.: A complete hydrostatically derived treatment procedure for the TMJ pain-dysfunction syndrome. J.A.D.A., *89:*1351, Dec., 1974.
88. Pomp, M. A.: Psychotherapy for the MPD syndrome. J.A.D.A., *89*:629, Sept., 1974.
89. Greene, C. S., and Laskin, D. M.: Long term evaluation of conservative treatment for MPD syndrome. J.A.D.A., *89*:1365, Dec., 1974.
90. Travell, J.: Ethyl chloride spray for painful muscle spasm. Arch. Phys. Med., *33*:291, Mar., 1952.
91. Jacobson, E.: *Progressive Relaxation.* Chicago, University of Chicago Press, 1952.
92. Jacobson, E.: *Tension in Medicine.* Springfield, Ill., Charles C Thomas, 1967.

92a. Benson, H.: *The Relaxation Response.* New York, William Morrow and Co., 1975.

92b. Bloomfield, H. H., Cain, M. P., Jaffe, D. T., and Kory, R. B.: *TM: Discovering Innery Energy and Overcoming Stress.* New York, Dell Publishing Co., 1975.

92c. Stone, R. A., and DeLeo, J.: Psychotherapeutic control of hypertension. New Eng. J. Med., *294*:80, Jan. 8, 1976.

92d. Smith, A.: The meditation game. The Atlantic, *236*:33, Oct., 1975.

93. Budzynski, T. H., and Stoyva, J. J.: An instrument for producing deep muscle relaxation by means of analog information feedback. J. Appl. Behav. Anal., *2*:231, Winter, 1969.

93a. Carlsson, S. G., Gale, E. N., and Ohman, A.: Treatment of temporomandibular joint syndrome with biofeedback training. J.A.D.A., *91*:602, Sept., 1975.

93b. Gangarosa, L. P., Merchant, H. W., No, H. P., and Hill, J. M.: Iontophoretic application of idoxuridine in recurrent herpes labialis: report of 18 clinical trials. To be published.

94. Anderson, D. C., and Ogle, R. C.: Facial pain of intracranial origin. Oral Surg., *37*:841, July, 1974.
95. Melrose, R. J.: Personal communication, May 15, 1975.
96. Schwartz, L. L.: Op. cit., p. 183.
97. Black, R.: Trigeminal pain. In *Pain and Suffering.* Edited by B. L. Crue, Jr. Springfield, Ill., Charles C Thomas, 1970, pp. 119–37.
98. Person, P.: Personal communication, May 15, 1975.
99. Medical Letter 15, No. 23, Nov. 9, 1973.
100. Bonica, J. J.: Op. cit., p. 798.
101. Nissen, K. I.: Plantar digital neuritis: Morton's metatarsalgia. J. Bone Joint Surg., *30*:84, Feb., 1948.
102. Rushton, J., Gibilisco, J., and Goldstein, N.: Atypical facial pain. J.A.M.A., *171*:545, Oct., 1959.
103. Bonica, J. J.: Op. cit., p. 137.
104. Rushton, J., *et al.*: Op. cit.
105. Moulton, R.: Oral and dental manifestations of anxiety. Psychiatry, *18*:261, Aug., 1955.
106. Walsh, J. P.: Psychogenic symptoms in dental practice. Oral Surg., *6*:437, Mar., 1953.
107. Borland, L. R.: Hysterical symptoms as a factor in oral disease. Oral Surg., *6*:444, Mar., 1953.
108. Engel, G. L.: Primary atypical facial neuralgia. Psychosom. Med., *13*:375, Nov.-Dec., 1951.
109. Webb, H. E., and Lascelles, R. G.: Treatment of facial and head pain associated with depression. Lancet, *1*:355, Feb. 17, 1962.
110. Lascelles, R. G.: Atypical facial pain and depression. Brit. J. Psychiatr., *112*:651, 1966.
111. Zung, W. W. K.: From art to science, the diagnosis

and treatment of depression. Arch. Gen. Psychiat., *29*:328, Sept., 1973.

112. Gayford, J. J.: The aetiology of atypical facial pain and its relation to prognosis and treatment. Brit. J. Oral Surg., 7:202, Mar., 1970.
113. Alvarez, W. C.: *The Neuroses.* Philadelphia, W. B. Saunders Co., 1951, Chapt. 3.
114. Boracchia, C., and Boracchia, B. M.: Personal communication, 1973.
115. Harris, W. E.: Endodontic pain referred across the midline: report of a case. J.A.D.A., *87*:1240, Nov., 1973.
116. Zung, W. W. K.: A self-rating depression scale. Arch. Gen. Psychiat., *12*:63, Jan., 1965.
117. Zung, W. W. K.: How normal is depression? Psychosomatics, *13*:174, June, 1972.
118. Holmes, T. H., and Masuda, M.: Life change and illness susceptibility. Separation and depression. A.A.A.S. Publication No. 94, pp. 161–86, 1973.
119. Holmes, T. H., and Rahe, R. H.: The social readjustment rating scale. J. Psychosomat. Res., *11*:213, 1967.
120. Wilson, D. C.: Atypical facial neuralgia. J.A.M.A., *99*:813, Sept. 3, 1932.
121. THE MEDICAL LETTER on Drugs and Therapeutics, 17, Jan. 3, 1975.
122. Bonica, J. J.: Op. cit., p. 947.
123. Elfenbaum, A.: Causalgia in dentistry: an abandoned pain syndrome. Oral Surg., 7:594, June, 1954.
124. Bonica, J. J.: Op. cit., p. 942.
125. Ibid., p. 980.
126. Agnew, G. R.; Personal communication.
127. Robinson, M., and Slavkin, H.: Dental amputation neuromas. J.A.D.A., *70*:662, 1965.
128. Bonica, J. J.: Op. cit., p. 980. Quoting Cooper, I. S., and Braceland, F. J.: Psychosomatic aspects of pain. Med. Clin. N. Amer., *34*:4, 1950.
129. Ibid., p. 982.
130. Bonica, J. J.: Op. cit., p. 982.
131. Moulton, R.: Op. cit., p. 262.
132. Reynolds, O. E., Hutchins, H. C., Werner, A. Y., and Philbrook, F. R.: Aerodontalgia occurring during oxygen indoctrination in the low pressure chamber. U.S. Naval Med. Bull., *46*:845, June, 1946.
133. Bonica, J. J.: Op. cit., p. 980.
134. Behrman, S.: Facial neuralgias. Brit. Dent. J., *86*:197, Apr., 1949.
135. Elfenbaum, A.: Op. cit., p. 597.
136. Rushton, J., *et. al.*: Op. cit., p. 546.
137. Elfenbaum, A.: Op. cit., p. 598.
138. Bonica, J. J.: Op. cit., p. 996.
139. Reynolds, O. E., and Hutchins, H. C.: Reduction of central hyper-irritability following block anesthesia of peripheral nerve. Am. J. Physiol., *152*:658, 1948.
140. Sluder, G.: The role of the sphenopalatine (or Meckle's) ganglion in nasal headaches. N.Y. Med. J., *87*:989, 1908.
141. Bickerstaff, E. R.: The periodic migrainous neuralgia of Wilfred Harris. Lancet, *1*:1069, May, 1959.
142. Wolff, H. G.: *Headache and Other Head Pain.* New York, Oxford University Press, 1950, pp. 410–429.
143. Eggleston, D. J.: Periodic migrainous neuralgia. Oral. Surg., *29*:524, Apr., 1970.
144. Giampaoli, A. V.: Stanford University Report of the 30th Congress of the American College of Allergists, 1974.
145. Scott, M.: Malar bone pressure test for evaluation of headache. J.A.M.A., *212*:1214, May 18, 1970.
146. Biofeedback in Action. Med. World News, *14*:27, Mar. 9, 1973.
147. Sicher, H.: Problems of pain in dentistry. Oral Surg., 7:149, Feb., 1954.
148. Ibid, p. 149.
149. Glick, D. H.: Locating referred pulpal pains. Oral Surg., *15*:613, May, 1962.
150. Ibid, p. 618.
151. Ray, B. S.., and Wolff, H. G.: Experimental studies on headache. Pain sensitive structures of the head and their significance in headache. Arch. Surg., *41*:813, 1940.
152. Ruch, T. C., and Fulton, J. F.: Op. cit., p. 369.
153. Hutchins, H. C., and Reynolds, O. E.: Experimental investigation of the referred pain of aerodontalgia. J. Dent. Res., *26*:3, Feb., 1947.
154. Ruch, T. C., and Fulton, J. F.: Op. cit., p. 370.
155. Wolff, H. G.: The nature and causation of headache. J. Dent. Med., *14*:3, Jan., 1959.
156. Holmes, T. H., Goodell, H., Wolf, S., and Wolff, H. G.: *The Nose.* Springfield, Ill., Charles C Thomas, 1950, p. 68.
157. Wolff, H. G.: *Headache and Other Head Pain.* New York, Oxford University Press, 1950, p. 452.
158. Ibid., pp. 457–458.
159. Orban, B., and Ritchey, B. T.: Toothache under conditions simulating high altitude flight. J.A.D.A., *32*:145, Feb., 1945.
160. Reynolds, O. E., *et al.*: Op. cit., p. 857.
161. Ibid., p. 8.
162. Sicher, H.: Op. cit., p. 159.
163. Nenzen, B., and Welander, U.: The effect of conservative root canal therapy on local mucosal hyperplasia of the maxillary sinus. Odontol. Rev., *18*:295, 1967.
164. Senia, E. S., and Clarich, J. D.: Arm pain of dental origin. Oral Surg., *38*:960, Dec., 1974.
165. Ruch, T. C., and Fulton, J. F.: Op. cit., p. 329.
166. Ibid., p. 332.
167. Matson, M. S.: Pain in orofacial region associated with coronary insufficiency. Oral. Surg., *16*:284, Mar., 1963.
168. Norman, J. E. de B.: Facial pain and vascular disease. Some clinical observations. Brit. J. Oral Surg., *8*:138, Nov., 1970.
169. Marcruz, R.: Pain in the neck, first sign of thrombosis. R. N., July, 1974.
170. Turner, G. O.: Alerting public to heart attack signs—without a stampede. Med. World News, *14*:18, Mar. 9, 1973.
171. Hall, S.: Aching jaw may warn of heart attack. Dent. Survey, p. 44, Apr., 1975.
172. Poliak, B.: Personal communication.

172a. Natkin, E., Harrington, G. W., and Mandel, M. A.:

Anginal pain referred to the teeth. Oral Surg., *40*:678, Nov., 1975.

173. Russel, H. I.: Role of heredity, diet and emotional stress in coronary heart disease. J.A.M.A., *171*:503, Oct. 3, 1959.

174. Friedman, M., and Rosenman, R. H.: Type A Behavior and your heart. Med. World News, *15*:512, May 17, 1974.

175. The Heart of the Type A Debate. Med. World News, *16*:103, Feb. 24, 1975.

176. Fredrickson, D. S.: Mutants, hyperlipoproteinaemia, and coronary artery disease. Brit. Med. J., *2*:187, Apr. 24, 1971.

177. Levy, R. I., Fredrickson, D. S., and Stone, N. J.: Cholestyramine in type II hyperlipoproteinemia: a double blind trial. Ann. Int. Med., *79*:51, July, 1973.

Chapter 12

Microbiologic Considerations in Endodontics

EDWARD WHITE

Bacteria are the primary contributors to pathogenesis of the dental pulp and periapical tissues (Fig. 12–1). It logically follows that procedures to eradicate offending microorganisms have high priority in therapy. For the last 30 or 40 years bacteriology has been a principal focus in endodontics for many reasons, only some of which are valid. During this time, determination of the microbial "status" of root canals has been the target of much research. As a result, an inordinate emphasis on microbiologic culturing of root canals has overshadowed proper consideration of more important therapeutic principles. To place this all in proper perspective, historical overview of the present state of the art will make it possible to identify those concepts which are no longer valid.

Infectious Etiology. The evidence is impressive that microbes cause pulp disease. Moreover, most pulp disease leads to an irreversible pulpitis that in turn leads to pulp necrosis and apical periodontitis. Clinical and experimental observations which strongly support the infectious etiology of pulp pathosis are:

1. When the pulp of a tooth is exposed to saliva contaminated with oral flora, pathologic changes occur within the pulp and periapical tissues.
2. Bacteria can usually be cultured from diseased, or exposed, necrotic pulp chambers. Paradoxically, bacteria may also be cultured from diseased pulps which have ***not*** been exposed to the oral cavity by fracture or caries.
3. The discomfort and swelling of periapical inflammation arising from diseased pulps are ameliorated by systemic antibiotics. The corollary—antibiotics act specifically against bacteria.
4. The removal of tissue, debris, ***and bacteria*** from root canals promotes healing and repair of affected periapical tissues.
5. Success of endodontically treated cases is somewhat greater for those with negative bacteriologic cultures than for those with positive cultures.

By deduction from the foregoing examples, one can argue in favor of bacterial involvement in pulp disease. More satisfying would be direct evidence for microbial involvement, but there is a paucity of information in this area. The report of Kakehashi, Stanley, and Fitzgerald is the first convincing evidence specifically implicating bacteria as etiologic agents of pulp inflammation.[1] Pulps of rat molar teeth were exposed by drilling into the pulp chamber, and the exposed pulps were left open to the oral cavity. These operative procedures were done on two groups of rats—***conventional*** rats, *i.e.,* rats housed under normal vivarium conditions with normal oral flora, and ***germ-free*** (gnotobiotic) rats, *i.e.* rats reared and housed in the absence of bacteria. Within eight days the regular animals developed intense inflammation and necrosis of the pulps and periapex. But in the germ-free groups, little or no inflammation developed within the full 42-day observation period. In this same gnotobiotic group, healing, evidenced by

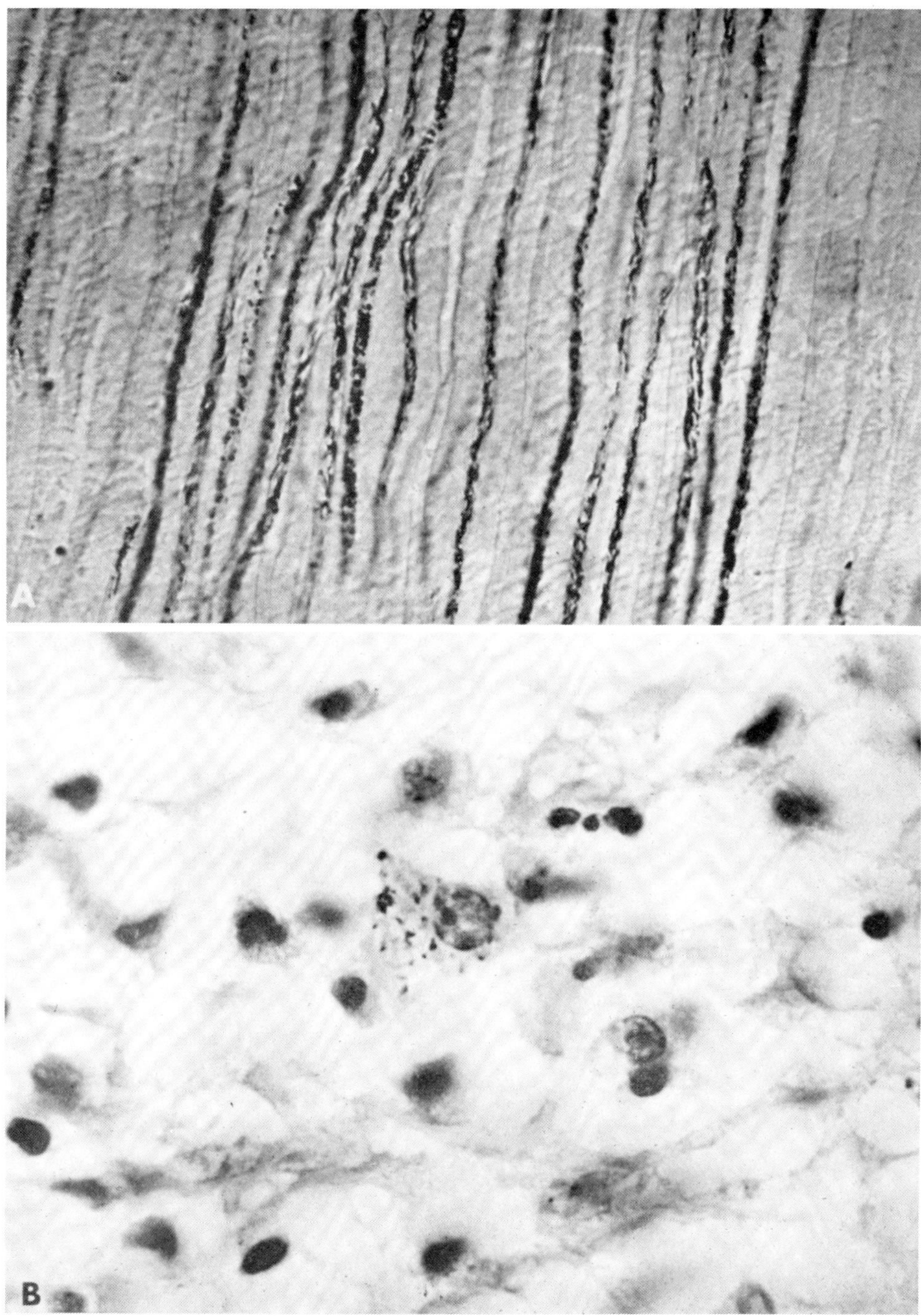

Fig. 12–1. Microorganisms are principal source of irritation to dental pulp. *A*, Bacteria descending dentinal tubules, between carious lesion and highly inflamed pulp. *B*, Pulp macrophage loaded with phagocytized bacteria. Coronal pulp inflammation is well advanced. (Orban collection.)

dentinal bridging, also occurred in spite of food and hair impactions. This classic study provides the basis for subsequent investigations to define and differentiate the role of trauma and microorganisms in pulp disease.

For the purpose of this discussion, let us assume that bacteria are the principal etiologic agents of pulp disease. It is then important to know which microorganisms, acting either independently or synergistically with other microorganisms, are pathogenic for pulp tissue. Can just any organism found in the mouth cause disease? Perhaps not, since the skin, mouth, intestine, and other orifices of the body contain countless microorganisms, but are not normally diseased.

Pathogenicity. Infection may be defined as a process whereby certain microorganisms gain access into a host, establish themselves, and multiply. Microorganisms are generally classified as pathogenic or nonpathogenic. Pathogenicity denotes the ability of organisms to cause disease; it is a relative quality dependent on inherent noxious factors of the microbe and resistance of the host. Virulence characterizes the degree of pathogenicity of organisms.

At present, scientific knowledge does not define exactly which bacteria are pathogenic for dental pulps. The presence of microorganisms within "infected" root canals does not necessarily mean these organisms directly contributed to the destruction of that organ. some organisms cultured from root canals are characterized as contaminants: organisms that entered from the oral cavity by caries, trauma, operative exposures, or leaking restorations. Normally, contaminants are considered to be nonpathogenic and not involved in the etiology of pulp disease. Based on present knowledge, however, this is a tenuous conclusion for any given organism. Surely some organisms colonize pulp chambers ***after*** the initial events of disease. Only further research will enable us to distinguish which organisms are etiologic agents and which organisms are casual contaminants.

Staphylococci are often cultured from pulpless teeth. *Staphylococcus aureus* is the virulent or pathogenic strain of these genera, and *Staphylococcus albus* is generally considered to be nonpathogenic, a common inhabitant of the skin. Both may be found in diseased pulp canals. This leads to the often-asked question, "Can *Staphylococcus albus*, a 'nonpathogen,' cause pulp inflammation and disease?" In an attempt to answer this question and to test the effects of

Table 12-1. Bacterial Exposure of Mice Following Trauma to Molars

Group	*Environment*	*Oral Flora*
I	Germ-free	None
II	Defined flora	Alpha streptococci
III	Defined flora	*Candida albicans*
IV	Defined flora	*Staphylococcus aureus*
V	Defined flora	*Staphylococcus epidermidis*
VI	Isolator conventional	Normal

different bacterial populations on pulp tissue, the following investigations were done by White et al.[2] Surgical excision of maxillary molar crowns exposed the pulps of several groups of mice raised in three different environments: (1) germ-free, (2) monocontaminated, and (3) isolator conventional environments, as noted in Table 12–1. Histologic evaluations were made at varying times postoperatively. The intensity of inflammation and healing response was evaluated and scored by microscopic examinations of both normal controls and the operated maxillae.

The four-day samples for group I (the germ-free mice) showed some focal necrosis and intrapulp hemorrhage. Specimens from subsequent sacrifice periods in group I consistently revealed overall repair and normal pulp architecture with a persistent odontoblastic layer.

Group II monocontaminated mice were raised germ-free, but were then inoculated with an indigenous strain of alpha streptococci isolated from the oral cavity of conventional mice. Group II had a slightly greater incidence of minimal cellular infiltrate and inflammation than did germ-free mice (group I), but this inflammatory response subsided after 21 days.

In group III monocontaminated mice inoculated with *Candida albicans* (a fungal organism commonly found in the mouth and often in pulpless teeth), the patterns of healing and repair were quite similar to those of group II mice infected with streptococci. In specimens from time periods greater than 21 days, little or no inflammation was noted for either group II or group III animals. This is important because, in humans, streptococci are the most frequently cultured organisms from diseased teeth. Twelve weeks after surgery, ***normal*** pulp architecture was histologically evident in both groups—those infected with streptococci and those with Candida (Fig. 12–2).

In contrast to the first three groups, significant

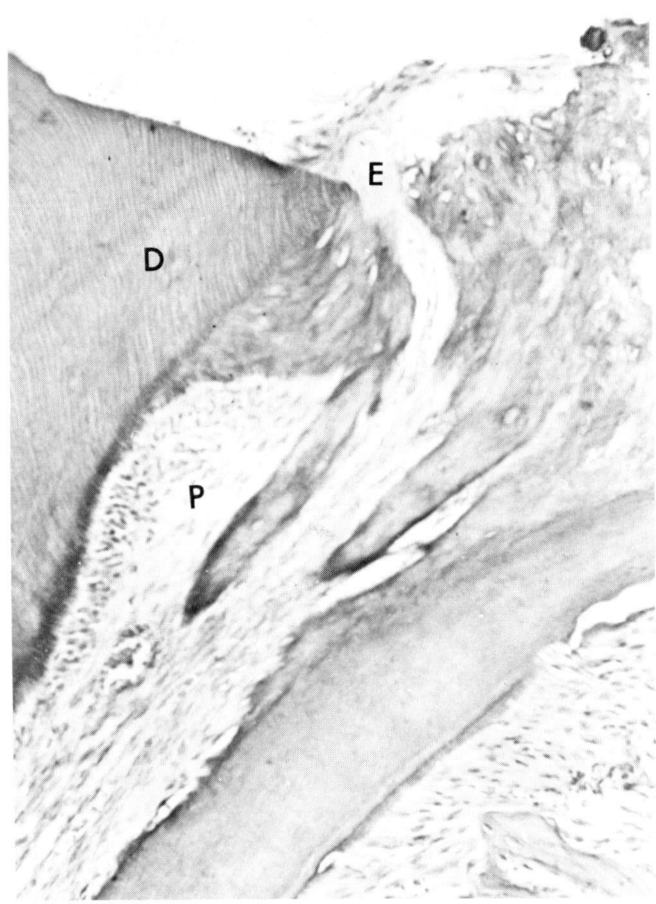

Fig. 12–2. Appearance of exposed rat molar pulp 12 weeks following infection with *Candida albicans*. Persistent odontoblastic layer and absence of inflammation and partial bridging of exposure (E) indicate normal pulp (P). (Courtesy Dr. Edward White.)

inflammatory response was seen in groups IV and V—animals inoculated with ***staphylococci.*** This resulted in high levels of inflammation represented by intense cellular infiltrate that appeared early and persisted throughout the experimental period. Two weeks after surgery, destructive inflammatory changes induced by staphylococci were quite apparent (Fig. 12–3). These typical changes were noted for animals inoculated with either *Staphylococcus albus* or *Staphylococcus aureus*. It appears, at least in mice, that either strain of staphylococci induces persistent pulp disease.

The isolator conventional mice, group VI, reared in a normal environment with normal flora, demonstrated the greatest degree of inflammation. Complete pulp necrosis was seen in several specimens in the later periods (Fig. 12–4). Periapical cellular infiltration was also present in groups III, IV, and V. In rodents, inflammatory responses are rarely of the intensity found in humans, but for mice the responses noted in Figure 12–3 were graded as "intense" and were seen in both staphylococci-inoculated and isolator conventional animals.

These data indicate that ***specific*** microbes are essential to initiate and sustain a vigorous inflammatory response in exposed dental pulps and periapical tissues of mice. Conversely, the pulps of ***germ-free*** mice had zero to minimal inflammation after cutting off the crowns of their molar teeth. These observations are consistent with other observations of inflammation in germ-free and monocontaminated animals.[3–7]

Recognizing the limitation of unconfirmed studies, one can say that in animals monocontaminated with staphylococcal organisms of ***either*** the pathogenic variety or the so-called nonpathogenic variety, a vigorous inflammatory response can develop. Organisms such as indigenous streptococci and Candida produce only mild to minimal inflammation in pulps, which tends to resolve within 21 days. Surgical trauma alone results in an initial transitory inflammatory reaction which tends to resolve rapidly in germ-free animals.

In view of this evidence, it could be said that, within the bounds of reason, surgical trauma *per se* does not cause irreversible pulp death. For that matter, trauma alone does not induce intensive and persistent inflammatory reactions in any tissue or organ. Microbial input and/or some suitable antigenic stimulus is essential for induction and maintenance of inflammation beyond the initial changes already noted. Pulp death in human beings would then be the result of an interplay between some form of trauma and microbial infection. Whether pulp death ultimately occurs or not will depend on host resistance and virulence of invading microorganisms.

Infection vs. Trauma. To distinguish between pulp inflammation from microbial insult and inflammation from traumatic insult creates a dilemma for the pulp biologist. Necrosis often occurs after pulp exposure from caries and/or operative procedures. In instances in which a pulp has not been exposed, inflammation and necrosis may occur from such traumatic insults as cavity preparation, mechanical forces associated with restorations, noxious restorative materials, and acci-

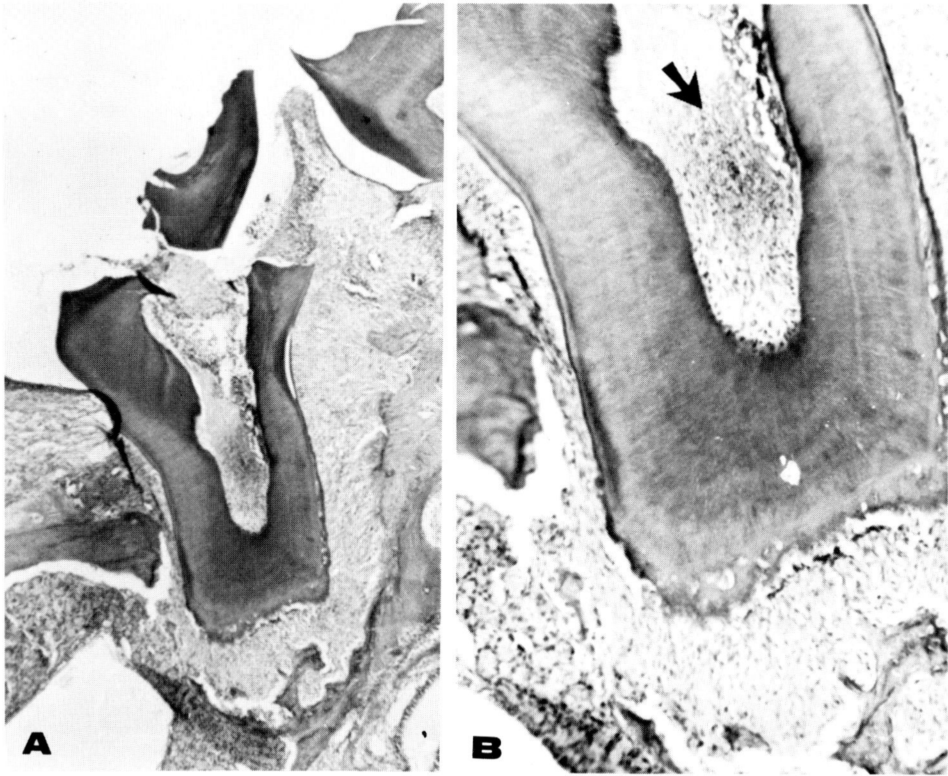

Fig. 12–3. *A,* Low-power view of severe inflammation in exposed rat pulp 2 weeks after monoinfection with *Staphylococcus aureus. B,* High-power view of Figure 12–3*A*. Inflammation *(arrow)* has advanced to apical third of pulp. (Courtesy Dr. Edward White.)

dental blows to teeth. Pulp biologists and endodontists may refer to these cases of pulp inflammation and necrosis as "sterile" death of the pulp. This, of course, implies that bacteria had no direct etiologic role, or if involved, in a secondary capacity.

This conclusion is based on the frequent inability to culture organisms from these cases. However, bacteria ***can*** be cultured from previously traumatized pulpless teeth whose pulps were not exposed to the oral cavity.[8–11] It would seem that the incidence of finding organisms in traumatized teeth increases with the diligence and sophistication of culturing techniques employed, especially anaerobic.[12,13] About 75 to 80% of non-exposed pulpless teeth yield bacteria by judicious culturing of pulp canals.

As a counter argument against "sterile" pulp death, it is necessary to point out that no evaluation has been made on traumatized teeth in germ-free environments. It is proposed that trauma in gnotobiotic environments, which would normally cause pulp death in conventional environments, would not lead to necrosis in the absence of bacteria. Broadly restated: no bacteria—no ***persistent*** inflammation. This heretical statement is made in spite of older concepts of the unique liability of dental pulps for irreversible injury due to constricted apical foramens, limited blood supply, stagnation of fluids, hypertension, lateral canals, and blocked lymph channels.

Experiments to bring to light the mechanisms of irreversible pulpitis are not yet complete in germ-free and conventional animals, but these experiments are in progress. Preliminary results indicate that severe trauma (*e.g.,* heat) induces extensive calcification of pulp tissue, osteodentin, in ***germ-free*** rats.[14] Similar trauma in ***conventional*** rats results in complete pulp necrosis. These findings, if confirmed by future investigation, may have a parallel with traumatized teeth in humans. In traumatized teeth, extensive pulp canal calcification by tertiary dentin may reflect minimal or no bacterial involvement in initial healing. Symptoms developing subsequent to calcification of pulp tissue may be the effect of bacteria lodging in

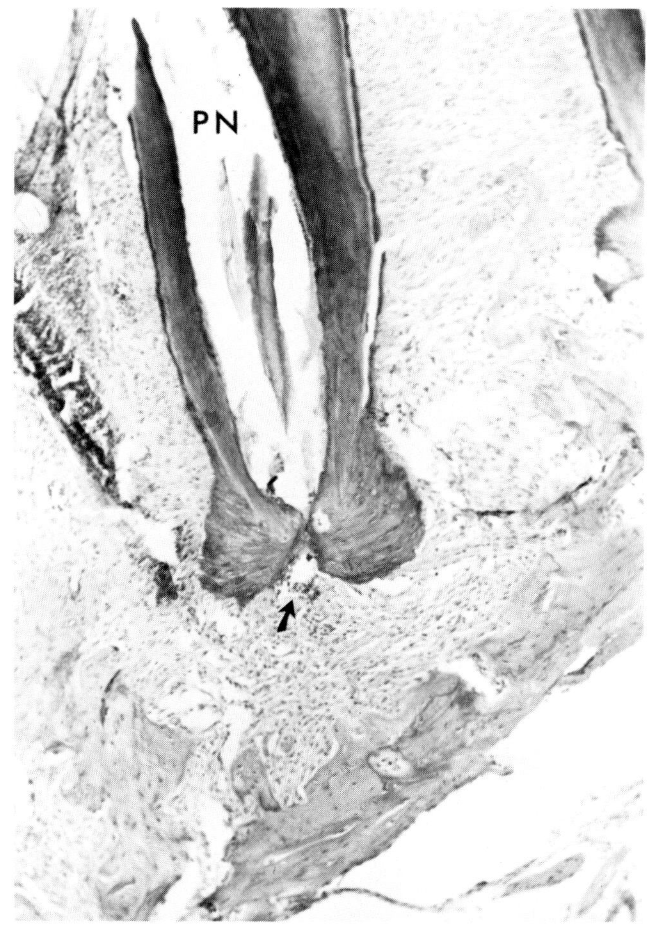

Fig. 12–4. Total pulp necrosis (PN) and initial periapical inflammation *(arrow)* 3 weeks following exposure of pulp in conventional control rat. Infection from normal mixed oral flora was responsible for this severe inflammatory response and pulp death. (Courtesy Dr. Edward White.)

the remaining pulp with diminished resistance to infection.

By contrast, early pulp necrosis reflects a major role for bacterial involvement. Pulp necrosis would obviously preclude further development of dentin, a condition frequently seen in adults who had a tooth traumatized as a child.

Portals of Entry. Against the background of hypotheses and evidence for bacterial involvement in pulp disease, it is useful to review the portals of entry for microorganisms into the dental pulp and periapical tissues.

Direct Pulp Exposure. This is the most obvious, the most frequent, and the least controversial avenue for microorganisms to gain access to a pulp. Access for bacteria can occur as the result of caries or through mechanical exposure from operative procedures or exposure from traumatic fracture of teeth.

Indirect Pulp Exposure. It has been proposed that microorganisms may gain entry to the pulp through the dentinal tubules, even though the carious process has not physically penetrated to the pulp chamber.[15] This issue is not clearly resolved. The pulp normally responds to caries by laying down reparative dentin, and some authorities consider reparative dentin relatively resistant to bacterial penetration. There is a substantial amount of information on the minimum thickness of dentin necessary to prevent irreversible inflammation with caries and/or operative procedures.[16,17] It would seem that bacteria within the dentinal tubules and more than 0.5 mm. from the pulp cause no pathosis. Irritant dentin is helpful in preventing pulp inflammation, but the carious process may progress faster than the deposition of this tertiary dentin, in which case the pulp is sure to be invaded by bacteria.

Lateral Canals. It has been proposed that lateral canals offer an avenue for entry of microorganisms into the pulp via the periodontal spaces.[18,19] Periodontal injury may also induce pulp inflammation.[20] This is a controversial issue, and to date, there is no information that this route is a ***substantial*** avenue for bacteria to enter healthy pulps and cause disease. Clearly, lateral canals are found anywhere on a root, and it seems reasonable that some organisms may gain access to the pulp through this pathway. It seems unlikely, however, that disease results without other contributing factors, because pulp inflammation through lateral canals rarely occurs.

Apical Foramen via the Periodontal Spaces. It has been proposed that if a tooth is dislodged or partially avulsed, organisms may traverse the periodontal spaces and gain access to the pulp via the apical foramen.[21] Even though experimental evidence tends to support this hypothesis, it does not exclude the entry of microorganisms by other means into pulps of teeth that have been dislodged or partially avulsed.

Retrogenic Infection. Retrogenic infection is pulp inflammation or death as a result of bacteria from adjacent diseased teeth which invade the pulp via the apical foramen. Even though some investigators may feel that retrogenic pulpitis rarely if ever occurs, this concept is frequently used in endodontic jargon to convince patients they should have a diseased tooth treated. The question commonly asked of clinicians is, "Can this infection spread to other teeth?" Some clinicians probably cringe a little and say, "Yes, it might affect your other teeth."

Hematogenic Anachoresis. In this instance, persistent blood-borne bacteria may be "attracted" to the pulp of a tooth which has been traumatized, but without exposure of the pulp to the oral cavity.[22] Initial inflammatory alterations occur within the pulp after trauma, and bacteria may be carried to this site by the blood stream. If the bacteria are virulent and the host-resistance is not sufficient to eradicate them, the bacteria, their toxic products, and antigens persist to induce a destructive inflammatory process. At least two factors are essential for this hypothesis to be accurate: (1) bacteria must enter the blood stream with some frequency; and (2) bacteria must be able to localize within the irritated pulp tissues.

Apparently transient bacteremias (bacteria detected in the blood stream through blood cultures) may occur after minimal trauma to oral tissues. Positive blood cultures have been found after eating, toothbrushing, bruxing, gingival surgery, extractions, or even endodontic procedures.[23–25] The potential for other sites of entry into the blood stream should not be excluded, such as the gut, skin, and genitalia. Perhaps the incidence of bacteremia is much more frequent than is assumed—a common daily occurrence with host defense mechanisms destroying the organisms without subsequent difficulty.

On the other hand, extensive reports show that bacteria become localized or colonized in areas of inflamed tissue. Following chemical irritation of skin and subsequent intravenous injection of bacteria, Rigdon demonstrated that bacteria could be isolated in substantial amounts in the area irritated by chemicals.[26] In a variety of animals, if teeth are traumatized without exposing pulps and subsequently bacteria are injected intravenously, the same bacteria can be isolated from the pulp tissue in a substantial number of cases.[8,27–29]

It is difficult to correlate these laboratory results to pulp necrosis in humans. In all of the animal studies, it was ***essential to inject*** microorganisms into the blood stream. In some animal research in which trauma was initiated and no organisms injected, no bacteria could be found in irritated or traumatized teeth. Although it is generally agreed that in human beings, bacteria can be found both in healthy pulps and in necrotic pulp chambers not exposed to the oral flora, the critical question is whether these organisms can play a role in the etiology of pulp disease.

Many factors associated with bacterial infection contribute to pathogenicity. The best known factors are toxins (*i.e.,* endotoxins and exotoxins), invasiveness, and enzymes produced by bacteria, such as hyaluronidase and collagenase. These toxic components play a major role in the colonization of bacteria and/or their destructive effect. Less well-known features are those associated with immune responses, which are usually thought of as protective, but may be destructive as well.

Immunologic Response. It may ***not*** be essential for viable bacteria to persist for a long time within the pulp to induce an irreversible inflammatory response. Bacterial degradation products can persist in tissues for substantial periods of time,[30] and these degradation products may act as ***antigenic*** stimuli to potentiate what histologically appears as an inflammatory response, but in reality may be an ***immunologic*** response. Even more important is the fact that an initial specific immune reaction may set the stage for persistent inflammation through nonspecific mediators. In addition, because of their potentially beneficial effects in the treatment of cancer,[31] these nonspecific destructive reactions assume greater importance.

It is essential to review a few principles and reactions to understand the cascading events currently postulated to explain immunologic response in pulp and periapical as well as periodontal pathogenesis.[32,33] All this can take place in the pulp where a rich supply of the cell mediators (plasma cells, lymphocytes, PMNs) are found.

Hypothetically, imagine that the pulp of a tooth is invaded by bacteria. The bacteria are antigenic and in a week or two induce detectable immune responses by the host. Antibodies in the form of immunoglobulins are produced from ***plasma*** cells (B cells) to react with antigens in the pulp. Antigen-antibody-complement complexes may form to induce inflammation in the tissue. Chemotaxis (the recruitment of ***neutrophils***) is also essential to, and a result of, these reactions. Other mediators which play a role are histamine (principally from mast cells), SRS, bradykinin, kallidin, and 5-hydroxytryptamine. The reactions here described are examples of ***immediate*** hypersensitivity (antigen-antibody), which is classically termed the Arthus reaction. It may take place in the pulp just as it might in the skin.

In contrast to immediate hypersensitivity, the other form of immunity is ***delayed*** hypersensitivity—cell mediated immunity (CMI). These reactions require specific antigenic stimulation of ***lymphocytes*** (T cells) which, in turn, liberate lymphokinins. These may be cytotoxic or influence other cells to participate in inflammatory reactions. Delayed hypersensitivity, CMI, may explain some forms of autoimmune disease—rejection of foreign grafts, for example. These reactions are not simple and in many instances require T cell and B cell interreaction as well as contributions from macrophages.

As mentioned earlier, the nonspecific potentiators of inflammation are becoming increasingly important in understanding the events in pulp and periapical disease. Several factors produced by immune reactions can nonspecifically amplify and exaggerate the destructive reactions in tissues. Among these are: chemotaxis, complement-fixation,[34,35] anaphylatoxin which affects smooth muscle contractibility and vascular permeability,[36] lysosomal enzymes, cathepsins,[37] and prostaglandins. The large group of substances previously discussed that are liberated from lymphocytes and may be dependent on macrophage interaction are the lymphokinins. Among these are: MIF—migratory inhibiting factor (keeps macrophages in the area of inflammation); MAF—macrophage activating factor (recruits macrophages to the area); LAF—lymphocyte activating factor (induces the nonsensitized lymphocytes to participate in the reaction); and OAF—osteoclastic activating factor (stimulates osteoclasts to destroy bone).[38]

Another reaction of interest is the localized Shwartzman reaction. This reaction lacks many of the features of an immune reaction—the lack of specificity of the inciting agent, the inability to demonstrate specific antibody participation, and the time sequence of events. To initiate the ***localized*** Shwartzman reaction, gram-negative bacteria (killed) or endotoxin is introduced into tissue followed by re-introduction 24 hours later. An inflammatory reaction similar to the Arthus reaction develops.

A ***generalized*** Shwartzman reaction requires that endotoxin or killed gram-negative bacteria be in the blood stream for both routes of adminstration. This results in bilateral cortical necrosis of the kidneys and endotoxic shock.

With this minimal list, one can readily see the complex factors involved in immunologic-inflammatory reactions. One should not lose sight of the fact that immune reactions and even inflammatory reactions can be destructive in the pathogenesis of disease, but may be beneficial in healing as well.

Iatrogenic Bacteremia. Another facet to consider is the possible hematogenous spread of organisms from infected teeth to other tissues or organs. This concept was in vogue as the "focal infection theory" during the first half of the twentieth century. It was then believed that infected teeth were a primary site from which bacteria spread causing a variety of systemic diseases. In that era extraction of all "infected" teeth was recommended.

That a bacterial "shower" from the oral cavity is possible is attested to by contemporary studies, which show an 88% incidence of bacteremia after scaling and curettage and 82% incidence after extraction. Moreover, endodontic instrumentation during which the apex has been perforated causes an 11% incidence of bacteremia. However, no bacterial isolations are demonstrated, if apical perforations have not occurred.[23,24] These figures are important when considering the spread of microorganisms into the circulation of patients with a history of rheumatic fever and mitral stenosis, since these patients are especially liable to develop subacute bacterial endocarditis. Bender and Seltzer have suggested that the incidence of bacteremia is much greater following extraction than from the more conservative endodontic treatment.[24] However, the incidence of normal seeding of microorganisms into the blood stream from the oral cavity or other sites is not known.

It is generally recommended that patients with heart valve damage be premedicated with antibiotics prior to dental treatment to prevent acute or subacute bacterial endocarditis. Often patients with a history of heart valvular damage are maintained on antibiotics for long periods of time. The beneficial effects of these antibacterial regimes are still subject to question.[39,40] About 50% of the organisms associated with initial bouts of endocarditis are streptococci that may have originated in the mouth. This concept of hematogenous spread of microorganisms leads us back to the era of focal infection and into the culturing of root canals.

Theory of Focal Infection. From a rather dim historical view, it would appear that bacteria were implicated as etiologic agents of pulp disease by Miller in the early 1900s.[41] Soon thereafter the medical and dental professions were warned that oral sepsis and infection could cause many disastrous systemic diseases. Hunter's classic report to the Faculty of Medicine of McGill University condemned diseased gingiva primarily and, to a lesser extent, pulpless teeth as the cause of many systemic diseases.[42] The overriding principle of what Hunter called oral sepsis, later to be extended to focal infection, was that organisms from diseased teeth would spread through the blood stream or lymphatics to other organs or tissues. It was even postulated that specific organisms had specific target tissues and that subsequent lesions could include almost any disease from neuritis to neurosis, nephritis, blindness, arthritis, or even cancer. Hunter's major criticisms were directed toward periodontal problems, but it soon became more popular to condemn pulpless teeth or teeth with pulpitis. Rampant extraction, accompanied by extensive alveolectomies, resulted from these fears. Rhein reported that 40 children exhibited at the International Medical Congress in London in 1913 had had every tooth removed as a prophylactic measure against oral sepsis.[43]

Such were the heroic, if misguided, attempts to rid the mouth of oral infection. Following World War I, Billings, Myers, and Rosenow, among others, fanned the focal infection fire with reports that streptococcal organisms could be isolated from tissues or blood of diseased patients.[44–46] If streptococci were injected into animals, a variety of bizarre and destructive pathologic events occurred. Unfortunately, this era was characterized by sloppy bacteriologic technical controls, and massive amounts of bacteria were injected into experimental animals. The limitation of bacteriologic classification and taxonomic controls clearly suggests that unknown kinds of organisms were being injected and many faulty conclusions were being publicized.

To recapture the sense of the times ***prior*** to 1911, endodontic procedures were being performed with no thought of a serious systemic threat. ***After*** 1911, however, all "infected" teeth were condemned. The persistent clinician had to prove he could eliminate ***all*** organisms from pulpless teeth. This practice, unfortunately, distracted attention from other critical factors that lead to successful treatment and brought about an era of culturing and overmedication.

BACTERIOLOGIC CULTURING

During this crucial era in the early 1900s, some conscientious practitioners, skeptical of the dogma of the day, were convinced that teeth could be saved through conservative endodontic procedures. To maintain an aura of respectability in a climate of extreme bacteriophobia, it became a quest to render root canals "sterile" in the course of treatment. Rhein, in a series of classic papers, laid the basis for removal of microorganisms as a model for acceptable treatment.[47–49]

One has to be impressed by the persistence and tenacity of the early advocates of endodontic therapy. To justify their treatment rationale, it was of primary importance to eliminate all microorganisms from the root canal. Considering the primitive culturing techniques of the day and the paucity of information about fastidious organisms, it is not surprising that many of the canals were found to be "sterile" before and after treatment.

Fortuitously, bactericidal and bacteriostatic agents had been used during canal instrumentation for a number of years before the focal infection scare. Sulfuric acid, for example, was used to decalcify dentin during canal enlargement. After Hunter's pronouncement, antimicrobial drugs were specifically incorporated into endodontic therapy for the purpose of killing microorganisms. Following reports that teeth could be rendered sterile, culturing became a fetish for some and a means unto itself for others.

From approximately 1926 to the present, reports of thousands of cases have appeared in the endodontic literature comparing the incidence of success or failure of treated cases based on positive or negative cultures prior to final obturation of root canals (Table 12–2). For example, Zeldow and Ingle reported approximately 95% success rate for teeth filled with negative cultures versus 83% for those filled with positive cultures.[51,52] Others, notably Bender and

Table 12-2. Correlation of the Positive Culture to the Prognosis of Endodontically Treated Teeth

			Success		*Failure*	
Investigators	*Culture**	*Cases*	*No.*	*%*	*No.*	*%*
Rhein, Krasnow,	+	152	129	84.8	23	15.2
and Gies[49]	–	340	320	94.1	20	5.9
Abramson[50]	+	38	32	84.2	6	15.8
	–	97	92	96.6	5	3.4
Zeldow and Ingle[51]	+	42	35	83.3	7	16.7
Ingle[52]	–	162	153	94.5	9	5.5

* = bacteriologic culture results of canal before filling
\+ = positive culture
– = negative culture

Failure rate of pulpless teeth filled in spite of positive bacteriologic culture is consistently *10% higher* than for those cases filled following negative culture. (Adapted from Zeldow, B. J., and Ingle, J. I.: J.A.D.A., *66*:24, 1963.)

Seltzer, did not find such disparity between success or failure based on positive or negative cultures.[53]

Culturing is still a controversial area in endodontics, but even 83% success with ***positive*** cultures leads one to question the real significance of culturing. Until the reasons for failure of endodontically treated teeth are more clearly defined and the distinction made between casual contaminants and true etiologic organisms, we must be careful not to put too much emphasis on the presence of bacteria in root canals. Culturing clearly has some advantages and may even enhance success. ***In itself, however, it does not provide the basis for success.*** The unfortunate aspect of culturing is that many clinicians may become preoccupied with achieving a negative culture to the detriment of other more important aspects of therapy, such as proper cleansing and obturation of the canal space.

Rationale for Culturing Endodontically Involved Teeth

1. There is some evidence that, prior to the obturation of canals, greater success is achieved in cases with negative cultures than in those with positive cultures.[51]

2. Antibiotic management in therapy can be better tailored to individual cases if antibiotic sensitivity testing is done for organisms isolated from root canals. Occasionally, acute inflammation does not respond favorably to local therapy, and complications or "flare-ups" occurring during treatment may be difficult to control. By early identification of the antibiotic sensitivity of organisms from canals, the clinician may better prescribe systemic antibiotic therapy for the needs of his patient.

3. As a teaching aid, the culturing technique offers the beginning student a yardstick for determining whether canal debridement has been thorough, whether leakage has occurred between visits, and whether an aseptic technique has been followed throughout the course of treatment. Although most experienced clinicians can readily follow an aseptic technique, students in the throes of learning should benefit from this check on technique. Bacteria in root canals are the simplest and easiest component of the root canal contents to monitor. Using bacteria as identifiable markers, the student can clean a canal until the markers are "gone." One should emphasize, however, that even in canals that are not thoroughly cleaned, the antimicrobial effects of intracanal medications may mask this bacterial marker. A negative culture can produce a false feeling of security and preclude proper consideration of other more important principles, including debridement.

Culturing Technique

Microbial etiology and culturing have been the subject of excellent articles and reviews,[54–56] and a variety of culturing techniques and materials are available. Before we discuss a detailed protocol for culturing root canals, an overview of the technique is appropriate. Basically, this procedure determines whether viable bacteria can be grown from a representative sample of root canal contents. The sample is inoculated into a suitable medium for bacterial growth, and the medium observed for growth of microorganisms. The procedure must be reasonably convenient for clinicians or it will not be utilized.

It is important that this procedure be done aseptically. Sommer and Crowley emphasized the importance of excluding extraneous organisms in culturing.[57] It is important to begin with sterile instruments and to eliminate organisms from the immediate environs of the operating field. Depending on the emphasis of a clinician, the culturing technique can be as sophisticated as desired, requiring even greater logistic support than outlined below.

Equipment. For the basic culture technique, the following items are needed: (1) liquid bactericidal agent, (2) sterile forceps, (3) sterile burs, (4) sterile paper points, (5) liquid culture medium (tube), *e.g.*, thioglycollate or trypticase soy broth, and (6) incubator.

Technique. The tooth to be evaluated is isolated with the rubber dam. The tooth surfaces and immediate dam area are scrubbed with a suitable bactericidal agent. In a dry field, access to the pulp chamber is achieved. For primary access, it is advisable to use two burs, one for gross tooth structure or restoration removal, and another for final entry into the pulp chamber. Once convenience form and canal access are established, a sterile paper point is inserted into the orifice of each canal. The points probably become moist by absorbing fluid from the canals. If not, the canals (only the canals) should be moistened with a sterile solution such as saline or anesthetic. These points are retrieved, the lip of the culture tube is flamed, and the points are introduced into the medium. The tube is incubated

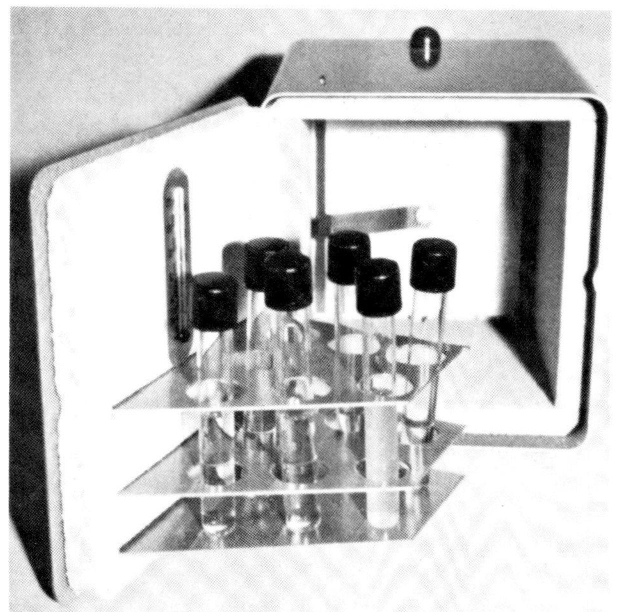

Fig. 12–5. Small, inexpensive, thermostatically controlled electric incubator adequate for average dental practice. Cloudy culture tube in right foreground is "positive." Remaining clear tubes are "negative." (Incubator courtesy of The Buffalo Dental Mfg. Co.)

for a minimum of 48 hours at 37° C in an inexpensive and convenient incubator suitable for office use (Fig. 12–5). After incubation, growth of bacteria is observed as cloudiness in the tube compared to non-inoculated tubes. Cloudy tubes are reported as positive cultures, and those remaining clear as negative cultures. Incubation longer than 48 hours is optimum. For cultures taken at subsequent appointments, the technique varies little except to realize that (1) a representative sample of the complete root canal system is essential, and (2) ***antimicrobial*** effects can be transferred to the media from canals that have been medicated. For subsequent cultures, the paper point should pass within a few millimeters of the apex and become moistened with root canal contents. For canals previously medicated, one should be aware that intracanal medication may be carried into the culture media, thereby inhibiting bacterial multiplication in the tube. Serene and McDonald detected a greater incidence of positive canals if sampling was done prior to saline irrigation, which has been used to wash the medication from the canals.[58]

For canals consistently positive after thorough debridement and medication, one must suspect defective restorations or a fractured root. On the other hand, a "false positive" result can be obtained with contamination of paper points by leakage of saliva during culturing or by contamination of points prior to transfer to the culture medium. Obviously, contaminated media may give a "false positive" reading as well. "False negative" results may be attributed to such causes as too few organisms in the sample to initiate discernible turbidity, inadequate sampling, or transference of intracanal medication to the culture medium. One must also consider that all organisms residing within root canals may ***not*** grow by present culture techniques.[13]

Bacterial and Antibiotic Sensitivity Identification. Bacteria may be identified and their susceptibility or resistance to antibiotic preparations may be determined by supplementary culturing and testing. For most dental offices, this would require the services of a microbiologic laboratory. Viable broth cultures or fresh samples of canal contents in a suitable "holding" medium should be sent to the laboratory for antibiotic sensitivity evaluation.[59] Briefly the technique is as follows:

The sample is streaked onto a suitable agar plate to allow for colony growth. The specific organisms may be identified by a microbiologist at this stage or may require further subculturing. For antibiotic sensitivity testing a representative sample of a positive culture is

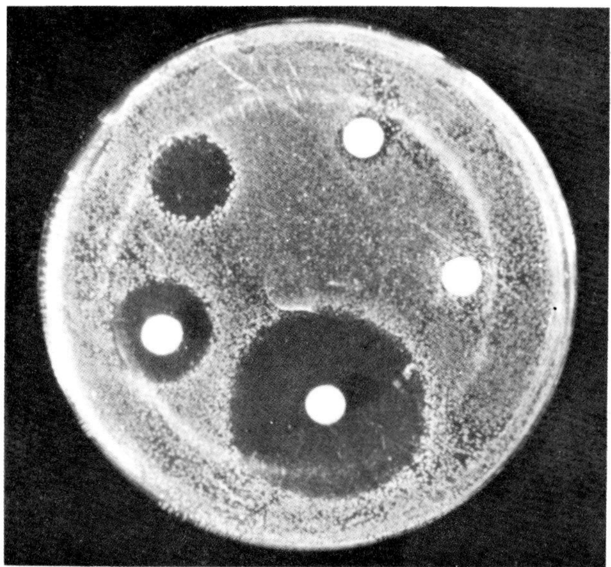

Fig. 12–6. Antibiotic disc-sensitivity test from routine root canal culture. Only effective antibiotic for these resistant staphylococci is chloramphenicol. Penicillin, erythromycin, and tetracyclines are ineffective.

streaked onto an agar plate, and antibiotic-impregnated disks are placed on the plate. The plate is then incubated for 24 hours, and inhibition of bacterial growth is recorded as sensitivity to any given antibiotic. The degree of sensitivity may be quantified for *in vitro* growth as illustrated in Figure 12–6.

Positive cultures may be the result of sampling organisms indigenous to the root canal, and this is the primary purpose of the culturing technique. Whether or not the organisms were the etiologic agents of pulp disease cannot be determined. They could be the organisms, however, to initiate an apical abscess in the event they are forced or carried into the periapex. These contaminants may be particularly dangerous if a stab inoculation is made, since streptococci are the bacteria most frequently isolated from root canals. These isolates are predominantly alpha streptococci, commonly identified as *Streptococcus viridans.* On further classification, many of these isolates are *Streptococcus mitis* and *salivarius,* common oral bacteria. Other streptococci may also be cultured: the gamma or nonhemolytic *Streptococcus faecalis* and group A, beta hemolytic *Streptococcus pyogenes. S. faecalis* are often quite resistant to antimicrobial regimes. A summary of several studies relative to the incidence of microbial isolates from root canals is presented in Table 12–3.

Microbial Status of Periapical Tissues

Although bacteria clearly may invade pulp tissue and become established in the root canal, the mechanisms of their involvement in the etiology of acute and/or chronic apical periodontitis are not well understood. The role of bacteria in radicular cyst formation is understood even less. There is little

Table 12-3. Classification and Incidence of Microorganisms Isolated from the Root Canals of Nonvital Teeth

Isolates	*MacDonald, Hare and Wood*[10]		*Mazzarella, Hedman and Brown*[60]		*Brown and Rudolph*[9]		*Winkler and Van Amerongen*[61]	
	Number							
Total Isolates	71		90		114		1,417	
	%							
Gram-positive	78.8		76.6		76.4		96.4	
Streptococci (all species)		28.1		27.8		28.1		62.9
Staphylococci		22.5		14.4		16.7		16.4
Corynebacterium (diphtheroids)		9.8		22.2		24.6		4.1
Other*		17.0		8.9		7.0		10.6
Yeast		1.4		3.3		—		1.6
Gram-negative	21.2		23.4		23.6		3.6	
Neisseria		5.6		3.3		2.6		1.1
Bacteroides		7.0		—		—		—
Pseudomonas		2.8		1.1		0.9		—
Coliform†		1.5		1.1		0.9		—
Fusobacterium		2.8		2.2		2.6		0.6
Other*		1.4		2.2		4.3		1.9
Spirochetes		—		8.9		12.3		
Unidentified		—		4.6		—		

— None reported
* Other includes unidentified organisms in each classification
† Gram-negative rods including *E. coli* and *A. aerogenes*

At least 75% of all microorganisms isolated from root canals are gram-positive. Streptococci and staphylococci constitute the most frequently isolated organisms. Spirochetes are frequently found in infected root canals, but are difficult to grow in the laboratory.

agreement as to whether bacteria invade, exist, or persist in periapical tissues prior to, during, or after endodontic therapy.

Theorizing begins about subsequent events in the pathologic process. One theory suggests that bacterial toxins and noxious products from pulp degradation pass from the root canal into the periapical spaces. These toxins initiate the destructive inflammatory responses observable within the alveolar bone. Much of the evidence to support this theory comes from the studies of Fish,[62] who reported that streptococcal organisms are never found in "living" tissues, even inflamed tissues, except in the early stages of acute inflammation. He proposed that bacteria colonized within necrotic pulp tissue serve as a depot for toxins to initiate periapical pathosis. His theory postulated that bacteria survive in periapical tissues only in centers of necrosis, walled off from host phagocytic cells. In this concept, bacteria survive primarily in the "privileged sanctuary" of the root canal,[55] cloistered from the host's defense mechanisms. It follows, therefore, that the bacteria and their toxins, as well as the noxious products of pulp degradation, must all be removed from the canal, followed by complete obturation of the space. This triad of treatment has evolved as being essential to successful therapy because the unclean underfilled canal harbors bacteria and/or stagnant tissue fluids. Endodontists convinced of this theory state that underfilled, debris-laden canals or voids or empty spaces in root canal fillings are the primary factors contributing to persistent periapical inflammation or failures following endodontic therapy. By contrast, it is here proposed that after endodontic therapy, more failures result from microorganisms gaining access to periapical tissues from the oral cavity via the ***crown*** of the tooth and poorly filled canals than from apical percolation of underfilled canals.

Alternatively, the survival of microorganisms or their antigenic components in periapical tissues may potentiate an inflammatory response and could account for many failures or flare-ups. Even though viable organisms are not often cultured from periapical tissues,[63] diligent microbiologic or histologic searching can often demonstrate the presence of organisms in this location. Winkler has reported that most periapical lesions associated with necrotic pulps exhibited uniform dispersion of bacteria.[64] The scarcity of bacteria in periapical lesions may be compared to the difficulty in isolating microorganisms in individuals with tuberculosis and late syphilis. It is generally conceded that the organisms are present, even though small in numbers, within the infected tissues of the host.

It is here proposed that bacteria are present in inflamed periapical tissues and that endodontic therapy should be directed at the elimination of microorganisms from root canals and from periapical tissues as well. Canal debridement and intracanal medication are quite effective in eliminating microorganisms from adequately cleaned root canals. It is suggested further that the apical foramen should be kept patent throughout treatment, until final obturation, to allow for diffusion of medication into the periapical spaces. The medication, on the other hand, should be beneficial and have no deleterious effect on periapical tissue in concentrations currently used in endodontic therapy. A patent apical foramen may: (1) allow for diffusion of medicaments into the periapical area;[65] (2) minimize postoperative pain by allowing exudate to drain into the root canal, the canal acting as a sump in this instance; and (3) provide an avenue for a modified "incision and drainage" of inflamed tissue. An endodontic instrument gently passed through a patent apical foramen may be compared to a scalpel incising a carbuncle.

With regard to the clinical success or failure of endodontically treated cases, it is suggested that periapical radiolucencies should vanish with time or at least decrease in size. Cases of failure, in which periapical radiolucencies persist or enlarge, or pain persists or recurs, might be explained by the presence of highly resistant organisms in the periapical tissues. These situations may require surgical curettage and/or vigorous systemic antibiotic therapy. A recent case report suggests that actinomyces in the periapical tissue caused a persistent fistula, which was resolved with apical surgery.[66] Streptococci seem well tolerated by human beings and may have evolved over a long period of time, living with human beings.[67] With lowered host resistance, bacteria may multiply and exacerbation of symptoms develop. If host resistance is enhanced, bacteria may be eliminated or diminished and repair may occur or symptoms vanish.

A simplified version of the events that might transpire in chronic periapical inflammation is as follows: bacteria gain entrance into injured pulp tissue; they initiate an inflammatory reaction by toxic or immune mechanisms; they may persist or be killed and antigenic fragments may become sequestered in chronically inflamed tissue serving as a depot for further stimulation; normal host proteins may become denatured and serve as further antigenic stimulation; the aforementioned events, coupled with systemic and localized antibody formation,[68] sensitized lymphocytes, and nonspecific inflammatory potentiators—all contribute to the complexity of chronic inflammation. It has also been proposed that "enhancing" antibodies allow for survival of bacteria in many chronic disease states, *e.g.*, syphilis, coccidiomycosis.[69] In some instances, antibodies to organisms in periapical tissues may allow for survival rather than destruction.

MICROORGANISMS OTHER THAN BACTERIA

The role of organisms other than bacteria in pulp disease is not known. One could guess that fungi, mycoplasmas, and even viruses may contribute to the pathogenesis of pulp disease. Two possible viral roles include: (1) as a phage infecting bacteria and contributing to the virulence of organisms, and (2) as a cytopathic infection. Clinical impressions suggest that during and immediately after influenza epidemics, many patients with the "flu" appear in dentists' offices with pulp and periapical disease. This may be the reflection of virus infecting the pulp or, more likely, the factors of lowered host-resistance allowing bacteria to gain an advantage in pulp infection. However, the possibility that viruses may exert a cytotoxic or cytopathic effect on pulp cells should not be dismissed without adequate investigation.

REFERENCES

1. Kakehashi, S., Stanley, H. R., and Fitzgerald, R. J.: The effects of surgical exposures of dental pulps in germ-free and conventional laboratory rats. Oral Surg., *20*:340, 1965.
2. White, E., Riley, D. P., Wiles, L., and Joyce, J.: Inflammation after pulp exposure of teeth in germ-free, defined flora and conventional mice. In *Germfree Research Biological Effects of Gnotobiotic Environments.* Edited by J. B. Heneghan. New York, Academic Press, 1973, p. 191.
3. Perkins, E. H., Nettesheim, P., Morita, T., and Walburg, H. E.: In *The Reticuloendothelial System and Atherosclerosis.* Edited by R. N. DiLuzio and R. Paoletti. New York, Plenum Press, 1967, p. 175.
4. Miyakawa, M.; In *Recent Progress in Microbiology.* Edited by G. Tunevall. Stockholm, Almquist and Wiksell, 1959, p. 299.
5. Gibons, R. J., Berman, K. S., Knoettner, P., and Kapsimalis, B.: Dental caries and alveolar bone loss in gnotobiotic rats infected with capsule forming streptococci of human origin. Arch. Oral Biol., *11*:549, 1966.
6. Korzen, B. H., Krakow, A. A., and Green, D. B.: Pulpal and periapical tissue responses in conventional and monoinfected gnotobiotic rats. Oral Surg., *37*:783, May, 1974.
7. Alter, E. A.: The effects of staphylococcus aureus on pulpal and periapical tissue in gnotobiotic rats. Master's Thesis, Indiana University, School of Dentistry, 1973.
8. Gier, R. E., and Mitchell, D. F.: Anachoretic effect of pulpitis. J. Dent. Res., *47*:564, 1968.
9. Brown, L. R., and Rudolph, C. E.: Isolation and identification of microorganisms from unexposed canals of pulp-involved teeth. Oral Surg., *10*:1094, 1957.
10. MacDonald, J. B., Hare, G. D., and Wood, A. W. S.: Bacteriological status of the pulp chambers of intact teeth found to be nonvital following trauma. Oral Surg., *10*:318, 1957.
11. Taklan, S.: A bacteriological study of the pulps of intact nonvital teeth. J. Brit. Endodont. Soc., *7*:75, July, 1974.
12. Kantz, W. E., and Henry, C. A.: Isolation and classification of anaerobic bacteria from intact pulp chambers of non-vital teeth in man. Arch. Oral Biol., *19*:91, Jan., 1974.
13. Wittgow, W. C., and Sabiston, C. B.: Microorganisms from pulpal chambers of intact teeth with necrotic pulps. J. Endodont., *1*:168, May, 1975.
14. White, E.: Unpublished data.
15. Bender, I. B., Seltzer, S., and Kaufman, I. J.: Infectibility of the dental pulp by way of dental tubules. J.A.D.A., *59*:466, 1959.
16. Hasler, J. F., and Mitchell, D. F.: Painless pulpitis. J.A.D.A., *81*:671, 1970.
17. Reeves, R., and Stanley, H. R.: The relationship of bacterial penetration and pulpal pathosis in carious teeth. Oral Surg., *22*:59, 1966.
18. Seltzer, S., Bender, I. B., and Ziontz, M.: The interrelationship of pulp and periodontal disease. Oral Surg., *16*:1474, 1963.
19. Rubach, W. C., and Mitchell, D. F.: Periodontal disease, age, and pulp status. Oral Surg., *19*:482, 1965.
20. Stahl, S. S.: Pulpal response to gingival injury in rats. Oral Surg., *16*:1116, 1963.
21. Grossman, L. I.: Origin of microorganisms in traumatized, pulpless, sound teeth. J. Dent. Res., *46*:551, 1967.
22. Csernyei, J.: Anachoretic effect of chronic periapical inflammation. J. Dent. Res., *18*:527, 1939.
23. Rogosa, M., Hampp, E. G., Nevin, T. A., Wagner, H. N., Briscoll, E. J., and Baer, P. N.: Blood sampling and cultural studies in the detection of postoperative bacteremias. J.A.D.A., *60*:171, 1960.
24. Bender, I. B., Seltzer, S., and Yermesh, M.: The incidence of bacteremia in endodontic manipulation. Oral Surg., *13*:353, 1960.
25. Sconyers, J. R., Crawford, J. J., and Moriarty, J. D.: Relationship of bacteremia to toothbrushing in patients with periodontitis. J.A.D.A., *87*:616, Sept., 1973.
26. Rigdon, R. H.: Localization of staphylococci in areas of

inflammation produced by Xylene. Arch. Surg., *41*:879, 1940.
27. Smith, L. S., and Toppe, G. D.: Experimental pulpitis in rats. J. Dent. Res., *41*:17, 1962.
28. Burke, G. W., and Knighton, H. T.: The localization of microorganisms in inflamed dental pulps of rats following bacteremia. J. Dent. Res., *39*:205, 1960.
29. Boling, L. R., and Robinson, H. B. G.: The anachoretic effects in pulpitis: II. histological studies. Arch. Oral Path., *33*:477, 1942.
30. Rickles, N., Ziberstein, Z., Kraus, S., Kaufstein, M., and Ginsburg, I.: Persistence of group A streptococci labeled with florescein isolthiocyanate in inflammatory sites in the heart and muscle of mice and rabbits. Proc. Soc. Exp. Biol. Med., *31*:525, 1969.
31. Morton, D. L., Eilber, F. R., Joseph, W. L., Trahan, E., and Ketcham, A. S.: Immunological factors in human sarcomas and melanomas. A rational basis for immunotherapy. Ann. Surg., *172*:740, 1970.
32. Good, R. A., and Fisher, D. W.: *Immunobiology.* Stamford, Sinauer Assoc., Inc., 1971.
33. Humphrey, J. H., and White, R. G.: *Immunology for Students of Medicine.* Philadelphia, F. A. Davis Co., 1970.
34. Snyderman, R., Shin, H. S., Phillips, J. K., Gewurz, H., and Mergenhagen, S. E.: A neutrophil chemotactic factor derived from C′5 upon interaction of guinea pig serum with endotoxin. J. Immunol., *103*:413, Sept., 1969.
35. Mergenhagen, S. E.: Complement as a mediator of the inflammatory response: interaction of complement with mammalian and bacterial enzymes. J. Dent. Res. (Suppl. No. 2), *51*:251, 1972.
36. Lichtenstein, L. M., Gewurz, H., Adkinson, N. F., Jr., Shin, H. S., and Mergenhagen, S. E.: Interactions of the complement system with endotoxic lipopolysaccharide: the generation of an anaphylatoxin. J. Immunol., *16*:327, 1969.
37. Bazin, S., and Delaunay, A.: Role of cathepsins in granulation tissue. J. Dent. Res. (Suppl. No. 2), *51*:244, 1972.
38. Horton, J. E., Oppenheim, J. J., Mergenhagen, S. E., and Raisz, L. G.: Macrophage-lymphocyte synergy in the production of osteoclast activating factor. J. Immunol., *113*:1278, Oct., 1974.
39. Doyle, E. F., Spagnuolo, M., Taranta, A., Kuttner, A. G., and Markowitz, M.: The risk of bacterial endocarditis during antirheumatic prophylaxis. J.A.M.A., *201*:129, 1967.
40. Wood, H. F., Feinstein, A. R., Taranta, A., Epstein, J. A., and Simpson, R.: Rheumatic fever in children and adolescents. Ann. Intern. Med., *60*:30, 1964.
41. Sommer, R. F., Ostrander, F. D., and Crowley, M. C.: *Clinical Endodontics: A Brief History of Root Canal Therapy.* Philadelphia, W. B. Saunders Co., 1961, p. 1.
42. Hunter, W.: The role of sepsis and of antisepsis in medicine. Lancet, *1*:79, 1911.
43. Rhein, M. L.: A prolonged study of the electrolytic treatment of dental focal infections—a preliminary report. Dent. Cosmos, *68*:971, 1926.
44. Billings, R.: Chronic focal infections and their etiologic relations to arthritis and nephritis. Arch. Intern. Med., *9*:484, 1918.
45. Myers, F. K.: The present status of dental bacteriology. N.D.A.J., *4*:966, 1917.
46. Rosenow, E. C.: The relation of dental infection to systemic disease. Dent. Cosmos, *59*:485, 1917.
47. Rhein, M. L.: Oral sepsis. Part 1, Dent. Cosmos, *54*:529, 1912.
48. Rhein, M. L.: The correct treatment of pulpless teeth. Must eliminate the possibility of periapical reinfection. Dent. Items of Interest, *37*:837, 1915.
49. Rhein, M. L., Krasnow, R., and Gies, W. J.: A prolonged study of the electrolytic treatment of dental focal infection—a preliminary report. Dent. Cosmos, *68*:971, 1926.
50. Abramson, I. I.: A frank appraisal of the present status of the bacterial culture test as a routine endodontic procedure. Paper presented at meeting of Amer. Assoc. Endodont., 1961, Chicago, Ill.
51. Zeldow, B. J., and Ingle, J. I.: Correlation of the positive culture of the prognosis of endodontically treated teeth: a clinical study. J.A.D.A., *66*:9, 1963.
52. Ingle, J. I.: A standardized endodontic technique utilizing newly designed instruments and filling materials. Oral Surg., *14*:83, Jan., 1961.
53. Bender, I. B., Seltzer, S., and Turenkopf, S.: To culture or not to culture? Oral Surg., *18*:527, 1964.
54. Morse, D. R.: The endodontic culture technique: a critical evaluation. Oral Surg., *30*:540, 1970.
55. Naidorf, I. J.: Inflammation and infection of pulp and periapical tissues. Oral Surg., *34*:486, 1972.
56. Sims, W.: Some comments on the microbiological examination of root canals. J. Dent., *2*:2, Oct., 1973.
57. Sommer, R. F., and Crowley, M.: Bacteriologic verification of roentgenographic findings in pulp-involved teeth. J.A.D.A., *27*:723, 1940.
58. Serene, T. P., and McDonald, E. D.: Endodontic culturing: a statistical study. J.A.D.A., *78*:1013, 1969.
59. Difco Supplementary Literature: Difco Laboratories, Detroit, Mich. Transport Media, p. 415, 1972.
60. Mazzarella, M. A., Hedman, W. J., and Brown, L. R., Jr.: Classification of microorganisms from the pulp canal of nonvital teeth. Research Paper, Project NM 008 015.10.01, U.S. Naval Dental School, National Naval Medical Center, Bethesda, Md., Aug. 1, 1955.
61. Winkler, K. C., and Van Amerogen, J.: Bacteriologic results from 4000 root canal cultures. Oral Surg., *12*:857, 1959.
62. Fish, E. W., and MacLean, I.: The distribution of oral streptococci in the tissues. Brit. Dent. J., *61*:336, 1936.
63. Hedman, W. J.: An investigation into residual periapical infection after pulp canal therapy. Oral Surg., *4*:1173, 1951.
64. Winkler, T. F., Mitchell, D. F., and Healey, H. J.: A bacterial study of human periapical pathosis employing a modified gram tissue stain. Oral Surg., *34*:109, 1972.
65. Wantulok, J. C., and Brown, J. I.: An *in vitro* study of the diffusibility of camphorated parachlorophenol and metacresylacetate in the root canal. Oral Surg., *34*:653, 1972.

66. August, D. S., and Levy, B. A.: Periapical actinomycosis. Oral Surg., *36*:585, Oct., 1973.
67. Rapaport, F. T., and Narkowitz, A. S.: Streptococcal antigens and antibodies in transplantation. Transplantation Proc., *1*:638, 1969.
68. Naidorf, I. J.: Immunoglobulins in periapical granulomas: a preliminary report. J. Endodont., *1*:15, Jan., 1975.
69. Medici, M. A.: The immunoprotective niche—a new pathogenic mechanism for syphilis, the systemic mycoses and other infectious diseases. J. Theor. Biol., *36*:617, 1972.

Chapter 13

Intracanal Medication and Systemic Antibiotic Therapy

EDWARD WHITE and THOMAS J. PALLASCH

Inasmuch as bacteria are the principal etiologic agents of pulp and periapical disease, antibacterial agents may be needed to control infection during endodontic therapy. Intracanal medication is the middle leg of the endodontic triad—cleansing, sterilizing (sanitizing), and obturating the root canal. From a practical point of view, bacteria may be effectively controlled or eliminated from diseased canals by two means: (1) debridement and proper irrigation while cleansing and shaping the canal, and (2) intracanal medication.

Canal Debridement. Proper cleansing of the root canal, with irrigation, is the most effective method for removing and/or killing bacteria. The importance of irrigation was emphasized by Ingle and Zeldow,[1] who showed that instrumentation alone, with sterile water irrigation, is ineffective in rendering positive canals negative. Irrigations of sodium hypochlorite or hydrogen peroxide, on the other hand, render approximately 75% of positive canals negative.[2,3]

Sodium hypochlorite is recommended for irrigation because (1) it acts as a solvent for pulp tissue and debris; (2) it mechanically flushes debris from canals and cutting surfaces of the instruments; (3) it kills bacteria; (4) it bleaches teeth; and (5) it acts as a lubricant for instruments within canals. Office solutions may be made by diluting household bleach, 5.25% sodium hypochlorite (Clorox or Purex), with an equal volume of water. This produces an irrigating solution of approximately 2.5% sodium hypochlorite. Many clinicians use the 5.25% solution as it comes from the manufacturer without noticeable ill effects. Spangberg, Engstrom, and Langeland suggested that 0.5 to 1.0% solutions be used to minimize toxicity and maintain bacteriostatic effects.[4] It is acknowledged, however, that the solvent properties of sodium hypochlorite are significantly diminished at these minimal concentrations.

The importance of irrigation in cleansing and shaping is discussed in Chapter 3, and so will be only briefly reviewed here. The solvent quality of sodium hypochlorite for pulp tissue was reported by Grossman and Neiman.[5] Apparently a pulp dissolves in 5% sodium hypochlorite within 30 minutes *in vitro*. Although this solvent property is especially beneficial in therapy, one should not rely too heavily on chemical dissolution of ***vital*** pulp tissue *in vivo*. Clinicians have detected large pieces of pulp tissue well beyond 30 minutes after instrumentation and sodium hypochlorite irrigation. Fibrotic pulp tissue may be quite resistant to thorough dissolution.

Although sodium hypochlorite provides a significant antibacterial effect,[2–4] Brown and Doran demonstrated that a maximal cleansing effect was achieved when sodium hypochlorite and hydrogen peroxide were used alternately as irrigating agents.[6] The effervescence of released oxygen, when the two solutions are mixed, accounts for increased efficiency. However, hydrogen peroxide irrigation has fallen in and out of favor. Criticism is based on the supposition that liberated oxygen causes pain and irritation in periapical tissues. Bhat has reported a case of emphysema presumed to be due to oxygen liberated from hydrogen peroxide which was forced into the loose infraorbital tissue during irrigation of a perforated maxillary lateral incisor (Fig. 13–1).[7] The complications cited in this case report should be viewed as an inappropriate application of hydrogen peroxide. Clinical experiences suggest that proper irrigation with hydrogen peroxide rarely, if ever, causes postoperative problems.

It is altogether possible that substantial advances in the removal of pulp and dentinal debris from root canals will be made through the use of enzymes and/or ultrasonic probes.

From a microbiologic viewpoint, proper canal debridement with irrigation is extremely important. It is axiomatic that the material taken out of a root canal is more important than the material put into it. Too often clinicians depend entirely on antimicrobial medication to eliminate bacteria, leaving in place a good deal of proteinaceous debris. This material, left within canals, may inhibit the bactericidal effects of intracanal medication and prevent proper obturation as well. It is therefore strongly recommended that the majority of the clinician's effort be directed toward cleaning the canal.

Although cleansing is the most important aspect of cleaning and shaping, the clinician must strive for obturation of the root canal system as well, to prevent ingress of organisms to the periapical area from the ***oral*** route by way of lateral canals, leaking restorations, or uncleaned areas of the canal itself.

Intracanal Medications. A second important aspect of bacteriologic control is the use of antibacterial intracanal medication, which should be (1) effective in eliminating or reducing bacteria within pulp canals and periapical tissues, and (2) nonirritating to the host.

The toxic, irritating, or inflammatory potential of intracanal medications is a much discussed (but little understood) topic. Most studies of toxicity have utilized relatively large quantities and high concentrations of medications in some soft tissue sites, *e.g.*, a patch test on the arm of a human being; intradermal or subcutaneous implantation in receptacles in ani-

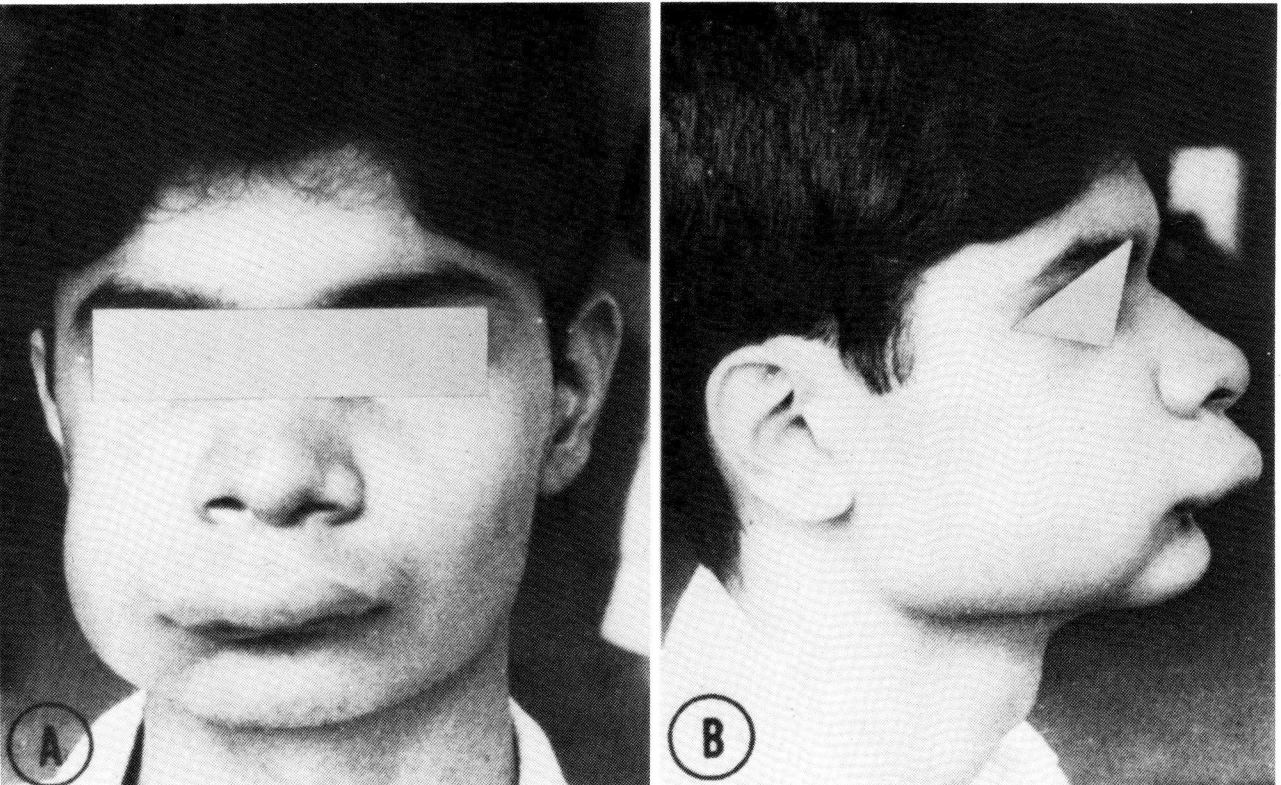

Fig. 13–1. Severe emphysema caused by injecting hydrogen peroxide irrigant into tissues. (From Bhat, K. S.: Oral Surg., *38*:304, Aug., 1974.)

mals. If misused, most of the intracanal medicaments produce inflammation. All other considerations of these drugs—based on shelf life, costs, staining qualities, and odor—can be evaluated with a little common sense.

Intracanal medications can be divided into two groups based on the host response. One group of caustic or highly irritating preparations includes compounds that were used primarily in the 1800s and early 1900s—arsenic trioxide, strong acids and alkalis, silver nitrate, metallic sodium, phenol and phenol derivatives, and formaldehyde. Interestingly, some of the drugs from this early group are still in use under certain conditions.

A second group have demonstrated minimal irritation to host tissues. Most of the preparations now in vogue fall within this group. The drugs are nonspecific in their bactericidal effects, *i.e.*, they kill a broad spectrum of microbial species. Probably the most commonly used drug in endodontics today is ***camphorated parachlorophenol.*** A concentration of 35% parachlorophenol in camphor is popular for minimal application, and recently a 2% aqueous solution that is less toxic has been evaluated for antibacterial effects.[4,8] Camphorated parachlorophenol is more effective than phenol in destroying bacteria *in vitro* and is moderately irritating to host tissues under experimental conditions.[9–11] Parachlorophenol may be used as a base line for comparison of other intracanal medicaments. The most irritating drugs are the derivatives of phenol and formaldehyde, such as ***formocresol;*** a moderately irritating drug is camphorated parachlorophenol; and the least irritating is ***Cresatin*** (metacresylacetate).[12] In the final analysis, the results of these toxicity studies and their interpretations must be tempered by clinical experience.

It is now popular to advocate using the ***least*** irritating intracanal medication, thereby excluding the use of formocresol. This would seem reasonable except that drugs have been compared for irritation potential in circumstances that cannot be equated with endodontic therapy. Empiric clinical observations suggest that formocresol is not an especially toxic drug when placed in pulp chambers in the amount and concentration recommended. These impressions are supported by reports that the ***deleterious*** effects of FMC are concentration-dependent,[13,14] as one would expect—high concentrations cause cellular damage and lower concentrations have minimal effects.

According to some techniques of applying intracanal medication, root canals are ***filled*** with minimal concentrations of less irritating drugs instead of ***minimal*** amounts of more concentrated drugs. The increase in efficacy claimed for the former method has not been borne out by clinical experience. Dilution of the concentrated medication within the tooth apparently is equally as effective—uncomplicated, successful treatment most of the time.

In recent years, the use of formocresol as an intracanal medication has been strongly criticized. It is, however, the most effective intracanal bactericidal agent against the broadest bacterial spectrum. Formocresol is acknowledged to be highly irritating to soft tissues when injected into or implanted in animals in high concentrations, but this fact should not rule out its use as an intracanal medication under certain conditions.

The ***safe use*** of formocresol is based on clinical experience, admittedly with minimal research evidence to support the recommendation. Formocresol may be used as an intracanal medication whenever: (1) a fistulous tract is present either periapically or through the periodontal spaces; (2) excessive weeping or drainage occurs on visits following the first visit; (3) pain persists for days after a visit; and (4) complete negotiation of all canals has not been successful. Formocresol may be indicated in these situations primarily because of the clinical impressions that fistulas close much more rapidly and weeping canals "dry up" much sooner than with other medicaments. Furthermore, formocresol seems to have an anodyne effect as well as being volatile and permeable. Hence it seems indicated if pain persists or canals are hard to negotiate. It has been shown to reduce an inflammatory response.[14]

In summary, formocresol offers the best potential bactericidal effect of drugs in current use and can be safely used ***in the amounts recommended*** (p. 585). There is at present a revival in the use of FMC. Perhaps in the near future it will be used as frequently as camphorated parachlorophenol.

Cresatin is the least toxic, but also the least effective, antimicrobial agent in current use. It is recommended primarily because of its minimal toxicity,[15] and more importantly, its anodyne effect. Clinical impressions again suggest that Cresatin is quite effective in ameliorating postoperative discomfort after the initial visit for therapy. It would seem to be particularly efficacious if pulp remnants were not entirely removed during limited emergency procedures at an initial visit.[16]

Diffusibility and Volatility. With utilization of present techniques, other qualities of intracanal medication are desirous. Among these are: ***diffusibility*** and ***volatility.*** The agent should permeate the entire root canal system, perhaps into dentin, lateral canals, and the periapex for maximum effectiveness.

A few years ago it was generally agreed that the ***effects*** of intracanal medication should be confined to the pulp canal spaces because of the potential toxic effect of these agents on periapical tissues. Current evidence indicates that the medication does penetrate the apical foramen and affects periapical tissues. These effects may be beneficial in destroying bacteria sequestered in the periapical region. Wantulok and Brown demonstrated that camphorated parachlorophenol and Cresatin diffused or volatilized through the apex of instrumented teeth *in vitro* and inhibited bacteria grown on agar plates.[17] The medications were applied to cotton pellets in concentrations similar to those used clinically. Several other groups have also reported that these agents, most notably formocresol, exert bactericidal effects through diffusion and volatilization.[18–20] Autoradiographic studies using tritium-labeled aqueous and camphorated para-

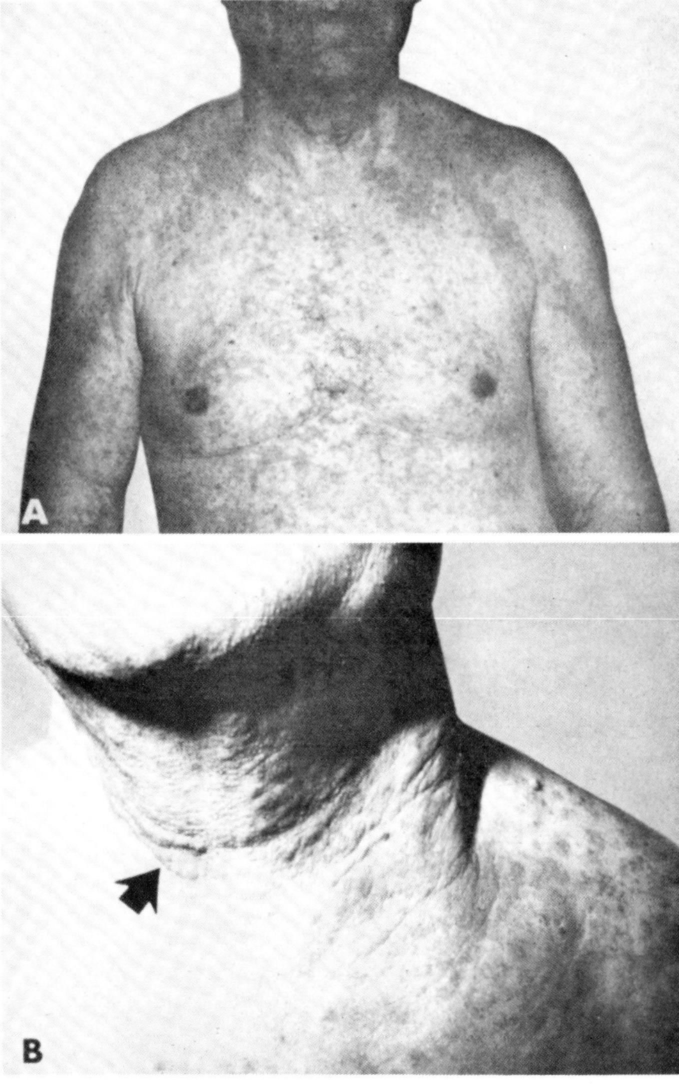

Fig. 13–2. Violent allergic response to camphorated parachlorophenol. *A,* Patient complained of rash and total body itching few hours following endodontic treatment. Rash persisted for ten days. Follow-up skin testing proved camphorated parachlorophenol to be allergen. *B,* Papular configuration *(arrow)* to eruption as well as overall macular reddening. (Courtesy Dr. Raymond G. Luebke.)

chlorophenol indicated that the aqueous solution penetrated the radicular dentin more effectively than the camphorated solutions.[21] If bacteria are sequestered and harbored in periapical lesions, it may be essential for a medication that is well tolerated and bactericidal to penetrate into these areas.

Effectiveness in the Presence of Organic Debris. Proteinaceous debris, that is, tissue, blood, and serum inhibit the antimicrobial effects of intracanal medication. Therefore, root canals should be effectively cleansed of organic debris before medication is used, to be certain that medication will not be inhibited. Volatile drugs, on the other hand, may have a better chance of penetrating debris to reach bacteria.

Medication and Culturing. The concept of interference with culturing arose some years ago when polyantibiotic pastes were popular for intracanal medication. It was noted that the "carry over" of penicillin into the culture medium would inhibit the growth of viable organisms, thereby giving false negative results. The addition of penicillinase (an enzyme which inactivates penicillin) to the medium helped to prevent a false negative result. A carry-over effect may be observed with other medications as well.

The use of polyantibiotic pastes has diminished in recent years for several reasons. For one thing, the validity of rendering canals "sterile," or bacteriologically negative, for successful therapy has been severely challenged. In addition, polyantibiotic pastes have not been demonstrated to be more effective than other preparations. Further, some concern has been expressed for the sensitizing potential of penicillin, although few allergic reactions have been attributed to the use of penicillin as an intracanal medication.[22,23] It would be more difficult, however, to verify how many patients have become sensitized to penicillin. Page, Trump, and Schaeffer demonstrated that labeled tetracycline placed in the pulp chamber of rat molars passed rapidly into the systemic circulation.[24] Another study has shown that antigens placed in pulp chambers sensitize experimental animals for immune response.[25] Taken together this evidence suggests that an immunizing potential for

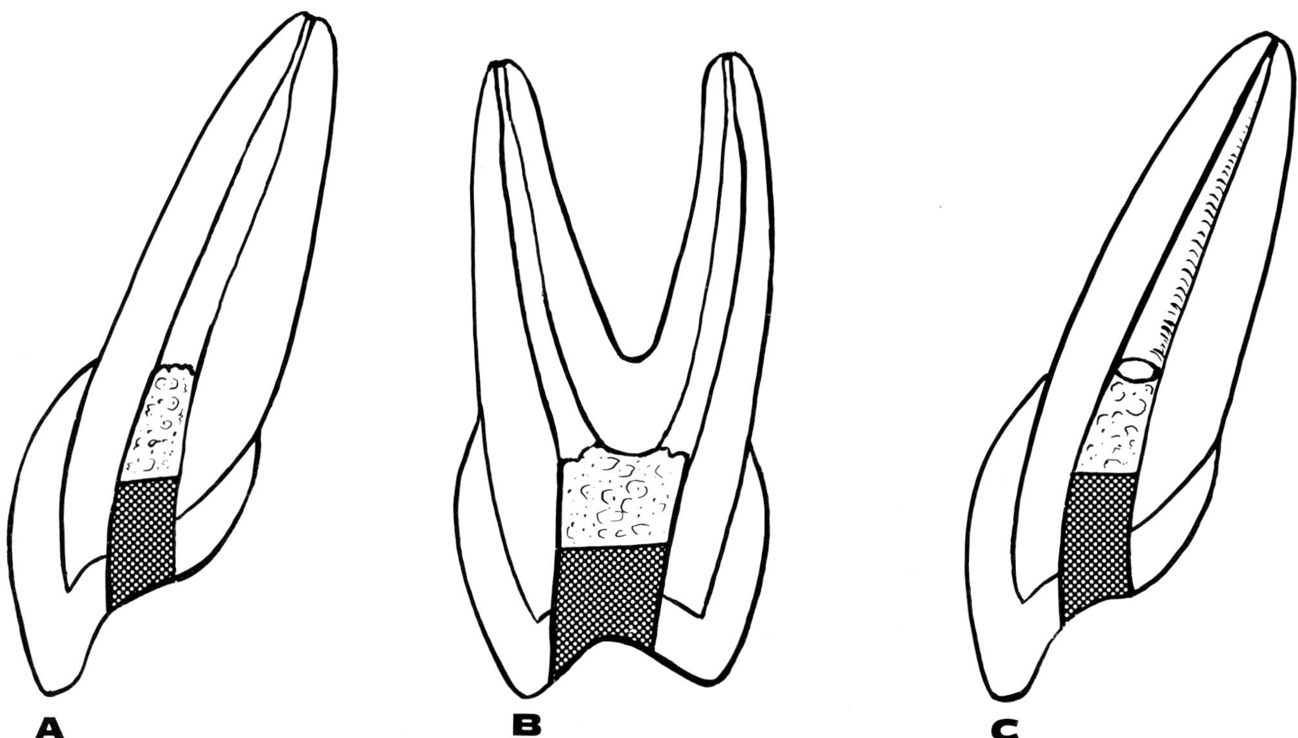

Fig. 13–3. Diagram of correct and incorrect root canal medication. *A*, Volatile medications—Cresatin, camphorated parachlorophenol, or formocresol—placed on small cotton pellet and covered with cotton, will permeate entire pulp space. *B*, Placement of medicaments and cotton only in pulp chamber leaves canals as overflow for small amounts of inflammatory exudate. *C*, Paper points should not be sealed in root canals. Even though they do not extend beyond apex they encourage percolation of medication into periapical tissues.

polyantibiotic preparations exists and that allergic reactions can occur. These preparations are not recommended when other drugs seem to be as effective in clinical treatment. Other medications may precipitate allergic reactions as well (Fig. 13–2), but they rarely do.

Glucocorticosteroids[26] and sulfathiazole[27] have both been suggested as intracanal medications for anodyne and anti-inflammatory effects. However, others have not found sulfathiazole to be effective in this regard.[28] Ingle has recommended that a polyantibiotic ophthalmic solution of neomycin, polymixin B, and bacitracin be used.[29] This is available as Neosporin ophthalmic drops or as Cortisporin with cortisone.

Methods of Application. The clinical methods of applying Cresatin, camphorated parachlorophenol, and formocresol are similar. Clinical experiences and experimental results suggest that minimal amounts of these medications are quite effective in medicating the entire root canal system.

The root canal should be dried with a paper point prior to application of the medication. A pledget of cotton, about one-third the size of the coronal pulp chamber, is moistened with appropriate medication and blotted ***dry*** with a cotton roll or sponge.

The ***dry*** medicated cotton pledget is then placed in the floor of the pulp chamber, covered with a large pellet of dry cotton, and a temporary filling is inserted (Fig. 13–3*A* and *B*). The medicament is volatile and has low surface tension. It will spread readily throughout the root canals between visits to the dentist. Numerous studies have shown that the minimal amount of medication applied to the cotton pledget in the manner described is adequate for bacteriologic control in therapy.

Great care is taken to leave within the root canal some space to act as a reservoir for exudate resulting from instrumentation. Paper points should not be used to carry medication deeply into the root canal. Sealing paper points in root canals not only reduces the effective volume of the root canal, but also encourages transfer of excess medication into the periapical spaces (Fig. 13–3*C*). Further, paper points have been lost within root canals or forced into the periapical spaces.[30]

SYSTEMIC ANTIBIOTIC THERAPY*

To this date, at least 40 different antibiotics have been developed with some degree of clinical efficacy. Those with immediate practical day-to-day use in dentistry number four: the penicillins, erythromycins, lincomycin and its congener clindamycin, and the cephalosporins. The following discussion will deal only with these four groups of antibiotics (oral preparations), along with the most basic principles of antibiotic therapy in oral and facial infections. A far more thorough discussion of the drug control of infection is available, particularly regarding antibiotic mechanisms of action, prophylactic antibiotic therapy, bacterial resistance, antibiotic combination therapy, bacterial sensitivity testing, and the entire spectrum of antibiotic agents.[31]

Principles. It is still probably true that the vast majority of oral and facial infections are caused by gram-positive organisms. The principal point of contention centers on the relative etiologic importance of the streptococcus and staphylococcus. In pulp infections, the principal pathogenic bacteria appear to be *Streptococcus salivarius* and *faecalis;* in periapical infections, the principal pathogens are alpha and beta streptococci and *Staphylococcus aureus.*[32] An acute cellulitis is most often caused by streptococci and localized abscesses by staphylococci.[32] A recent study by Goldberg raises the possibility that a substantial number of potentially pathogenic staphylococci may be isolated from oral abscesses that exhibit resistance to penicillin G, erythromycin, and even lincomycin.[33] Therefore it is conceivable that the oral bacterial flora is shifting from an overwhelming preponderance of routinely antibiotic-sensitive streptococci to a greater number of routinely insensitive staphylococci. If such a change in oral microbial pathogens is in fact occurring, a much more sophisticated level of knowledge regarding antibiotic therapy will be required. Certainly one factor in the changing patterns of pathogenic oral bacteria is the still too prevalent overuse of antibiotics, especially prophylactically. Tarsitano has aptly illustrated the fallacy as well as the high cost of such measures.[34] Antibiotics have not been shown to promote wound healing and are not to be employed to mask sloppy surgical procedures.

Indications. Antibiotics are most properly employed in the ***treatment of an established, active oral or facial infection,*** as determined by the presence of one or more symptoms of fever, malaise, edema, purulence, lymphadenopathy, and an elevated leukocyte count. Antibiotics are not a substitute for surgical drainage nor are they to be employed prophylacti-

*See *Clinical Drug Therapy in Dental Practice,* Thomas J. Pallasch, Philadelphia, Lea & Febiger, 1973.

cally, except in established situations (rheumatic heart disease, congenital heart disease, and intracardiac prostheses). The promiscuous prophylactic use of antibiotics only encourages the selection of, and eventual dominance of, resistant bacterial strains.

Route of Administration and Dosage. It is not possible to state absolute dosages, as the amount of drug administered depends on: (1) the offending organism; (2) the success (or lack) of surgical drainage; (3) the nature, virulence, and natural course of the infection, (4) the pharmacologic properties of the drug; and (5) the physical status of the patient. With oral antibiotic therapy, the most common dosage intervals are four to six hours. ***The duration of therapy is determined solely by the clinical remission of disease.*** In the case of oral and facial infections this remission is likely to occur in five to seven days, sooner if the surgical drainage is successful. Prolonged antibiotic therapy beyond that which is clinically necessary only promotes the emergence of resistant bacterial strains and increases the possibility of antibiotic toxicity and sensitization. The question of oral versus parenteral therapy is moot. Either route of administration is usually effective. However, it must be remembered that many patients do not take their oral medication as directed.

Toxicity. The toxic effects of antibiotics fall into three categories: (1) direct toxicity, (2) sensitization (allergy), and (3) host alterations. Direct toxicity may take the form of deafness with streptomycin, liver damage with the tetracyclines, and the increasingly important pseudomembranous colitis associated with clindamycin. Allergy to the antibiotics is rare, with the exception of penicillin and the sulfonamides. Anaphylaxis with penicillin has occurred by every route of administration and occurs most often in patients who have experienced a prior skin reaction. Alterations in the bacterial flora of the host include superinfections (defined as the occurrence of a new infection during the treatment of a primary one) such as staphylococcal enteritis and candidiasis (moniliasis).

Choice of Antibiotic Agent. The initial agents of choice in oral and facial infections are those with a predominant gram-positive spectrum: penicillin G or V, erythromycin, or lincomycin and its congener, clindamycin (Table 13–1). The cephalosporins, as exemplified by Cephalexin, should be reserved primarily for the treatment of severe facial infections

Table 13-1. Proprietary (Brand) Names

Penicillins	
Oral Penicillin G:	Pentids, Kesso-Pen, Pfizerpen
Penicillin V:	Compocillin V (VK), V-cillin (K), Pen-Vee (K), Ledercillin VK
Phenethicillin:	Darcil, Maxipen, Syncillin
Ampicillin:	Amcill, Polycillin, Principen, Totacillin
Erythromycins	
Erythromycin Base:	E-Mycin, Ilotycin
Erythromycin Succinate:	Erythrocin, Pediamycin
Erythromycin Stearate:	Erythrocin
Erythromycin Estolate:	Ilosone
Lincomycin Group	
Lincomycin	Lincocin
Clindamycin	Cleocin
Cephalosporins	
Cephalexin	Keflex

and those due to penicillinase-producing staphylococci. The tetracyclines are not the initial drugs of choice in oral infections. The choice between the penicillins, erythromycins, and the lincomycin group is determined by clinical experience, suspected bacterial pathogens, history of allergy, and the desirability of a bactericidal over a bacteriostatic agent. Of these three only penicillin is bactericidal; however, all three are usually effective against most oral infections. The lincomycin group are at present still quite effective against penicillinase-producing staphylococci. The penicillins are associated with a high incidence of allergy, including anaphylaxis, whereas the other agents are not.

The question of combination antibiotic therapy has received extensive attention and the work of Jawetz[35] and of Chang and Weinstein[36] has clarified the issue to some extent. The combination of two bactericidal or two bacteriostatic agents may be synergistic, but usually is not antagonistic. The combination of a bacteriostatic (bacterial protein synthesis suppressor) with a bactericidal (bacterial cell wall or cytoplasmic membrane inhibitor) results in diminished effectiveness of the latter. The combination of penicillin and erythromycin is therefore irrational. The most common clinical occurrence in antibiotic combination therapy is antibiotic "indifference," in which the resultant effect is equal to the single most active drug or equal to the arithmetic sum of the effects of the two drugs.[35]

Specific Antibiotic Agents

Penicillins. The four basic penicillins (oral) in present use in the treatment of dental infections are:

benzyl penicillin (penicillin G), phenoxymethyl penicillin (penicillin V), phenoxyethyl penicillin (phenethicillin), and alpha-aminobenzyl penicillin (ampicillin). These agents differ in their rate of oral absorption and the bacterial spectrum against which they are effective. All are readily inactivated by penicillinase. All are bactericidal and suppress the formation of the rigid bacterial cell wall. Oral penicillin G is poorly absorbed with two-thirds to three-quarters of an oral dose destroyed in the stomach and small intestine.[37] To obtain comparable blood levels orally, penicillin G must be taken in doses four to five times those employed intramuscularly. Penicillin V, phenethicillin, and ampicillin are much better absorbed orally; approximately 65% of a dose of penicillin V is absorbed orally.[38] On an equivalent oral dose basis, the blood levels attained with penicillin V are two to five times greater than with penicillin G.[36,38] The antibacterial spectrum of penicillin V and phenethicillin are virtually identical to penicillin G.[37] Ampicillin possesses a greater gram-negative spectrum than does penicillin G, but is slightly less effective against gram-positive organisms. Penicillins such as dicloxacillin and methicillin should be reserved solely for the treatment of infection due to penicillinase-producing microorganisms. The penicillins are prepared in 125 mg., 250 mg. and 500 mg. tablets.

Erythromycins. Erythromycin is the classic substitute for the patient who is allergic to penicillin, because its antibacterial spectrum closely approximates that of penicillin G. Erythromycin is also effective against some strains of penicillinase-producing staphylococci. The primary differences between penicillin G and erythromycin is that the latter is bacteriostatic and the former is highly allergenic. Erythromycin is prepared as a free base form as well as the stearate, succinate and estolate salts. An unusual form of allergic reaction, cholestatic hepatitis, occurs only to the estolate salt (Ilosone) and is probably rare. The estolate salt produces a higher and more persistent peak blood level than the other preparations, but this is not an important factor in successful therapy with the erythromycins.[39] Erythromycin is an acceptable substitute for penicillin G, particularly if there is concern about penicillin allergy and anaphylaxis. The erythromycins are formulated in 250 mg. capsules and tablets.

Lincomycin and Clindamycin. These two congeners possess an essentially gram-positive spectrum but also possess considerable activity against penicillinase-producing staphylococci and are highly effective against anaerobic organisms, particularly bacteroides. They are bacteriostatic and inhibit bacterial protein synthesis. They are adequately absorbed orally, but only about 20 to 30% of an oral dose of lincomycin is absorbed, and this can be considerably reduced by meals.[40] Clindamycin is much better absorbed than lincomycin and erythromycin in the presence of food.[41] Of critical importance is the increasing evidence of severe colitis associated with their use. Symptoms include diarrhea, abdominal pain, fever, and friable, edematous intestinal mucosa associated with yellowish-white plaques.[42] Several deaths have been reported, usually in severely debilitated patients.[43] The actual incidence of this colitis is still unknown, but until the entire issue is resolved, the use of lincomycin and clindamycin should be restricted in dentistry. The ***Medical Letter*** has recommended that these antibiotics be reserved for severe anaerobic infections caused by *Bacteroides fragilis* and some staphylococcal infections in penicillin-allergic patients.[43] Lincomycin is prepared in 500-mg. capsules and clindamycin in 75- and 150-mg. capsules.

Cephalosporins. This superb group of antibiotics is related in chemical structure to penicillin, but is classically broad-spectrum and highly resistant to penicillinase. They are bactericidal and probably possess a mechanism of action similar, if not identical, to that of penicillin G. Due to their similarity in chemical structure, cross-allergenicity with penicillin is possible and must be suspected until proved otherwise. Fortunately, in most cases this cross-allergenicity has not developed, and the cephalosporins have been safely administered to many penicillin-allergic patients. Cephalexin is the oral preparation of choice and is well absorbed from the gastrointestinal tract even in the presence of food. Because these drugs are effective against many gram-positive and gram-negative organisms, in addition to penicillinase-producers, they should not be used indiscriminately, since selection out of resistant strains can occur. They should be used only when clearly indicated for severe facial infections. They are our last line of antibiotic defense. The cephalosporins, however, are drugs of choice in the prophylactic treatment of patients with rheumatic heart disease who are receiving daily doses of penicillin.[31] Cephalexin is prepared in 250 mg. capsules.

REFERENCES

1. Ingle, J. I. and Zeldow, B. J.: An evaluation of mechanical instrumentation and the negative culture in endodontic therapy. J.A.D.A., *57*:472, 1958.
2. Stewart, G. G.: Importance of chemomechanical preparation of the root canal. Oral Surg., *8*:993, 1955.
3. Auerbach, M. B.: Antibiotics vs. instrumentation in endodontics. New York State Dent. J., *19*:225, 1953.
4. Spangberg, L., Engstrom, B., and Langeland, K.: Biologic effects of dental materials. Oral Surg., *36*:856, Dec., 1973.
5. Grossman, L. I., and Neiman, B. W.: Solution of pulp tissue by chemical agents. J.A.D.A., *28*:223, 1941.
6. Brown, J. I., and Doran, J. E.: An in vitro evaluation of the particle flotation capability of various irrigating solutions. Calif. Dent. Asso. J., *3*:60, Jan., 1975.
7. Bhat, K. S.: Tissue emphysema caused by hydrogen peroxide. Oral Surg., *38*:304, Aug., 1974.
8. Kawahara, C. M., Regan, P. F., Tenca, J. I., and Pelleu, Jr., G. B.: Antimicrobial efficacy of reduced concentrations of parachlorophenol in extracted teeth. J. Endodont., *1*:48, Feb., 1975.
9. Harrison, J. W., and Madonia, J. V.: The toxicity of parachlorophenol. Oral Surg., *32*:90, 1971.
10. Torneck, C. D.: Reaction of hamster tissue to drugs used in sterilization of root canal. Oral Surg., *14*:740, 1961.
11. Powell, D. L., Marshall, F. J., and Melfi, R. C.: A histopathologic evaluation of tissue reactions to the minimum effective doses of some endodontic drugs. Oral Surg., *36*:261, Aug., 1973.
12. Schilder, H., and Amsterdam, M.: Inflammatory potential of root canal medicaments. Oral Surg., *12*:211, 1959.
13. Loos, P. J., and Han, S. S.: An enzyme histochemical study of the effect of various concentrations of formocresol on connective tissues. Oral Surg., *31*:571, 1971.
14. Straffon, L. H., and Han, S. S.: The effect of formocresol on hamster connective tissue cells, a histological and quantitative radioautographic study with Proline-H. Arch. Oral Biol., *13*:271, 1968.
15. Brown, J. I.: An evaluation of the antimicrobial effectiveness of intracanal medicaments. J. Southern California Dent. Assoc., *40*:845, 1972.
16. Lance, J. R., and Marshall, R. J.: Emergency endodontic therapy: report of case. J.A.D.A., *85*:1119, 1972.
17. Wantulok, J. C., and Brown, J. I.: An *in vitro* study of the diffusibility of camphorated parachlorophenol and metacresylacetate in the root canal. Oral Surg., *34*:653, 1972.
18. Treanor, H. F., Jr., and Goldman, M.: Bactericidal efficiency of intracanal medication. Oral Surg., *33*:791, 1972.
19. Vanderwall, G. L., Dowson, J., and Shipman, C.: Antibacterial efficacy and cytotoxicity of three endodontic drugs. Oral Surg., *33*:230, 1972.
20. Wesley, D. J., Marshall, F. J., and Rosen, S.: The quantitation of formocresol as a root canal medicament. Oral Surg., *29*:603, 1970.
21. Avny, W. Y., Heiman, G. R., Madonia, J. V., and Wood, N. K.: Autoradiographic studies of the intracanal diffusion of aqueous and camphorated parachlorophenol in endodontics. Oral Surg., *36*:80, July, 1973.
22. Grossman, L. I.: Sterilization of infected root canals. J.A.D.A., *85*:900, 1972.
23. Fox, J., and Moodnik, R. M.: Systemic reaction to polyantibiotic root canal dressing. New York State Dent. J., *30*:282, 1964.
24. Page, D. O., Trump, G. N., and Schaeffer, L. D.: Pulpal studies. I: Passage of 3H-tetracycline into circulatory system through rat molar pulps. Oral Surg., *35*:555, 1973.
25. Barnes, G. W., and Langeland, K.: Antibody formation in primates following introduction of antigens into the root canal. J. Dent. Res., *45*:1111, 1966.
26. Barker, B. C. W., and Ehrmann, E. H.: Human pulp reactions to a glucocorticosteroid compound. Aust. Dent. J., *14*:104, 1969.
27. Frank, A. L., Glick, D. H., Weichman, J. A., and Harvey, H.: The intracanal use of sulfathiazole in endodontics to reduce pain. J.A.D.A., *77*:102, 1968.
28. Seltzer, S., Bender, I. B., and Ehrenreich, J.: Incidence and duration of pain following endodontic therapy: relationship to treatment with sulfonamides and to other factors. Oral Surg., *14*:74, Jan. 1961.
29. Ingle, J. I.: Personal communication, 1972.
30. White, E.: Paper point in mental foramen. Oral Surg., *25*:630, 1968.
31. Pallasch, T. J.: *Clinical Drug Therapy in Dental Practice.* Chapter V, Drug Control of Infection. Lea & Febiger, Philadelphia, 1973.
32. Burnett, G. W.: The microbiology of dental infections. Dent. Clin. N. Amer., *14*:681, 1970.
33. Goldberg, M. H.: The changing biologic nature of acute dental infection. J.A.D.A., *80*:1048, 1970.
34. Tarsitano, J. J.: The use of antibiotics in dental practice. Dent. Clin. N. Amer., *14*:697, 1970.
35. Jawetz, E.: The use of antimicrobial combinations. Ann. Rev. Pharmacol., *8*:151, 1968.
36. Chang, T. W., and Weinstein, L.: Inhibitory effects of other antibiotics on bacterial morphologic changes induced by penicillin G. Nature (Lond.), *211*:763, 1966.
37. Weinstein, L.: Antibiotics. I. The Penicillins. In *The Pharmacologic Basis of Therapeutics.* Edited by L. S. Goodman and A. Gilman. 4th Ed., The Macmillan Company, New York, 1970.
38. Farrar, W. E., Jr., and Sellers, T. F., Jr.: *Chemotherapy of Bacterial Infections V: The Penicillins and Cephalosporins.* In *Drill's Pharmacology in Medicine.* Edited by J. R. DiPalma. 4th Ed., McGraw-Hill, New York, 1971.
39. Ross, S.: *Erythromycin, Oleandomycin and Triacetyloleandomycin.* In *Antimicrobial Therapy.* Edited by B. M. Kagan. W. B. Saunders Company, Philadelphia, 1970.
40. Kaplan, J., and Weinstein, L.: Lincomycin. Pediat. Clin. N. Amer., *15*:131, 1968.
41. The Medical Letter on Drugs and Therapeutics: Clindamycin (Cleocin). *12*:85, 1970.
42. Stroehlein, J. R., Sedlack, R. E., Hoffman, H. N. II, and Newcomer, A. D.: Clindamycin-associated colitis. Mayo Clin. Proc., *49*:240, 1974.
43. The Medical Letter on Drugs and Therapeutics: Colitis associated with clindamycin. *16*:73, 1974.

Chapter 14

Endodontic Instrument Sterilization and Operative Field Disinfection

EDWARD WHITE

The primary objective of sterilization and disinfection in the dental office is the prevention of disease transmission between patients and between patients and dental personnel. Transmission of infectious disease between individuals is cross-contamination. Sterilization and aseptic requirements in endodontic practice are not unlike disinfection for other areas of clinical practice. Patients are asked about their medical history at the initial appointment. Although this practice alerts a dentist to possible health problems, patients may unknowingly harbor a variety of infectious diseases, any one of which can be transmitted to other individuals, including the dentist and staff, if aseptic techniques are not carefully observed.

Transmission of Infectious Disease. The need for, and value of, microbiologic control with therapy was demonstrated in the late 1800s by Lister.[1] The implications of cross-contamination, however, were not fully realized until the early 1900s. Over the years, injection of drugs and vaccines for such diseases as malaria, diabetes mellitus, and yellow fever led to an unusually high incidence of hepatitis.[2] The consistent association of hepatitis with parenteral injection demonstrated the need for adequate microbiologic control. Bacterial disease could be controlled with relative ease, but control of viral hepatitis required strict observance of the basic principles of sterilization.

A brief review of the transmission of hepatitis may serve as a model for the dental practitioner in considering the importance of sterilization and aseptic techniques. Viral hepatitis may be limited to those diseases commonly designated as "infectious" hepatitis and "serum" hepatitis.[2] Identification of the hepatitis B antigen (Australian antigen), and its correlation with the disease formerly termed ***serum*** hepatitis, has simplified and sharpened the diagnosis of viral hepatitis. Now serologic identification of the hepatitis B agent confirms the diagnosis of hepatitis B virus disease (HBV serum hepatitis) and distinguishes it from hepatitis A (infectious hepatitis).

It was mistakenly thought that transmission of (serum) hepatitis, HBV, occurred only by parenteral inoculation with blood or serum products, through transfusion, injection, or surgery with inadequately sterilized equipment. Now, however, it appears that other routes or mechanisms of infection must be operative. An individual who has experienced either subclinical or overt HBV may be antigen-positive and a carrier for this viral disease. When carriers have been identified, they are usually instructed by their physician in procedures designed to protect their normal daily contacts. However, a significant increase in the incidence of HBV, with an attendant increase in the carrier reservoir among young adults, has occurred in the last few years. Many authorities believe that this increase is directly correlated to an increase in the use of self-injected drugs among communal users of drug injection equipment.[3] These individuals may appear in dental offices and the professional staff, or subsequent patients, could unknowingly become infected with HBV if great care in disinfection and prevention is not taken routinely.

Concern has been expressed about the hazard of

hepatitis for dentists and auxiliary personnel.[4–6] It would appear that a number of dentists and staff have experienced hepatitis without recent history of injections of any kind. A study at the University of Southern California suggested that dentists and some specialists, notably oral surgeons, experienced a higher incidence of hepatitis than did random populations.[4] In addition, serologic evaluation of 1,245 general dentists attending the 1972 meeting of the American Dental Association revealed that 0.9% of those tested were HBV positive and 12.7% had the corresponding anti-HBV antibodies, which indicated a moderately increased risk over the general population.[5] Another study of oral surgeons (unpublished data) indicated high liability to infection. The higher incidence of hepatitis in oral surgeons was also found by Feldman and Schiff.[6a] In Dade County, Florida (Miami) 21% of the oral surgeons had had hepatitis compared with 6.7% for dental general practitioners and 2.4% for lawyers. There was also a positive correlation between dentists with hepatitis and the treatment of drug addicts. Other specialities, notably those with a surgery component such as endodontics, may be at a greater risk as well.

Clearly, practitioners and staff are in some danger of infection with HBV. Infection may result from percutaneous introduction of virus through accidental skin penetrations and skin microabrasions while handling contaminated material in treatment or in clean-up or preparatory procedures. Infectivity of saliva and pulmonary exposure through aerosols are possible,[7–9] but further study is required to clarify this issue. It has been suggested that dental personnel may be carriers of infection.[10] Caution must be exercised before final scientific judgment is passed on this issue in spite of the fact that several judicial decisions have been rendered adverse to dentists. Both in California and Maryland general dentists have been legally barred from practice as asymptomatic carriers of hepatitis B virus. The same fate befell a Pennsylvania oral surgeon.[11–14]

The possibility that dentists may inadvertently transmit viral hepatitis from one patient to another because of faulty procedures for sterilization has been considered for several years. Consequently, one must prevent transmission of hepatitis and other infectious diseases by all practical methods. Every precaution also must be taken to prevent nosocomial cross-contamination from the infected root canals of one patient to those of another.

Sterilization Methods. In modern dental practice, all dental facilities should include an autoclave. Autoclaving permits the complete destruction of microorganisms by heat, usually steam under pressure at 121° C for 20 minutes at 15 pounds pressure. A properly loaded autoclave is the most reliable method of sterilization. Certain types of large institutional autoclaves operate at even higher temperatures and pressures reducing even more the time required for sterilization of instruments.

An alternative to the autoclave is the dry heat sterilizer, in which sterilization may be achieved by maintaining a temperature of 170° C for one hour. Formerly dry heat sterilization was the most popular endodontic method because endodontic carbon steel intracanal instruments, that is, files and reamers, rusted in the steam of an autoclave. With the

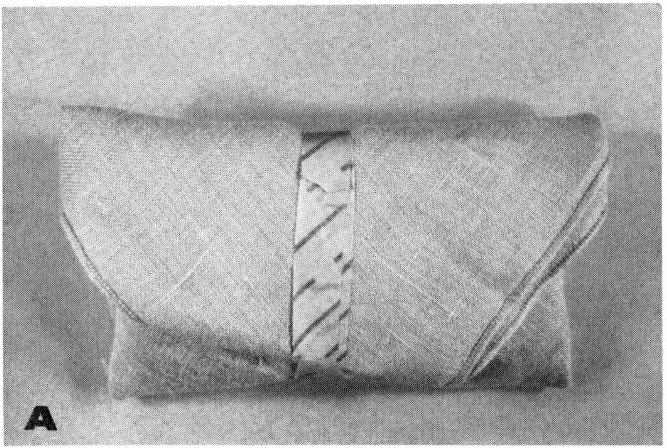

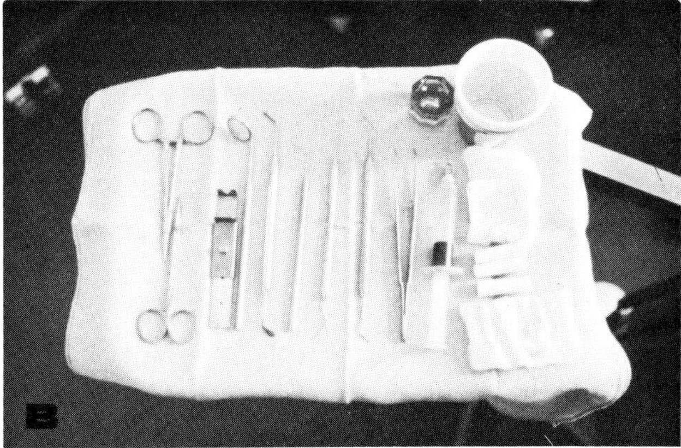

Fig. 14–1. *A,* Towel kit containing instruments, wrapped in double towel bound with autoclave tape. Sterilization temperature changes color of tape. Sterile kits may be stored months at a time. *B,* Towel kit opened on Mayo stand. Working surfaces, instruments, and cotton products are sterile.

availability of stainless steel endodontic instruments, however, rusting is no longer an autoclaving problem. Dry heat sterilization is less popular today because it is time-consuming and frequently chars the paper and cotton products used in endodontic therapy. Ethylene oxide is currently being employed extensively in several dental colleges in this country to sterilize handpieces and other dental items, including endodontic instruments. This procedure requires equipment not usually found in dental offices and may not be appropriate here.

Bactericidal and bacteristatic liquid chemicals such as Zephiran chloride are not reliable agents as ***initial*** sterilizing solutions.[15] Disinfection denotes destruction of pathogenic microorganisms. Some disinfectants destroy only vegetative organisms, but not spores of microorganisms or some virus. Chemical disinfectants may be quite effective, however, to preserve and ***maintain*** sterility of instruments in storage after thorough sterilization by autoclaving. When used as holding solutions, chemical disinfectants should be changed every two weeks because the bactericidal effect is reduced on standing.

Aseptic Protocol. The hands of the operator should be thoroughly scrubbed with soap and water. If absolute sterility is required, the operator should wear rubber gloves although this is rarely required. For the protection of the dental personnel, rubber gloves should always be used when treating patients with a history of hepatitis or other infectious diseases.

After the rubber dam is applied, the operating field is sanitized with a chemical disinfectant. If culturing is to be done, outside bacterial contamination of instruments must be prevented to avoid "false positive" results. Fortunately, the autoclaving used to prevent exogenous contamination is the same as that used to prevent disease transmission.

Another preventive measure against disease transmission deals with the contaminated instruments after their use. Dentists and their staff must be alert to the great hazard from puncture by these sharp materials. In removing instruments from the chairside, the greatest problems are haste and the use of bare hands to carry them to the cleaning area. An endodontic assistant who pricked her finger while cleaning files prior to sterilization subsequently experienced a severe case of HBV, antigen positive, requiring hospitalization and a long convalescence period.

Therefore, ultrasonic cleaners, in combination with detergent, are strongly preferred over hand washing with a brush for removing contaminating protein. For sterilization, therefore, all instruments are collected, cleaned ultrasonically, rinsed, sorted, and prepared for the autoclave. Many clinicians find it expedient to organize instruments and material for endodontic therapy into kits or packs.

Endodontic Kits. Kits or packs may vary from elaborate and personalized trays to simple towel kits. Within dental school environments, it is often convenient to sterilize and store instruments in metal boxes. It is also convenient to utilize a simple towel kit (Fig. 14–1). The kit contains everything needed for endodontic therapy, such as mouth mirror, endodontic explorer, periodontal probe, cotton pliers, excavator, scissors, spreaders and pluggers, measuring device, plastic instrument, irrigation syringes and needles, cotton rolls, sponges, and any favorite instruments. The entire kit is autoclaved and subsequently stored in double wrapping of towels, which maintains sterility.

Such items as rubber dam clamps, files, reamers, finger spreaders, and burs are not convenient to manage in a towel kit. It is important, however, to sterilize and store each of these items. Files and reamers may be stored in a sterile metal or plastic box. Stainless instruments are sterilized right in the metal box in an autoclave (Fig. 14–2). Sterile instruments may also be stored in an inexpensive plastic box containing a chemical disinfectant (Fig. 14–3).

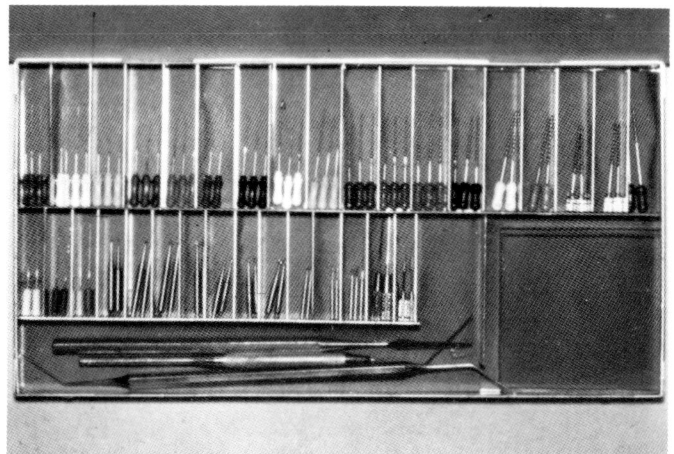

Fig. 14–2. Instrument case with lid opened. All instruments are stainless or carbide and can be autoclaved. Sterile pliers are used to retrieve instruments. Case remains sterile and need only be resterilized when instrument size is depleted.

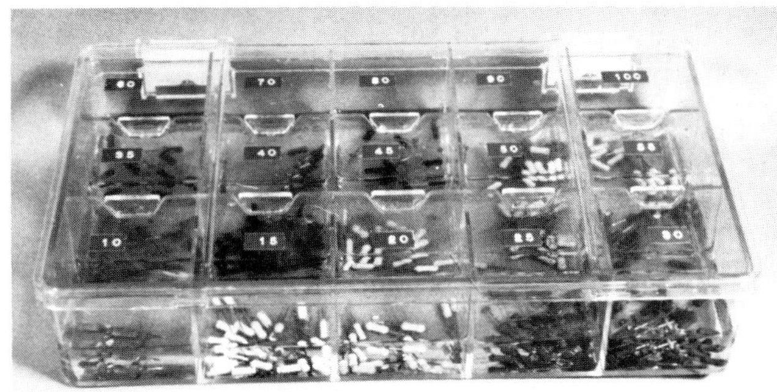

Fig. 14–3. Plastic organization box for storage of sterilized intracanal instruments. Chemical disinfectant maintains sterility. (Courtesy Dr. Edward White.)

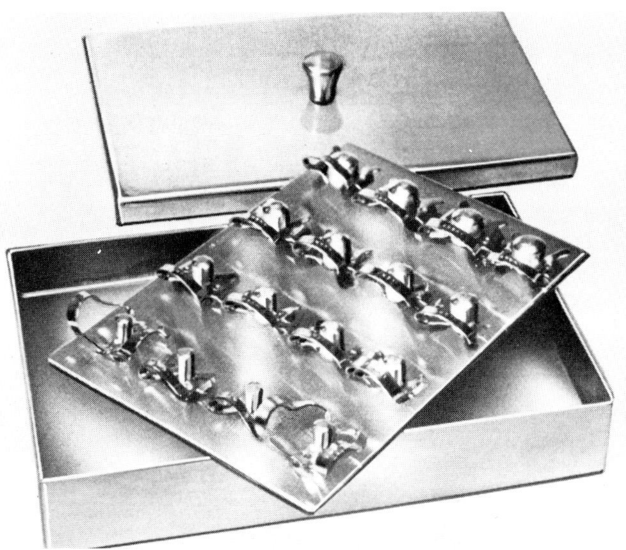

Fig. 14–4. Rubber dam clamp holder and sterilizing pan designed by Dr. J. B. Freedland. Clamps attach to graduated-size pegs. Pan is filled with disinfecting solution to maintain sterility of autoclaved clamps. (Courtesy J. W. Ivory Dental Manufacturing Co.)

Traditionally, many practitioners do not autoclave rubber dam clamps. However, contaminated clamps have a strong potential for transmitting disease because clamps often penetrate the gingiva and are contaminated with blood and serum. After use, clamps and other miscellaneous instruments can be scoured in an ultrasonic cleaner, placed in a container, and autoclaved. After sterilization, clamps may be transferred to a divider kept in a pan to which a chemical disinfectant has been added for "holding" (Fig. 14–4).

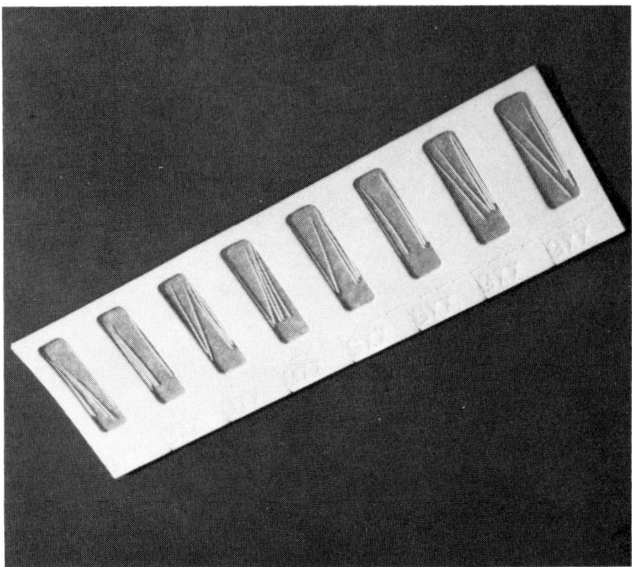

Fig. 14–5. Packaged and sterilized paper points. Each section of 6 points may be separated at perforation. Points are reached by breaking plastic window. (Courtesy Johnson & Johnson Co.)

For chairside use, a "banker's" sponge which has been thoroughly saturated with an appropriate chemical disinfectant (for example, Zephiran chloride) will maintain sterility and provide ready access to fresh sterile instruments. No used or infected instruments are placed in the sponge, and as previously stated, the disinfectant must be changed regularly.

Currently, some items used in endodontic practices—such as paper points, cotton pellets, and anesthetic needles—are pre-sterilized by the manufacturer (Fig. 14–5). Handpieces and attached syringe tips on the dental unit are difficult, if not impossible, to completely sterilize. Wiping or scouring them with chemical disinfectants is currently recommended.

Electrically heated sterilizers containing molten metal, metal beads, glass beads, or salt are especially designed for use in sterilizing intracanal instruments. This type of sterilizer is ***not*** predictably effective, however, in eliminating all microorganisms, and consumes more time in a less efficient procedure than using presterilized "packaged" supplies and equipment.

In summary, a dental practitioner must have two concerns in the areas of sterilization and disinfection: (1) prevention of disease transmission, both systemic and localized, from patient to patient and from patient to dental personnel and (2) contamination during the culturing technique. Prevention of disease is possible by careful handling of contaminated instruments followed by proper sterilization. Patients and office staff alike deserve the highest standards of protection in a dental practice.

REFERENCES

1. Lister, J.: Demonstrations of antiseptic surgery before members of the British Medical Association. Edinburgh Med. J., *21*:193, 1875.
2. Mosley, J. W., and Galamabos, J. T.: Viral hepatitis. In *Diseases of the Liver.* Edited by L. Shiff. Philadelphia, Lippincott, 1969, p. 410.
3. Mosley, J. W.: Epidemiologic implications of changing trends in type A and type B hepatitis. In *Hepatitis and Blood Transfusion.* Edited by G. N. Vyas, H. A. Perkins, and R. Schmid. New York, Grune and Stratton, 1972, p. 23.
4. Mosley, J. W., and White, E.: Viral hepatitis as an occupational hazard of dentists. J.A.D.A., *90*:992, May, 1975.
5. Mosley, J. W., Edwards, V. M., Casey, G., Redeker, A. G., and White, E.: Hepatitis B. Virus Infection in Dentists. N. Engl. J. Med., *293*:729, Oct. 9, 1975.
6. Feldman, R. E., and Schiff, E. R.: Hepatitis in dental professionals. Gastroenterology, *65*:539, Sept., 1973.

6a. Feldman, R. E., and Schiff, E. R.: Hepatitis in dental professionals. J.A.M.A., *232*:1228, June 23, 1975.

7. Heathcote, J., Cameron, C. H., and Dane, D. S.: Hepatitis B antigen in saliva and semen. Lancet, *1*:71, Jan. 19, 1974.
8. Kistler, G. S., Sommabend, W., and Krech, U.: Hepatitis B antigen (HB-Ag, Australia Antigen) in mixed saliva of patients with HB antigenemia. Path. Microbiol., *39*:313, 1973.
9. Ward, R., Borchert, P., Wright, A., and Kline, E.: Hepatitis B antigen in saliva and mouth washings. Lancet, *2*:725, Oct. 7, 1972.
10. Levin, M. L., Maddrey, W. C., Wands, J. R., and Mendeloff, A. I.: Hepatitis B transmission by dentists. J.A.M.A., *228*:1139, 1974.
11. Mosley, J. W.: The HBV carrier—a new kind of leper? N. Engl. J. Med., *292*:477, Feb. 27, 1975.
12. Williams, S. V., Pattison, C. P., and Berquist, K. R.: Dental infection with hepatitis B. J.A.M.A., *232*:1231, June 23, 1975.
13. Vaisrub, S.: Editorial. Hepatitis B—traffic in the dentist's office. J.A.M.A., *232*:1270, June 23, 1975.
14. Editorial: Must hepatitis carriers stop treating patients? Med. World News, *16*:19, Dec. 15, 1975.
15. Lyon, T. C.: Quaternary ammonia compounds; should they be used for disinfection in the dental office? Oral Surg., *36*:769, Nov. 5, 1973.

Chapter 15

Endodontic Surgery

JOHN I. INGLE, EDWARD E. BEVERIDGE, RALEIGH R. CUMMINGS, ALFRED L. FRANK, DUDLEY H. GLICK, and BERTRAM L. WOLFSOHN

Endodontic surgery was first recorded 1500 years ago when Aetius, a Greek physician-dentist, first excised an acute apical abscess with a small scalpel.[1] In more recent times the procedure has been refined and popularized, although one may question whether Hullihen's contribution in 1839 was refinement over Aetius.[2] "Make an incision through the gum, along the entire length of the fang," stated Hullihen, "then apply a roasted fig or bruised raisins to the gum."

In 1884 Farrar described a "radical and heroic treatment of alveolar abscess by amputation of roots and teeth,"[3] and Rhein, in 1897, was advocating "amputation of roots as a radical cure in chronic alveolar abscess."[4] G. V. Black, in 1886, was also advocating the total amputation of the individual roots of molars that were severely involved in periodontal diseasé, and root canal filling of the remaining healthy roots.[5] In 1919, Garvin was demonstrating retrofillings radiographically.[6]

Today, endodontic surgery is a successful, and often necessary, part of comprehensive endodontic services. As with all successful methods, however, part of its success is due to its simplification, and therein lie the seeds of its abuse. The surgical approach to endodontics has been badly misused. In some hands periapical surgery follows the root canal filling of virtually every anterior tooth treated. Other dentists refuse to perform any endodontic surgical procedures. Both groups lack an appreciation of comprehensive dental care.

The mistaken impression that surgical endodontics is "radical" therapy must be dispelled. The controversy over "surgical" versus "conservative" endodontics is misleading, for often the surgical approach ***is*** the conservative approach—the procedure saves the tooth, the height of conservatism. Radical therapy is extraction and tooth loss.

There are definite indications for endodontic surgery, just as there are definite contraindications. In order to understand these indications, one must first know the available procedures and their application. This calls for a classification of endodontic surgical techniques and a short explanation of each. A detailed description is presented later in the chapter.

Methods of Endodontic Surgery

- I. Surgical fistulation
  - A. Incision
  - B. Trephination
- II. Periradicular surgery
  - A. Periapical surgery
    - 1. Apicocurettage
    - 2. Apicoectomy
    - 3. Retrofilling
  - B. Corrective surgery
    - 1. Periodontal defect
      - a. Curettage
      - b. Total root amputation
        - i. Single or multiple roots
        - ii. Hemisection of the tooth
    - 2. Root resorptive defect
    - 3. Fracture defect
    - 4. Carious defect
    - 5. Anomalous defect
- III. Intentional replantation

Surgical drainage by ***incision,*** occasionally by ***trephination,*** is a time-honored method of evacuating frank pus from an acute abscess.

Periradicular surgery includes both ***periapical surgery*** and ***corrective*** surgical measures, and constitutes the great majority of endodontic surgical cases. ***Apicocurettage*** and ***apicoectomy*** are basic techniques, which are seldom done *per se,* but serve as the initial step of retrofilling and most corrective surgery. ***Retrofilling*** involves root end resection and the placement of an apical filling.

Total root amputation and ***hemisection*** have become increasingly valuable as the horizons of periodontal therapy and periodontal prosthesis are extended. It is differentiated from apicoectomy wherein only the root tip is resected. ***Intentional replantation*** is one of those rare surgical techniques that are utilized as a last resort.

INDICATIONS AND CONTRAINDICATIONS FOR ENDODONTIC SURGERY

Over the past ten years there have been marked improvements in ***non***surgical endodontics which have sent success rates soaring. Those hopeful signs have materially affected the incidence of surgery in that most dentists initially treat most cases nonsurgically. Only if the nonsurgical approach fails is surgery employed. Consequently, a good deal less surgery is now being done and the list of indications for surgery has diminished. True, there are "black and white" cases in which the tooth cannot be saved without surgery, and these constitute the core of "indications." But there are also a number of situations in the "grey area" where the "wait and see" philosophy follows nonsurgical therapy. We have finally passed the era in which small lesions were treated nonsurgically and large lesions routinely managed surgically. The surgical criterion of area size has been relegated to the dust heap as one realizes that large rarifying lesions heal as completely (if not as rapidly) as small ones if the noxious agents from the pulpless canal are eliminated.

Concern over developing apical cysts is materially reduced. One must conclude that most apical cysts will heal following root canal filling and without surgical intervention. Exceptions to this "rule of thumb" are discussed in Chapter 10. The anxious and fearful anticipation of surgery common to most patients and the ever-present possibility of postoperative pain and swelling also serve as deterrents to indiscriminate surgery.

General Indications for Endodontic Surgery

The following are ***general*** indications and should not be considered "automatic" indications:

A. Necessity for drainage
   1. Elimination of toxins
   2. Alleviation of pain
B. Failure of nonsurgical therapy
   1. Obviously inadequate filling
   2. Apparently adequate filling
   3. Persistent post-procedural discomfort
C. Predictable failure with ***non***surgical therapy
   1. Flaring open apex, unresolved
   2. Severely curved root end
   3. Internal, external, or apical resorption
   4. Fractures in the apical third
   5. Apical cyst
   6. Need for biopsy
D. Impracticality of ***non***surgical therapy
   1. Jacket crowns
   2. Fixed partial denture attachment
   3. Dowell-retention crown
   4. Excessive calcification or irretrievable root fillings
   5. Associated periodontal lesion
E. Procedural accidents
   1. Instrument fragmentation
   2. Perforation
   3. Overinstrumentation
   4. Gross overfilling

Necessity for Drainage

In dealing with the acute apical abscess, it is often necessary to establish drainage of the lesion for two reasons: (1) to evacuate the pus and toxins gathered in the area of cellulitis, and (2) to afford the patient some degree of comfort.

Elimination of Toxins. The toxic exudate that accumulates in the soft tissue and bony lesion of an acute apical abscess should be drained. First and foremost, early drainage speeds healing and is preferred to the slow removal of pus and toxins by the vascular and lymphatic systems. The latter—so-called "blind" drainage by the body—sometimes takes weeks, unless the lesion ruptures and drains spontaneously.

Prevention of spontaneous drainage is the second reason for surgical intervention. The possibility of a disfiguring cutaneous fistula always exists, hence the insistence upon intraoral incision to control the location of the drainage site (Fig. 15–1).

Alleviation of Pain. The tremendous pressure, and attendant pain, which builds in an acute apical abscess

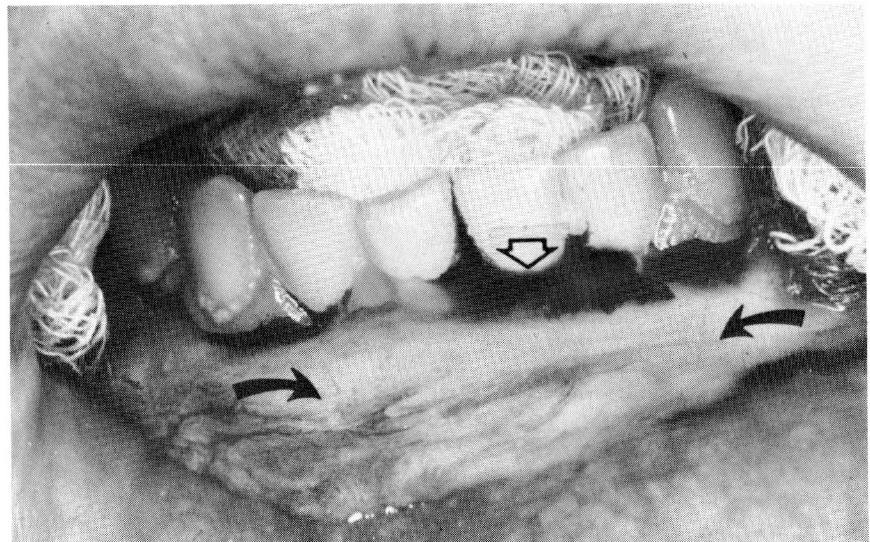

Fig. 15–1. Intraoral incision releases accumulated pus *(arrows)* and blood *(open arrow)* into vestibule preventing disfiguring extraoral fistula of chin. (See Fig. 9–15.)

can best be relieved by surgical drainage. With the drainage comes relief from discomfort. Although the gross swelling from the cellulitis may persist, the patient usually reports comparative comfort even as the local analgesia wears away.

Failure of Nonsurgical Therapy

Persistently enlarging or newly developing radiolucencies associated with previously filled canals are a sign of failure, and indicate that an irritant of some kind is interfering with normal bone metabolism. The area of pathosis may result from five possible sources of irritation: (1) from persistent localized infection or trauma, (2) from biochemical irritation by noxious tissue-fluid percolating through voids in the filling in the incompletely obturated main canal, (3) from patent, unfilled accessory canals, (4) from filling materials ***grossly*** extruded through a perforation or through the apical foramen or (5) from a vertical root fracture. Regardless of etiology, these failure cases may be divided into two groups on the basis of roentgenographic evidence: (1) those in which the root canal fillings appear to be inadequate, and (2) those in which the fillings appear to be adequate. A third group includes all those cases in which failure must be concluded from the prolonged persistence or recurrence of ***pain*** or ***swelling*** following completion of treatment.

Obviously Inadequate Filling. When a roentgenogram reveals the canal to be inadequately obturated and periapical pathosis develops or persists, the lack of obturation can first be assumed to be the cause of failure. If at all possible, ***retreatment*** and ***refilling*** the canal constitute the corrective treatment of choice. Surgical intervention is required if the faulty filling cannot be removed from the canal, and the retrosurgical approach is the only recourse. Retrofilling is necessary when silver points are irretrievable, in the case of certain cements too hard and insoluble to be removed with files or reamers, or when a mass of gutta percha or cement has been forced beyond the apical foramen and serves as a severe irritant (Fig. 15–2). Actually, the grossly overfilled canals often are not totally obturated because of a lack of filling compression against an open apex.

Apparently Adequate Filling. On occasion an endodontic case may fail in spite of what appears in the roentgenogram to be a sound and adequate root canal filling. In such cases a four-stage examination should be conducted in an attempt to learn the true cause of failure. First, a ***thorough*** roentgenographic study should be made to eliminate the possibility of inadequate filling. Second, the tooth should be checked for occlusal trauma. Third, the vitality of the adjacent teeth should be checked. Finally, the sulcus should be painstakingly explored to see if an associated periodontal pocket or vertical root fracture can be found (see p. 647).

If none of these factors can be indicted, the apparently adequate filling should be removed and the canal carefully retreated and thoroughly obtu-

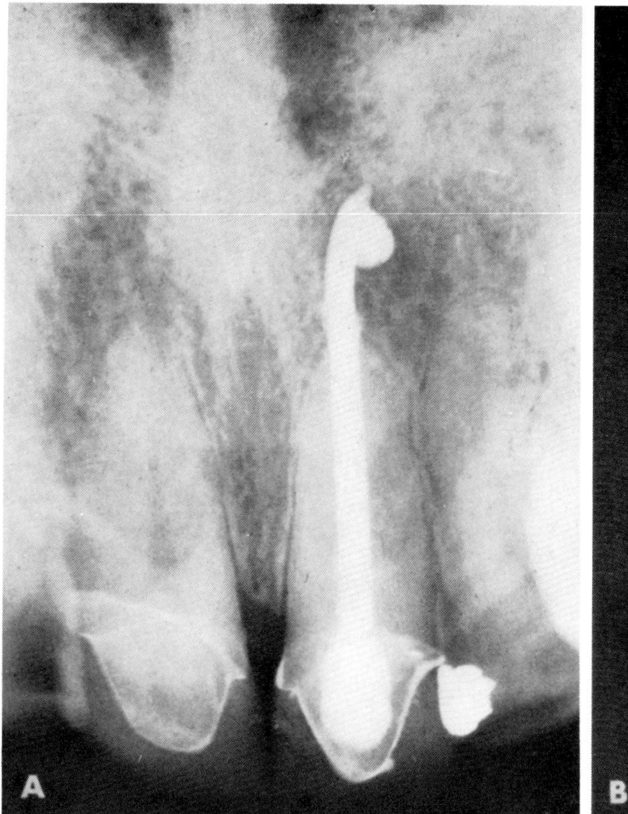

Fig. 15–2. *A,* Gross overfilling with gutta percha which could have been corrected surgically. *B,* Unfortunately, tooth was extracted before corrective surgery was attempted.

rated. If healing still fails to occur, a surgical exposure should be made to see what unusual cause of persistent inflammation is present. An undisclosed vertical fracture might be such a cause. One might also be surprised to find a perforation. Also, a root end that inclines sharply toward or away from the central x-ray beam may create the illusion of being filled to the apex, when in reality a perforation short of the apex exists, and the apical third of the canal remains uncleansed and unfilled.

If it is found necessary to make a surgical exposure to evaluate these problem cases, a fine, sharp right-angle explorer should be used to probe carefully and explore the entire apex of the root in a check of the density of the root canal filling, or in the case of a silver point filling, the fit of the point in the prepared apical cavity. Accessory foramens that are not obvious to the eye may be discovered by exploration. Once diagnosis is made, retrofilling may be completed at the same appointment.

Persistent Post-procedural Discomfort. Nonsurgical therapy *per se* must be considered inadequate when discomfort persists at the periapex long after therapy is completed, and in spite of a well-filled canal. These cases usually involve maxillary canines or premolars with lingual inclination of the crown, thus tipping the root end out through the buccal plate of bone. The patient invariably complains of pain on palpation of the area. The solution to the problem may be apicocurettage of the inflammatory tissue and a beveled resection of the root apex to position it back within the bony case. Sometimes even surgery fails to cure the persistent pain.

Predictable Failure with Nonsurgical Therapy

Under ***certain*** circumstances, a higher percentage of nonsurgical cases may be expected to fail. Typical of these are: (1) teeth with flaring open apices, (2) severely curved root ends, (3) perforating internal or external resorption, (4) fractures in the apical third with displacement of the separated portions, (5) keratinizing or globulomaxillary cysts associated with pulpless teeth.

Open Flaring Apex. If the root formation of a tooth has been arrested by death of the pulp prior to

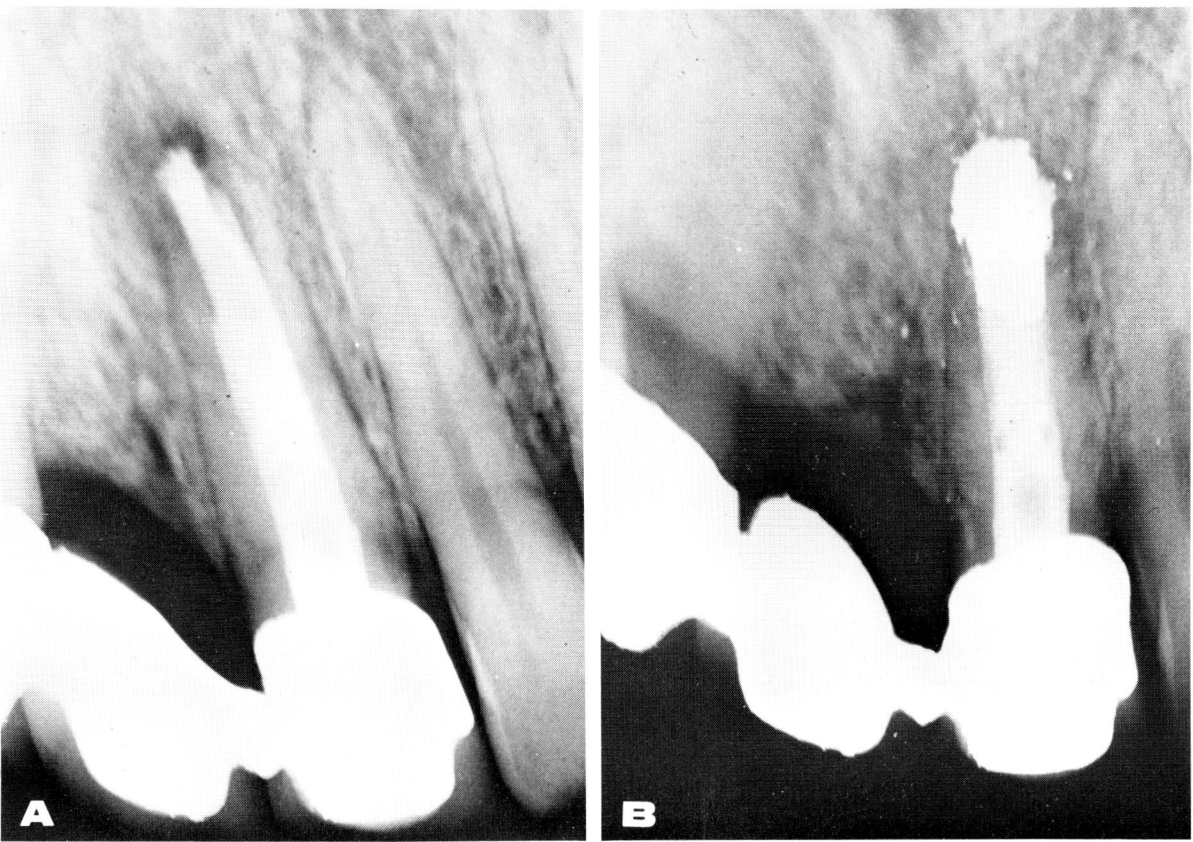

Fig. 15–3. *A*, Incomplete obturation of blunderbuss-shaped canal. Bridge abutment is a porcelain-faced crown. *B*, Three-year recall radiograph following retrofilling. (Courtesy Dr. Joe Merrell.)

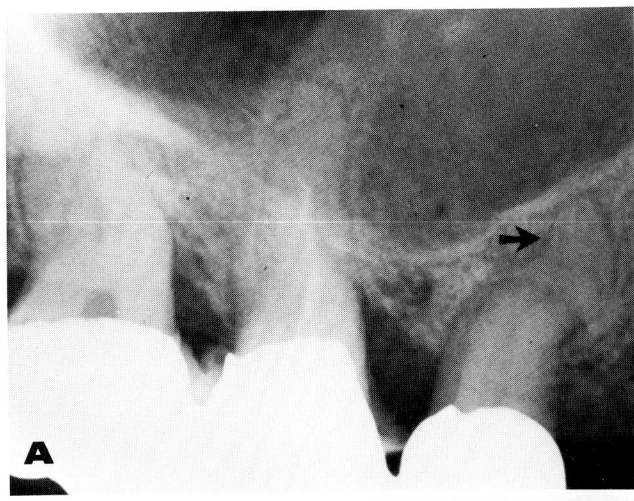

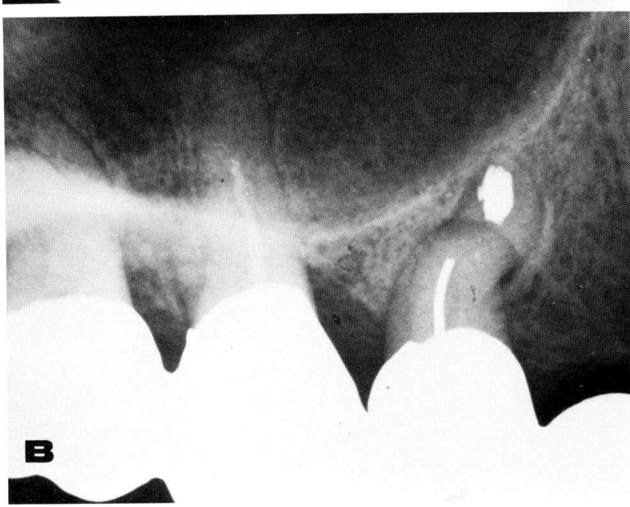

Fig. 15–4. *A*, Bayonet-curved first premolar in periodontal prosthesis. Curve could not be negotiated and silver point filling was placed to elbow. *B*, Periapical lesion continued and so retrofilling was placed. Three-year recall radiograph shows healing. Partially filled second premolar asymptomatic. (Courtesy Dr. Alfred L. Frank.)

closure of the apex, it may usually be corrected by cementogenesis (p. 689). The root may be stimulated to regrowth and the apex "sealed over" with new cemento-dentin—apexification. In the event this procedure fails, surgical exposure and retrofilling may be the only alternative means of saving the tooth (Fig. 15–3).

Severely Curved Root End. A pulpless tooth, with apical defalcation so severe that conventional instrumentation is impossible or inadequate, may be a candidate for surgical therapy (Fig. 15–4). Before surgery is considered, every effort must be expended to cleanse, reshape, and obturate the canal by nonsurgical methods. Filling by the softened gutta percha technique or intentionally using "broken instruments" for filling must first be attempted. If these attempts fail and a periapical lesion develops or persists, the option for surgical intervention and retrofilling should be exercised.

Resorption. The surgical approach and retrofilling may be used where communication has developed between the periodontium and the root canal through an area of internal or external resorption. This resorption may occur along the side of the root or at the apex. Consider first the lateral resorptive defect. Before surgical exposure is employed to reach and effect a repair, a nonsurgical effort should be made to narrow the defect and obturate the canal. Utilizing calcium hydroxide as a biologically active agent, the bony lesion may be stimulated to fill in the defect and serve as a matrix for obturation from within the canal (p. 696). This failing, the lateral defect may be exposed surgically and repaired with an external filling (Fig. 15–5). In the case of resorption in the sulcular area, where bone is not present to be stimulated to fill in the defect, surgical exposure is first used and the defect repaired at the time the canal is obturated (Fig. 15–6).

In the case of advanced external resorption of the apex, apicoectomy may be necessary to remove that portion of the root which cannot be adequately instrumented and filled (Fig. 15–7). This is not to say that ***every*** root apex showing resorption must be resected. Calcium hydroxide stimulation of apical resorption areas should first be attempted before surgical intervention and retrofilling are used.

Apical Fractures. Many teeth have been condemned because of horizontal fractures near the apex. Patience on the part of the dentist is frequently the best therapy, since without endodontic treatment in such cases, vitality may be maintained and the fractured segments fused by cementum and osteodentin (see Fig. 16–27). If death of the pulp occurs and a ***pathologic lesion*** develops in and around the fractured tip, it is a relatively simple matter to remove surgically the apical root fragment at the time root canal therapy is completed (see Fig. 16–27).

Apical Cyst. The keratinizing apical cyst or globulomaxillary cyst associated with a pulpless tooth can sometimes be diagnosed with considerable accu-

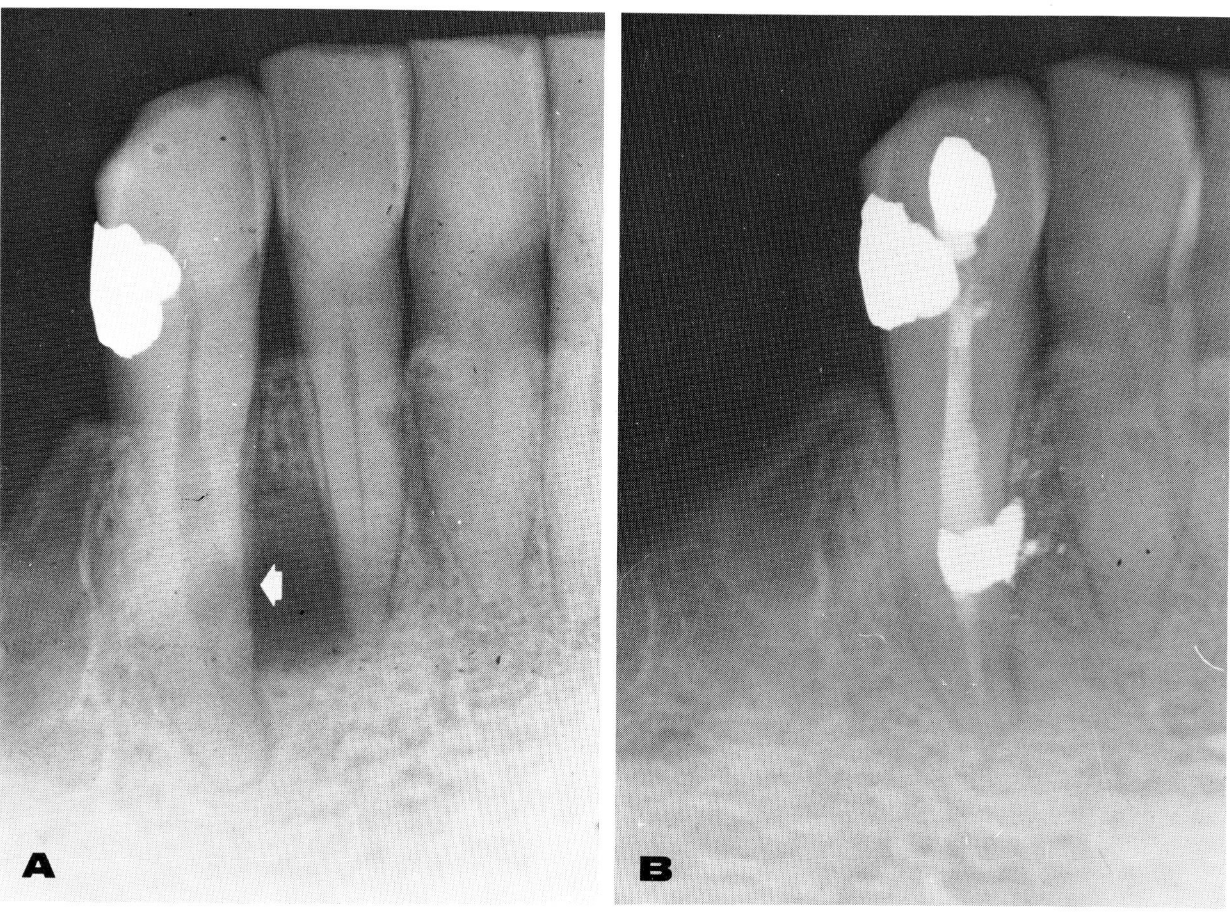

Fig. 15–5. Surgical sealing of perforative defect of internal resorption with amalgam. *A,* Preoperative radiograph. *B,* One-year recall radiograph. Calcium hydroxide therapy should first be attempted in similar cases. (From Frank, A. L.: Dent. Clin. N. Amer., *18*:465, Apr., 1974.)

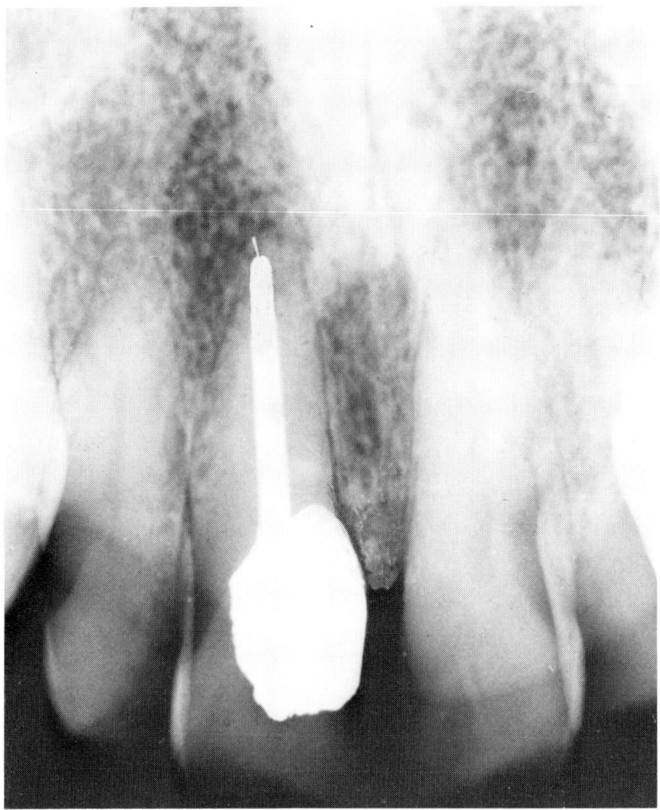

Fig. 15–6. Huge resorptive defect surgically exposed and repaired by amalgam filling.

racy prior to treatment (see Fig. 9–32). The pathognomonic characteristic of a cyst to separate the roots of the teeth as the cyst expands is an indication for surgical intervention (see Fig. 10–31).

Need for Biopsy. On rare occasions a periapical lesion associated with a pulpless tooth may be suspected as something other than an inflammatory lesion—a malignancy for example (see Fig. 9–42). In this case a biopsy of the tissue, removed in its entirety by apicocurettage, is in order. If the biopsy report is ***negative,*** root canal filling should then be completed without additional surgical intervention.

Impracticality of the Nonsurgical Approach

Impracticality of the conventional approach exists when restorations or calcifications interfere with a coronal approach to the root canal. Jacket crowns, fixed partial denture attachments, retentive dowels, or excessive calcification in canals may preclude a nonsurgical procedure. Careful evaluation from an operative point of view is required, with thought for the physical, mental, and economic well-being of the patient.

Jacket Crowns. The gross reduction of tooth structure for jacket crowns, both porcelain and porcelain baked on metal, materially weakens the crown of the tooth. Endodontic cavity preparation further weakens these preparations, making the tooth highly subject to fracture at the gingiva (Fig. 15–8*A*). In addition, porcelain jacket crowns themselves, once penetrated, are easily split. Retrofilling may be the answer—a retrosurgical approach and apical retrofilling (Fig. 15–8*B*).

It is not advocated that poorly fitting or unattractive jacket crowns be protected by retrofilling. The patient could be forewarned that the crown might split or come loose, in which case it would be replaced

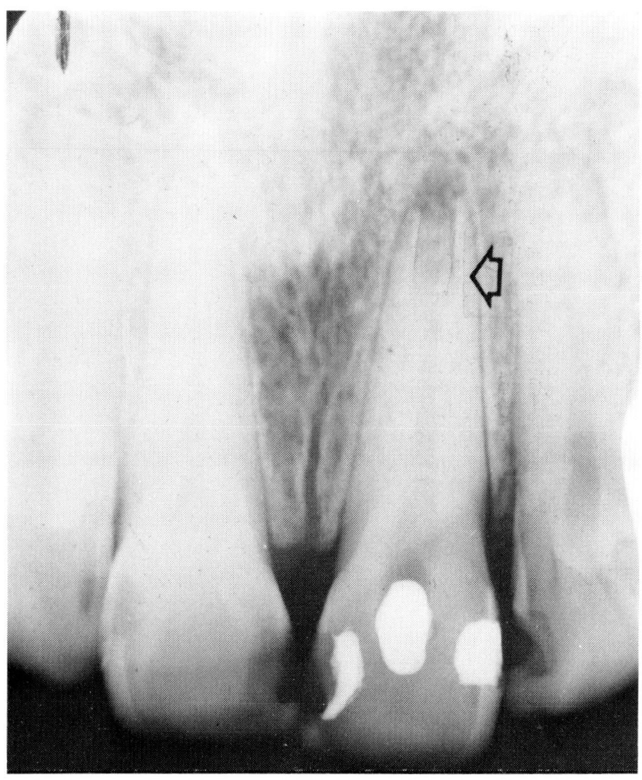

Fig. 15–7. Internal resorption in apical third of central incisor *(arrow)* indicates presence of vital tissue. Calcium hydroxide therapy should be attempted to stimulate apical repair. If resorptive process continues, root canal should be filled and apicoectomy done (retouched for clarity). (From Luebke, R. G., Glick, D. H., and Ingle, J. I.: Oral Surg., *18*:97, July, 1964.)

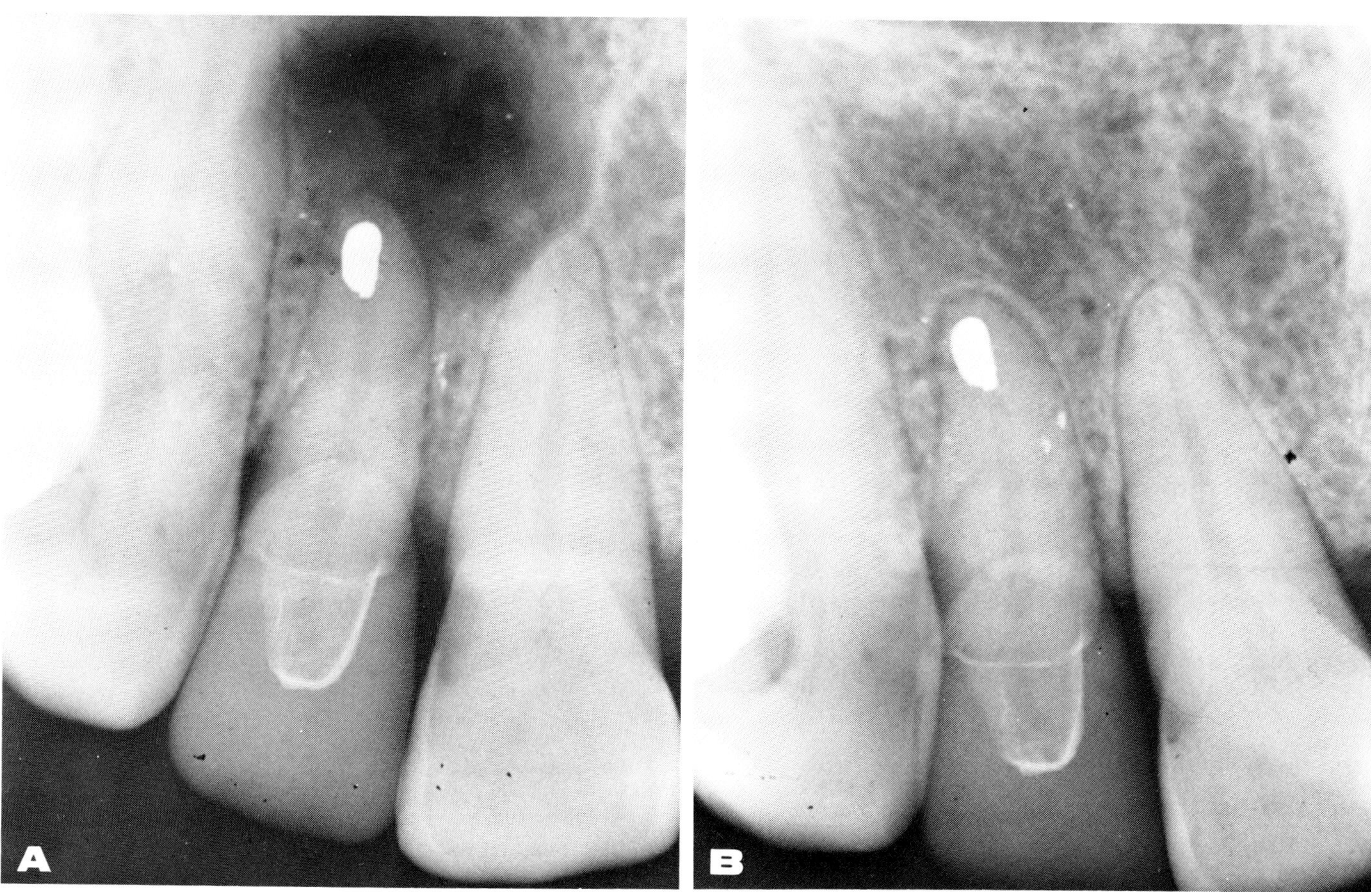

Fig. 15–8. *A,* Access through lingual of esthetic well-fitting porcelain jacket crown might well have split crown and destroyed remaining tooth structure as well. Retrofilling has just been placed. *B,* Two-year recall radiograph. (Courtesy Dr. Alfred L. Frank.)

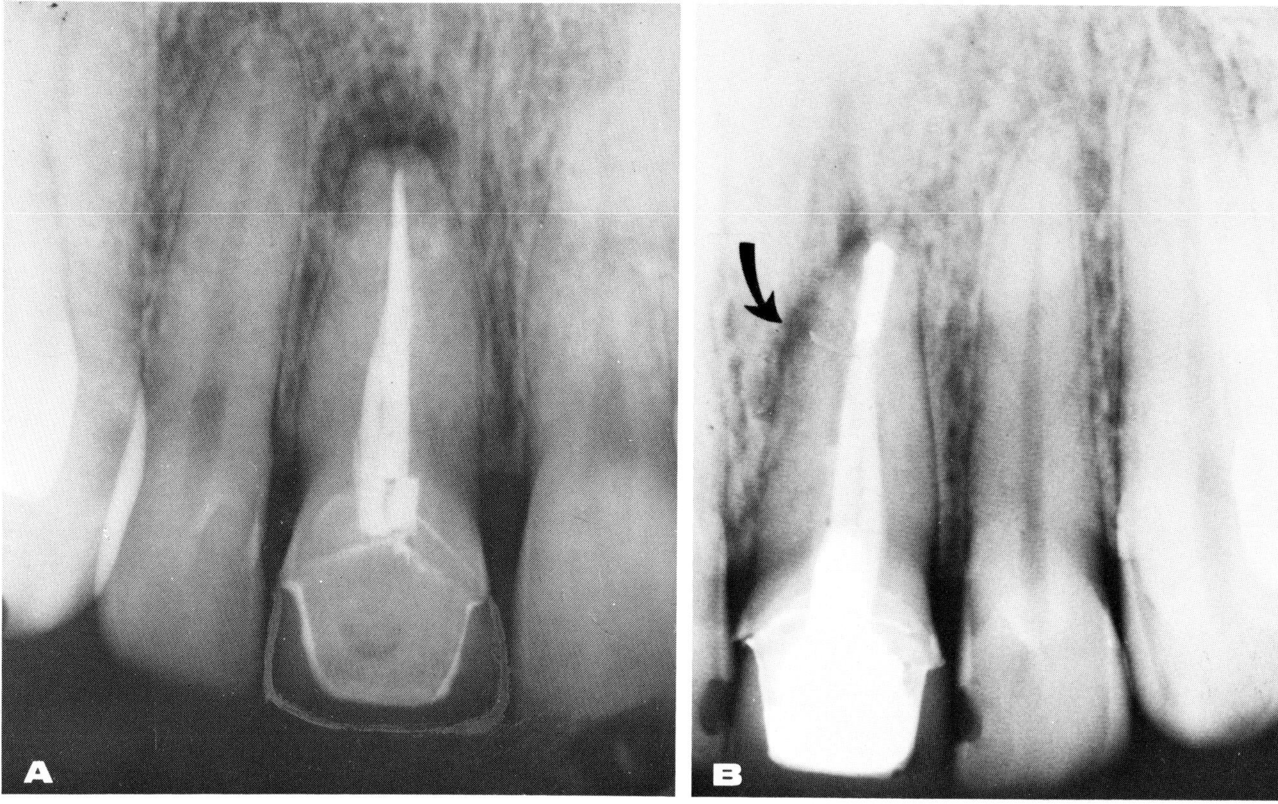

Fig. 15–9. *A,* Jacket crown undoubtedly placed at early age, hence obviously short proximal extension now that tooth has erupted. Broad remaining tooth structure is perfectly adequate to sustain endodontic cavity preparation without fracturing. Cases of this type should be retreated nonsurgically, not retrofilled, and short defective crown replaced. (Crown retouched for clarity.) *B,* Failure related to unfilled, lateral, accessory canal, although apical foramen has been successfully obturated with retrofilling. Noting lateral lesion, entire canal should have been either obturated or filled conventionally from crown. (From Luebke, R. G., Glick, D. H., and Ingle, J. I.: Oral Surg., *18*:97, July, 1964.)

following root canal therapy. Also, in the event a lateral lesion is seen in the radiograph, signifying a patent and necrotic accessory canal, a retrofilling is ***not*** indicated (Fig. 15–9), but rather the canal must be filled in the conventional nonsurgical manner.

Fixed Partial Denture Attachments. If root canal therapy is necessary for fixed partial denture abutment teeth, special assessment of the attachments should be made before treatment is begun. If, for example, the bridge attachments are inlays, the endodontic access preparations will probably destroy the retention of the castings. Extensive coronal preparation also may weaken the crown with resultant fracture. In these cases the retrosurgical approach could be used ***if indicated,*** leaving the restoration undisturbed.

Dowel-Retention Crowns. Endodontic failure under retentive dowels is a common indication for retrosurgical filling. The dowel may be in an abutment tooth, and an entire bridge would have to be removed to provide access to the involved canal (Fig. 15–10). In other cases, removing the dowel may split the root. Some dowels are so well retained that they cannot be removed. In such cases, the surgical approach and retrofilling may be the only approach (Fig. 15–11).

Excessive Calcification or Irretrievable Root Filling. Roentgenograms may reveal a canal so thoroughly obliterated in its coronal half or two-thirds that a conventional approach is contraindicated. The crown could be hopelessly "gutted" in the attempt to establish access to the distant canal orifice.

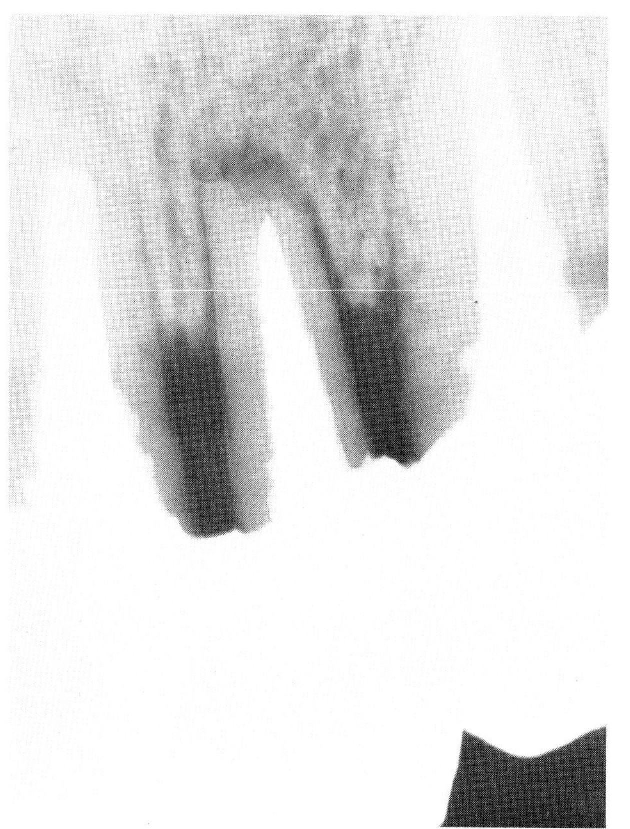

Fig. 15–10. Indication for retrosurgical filling. Attempt to remove retentive dowel for treatment will require removal of entire prosthesis. Fracture of roots could result. Retrofilling should be reserved for well-fitting esthetic crowns.

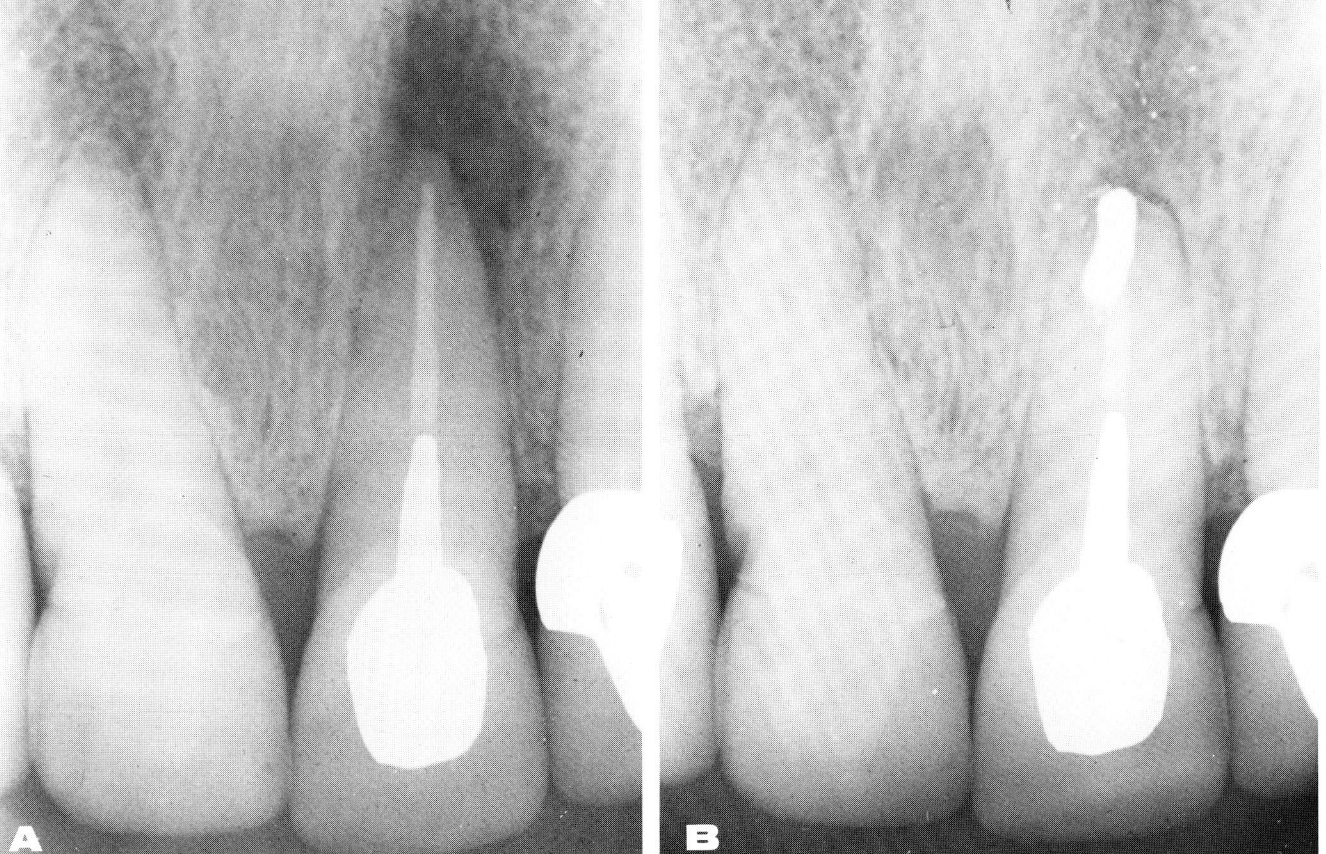

Fig. 15–11. *A,* Well-fitting, esthetic dowel crown restoring incisor with poorly obturated canal. *B,* One year postoperative recall radiograph following retrofilling. Matched anterior crowns have not been disturbed. (Courtesy Dr. Alfred L. Frank.)

The same problem obtains when the canal is blocked by an irretrievable filling. This is a prime indication for a surgical approach to the apex and a retroamalgam filling placed in the remaining canal (Fig. 15–12).

Associated Periodontal Lesion. Hiatt has shown that a secondary periodontal lesion associated with a primary periapical lesion will be repaired following concomitant treatment of both lesions.[7,8] However, experience has proved that many lesions involving both periapical and periodontal tissues will heal spontaneously and require no surgical intervention. As discussed in the section on endodontal-periodontal surgery, these spontaneously healing lesions are of primary endodontal origin. As the cases become more complex, with an increasing overlay of periodontal disease, the need for corrective surgery increases. Complete bone loss from periodontal disease may require total amputation of the pathologic root in multirooted teeth (Fig. 15–13) if

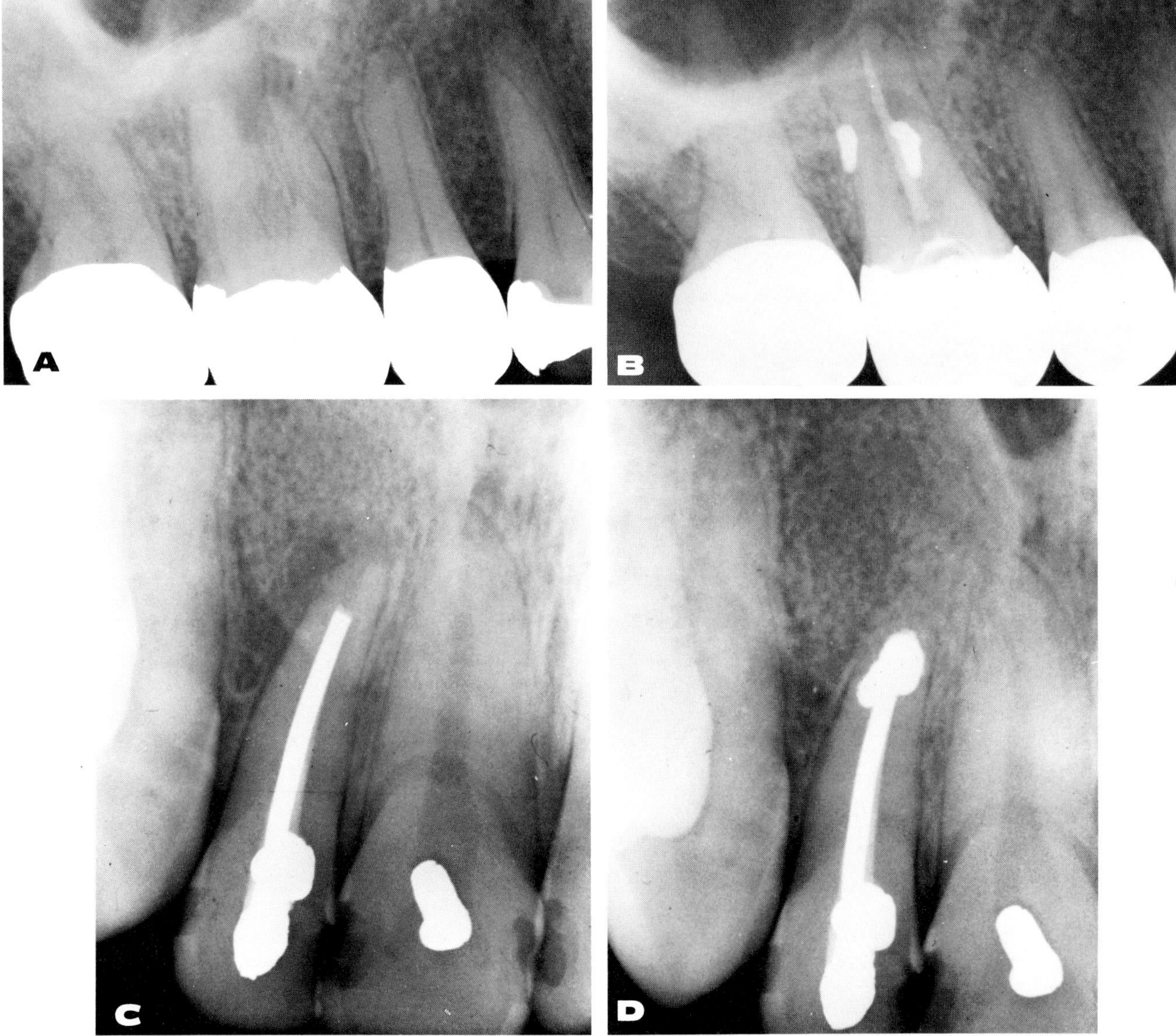

Fig. 15–12. *A,* Calcified buccal canals of pulpless first molar in well-restored arch. *B,* Recall radiograph, 18 months after retrofilling. *C,* Irretrievable silver point which does not adequately obturate canal. Note lateral as well as periapical lesion. *D,* One-year recall radiograph shows complete healing. Both apical foramen and lateral perforation were obturated. (Courtesy Dr. Alfred L. Frank.)

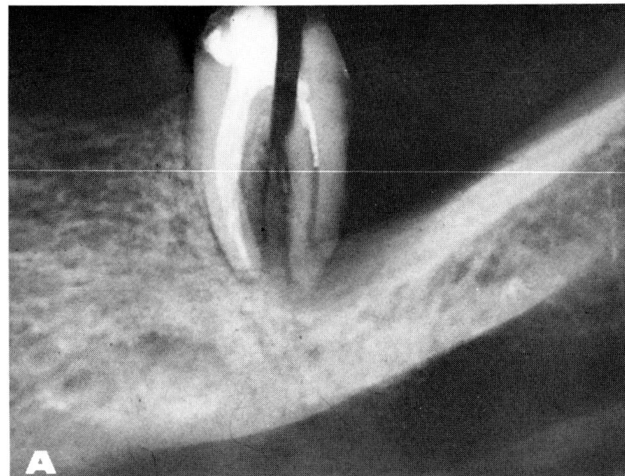

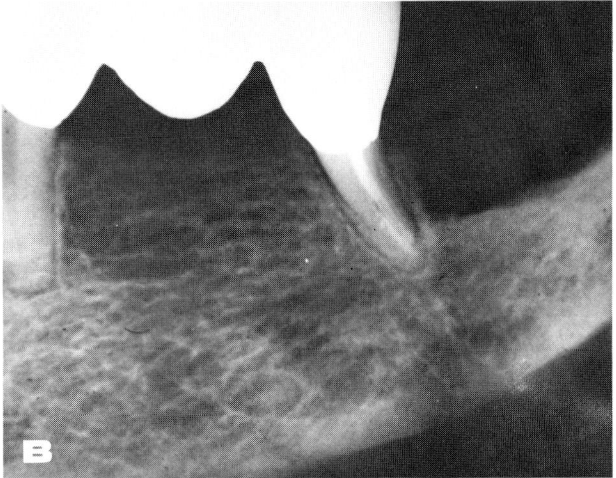

Fig. 15–13. *A*, Advanced periodontal lesion and resorption involving distal root in 68-year-old patient. Amputation is made at expense of root to be removed. *B*, Bicuspidized molar root becomes abutment for well-restored bridge. (Courtesy Dr. Alfred L. Frank.)

combined treatment fails. Scaled down from this advanced surgery is curettage, done with or without a flap, in lesser involved cases.

Procedural Accidents

Procedural accidents or inadequacies create circumstances which, if not corrected, increase the probability of failure. Broken instruments, perforation, overinstrumentation, and gross overfilling may lead to an unfavorble prognosis.

Instrument Fragmentation. Most broken instruments are firmly locked in the canal, and their removal is difficult, if not impossible. After a reasonable effort at removal has proved fruitless, the operator is justified in leaving the firmly locked instrument in place where it may act as an apical seal. Ingle has shown that less than 1% of endodontic failures result from broken instruments.[9] Crump and Natkin have shown that "broken instrument" cases were as successfully filled as a matched series of cases obturated in the conventional way.[10]

In the case of failure, however, surgical intervention with resection of the root end containing the broken instrument is indicated. In those rare cases in which the fragment is central in the canal and cannot be by-passed, the retrosurgical approach may be used and a retrofilling placed (Fig. 15–14). If the fragment protrudes through the foramen, and periapical inflammation persists, the apex may be exposed and a retrofilling placed (Fig. 15–15).

Perforation. Perforation near the apex usually makes instrumentation and filling of the true canal virtually impossible. If a periapical lesion develops, the first attempt at repair should be with intracanal calcium hydroxide to stimulate new bone in the defect. This may serve as a matrix against which the canal may be reobturated without gross overfilling (Fig. 15–16). In the event this approach fails, a surgical approach should be used. The root canal filling can be completed and the root tip resected to the point at which the instrument deviated from the canal. If the perforation is more centrally located on the root, retrofilling of the defect is indicated.

Overinstrumentation. The use of instruments too large for the bulk of root structure will lead to fracture of the root tip. If pathosis develops and persists, this tip must then be removed surgically (Fig. 15–17). As previously discussed, overinstrumentation can easily go undetected by roentgenogram, but will become apparent when filling material is extruded through it.

Gross Overfilling. On occasion, even the most skillful operator can overfill at the apex. ***Gross*** overfilling ***may*** result in postoperative pain, a persistent foreign body reaction, and incomplete healing at the apex (Fig. 15–18). If a mass of cement is present it may be removed by apicocurettage, and a retrofilling is placed to seal the apex. Overfilling with a silver point can mean that the point does not thoroughly obturate the apex. If a lesion develops, it should be removed and retreated, but failing this, it should be

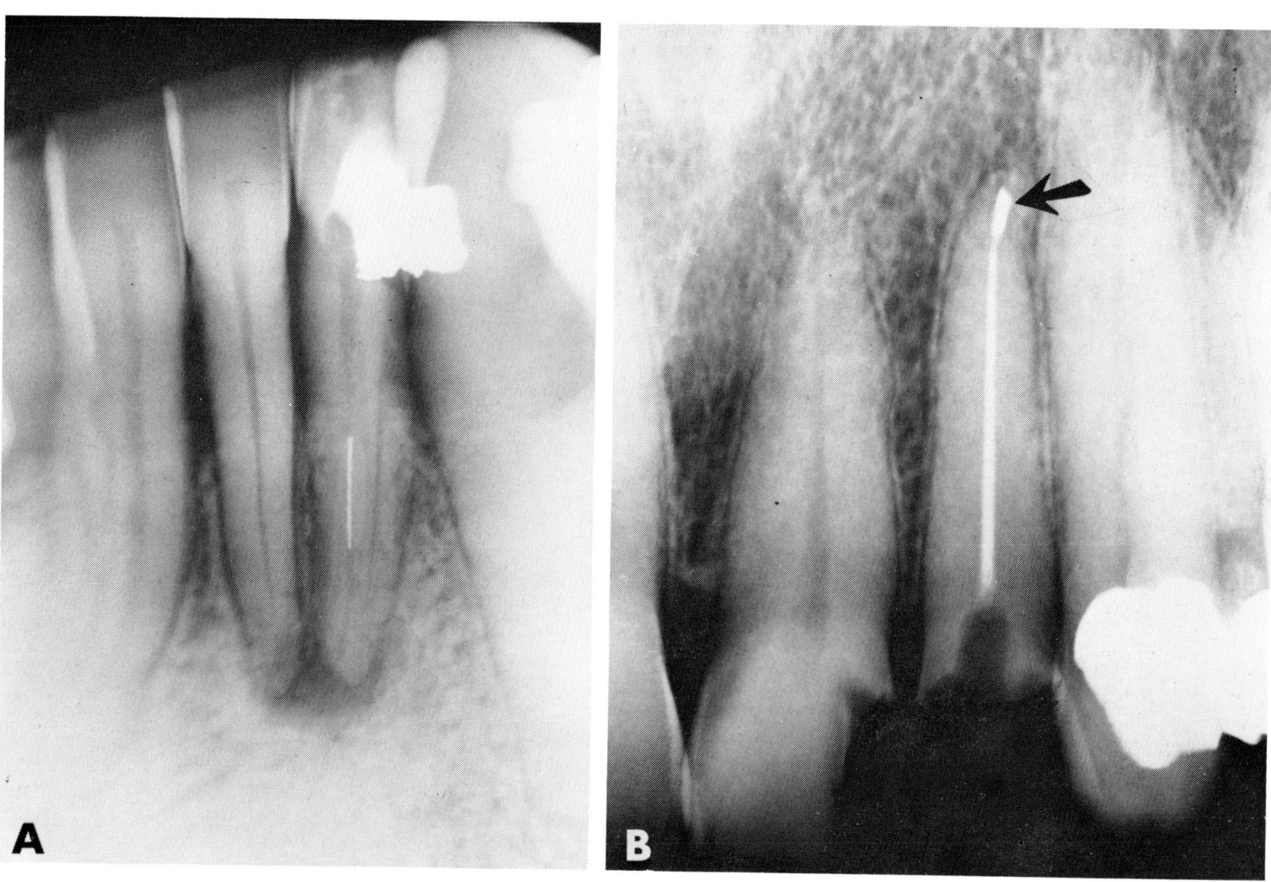

Fig. 15–14. *A,* Broken instrument firmly locked centrally in canal cannot be by-passed. Periapical pathosis persists. Approach to apex for filling must be surgical. *B,* Successful retrofilling *(arrow)* placed six months previously to obliterate apical canal following instrument fragmentation. (Luebke, R. G., Glick, D. H., and Ingle, J. I.: Oral Surg., *18*:97, July, 1964.)

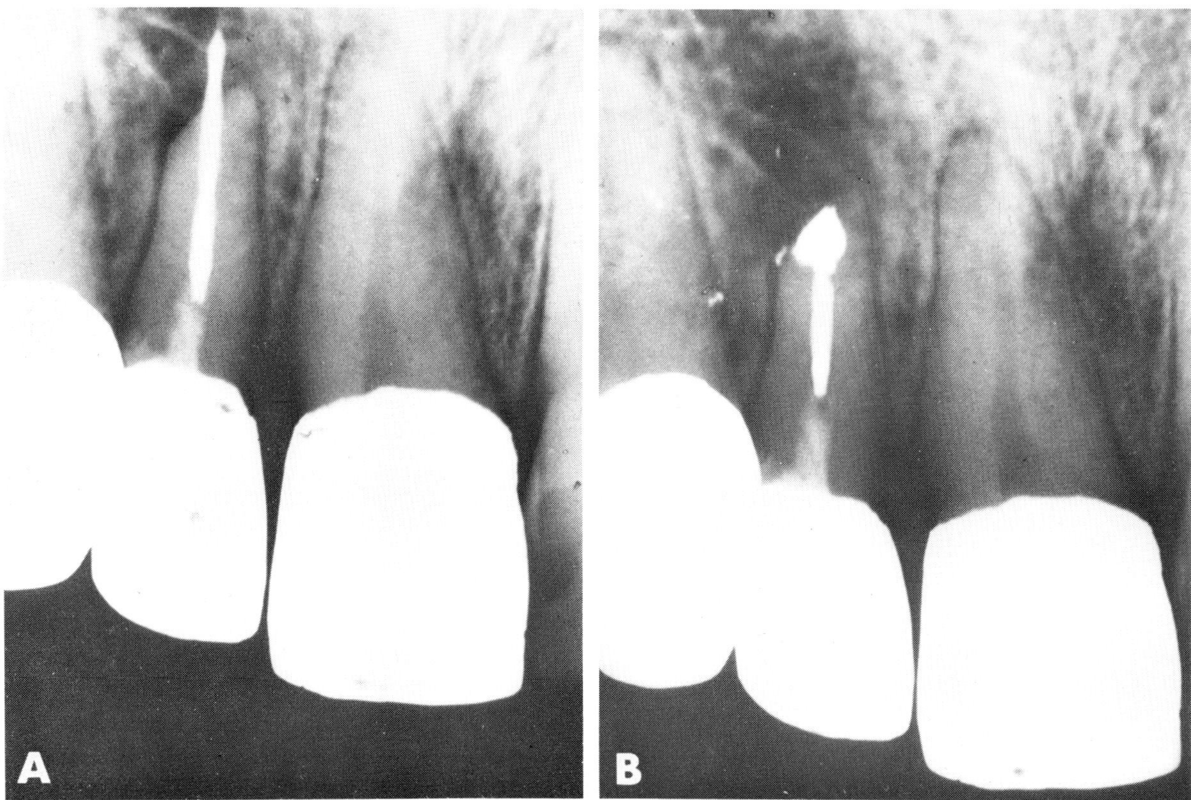

Fig. 15–15. *A*, Broken instrument protruding through apical foramen but not obliterating canal. Periapical pathosis persists. *B*, Broken instrument could not be pulled through apex with hemostat. Retrofilling was placed to insure obturation.

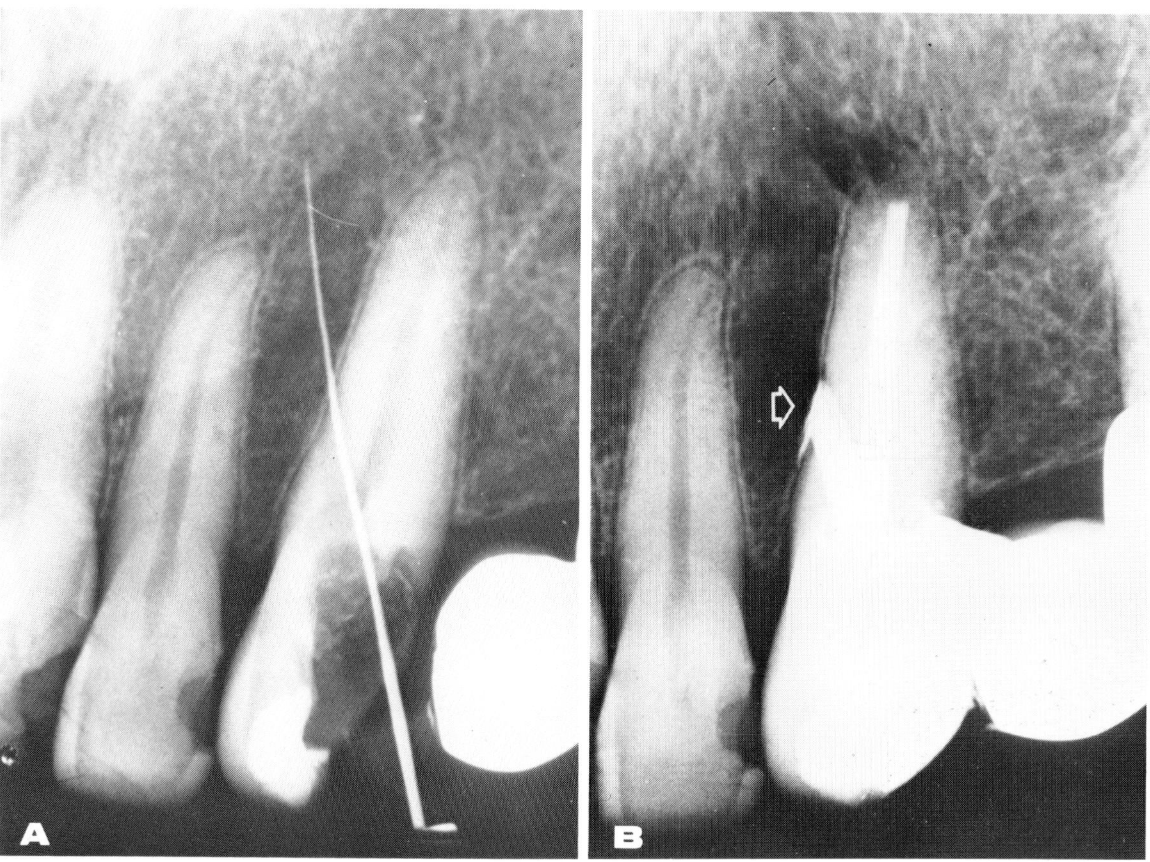

Fig. 15–16. Repair of mechanical perforation following calcium hydroxide therapy. *A,* Preoperative radiograph. Gross perforation is caused by misdirected bur. Main canal was located, cleansed, and shaped in addition to perforated "canal" prepared with large blunted files. Thick paste of calcium hydroxide was inserted. Patient was reappointed 6 weeks later. *B,* Post-filling radiograph. Gutta percha point was fitted for each canal and well condensed. Note how new matrix of healing is demonstrated by form of sealer and gutta percha at site of perforation *(arrow).* (From Frank, A. L.: Dent. Clin. N. Amer., *18*:465, Apr., 1974.)

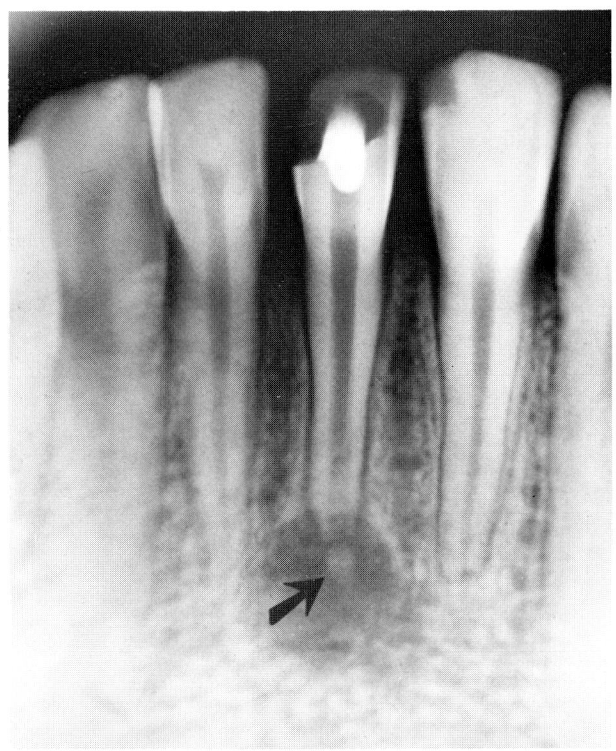

Fig. 15–17. Overinstrumentation has led to apical perforation and fracture of root tip *(arrow)* which must be removed surgically.

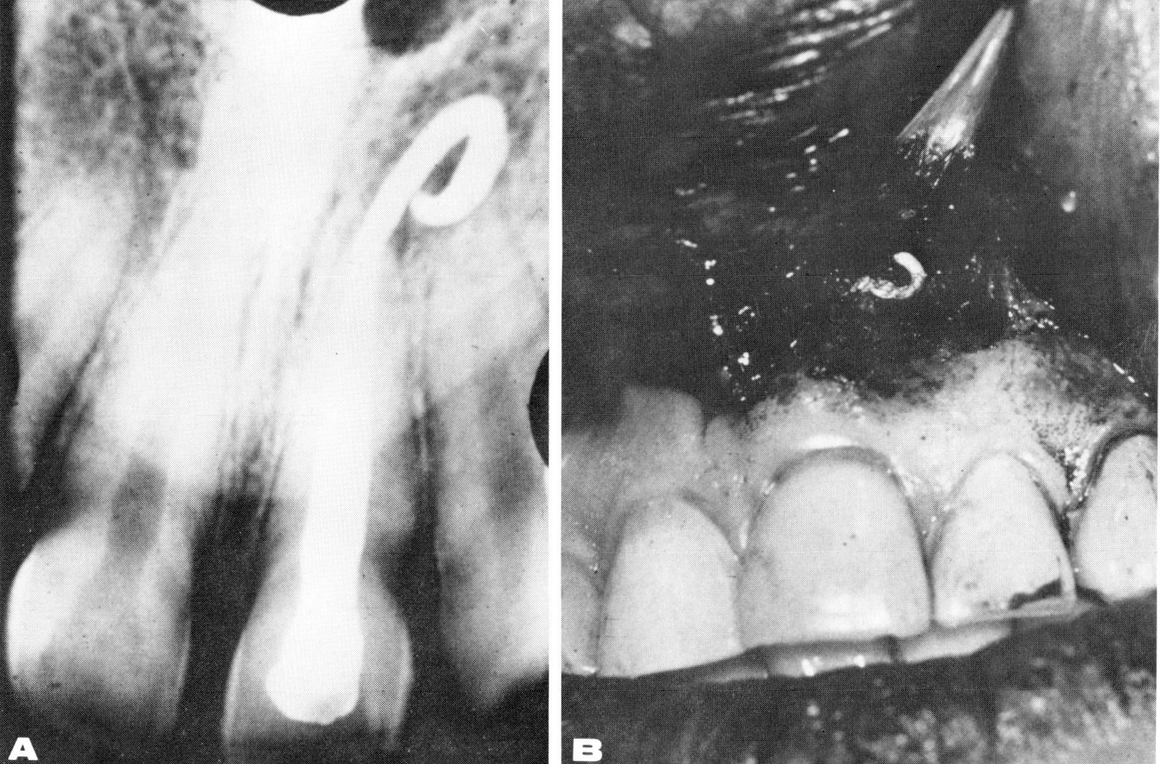

Fig. 15–18. *A*, Gross overfilling with gutta percha causes constant pain and inflammation. *B*, Surgical exposure of filling. Excess may be seared off. If canal is not sealed by heat, retroamalgam filling should be placed.

severed at the apex and a retrofilling placed. If the excess filling is gutta percha, it may be "seared flush with the cut root end" with a heated instrument and "visually checked for obturation."[11] A retroamalgam filling may be placed if the gutta percha appears inadequate.

Contraindications to Endodontic Surgery

There are five main contraindications to endodontic surgery: (1) indiscriminate surgery, (2) psychologic impact upon the patient, (3) systemic health problems, (4) anatomic considerations, and (5) postsurgical sequelae.

Indiscriminate Surgery

Some of the contraindications to endodontic surgery have already been spelled out. That is, surgery should not be a catch-all for every endodontic case or a cover-up for lack of skill in nonsurgical endodontic techniques. It is not indicated (except as previously outlined) simply because a periapical lesion is present at the time of treatment. It is not necessarily indicated because a large lesion is present or because the operator believes a lesion ***may become*** cystic.

Psychologic Impact

Patients facing endodontic surgery range in their psychic response from the person terrified by the mere suggestion of surgery to the masochist addicted to polysurgery who is seeking the experience. In between is the great mass of patients who would "rather not, but if it is necessary, you have my permission to go ahead." Patients should be allowed to verbalize their thoughts and fears after they have been thoroughly informed of the operation itself, the options, and the possible consequences. They should then willingly consent, not being wheedled into a procedure they dread unless there is no apparent alternative.

One is well advised to avoid surgical intervention for the highly emotional or extremely apprehensive patient. Surgery to the very young or very old can be a psychic trauma as well. If ataraxics or hypnotic drugs are used for tranquility or sedation, the very young and the very old must be considered poor risks. Extraction could be an even greater risk.

Poor Health

As detailed in Chapter 10, a complete medical history must be taken. The patient's blood pressure should be determined and recorded. If any question exists about the patient's health, medical consultation must be sought, preferably through the patient's physician. Contraindications would include depressive reactions such as extreme fatigue, blood dyscrasias, and neurologic problems such as a cerebral palsy or "brittle" epilepsy. If the patient has a debilitating or terminal disease, any surgery is contraindicated. Diabetes, heart disease, adverse drug reactions, and pregnancy in the first or last trimester often are considered contraindications to surgery.

Anatomic Considerations

An awareness of important structural relationships allows one to determine whether anatomic hazards contraindicate or limit endodontic surgery.[12]

Maxilla. ***Anterior Facial Region.*** The maxillary incisors and the alveolar process are closely related to the floor of the nose. In some individuals a combination of a short alveolar process and long roots allows the incisor apices to contact the thin bony plate of the nasal floor, particularly if the teeth are vertically erect in the alveolar process. The lateral incisors are seldom as close to the nasal floor as the central incisors. In any case, careful roentgenographic examination is essential to avoid nasal perforations. The canine occupies a "neutral" position between the maxillary sinus and the nasal cavity and has no intimate relationship to either cavity. In rare instances the maxillary sinus extends forward to the canine alveolus, and sometimes the nasal cavity approaches the mesiolingual surface of the canine.[12a]

In addition to problems with the nasal floor, the maxillary incisors and canines often exhibit little labial cortical plate and usually no medullary bone between the labial root surface and the overlying soft tissue (Fig. 15–19). In individuals with particularly prominent roots, labial fenestrations or dehiscences are sometimes present in the alveolar bone, for virtually the entire length of the root.

Missing cortical bone is a considerable problem for the endodontist, as well as the orthodontist and the periodontist. The orthodontist has long been accused of producing a root fenestration or dehiscence in the incisor region, a process orthodontists refer to as

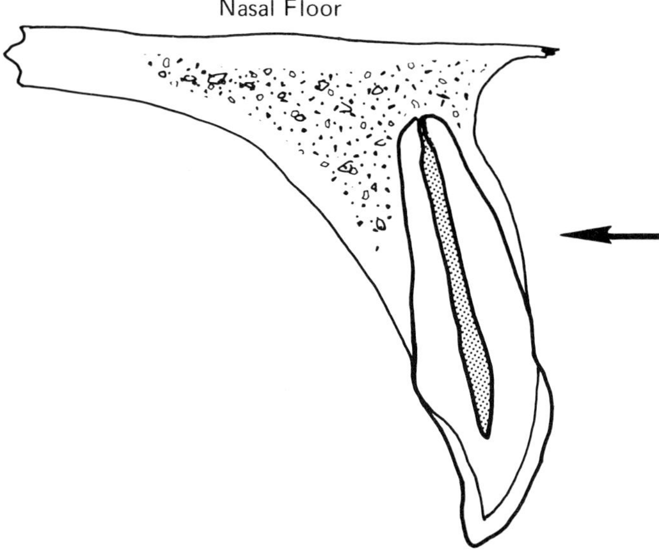

Fig. 15–19. Long axis of maxillary incisor is more nearly vertical than premaxilla alveolar process. Thin labial cortical plate *(arrow)* with no supporting bone is result. (Courtesy Dr. Raleigh R. Cummings.)

"gingival stripping." The periodontist who deals with this lesion has found that attempting to repair one dehiscent area often creates another nearby.[13] The clue to development of this aberration lies in the missing or paper-thin buccal cortical plate. Any surgical intervention (including endodontic) in the region may well develop into a fenestration (Fig. 15–20). Where the cortical plate is missing, the gingiva may fail to reattach directly to the root surface. Further surgical intervention or a developing gingival inflammation may cause the fenestration to become an irreparable dehiscence (Fig. 15–21).

Posterior Fenestration and the Maxillary Sinus. As with anterior teeth, a minimal amount of alveolar bone overlies premolar and molar buccal eminences, and fenestrations may exist, particularly in the apical portion (Fig. 15–22). Special attention should be given to the molar whose mesiobuccal root is prominently located to the buccal. Moreover, less than adequate blood supply may exist between the buccal root surface and mucosa at points of bony fenestration.

As the floor of the nose, the maxillary sinus could be a source of embarrassment to the surgeon. Although the sinus can be safely entered, it should be avoided if possible. First premolars are generally further removed from the floor of the maxillary sinus than are second premolars and molars, at which site perforation is more frequent. Second premolars grow closer to the maxillary sinus ***wall,*** whereas molars sometimes reach the floor and sometimes protrude into the sinus (Fig. 15–23). The maxillary sinus normally expands with age and into areas of nonfunctional bone. In certain instances it can be seen expanding into an area of a previous extraction (Fig. 15–24). A similar situation may exist where the sinus dips between the divergence of molar roots, or where the periapical tissue of the root directly contacts the lining membrane of the sinus. These conditions complicate surgical access and can lead to sinus perforation.

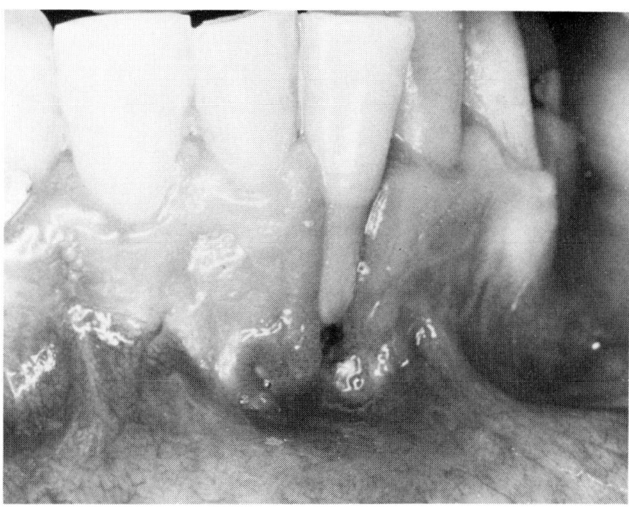

Fig. 15–20. Dehiscence which developed from endodontic surgery. Extreme labial and rotated position of tooth provided clue of root fenestration through cortical plate. Failure from circular incision should have been prognosticated and rectangular flap used instead.

Palate. Should palatal surgery be indicated, the palatal flap design must be such that the greater palatine vessels and nerve are not severed. The greater palatine foramen itself is rarely disturbed in that it is located lingual to the third molar. Severance of the greater palatine artery and resultant profuse hemorrhage can be avoided by utilizing an extensive flap loosened at each interproximal space or modified into a triangular flap with a vertical incision in the anterior or midpalate. The height of the palatal vault,

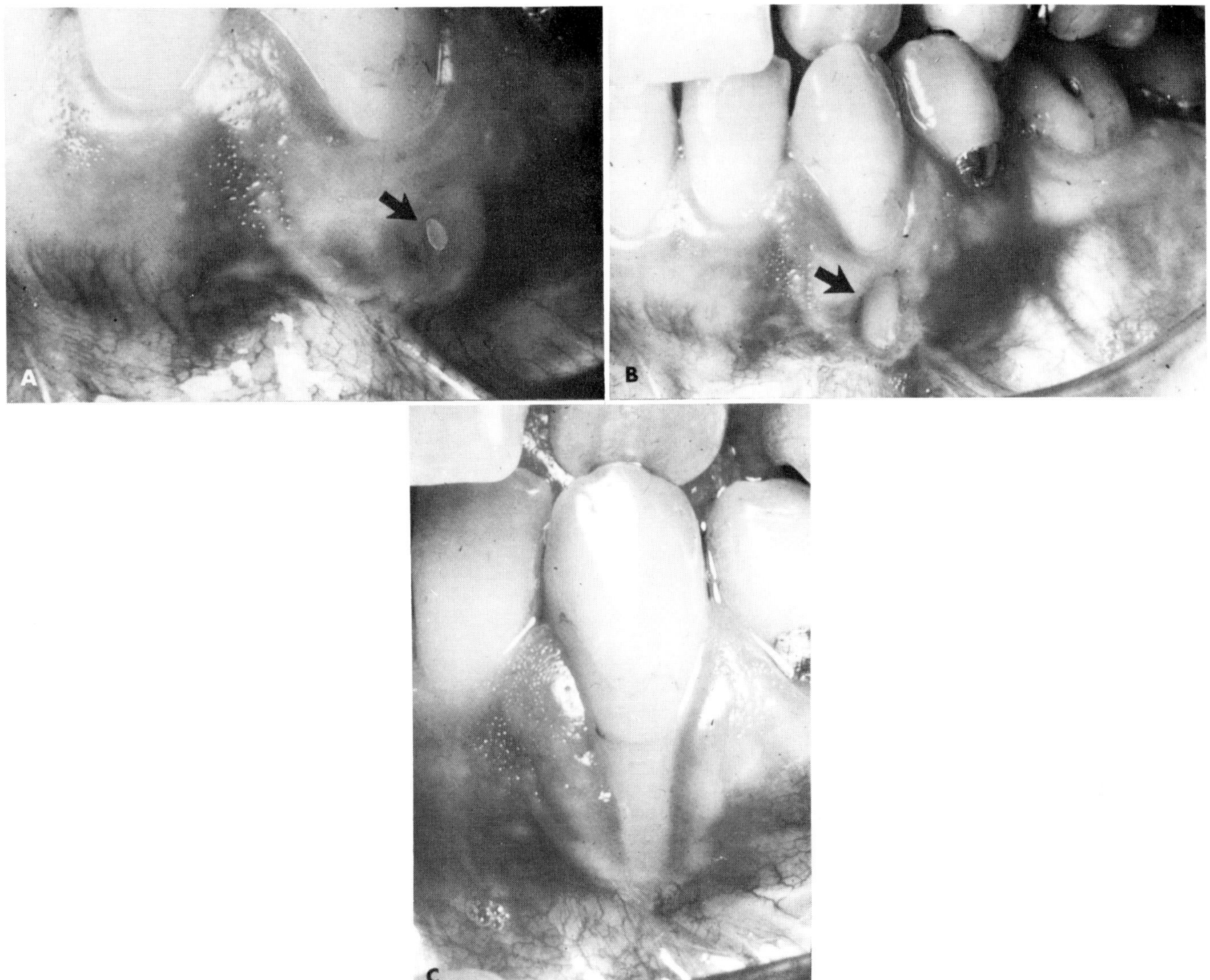

Fig. 15–21. Chronology of dehiscence developing out of root fenestration following endodontic surgery. *A,* Small fenestration *(arrow)* has developed on root of mandibular canine in line of incision of circular flap. *B,* Attempts to surgically repair minor fenestrations have failed and large fenestration has developed *(arrow).* Buccal position of root indicates it is unlikely to have labial bony housing. *C,* Following loss of isthmus of gingival tissue fenestration developed into complete dehiscence within six months. Root caries developed within one year. (Courtesy Dr. A. L. Ogilvie.)

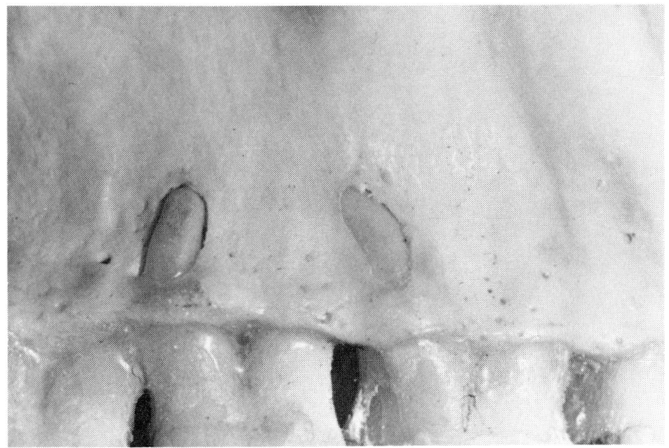

Fig. 15–22. Human skull with two large bony fenestrations over distal buccal roots of maxillary molars. Horizontal incision across these root surfaces would lead to tissue dehiscence. If, following root canal therapy, tenderness persists in this region, horizontal flap may be raised and roots beveled back to within bony housing. (Courtesy Dr. Raleigh R. Cummings.)

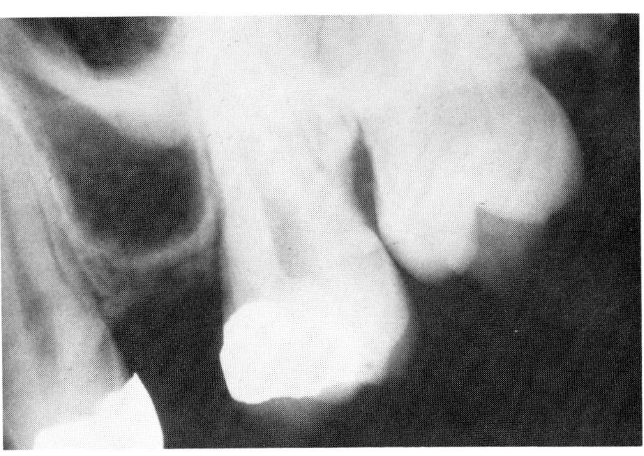

Fig. 15–24. Maxillary sinus has expanded into region of alveolar process formerly occupied by second premolar. (Courtesy Dr. Raleigh R. Cummings.)

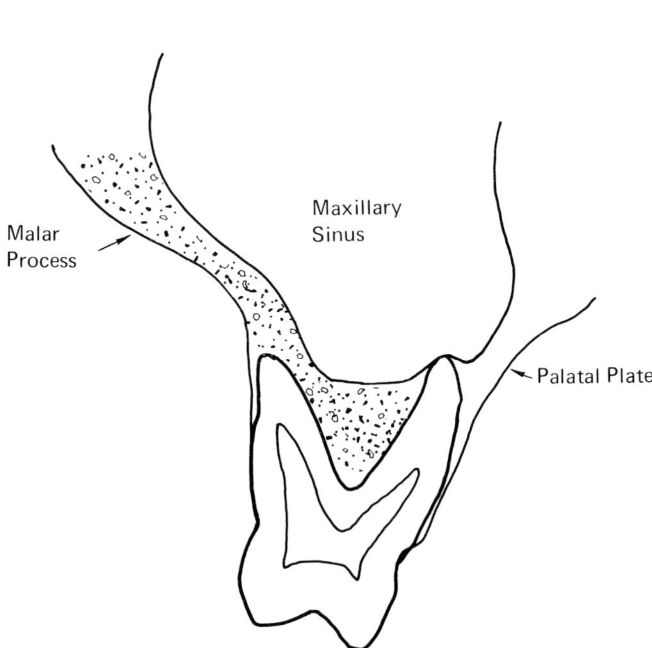

Fig. 15–23. Relation of maxillary molar to maxillary sinus. Palatal root at times will protrude into sinus. (Courtesy Dr. Raleigh R. Cummings.)

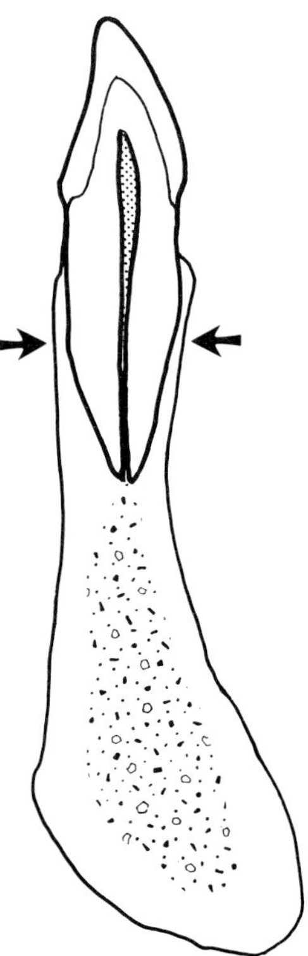

Fig. 15–25. Extremely thin labial and lingual cortical plates *(arrows)* in anterior region with no intervening spongiosa. (Courtesy Dr. Raleigh R. Cummings.)

the length of the palatal root, and its degree of divergence are the three factors determining the ease of access in palatal root surgery. A shallow vault, for example, coupled with a long palatal root with little lingual divergence can make the palatal approach most difficult.

Mandible. ***Anterior Region.*** The anterior alveolar process is quite narrow in its labiolingual dimension. The labial and lingual cortical plates are usually contiguous to the roots of the incisors and canines for their entire length with no intervening cancellous bone (Fig. 15–25). In gaining surgical access and isolating the apex, one must take care that the ***lingual*** alveolar plate is not also perforated.

Dehiscence and fenestration is another serious problem in the anterior mandible. Frequently, the incisors "show through" the alveolar plate, and horizontal or circular flaps are absolutely contraindicated. A third problem relates to the labial "bow shape" of the mandibular canine, its apex lying deeper to the lingual than the incisors. In certain cases a discouraging amount of labial cortical bone must be removed to reach the apex while at the same moment the greater curvature of the root may fenestrate through its bony housing (see Figs. 15–20 and 15–21).

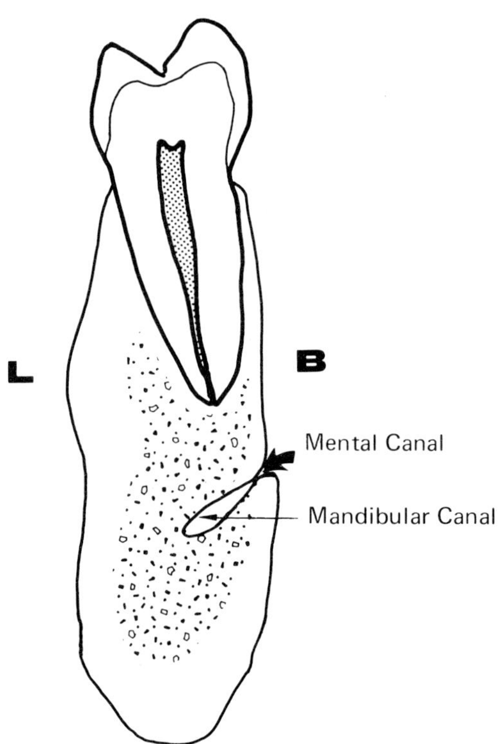

Fig. 15–26. Apex of mandibular premolar is much closer to buccal cortical plate than to lingual. (Courtesy Dr. Raleigh R. Cummings.)

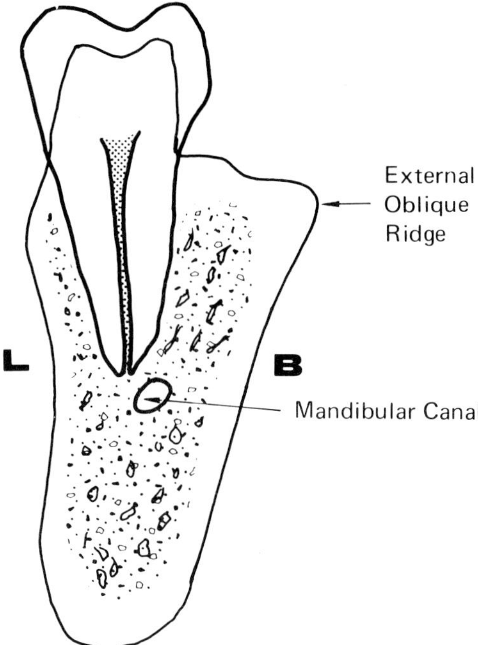

Fig. 15–27. External oblique ridge, buccal to second and third molars, provides thick bulk of buccal bone. Mandibular canal is closer to apices than in first molar-premolar region. (Courtesy Dr. Raleigh R. Cummings.)

Posterior Region. The outer and inner plates of alveolar bone thicken in the posterior portion of the arch. Premolars and first molars are generally close to the buccal alveolar plate (Fig. 15–26), whereas second and third molars are closer to the lingual plate (Fig. 15–27).

On occasion, therefore, swelling and tenderness can be detected on the lingual aspect of second and third molars developing acute apical abscesses. Considerable concern and early treatment must be given in these instances as an acute exacerbation in this area can cause infection to spread rapidly via the submaxillary fascial space below the mylohyoid muscle. There are still a few deaths each year from Ludwig's angina spread into the superior mediastinum. Infections requiring incision and drainage in this area should be managed by a skilled oral surgeon.

As for the buccal surgical approach for second and third molars, the buccal thickness of bone in this area makes for deep if not impossible apical access through both cortical and spongy bone.

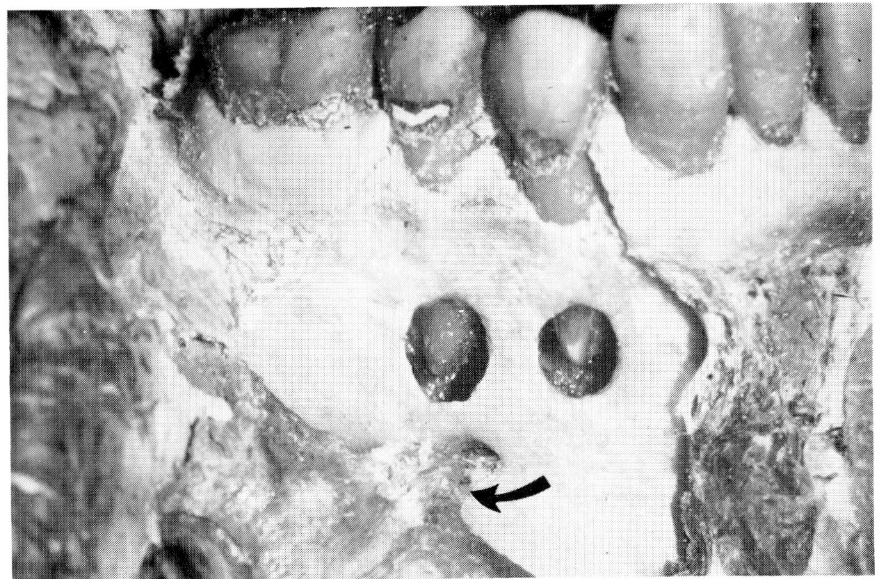

Fig. 15–28. Neurovascular bundle is seen in cadaver dissection exiting *(arrow)* from mental foramen. Notice its close relation to both premolars. (Courtesy Dr. Raleigh R. Cummings.)

The relationship of the mandibular canal, with its nerve and vessels, to the premolars and molars is dependent on the height of the mandibular body and the length of the roots. For example, a combination of a low mandibular body and relatively long roots allows for close proximity of the molars and second premolar to the mandibular canal. The first premolar will in turn be close to the mental canal. One must be cognizant of the path of the mental canal, so that a seemingly safe access through bone anterior to the mental foramen does not result in a frank exposure of the mental canal itself. The mandibular canal and mental foramen must be avoided at all costs (Fig. 15–28).[13a]

Access for mandibular endodontic surgery from the lingual aspect is extremely clumsy and unnecessary. In addition, damage to the lingual nerve or artery may occur as well as the possibility of confronting a wide mylohyoid ridge.

There are some additional anatomic considerations. ***Short root length*** precludes root resection if the crown-root ratio would become so disproportionate as to limit the useful future of the tooth. Apicocurettage is ***not*** contraindicated, however, and shortened root length could be corrected by an endodontic implant, although anatomic landmarks, such as the mandibular canal and maxillary sinus, must be considered.

Poor bony support, a result of advanced periodontal disease, may well dissuade one from endodontic surgery, although loss of alveolar support from an advanced ***periapical*** lesion is not necessarily a contraindication to endodontic surgery. If such cases are treated endodontically, full alveolar support can be expected to develop within a year or two (see Fig. 10–41). Stability of teeth with poor bony support may be materially improved by the endodontic implant. At least one-third of the bone must remain, however, before an implant is used (see pp. 664–669).

Postsurgical Sequelae

In addition to tissue dehiscence, there are other sequelae of which the student should be aware. After surgery there is always the possibility of swelling. This is not the swelling of infection, but rather that which accompanies any surgical trauma. It may be held to a minimum by gentle consideration of the tissues during treatment.

Gross swelling may also develop from a "hematoma"—hemorrhage into the tissue, usually the upper lip, from a vessel ruptured after the procedure. Although the swelling is relatively painless, the patient is unsightly for a few days (Fig. 15–29). Ecchymosis around the eye may also develop and pass through the various stages of black and blue, to purple, yellow, and green (Fig. 15–30).

Another interesting postsurgical development has been experienced by all, and reported by Everett.[14] This is a palatal osseous defect that remains forever radiolucent, although it is not considered pathologic (Fig. 15–31). Biopsies have shown the bony defect to

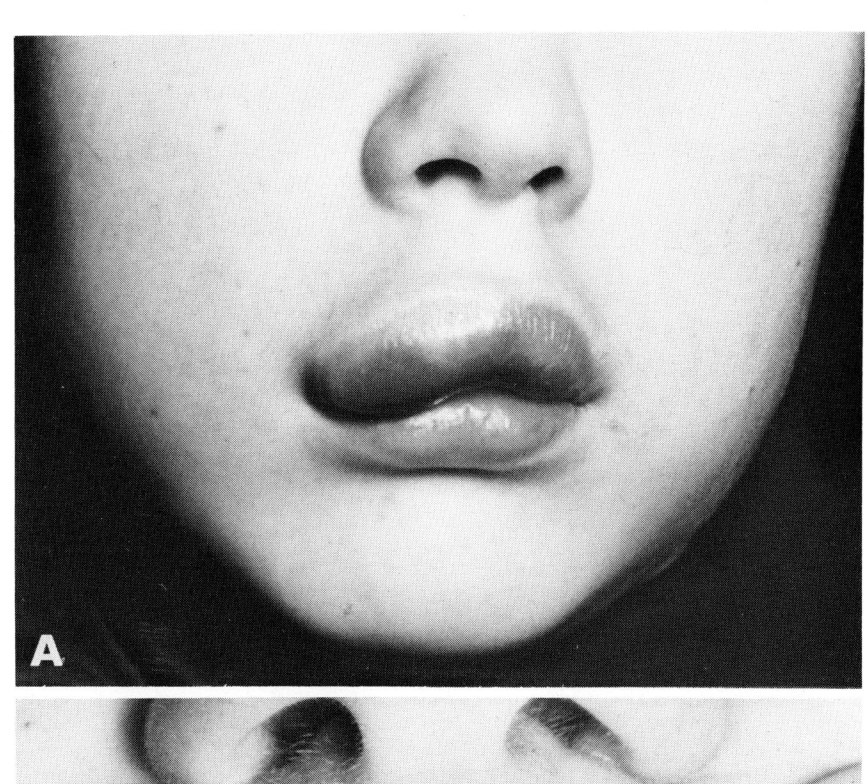

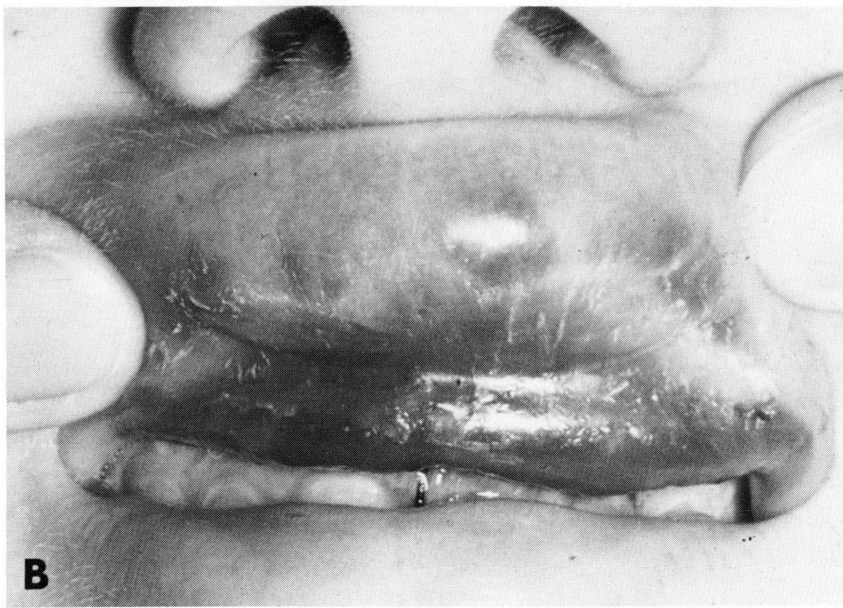

Fig. 15–29. Ecchymosis of upper lip following endodontic surgery. *A*, Although unsightly, swelling is relatively painless. *B*, Blue-black color inside lip indicates ruptured vessel rather than inflammation from infection.

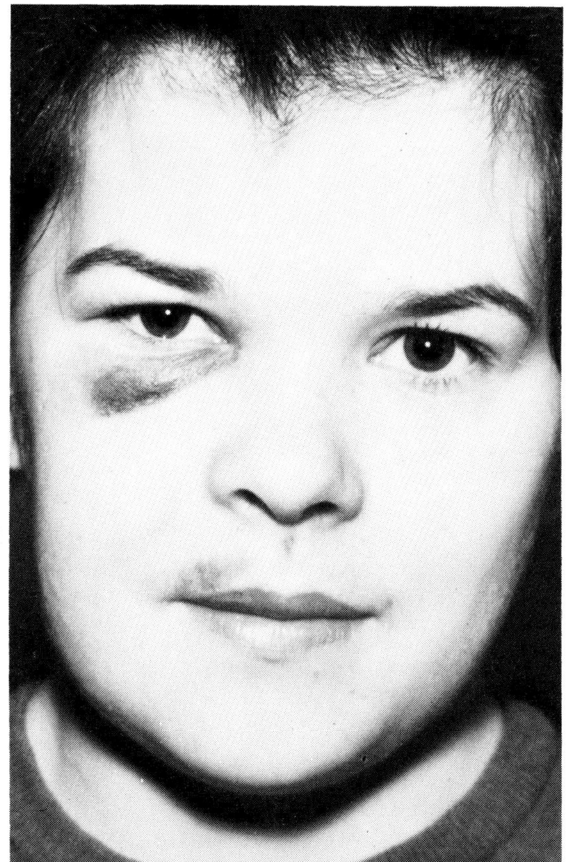

Fig. 15–30. "Black eye" ecchymosis following periapical surgery. Also note discoloration of upper lip.

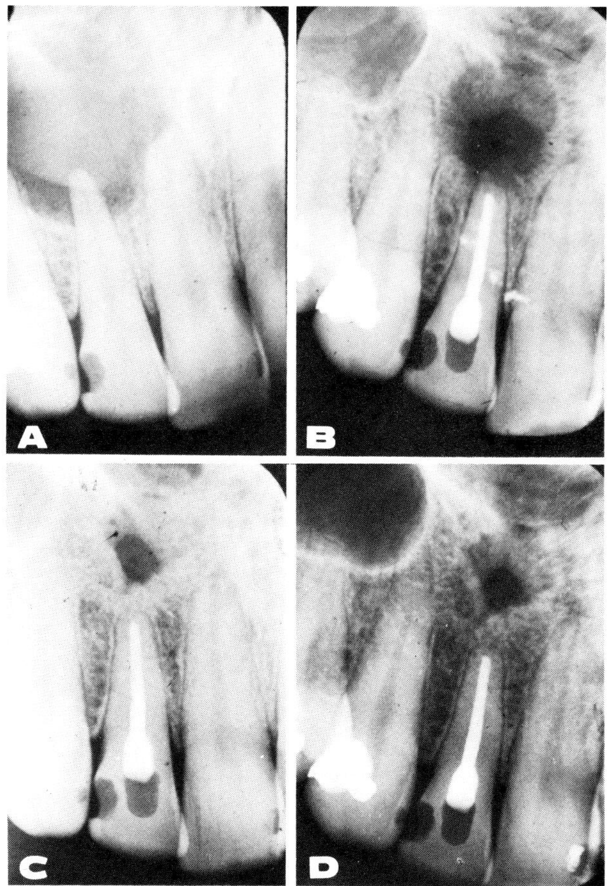

Fig. 15–31. Progressive development of periapical scar over two-year period. This permanent artifact frequently follows through-and-through osseous destruction of both labial and palatal cortical plates. Nonpathologic radiolucency is filled with fibrous connective (scar) tissue. (Courtesy Dr. Murray Krasnoff.)

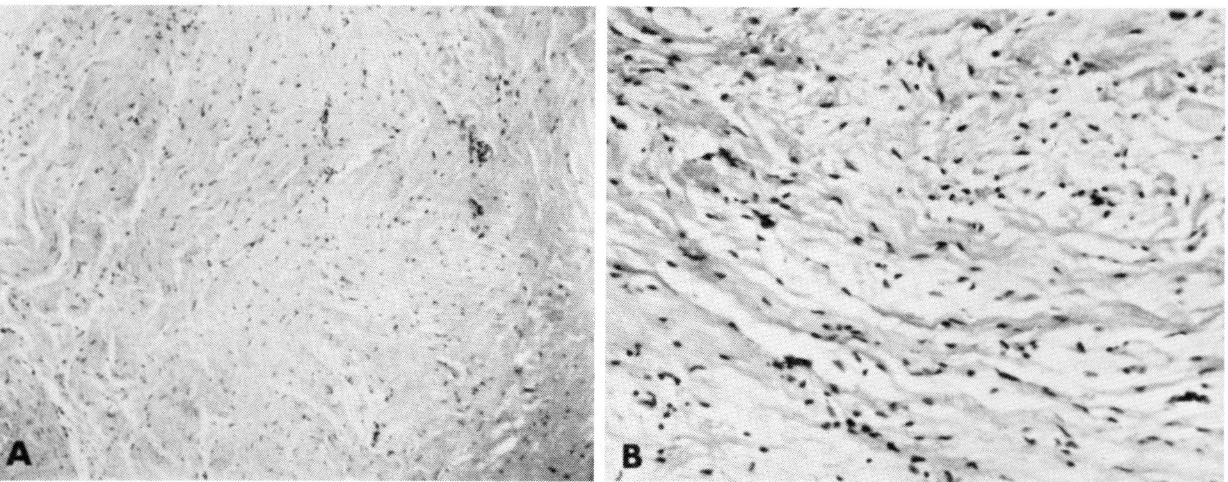

Fig. 15–32. Biopsy of periapical scar where calcification had failed to develop. *A*, Lower power of dense connective tissue fibers. No demonstrable inflammation is present. *B*, High power. Dense collagenous fibers and fibrocytes from same specimen. No inflammatory cells are present. (Courtesy Dr. S. N. Bhaskar and U.S. Army Research Institute.)

be filled with fibrous connective tissue, not inflammatory tissue (Fig. 15–32). It appears to be a region of failure of calcification in the premaxilla when the pathologic or surgical defect destroyed both ***labial*** and ***palatal*** cortical plates of bone. The reason for this incomplete osseous repair remains a mystery.

If surgical exposure reveals the absence of labial and palatal cortical bone, the patient should be made aware of the eventual consequence. He should not be frightened by the revelation, but should be instructed to report this fact to anyone considering further surgery or extraction. The final roentgenogram should always be retained by the dentist for future comparison.

METHODS OF ENDODONTIC SURGERY

Endodontic surgery may be defined as any surgery relating to problems of the pulpless tooth or periodontally involved tooth requiring root amputation and endodontic therapy. The various methods of endodontic surgery may be classified as follows:

- I. Surgical fistulation
  - A. Incision
  - B. Trephination
- II. Periradicular surgery
  - A. Periapical surgery
    - 1. Apicocurettage
    - 2. Apicoectomy
    - 3. Retrofilling
  - B. Corrective surgery
    - 1. Periodontal defect
      - a. Curettage
      - b. Total root amputation
        - i. Single or multiple root
        - ii. Hemisection of tooth
    - 2. Root resorptive defect
- III. Intentional replantation

SURGICAL FISTULATION

Incision

Incision and drainage is the standard method used to drain the acute apical abscess. Although the technique is relatively easy, two problems always accompany an "I & D." First is the problem of timing, the optimal time at which to intervene. Second is the problem of obtaining adequate local analgesia.

Learning the correct moment for surgical intervention is gained by experience, often at the patient's expense. ***Ideally,*** the immediate area to be incised, the "pointed" area, should feel ***soft*** and ***fluctuant*** under the examiner's fingertips. That is, the tissue should feel watery under gentle palpation, and if pressure is exerted on one side of the swelling, the feeling of pressure is transmitted through the fluid and is felt as a "wave" on the opposite side of the swelling. The apex of the swelling may appear whitish or yellowish. This is the ideal time at which to anesthetize, incise, and drain.

Rarely is a lesion first seen in the fluctuant stage, but rather as an ***indurated,*** or very hard, swelling. This is the time when the pain is most severe and the cellulitis at its peak. The condition may have developed overnight.

It is during this indurated stage that decisions are made and, along with decisions, the greatest number of errors. Should the patient be given systemic antibiotics and sent home with instructions to use hot intraoral rinses (hot-holds) every half hour until the abscess points? Or should the lesion be incised at that moment? There is no rule of thumb in this matter, and occasionally it is wiser not to wait for the lesion to become fluctuant, but to incise and drain while it is still indurated. If the timing is right, a great flow of pus and broken-down blood can be evacuated, much to the relief of both patient and dentist (see Fig. 15–1). If the timing is wrong, only hemorrhage results and the cellulitis persists.

Whether to incise when the lesion is ***indurated*** depends somewhat on intuition backed by experience. It may be said, however, that the signs and symptoms that call for an "I & D" ***at that moment*** are rather vague—not at all well defined. Possibly it is the slight difference in color that prompts the decision. The area may be purplish rather than bright red, and blood that is evacuated from such a lesion looks like "grapejuice."

In some cases the lesion may come to a rather sharp "point," not necessarily rounded out and hard, but actually to a "peak." Right at the apex, this "peak" is exquisitely painful to palpation.

These slight differences in color and form are indications for incision in spite of induration. If the aforementioned signs are absent, the intraoral application of heat should be prescribed to speed up the "gathering" of the necrosis. In any case, ***antibiotic therapy should begin at once*** to reduce the bacteremia that accompanies the acute apical abscess.

The second problem, that of obtaining local analgesia, exists because (1) it is almost impossible to

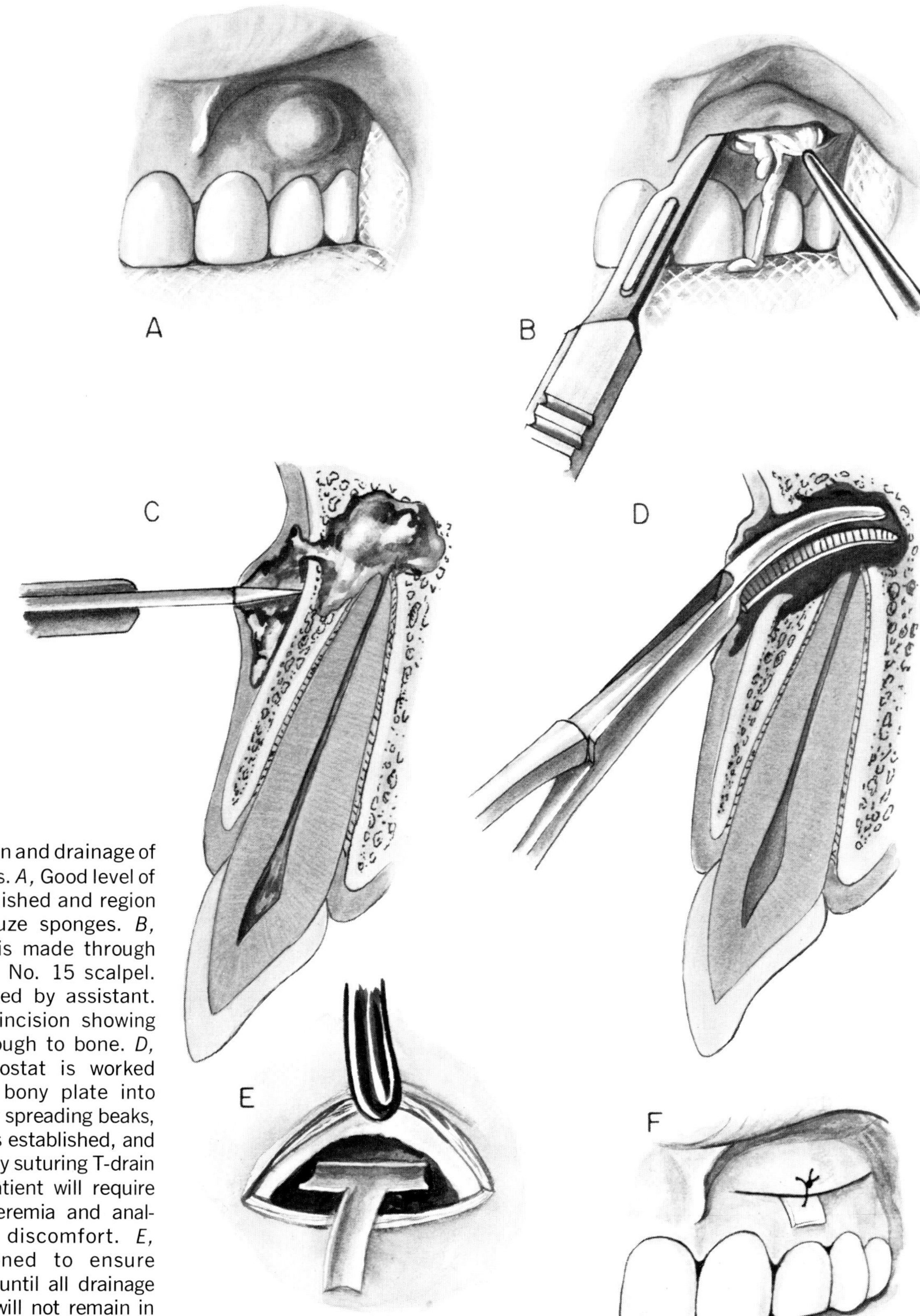

Fig. 15–33. Incision and drainage of acute apical abscess. *A,* Good level of anesthesia is established and region is packed with gauze sponges. *B,* Sweeping incision is made through core of lesion with No. 15 scalpel. Drainage is aspirated by assistant. *C,* Profile view of incision showing scalpel carried through to bone. *D,* Small curved hemostat is worked through defect of bony plate into body of infection. By spreading beaks, adequate drainage is established, and may be maintained by suturing T-drain through incision. Patient will require antibiotics for bacteremia and analgesics to control discomfort. *E,* T-drain is positioned to ensure patency of incision until all drainage ceases. *F,* If drain will not remain in place, it may be sutured there.

establish perfect analgesia for an acutely inflamed and abscessed area, and (2) there is some reluctance to inject into the area. Not only is it initially very painful to increase the fluid pressure by injecting into the region, but it is also unwise to risk spreading the infection by the pressure of injection. One might argue this last point by stating that the patient is taking an antibiotic. This argument is not valid, for the infecting bacteria could be resistant to the initial antibiotic, or the patient may not bother to fill the prescription or take the drug.

In any case, ***conduction*** analgesia, as far from the site of infection as possible, should be given initially. Bilateral "mental" injections will anesthetize the anterior mandible. If the premaxilla is involved, an infra-orbital injection can be used, entering the fornix of the vestibule in the region of the ***maxillary second premolar*** and depositing the solution on a mid-pupillary line under the infra-orbital ridge. A nasopalatine injection should be given as well. Lidocaine 2% with epinephrine 1:50,000 is preferred. Following block analgesia, intramucosal wheal infiltration around the perimeter of the lesion should be used. All injections are made slowly with little pressure. The area should now be ready for ***surgical fistulation.***

If a rupture of the bony plate by the abscess is suspected, it is advisable to develop "through and through" drainage. This may be done through an anatomic pathway established through the pulp canal, the root apex, and the incised area. The first step is to prepare an access cavity into the pulp chamber of the involved tooth. The canal should then be irrigated with sodium hypochlorite, and if the canal is very fine, it should be enlarged and the apex perforated with the enlarging reamer. Then the surgical phase follows.

A regular incision and drainage (I & D) sterile towel kit should always be kept in readiness. The kit should contain:

10 2″ by 2″ gauze sponges
3 cotton swabs
1 pair cotton pliers
1 scalpel with #15 blade
1 small curved hemostat
1 10-cc. Luer syringe with 23 g needle
1 cup with 20-cc. sterile saline solution
1 needle forcep
1 #1, half curved needle mounted with 000 silk thread
1 suture scissors
1 aspirator tip
a selection of rubber dam "T" drains in alcohol

Order of the operation following preparation of the root canal:

1. Arrange the instruments.
2. Place the gauze sponges to catch the flow (Fig. 15–33*A*).
3. Swab the area with disinfectant.
4. Test the depth of anesthesia with the end of the swab stick.
5. Perform a sweeping horizontal incision through the pointed area down to the bone (Fig. 15–33*B* and *C*).
6. Have assistant aspirate immediately (Fig. 15–33*B*).
7. Take a culture with a sterile swab and inoculate a tube of medium.
8. Open the incised area widely by following out the tract with a hemostat. Spread the handles of the hemostat to separate the beaks (Fig. 15–33*D*).
9. Irrigate with 10 cc. of a saline solution through the pulp-canal, recovering the irrigant with the aspirator at the incision.
10. Place a "T" drain with the bar of "T" inside the incision (Fig. 15–33*E*).
11. Suture the drain in place if necessary (Fig. 15–33*F*).
12. Medicate and seal the pulp cavity.

In spite of all preparations, this can still be a momentarily painful operation. It should be done deftly, with speed and with "tender loving care," for the patient may be near the breaking point from pain and sleepless nights. The incision may be the final insult, bringing the patient to tears. This is an excellent indication for nitrous oxide-oxygen analgesia to potentiate the injected analgesic. If the drainage is productive, every patient is greatly relieved and most grateful, either the same or the next day.

Patients treated in this rather heroic manner usually recover in a remarkably short time. Full alleviation of all symptoms can be achieved in four or five days (Fig. 15–34). Nonetheless, antibiotic therapy should be continued for four days to prevent bacteremia. The culture taken at the time of the incision should be used for an antibiotic sensitivity test. In view of the problems that might develop from bacteremia, it is best to ascertain the effectiveness of an antibiotic. If the initial choice is incorrect, a change in drug can be made when results from the test are learned in twenty-four hours (see Chapter 12, p. 574).

The patient should return each day for a checkup

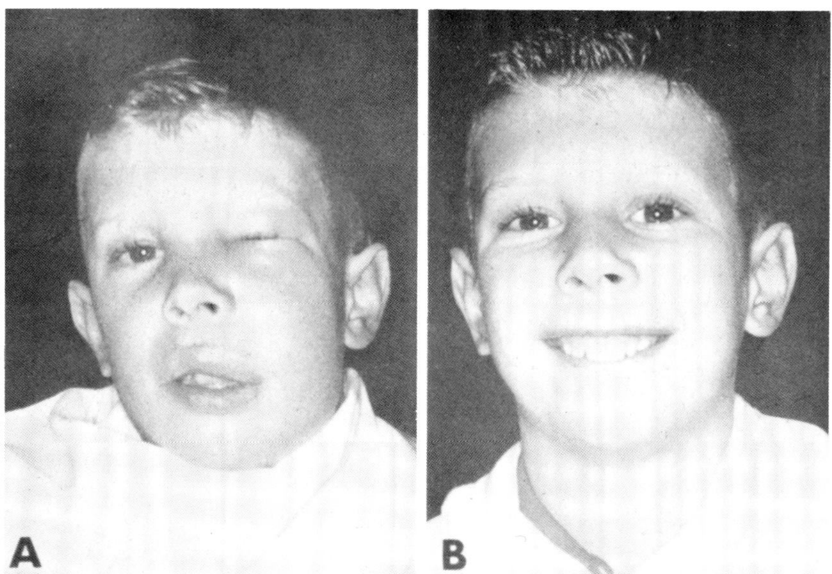

Fig. 15–34. Rapid dissolution of massive cellulitis following incision and drainage and antibiotic therapy. *A,* Unilateral facial asymmetry and eye closure indicate severity of inflammatory edema from abscess apical to maxillary lateral incisor. *B,* Five days later all signs of inflammation have vanished and patient is ready for root canal therapy. (Courtesy Dr. Bertram L. Wolfsohn.)

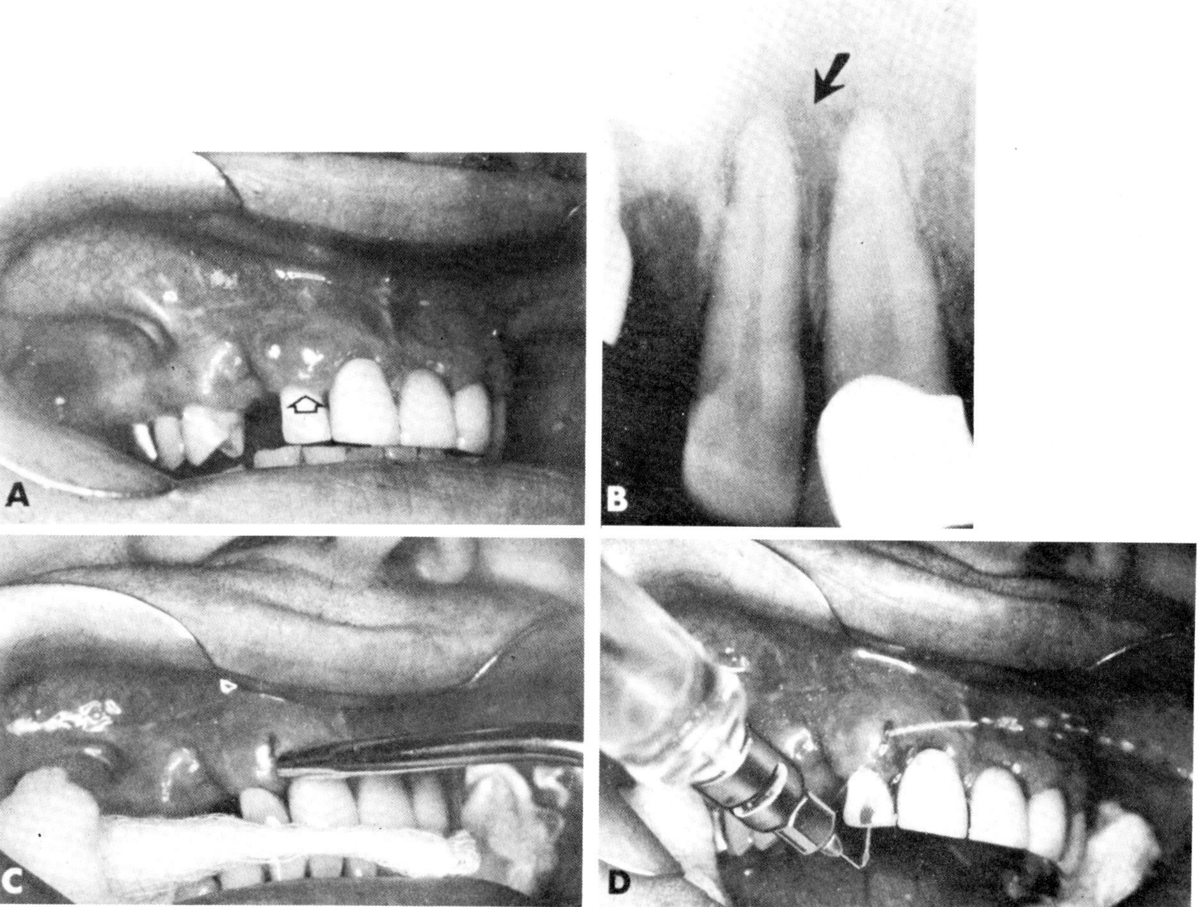

Fig. 15–35. Surgical drainage of "phoenix" abscess. *A,* Recurrent apical abscess *(arrow)* associated with pulpless tooth. *B,* Chronicity of lesion is indicated by periapical radiolucency *(arrow).* *C,* Area is anesthetized and pulp chamber opened with high-speed burs. Irrigation of canal removes pulp debris. Incision is made through abscess and contents are aspirated. *D,* Through-and-through saline irrigation of lesion greatly reduces bacteria and toxic contents. (Courtesy Dr. Bertram L. Wolfsohn.)

and reassurance. The drain can usually be removed on the second day. Root canal therapy for the involved tooth may be completed as soon as the region is comfortable. Periapical surgery is seldom indicated following an acute apical abscess.

This same approach of interceptive therapy may be used for relief during the subacute phase of an apical abscess or for the phoenix abscess. The signs and symptoms of the ***subacute abscess*** are less severe than the acute apical abscess. Cellulitis is not present although the gingival swelling has pointed. The discomfort is much less severe since the bony cortical plate has usually been perforated by the chronic process (Fig. 15–35*A* and *B*).

Again, under local anesthesia the canal is opened through an access cavity and cleansed by sodium hypochlorite irrigation. The abscess is then incised. Saline solution, injected through the canal and out the apex, is aspirated at the surgical fistula (Fig. 15–35*C* and *D*). A drain is placed, to be removed within two days. Healing is uneventful, and within three or four days, root canal therapy may be undertaken.

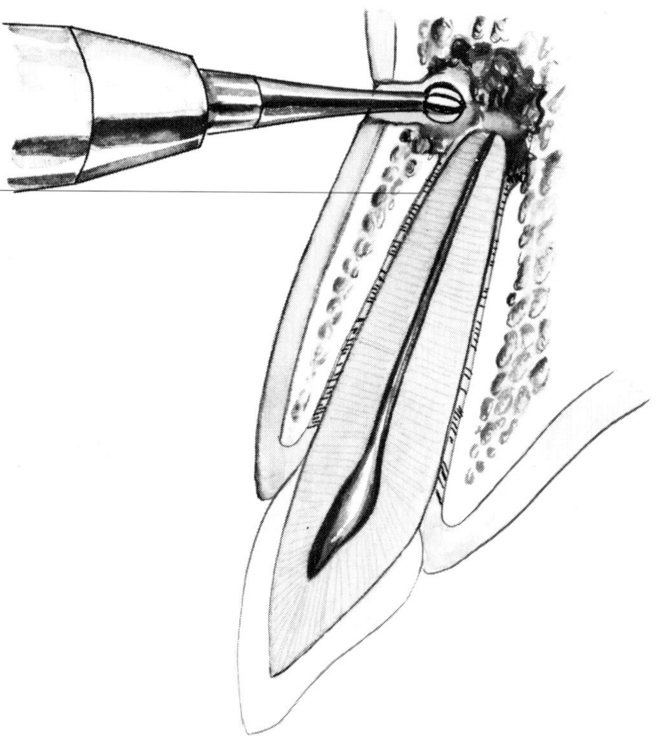

Fig. 15–36. Surgical fenestration of intact labial cortical plate to relieve liquid and gas pressure of acute apical abscess. Accuracy in pinpointing lesion is done by radiograph.

Trephination and Drainage

Trephination in the Western Hemisphere is at least as old as the Inca civilization. This surgical form is used to secure drainage and alleviate pain when exudate in the cancellous bone is dammed up behind the cortical plate (Fig. 15–36). The tremendous pressure leads to the excruciating pain of acute apical periodontitis or acute apical abscess. Again, under anesthesia, the root canal is opened through an access cavity, and if necessary, the canal is enlarged.

The focal area of the lesion is then pinpointed by examination. Working through an incision of the soft tissue, the overlying cortical plate of bone is penetrated at the region of the involved root apex. The bone is scored with a heavy punch (Fig. 15–37), which in itself may penetrate through to the cancellous bone of the involved area. If penetration of the cortical plate is not possible, the scored area is enlarged with a small round bur used under a copious flow of water (Fig. 15–37). "Through and through" irrigation, via the anatomic pathway of the pulp canal and trephined fistula, speeds relief and healing. Oftentimes the dentist is disappointed because no great flow of exudate or pus appears. When the anesthesia wears off, however, the patient will report relief, for a "safety valve" has been developed through the surgical fistula.

Trephination is not always as easy as this discussion might indicate. Locating the exact point to enter the bone is the first problem. One must also be careful to avoid structures such as the inferior alveolar nerve, the mental foramen, or the roots of vital teeth in the area. Knowing when the buccal plate has been penetrated is important to prevent drilling through both plates. The dentist must be sure of his location and action. Using a No. 7 lead shot, a broken bur head, or a pellet of gold foil in the incision is one way to pinpoint by x-ray the exact location for entrance.

Trephination, when indicated and done well, gives great relief to a suffering patient.

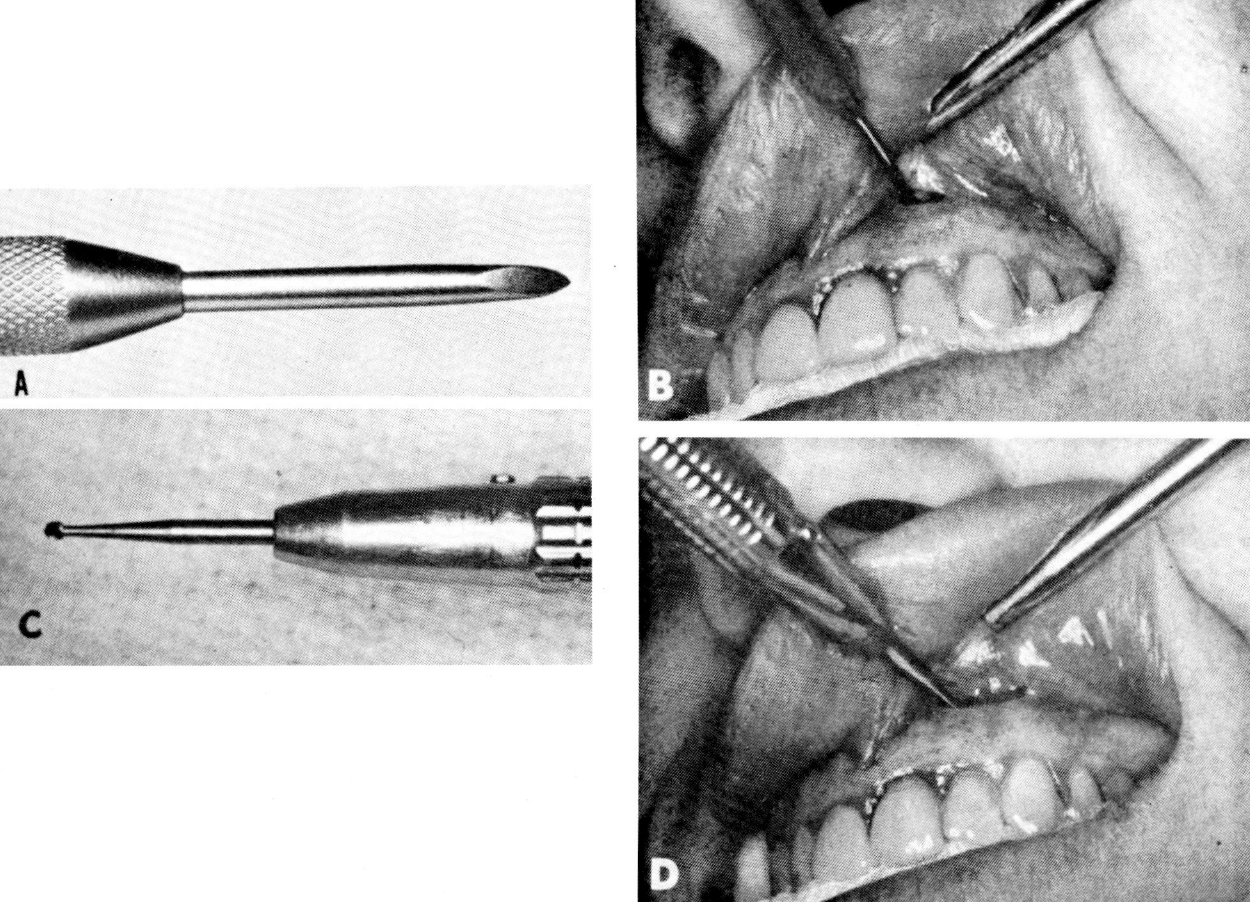

Fig. 15–37. Trephination and drainage of nonperforating apical abscess. Dramatic reduction in discomfort is achieved by relieving pressure of edema and pus. *A,* Heavy punch fashioned from shaft of broken instrument used to score and often penetrate buccal plate. *B,* View of punch being used through small apical incision. *C,* Straight handpiece mounted with a No. 4 or No. 6 round bur is used when necessary to perforate thick buccal plate. *D,* Accuracy in trephination. Bur must enter bony cavity and not gouge root end. (Courtesy Dr. Bertram L. Wolfsohn.)

PERIRADICULAR SURGERY

The technique for incision and drainage differs enough from apicocurettage, apicoectomy, and retrofilling to be discussed separately. Four basic steps are common to these remaining surgical procedures whether one stops at curettage or goes on to perform a root resection or complete the spectrum by placing a retrofilling.

Periapical Surgery

The first step is adequate flap design, second is the proper location of the apex in question, third is curettage of the chronic inflammatory tissue, and fourth, adequate suturing of the flap.

Surgical Instruments. The listed instruments, or acceptable substitutes, constitute the surgical kit. They are most conveniently wrapped in double towels, labeled, and autoclaved. A sterile technique is utilized to make the sterilized tray set up (Fig. 15–38).

Suggested Surgical Instrument Set

1 Scissors, Misdom-Frank D701
1 Hemostat, 4¾″ mosquito, Halstead 1
1 Needle holder, Misdom-Frank D600
1 Knife handle, #3 Bard-Parker
2 Knife blades, #15 " "
1 Periosteal elevator, D.E. #9H, Hu-Friedy
1 Retractor
1 Curette, periodontal, #1-2P, Eastern
1 Curette, #33L D.E., Starlite M.G.
1 Curette, #36 D. E., SSW
1 File, periodontal, #11-12P, Eastern
1 Retro amalgam carrier
1 Amalgam plugger, #2T D.E., Eastern
1 Burnisher, beavertail
1 Aspirator handle

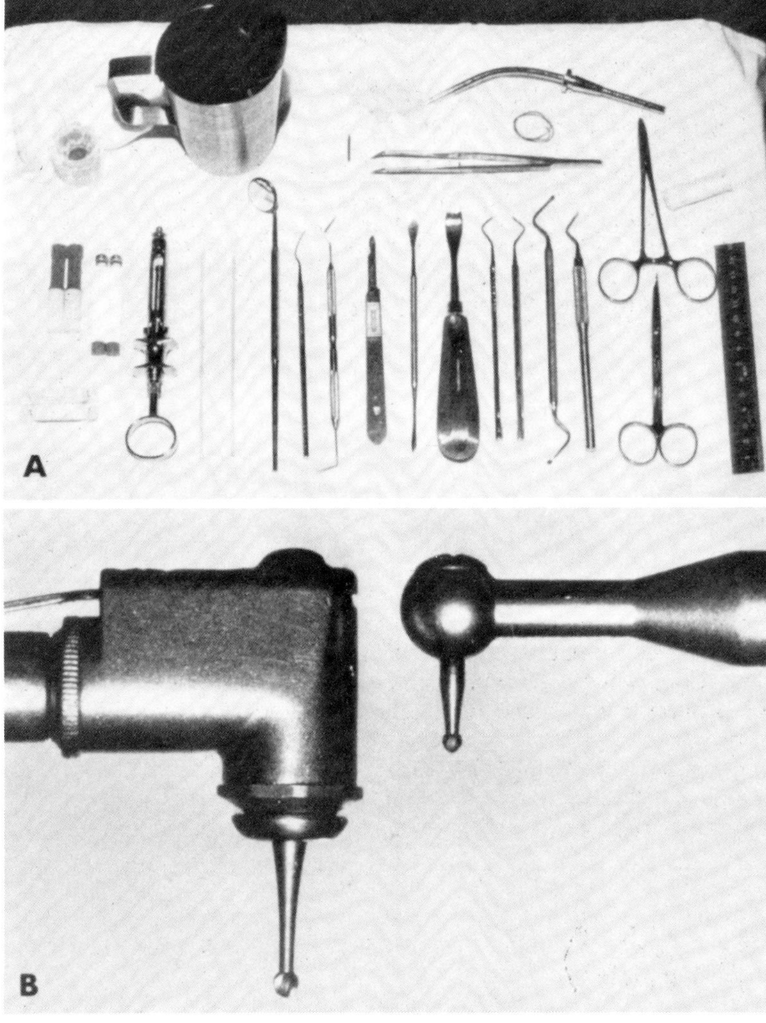

Fig. 15–38. Instruments required for endodontic surgery. *A,* Prearranged surgical tray with logical placement of instruments ranging from anesthetics on left through suturing equipment on right. Prearranged tray is kept in sterilized readiness for immediate use. *B,* Regular contra-angle handpiece with regular length bur compared with miniature handpiece used for apical preparation in retrosurgical filling technique.

2 Aspirator tips, Coupland #2 and 4
2 Burs, S.H.P., carbide; #½, 1,2,8,35,700,701
2 Burs, A.H.P., carbide; #8, 702
2 Burs, A.H.P. (long shank), carbide, #701, 702
2 Sutures, 0000 silk, with ½ round needle attached, J. & J. FS-2
12 Gauze sponges 2″ × 2″
12 Cotton pellets, #4
1 Handpiece, straight
1 Handpiece, contra-angle, Kaltenbach-Voigt

Caveats. It is assumed that in all cases the best quality of root canal filling has been completed, a postoperative radiograph taken, adequate premedication administered when indicated, and adequate regional anesthesia obtained.

Flap Design. The following are guidelines for flap design and its execution: (1) Previously mentioned anatomic considerations must be thoroughly studied. (2) Generally, the incisions of the flap should extend at least one full tooth to each side of the tooth undergoing operation. When loss of a large amount of labial cortical plate is predicted, the flap should be located to be sutured back over ***sound*** bone. The rectangular and trapezoidal flaps allow for a good vascular base to the flap, yet avoid exposed root surfaces and fenestrations of bone. (3) If the flap is raised vertically, apical extension to allow placement of the retractor on solid bone is necessary to minimize trauma and postoperative bruising. (4) Incisions must be located so that sutures are placed in durable tissue, preferably attached gingiva. (5) The periosteum must be reflected with a full-thickness flap.

Failure to consider these guidelines is the greatest cause of postoperative sequelae of swelling and ecchymosis. Working through too small a flap opening or abusing the flap with the retractor increases the traumatic after-effects. Ease and rapidity of treatment also keep swelling to a minimum.

Five different types of mucoperiosteal flap may be used: (1) curved, (2) triangular, (3) trapezoidal, (4) rectangular, and (5) scalloped.

1. The Curved Flap. The curved (semilunar) flap was at one time the most commonly used flap; the curved, horizontal incision being made completely through the gingival tissue and periosteum. The apogee of the curve should be toward the incisal; that is, down in the maxilla and up in the mandible (Figure 15–39*A*). Preferably the incision is made at a right angle to the tissue in the tough attached gingiva, which may then be approximated more easily for suturing. In length it should include at least one adjacent tooth on either side of the involved tooth or teeth, and should be curved enough so that when retracted the involved periapical area is well exposed (Fig. 15–39*A*). If it is necessary to cross the labial frenum, the curved incision should notch down around the frenal attachment (Fig. 15–39*B*). When repositioning this flap, the "tit" of the frenum is first sutured to place. This positions the entire flap (Fig. 15–39*B*).

The curved flap may be retracted, periosteum and all, with a sharp periosteotome or a No. 7 wax spatula used for this purpose. During surgery it is held retracted with a flat or claw retractor held firmly in the left hand (Fig. 15–39).

In making these incisions, one must be careful to avoid the free gingiva at the height of the marginal gingiva. If the incision is made too closely to the free

---

Fig. 15–39. Surgical flap design and geometric nomenclature for flaps. *A, (Above)* ***Circular*** flap frequently used for periapical surgery. Involved tooth *(arrow)* is lateral incisor. *(Below)* Full curve to flap allows broad tissue retraction and easy access to periapical area. *B, (Above)* ***Circular*** flap modification avoids labial frenum. Central incisor *(arrow)* is involved tooth. *(Below)* Adequate retraction is gained in area of midline. *C, (Above)* ***Triangular*** flap relaxing incision is vertical or oblique. Base incision may cut across or include all of central papilla. Flap is folded back on diagonal "hinge." *(Below)* Adequate access reaches periapical region of central incisor *(arrow)*. More retraction is gained by elongating vertical incision. *D, (Above)* ***Trapezoidal*** flap oblique-relaxing incisions broaden base and provide greater blood supply. Central incisor *(arrow)* is involved tooth. *(Below)* ***Trapezoidal*** flap fully retracted provides excellent access. *E, (Above)* ***Rectangular*** flap is recommended if bony fenestration is expected. Vertical relaxing incisions are placed on interproximal bone and not across fenestrated root surfaces. *(Below)* Vertical retraction of ***rectangular*** flap reveals fenestration of roots of central incisors. Lateral incisors could also be fenestrated. Circular or trapezoidal incision across these surfaces could lead to future dehiscence. *F, (Above)* ***Scalloped*** flap avoids interference with architecture of free gingiva and interdental papillae. Scalloped incision in attached gingiva parallels free gingiva groove. *(Below)* Flap is easily repositioned for accurate suturing. (Luebke, R. G., and Ingle, J. I.: J. Amer. Soc. Periodon., *2*:301, Jan.-Feb., 1964, and Luebke, R. G.: W. B. Saunders Co. Dent. Clin. N. Amer., *18*:379, April, 1974.)

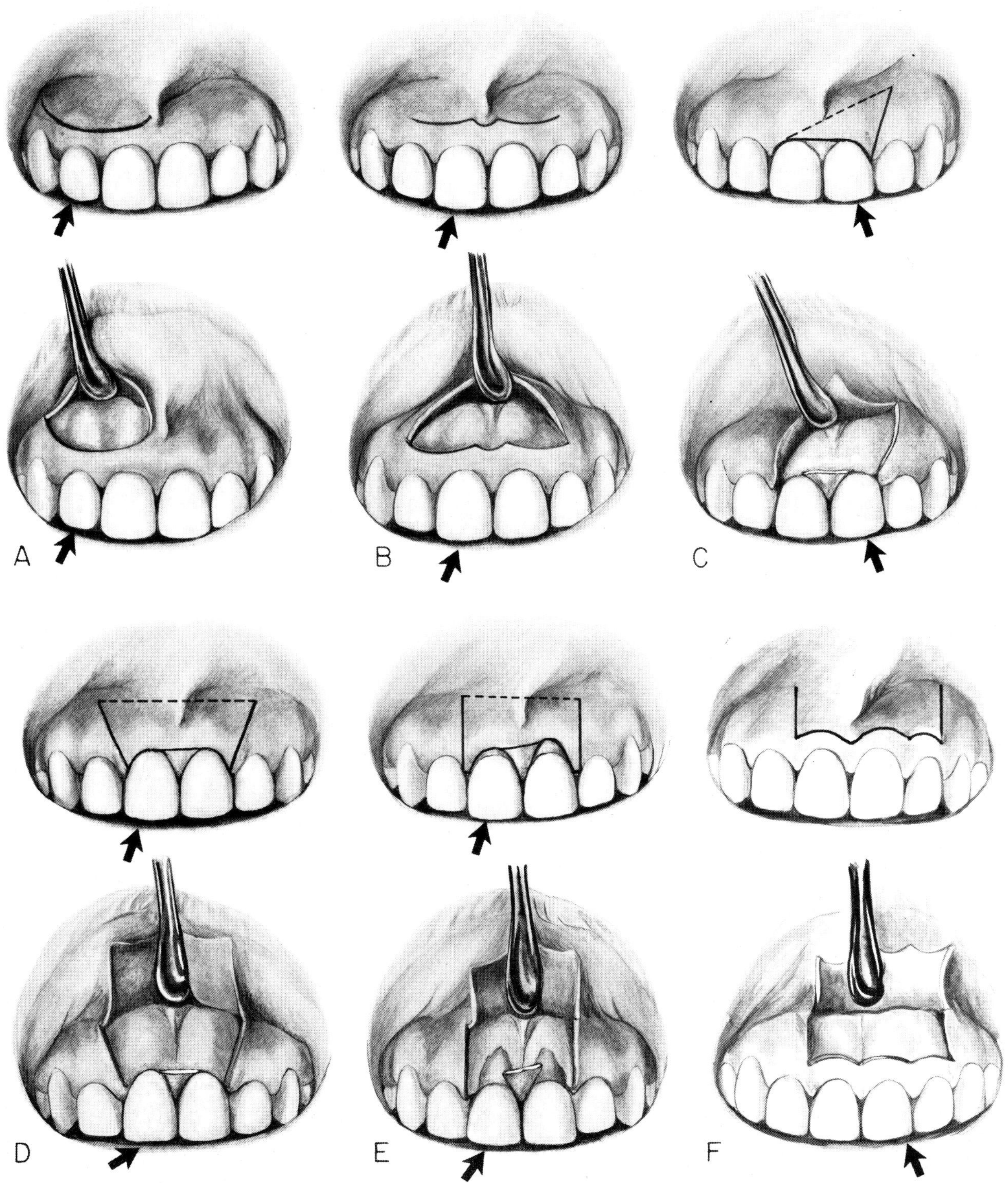

Fig. 15–39. *(Legend on opposite page)*

marginal gingiva, it is possible that the thin isthmus may degenerate and a dehiscence begin at the neck of the tooth (see Fig. 15–21*B*). The same might happen if a ***suture*** is placed in the ***marginal gingiva*** rather ***than into the interproximal papillae where it should be placed.***

The curved incision is not recommended if one suspects that buccal cortical bone is missing and a dehiscence might develop (see Fig. 15–21). This judgment can usually be made by determining the prominence of the roots and their relative position to the buccal plate of bone. Permanent irreparable scars may develop from faulty preoperative evaluation of these cases (see Fig. 15–20). A rectangular flap should be used if the possibility of a dehiscence is present.

2. The Triangular Flap. This flap is well recommended for surgery involving short-rooted teeth. Incision along the gingival border forms the base of a triangle whose altitude is the relaxing vertical or oblique incision and whose hypotenuse is the "hinge" (Fig. 15–39*C*). The vertical incision ends at the labioproximal line angle of the tooth, leaving the tip of the papilla intact (Fig. 15–39*C*). The horizontal incision should also include one full papilla, and to facilitate final suturing, the tip of this papilla should be left intact by incising across from the ***labiocervical*** of one tooth to ***this*** same point on the approximating tooth. The flap may then be released with a sharp periosteotome and held back with a retractor (Fig. 15–39*C*).

This type of incision is not recommended if a long-rooted tooth is involved. In this case, the single vertical incision of the triangular flap would have to be carried far into the alveolar mucosa, and the tugging at the flap, in order to reach the apex, would increase tissue trauma.

3. The Trapezoidal Flap. The full trapezoidal flap is actually a double triangular flap, in that two oblique incisions are made rather than one, and the entire flap is retracted toward the vestibule. The incisions are designed to leave the flap wider at its base than at the gingival margin thus improving the blood supply to the flap.

Th oblique incisions are made to include at least one full tooth and papilla to one side of the involved tooth. Then the papilla between the two teeth is separated with a horizontal incision through the labial (Fig. 15–39*D*). The entire labial flap is then retracted with a periosteotome and held in position with a retractor (Fig. 15–39*D*).

The trapezoidal flap has a decided advantage over the triangular flap if the tooth to be operated has a long root. It also has an advantage over the curved incision if a chance for dehiscence is present.

4. The Rectangular Flap. The broad classification of "vertical" includes two flaps of vertical design. Since it is possible to describe the exact shape of each with a geometric expression, the term "rectangular" is logical for this particular flap (Fig. 15–39*E*).

Usually the trapezoidal vertical flap is preferred to the rectangular flap. On the other hand, if root fenestration through the alveolar cortical bone is suspected, vertical incisions upon a base of interproximal bone should be used to preclude crossing a root surface with the incision (Fig. 15–39*E*). The oblique incision of the trapezoidal flap, if carried across a

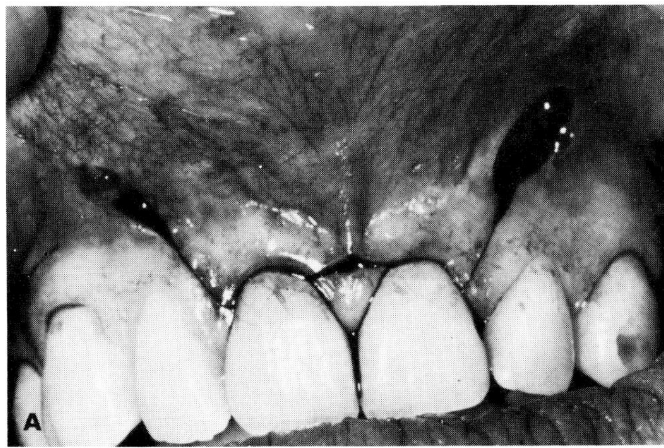

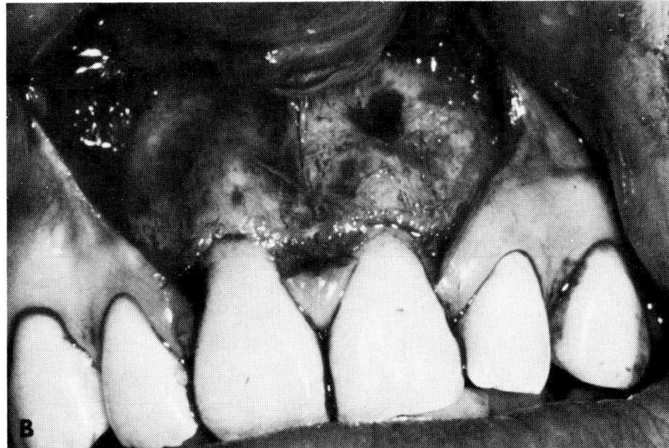

Fig. 15–40. ***Trapezoidal*** flap used at maxillary midline. *A*, Oblique relaxing incisions and horizontal base incision across central papilla are apparent. *B*, ***Trapezoidal*** flap fully retracted. Horizontal incision across central papilla allows for suturing through anesthetized labial tissue. If entire papilla is retracted, suturing must be carried through unanesthetized lingual papilla. (Courtesy Dr. Edward E. Beveridge.)

fenestrated root, may never heal, and may eventually lead to a dehiscence in the area (Fig. 15–40).

5. The Scalloped Flap. The scalloped flap has become the flap of choice in the majority of periradicular surgery cases.[15] It combines the great visual access and tissue relaxation of the trapezoidal or rectangular flaps while overcoming the undesirable reparative defects in the interdental papilla the latter two designs might create. As with the curved flap, however, areas of root fenestration are to be avoided.

The scalloped flap is produced by first making a continuous scalloped incision in the firm attached gingiva, beyond and parallel to the free gingival groove. At both ends of the curved incision vertical or oblique relaxing incisions are made (Fig. 15–39*F*).

The scalloped flap has the advantage of suturing into the dense attached gingiva. It can also be more accurately returned to its proper position by aligning the points of the flap where the vertical and horizontal incisions join. A suture may be placed in each tip of tissue in the incision.

Location of the Apex. Following reflection of the flap (Fig. 15–41*A*,*B*,*C*), the apex must be correctly located. In many instances where the cortical plate is destroyed, the underlying chronic inflammatory tissue is readily observable. In other instances, probing with a small, sharp periodontal curette allows the operator to pierce the thin, fragile, undermined cortical plate of bone (Fig. 15–41*C*). Where the bony plate is intact, it must be perforated with a fissure or round bur in a copious water coolant (Fig. 15–41*D*).

Three methods may be employed to assure proper location of the window as mechanical perforation is made through the bony plate. First, the tooth is measured in the radiograph and then a sterile rule is lined up at this length alongside the long axis of the tooth, to mark off the apex. The measurement of the last file used for canal enlargement may also be used. Another technique is to cut a small bony window and take a radiograph with a broken-off head of a sterile bur or a piece of silver point placed in the bony depression. If progress is uncertain, a third method used to avoid damaging adjacent roots is to take confirmatory radiographs, particularly if the apex is located far to the lingual. Failure to assure oneself of apical location can result in serious consequences.

Apicocurettage. Once the apex has been properly located and the window properly enlarged, curettage should be performed by means of a sharp, small, curved curette. At this time it is not uncommon to encounter painful areas within the periapical tissues in an otherwise insensitive surgical area. Pressure injection of lidocaine with 1:50,000 epinephrine directly into the painful tissue will generally control it (Fig. 15–41*E*). On rare occasions in the maxilla, proper palatal anesthesia is necessary to ensure complete comfort.

The curettage and debridement of the inflammatory tissue is accomplished with the surgical curette. First, the back side of the curette is used to loosen the fibrous capsule from the wall. Then the loosened inflammatory tissue is "scooped" out of the cavity with the curette (Fig. 15–41*F*). One often wonders how much of the chronic inflammatory lesion must be removed. To curette away every shred is difficult, time consuming, frustrating, painful, and impossible. Clinical experience has shown that it is not necessary to remove it entirely. The periphery is, after all, defensive reparative tissue. The old concept that the cementum must be curetted away is also not based on scientific fact.

When a periapical lesion is so large that it includes the apices of adjacent vital teeth, curettage around these teeth is avoided to prevent their devitalization. Once again, clinical evidence reveals this type of sacrifice unnecessary.

Where a gutta percha overfilling exists, the excess may be removed with a plastic instrument heated to instantaneously sear the gutta percha. If it is not adequately heated, it will just soften and pull the gutta percha, disrupting a good fit. When a silver point extends into the periapical space, the excess should be severed with a high-speed fissure bur with water irrigation and a light brushing motion. The use of the bur for trimming excess gutta percha is avoided as it tends to pull the gutta percha.

Following the removal of all excess filling material, the area should be thoroughly irrigated. Then the apical root structure should be carefully examined with a fine, sharp explorer to determine the adequacy of the remaining root canal filling or the presence of any unfilled accessory canals (Fig. 15–41*G*). This is also the time to determine whether any horizontal or vertical root fractures are present. If continued bleeding makes inspection impossible, surgical bone wax may be packed against the surrounding alveolar bone with a small moistened cotton pellet held in tweezers. If inspection reveals the root canal adequately filled and no accessory foramen or fractures, the bone wax is removed and a radiograph

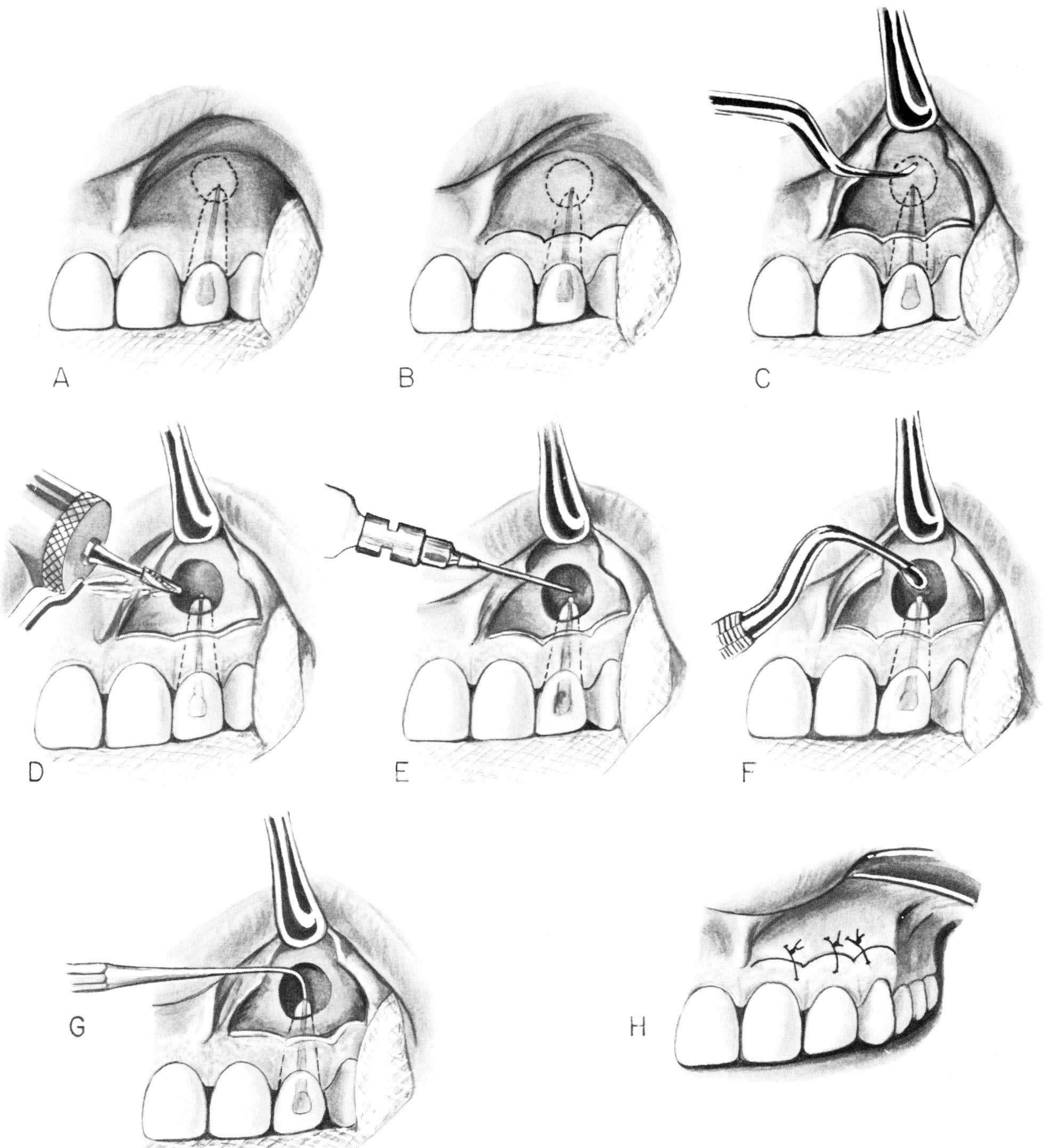

Fig. 15–41. Step-by-step procedure of periapical surgery. *A,* Immediate root canal debridement and filling are completed, area anesthetized and packed with gauze sponges. Surgical tray is arranged by assistant. *B,* Scalloped incision is made involving teeth adjacent to pulpless tooth. *C,* Flap is retracted and sharp curette used to determine density of cortical plate. If bone is perforated, it may be removed with curette. *D,* If buccal plate is solid it is removed with high-speed fissure bur with water coolant. *E,* Inflammatory tissue is probed with sharp curette and if painful it is injected with lidocaine. Needle is forced through inflammatory tissue into bone in areas of discomfort, where anesthetic is deposited under pressure. This will guarantee full anesthesia. *F,* Curettage and debridement of inflammatory tissue by surgical curette. Tissue is loosened with back of curette and then removed by curettage. Lesion is thoroughly irrigated and aspirated. *G,* Efficacy of obliteration is checked with sharp, right-angle explorer. Filling should be dense, but if found wanting retrofilling is placed. *H,* Flap is sutured to position with two or three interrupted sutures. Final roentgenogram shows no excess filling material and well-obliterated canal. Patient is instructed not to inspect area and to return in three days for suture removal. (Scalloped flap design from Luebke, R. G.: Dent. Clin. N. Amer., *18*:379, April, 1974.)

taken of the operative site. This must always be done prior to suturing the flap (Fig. 15–41*H*).

Apicoectomy. If there is indication for root resection, a No. 702 bur in a high-speed handpiece is used to bevel the root end to a level at which the fractured apex, the unfilled apex, the resorptive defect, or the perforative defect is removed, or a level of satisfactory root canal filling is exposed (Fig. 15–42). Root ends must sometimes be resected to overcome persistent periapical pain (Fig. 15–43). Before suturing, a final radiograph is taken (Fig. 15–44).

Marsupialization. Freedland,[16] among others,[17,18] has suggested a conservative method to stimulate healing of massive periapical areas, particularly when a cyst is involved. After root canal therapy is complete, an incision is made directly into the lesion, which is then aspirated and irrigated. A short section of plastic tubing is then inserted into the incision to act as a continuous drain (Fig. 15–45). This tubing,

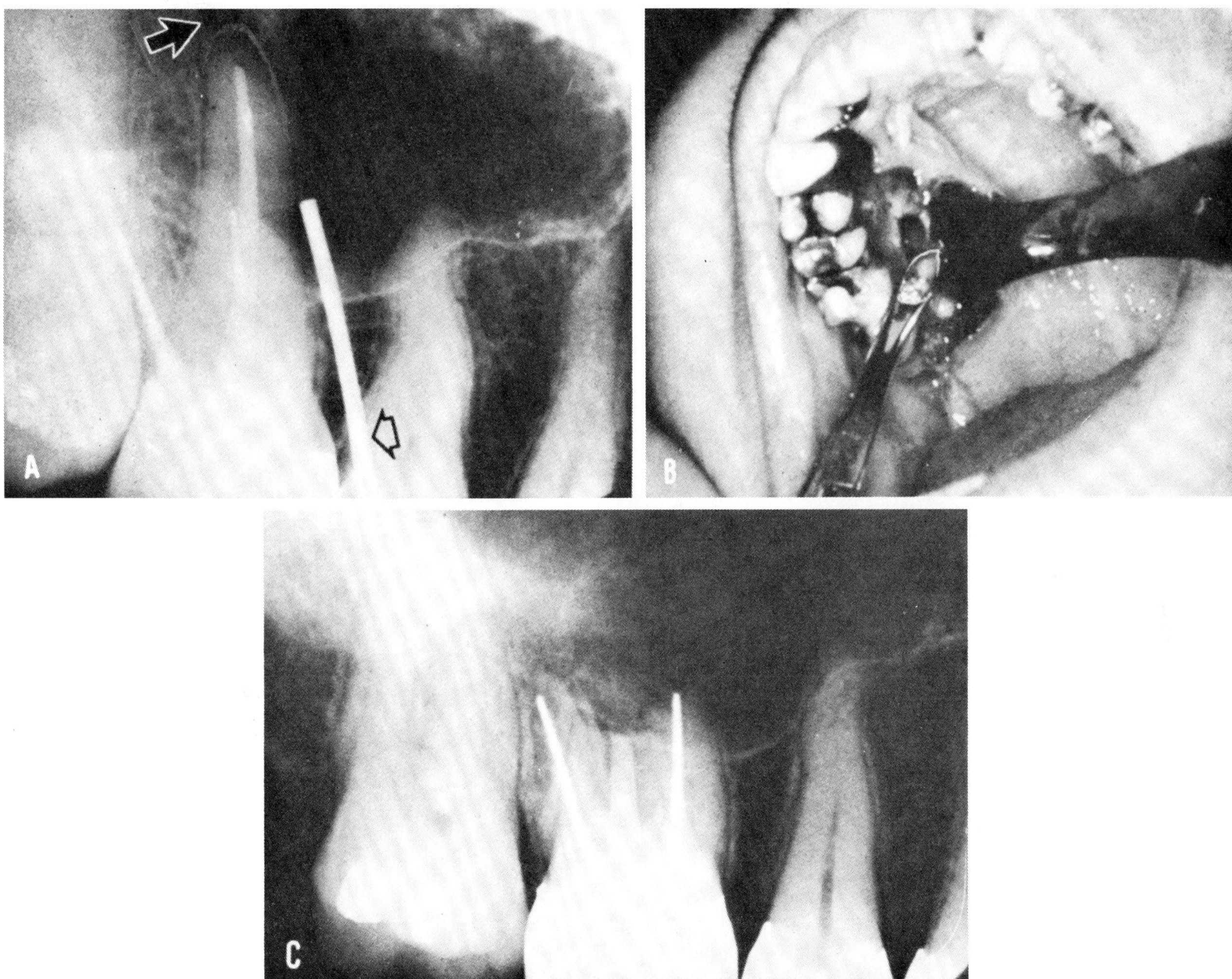

Fig. 15–42. Apicoectomy is necessary to correct persistent postoperative discomfort, severely curved and unfilled root ends, apical external resorption, and procedural accidents. When indicated, apicoectomy may be done on any tooth regardless of location. *A,* Persistent postoperative discomfort following root canal therapy for maxillary first molar. Periapical lesion *(arrow above)* drains into the sulcus *(open arrow)*. Apicoectomy of the palatal root is indicated. *B,* Palatal triangular flap exposes bony perforation at apex of lingual root. Root end is resected and removed with hemostat. *C,* Roentgenogram six months following apicoectomy. Discomfort is alleviated and osseous repair completed. (Courtesy Dr. Dudley H. Glick.)

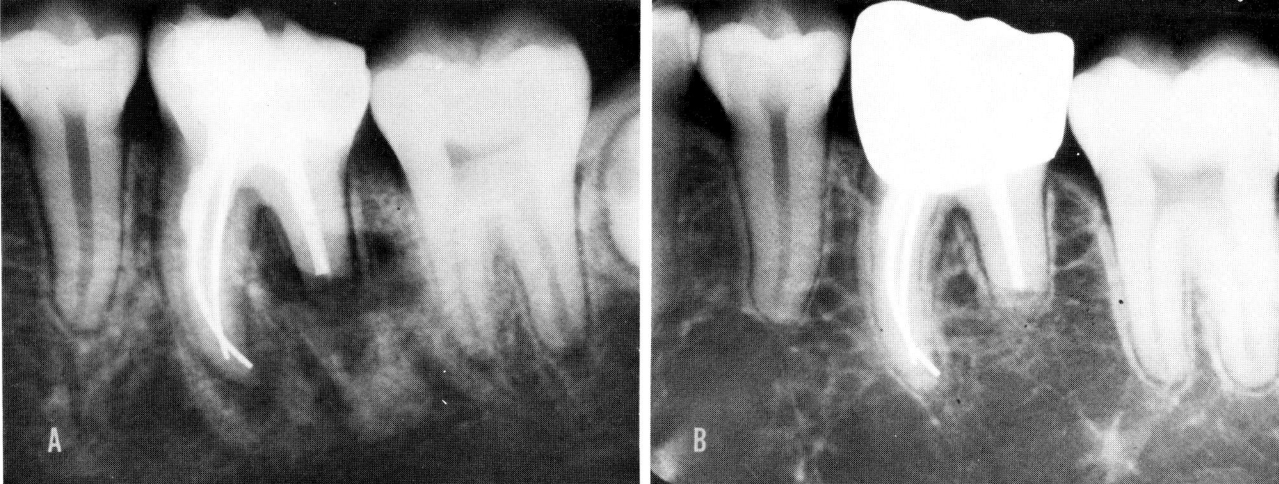

Fig. 15–43. Apicoectomy of mandibular molar to relieve persistent discomfort. *A,* Buccal flap is laid and distal root amputated through buccal plate. Notice condensing osteitis related to the pre-existing chronic pulp disease. *B,* Complete repair and osseous remolding one year following apicoectomy. Discomfort was entirely relieved by surgery. (Courtesy Dr. Alfred L. Frank.)

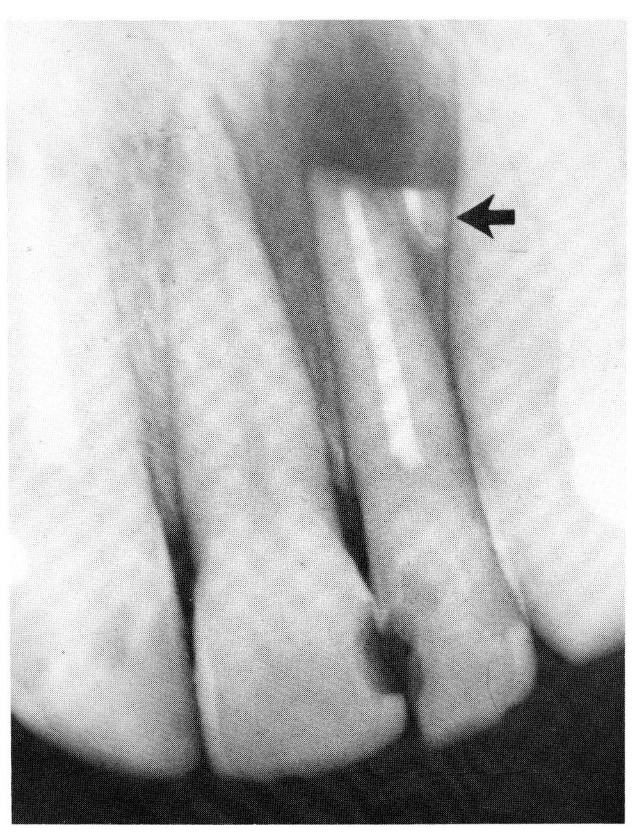

Fig. 15–44. Roentgenogram, taken ***after*** suturing, revealed amputated root tip. Roentgenogram should always be taken ***prior*** to suturing and dismissal.

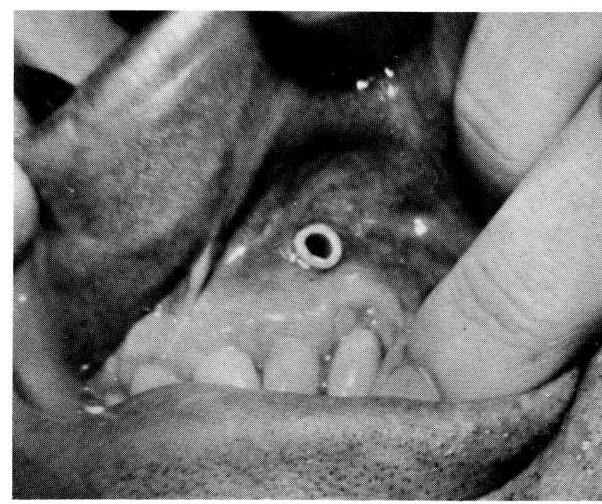

Fig. 15–45. Marsupialization of apical cyst. Surgical plastic tubing maintains opening and drainage as healing progresses behind tubing. (From Freedland, J. B.: Oral Surg., *29*:455, Mar., 1970.)

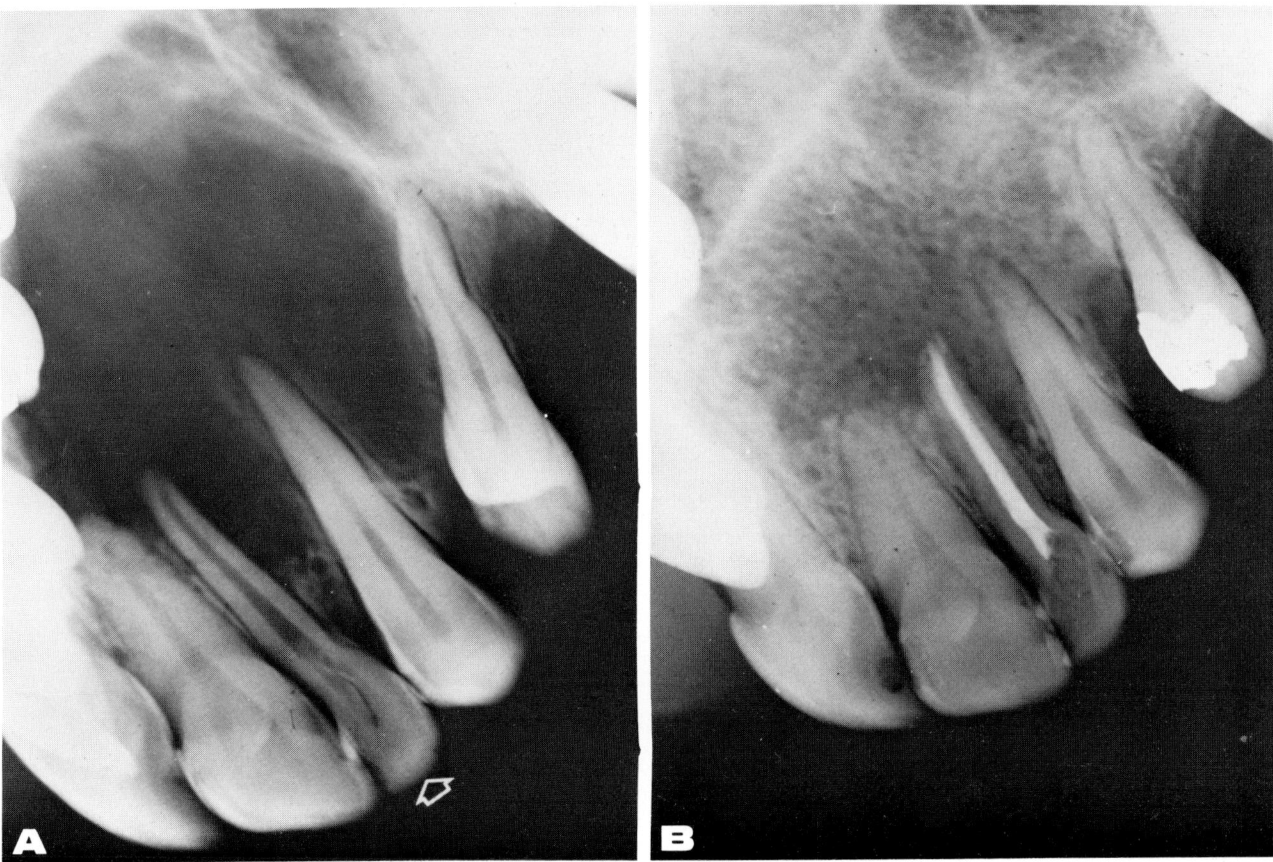

Fig. 15–46. *A,* Enormous cyst extending from pulpless lateral incisor to second premolar that has been radically moved by pressure of constantly enlarging cyst. *B,* Root canal therapy completed and marsupialization by surgical tubing was done. Four-year recall radiograph shows dramatic repair of osseous lesion. (Courtesy Dr. E. H. Ehrmann, Melbourne, Australia.)

which is used in cardiovascular procedures and is readily available from a medical supply company, is 0.184 inches in diameter. "Epithelization of the margins of the surgical window takes 5 to 7 days. The patient is instructed in the use of a hand syringe to flush the lesion with saline and in removing and replacing the tube."[16] Each month, healing is evaluated and the tube shortened as new tissue forms behind it. Ehrmann has shown the unusual repair of a huge lesion using this technique (Fig. 15–46).[19]

Retrofilling. If the apex is not adequately sealed, a retrofilling is indicated. In this case the root is resected from mesial to distal, so that the bevel faces the operator working from the labial (Fig. 15–47). Cummings has noted that resecting 2 to 3 mm. of the apex will remove all the accessory canals found there (Fig. 15–48).[19a] The bevel will result in the lingual aspect of the root being longer than the labial. This may present a bizarre radiographic appearance in which the filling appears short, but the bevel does permit greater visibility of the apical foramen.

The apical resection preparation and filling demand all the considerations of good surgical and operative dentistry (Fig. 15–49). If a lateral accessory canal is present with an associated lateral lesion, then the entire canal should be thoroughly obturated. This calls for the use of long instruments down the canal and repeated irrigation and drying before filling. Leakage through accessory canals has led to failure (see Fig. 1–55).

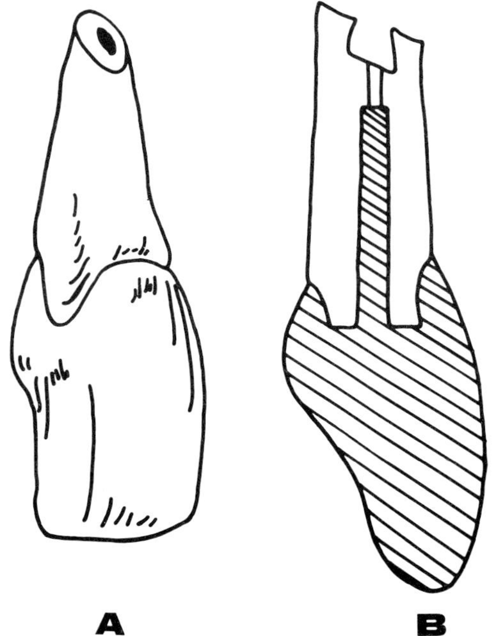

Fig. 15–47. *A*, Oblique amputation of apex facing toward labial. *B*, Undercut cavity prepared to receive retroamalgam filling. (Courtesy Dr. Alfred L. Frank.)

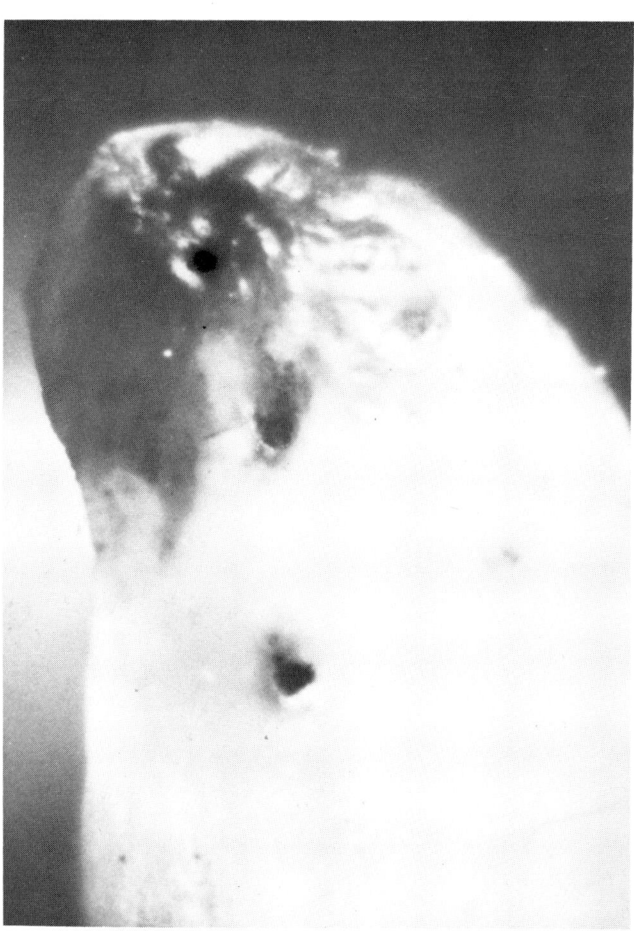

Fig. 15–48. Photomicrograph of root apex showing accessory foramens that penetrate to main canal in 12% of unresected cases. Amputating 2 to 3 mm. of apex will eliminate these communications. (Courtesy Dr. Raleigh R. Cummings.)

The first phase of retrofilling therapy deals with coronal filling (Fig. 15–50*A, B, C, D*), if the crown is not already filled with a dowel or well-condensed filling. This second phase of the retrosurgical approach has been described above—the curettage and oblique resection of the apex (Fig. 15–50*E, F*). This presents the opening to the root canal in plain view (Fig. 15–50*G*). The bony cavity is then packed for four minutes with racemic epinephrine (Orostat)* 2:100 (2%) which will arrest bleeding (Fig. 15–50*H*).

*Orostat—Belport Co., 553 Dawson Drive, Camarillo, Calif. 93010.

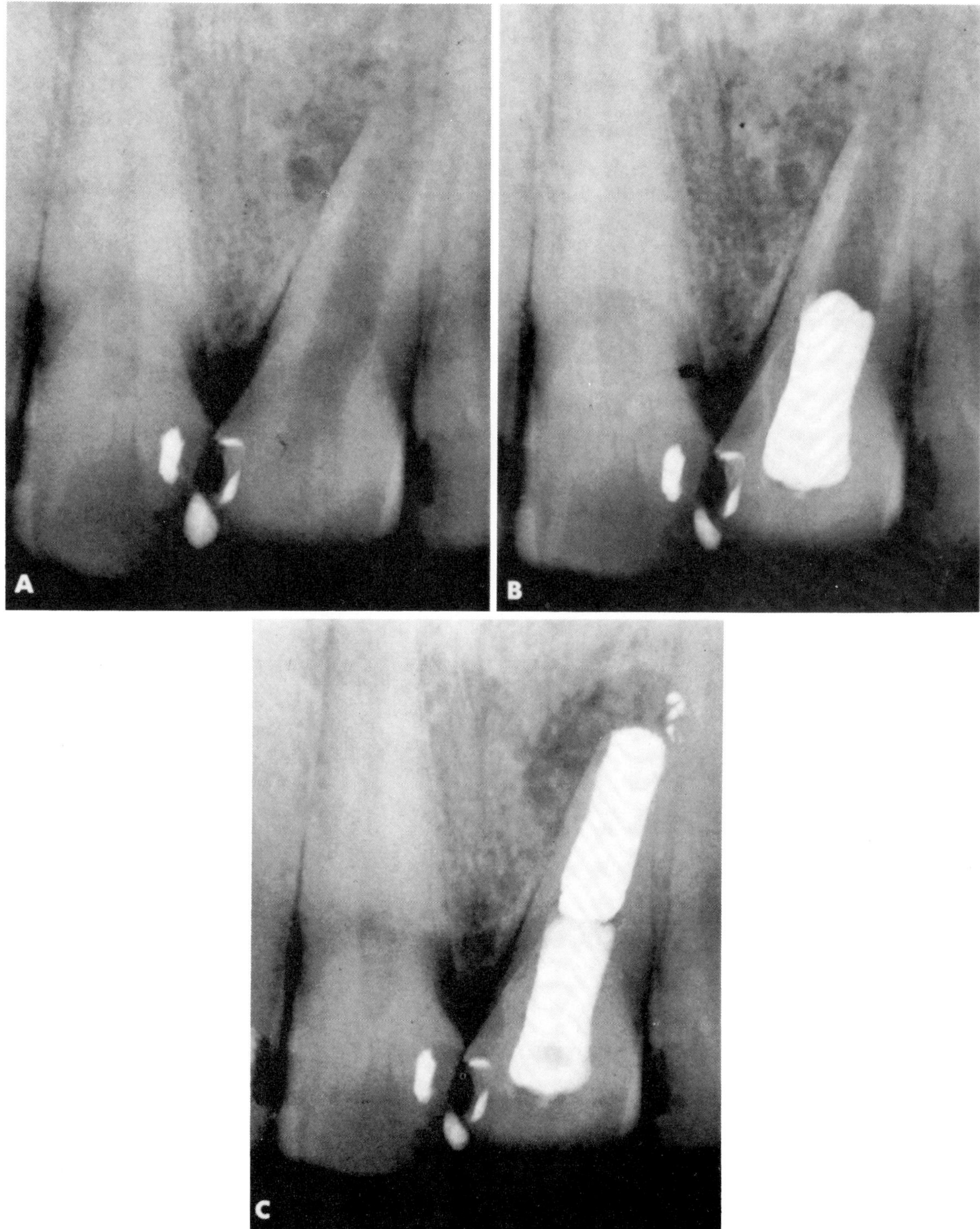

Fig. 15-49. It is important to debride and fill entire pulp canal and chamber of pulpless tooth with open flaring apex. Apexification should first have been attempted in this case using calcium hydroxide over a period of one year. *A,* Central incisor devitalized at age 9. Blunderbuss shape of canal is readily apparent. *B,* Through conventional approach coronal half of tooth is debrided and filled above gingival with nonstaining cement. This serves as matrix for retrofilling to be placed. *C,* Apical half of canal is debrided, filed, and obturated with amalgam condensed against coronal cement filling. "Question mark" of amalgam remaining at apex in no way questions successful outcome of case.

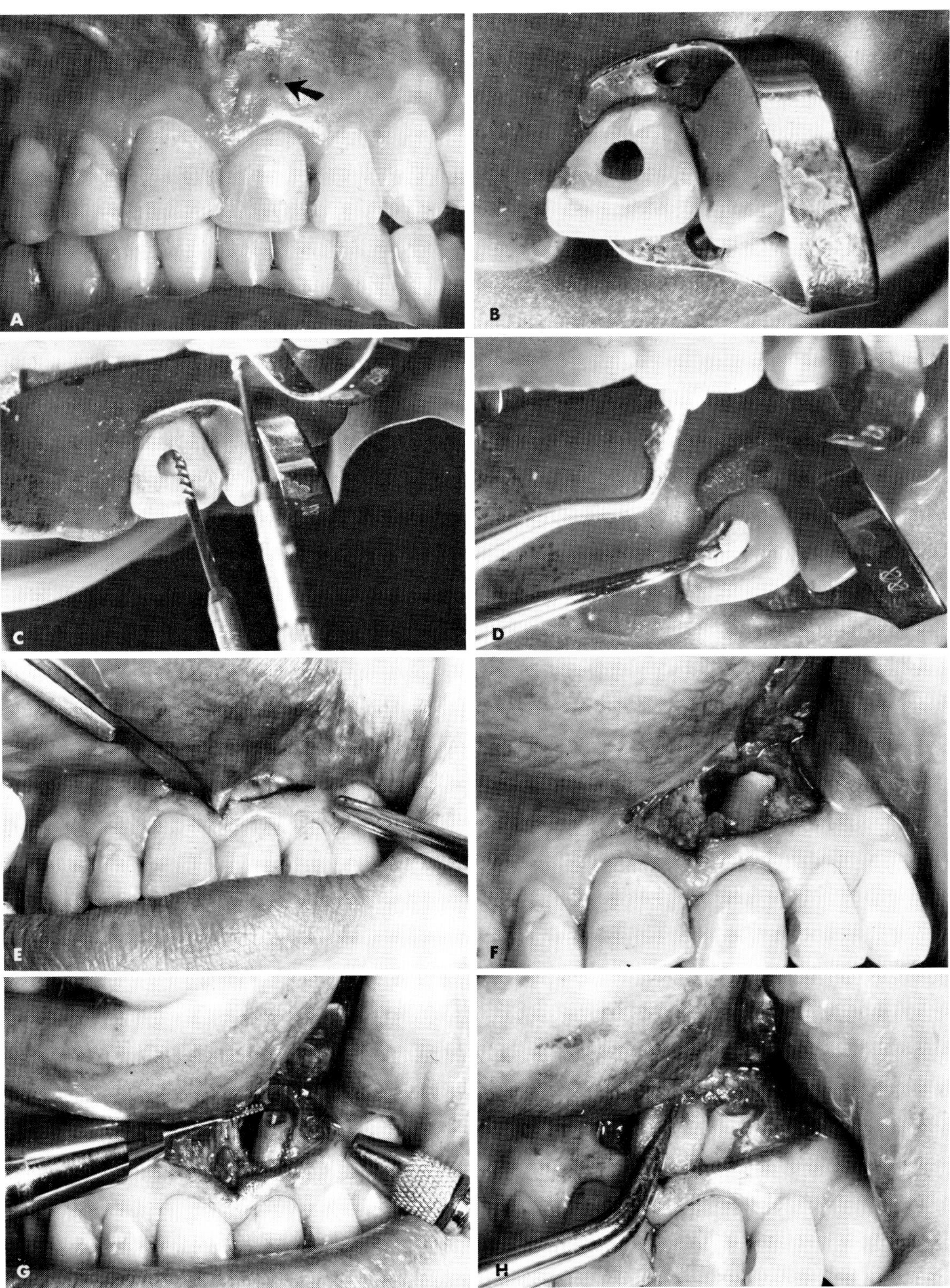

Fig. 15–50. Retrofilling through surgical approach of case shown in Figure 15–49. *A,* Constant draining fistula *(arrow)* signifies periapical lesion is present. *B,* Conventional lingual approach showing access necessary to debride and fill coronal half of tooth. *C,* Mirror view of canal debridement and enlargement. All instrumentation is done in presence of sodium hypochlorite. *D,* After irrigation and drying, coronal cement restoration, putty-like in consistency, obliterates crown. *E,* Midline modification of circular incision includes frenum "tit." Fistula is within flap. *F,* Curettage of chronic inflammatory tissue reveals stunted root curved toward labial. *G,* Amputation of apex on bevel toward labial provides ready access into canal. High-speed tapering burs and water coolant should be used for amputation. *H,* Two per cent racemic epinephrine arrests hemorrhage prior to canal debridement and filling.

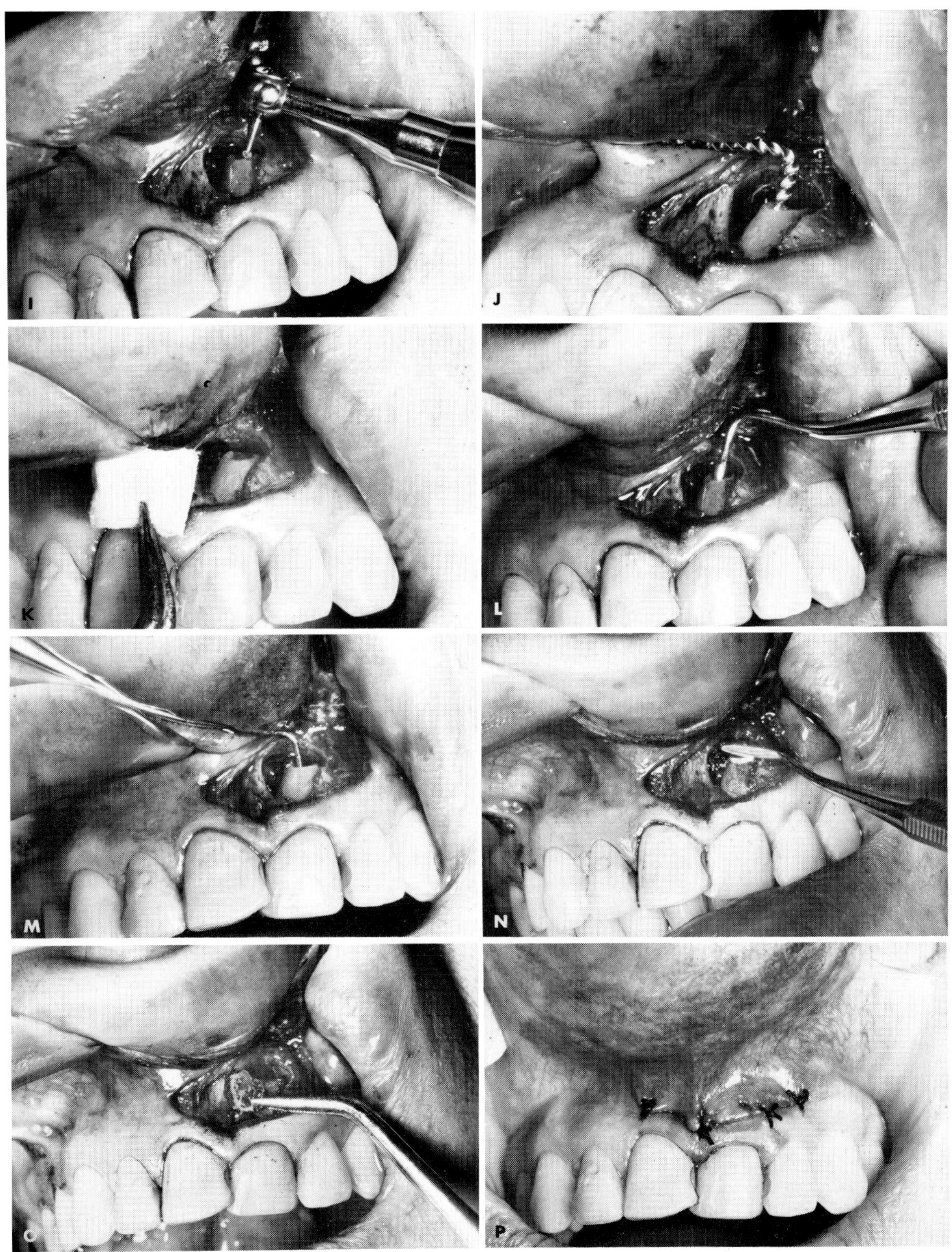

I, Canal debridement by miniature handpiece mounted with No. 2 round bur. This handpiece may also be used to prepare apical cavity in closed canal. *J,* Large file debriding apical canal. File should be bent at acute angle or locked in hemostat at acute angle and used to file apical portion of canal. *K,* Following debridement and irrigation bony cavity is packed with Gelfoam gelatin sponge or bone wax to take up amalgam particles. *L,* Zinc-free amalgam may be condensed into open apex with conventional amalgam pluggers. *M,* Fine pluggers devised from broken instruments are used for retrofilling in finer canals. *N,* Excess amalgam is carved away under water spray with fine Hollenback carver. Amalgam crumbs are aspirated from region. *O,* Final removal of gelatin sponge and epinephrine-soaked cotton pellets. Fine amalgam particles are removed with sponge. *P,* Suturing of flap. First sutures are placed through the midline frenum and followed by interrupted sutures to each side. Sutures are removed in three days and full recovery should occur within one week. Care must be exercised to remove all cotton fibers.

The third phase of the retrofilling is the preparation of the apical canal, which may be done in one of three ways. It may be enlarged directly with a No. 2 round bur (Fig. 15–50*I*) (see also Fig. 15–38*B*), or it may be enlarged with progressively increasing sizes of files, either bent at an acute angle or cut off and held in a hemostat (Fig. 15–50*J*), or an unusual "slot" preparation, which is discussed below, may be used. Preparation should extend as far down the canal as possible. Perimeter enlargement is carried well back into sound, clean dentin. No matter which method of enlargement is used, the clinician must bear in mind that the ***tooth is rarely erect,*** but rather slopes to the lingual.

During any of the three types of preparation, irrigation should be used with constant aspiration by the assistant. If bleeding has started again, it should be controlled with more racemic epinephrine (Orostat). The canal may be dried with bent paper points or a constant stream of ***very low***-pressure warm air.

The preparation is now ready for filling. If there is any bleeding, the racemic epinephrine should again be applied and the hemorrhage controlled. While the assistant is readying the filling material, the clinician is packing the cavity with gelatin sponge or bone wax to catch the excess particles of filling material and facilitate their final removal (Fig. 15–50*K*).

Zinc-free silver amalgam has become a rather universally used filling material for retrofilling. Marcotte and Dowson compared zinc-free alloy amalgam to gutta percha and found "both materials equally well tolerated" by periapical tissue in monkeys.[11] Using a dye penetration method, Barry and his associates tested a number of materials as retrofillings.[21] They found amalgam to be the most dependable, and Durelon, a polycarboxylate cement, to be the least. They also had no confidence in "heat-sealed" gutta percha as an apical obliterating agent. The best filling, according to Barry, was not a retrofilling, but gutta percha and cement placed by lateral condensation from the coronal approach. Omnell has shown ***electrolysis around regular*** zinc-containing silver alloy amalgam used as a retrofilling.[22] The electrolysis of the tissue is caused by a constant electrical flow between zinc and the other metals in the amalgam. Zinc carbonate is precipitated in the tissue and the periapical lesion is slow to heal. Cements and gutta percha have also been used, but none seems as efficient as amalgam. Persson compared amalgam to Cavit in retrofilling and, after one year, achieved "significantly better" results with amalgam.[23]

The amalgam is carried to the apical cavity with a midget amalgam carrier (Messing carrier) made for this purpose. Condensation is done with either standard amalgam pluggers, if space permits (Fig. 15–50*L*), or specially devised instruments (Fig. 15–50*M*). The successful outcome of the case will depend on the condensation of the amalgam and complete apical seal.

The excess amalgam is removed with a fine carver, the small loose pieces being removed by saline or water irrigation and aspiration (Fig. 15–50*N*). One must be careful not to press the amalgam particles into the marrow spaces of the bone.

The next step is the removal of the bone wax or gelatin sponge (Fig. 15–50*O*) and a thorough irrigation and aspiration (Fig. 15–50*P*). Before suturing, the final roentgenogram is made to locate loose amalgam particles. Remember to look under the edge of the flap if a radiopaque particle cannot be found in the periapical area. The tissue will tolerate small particles of amalgam; however, if left under a thin gingiva these particles show through, giving the appearance of a tattoo.

Apical preparation, when the foramen is quite inaccessible to bur or instrument use, may be accomplished by a slot preparation suggested by Matsura,[20] Glick, Dow, and others (Fig. 15–51). To accomplish this preparation, a fine cross-cut fissure bur in a straight handpiece is used to make a ***vertical*** cut of approximately 3 to 5 mm. in length (Fig. 15–51*B*). A dovetailed lock is then prepared with a round or inverted cone bur which is slightly larger than the previously used fissure bur. The dovetail must completely eliminate the root canal and extend the full length of the initial vertical cut (Fig. 15–51*C*). The retrofilling may then be packed from the ***labial,*** not the apex, which is a distinct advantage where access is limited.

The importance of checking the apical seal of any root canal filling, whenever the root end is surgically exposed, must again be emphasized. A sharp right-angle explorer is used to search out the apical foramens. The density of the apical filling is then carefully probed, and if found wanting, a retrofilling should be done right at that time.

The patient should be shown the final roentgenogram if the filling appears to be considerably short of the apex (Fig. 15–52). This appearance is related to

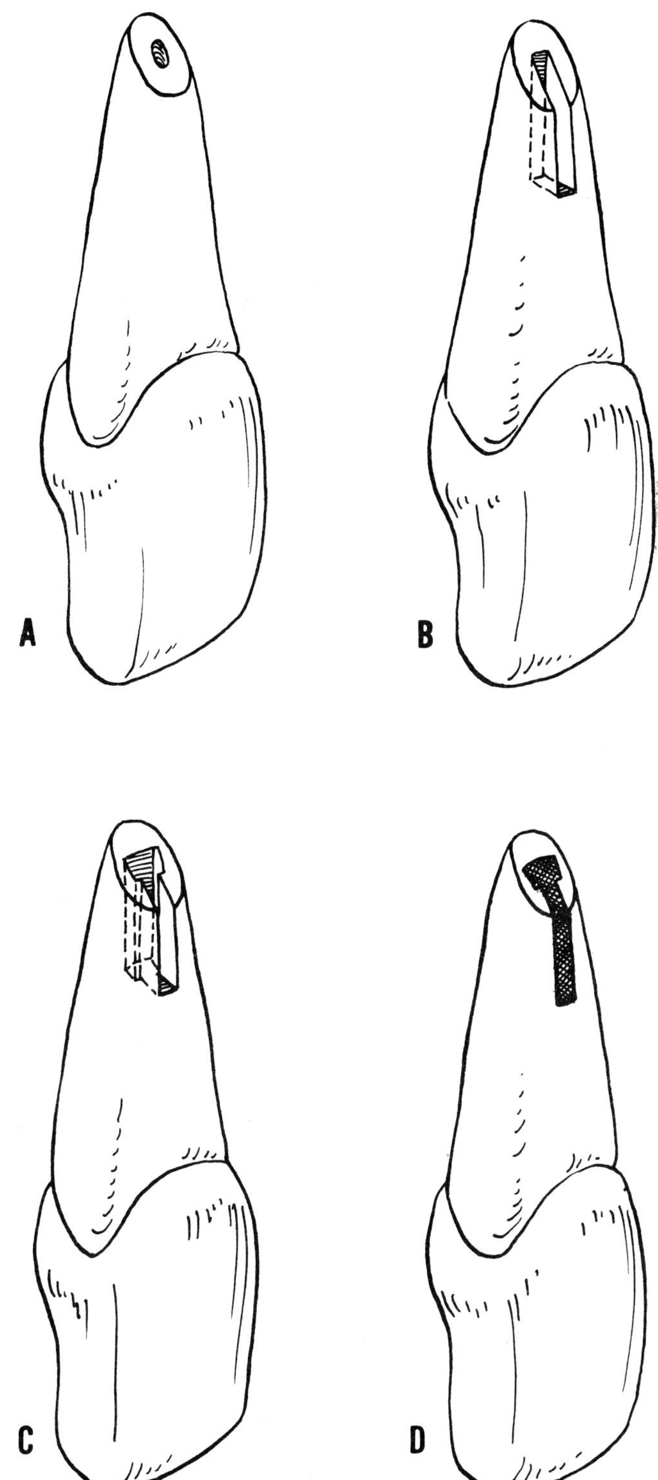

Fig. 15–51. Apical preparation and retrofilling when canal is virtually obliterated by calcification. *A,* Root beveled toward labial by high-speed burs. *B,* Slot is prepared with fine fissure bur to involve fine remaining canal. *C,* Dove-tailed lock is cut at base of slot with inverted cone bur. *D,* Retro-amalgam filling is placed into undercut, keyed slot preparation. Excess is trimmed away to complete preparation. (Courtesy Dr. Pierre R. Dow.)

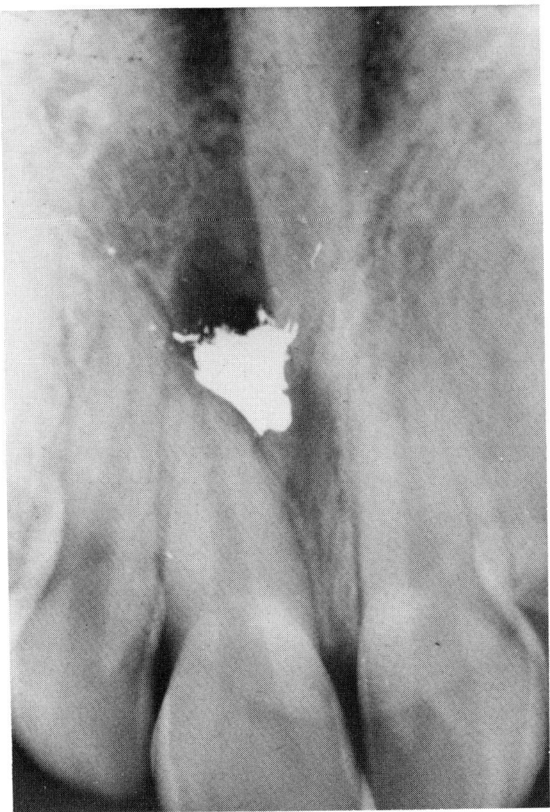

Fig. 15–52. Continued failure following ineffective retrofilling. Floor of nose has been perforated by lesion. Possibility of malpractice lies not with inadequate filling, but with not retreating or informing the patient.

the fact that the root is beveled to the labial and a considerable portion of the root extends beyond the apical orifice. This fact should be explained to the patient for any future discussion he may have, and a note of the discussion is made in the chart.

Suturing. The final step in either curettage, root resection, or retrofilling is to replace the periosteal flap and secure it to its original position by sutures. Presterilized atraumatic needles in varying sizes and shapes are available with preattached, knotless nylon or silk material of varying diameters. A common choice is the Ethicon FS-2 needle mounted with a 0000 braided black silk suture.

Where either the curved or scalloped flap has been employed, an adequate number of "interrupted" sutures is indicated. Care must be exercised to ***place the sutures into the interproximal tissue.*** The ***marginal gingiva*** overlying a root prominence is avoided to prevent the development of a V-shaped defect in the marginal gingiva caused by the tug of the suture. This defect could mark the beginning of a future dehiscence.

Where the triangular, trapezoidal, or rectangular flap has been employed, a "suspensory periodontic" suture offers the advantage of the greatest assurance of the retention and reattachment of the flap at its proper, most coronal position. The suspensory suture(s) embraces the labial gingiva in close approximation to the alveolar process and is passed circumferentially and knotted on the labial surface of the involved tooth. Interrupted sutures are used for the balance of the vertical segment of these flaps (Fig. 15–53). This improvement in suture technique has decreased the incidence of unfavorable periodontal defects following the total reflection of interdental papilla. In most instances, sutures are left in place a minimum of three days. Sutures left much longer than five days become secondarily infected and are extremely uncomfortable. Following final oral irrigation, the patient is ready for instructions.

Postoperative Care. The patient should be thoroughly instructed about postoperative care and sent from the office with a printed set of instructions.

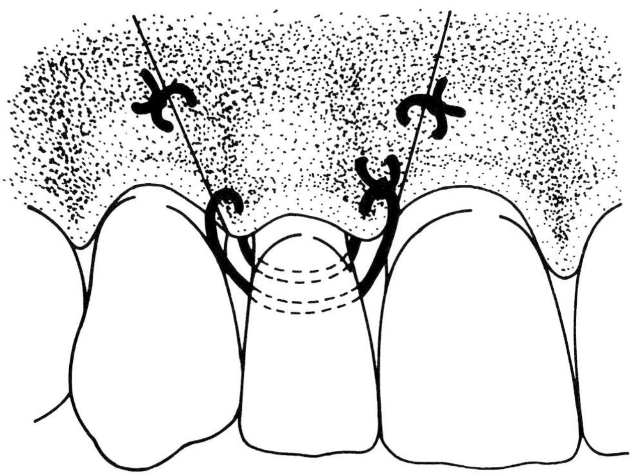

Fig. 15–53. Periodontal suspensory suture. Both passes of suture are to palatal, which gives lingual tug to labial tissue providing for better adaptation. (Courtesy Dr. Alfred L. Frank.)

Home Instructions Following Endodontic Surgery

A. *What to do Following Surgery:*

1. After leaving this office, rest and avoid strenuous activities for the remainder of the day.
2. Take 2 aspirin or Tylenol every 2 to 4 hours until you retire, to maintain comfort.
3. Apply an ice bag or cold compress to the outside of your face over the operated area. Apply for 10 minutes, then remove for 10 minutes. Continue the applications for the first 4–6 hours of the first day only. This can help keep swelling and discoloration to a minimum.
4. Eat soft foods only for the first 24 hours.
5. Avoid chewing in the operated area until the sutures are removed.
6. Brush ***all*** of your teeth after each meal. In the area of the operation, take care to avoid touching the sutures.
7. A solution of a half teaspoon of salt in a full cup of hot water ***held*** in your mouth for 2 to 3 minutes every hour may make your mouth more comfortable.
8. Do not rinse vigorously, nor employ a "Water Pic."
9. Avoid lifting or unnecessarily exercising your lip. It is possible to accidentally tear the sutures, open the incision, and delay healing.
10. Return to this office for suture removal as directed.
11. If a surgical dressing has been used, notify this office immediately if it should loosen or fall out in the first 48 hours.

B. *What to Expect Following Surgery:*

1. Some discomfort is usually present. Severe pain seldom occurs. If aspirin or Tylenol does not restore comfort, please phone for a prescribed pain reliever.
2. There will be some swelling and discoloration present for three to five days following surgery. This is a normal part of the healing process.
3. There is often a temporary loss of feeling in the operated area.
4. The operated tooth may feel loose for a time.
5. (Insert instructions specific for this case).

C. *Should Any Condition Arise Which Causes You Concern, Please Call This Office*

One of the most thoughtful considerations that can be given your patient, other than the highest standards of surgical skill, is to show your concern during the first 24 hours following surgery. This is best done by telephoning the patient the evening of, or morning after, surgery. This practice affords the dentist the opportunity to check his patient's progress and is greatly appreciated by all patients.

Corrective Surgery

Periodontal-Endodontal Defects. Concomitant periapical and periodontal lesions often condemn the involved teeth to extraction. On the other hand, concurrent endodontic and periodontic therapy may be used to save apparently hopeless teeth. These cases should be carefully examined to determine the primary source of the communicating lesion, for the origin of the lesion is the determining factor in prognosis. These lesions will be primarily ***endodontal*** in origin, primarily ***periodontal*** in origin, or a ***combination*** of both.

Simon, Glick and Frank have classified these lesions into five types: (1) primary ***endodontal*** lesion, (2) primary endodontal lesion with secondary periodontal involvement, (3) primary ***periodontal*** lesion, (4) primary periodontal lesion with secondary endodontal involvement, (5) "true" combined lesion.[24] Each division deserves further explanation.

Primary Endodontal Lesions. These lesions may appear as drainage from the gingival sulcus or swelling of the facial attached gingiva. The initial impression is that these are periodontal in origin. In reality, they are merely fistulas draining periapical or accessory root canal lesions related to pulp disease (Fig. 15–54*A*, *B*). Instead of pointing immediately opposite the periapex, the infection has worked its way through the space of the periodontal ligament to drain in the sulcus. In the case of lateral root canals, the infection will drain opposite the accessory foramen, which could be in the furca or sulcus.

Three tests are used to determine the origin of the lesion, the first being a radiograph with a gutta percha point placed in the stoma of the fistula and gently teased to the full depth of the lesion. The second test, of course, is with a pulp tester, which differentiates between a pulpless tooth and vital tooth with a periodontal lesion. The third test is a periodontic probe and x-ray examination—does the patient have other similar periodontal lesions?

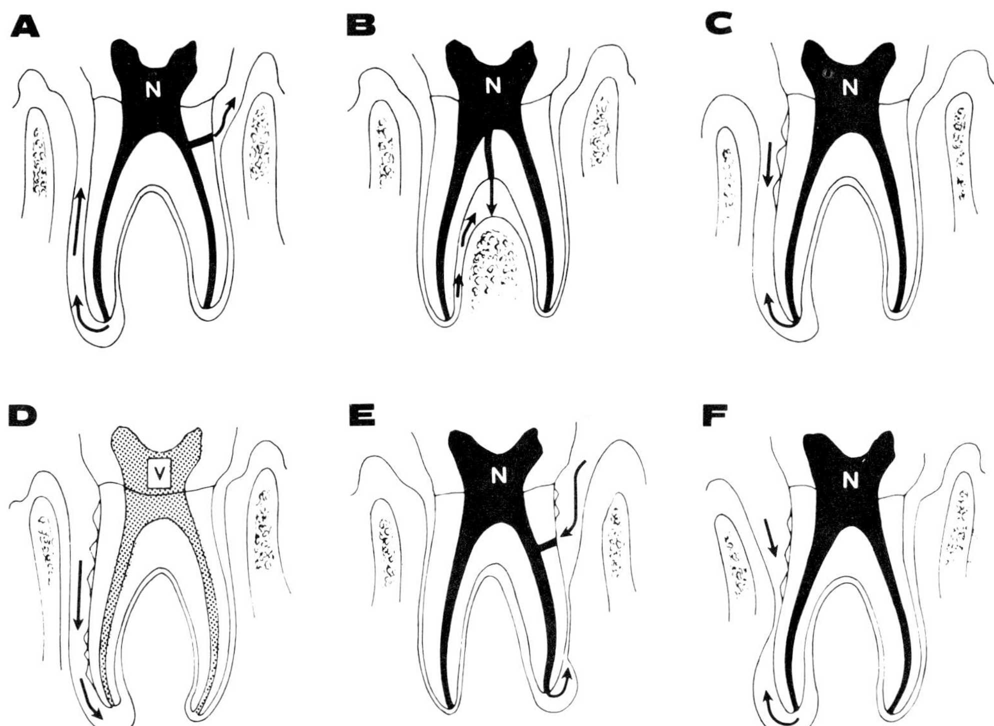

Fig. 15–54. *A,* Primary endodontal lesion—lateral accessory canal. *B,* Primary endodontal lesion—furcation accessory canal. *C,* Primary endodontal lesion with secondary periodontal involvement. *D,* Primary periodontal lesion. Pulp is vital. *E,* Primary periodontal lesion with secondary endodontal involvement. Pulp has become necrotic by retrogenic infection. *F,* True combined lesion wherein primary pulp disease and its periapical sequelae and primary periodontal disease meet. (From Simon, J. H., Glick, D. H., and Frank, A. L.: J. Periodontol., *43*:202, April, 1972.)

The importance of differentiating the endodontal-only lesion is that the prognosis is excellent—healing by ***nonsurgical*** endodontic therapy alone. Using periodontal curettes, the root surface should be planed to be sure it is free of deposits (Fig. 15–55).

Primary Endodontal Lesions with Secondary Periodontal Involvement. This type of lesion is merely an extension of the ones just described, but these fistulas are ignored by the patient and chronic periodontal disease extends into the lesion with plaque and calculus formation (Fig. 15–54*C*). The localized periodontitis complicates the prognosis, and the tooth now requires both endodontic and periodontic therapy. Assuming the endodontic therapy is successful, the outcome depends on the success of the periodontic therapy. Following endodontic therapy alone, the periapex may heal spontaneously, but not the ***secondary*** pocket which requires curettage and root planing at the very least.

Primary Periodontal Lesions. Unchecked periodontitis or periodontosis progresses along the root surface until the periapex is reached. A perfectly normal pulp response with the pulp tester will prove the lesion to be singularly periodontal (Fig. 15–54*D*). This does not mean, however, that the pulp could not become involved through retrogenic infection. Treatment is wholly periodontic, and care must be taken not to devitalize the pulp during deep therapy.

Primary Periodontal Lesions with Secondary Endodontal Involvement. Progression of a periodontal lesion may involve lateral or accessory canals leading to the pulp or they may extend to the very apex. When the lesion involves the primary pulp vessels at the apex, retroinfection is a distinct possibility, with the pulp becoming inflamed and eventually necrotic (Fig. 15–54*E*). As mentioned, periodontal therapy may also lead to pulp death if important vessels are severed. Quite obviously, both endodontic and periodontic therapy will be necessary to provide a successful result. The endodontic treatment should be completed first or the pulp toxic reservoir will continue to abort the desired periodontal healing.

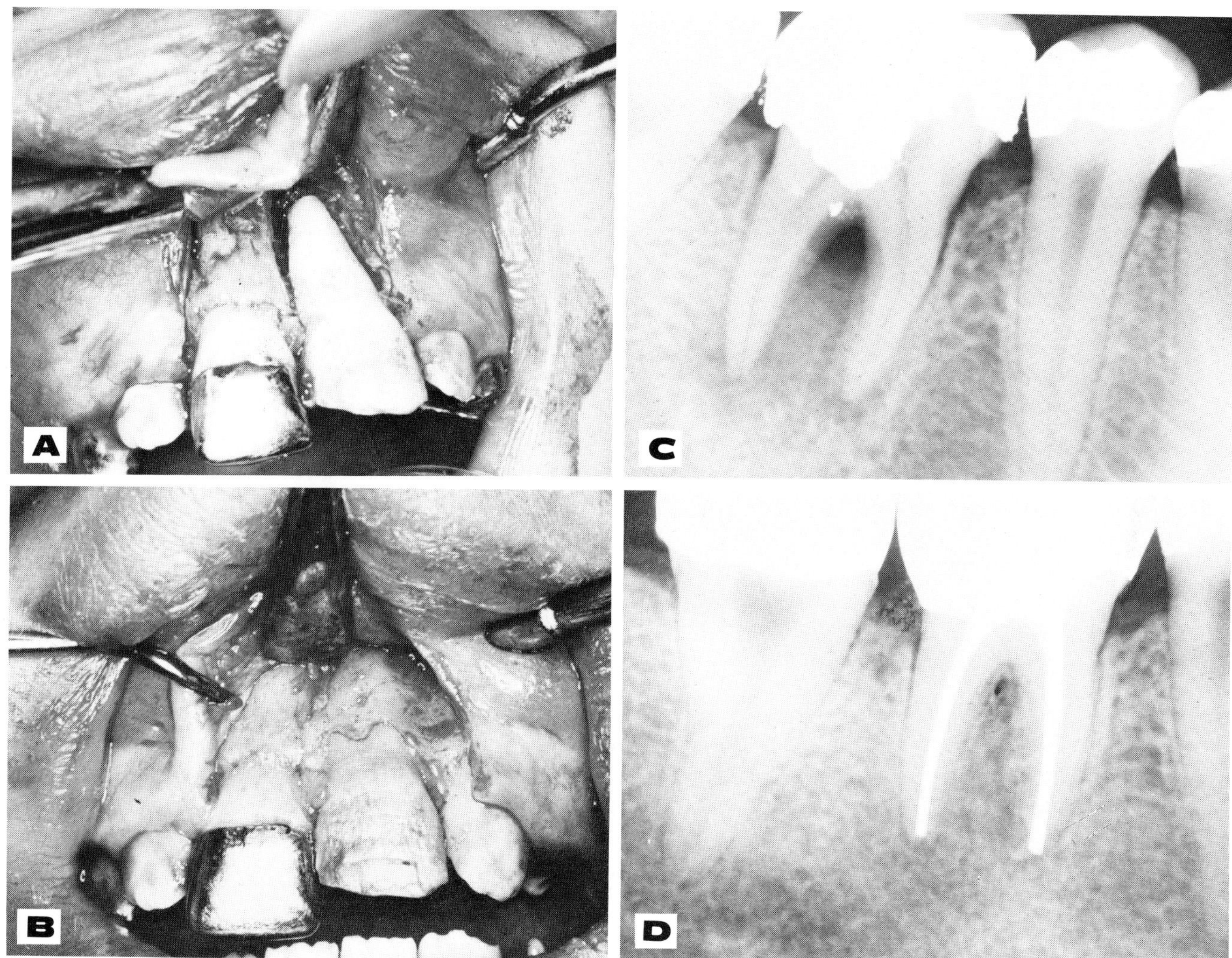

Fig. 15–55. Osseous repair of primary endodontal lesions. *A,* Following root canal therapy, the surgical approach was not necessary to achieve repair. These are the cases that heal with root canal treatment alone. *B,* "Reentry" two years later reveals excellent regrowth of alveolar bone, cementum, and ligament. (From Hiatt, W.: J. Amer. Soc. of Periodont., *1*:152, July-Aug., 1963.) *C,* Preoperative radiograph of pulpless molar with periapical as well as furcal osseous destruction. Drainage was through buccal and lingual sulcus. *D,* Thirty-month recall radiograph showing complete healing of primary endodontal lesions following canal obturation. No surgical intervention. (Courtesy Dr. Alfred L. Frank.)

Prognosis in these cases of primary periodontal etiology is not so good as if the primary lesion is endodontal. This can be said of all periodontic therapy, with which the prognosis is much more guarded than with endodontic therapy.

"True" Combined Lesions. These lesions occur where a pulpally induced periapical lesion exists on a tooth that is also periodontally involved. The infrabony defect occurs when the two lesions meet and merge (Fig. 15–54*F*). Again, the endodontic treatment should precede the periodontic. Prognosis, of course, is more dependent upon the periodontal outcome. If a three-wall infrabony pocket is present, Prichard has shown that success is much more predictable (see Fig. 1–11).[25]

If a combined lesion is found in a mouth that is otherwise free of periodontal disease, one should be suspicious of a vertical root fracture, particularly if the lesion does not respond to combined therapy. It may be necessary to lay a flap to find this defect, which has a rather hopeless prognosis.

In summary, it can be said that prognosis of endodontal-periodontal lesions is a sliding scale descending from the primary ***endodontal*** lesion through the primary ***periodontal*** lesion to the true combined lesion (Fig. 15–56). Of course, some of these apparently hopeless cases may be salvaged by totally amputating the involved root (Fig. 15–57).

Surgical Treatment

Endodontal-periodontal lesions may be treated by a variety of approaches, simplistic to sophisticated. For the extended lesion, but purely endodontal in origin,

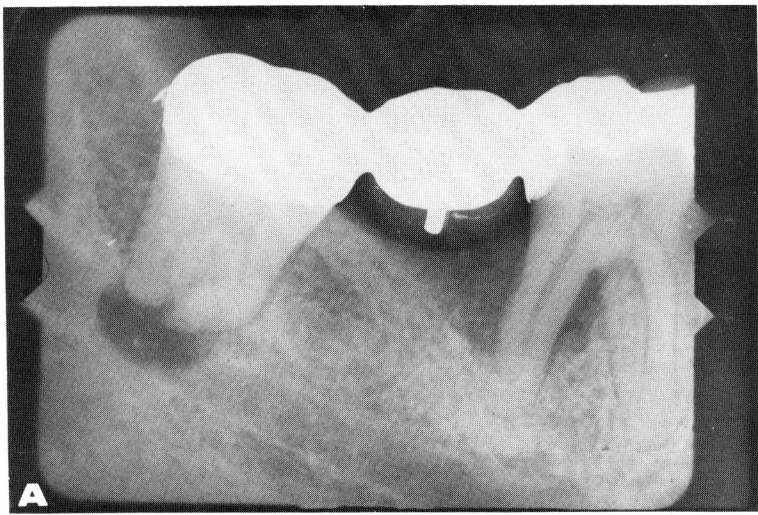

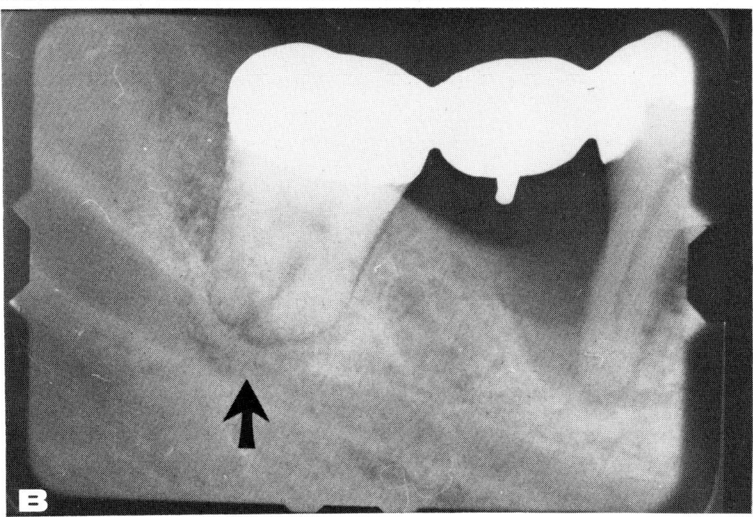

Fig. 15–56. Two primary periodontal lesions. *A,* Third molar with apparent periapical lesion responds positively to electric pulp tester. Occlusal equilibration is the only treatment. Pocket distal to ***first*** molar was curetted. *B,* Two and one-half years later third molar "periapical" lesion has healed, but first molar lesion has worsened and could develop into combined lesion. Notice apparent proximity of third molar lesion to mandibular canal. (Courtesy Dr. Nguyen Nguyen.)

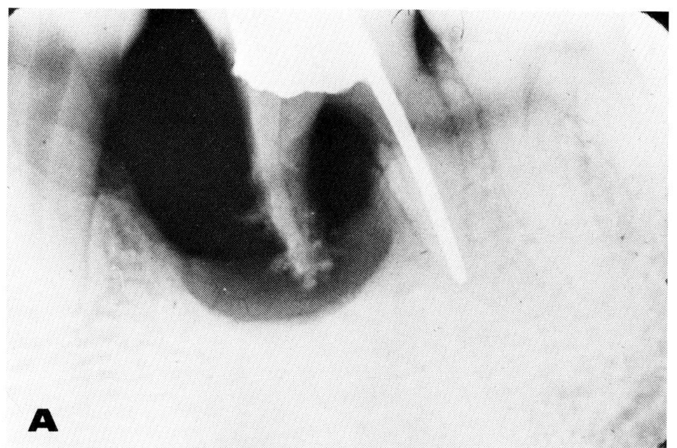

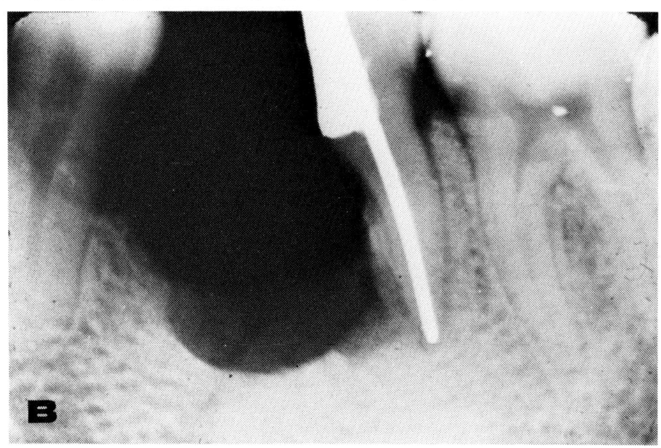

Fig. 15–57. True combined lesion associated with sugar cane chewing habit. *A*, Immediately following endodontic treatment and prior to surgical hemisection. *B*, Following hemisection of periodontally hopeless root. Restoration by bridge is necessary. (Courtesy Dr. Robert Mendel.)

nonsurgical root canal therapy eliminating canal toxins will suffice to produce complete repair. For the complex combined lesion, primarily involved periodontally, curettage, or even bone marrow transplants might be required for healing, or it may be that only total root amputation will suffice.

Subgingival Curettage. In order to ***speed*** and ***improve*** healing of a chronic fistulous tract draining from the periapex to the sulcus, subgingival curettage may be employed. Following completion of the root canal filling, the area may be anesthetized and sharp periodontal curettes used to remove the inflammatory tissue lining the fistula (Fig. 15–58). To provide support to the tissue being curetted, a finger is placed against the gingiva overlying the track, and curettage is carried out against this pressure. In the same procedure, the root surface should be curetted free of all plaque and deposit and the area thoroughly irrigated. A covering of adhesive foil may then be placed to protect the organizing blood clot. Complete repair, with reattachment and new bone, should be expected within a matter of weeks.

Flap Approach. In the event the endodontal lesion is thought to have a serious periodontal overlay, either secondary or primary in nature, a vertical flap may be laid over the involved area and thorough curettage carried out (Fig. 15–59). A full vertical flap, either horizontal or trapezoidal in design, should be used in order to involve the free gingiva in the curettage. The inflammatory tissue from the underside of the flap is first removed, and the thin epithelial margin of the free gingiva is then curetted away or trimmed away with curved scissors. This slows the downgrowth of the oral epithelium back into the fistulous pocket, which could separate the organizing clot from attachment to the root surface.

The curettage is then turned against the root surface and the inflammation and deposits are removed from the root. The area is irrigated with water and the flap sutured into position. Again, adhesive foil may be used to cover the entire surgical area and teeth, in order that healing may better organize. The sutures are removed in three to five days.

If total periapical healing is obtained through this procedure, but only partial periodontal healing, the remaining periodontal defect may be maintained by subgingival curettage two or three times a year. The compromised result is preferable to the former lesion, which was infected and constantly draining pus from the periapex out the gingival sulcus.

Gingival Repair of a Periodontal Defect. In the event a gingival dehiscence develops as a result of endodontic surgery (see Fig. 15–20 and Fig. 15–21), corrective periodontic surgery must be used to overcome the defect. The most common methods utilize either a vertical sliding flap with a supplementary relaxing incision (Fig. 15–60) or a lateral sliding flap. Even free gingival grafts should be considered. Fenestration of the root surface through the overlying bone complicates any of these approaches, which are well described in any standard periodontic text.

In cases of horizontal tooth fracture, just at or below the gingiva, periodontic surgery may be combined with root canal treatment to save the

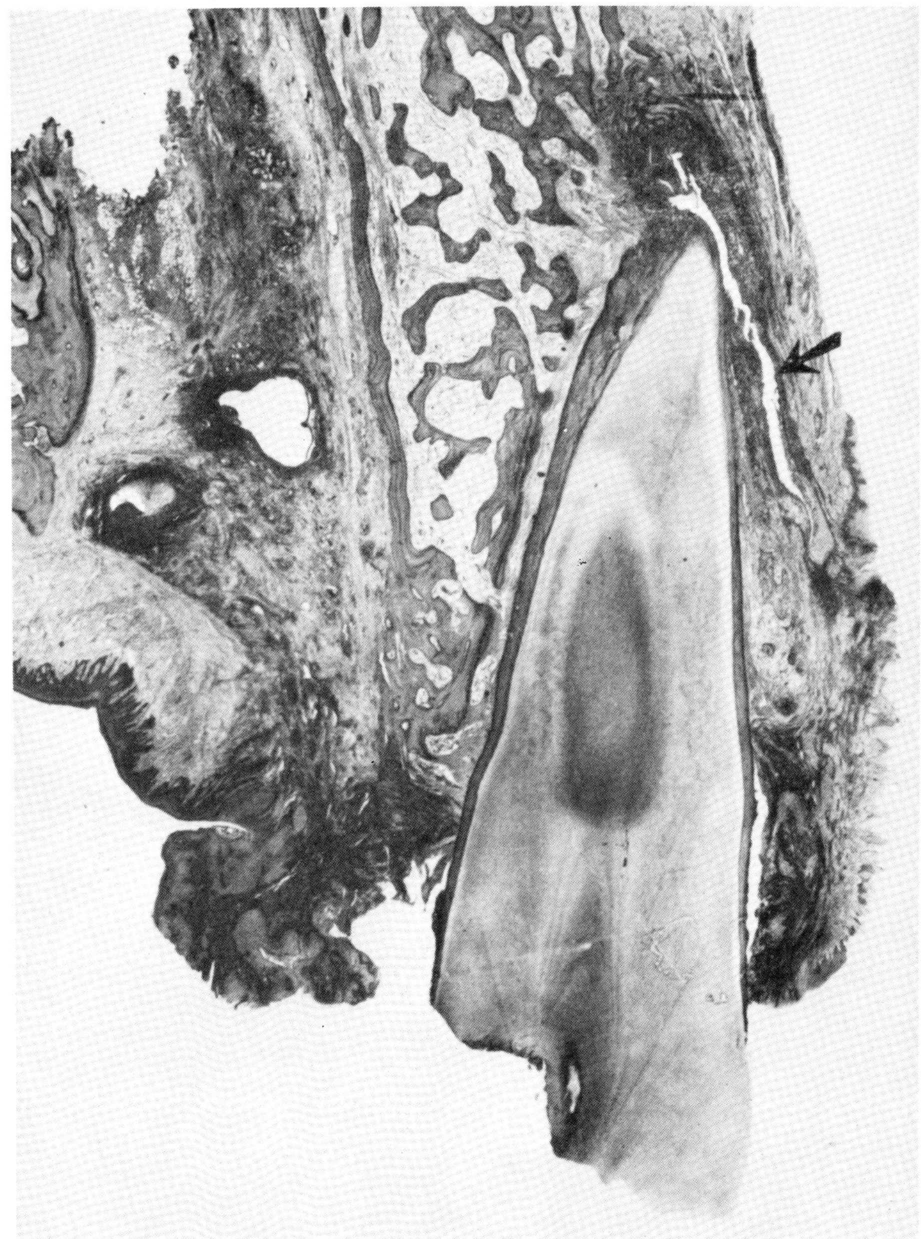

Fig. 15–58. Suppurative apical periodontitis and its path of drainage in anterior mouth. Purulent exudate has reached for surface along route offering least resistance. Characteristically, this route is through thin labial bone to surface of mucosa, opposite apical half of root. This section shows almost entire length of epithelialized fistula *(arrow)*. Human maxillary central incisor. (From Matsumiya, S.: *Atlas of Oral Pathology*. Tokyo Dental College Press, 1955.)

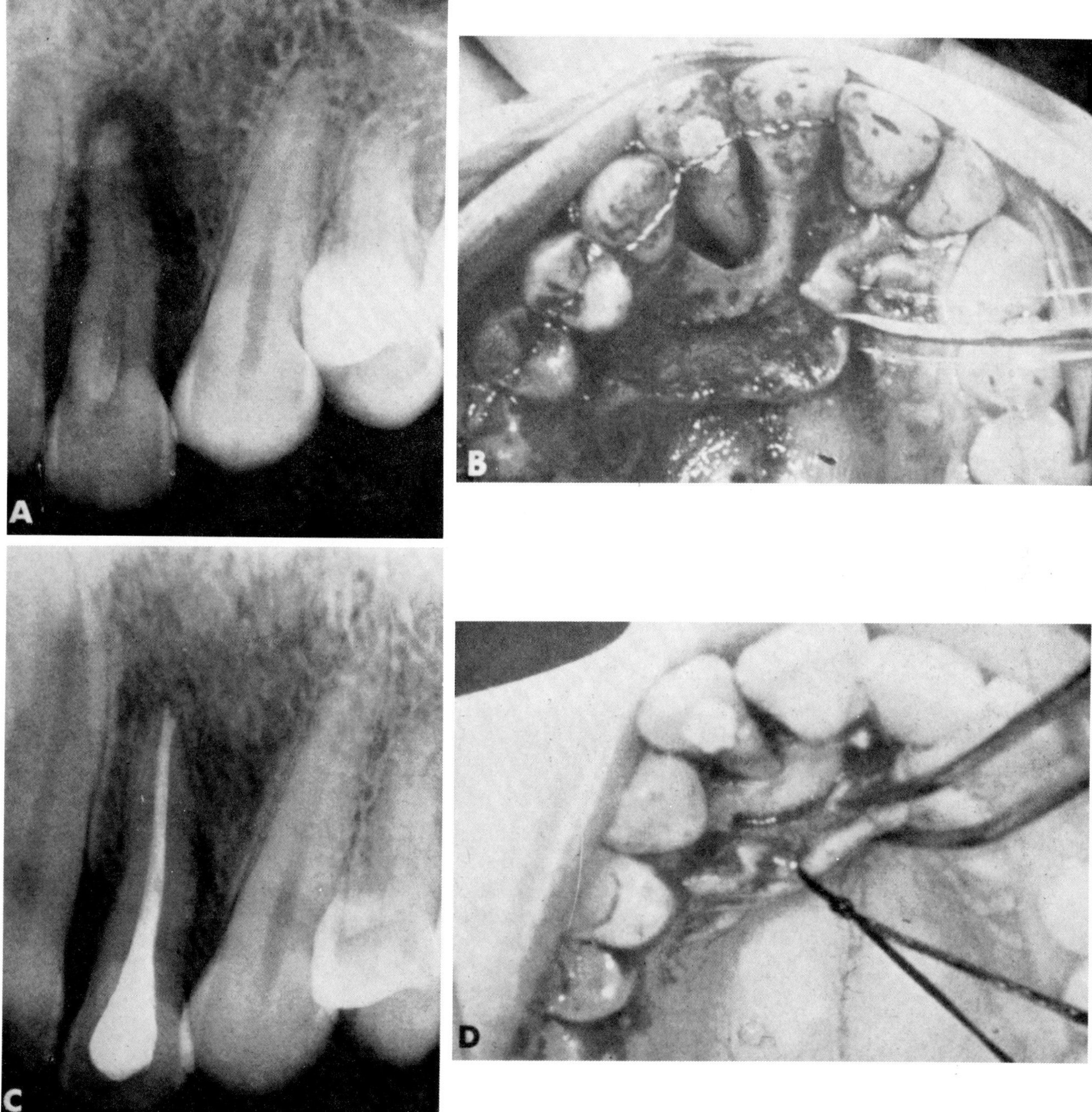

Fig. 15–59. Osseous repair following endodontic therapy and corrective periapical-periodontal surgery of primary periodontal lesion with secondary endodontal involvement. One would suspect periodontal lesion first developed from root defect apparent in *A*. *A,* Periodontal-periapical bony lesion involving pulpless lateral incisor with invaginated anomaly at cingulum which probably extends onto root. Reattachment will not occur unless root defect is ground away and root surface smoothed. *B,* Palatal surgical flap exposes huge bony lesion which was then thoroughly curetted. Root canal treatment preceded surgery. *C,* Six months following therapy, osseous repair is revealed in recall roentgenogram. *D,* Bony regrowth and reattachment are seen one year after therapy when palatal flap is again raised. (Courtesy Dr. Ernesto Meuller, Caracas, Venezuela.)

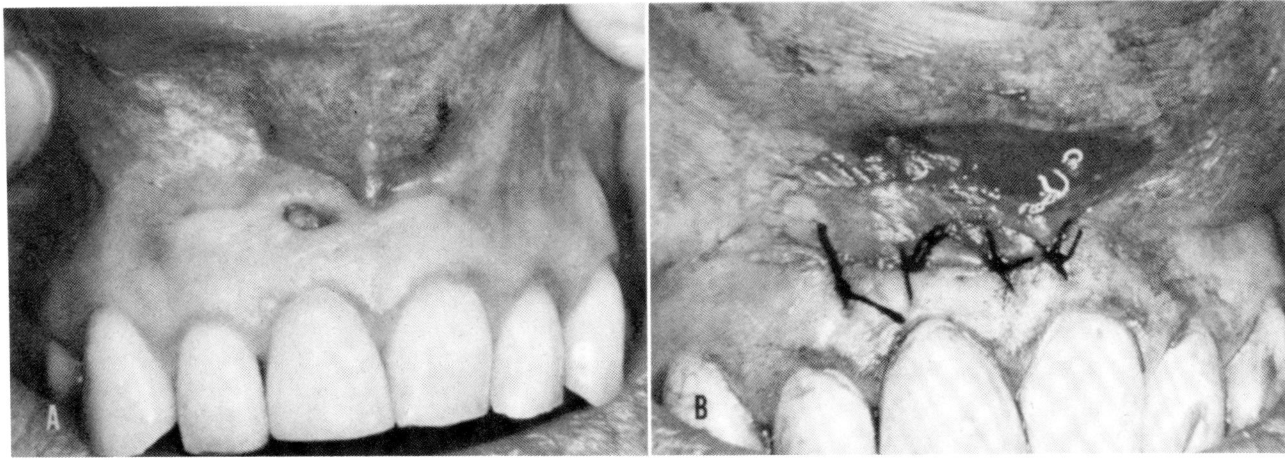

Fig. 15–60. Corrective surgical procedure for fenestrating defect following periapical surgery. *A,* Fenestrating lesion apical to treated pulpless tooth. *B,* "Freshening" incision across defect, and relaxing incision above in alveolar mucosa allow new coaptation of margins of defect. Protruding root is beveled back into depths of defect. (Courtesy Dr. Dudley H. Glick.)

remaining root structure and prepare it for reception of a dowel restoration. Gingival surgery in these cases may utilize apically repositioned flaps or in some cases a regular old time gingivectomy (Fig. 15–61). In either case, osseous recontouring of the alveolar crest is frequently necessary (Fig. 15–61*B*) to free up enough of the root to transform it into a clinical "crown." Once the root is "elongated" adequate tooth structure is available for rubber dam placement and root canal treatment (Fig. 15-61*C*). The surgical site may be protected by a periodontal pack during healing, and a provisional esthetic crown may be placed as well (Fig. 15–61*D*). To salvage roots involved in deeper horizontal fractures, orthodontic elongation may be employed as discussed in Chapter 16.

Gingival surgery in conjunction with crown amputation and root canal therapy in preparation for overdenture construction is also vitally needed. All retained roots supporting an overdenture are dependent on a collar of firm attached gingiva to ensure their long-term retention (Fig. 17–22*D*). Again, the root canal therapy can be done immediately after the crown is amputated and before the gingival surgery is completed.

Total Root Amputation and Hemisection. In 1894, Doctor W. J. Younger, addressing the meeting of the American Medical Association on "pyorrhea alveolaris," had this to say about hopelessly involved roots of molar teeth: "My treatment in these cases has been to open into these roots, remove their pulps, fill them and amputate (the involved root); then grind away enough of the articulating surface of the crown, immediately over the removed root, in order to bring the pressure in the effort of mastication upon the (solid) roots. By these means, these teeth can be made comfortable and serviceable for years, if not for a lifetime."[26]

It is difficult today to add to Doctor Younger's description of total root amputation made over three-quarters of a century ago. Discussions of prior authorship of root amputation overlook the past. G. V. Black dealt at some length with total root amputation in 1886 (Fig. 15–62).[5]

Root amputation is such a logical procedure when an individual root is hopelessly involved with caries, internal resorption, or periodontal disease (Fig. 15–63). Molars may be narrowed mesiodistally or buccolingually to premolar size and still be perfectly serviceable. Maxillary first premolars with two roots and hopeless mesiodistal furca involvement may be sectioned to become canine in size and be restored to an esthetic, serviceable condition. There is no reason why the remaining portion of any of these teeth cannot serve as fixed partial denture abutments or be included in a full arch restorative prescription (Fig. 15–64). And quite often, amputation of a hopelessly involved root of an abutment tooth will save remaking an entire fixed prosthesis, even full arch in extent

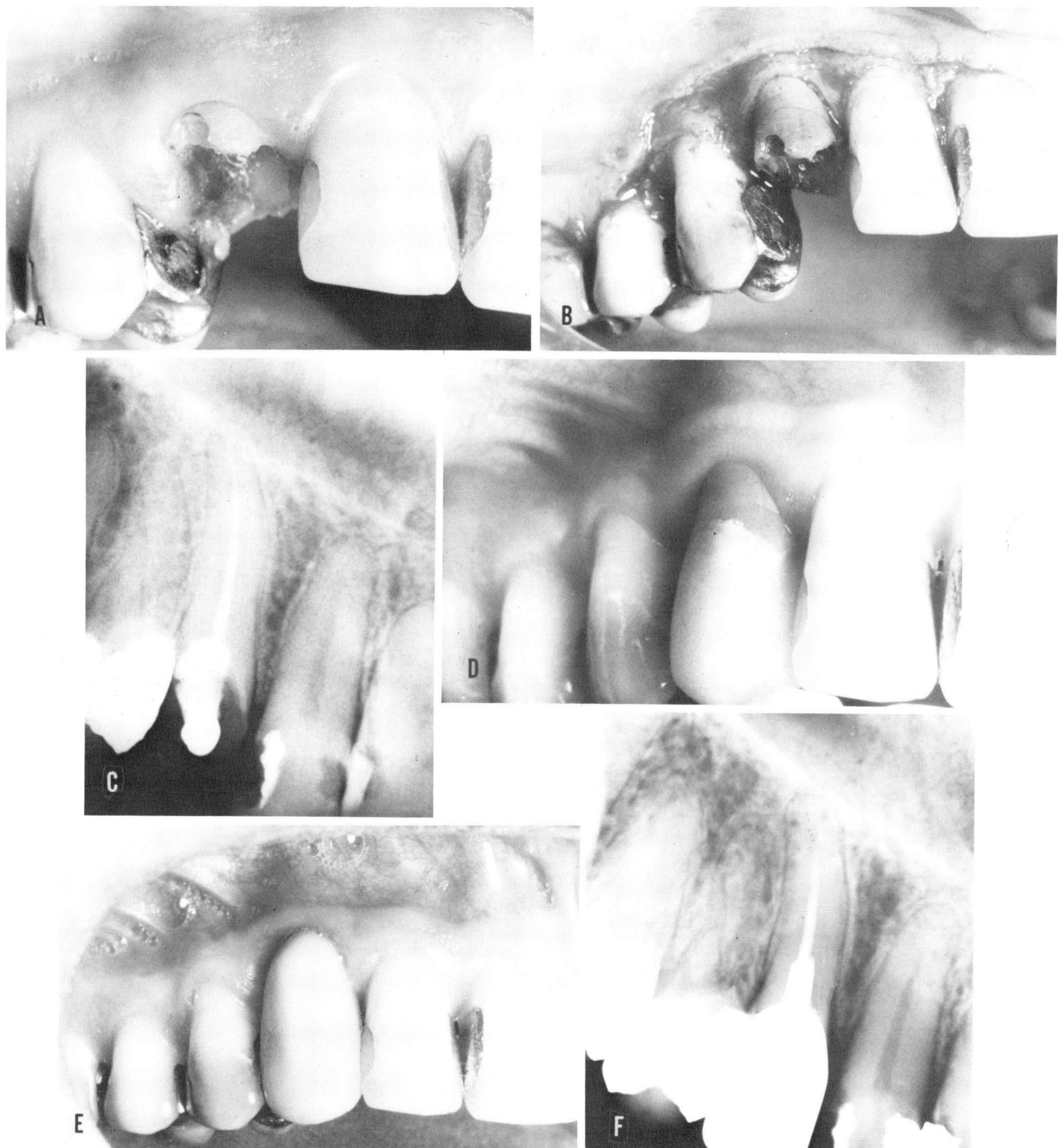

Fig. 15–61. Use of corrective surgery and endodontic therapy to salvage apparently hopeless fractured tooth. *A*, Maxillary canine fractured through pulp and well below gingival level. *B*, Corrective periodontal surgery is initiated with lingual and labial gingivectomy which leaves a small margin of attached gingiva. Apically repositioned flap could also have been used. Osseous recontouring raises labial bony level around fractured tooth as well as adjacent teeth. Interdental grooving is deepened. Following immediate root canal therapy, periodontal dressing and temporary crown are placed. *C*, Immediate pulpectomy and gutta percha root canal filling are completed at surgical appointment. *D*, Periodontal healing at end of two months: firmly attached gingiva with knife edge margins. Elongation of crown is realized by comparing this photo with *A*. Temporary crown has been placed. *E*, Final restoration with baked-on porcelain dowel crown. *F*, Roentgenogram of dowel crown in place. This single restoration is far superior, less time-consuming, and less expensive than extracting tooth and placing fixed prosthesis.

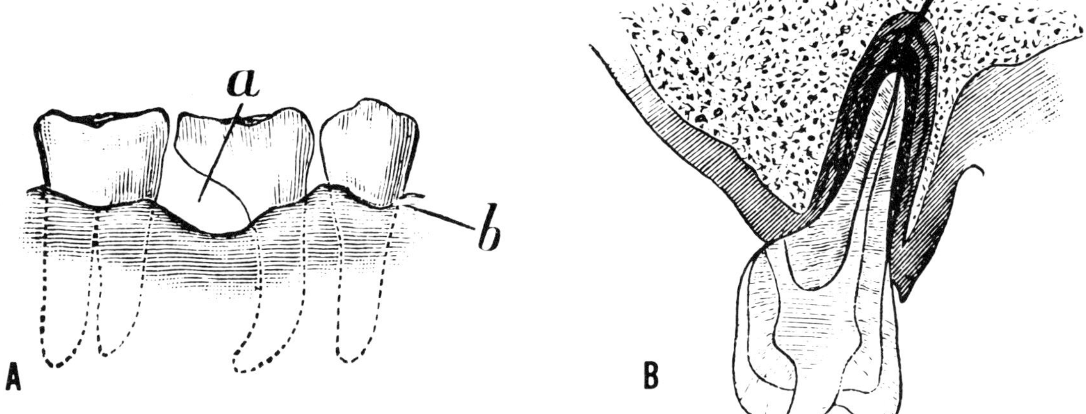

Fig. 15–62. In 1886 G. V. Black discussed technique of total root amputation in Litch's *Textbook of Operative Dentistry. A,* Black's illustration of root amputation for mandibular molar. *B,* Black's illustration of amputation of lingual root of maxillary molar.

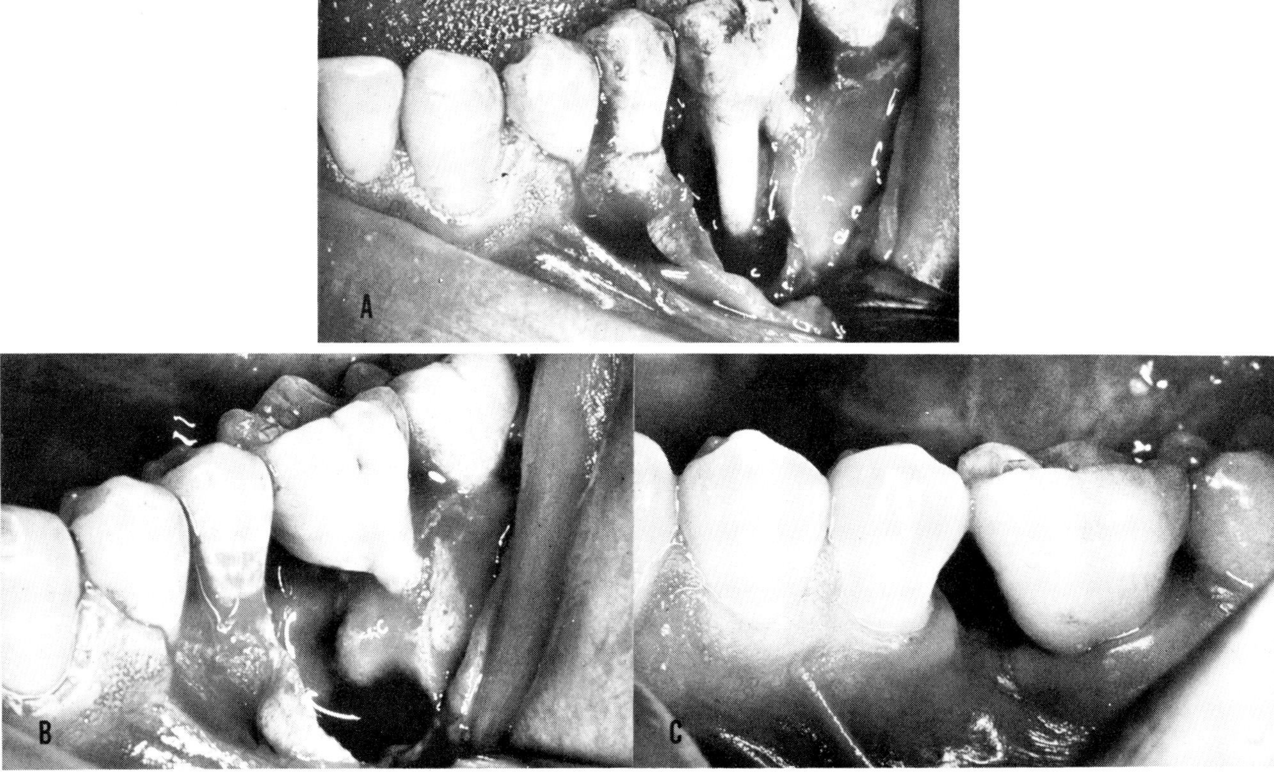

Fig. 15–63. *A,* Total amputation of mesial root involved with cavernous periodontal lesion. Tight contained arch supports tooth from mesial and distal. Root canal therapy of distal canal has been completed before surgery. *B,* Total amputation of involved root. Stump has been filled with amalgam and amputation cuts across amalgam. *C,* Appearance, six months after surgery. Patient is instructed in special oral hygiene for well-contoured stump. Minor periodontal corrective surgery could improve tissue contour in area.

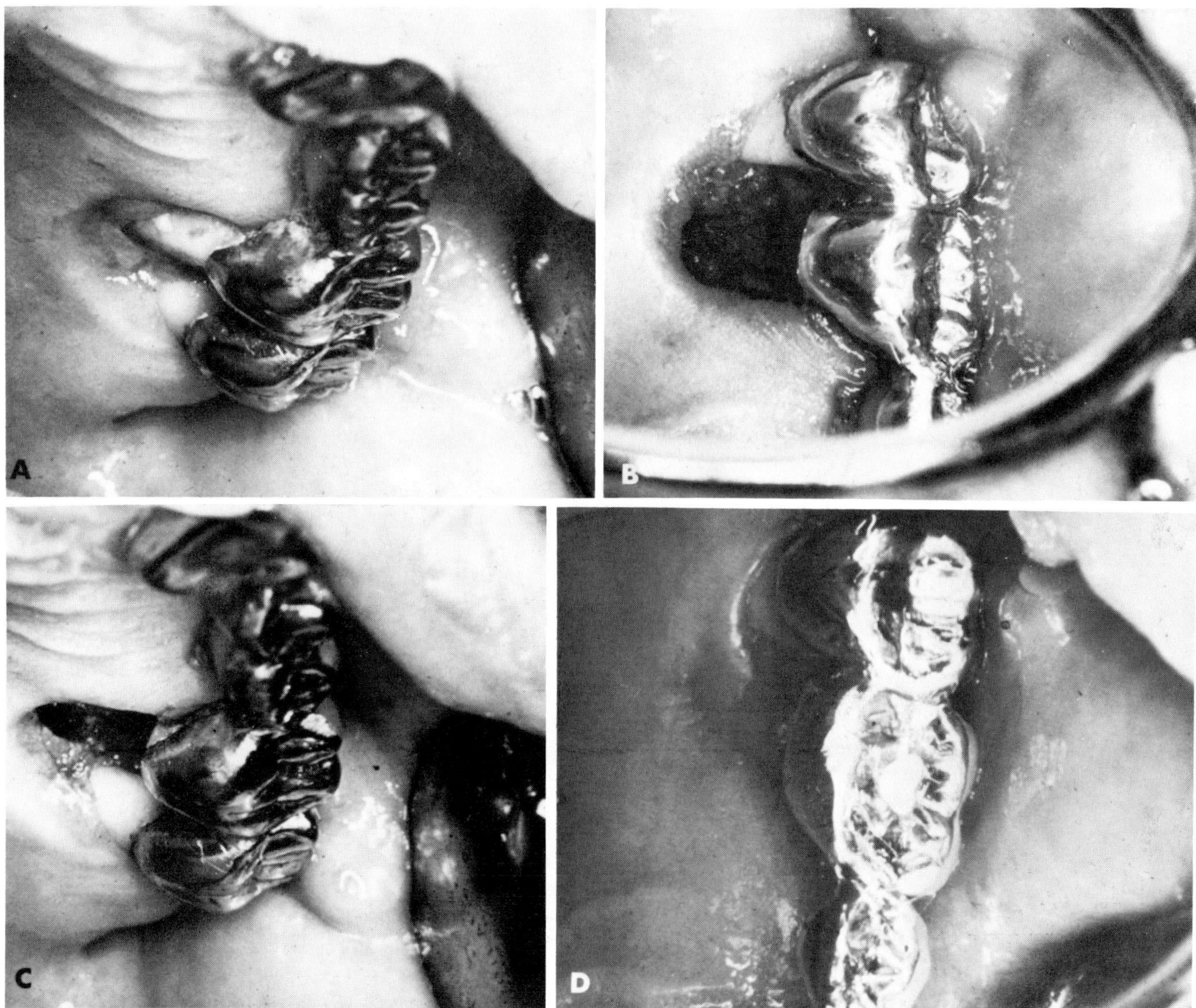

Fig. 15–64. Importance of recontouring the tooth structure in area of amputation. *A,* Hopelessly involved lingual root of maxillary molar abutment of extensive fixed prosthesis. *B,* Mirror view of amputated area. Sharp edges must be recontoured. Either amputated root should be left in place during recontouring or cavity should be packed with Gelfoam to prevent metal particles from filling space. *C,* Recontour of lingual portion of root and crown. Buccal-lingual narrowing of occlusal table was completed at later appointment. If deep periodontal defect remains after healing, tissue should be recontoured by gingivoplasty. *D,* Healing, 19 months later. Occlusal table has been narrowed buccal-lingually. Final inlay to be placed. (Courtesy Dr. Dudley H. Glick.)

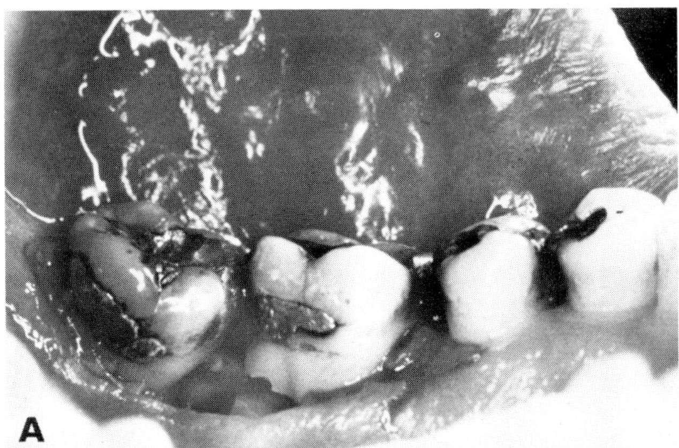

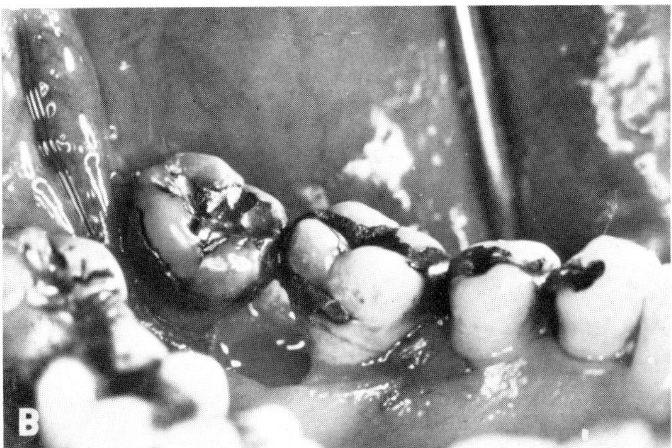

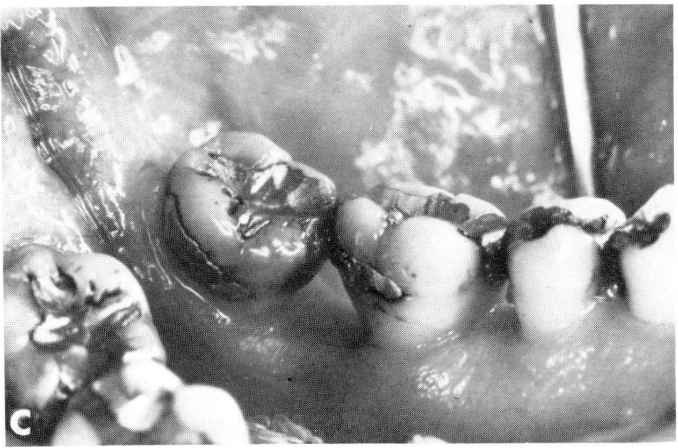

Fig. 15–65. Careful preparation of amputation stump is vital to success. *A*, Distal root amputated. Jagged stump must be recontoured. *B*, Stump recontoured to provide adequate access for oral hygiene. Root remains in socket during reshaping to block debris. *C*, Health of tissue one year after amputation. Unrestored tooth is subject to fracture and should not only be restored but splinted. (Courtesy of Dr. Edward E. Beveridge.)

(see Fig. 1–12). Common sense in evaluating the remaining bony support and the future usefulness of the involved member, all figure into the predictability of outcome.

Two different approaches to the problem are available. One approach is merely to amputate and remove the involved root at the point where it joins the crown—***root amputation.*** The other approach is to cut the entire tooth in half, from mesial to distal in maxillary molars and premolars, and from buccal to lingual in mandibular molars, removing in either case the pathologic root—***hemisection.*** The secret to the future in any case is the careful preparation and restoration of the remaining portion of the tooth so that no possibility exists for future entrapment of bacteria or food particles (Fig. 15–65).

Single- or Multiple-Root Amputation. If at all possible, the root canal therapy of the roots to be retained should be completed prior to the surgical appointment. Coronal reshaping and buccal-lingual narrowing should preferably be done first, to "bring the pressure in the effort of mastication upon the solid roots."[26] This can be quite effective in the case of the maxillary molar with lingual root amputation. Lingual narrowing of the buccal-lingual width of the occlusal table will bring the forces of mastication directly over the axis of the retained buccal roots. The occlusion should also be adjusted so that the trauma of lateral excursion is eliminated (Fig. 15–66).

Buccal-lingual narrowing is not advised for mandibular molars. Their greatest support comes from the contained arch which does not allow for mesial or distal drifting (see Fig. 15–63). If advisable, the involved tooth should also be splinted to adjacent teeth (Fig. 15–67), or may become a member of a full arch prosthesis which will ensure its position and stability. This is particularly true in the mandible.

Following coronal reshaping, attention is turned to the endodontic procedures. Since one is usually dealing with a vital tooth, pulpectomy, canal enlargement, and filling are in order. Intracanal medication is not necessary in these cases.

The ***root to be amputated*** should have the pulp removed and bleeding controlled. Then a cavity is prepared through the coronal opening well down into the root, using a surgical-length bur. Usually a No. 4 bur will suffice. The cavity is then filled with amalgam, firmly condensed. When the root canals of the roots to remain have been instrumented and filled, a coronal temporary filling is placed and preparation made for amputation.

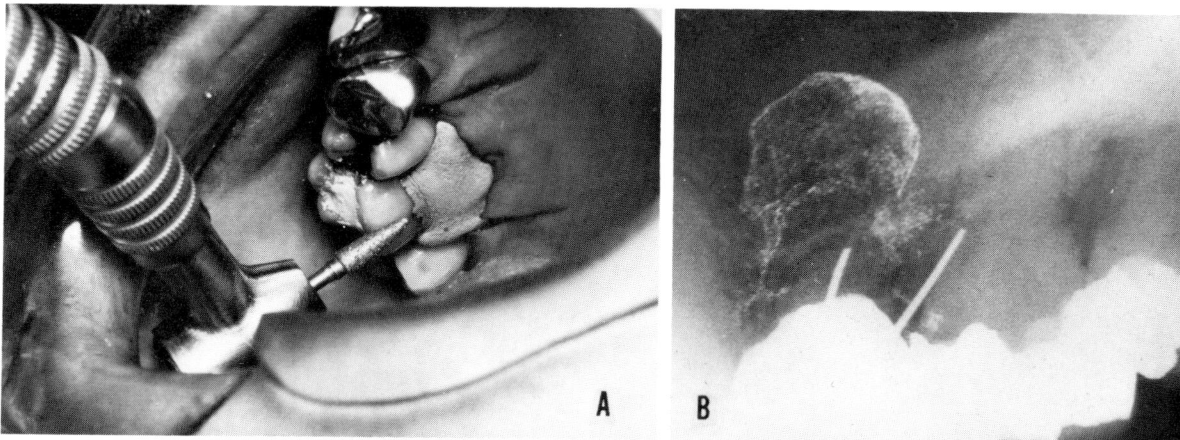

Fig. 15–66. Importance of recontouring to place forces of mastication more nearly over remaining root structure. *A*, High-speed diamond stones are used to narrow occlusal table and recontour stump. Placement of periodontal dressing precludes debris from entering surgical area. *B*, Another case illustrating debris forced into huge periodontal defect at time of amputation and recontour of metal restoration. As much reshaping as possible should be done ***before*** amputated root is removed.

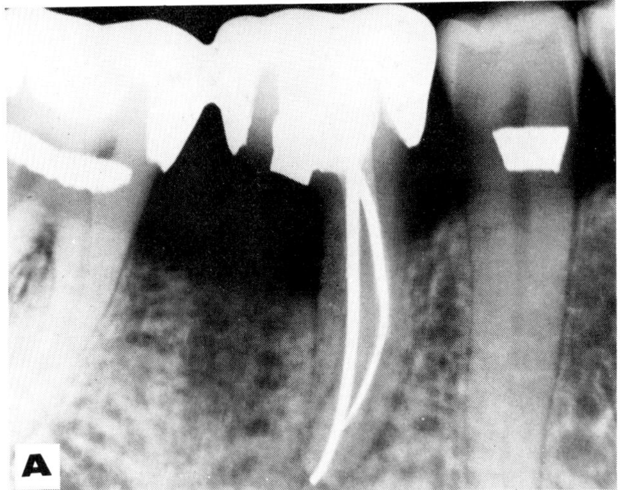

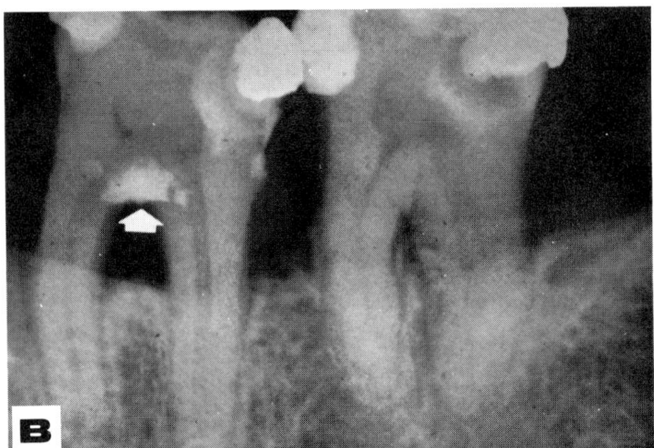

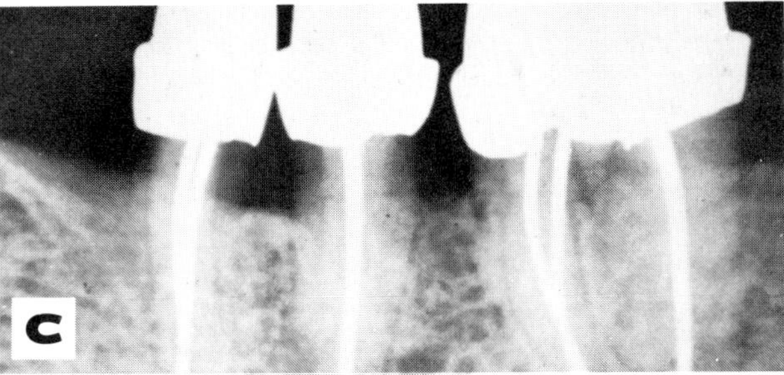

Fig. 15–67. *A*, Splinting to adjacent tooth following amputation of distal root was necessary because of diastemas between these teeth. Also note amalgam restoration which fills amputated distal canal. *B*, Necessity of splinting two pulpless molars with advanced periodontitis to be used as terminal abutments of full arch periodontal prosthesis. Note furcal caries *(arrow)* as well. *C*, Root canal therapy is followed by hemisection of first molar. Telescopic copings are placed to receive prosthetic splint. (From Abrams, L. and Trachtenberg, D.: Dent. Clin. N. Amer., *18*:415, Apr., 1974.)

Ultraspeed equipment has made root amputation a relatively simple procedure. The bifurcation of the root to be amputated must be well explored with a probe and cowhorn explorer prior to amputation, and if full determination of the anatomy of the region cannot be made, a flap should be laid to make visible the problem at hand. Frequently, osseous recontouring is *de rigueur* in any event, and both phases of the operation can be accomplished under one flap (Fig. 15–68).

The cut to amputate the root is made with a bur long enough to reach from one side of the root to the other (Fig. 15–69*A*). In sectioning a mandibular molar a No. 701 XL bur is used for this long reach. Care is exercised in maintaining the correct angulation of the bur so as not to gouge into the remaining root or the crown.

When the root is completely severed, there may be enough destruction of supporting bone to permit the root to be lifted from its socket (Fig. 15–69*B, C*). On the other hand, there may be enough cortical bone remaining to allow the buccal plate to be removed and the root extracted to the buccal. Insofar as possible, before the amputated root is removed, the reshaping and polishing of the crown begins. This procedure is most important, and a good deal of attention and time should be spent in perfecting the preparation. Diamond stones in ultraspeed equipment are ideal for reshaping. The outline of a well-designed bridge pontic should be kept in mind while reshaping. No semblance of a stump should be left (Fig. 15–70), and enough clearance between the undersurface of the crown and the tissue should be established to facilitate oral hygiene (Fig. 15–71).

Another case of total root amputation applies to a tooth hopelessly involved periodontally and a non-terminal member of an ***extended*** fixed prosthesis. Premolars are the commonly involved teeth in this situation. The method of treatment for these cases is quite simple. The tooth is anesthetized and a small coronal cavity is developed through the full or three-quarter crown. A pulpectomy is done and bleeding arrested. The crown is cleaned completely of pulp tissue, and a cavity is prepared with a round bur down into the root to below the gingival level. The entire cavity is filled with amalgam if a full veneer crown is in place or if the involved tooth is a premolar. Anterior teeth with three-quarter crowns should be restored coronally with silicate cement. A buccal flap is raised opposite the involved root and the ***entire root*** is amputated at a level ***well below*** the

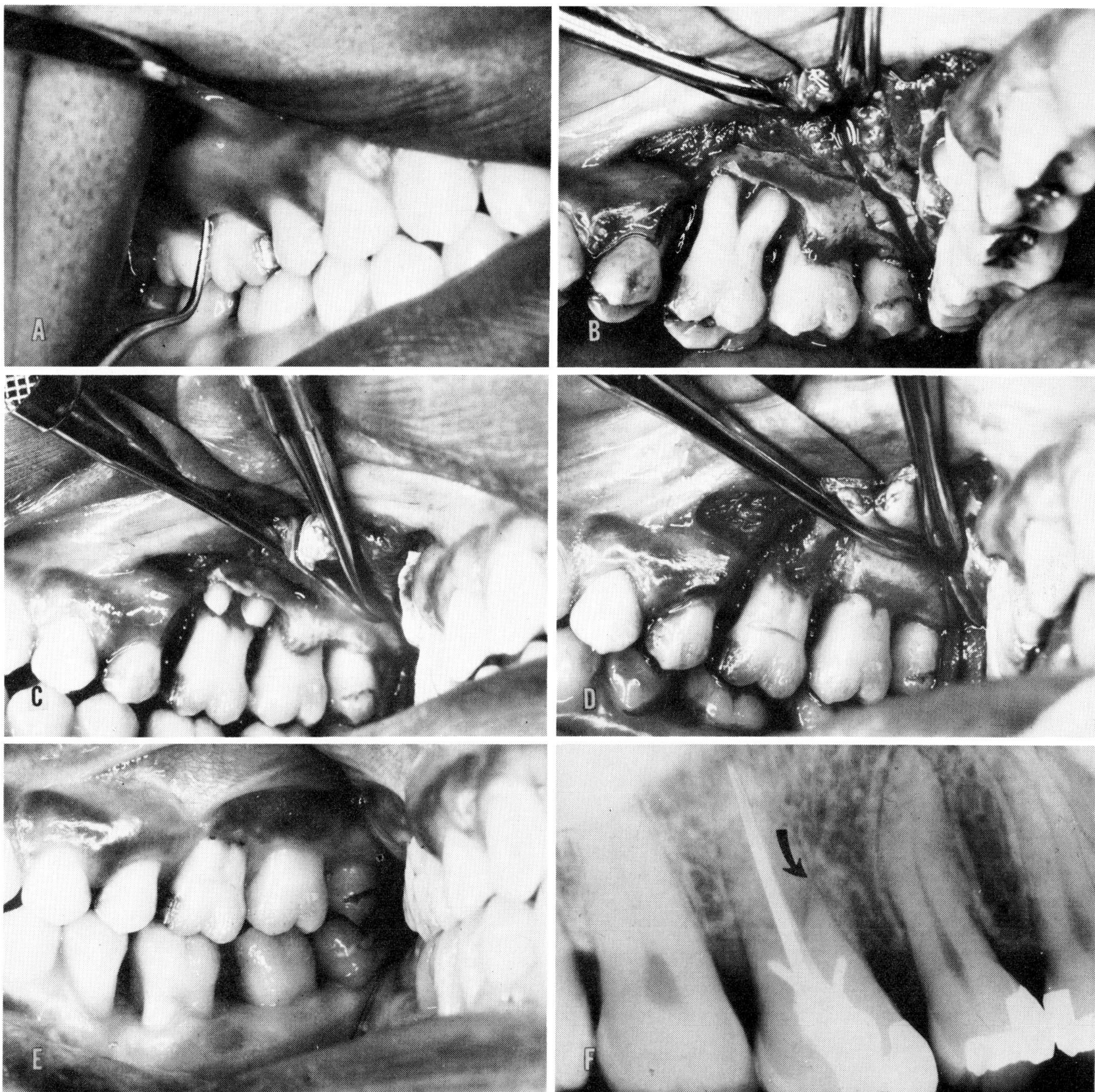

Fig. 15–68. Importance of elevating surgical flap to determine extent and direction of periodontal involvement. *A*, Periodontal probe reveals 5 mm. pocket buccal to maxillary first molar. Interpoximal pockets are even deeper. *B*, Mirror view following flap elevation. Reverse architecture of periodontal lesion as well as furca involvement of buccal roots of molar are seen. Acceptable result can be achieved by osseous recontouring and amputation of two buccal roots. *C*, Because of high furca, roots are amputated on long bevel retaining some of their support to lingual. *D*, Osseous recontouring around all three molars is apparent. Root canal therapy was completed after amputation. *E*, Final periodontal result six months following surgery. Root canal therapy has been completed in all three roots. Amputated buccal roots were filled with silver points pulled by hemostat through apex and then severed and polished. *F*, Final results in recall roentgenogram. Because buccal roots were amputated on long bevel mesiobuccal root appears to be filled far short of apex *(arrow)*. This roentgenographic phenomenon should be explained to patient. (Periodontal therapy by Dr. Alex Drennan.)

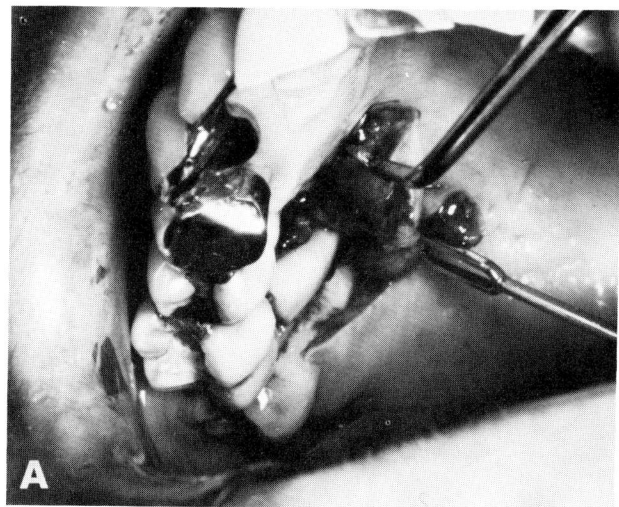

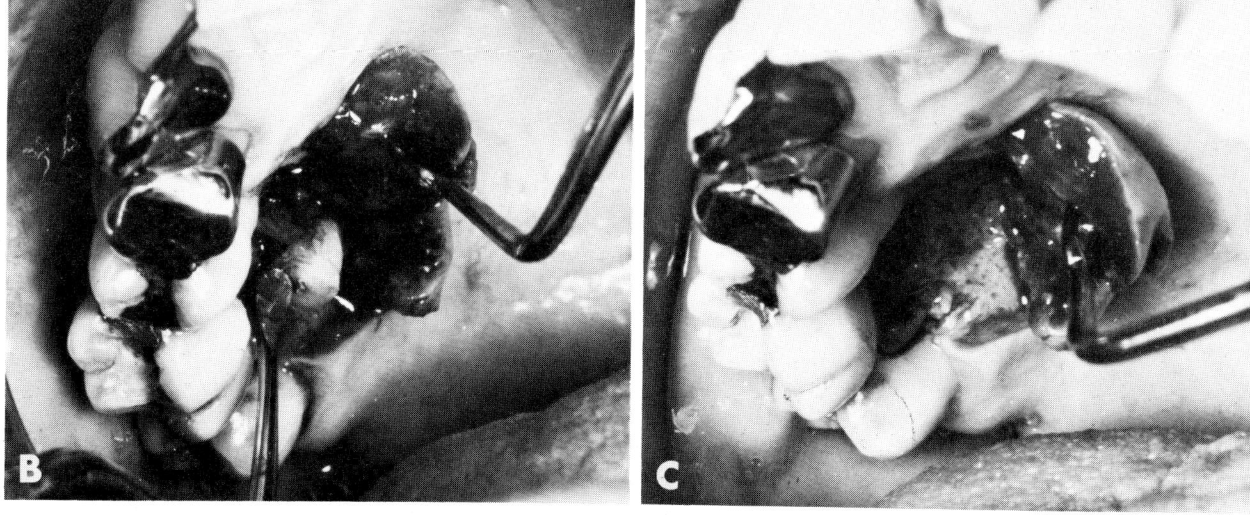

Fig. 15–69. Amputation procedures of lingual root of maxillary molar. *A,* After careful exploration for position of furca, lingual root is amputated with high-speed, extra long, fissure bur. *B,* Removal of root tip. Endodontic therapy had previously been completed. Amalgam filling in lingual canal is apparent in amputated root tip. Buccal-lingual narrowing of occlusal table and recontour of lingual stump should be completed before the root is removed. Stump may be recontoured and polished without leaving any spicules of tooth structure. Final finish is with fine diamond points. *C,* Adequate surgical access allows excellent view of amputated area.

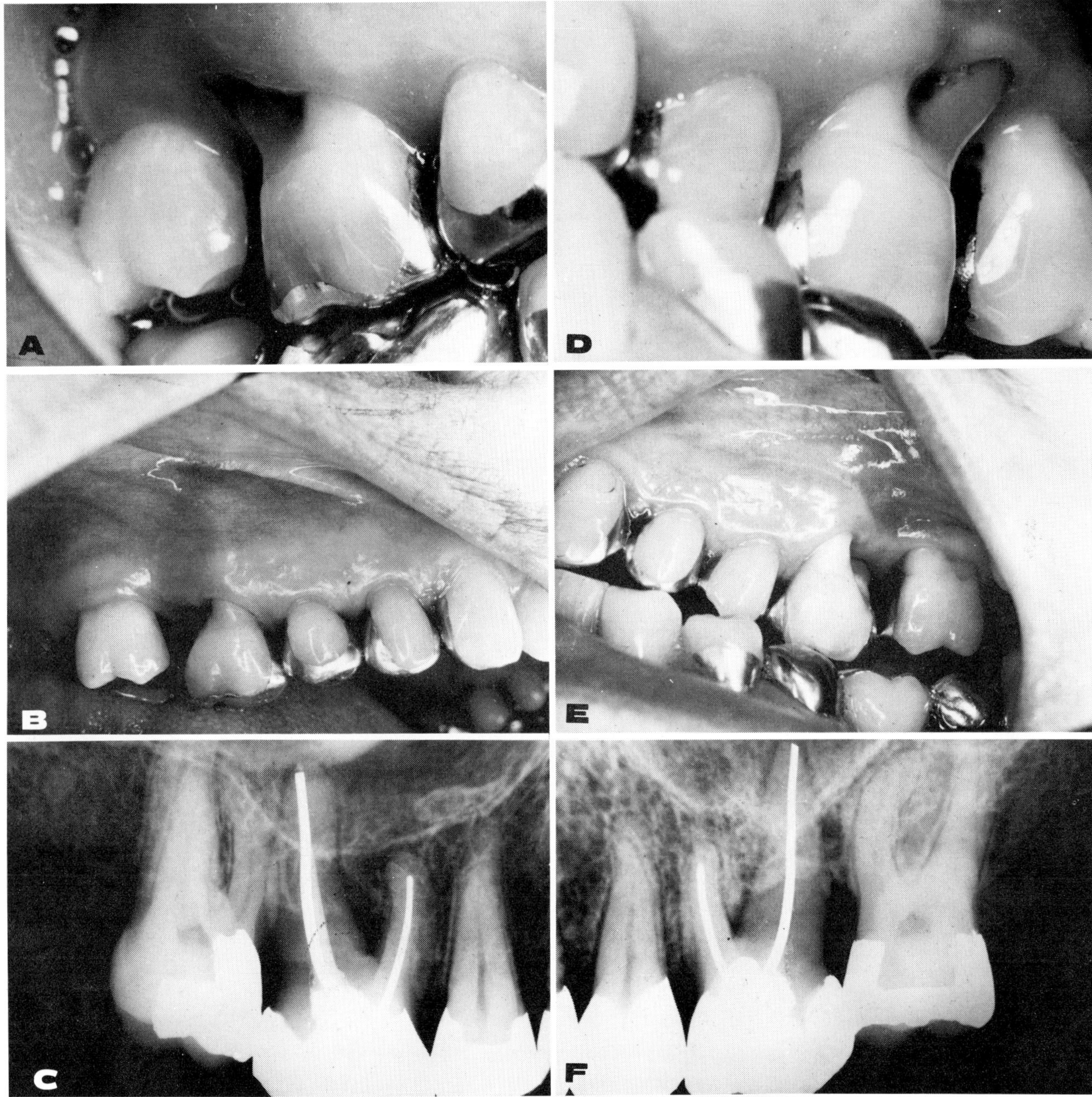

Fig. 15–70. Excellent bilateral examples of importance of shaping amputated area. *A,* Right maxillary first molar prior to root canal therapy and amputation. Distobuccal root has lost its entire bony support. Because furca is exposed, flap need not be raised to amputate this root. *B,* Result six years after amputation. Occlusal table has been narrowed considerably. *C,* Root canal therapy for remaining mesiobuccal and lingual roots. Furca area is easily maintained from distal. *D,* Left maxillary first molar in same patient with bony housing of distobuccal root completely destroyed. *E,* Result six years following root canal therapy and amputation. Patient is meticulous in home care. *F,* Root canal therapy for remaining mesiobuccal and lingual roots.

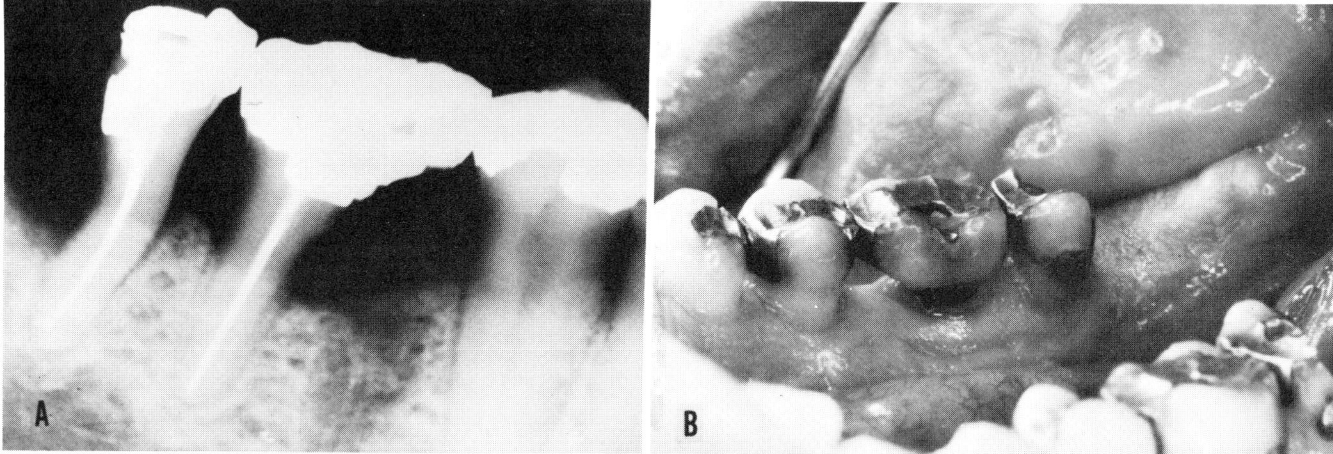

Fig. 15–71. Total root amputation and hemisection for treatment of hopelessly involved molar teeth. *A*, Mesial root of first molar has been amputated and root canal therapy completed for remaining distal root. Second molar has been bicuspidized by hemisection. *B*, Mirror view of result one year following surgery. In spite of failing restorative dentistry, teeth are serviceable. Excellent oral hygiene is maintained by patient. Both amputated first molar and bicuspidized second molar must be crowned and should be splinted.

gingival margin. It should be contoured in a convex, not a concave, shape. The severed root is then removed to the buccal and the flap sutured. The former bridge abutment has now become a bridge pontic.

Hemisection. On occasion it may be necessary to section completely through the crown of a tooth, this half of the crown to be removed with the involved root. Hemisection is the preferred technique if the tooth is to be included in a fixed prosthesis.

The method of approach to hemisection does not materially differ from that of single-root amputation. In this case it is not necessary to place an internal amalgam filling in the root to be amputated, for the entire side of the tooth is to be removed, whereas the remaining half is treated and restored. Molars may be reduced to bicuspid size and still serve a most useful function (Fig. 15–72). Molars with periodontal disease invading the bifurcation may be "bicuspidized" by hemisection. The furca is then turned into an interproximal space where the tissue is more manageable by the patient (Fig. 15–73).

Again, the ultraspeed equipment mounted with a long fissure bur (No. 702 XL) is perfect for sectioning the tooth into two halves; buccal from lingual in the case of maxillary molars and mesial from distal in the mandibular molars (Fig. 15–74). Care must be exercised not to gouge the remaining stump. When the cut is complete, the pathologic half of the tooth is extracted with forceps or eased out with an elevator.

It is important to finish the overhang of the crown at the bifurcation and to smooth the cut surface of the stump down completely to the furca. The remaining half of the tooth may be immediately treated by root canal therapy. A premolar clamp may be placed along with the dam, and pulpectomy, canal shaping, and filling carried out at the same appointment (Fig. 15–75*B*). Final restoration should follow shortly, so that the remaining root has no opportunity to drift (Fig. 15–75*C*).

Long-term excellent prognosis of teeth with roots totally amputated or hemisected is dependent upon the quality of the original surgery and recontouring of the stump, upon the quality of the root canal filling in the remaining roots, and upon the quality of the final restoration. Any one of these can be the "horseshoe nail" that causes the failure of the case. When all these elements are well executed, a superb and lasting result will be achieved (Fig. 15–75*D*).

It may be necessary to recontour a soft tissue defect that may develop after the amputated root is removed. The healed socket should not necessarily be accepted as the final tissue contour. In the case of the palatal root of the maxillary molars, for example, healing usually leaves a deep "dimple" where the root was removed, a defect in form which will be difficult for the patient to maintain following restoration. A

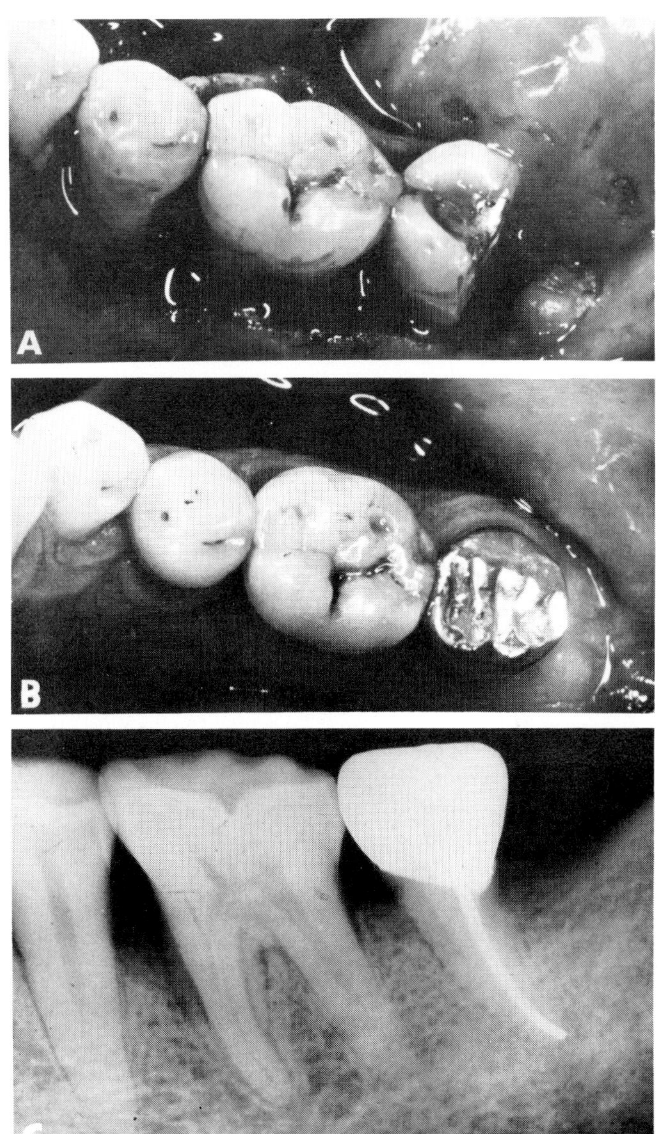

Fig. 15–72. Terminal molar, hemisected and bicuspidized. *A,* Distal half of tooth removed. *B,* Final full crown restoration contacts both adjacent and opposing molars. *C,* Osseous repair around well-restored mesial root one year following therapy.

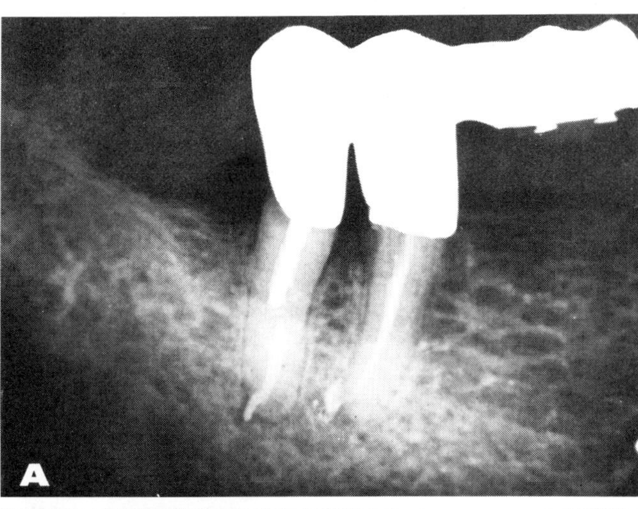

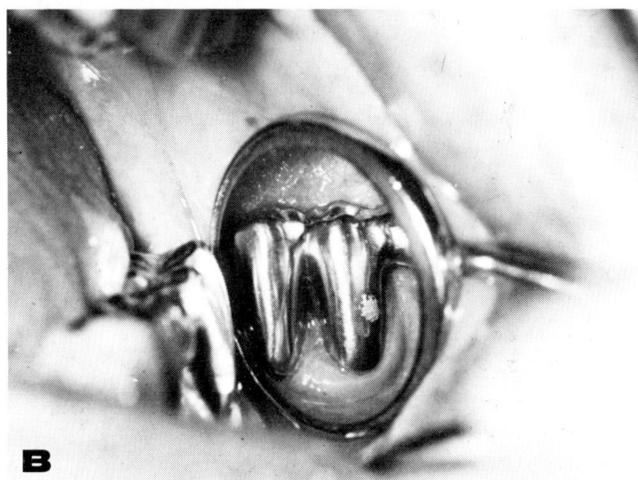

Fig. 15–73. Terminal molar to be used as bridge abutment with periodontal disease involving furca. *A,* Canals obturated with softened gutta percha and tooth hemisected or bicuspidized. *B,* Mirror view of buccal shows how tissue may now be maintained as interdental papilla. (Courtesy Dr. James D. Zidell.)

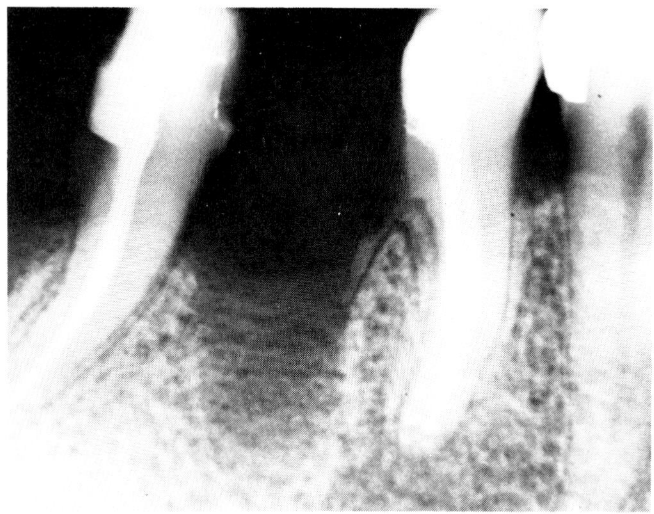

Fig. 15–74. Double hemisection—two molars bicuspidized to serve as abutment teeth. Note that cut has been made at expense of removed portion of tooth. (Courtesy Dr. Alfred L. Frank.)

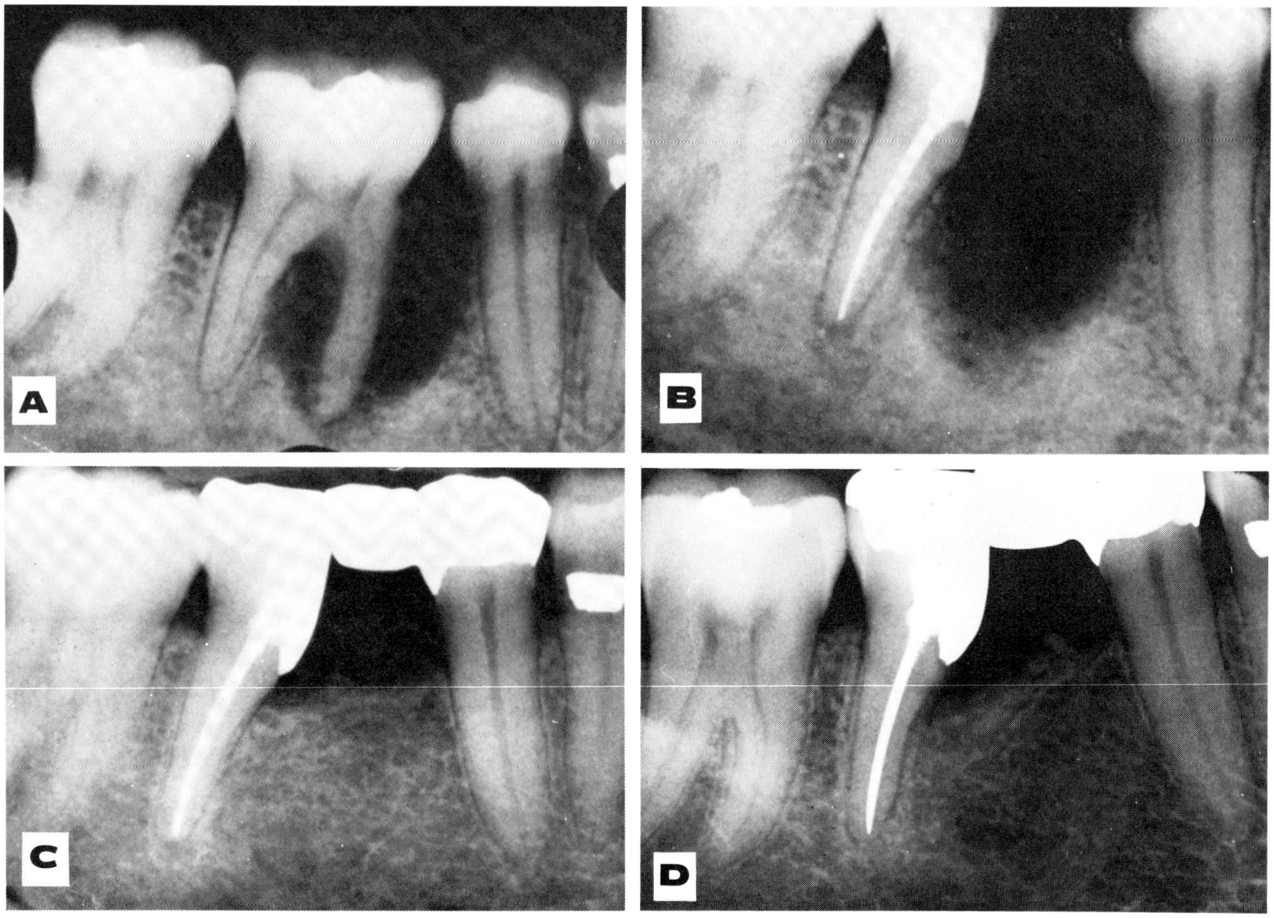

Fig. 15–75. Hemisection of mandibular molar. *A,* Decision to hemisect molar and restore space relates to open contacts and future drifting. *B,* Tooth is cut in half through furca, and pathologic root removed. Root canal therapy for remaining distal root is done at same appointment through exposed pulp chamber. *C,* Final restoration of space converts first molar into bicuspid. *D,* ***Twenty-year*** recall film attests to meticulous therapy and long-range efficacy of this case. (Endodontic therapy and restoration by Dr. James L. McPherson.)

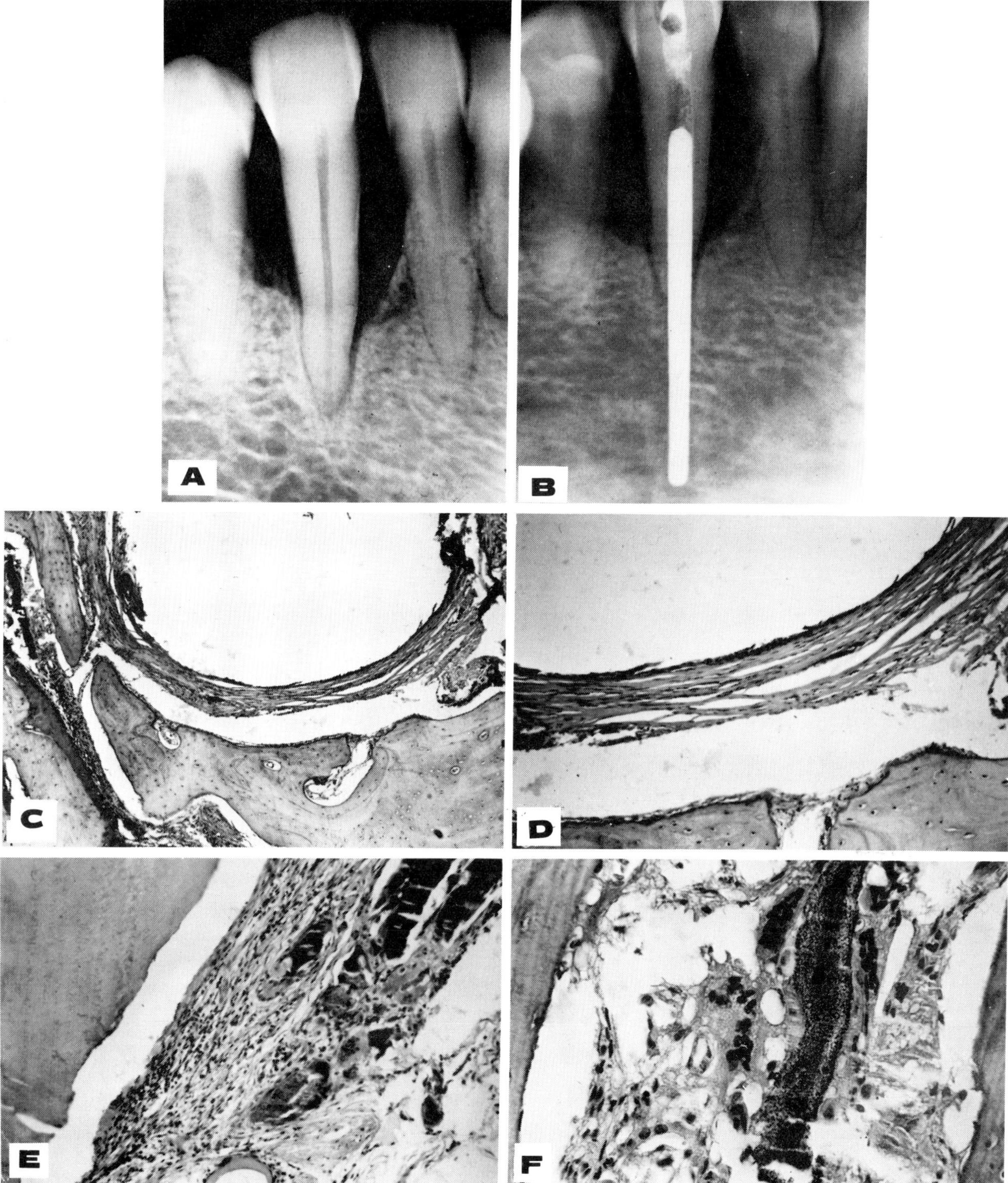

Fig. 15–76. Histologic study of implant failure. *A,* Canine, mobile from periodontal bone loss. Endodontic implant placed and periodontal treatment scheduled. *B,* Forty-four month recall, case failing for lack of periodontal therapy or patient maintenance. Patient agrees to block section removal for histologic examination. *C,* High-power photomicrograph of transverse section through region of implant. Dense strands of fibrous connective tissue separate implant from bone. No inflammation. (Space is histologic preparation artifact.) *D,* Higher power showing mature fibrous capsule and bone with no inflammation or foreign body reaction. *E,* Section of apical root *(left)* with Diaket sealer *(upper right),* foreign body reaction to sealer, and slight chronic inflammation—not adjacent to implant. *F,* High-power photomicrograph of marrow space with Diaket sealer and foreign body reaction. (From Frank, A. L., and Abrams, A. M.: J.A.D.A., *78*:520, Mar., 1969.)

gingivoplasty designed to recontour this tissue will materially add to the assured future of the case (see Fig. 16–26). Extra "rolls" of tissue or vulva-like creases, which would serve as a future bacterial trap, may also have to be removed by gingivoplasty.

All in all, total root amputation and hemisection should be considered only one more weapon in the arsenal of the dentist determined to retain and not remove the dentition. Here more than in any other area, endodontics, periodontics, and restorative dentistry conjoin to maintain the dentition.

ENDODONTIC IMPLANT

Another contributor to this sophisticated armamentarium is the endodontic implant. Teeth that have lost a good portion of their alveolar support through periodontal disease may be stabilized and maintained by the use of the chrome-cobalt endodontic implant. Before the rather heroic endodontic procedures are undertaken, the periodontal disease must be controlled and the cause of the marginal periodontitis eliminated. Then, and only then, should implants be considered.

Chrome-cobalt alloys have long been used for body replacement parts—hip joints, orthopedic plates and screws, and partial dentures. Venable et al. established the fact that in order for an implant to be satisfactory, it would have to be inert and nonelectrolytic.[27] Bernier and Canby demonstrated histologically that these surgical chrome-cobalt alloys are well accepted by soft tissue and bone as alveolar bone implants.[28]

More recently, Seltzer and his associates demonstrated corrosion and inflammation around endodontic implants placed in the molars of a dog.[29] However, it was pointed out subsequently by Weissman that a great difference exists in the chrome-cobalt alloys and that the composition of the alloy tested by Seltzer was not the standard surgical or dental alloy.[30] Sandrik et al., in demonstrating corrosion in alloys used in dentistry, discussed the influence dissimilar metals have in initiating corrosion.[31] From this experience one would suspect that the portion of an endodontic implant that extends into bone should not be handled with metal instruments that may leave microscopic fragments of dissimilar metal to serve as a nidus for future corrosion. Orthopedic surgeons have also learned to use chrome-cobalt screwdrivers to set chrome-cobalt screws. To overcome this possibility, Hodosh has suggested coating endodontic implants with a polymer.[32]

Frank and Abrams were able to examine histologically the tissue surrounding an endodontic implant and found ***no inflammation*** in the collar of dense fibrous connective tissue that separated the metal implant from the bone.[33] They did find inflammation, however, and foreign body reaction in relation to the cement, Diaket, which extruded into the tissue when the implant was cemented (Fig. 15–76).

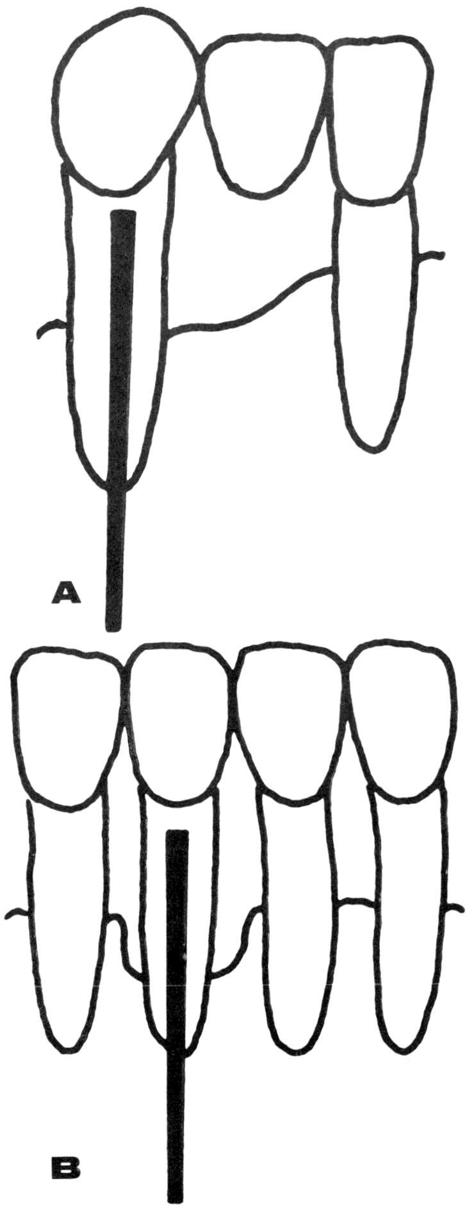

Fig. 15–77. Indications for endodontic implant. *A*, As bridge abutment. *B*, Considerable restorative effort to replace, and adjacent teeth would be poor abutments. (From Frank, A. L.: Dent. Clin. N. Amer., p. 675, Nov., 1967.)

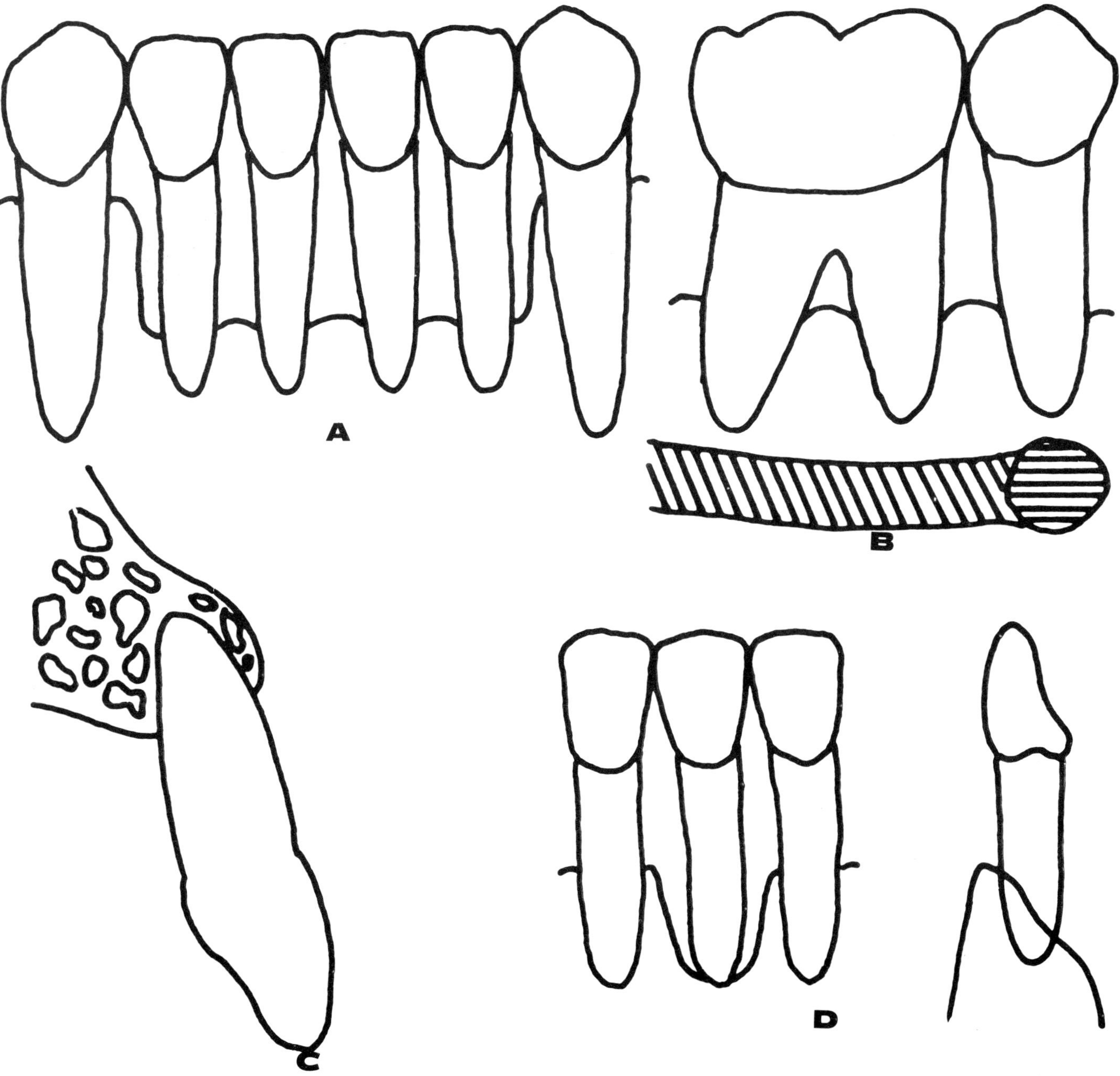

Fig. 15–78. Contraindications for endodontic implant. *A,* Multiple incisors periodontally involved with good canine abutments. *B,* Danger of invading anatomic structures. *C,* Implant would perforate into soft tissue. *D,* Inadequate bony support. (From Frank, A. L.: Dent. Clin. N. Amer., p. 675, Nov., 1967.)

A number of authors have demonstrated the successful use of endodontic implants,[39,40] which are not to be confused with the metallic endosseous post or blade abutment implants. This latter implant pierces the oral mucosa and provides a potential bacterial pathway between the oral cavity and the underlying bone. The endodontic implant is much more predictable of success because it passes through the pulp canal of the tooth to reach the bone and can be completely sealed off.

To stabilize teeth that have lost alveolar support, Frank has listed the indications and contraindications for the endodontic implant.[41,42] At the same time, he has warned against its abuse. He also points out the use of this implant to restore length and stability to fractured teeth, a procedure to be discussed in Chapter 16.

Indications

The candidate for endodontic implant is the patient whose crown-root ratio is unfavorable and can be improved by means of this procedure:

1. When it is necessary to have additional root length for a tooth to serve as a satisfactory bridge abutment (Fig. 15–77*A*).
2. When the extraction and replacement of an isolated periodontally involved tooth would necessitate a considerable restorative effort (Fig. 15–77*B*).
3. When a periodontally involved tooth is present and the adjacent teeth would not be satisfactory abutments (Fig. 15–77*B*).

Contraindications

Endodontic implant is contraindicated:

1. When multiple incisors are periodontally involved and the adjacent teeth would serve as satisfactory abutments (Fig. 15–78*B*).
2. When anatomic structures are in close proximity to the apex and could not be avoided by an implant procedure (Fig. 15–78*B*), for example: mandibular canal, mental foramen, maxillary sinus, the nose.
3. When the inclination of the tooth is such that an implant through the canal would extend out of the facial bone into the soft tissues (Fig. 15–78*C*).
4. When there is a periodontal pocket in close proximity or communicating to the apex of the involved tooth. Special consideration should be given to the buccolingual aspect. It is necessary to appraise the supporting structure with the periodontal probe. The radiograph alone is not adequate (Fig. 15–78*D*).

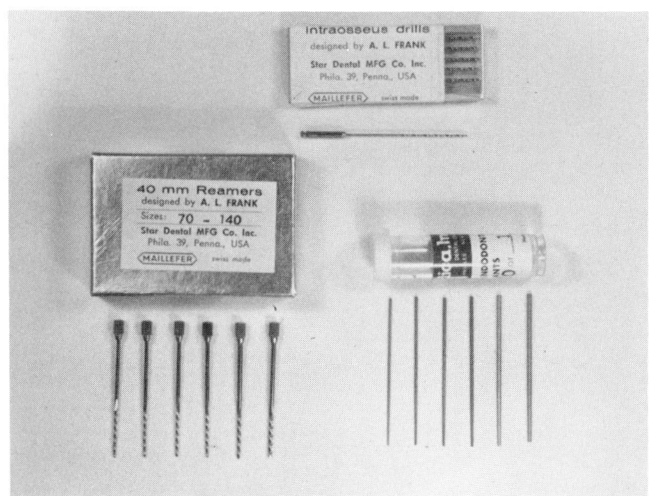

Fig. 15–79. Specialized instruments and selection of endodontic implants. *Top,* Intraosseous drill. *Left,* 40-mm. reamers in standardized sizes 70–140. *Right,* Chrome-cobalt implants. (Courtesy Star Dental Manufacturing Co.)

5. When the patient has had a history of bleeding problems.
6. When the patient has a history of previous bone infection, either in the mouth or in the extremities.
7. When the patient has a history of rheumatic heart disease, diabetes, and other systemic illnesses.

Frank has pointed out that this procedure is not meant as a means of temporary stabilization nor for the terminal periodontal case.[41] He has condemned the misuse of the technique.

Instruments. Special instruments and filling materials are required for the successful outcome of these cases: (1) Extra long (40 mm.) reamers in standardized sizes 70–140, (2) a special intraosseous drill, and (3) standardized chrome-cobalt endodontic implants sizes 70 to 140 (Fig. 15–79). Powell and Bjorndal have shown, however, a lack of conformity of the endodontic implants and special instruments to the system of standardization developed by Ingle.[43] Because of these inaccuracies, the authors warned that an adequate apical seal cannot automatically be expected.

Basic Technique for the *Vital* Periodontally Involved Tooth

One must remember that the implant is being placed for periodontal reasons, not endodontal, and that the vital pulp, in virtually every case, is being sacrificed by intentional extirpation. A final caveat—long-lasting success will be no better than the obturation of the canal by the implant as it passes into the bone. An absolutely round tapered preparation must be made at the apex to be sealed by the round, unyielding implant. Anything less is doomed. Also again, the periodontal disease must be controlled, and at least one-third of the bony support must remain for the tooth under treatment.

Under lidocaine anesthesia with epinephrine 1:50,000, the rubber dam is placed and an access cavity prepared to the pulp. Strict asepsis is maintained. One must bear in mind the rigidity of the chrome-cobalt implant. So to achieve absolutely direct apical approach, the incisal edge of anterior teeth may have to be invaded (Fig. 15–80). Composite final restoration has made repair of this incisal damage much less a problem.

Using an endodontic instrument, the exact tooth length is radiographically established. The vital pulp is then removed by barbed broach and the canal is flooded with 5% sodium hypochlorite, which is allowed to remain. To the actual length of tooth, 2 or 3 mm. are added so that instrumentation will

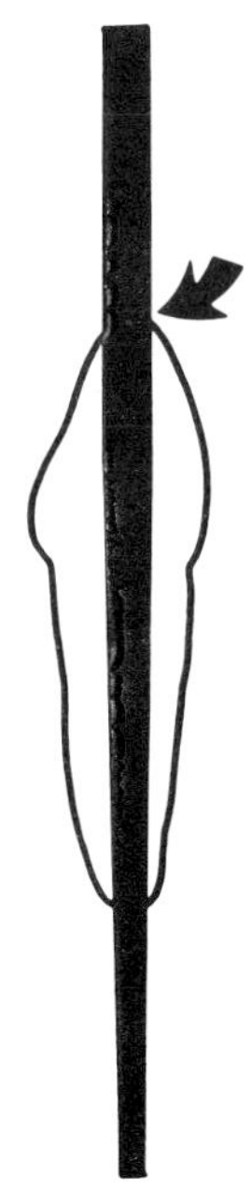

Fig. 15–80. Rigid instruments and implants require invasion of inciso-labial in coronal cavity preparation. It is later restored with composite filling. (From Frank, A. L.: Dent. Clin. N. Amer., p. 675, Nov., 1967.)

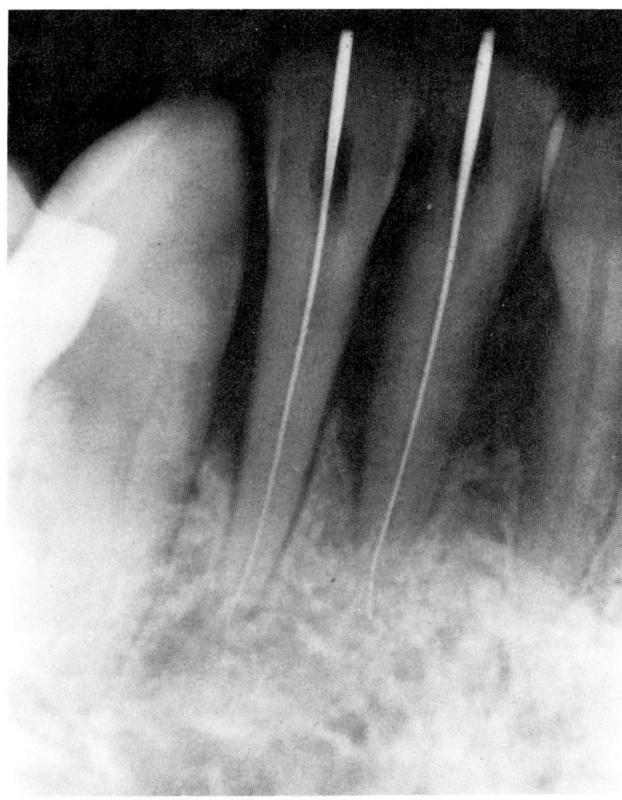

Fig. 15–81. Mandibular incisors to be stabilized with endodontic implants. Vital pulpectomy and canal enlargement with perforation of apex are initial steps. (Courtesy Dr. Alfred L. Frank.)

purposely perforate the apex (Fig. 15–81). This intra- and extracanal enlarging and shaping is carried to at least a size 60 instrument, reaming out through the foramen. The coronal portion of the canal is filed free of the pulp remnants. Constant irrigation is imperative to remove the debris.

At this time, the ***intraosseous*** preparation is begun to receive the implant. The 40-mm. reamers are employed, starting with an instrument three numbers smaller than the last number used in the canal (Fig. 15–82*A*). The bone is carefully reamed up to 10-mm. beyond the apex, advancing through the sizes until one is certain the apical perforation is perfectly round and any ovoid canal has been eliminated at the apex (Fig. 15–82*B*). In treating mandibular incisors (or any teeth for that matter), one must be certain there are not two canals and two orifices to contend with.

In the event the bone is extremely dense and impenetrable to hand instrumentation, it will be necessary to start the osseous preparation with the

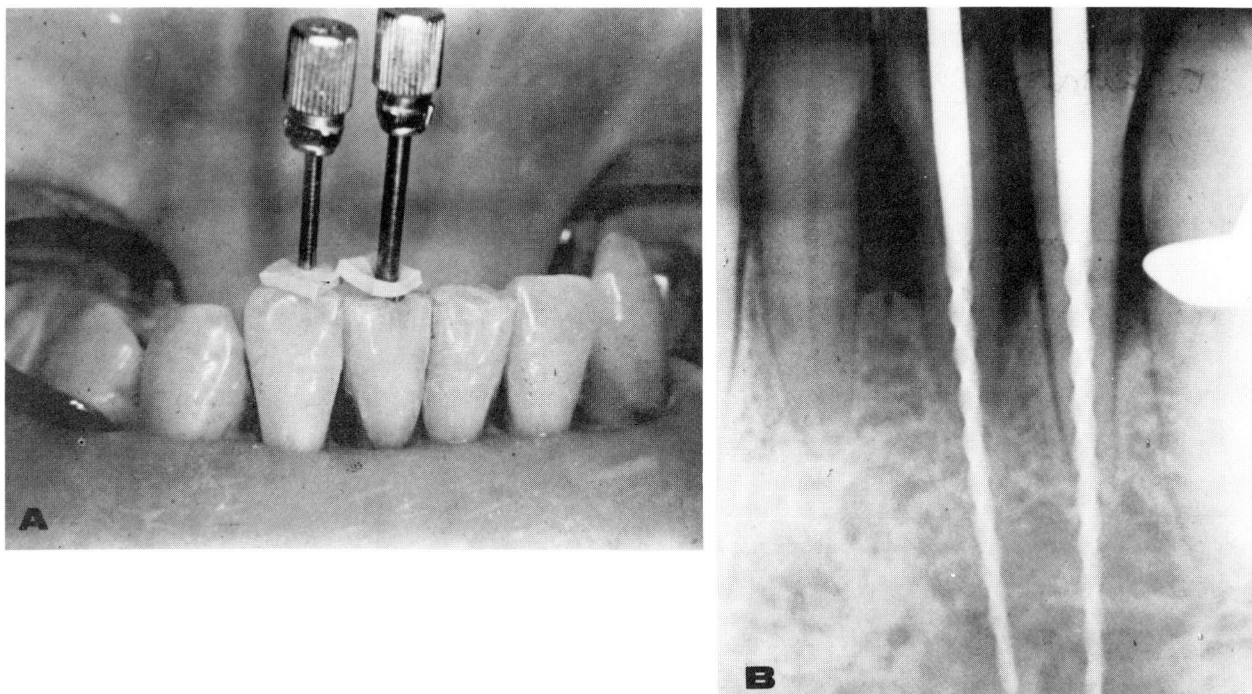

Fig. 15–82. Intraosseous preparation. *A,* Bone apical to lateral incisor is starting to be enlarged with 40-mm. instrument, size 45. Central incisor is being enlarged with size 80 instrument. *B,* Instruments preparing intraosseous cavities. (Courtesy Dr. Alfred L. Frank.)

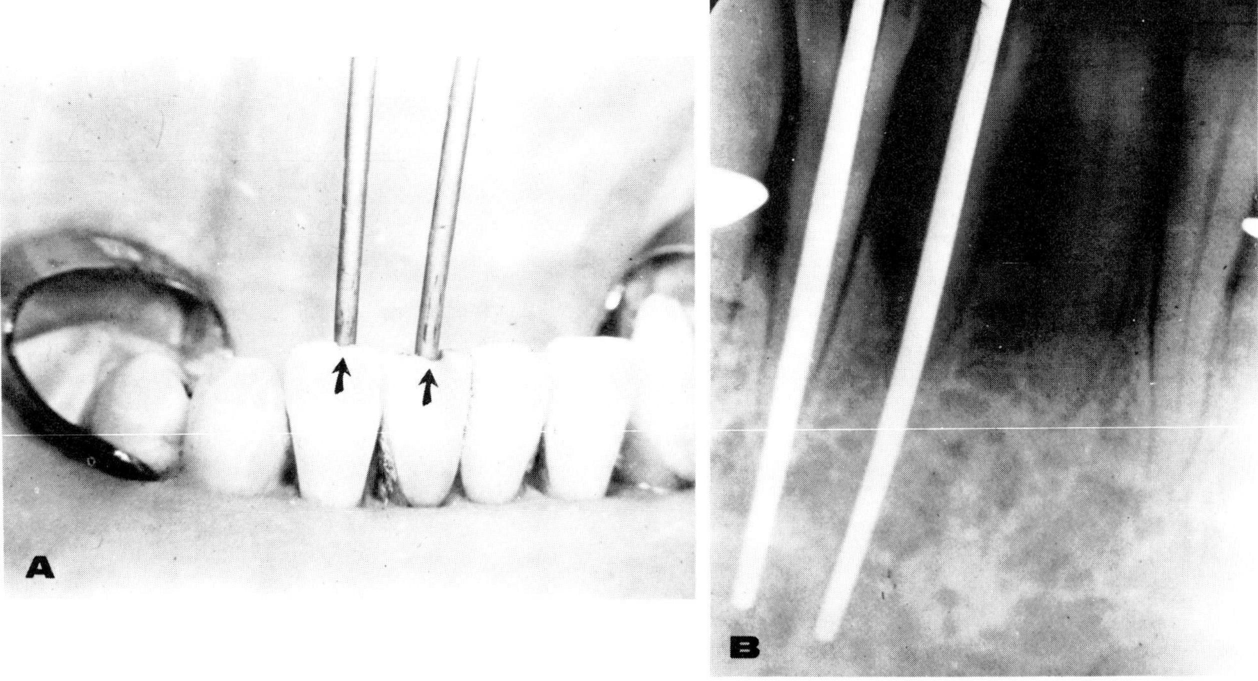

Fig. 15–83. *A,* Trial point implants in place. Notice that both coronal preparations have invaded inciso-labial to gain direct access. *B,* Trial implants in place. To ensure firm seating at tooth apex, both must be shortened by 1 mm. from tip. (Courtesy Dr. Alfred L. Frank.)

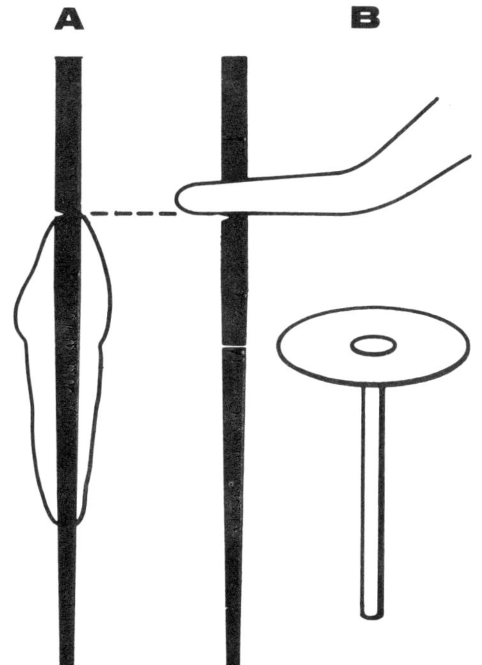

Fig. 15–84. *A,* Fitted implant is nicked at incisal to record length. *B,* Upon removal, implant is sectioned at desired length with carborundum disk. (From Frank, A. L.: Dent. Clin. N. Amer., p. 675, Nov., 1967.)

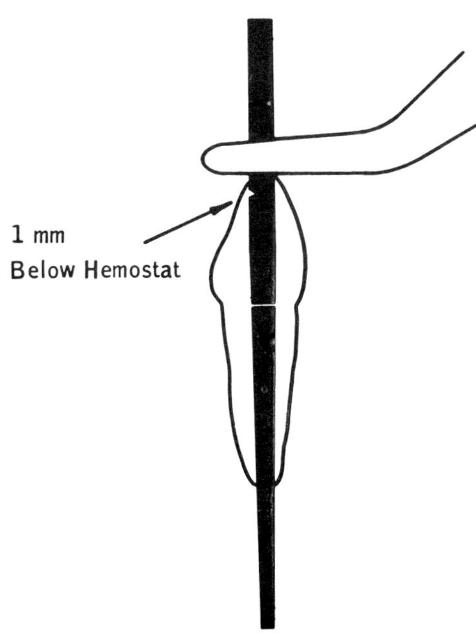

Fig. 15–85. One millimeter is added to "plugger" length of sectional implant to compensate for width of carborundum disk. (From Frank, A. L.: Dent. Clin. N. Amer., p. 675, Nov., 1967.)

extra-long cylindrical drill used in the contra-angle handpiece. It is imperative that an instrument stop be used on the drill just as it was on the long reamers. This is set at the tooth length plus the length of the desired osseous preparation.

The drill is used only to prepare a "starter-hole" in the bone and must be smaller than the prepared apex to avoid binding there. Returning to the 40-mm. reamers, the continuous intracanal-extracanal preparation is completed to at least a size 70 instrument, or until the apex is reamed round.

Paradoxically, bleeding has not been a particular problem. If hemorrhage is encountered, the preparation may be flooded with Orostat, racemic epinephrine (2%), and time allowed for clotting. The canal is dried and the flame-sterilized implant is now tested for fit.

The fit must be firm and tight. A heavy beaked hemostat must be used to seat and remove the implant; cotton pliers are not adequate. The first trial of the implant is to determine whether it will go completely into place at full working length. Fric-

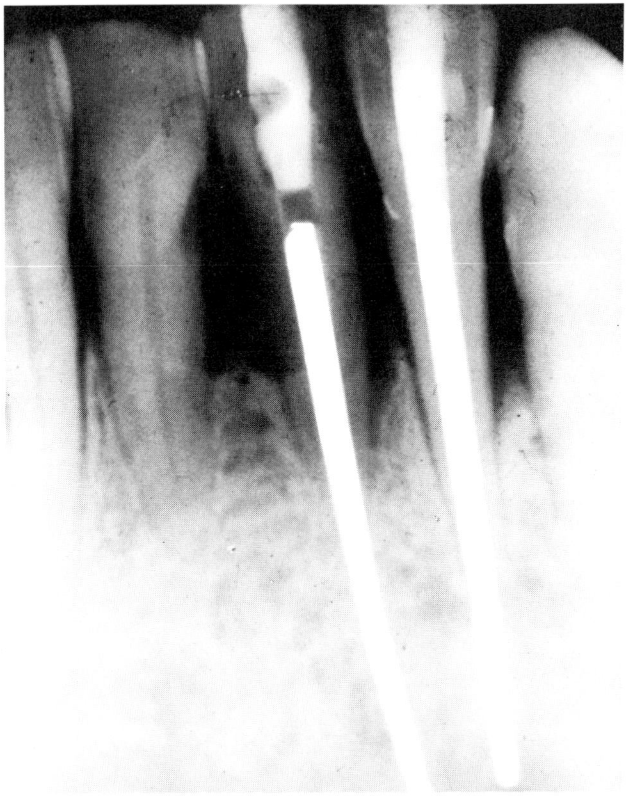

Fig. 15–86. Final treatment film of endodontic implants. Periodontal followup is imperative. (Courtesy Dr. Alfred L. Frank.)

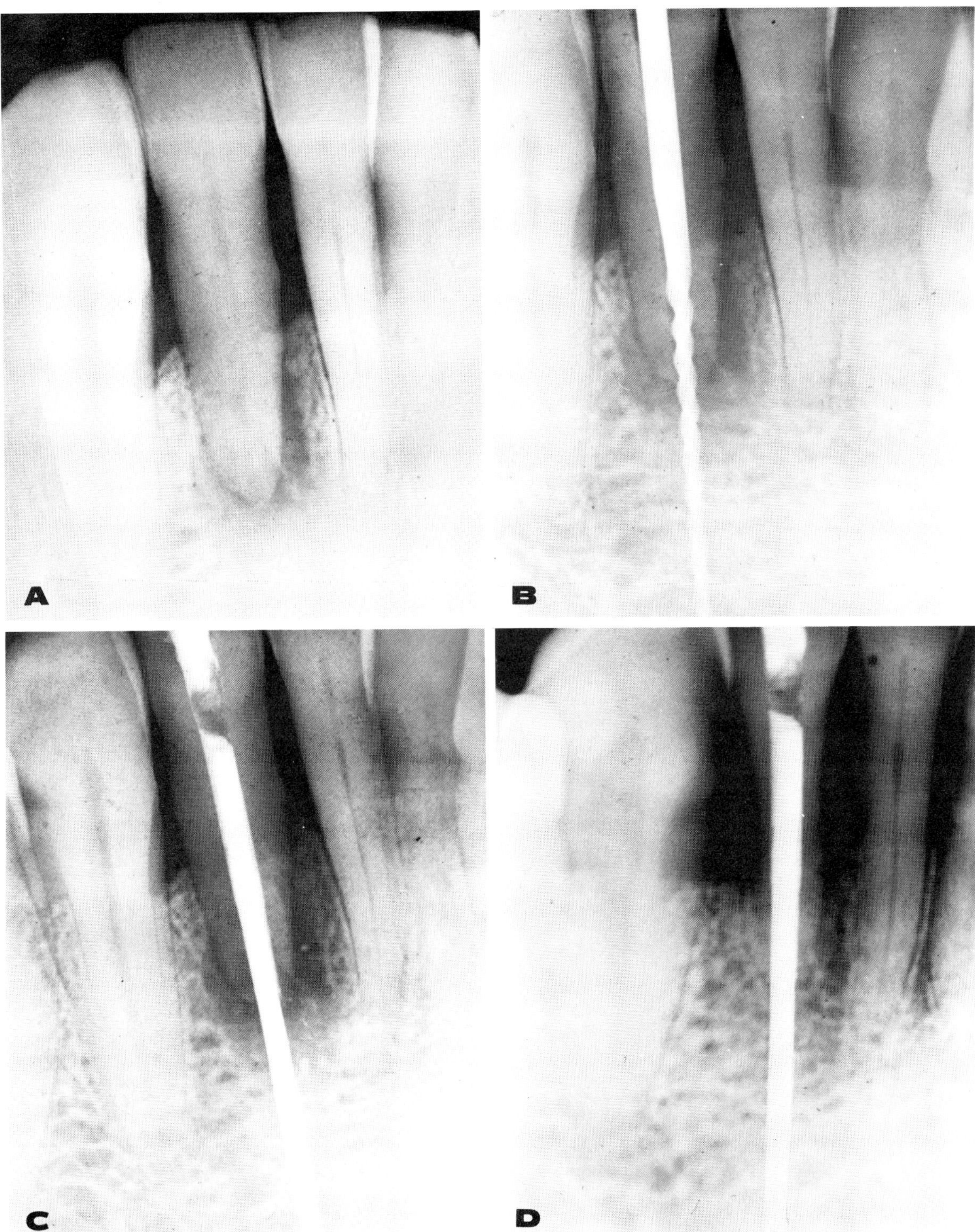

Fig. 15–87. Endodontic implant to stabilize pulpless tooth with combined periodontal lesion. *A,* Preoperative radiograph showing endodontal-periodontal lesion. *B,* Intraosseous preparation. *C,* Cementation of endodontic implant. *D,* Recall radiograph at 18 months. Healing is complete. (From Frank, A. L.: Dent. Clin. N. Amer., p. 675, Nov., 1967.)

tional fit is tested by "tug-back" (Fig. 15–83*A*). The implant is removed and one millimeter is then cut from the tip of the implant and is reseated. This is to ensure that the implant is sealing the apex as it passes through and is not being stopped short by butting against the bone. The final fitted implant should bind firmly at the apex and end ***1 mm. short of the prepared intraosseous length*** (Fig. 15–83*B*). The implant is then marked with a carborundum disk at the incisal edge and withdrawn (Fig. 15–84*A*). The canal is thoroughly irrigated with dilute sodium hypochlorite and dried thoroughly with blunted absorbent paper points. The points are premeasured to be used only within the canal and not disturb the intraosseous blood clot. If hemorrhage persists, a blunted paper point is left in the canal for a clot to form against. Cementation is delayed until the blood clot has formed.

The implant must be completely separated with a carborundum disk at a point below the gingival level or even further if a dowel restoration is to be used (Figure 15–84*B*). Care is then taken to thoroughly coat with cement only the portion of the flame-sterilized implant that will be in the canal. The implant is dropped to place and forced into position, its remaining portion serving as a plugger. One millimeter is added to the implant "plugger" to compensate for the 1 mm lost in separating the implant with the carborundum disk (Fig. 15–85). When the incisal mark is 1 mm. below the incisal edge, a final confirmatory radiograph is taken (Fig. 15–86). Gutta percha is placed to seal off the implant and a final coronal composite restoration is inserted.

Modifications

There are modifications of the ***vital*** pulp technique just described. One deals, of course, with the necrotic rather than the vital pulp. In the latter case, the implant is placed in one appointment. In the necrotic case, basic endodontic procedures are followed in cleaning, shaping, and sanitizing the canal before the apex is perforated. These preliminaries necessitate at least one extra appointment before implantation procedure is begun. Placement of the implant will materially stabilize a mobile root. At the same time, a preexisting periapical lesion should be expected to heal (Fig. 15–87).

Another modification concerns the situation in which the implant would perforate the cortical bone because of the position of the tooth in the alveolus

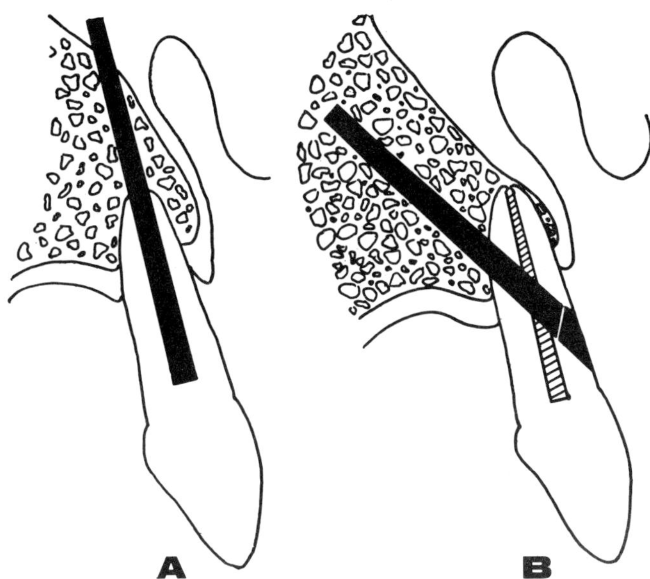

Fig. 15–88. *A,* It is imperative that replant be entirely intraosseous. *B,* Modification of conventional implant placement to take advantage of palatal bone for stabilization. (From Frank, A. L.: Dent. Clin. N. Amer., p. 675, Nov., 1967.)

(Fig. 15–88*A*). If such is the case in the maxilla, the large mass of cancellous bone in the palate may be used for support (Fig. 15–88*B*). As a first step, the entire root canal must be cleaned, shaped, and obturated in the usual manner (Fig. 15–89). Then a labial flap is raised and a nick is made with a round bur in the proper position on the labial of the root. This countersink is to better position the cylindrical drill which is used to cut from labial to lingual, right through the center of the gutta percha filled canal, and about 10 mm. into the palatal bone. The drill must be carefully oriented to accurately make this initial cut (Fig. 15–90). Hand instruments are then employed to enlarge both the tooth and the intraosseous preparation to a large size—at least number 70. The implant is then cemented into place (Fig. 15–91*A*), and the labial cavity is filled with composite cement before the flap is replaced (Fig. 15–91*B*).

The treatment of the curved canal is similar to the technique just described. The curved root is shaped and filled in the conventional manner, using lateral or vertical compaction of the gutta percha filling. The implant is then made, bypassing the apical filling, perforating the root at the elbow, and extending the implant out into the cancellous bone (Fig. 15–92).

If the treated teeth are exceptionally mobile, they

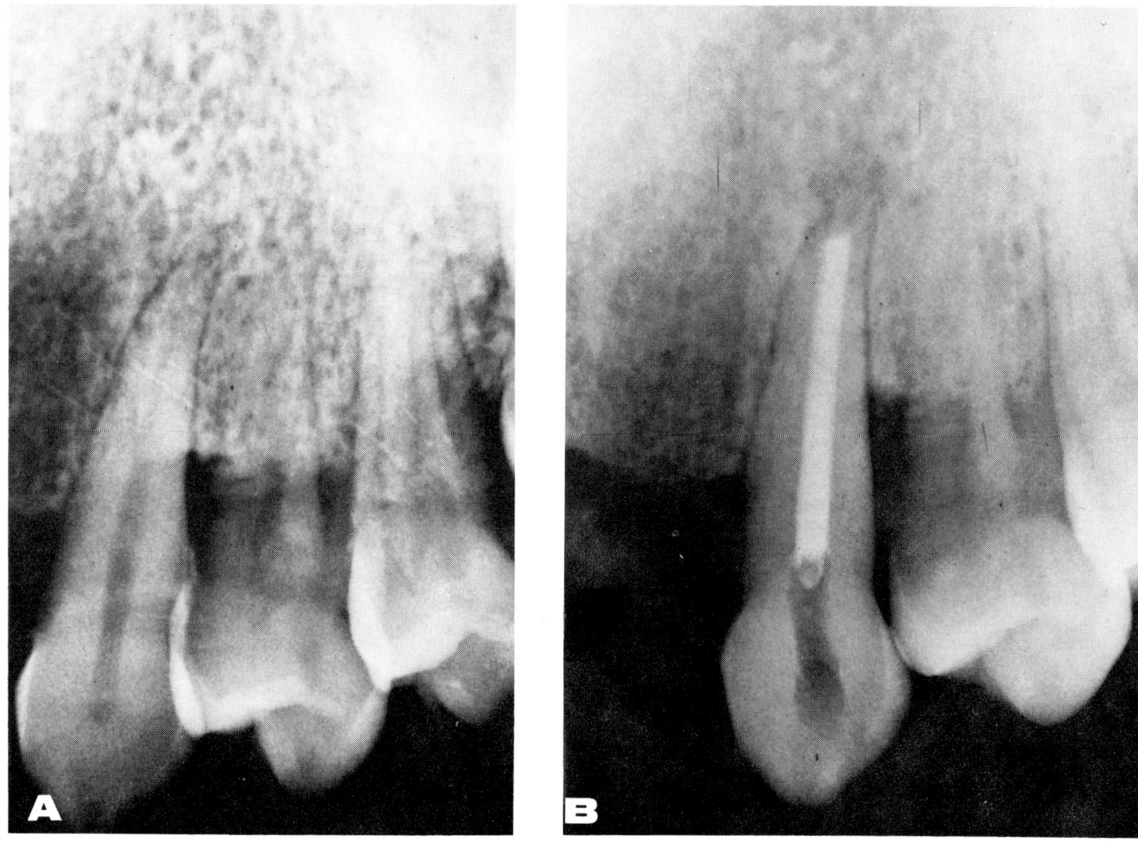

Fig. 15–89. *A,* Periodontally involved canine needs stabilization to become effective abutment. *B,* Pulpectomy, canal preparation, and obturation with gutta percha. (From Frank, A. L.: J.A.D.A., *74*:451, Feb., 1967.)

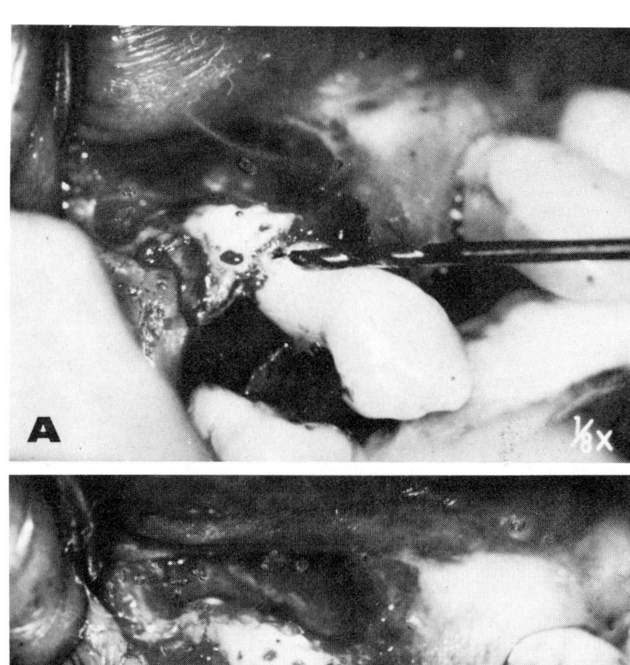

Fig. 15–90. *A,* Cylindrical drill preparing pathway for intraosseous preparation into palatal cancellous bone. *B,* Trial fit of endodontic implant. (From Frank, A. L.: J.A.D.A., *74*:451, Feb., 1967.)

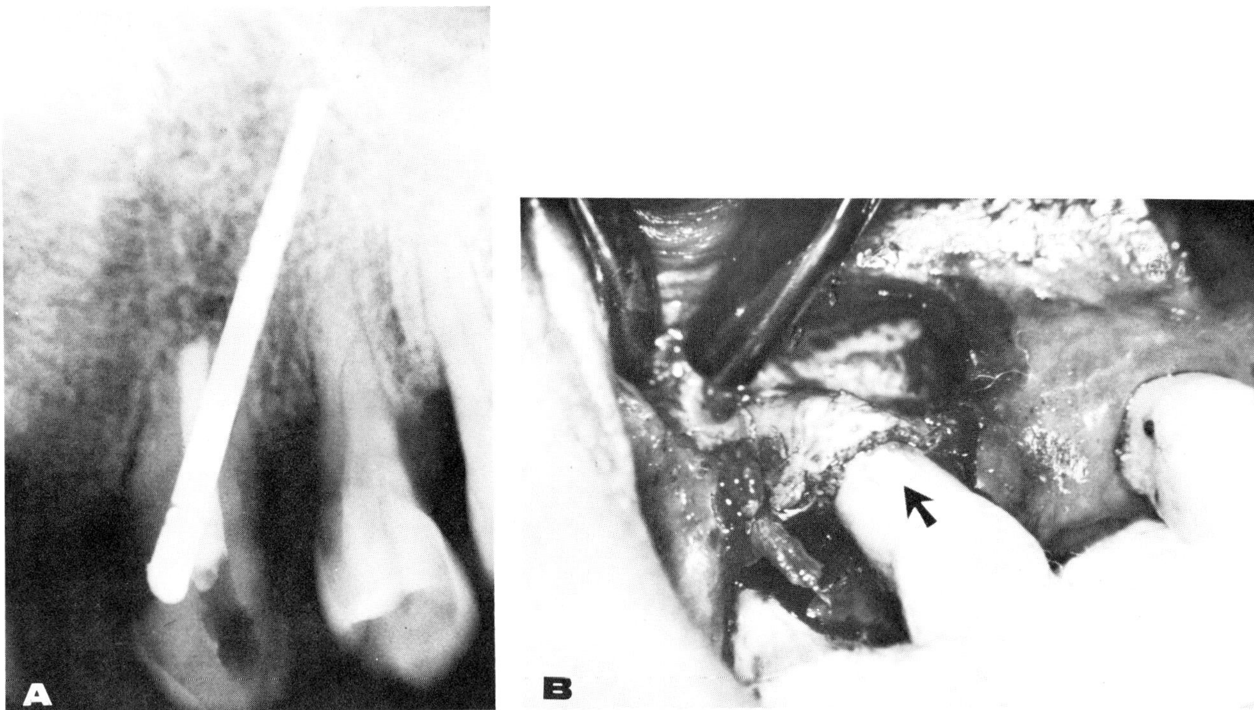

Fig. 15–91. *A*, Final radiograph of endodontic implant extending from labial of canine into palate. Weird appearance of radiograph should be explained to patient for future reference. *B*, Composite restoration *(arrow)* is placed in labial cavity before flap is sutured. (From Frank, A. L.: J.A.D.A., *74*:451, Feb., 1967.)

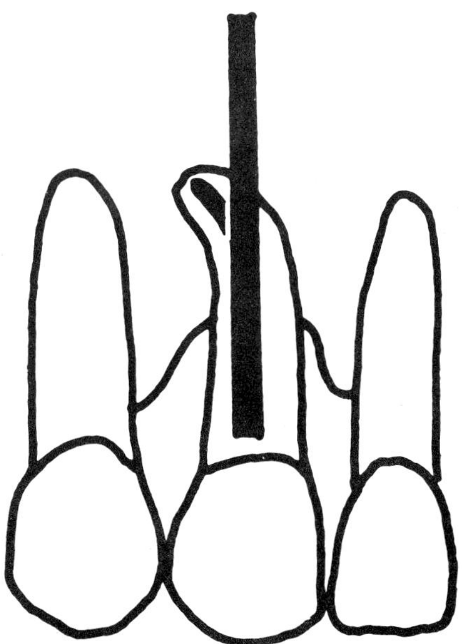

Fig. 15–92. Modification of use of endodontic implant for curved root. Canal is sealed with gutta percha and intentional perforation for implant is at "elbow" into bone. (From Frank, A. L.: Dent. Clin. N. Amer., p. 675, Nov., 1967.)

should be temporarily stabilized for three or four weeks while healing takes place. Frank has also found it advisable to permanently splint the involved tooth to an approximating tooth, if at all possible.[44]

ROOT-RESORPTIVE DEFECT

Eventual repair of a defect on the root surface from either internal or external resorption will depend, in large part, on whether there is a complete communication from the pulp to the oral cavity. If the lesion has destroyed an area of the root into the periodontal structures, but has not communicated with the oral cavity, it can generally be repaired by inserting a material such as calcium hydroxide into the cleaned and prepared root canal in an attempt to promote cementogenesis. One should expect cementification and bone repair to follow, and finally the internal and external defects may be obturated by nonsurgical root canal filling alone (see Cementogenesis, pp. 696–700).

In the event cementogenesis and new bone formation do not occur to serve as a matrix for the internal filling of the canal and defect, or in the event the lesion has broken through to communicate with the oral cavity (Fig. 15–93*A*) and will not respond by cementogenesis, corrective radicular surgery is in order.

If the clinician is at all unsure about the lesion, it is suggested that a flap be raised to inspect the defect visually. Plans to proceed will then be much clearer (Fig. 15–93*A,B*). Circular or scalloped flaps are seldom used in corrective surgery, for the full length of a root must be inspected. If the lesion is near the gingiva, a triangular flap may be used. Either a trapezoidal or rectangular flap must be used, however, if the defect extends to or beyond the apex.

If the decision is made to fill the root defect before filling the canal, an internal matrix must be used in the canal after the suggestion by Dow.[45] The standard coronal preparation is completed and the pulp is removed. A silver point is then temporarily placed in the canal, and the lesion on the root is smoothed and undercut to receive an amalgam filling (Fig. 15–93*C,D*).

The zinc-free alloy amalgam is condensed and trimmed with a sharp carver. Loose amalgam particles are irrigated and aspirated away. The temporary silver point may then be removed and the flap sutured back to position (Fig. 15–93*E,F*).

Either at this appointment or subsequently, canal enlargement and filling are completed. If the pulp canal is thought to be infected, intracanal medication should be used and the root canal therapy completed at a later date. The final result should be full repair in the area of the defect and normal periapical health as well (Fig. 15–93*G,H*).

In the case of the defect which opens into the sulcus, the approach will depend to a great extent upon the location of the lesion. If the defect is approachable from the labial, a flap should be raised. This is less disfiguring after surgery than a gingivectomy (see Fig. 1–32). Here again, the root canal filling may be completed before the defect is restored with composite filling material, or a temporary silver point may be used to keep the canal patent during repair. Reattachment of the tissue should develop to the very margin of the filling. This deep sulcus may be maintained by periodontal curettage of the soft tissue lining two or three times a year. The patient should be shown how to care for the area with toothbrushing.

If the resorptive defect is into the sulcus on the lingual, it is better to do a gingivectomy in the area, exposing the entire margin of the lesion (Fig. 15–94). The root canal therapy is completed and the defect restored with a well-condensed amalgam which can later be polished (Fig. 15–94*C*). If the amalgam shows through the labial enamel of the crown, care should be taken to place a cement base toward the labial.

Some cases of resorption are so extensive nothing can save the tooth or one of its roots. Extraction may be the solution for some cases or total root amputation or hemisection for others. A case in point, calling for hemisection, is illustrated in Figure 15–95. Internal-external resorption has destroyed virtually one-half of a lower first molar, a terminal tooth in the arch with an excellent opponent molar as well. Probing with a cowhorn explorer and viewing the radiograph reveals the massive lesion and defect (Fig. 15–95*A,B*). The crown of the tooth is sectioned buccolingually with a high-speed fissure bur (Fig. 15–95*C,D,E*). The mesial crown and root are then extracted, and immediate root canal therapy is completed in the remaining distal root (Fig. 15–95*F,G.*). A premolar clamp may be used on the "bicuspidized" remaining half of the molar. Finally, the tooth and the space should be restored very soon to avoid tipping of the free section (Fig. 15–95*H*). Function against the maxillary opponents prevents their continual eruption.

Much of the treatment in correcting resorptive defects is applied ingenuity with standard methods of treatment. It is important not to consider a case necessarily hopeless without first investigating the possibilities of treatment.

FRACTURE DEFECT

Teeth suffering coronal fractures that involve both the pulp and periodontal structures often may be saved by combined endodontic-periodontic corrective surgery. If, by examination, it appears practical to undertake therapy, the periodontal surgery is first completed to establish enough "crown" length for a rubber dam clamp. This was thoroughly discussed under "Endodontal-Periodontal Defects," page 641.

Repair of root fractures, both horizontal and vertical, is usually a nonsurgical procedure. Normal biologic repair of ***horizontal*** root fractures should first be sought (Fig. 15–96), and this failing, cementogenesis should be attempted by packing a cleansed and shaped canal with a material such as calcium hydroxide. Good results have been achieved by this

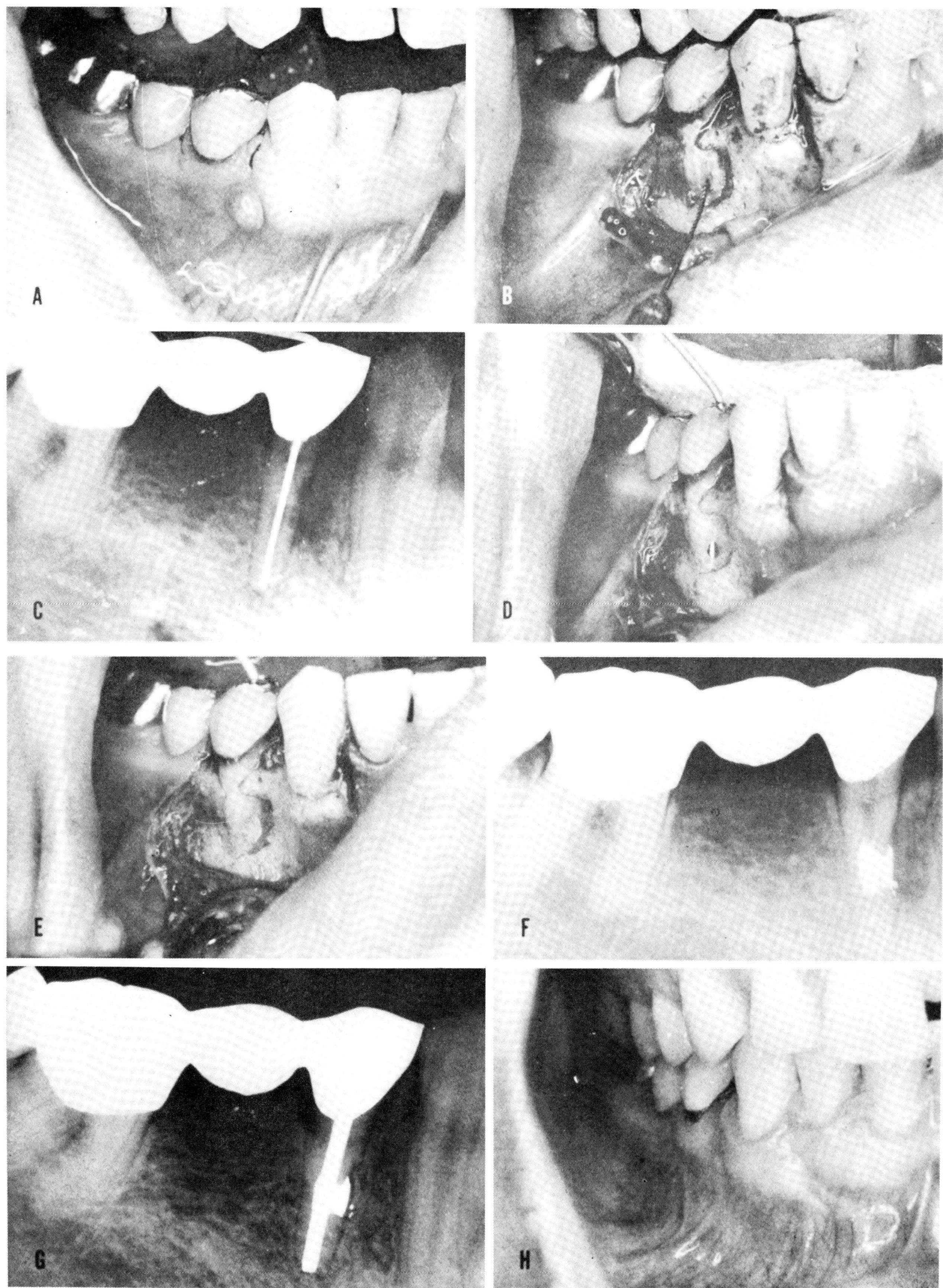

Fig. 15–93. *(Legend on opposite page)*

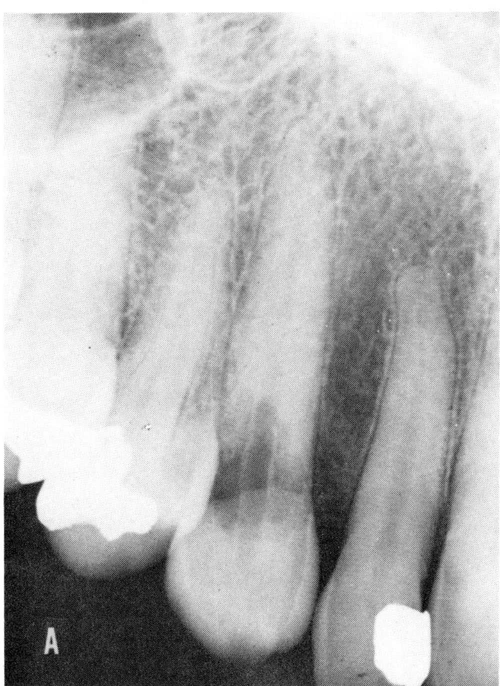

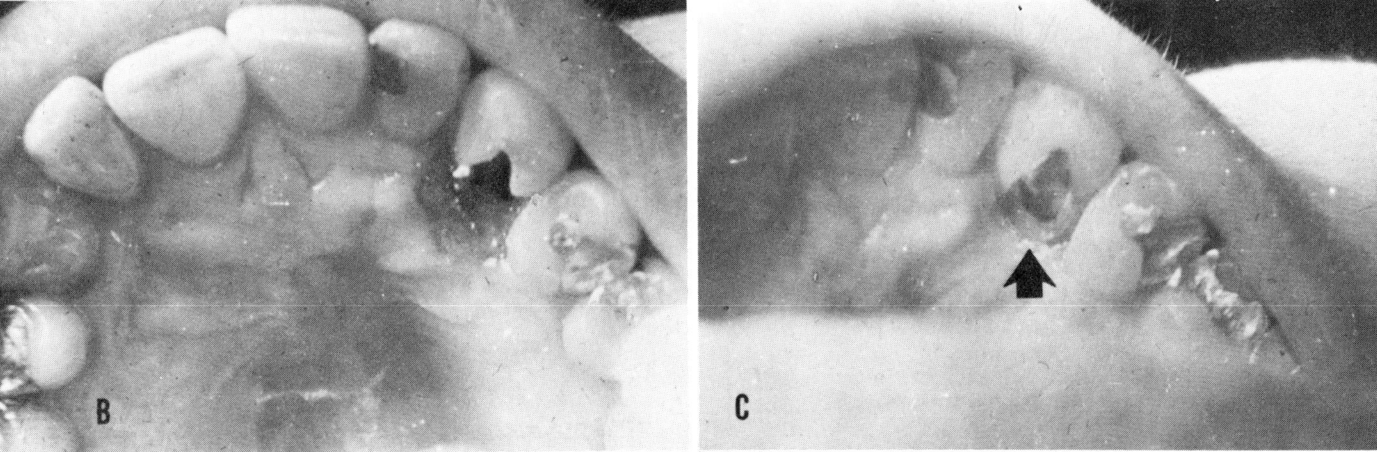

Fig. 15–94. Surgical correction of internal resorptive defect which has opened into lingual sulcus. *A,* Roentgenogram of defect. *B,* Palatal gingivoplasty exposes margins of defect. Cavity preparation extends to central axis allowing unstrained approach to canal and apex. Pulpectomy, canal enlargement, and root canal filling complete therapy. Labial cement base prevents lingual amalgam from showing through. *C,* Tissue adaptation to polished amalgam filling *(arrow)* is apparent in three months.

Fig. 15–93. Corrective surgical repair of root-resorptive defect. *A,* Constant drainage mesial to first premolar bridge abutment. Internal and external resorption were revealed in roentgenogram. *B,* Elevating rectangular flap reveals huge dehiscence and resorptive defect. Instrument placed into defect proves connection with pulp lesion. *C,* Conventional occlusal endodontic cavity is prepared and pulpectomy is performed. Internal matrix of endodontic silver point is placed. *D,* Internal matrix in place and hemorrhage controlled. *E,* Amalgam filling inserted into external resorptive defect. Non-zinc alloy is used. *F,* Silver point is immediately removed and flap repositioned and sutured. Because of time constraints in this particular case, canal enlargement and obliteration are completed at subsequent appointment. *G,* Roentgenogram 9 months following therapy. Repair of bone is apparent. *H,* Photograph nine months following therapy. Note complete repair of draining fistula and incisions. (Courtesy Dr. David Yankowitz.)

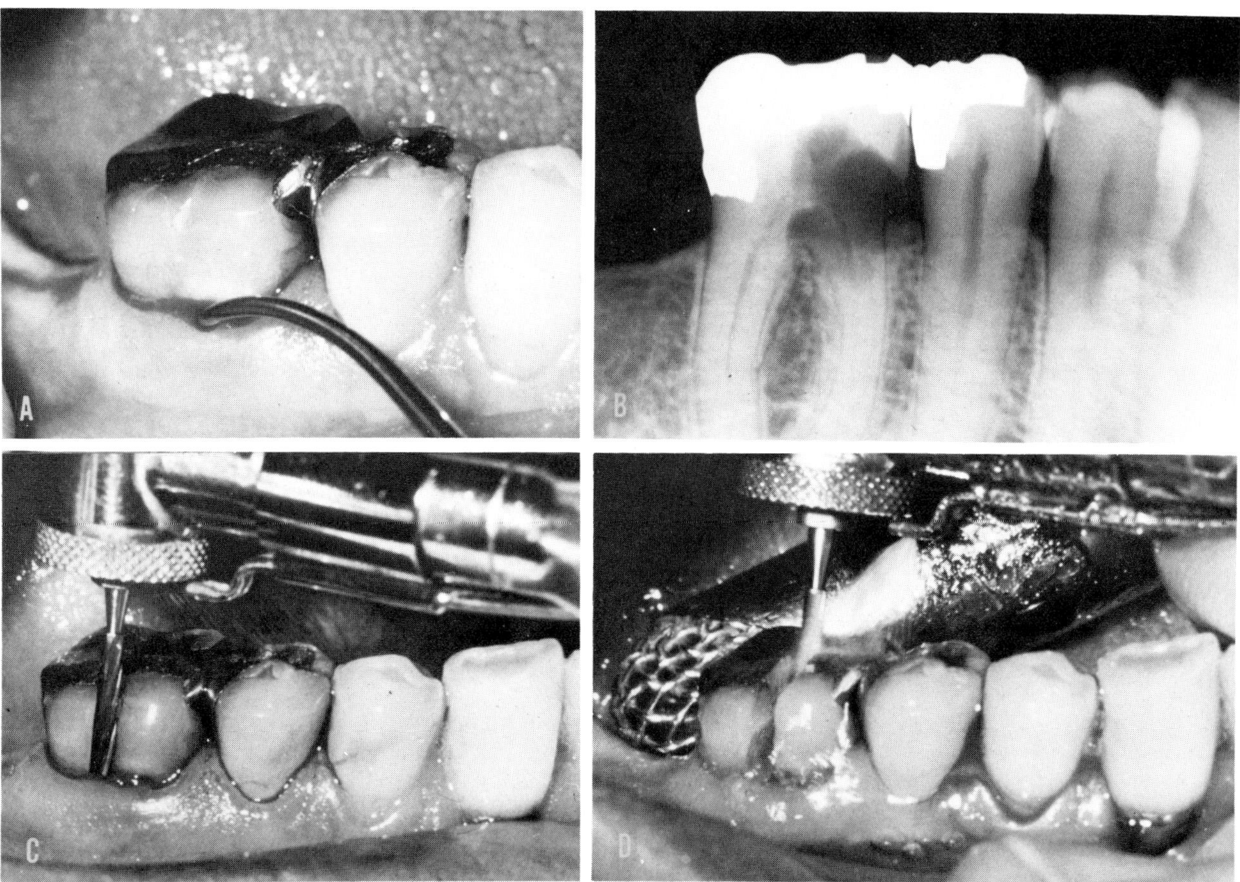

Fig. 15–95. Technique for hemisecting and restoring mandibular molar. *A,* Using cowhorn explorer, resorptive lesion and relation to crest of alveolar process are established. *B,* Huge area of internal resorption involving mesial half of molar. *C,* An extra long, No. 559-XL fissure bur has length of reach necessary to cut entirely through crown to furca. *D,* Tooth is sectioned from buccal to lingual with copious water coolant and aspiration. Extra long bur, in metal chuck high-speed handpiece, spins with absolute concentricity.

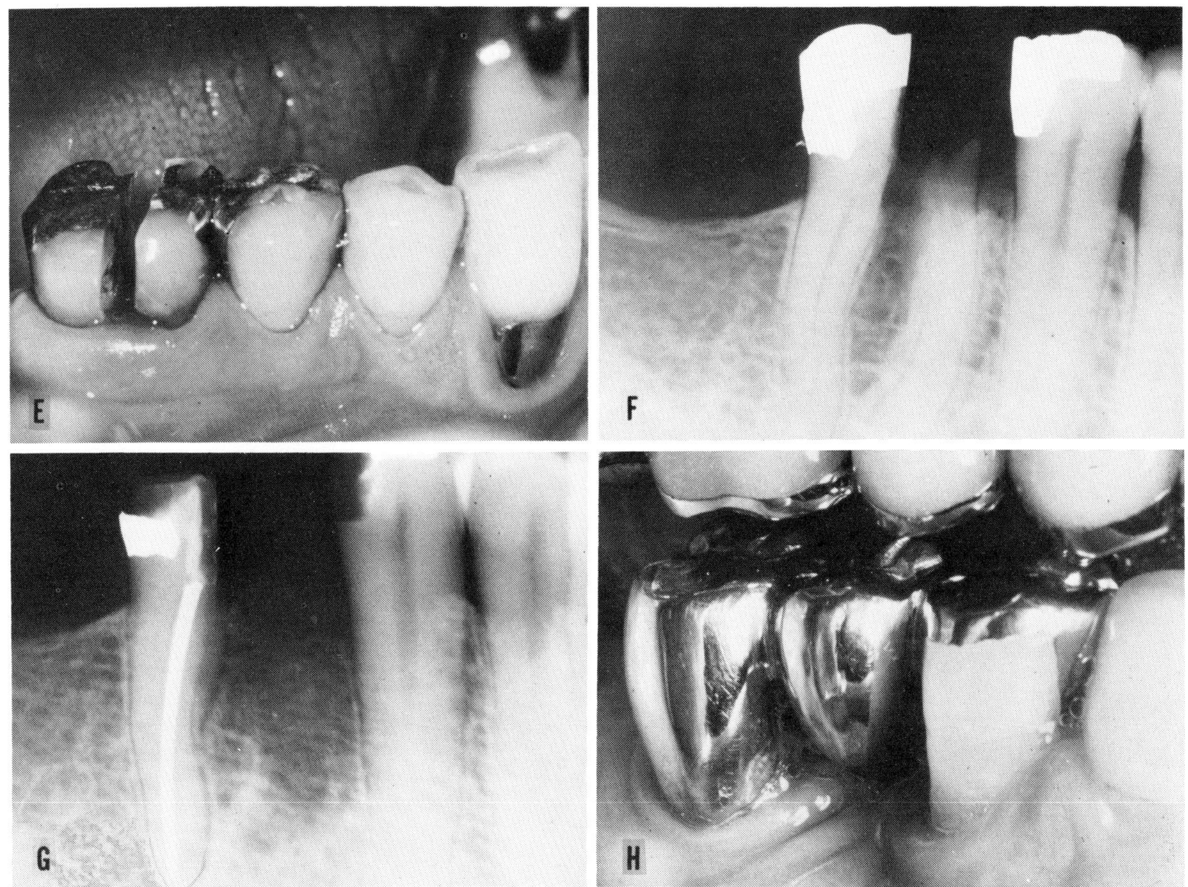

Fig. 15–95. *(Continued)*

E, Sectioning completed. Base of cut must terminate at alveolar crest. *F,* Hemisected mandibular molar. Pathologic mesial half is ready for extraction. Accuracy of sectioning is shown by roentgenogram. *G,* Care must be exercised not to gouge remaining distal portion. Root canal therapy is completed at same dental appointment. Teeth are ready for immediate restoration. *H,* Importance of restoration for contact with opposite arch is here demonstrated. (Restoration by Dr. Milan V. Starks.)

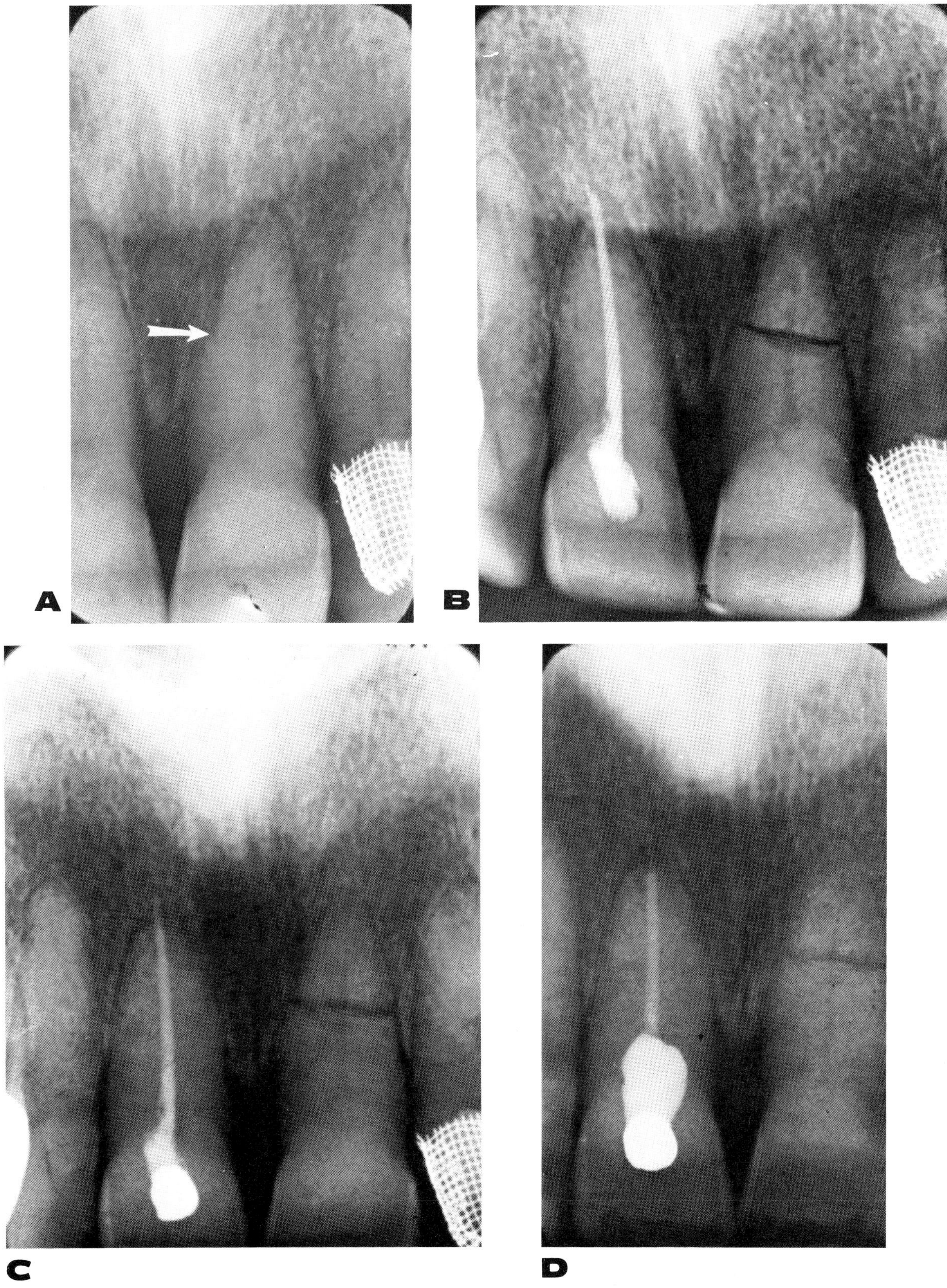

Fig. 15–96. *(Legend on opposite page.)*

approach as reported in the section on cementogenesis, page 696.

The vertical root fracture is something else and most dentists are quite pessimistic about a good prognosis for these cases. Some fracture cases are so badly infected and phoenix-like in nature that nothing will suffice but extraction. In some cases, cementification should be attempted. If mastication constantly separates the two halves for bacterial ingress, nothing will work. If an attempt at cementogenesis fails, and an abscess recurs at the fracture site, the prognosis is bleak and extraction or total root amputation (in the case of multirooted teeth) should be done before a large bony defect forms.

CARIOUS DEFECT

Dental caries often may extend below gingival level and into the pulp as well. The tooth involved could be most important; a bridge abutment, for example (Fig. 15–97*A,B*). Corrective surgery is often the answer to retaining an important tooth.

A huge roll of gingival tissue may be removed by gingivectomy, freeing the margins of the cavity and "elongating" the crown so that a rubber dam clamp can be positioned (Fig. 15–97*C*). Following root canal therapy and gingival healing, a new restoration may be placed (Fig. 15–97*D*).

Dow has recommended the use of gingival surgery for Class V carious defects that invade the pulp and must be restored before root canal therapy is undertaken.[45]

ANOMALOUS DEFECT

The most common tooth anomaly requiring corrective surgery is the invaginated maxillary lateral incisor in which the "second" pulp may become necrotic, the so-called *dens invaginatus* or *dens in dente.* In the event the peculiarly shaped canal cannot be properly obturated or even properly cleansed or prepared, surgical exposure of the root surface may be in order to evaluate the aberrant foramens and obturate the openings with retrofillings (Fig. 15–98). Attempts at cementogenesis and canal filling with softened gutta percha should be tried first, however.

INTENTIONAL REPLANTATION

(See also, Chapter 16)

There are some teeth requiring root canal therapy which are absolutely inoperable *in situ.* Pulpless molar teeth in mouths with such a small orifice that finger manipulation is impossible in the posterior mouth are examples of candidates for extraction and intentional replantation.

Pulpless teeth have also been encountered with so many perforations or lateral aberrations of the canal that repair *in situ* was impossible (see Fig. 16–50). If extraction appears to be the only answer to these cases one is right to pose, "What have we to lose?" by attempting replantation (Fig. 15–99).

Before the tooth is extracted a method of retaining the tooth during reattachment should be devised. One possibility is to take impressions prior to extraction and to construct a banded splint. Bands also may be adapted in the mouth and welded together to be ready for cementation at the time of replantation. In the anterior mouth the "boxer's guard" type of splint can be used (see Fig. 16–45). However, this is an emergency approach and intentional replantation should not be emergent, but rather elective and well planned.

After the splint is constructed, the tooth is anesthetized and carefully extracted. The patient should not only be warned that the tooth might fracture during extraction, but should give and sign informed consent for treatment. He should also be properly informed of the guarded prognosis any replanted tooth carries with it. The tooth should be received in a gauze sponge soaked in sterile saline and should be held in this sponge throughout treatment. Prognosis is greatly improved if the tooth is out of the alveolus a relatively short time.

Fig. 15–96. Biologic repair of horizontal root fracture. *A,* Accident fractures left central incisor *(arrow)* which remains vital. Right central incisor devitalized. *B,* Five months later pulpless tooth has been filled, and fracture line of vital tooth has separated. No discoloration nor discomfort. *C,* Recall radiograph 2½ years later, fractured root is repairing. *D,* Ten years after accident, fractured root has completely repaired and tooth has remained vital. (Courtesy Dr. Bernard H. Poliak.)

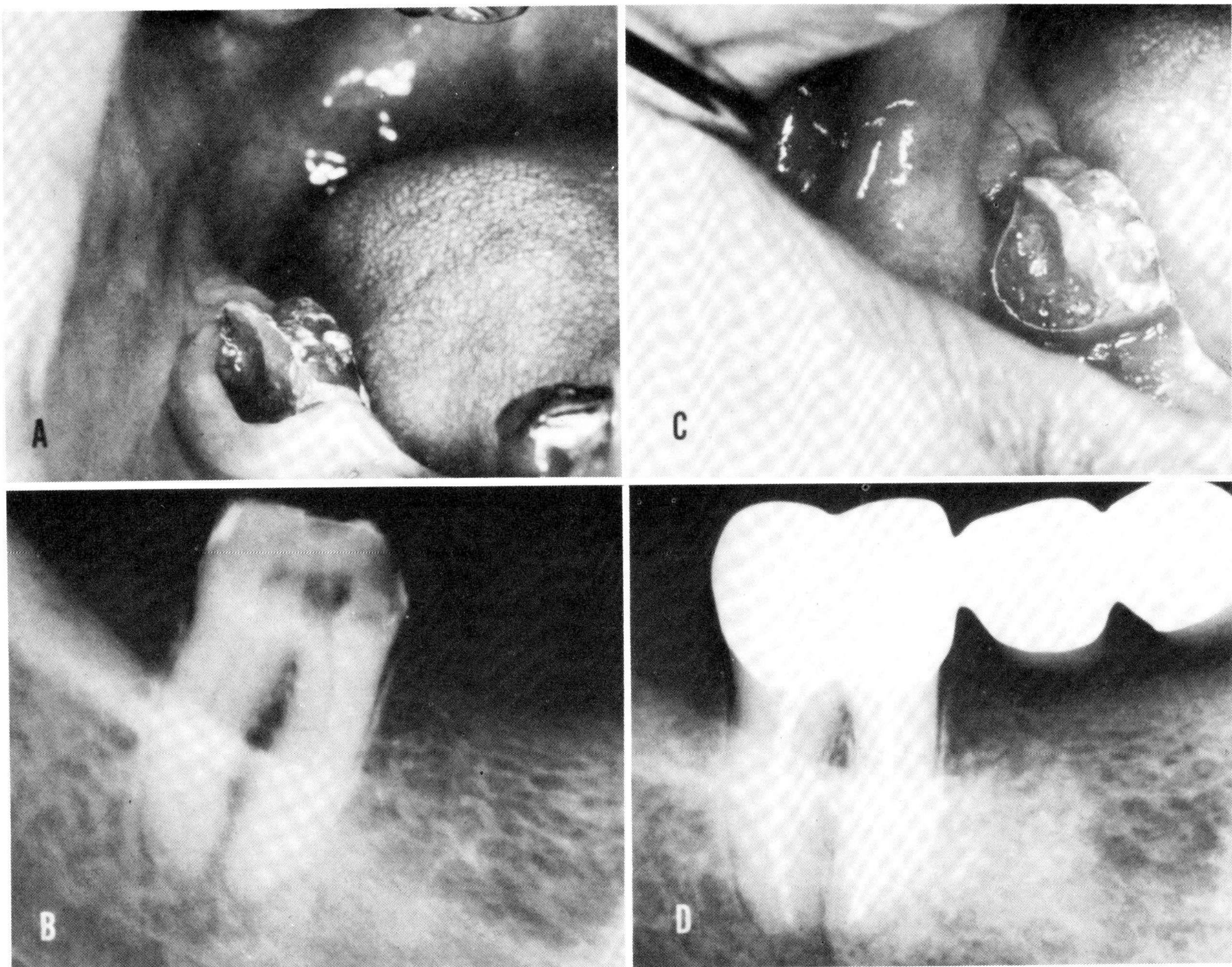

Fig. 15–97. Corrective surgery and endodontic therapy for large carious defect involving terminal molar bridge abutment. *A,* Recurrent caries involves pulp and extends far under heavy rolled gingiva. *B,* Excellent bony support for tooth and extent of carious lesion. *C,* One week healing after gingivectomy. Margin of carious lesion is completely exposed, and crown "elongated" for rubber dam clamp placement and root canal therapy. *D,* Fixed prosthesis following combined periodontic-endodontic procedures. Otherwise hopelessly destroyed bridge abutment has been saved. (Courtesy Dr. Eugene Natkin.)

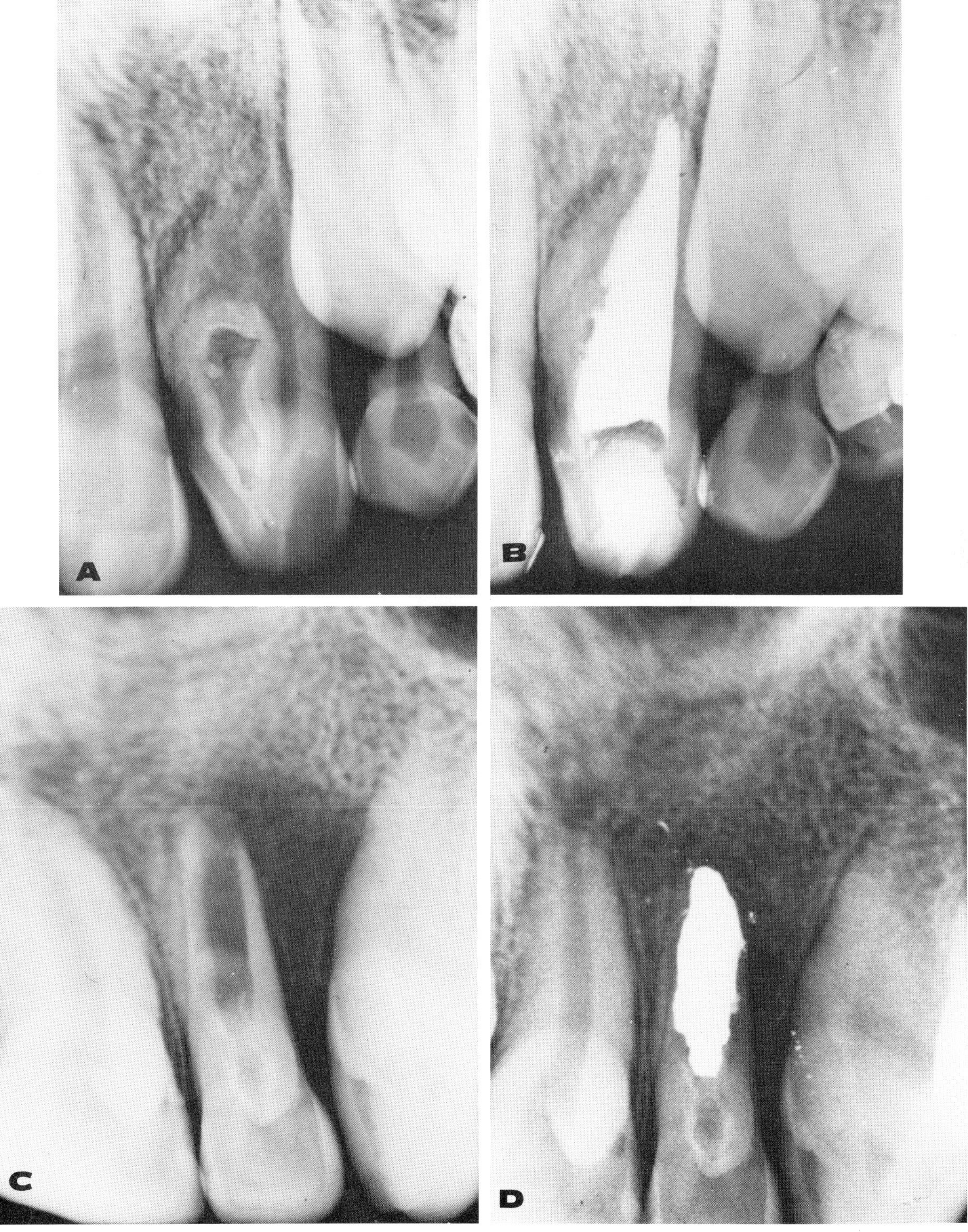

Fig. 15–98. *A,* ***Dens in dente*** of maxillary lateral incisor leading to pulp necrosis and periapical inflammation. *B,* Nonsurgical obturation of anomalous canals—one-year recall. (Courtesy Dr. Frank Gruchalla.) *C,* ***Dens invaginatus*** with massive periapical and lateral lesion. Did not respond to calcium hydroxide therapy. *D,* Surgical retrofilling necessary to properly obturate open tube canal. (Courtesy Dr. Alfred L. Frank.)

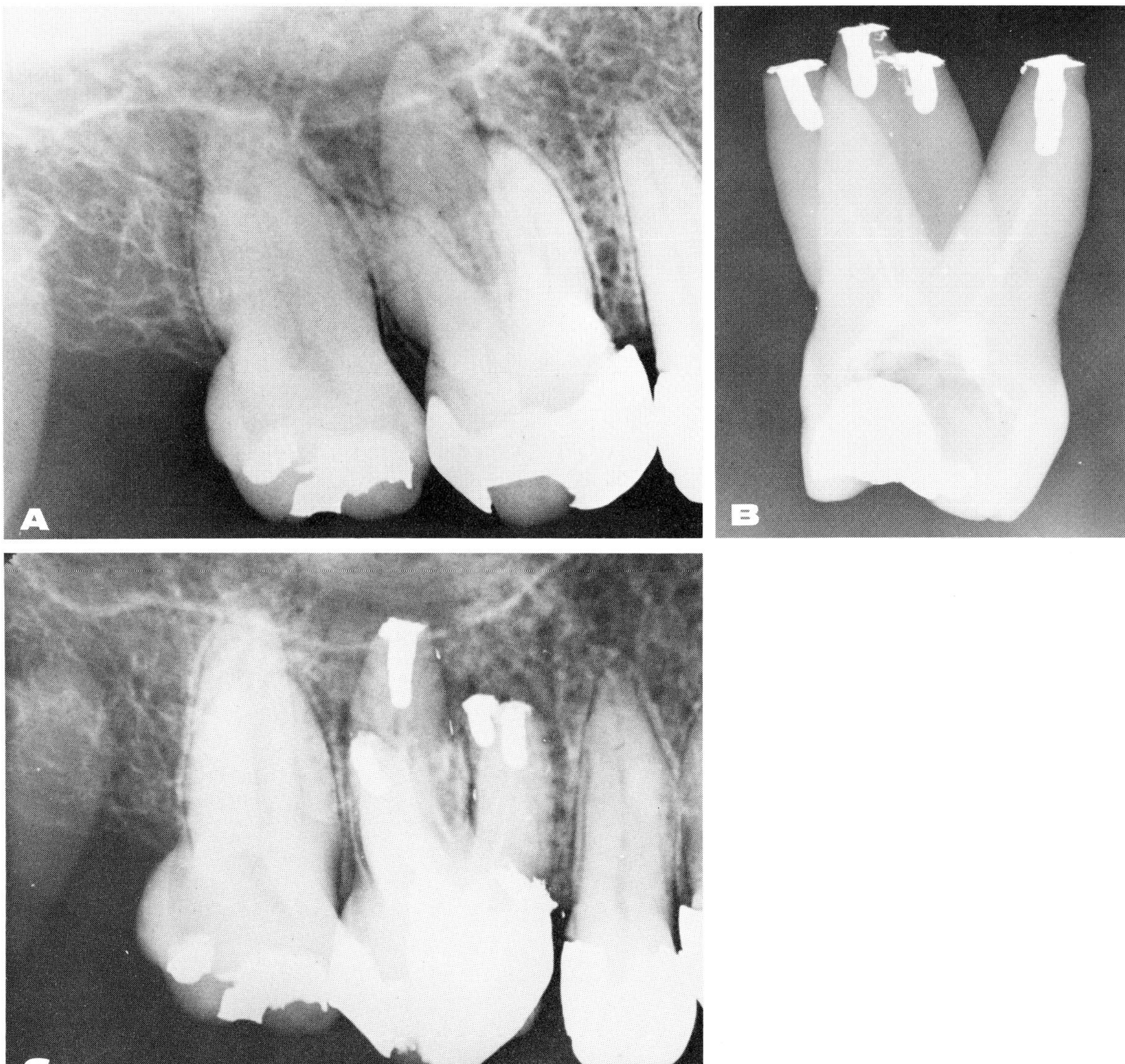

Fig. 15–99. *A,* Maxillary first molar with periapical lesions at each root end, but canals calcified into roots. Extraction, retrofilling, and intentional replantation appear to be solution. *B,* "Bench-top" radiograph showing retrofillings. *C,* Six-month recall radiograph. Four root canals were surprise. (Courtesy Dr. Antonio Rothier, Rio de Janeiro, Brazil.)

A standard coronal cavity is developed and the canal or canals prepared in hand as carefully as *in situ*. Saline solution irrigation is recommended. The root canals are filled, and if necessary, the perforations or lateral canals are filled with non-zinc amalgam.

The root canal filling is complete and a filling is placed in the crown. The tooth is now ready for replanting. The alveolus should be ***gently*** curetted to remove the clot and packed to prevent bleeding. The other teeth involved in the splint are then dried and covered with zinc oxide-eugenol cement. The involved tooth is cemented to the splint in hand, and while all the cement is soft, the splint is carried to place and the involved tooth positioned into its exact position. The excess cement is finally chipped away and an adhesive tinfoil dressing is placed over the entire area for twenty-four hours.

In three weeks to one month the splint may be carefully removed. During the recovery period the patient is admonished to keep the region scrupulously clean to prevent gingivitis. Reattachment will not occur in the face of gingival inflammation.

If a reattachment without ankylosis develops, the patient should retain the tooth for a lifetime. If ankylosis and root resorption develop, the future of the tooth is limited. Even a short life, however, may justify the expense in time and money to replant an otherwise hopeless tooth.

REFERENCES

1. Guerini, V.: *A History of Dentistry*. Philadelphia, Lea & Febiger, 1909, pp. 117–118.
2. Hullihen, S.: Observations on toothache. Amer. J. Dent. Sci., *1*:105, 1839.
3. Farrar, J.: Radical and heroic treatment of alveolar abscess by amputation of roots of teeth, with description and application of the cantilever crown. Dent. Cosmos, *26*:135, 1884.
4. Rhein, M.: Cure of acute and chronic alveolar abscess. Dent. Items Interest, *19*:688, 1897.
5. Black, G. V.: *The American System of Dentistry*. Edited by W. Litch. Philadelphia, Lea Brothers, 1886, pp. 990–992.
6. Garvin, M. H.; Foci of infection in relation to nonvital teeth. J. Nat. Dent. Assoc., *6*:195, Mar., 1919.
7. Hiatt, W.: Regeneration of the periodontium after endodontic therapy and flap operation. Oral Surg., *12*:1471, 1959.
8. Hiatt, W.: Periodontal pocket elimination by combined endodontic-periodontic therapy. J.A.S.P., *1*:152, Aug., 1963.
9. Ingle, J. I.: Exitos y Fracasos en Endodoncia. Revista de la Asociacion Odontologica Argentina, *50*:67, 1962.
10. Crump, M. C., and Natkin, E.: Relationship of broken root canal instruments to endodontic case prognosis: a clinical investigation. J.A.D.A., *80*:341, June, 1970.
11. Marcotte L. R., Dowson, J., and Rowe, N. H.: Apical healing with retrofilling materials amalgam and gutta percha. J. Endodont, *1*:63, Feb., 1975.
12. Cummings, R. R.: Endodontic considerations in endodontic surgery. Unpublished paper, Loma Linda University, 1970.

12a. Sicher, H., and Du Brul, L. E.: *Oral Anatomy*. 6th Ed., St. Louis, C. V. Mosby Co., 1975, pp. 413–430.

13. Luebke, R., and Ingle, J. I.: Geometric nomenclature for mucoperiosteal flaps. J. Am. Soc. Periodont., *2*:301, Jan.-Feb., 1964.

13a. Panella, A. S.: A study of the relationships of the mandibular canal to the apices of posterior teeth. Research report, University of Southern California, 1974.

14. Everett, F. G.: Apicoectomy followed by unusual radiologic finding. Oral Surg., *4*:1531, Dec., 1951.
15. Luebke, R. G.: Surgical endodontics. Dent. Clin. N. Amer., *18*:379, Apr., 1974.
16. Freedland, J. B.: Conservative reduction of large periapical lesions. Oral Surg., *29*:455, 1970.
17. Partsch, C.: *Bericht de Poliklinik fuer Zagnkeil-kunde*. Leipzig, 1899.
18. Sommer, R. F., Ostrander, F. D., and Crowley, M. C.: *Clinical Endodontics*. 2nd Ed. Philadelphia, W. B. Saunders, 1961, pp. 471–7.
19. Ehrmann, E. H.: Personal communication. August, 1972. (From Melbourne, Australia.)

19a. Cummings, R. R.: The rationale of apical resection in retrofilling procedures. Master's Thesis, Loma Linda University, 1970.

20. Matsura, S. J.: A simplified root-end filling technic. J. Mich. State Dent. Assoc., *44*:40, Feb., 1962.
21. Barry, G. N., Heyman, R. A., and Elias, A.: Comparison of apical sealing methods. Oral Surg., *39*:806, May, 1975.
22. Omnell, K. A.: Electrolytic precipitation of zinc carbonate in the jaw. Oral Surg., *12*:846, July, 1959.
23. Persson, G., Lennartson, B., and Lundstrom, I.: Results of retrograde root filling with amalgam and cavit as materials. Swedish Dent. J., *67*:123, 1974.
24. Simon, J. H. S., Glick, D. H., and Frank, A. L.: The relationship of endodontic-periodontic lesions. J. Periodont., *43*:202, Apr., 1972.
25. Prichard, J.: The infrabony technique as a predictable procedure. J. Periodont., *28*:202, July, 1957.
26. Younger, W. J.: Pyorrhea alveolaris. J.A.M.A., *23*:790, Nov., 1894.
27. Venable, C. S., Stuck, W. G., and Beach, A.: Effects on bone from the presence of metals; based upon electrolysis; experimental study. Ann. Surg., *105*:917, 1937.
28. Bernier, J. L., and Canby, C. P.: Histologic studies on the reaction of alveolar bone to vitallium implants. J.A.D.A., *30*:188, 1943.
29. Seltzer, S., Green, D. B., de la Guardia, R., Maggio, J., and Barnett, A.: Vitallium endodontic implants: a scanning electron microscope, electron microprobe, and histologic study. Oral Surg., *35*:828, June, 1973.
30. Weisman, S.: Letters to the Editor. Oral Surg., *37*:288, Feb., 1974.
31. Sandrik, J. L., Bapna, M. S., and Rysiekjo, M. R.:

Demonstration of corrosion of dental alloys. J. Dent. Ed., *38*:106, Feb., 1974.
32. Hodosh, M., Shklar, G., and Povar, M.: Polymer-coated metal endodontic stabilizers. Oral Surg., *38*:804, Nov., 1974.
33. Frank, A. L., and Abrams, A. M.: Histologic evaluation of endodontic implants. J.A.D.A., *78*:520, 1969.
34. Strock, A. E., and Strock, M. S.: Method of reinforcing pulpless anterior teeth—preliminary report. Oral Surg., *1*:252, 1943.
35. Souza, M.: El uso de estabilizadores intro-oseo en apicectomias y en organos para-dentosicos. Odont. Urug., 7:13, 1953.
36. Bruno, B. J. A.: Estabilizacion intraosea. Odont. Urug., *8*:311, 1954.
37. Guntert, V. G.: Uber stiftimplantate-eine stellugnahme. Zahnaerztl. Rundsch., *66*:519, 1957.
38. Staegemann, V. G.: Die stifverbolzung gelockerter zahne. Zahnaerztl. Rundsch., *67*:263, 1958.
39. Orlay, H. G.: Endodontic splinting treatment in periodontal disease. Brit. Dent. J., *108*:118, 1960.
40. Kaiser, J. H.: Personal communication, 1961.
41. Frank, A. L.: Endodontic endosseous implants and treatment of the wide open apex. Dent. Clin. N. Amer., p. 675, Nov., 1967.
42. Frank, A. L.: Improvement of the crown root ratio by endodontic endosseous implants. J.A.D.A., *74*:451, Feb., 1967.
43. Powell, W. D., and Bjorndal, A. M.: An evaluation of the standardization of endodontic endosseous implant instruments. Oral Surg., *36*:101, July, 1973.
44. Frank, A. L.: Personal communication, June, 1975.
45. Dow, P.: Control of gingival seepage prior to endodontic therapy. Oral Surg., *12*:497, April, 1959.

Chapter 16

Diagnosis and Treatment of Traumatic Injuries and Their Sequelae

JOHN I. INGLE, ALFRED L. FRANK, EUGENE NATKIN
and EDWIN B. NUTTING

Traumatic injury to the teeth is a common dental problem, usually an emergency requiring prompt attention. This attention may consist of diagnosis and simple palliative treatment of soft tissues or protection of exposed coronal dentin. In more extreme circumstances, repositioning or replantation of luxated teeth may be required, and in many instances pulp therapy ranging from pulpotomy to root canal filling will be necessary[1] (Fig. 16–1).

Unfortunately, inexperience or the pressures of the emergency situation may affect the practitioner's ability to distinguish between cases requiring prompt and definitive pulp therapy and those in which the need for pulp therapy is best postponed. In young teeth especially, pulps that have been apparently devitalized by trauma often return to normal vitality after a short period of time. Judicious delay for the purpose of re-evaluation does not imply an indefinite wait for the rejuvenation of a pulp that shows no signs of recovery. Once death of the pulp has been ascertained, root canal therapy should be started promptly to prevent acute sequelae as well as the progressive discoloration so common to traumatic cases.

HISTORY

The history obtained from the patient involved in a traumatic accident is essential to arriving at a proper diagnosis and treatment plan, and should include the following information:

1. Time of occurrence of the accident
2. Nature of the accident
3. Previous accidents involving the teeth
4. Prior treatment for the present injury

Generally, patients seek prompt dental care following traumatic injury to the teeth. However, if the injury does not involve fracture or displacement of teeth, the patient may see no need to seek treatment until prompted by the later occurrence of swelling, pain, or tooth discoloration. Patients may even delay seeking treatment in cases of traumatic pulp exposure, root fracture, or displacement of teeth if they are not in great discomfort. Decisions concerning the possible recovery of apparently devitalized teeth or the prognosis for pulpotomy depend to a great extent on the time that has elapsed since the accident.

Information concerning the nature of the accident may provide the dentist with clues about the type of injury to be expected. A soft or padded blow is likely to result in root fracture, whereas contact with hard objects usually causes coronal fracture.[1a]

The patient should be questioned about previous accidents involving the teeth. Some patients are accident prone, and if this is the case, it should alert the dentist to the possible presence of previously devitalized pulpless teeth. In addition, accident

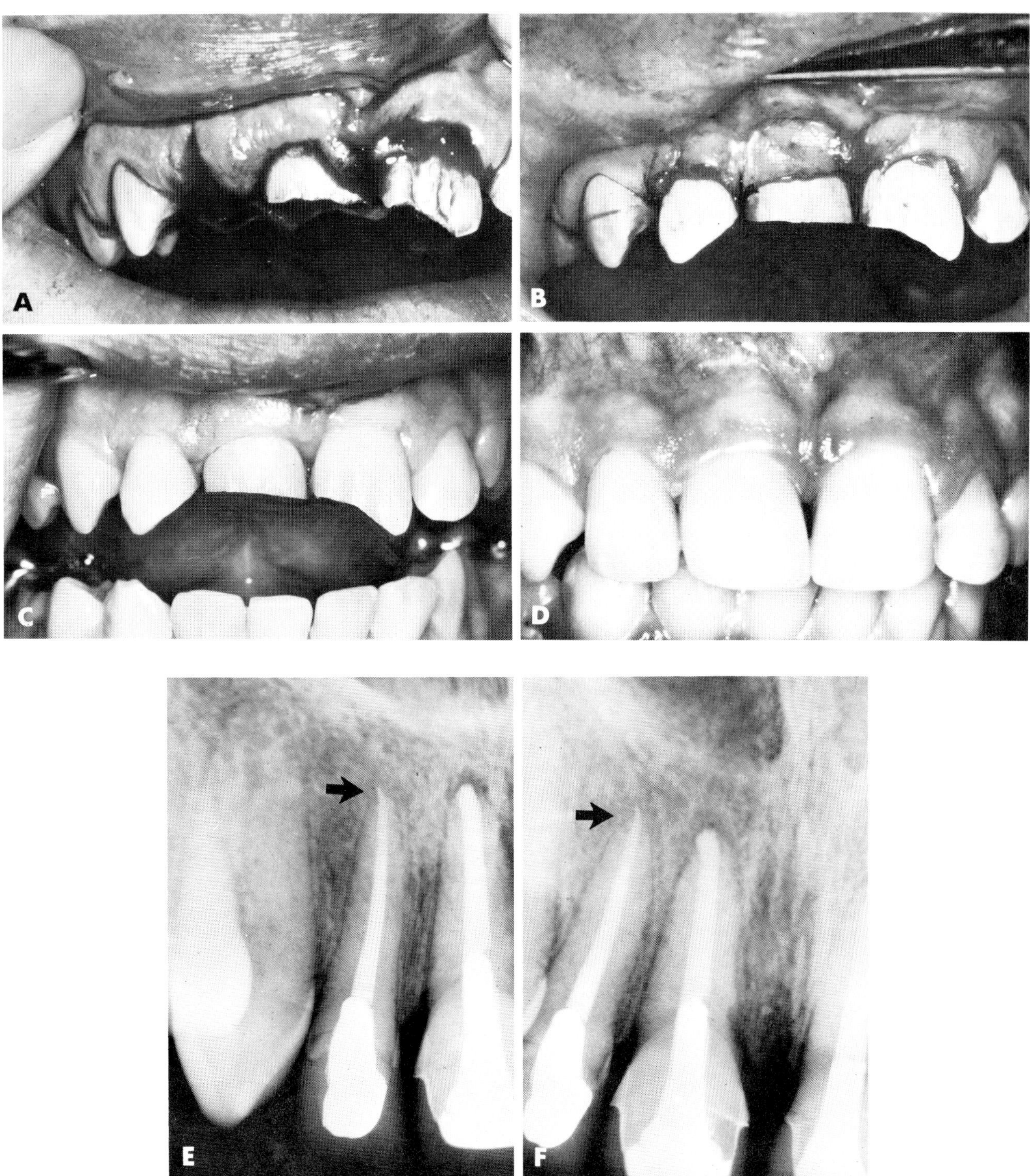

Fig. 16–1. Impact injury to maxillary incisors and soft tissues of 11-year-old girl. *A,* Coronal fractures of central incisors and total avulsion of lateral incisor. *B,* Lateral incisor immediately following replantation. Jagged incisal edges have been smoothed. *C,* One month after accident. Replanted lateral incisor is firm in alveolus and soft tissue healing is complete. *D,* Final restoration of central incisors and right lateral incisor with porcelain jackets. (Restoration by Dr. Ralph Yuodelis.) *E,* One month roentgenogram. Note slight resorption beginning at apex of replanted tooth. Root canal therapy has been completed for central incisors. *F,* Six months after accident. No further resorption of lateral incisor has developed.

proneness should be considered in planning restorations for fractured teeth. Porcelain jacket crowns, for example, are not indicated for an individual who frequently sustains injuries to the teeth or who engages in contact sports.

Treatment for injuries to the teeth may have been rendered by another dentist subsequent to the accident, and the precise nature of this treatment should be determined.

Subjective Symptoms

The patient should be questioned about the following: (1) spontaneous pain from the teeth; (2) discomfort of the teeth to touch, or pain during mastication; (3) pain from thermal stimuli and sweet or sour foods; (4) mobility or displacement of teeth.

CLINICAL EXAMINATION

The clinical examination should provide the bulk of information necessary for proper diagnosis and treatment. Careful determination of the following should be made:

1. Injury to the soft tissues.
2. Presence of foreign material in the tissues.
3. Injury to alveoli.
4. Fracture of crowns.
   (*a*) Extent of tooth structure lost.
   (*b*) Pulp exposure.
5. Displacement of teeth (labial, lingual, intrusion, extrusion, complete avulsion).
6. Mobility.
7. Reaction to percussion and palpation.
8. Reaction to vitality tests (heat, cold, electric pulp tester).
9. Abnormalities in occlusion.
10. Discoloration of the crown.
11. Pocket depth around traumatized teeth and adjacent uninjured teeth.
12. Radiographic appearance.
    (*a*) Presence of root fracture.
    (*b*) Degree of extrusion or intrusion.
    (*c*) Presence of periapical rarefaction.
    (*d*) Extent of development of root apex.
    (*e*) Size of pulp chamber and root canal.

In addition to the initial roentgenograms, recorded results of periodontal probing and vitality tests must be maintained as part of the permanent record. Recording the findings of vitality tests is most important. Progressive decreases in vitality responses at subsequent visits will indicate the need for root canal therapy, whereas a return of vitality responses will indicate that root canal treatment is unnecessary.

CLASSIFICATION OF TRAUMATIC INJURIES

In formulating a classification for traumatic injuries to the teeth, the author has leaned heavily on the excellent classification of Ellis.[2] This has been modified in certain respects because of the particular orientation of emphasis demanded in a textbook of endodontics. To a great extent this modification closely resembles the World Health Organization classification of injuries of oral hard tissues formulated in 1969.[2a]

Class I Tooth traumatized—crown and root are intact
  A. Pulp may be devitalized
  B. Internal resorption may develop
  C. External resorption may develop
Class II Coronal fracture—pulp not exposed
Class III Coronal fracture—pulp exposed
Class IV Coronal fracture—extending subgingivally
Class V Root fracture with or without loss of crown structure
  Division 1—Horizontal fractures
  Division 2—Vertical and chisel fractures
Class VI Displacement of teeth with or without fracture
  Division 1—Partial displacement
    A. Labial or lingual displacement
    B. Extrusion
    C. Intrusion
  Division 2—Complete avulsion
Class VII Injuries to deciduous teeth

Class I: Tooth Traumatized—Crown and Root Are Intact

Paradoxically the severest pulp injury often occurs in traumatized teeth that have suffered the least apparent injury. It is, in fact, often observed that teeth sustaining fractures of the crown or root retain their pulp vitality, whereas the pulps of unfractured but similarly traumatized adjacent teeth are devitalized. Apparently the force of a blow is greatly dissipated in the process of fracture, thus diminishing the shock to the pulp. On the other hand, the pulp and apical vessels of the unfractured tooth receive the full force of the blow and tend thus to be more seriously injured.

Occasionally one sees an adult dental patient who remembers a childhood accident to the teeth which at the time was dismissed as trivial. At present one of the

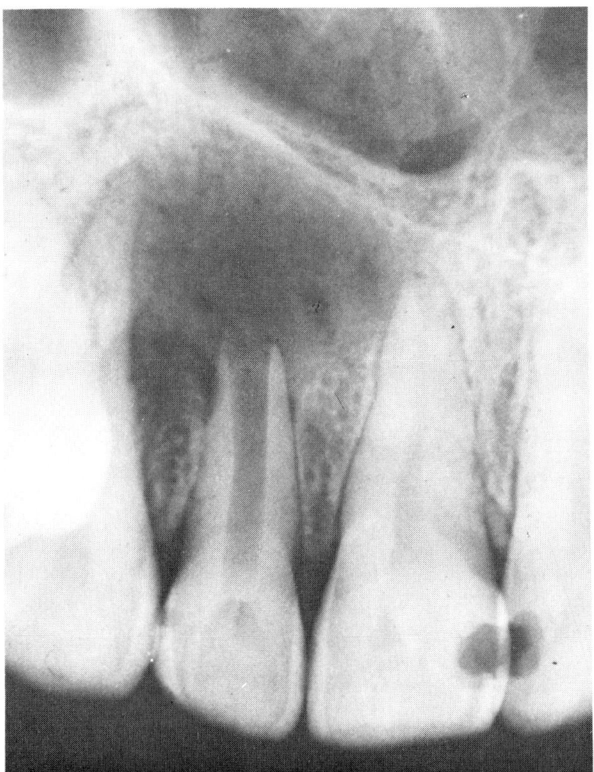

Fig. 16–2. Enormous root canal and open apex of maxillary lateral incisor indicate early devitalization of pulp. Normal adjacent teeth have completed root development.

traumatized teeth is nonvital. A roentgenogram shows that the pulp chamber and root canal of the devitalized tooth are enormous, and that the root-end is not completely formed (Fig. 16–2). It may be assumed that devitalization of the pulp of this tooth probably occurred at the time of injury and that further development ceased. The adjacent vital teeth meanwhile continued normal development.

Even more striking is the case in which devitalization of the pulp of one young tooth occurred, while the pulp of an adjacent tooth was stimulated by the injury to produce excessive reparative dentin (Fig. 16–3). In the latter instance, the pulp may appear roentgenographically as a barely perceptible line or may, in fact, be completely obliterated. Barker and Mayne have shown the bizarre forms of root closure and/or continued twisted root formation subsequent to trauma.[3]

After a traumatic accident the diagnosis of pulp vitality is made on the basis of thermal and electric pulp tests. If pulp test responses are negative and root development of the traumatized tooth is complete, there is little justification for anticipating future return of vitality. Immediate pulpectomy and root canal filling are the indicated treatment procedures.

In the case of the recently erupted tooth whose root development is not complete, one is faced with a more complex diagnostic problem. In most instances such teeth give erratic responses to pulp tests and, in fact, a recently erupted tooth which ***has never been traumatized*** may yield ***negative responses to all pulp tests.*** In addition, the large apical opening and the more abundant pulp blood supply make it more likely that the young tooth will recover from the shock of traumatic injury. This initial shock, which may have damaged the ability of the tooth to respond to sensory stimuli, may not have been sufficient to destroy the pulp circulation. There is good evidence that bacteria must also be involved for necrosis to develop (see Chapter 12). After a period of time the sensory responses may return.

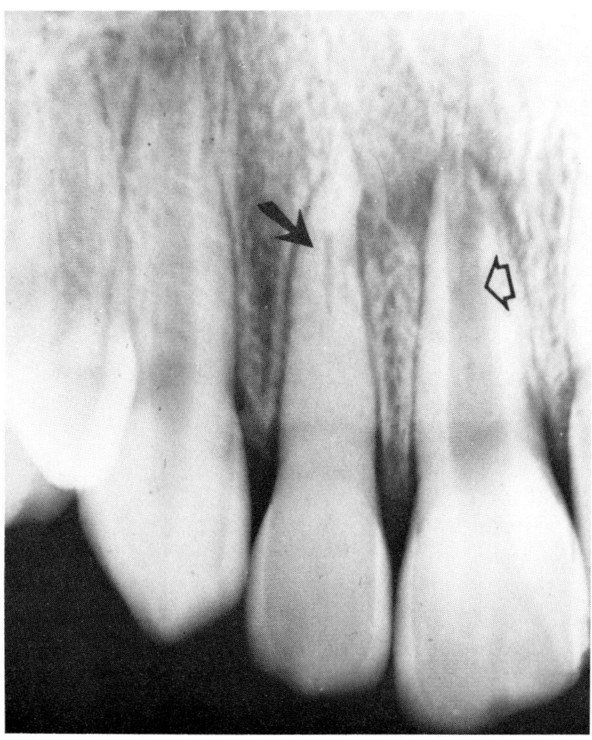

Fig. 16–3. Impact injury resulted in devitalization of pulp of maxillary central incisor *(open arrow)* and almost complete calcification of pulp of lateral incisor. Note small segment of patent root canal which can still be seen roentgenographically in root of lateral incisor *(black arrow).* Also note bony lesion mesial to this canal, indicating presence of lateral accessory canal.

Thus in young permanent teeth, the unreliability of pulp tests and the increased likelihood of recovery justify delay of treatment for later re-evaluation of pulp vitality. Many young teeth that are apparently devitalized by trauma gradually return to normal over a period of six to ten weeks. Discoloration of the crown due to initial pulp hemorrhage may slowly disappear as the vascular system repairs and the elements of hemorrhage are removed from the dentin.

Lack of vital response at the end of a ten-week period does not mean that pulp death has definitely occurred, since even a ***normal, recently erupted*** tooth may not respond to pulp-test stimuli. It is therefore reasonable to wait for additional indications of true pulp death while keeping in mind, of course, that the "waiting game" must be carefully controlled. The signs of necrosis include the appearance or progressive increase of coronal discoloration, symptoms of pulpitis, development of a periapical radiolucency, or cessation of further root development. If, in spite of a nonvital pulp response, the root apex continues its development, pulp vitality should be assumed and root canal therapy should ***not*** be instituted. If the evidence for nonvitality of the pulp ***is*** clear-cut, complete endodontic therapy should be carried out as soon as possible in order to prevent the development of serious acute or chronic sequelae such as abscesses and cysts. In addition, prompt treatment will forestall the possible development of intense coronal discoloration and will increase the chance of successful bleaching if discoloration is already present.

In the event the pulp expires, root growth ceases and tooth formation is left incomplete. The mass of necrotic pulp serves as a periapical tissue irritant, and the apex gapes open in a blunderbuss or tubular shape. If the tooth is to be saved, root growth must be charged-up once again to close the apex, or the canal will have to be filled from the apex—the retrofilling.

Apexification

For most cases it has been found possible to induce continued root formation and apical closure (Fig. 16–4). This phenomenon was observed by Nygaard-Ostby after stimulation of periapical bleeding by overinstrumentation.[4] Successful apical closure has also been induced with a calcium hydroxide paste, noted by Kaiser as early as 1956 (Fig. 16–5),[5] and reported by him in 1964.[6] Also in 1964, Frank demonstrated that the prime effort, in what has been termed "apexification," must be directed toward removing the contaminants from within the canal by careful instrumentation and medication, to be followed by a partial filling of the canal space with a temporary filling material, in this case calcium hydroxide, which is thought by some to be a biologic activator.[7,7a,8] To control possible infection, the calcium hydroxide is mixed with camphorated parachlorophenol to a thick putty-like consistency. Since the mixture does not chemically set, it slowly resorbs and must be replaced every three to six months. Progress of root development is periodically measured radiographically.

There are two schools of thought about the biologic phenomenon of cementification which leads to apical closure. The first is that no chemical activator need be placed in the canal to stimulate cementum production and fire up the genetic memory of the tooth. This group holds that by merely removing the toxic debris and bacteria from the canal, and temporarily filling the space to nearly the interface with the tissue, the producing cells will be charged-up once again and fulfill their original obligation of completing the tooth root. Calcium hydroxide is used only because it is handy and does not set-up to block the canal.

The second school of thought believes that this process is natural, but that it must be stimulated by a biologic activator—in this case calcium hydroxide. The rationale is as follows: calcium hydroxide will stimulate odontoblasts to produce dentin; why not the cementoblasts, fibroblasts, and osteoblasts as well? The truth will not be known until someone completes a study matching calcium hydroxide against empty-canal controls or canals filled with an inert material such as Aquaphor. This number of cases is hard to come by.

In either event, what finally happens at the apex, that is, what does the histologic picture show? For an answer we can turn once again to Kaiser,[5] and a histologic evaluation of his 1956 historic case of apexification removed in block section 10 years after treatment (Fig. 16–6*A*). A medium-power photomicrograph of the same area shows the organization of the fibroblasts attaching to the cementum, but giving way to inflammatory tissue rather than alveolar bone proper (Fig. 16–6*B*). The high-power picture (Fig. 16–6*C*) dramatizes the cellularity of the cementum, the periodontal fibers, and the lymphocytes, plasma cells, and foam cells.*

*Histologic evaluation by Major General Surindar N. Bhaskar.

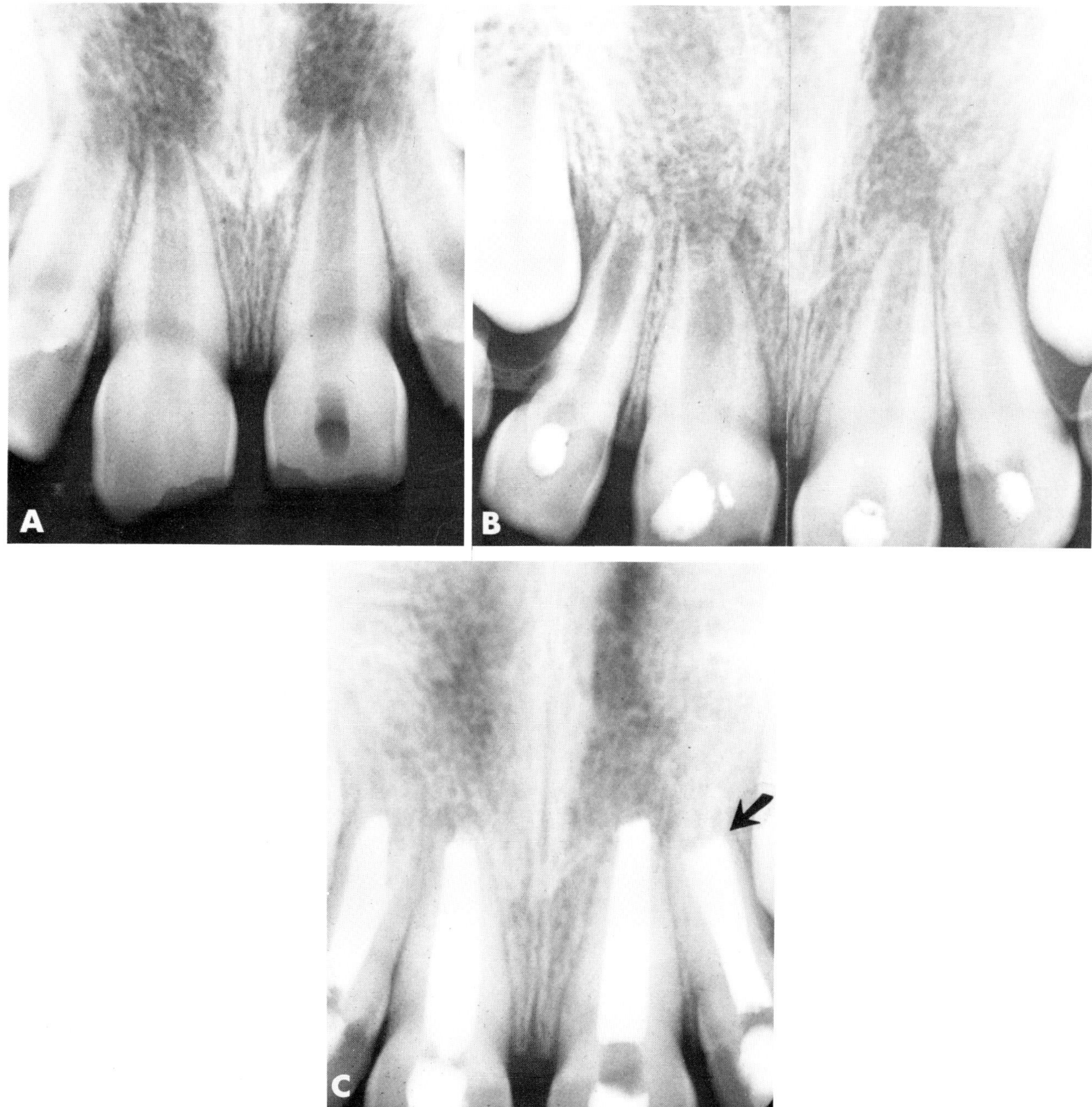

Fig. 16–4. Induction of root-end closure with calcium hydroxide paste. *A,* Pulps of all four maxillary incisors have been ***devitalized*** by traumatic accident. Apices are wide open. *B,* Seven months after filling with calcium hydroxide paste, root apices have closed sufficiently to allow root canal filling. *C,* Root canals filled with gutta percha by lateral condensation technique without surgery. Total apical closure is shown by dense blunted fillings *(arrow)*. (Courtesy Dr. Alfred L. Frank.)

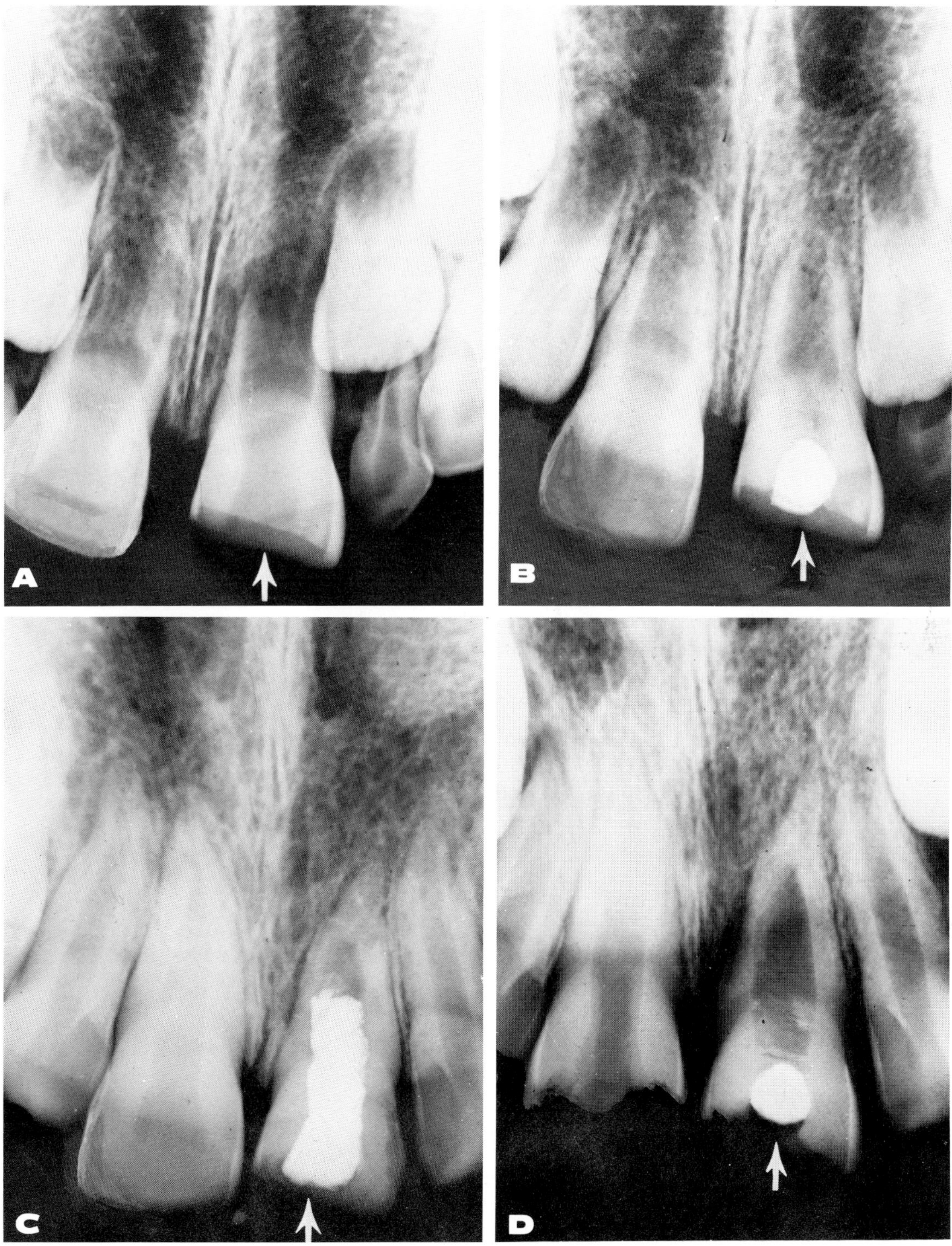

Fig. 16–5. Historic case of apexification. *A,* Male, age 7, presented himself May 29, 1956 with fractured pulpless left central incisor *(arrow).* Pus exuding from gingival crevice. *B,* One year later, after five changes of calcium hydroxide-camphorated parachlorophenol paste. Note increased root length and beginning closure. *C,* Fifteen months later—root tip has now formed. Calcium hydroxide used twice during year. Sinus track not draining so canal not filled. *D,* Radiograph taken 3½ years following initial appointment. Canal filled with calcium hydroxide and patient asked to return in six months—returned 6½ years later, May 1966, with crown decayed away and part of root intact. Right central incisor has subsequently been fractured and decayed. Root removed in block section for histologic study (Fig. 16–6). (Courtesy Dr. J. Henry Kaiser.)

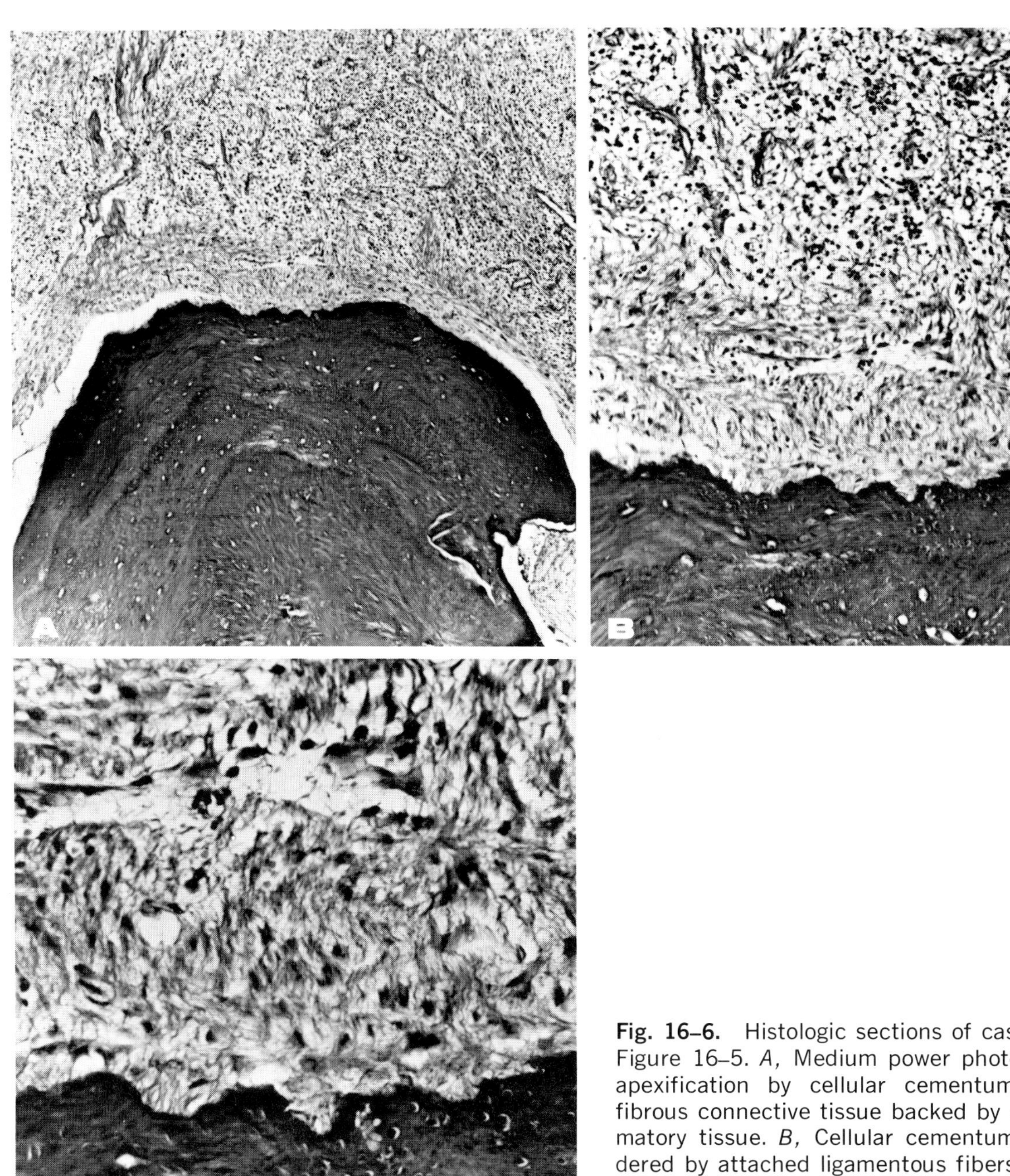

Fig. 16–6. Histologic sections of case presented in Figure 16–5. *A,* Medium power photomicrograph of apexification by cellular cementum. Attached is fibrous connective tissue backed by chronic inflammatory tissue. *B,* Cellular cementum (bottom) bordered by attached ligamentous fibers. Lymphocytes and foam cells from CAP are infiltrating connective tissue. *C,* High power photomicrograph of cellular cementum, periodontal fibers, lymphocytes, plasma, and foam cells. (Courtesy Dr. J. Henry Kaiser.)

A great deal may be drawn from Kaiser's clinical history, radiographs, and histologic report. Apparently an unfilled canal, even thought it appears to be sealed off at the apex, may still be microscopically open to allow fluid and bacterial passage from canal to periapical tissue and *vice versa.* It clearly says that canals of apexification cases should be finally obturated and the crown properly restored. Other cases, thought to be completely calcified at the apex, have shown a slight extrusion of sealer when the canal is filled, proving the existence of a fine opening. Even the cellular cementum could be "Swiss cheese" porous.

Nevins and his associates believe they may have the answer to this problem.[8a] They have set out deliberately to produce a material containing the constituents necessary to produce calcified structures both within and outside the open canal. This new material appears to be capable of inducing rapid physiologic root closure. Gelable in composition, this material consists of a buffered solution of colloidal collagen as matrix, calcium and phospate salts as apatite, and potassium iodide (5% Lugol's solution) as a bacteriostat.

To date, this material has been used experimentally in young monkeys. The pulps are extirpated from immature permanent incisors with open apices. Then this highly viscous solution is syringed into the canal, making contact with periapical tissues. A tight temporary coronal seal of gutta percha and Cavit is placed, and within 15 minutes the gel is set at body temperature.

During gelation, tropocollagen molecules spontaneously polymerize to form collagen fibers, the normal matrix of bone, cementum, and dentin (Fig. 16–7*A*). Calcium-phosphate aggregates within the gel transform from an amorphous state to the stable hydroxyapatite phase.

Initial healing at the apex consists of a chemotactic attraction of fibroblasts by the collagen gel material. The gel's fibers form a three-dimensional matrix within the canal capable of supporting periapical connective tissue ingrowth (Fig. 16–7*B*).

At 12 weeks, new connective tissue, containing sizeable blood vessels, may be demonstrated within the canal (Fig. 16–8*A*). The new connective tissue (Fig. 16–8*B*), which is replacing the collagen-chemical gel, is also rapidly depositing a new cementum-like tissue at the apex (Fig. 16–8*C*), as well as an internal attachment of the new connective tissue into an internal cementum-like repair (Fig. 16–8*D*). Using this new collagen chemical gel, full apexification has been achieved in monkeys in a matter of weeks (Fig. 16–8*E*).

From these results, it seems possible to induce a desired tissue differentiation. This may be a step in the direction of re-establishing vital healthy tissue within the treated root canal resulting in a true physiologic seal.

Clinical Technique. The following technique for inducing closure has been described by Frank as a predictable procedure.[7,8]

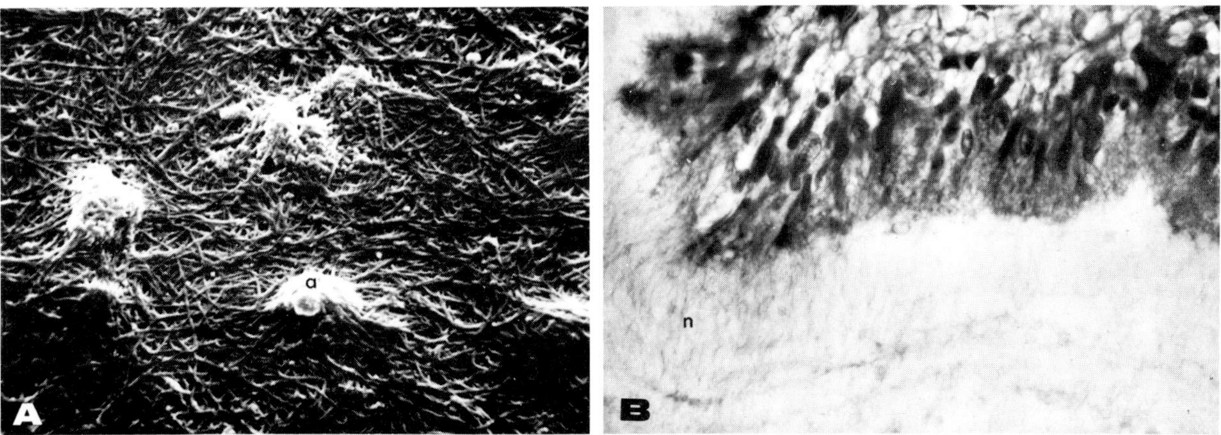

Fig. 16–7. *A,* Collagen-calcium phosphate gel after gelation. Disoriented collagen fibrils and calcium phosphate aggregates (a) are apparent. *B,* Calcified collagen gel (bottom) and palisading row of fibroblast-like cells at interface and new collagen fibrils (n). Connective tissue ingrowth produced in eight weeks. (From Nevins, A. J., Finklestein, F., Borden, B. G., and Moodnik, R. M.: J. Endodont., *1*:303, Sept., 1975.)

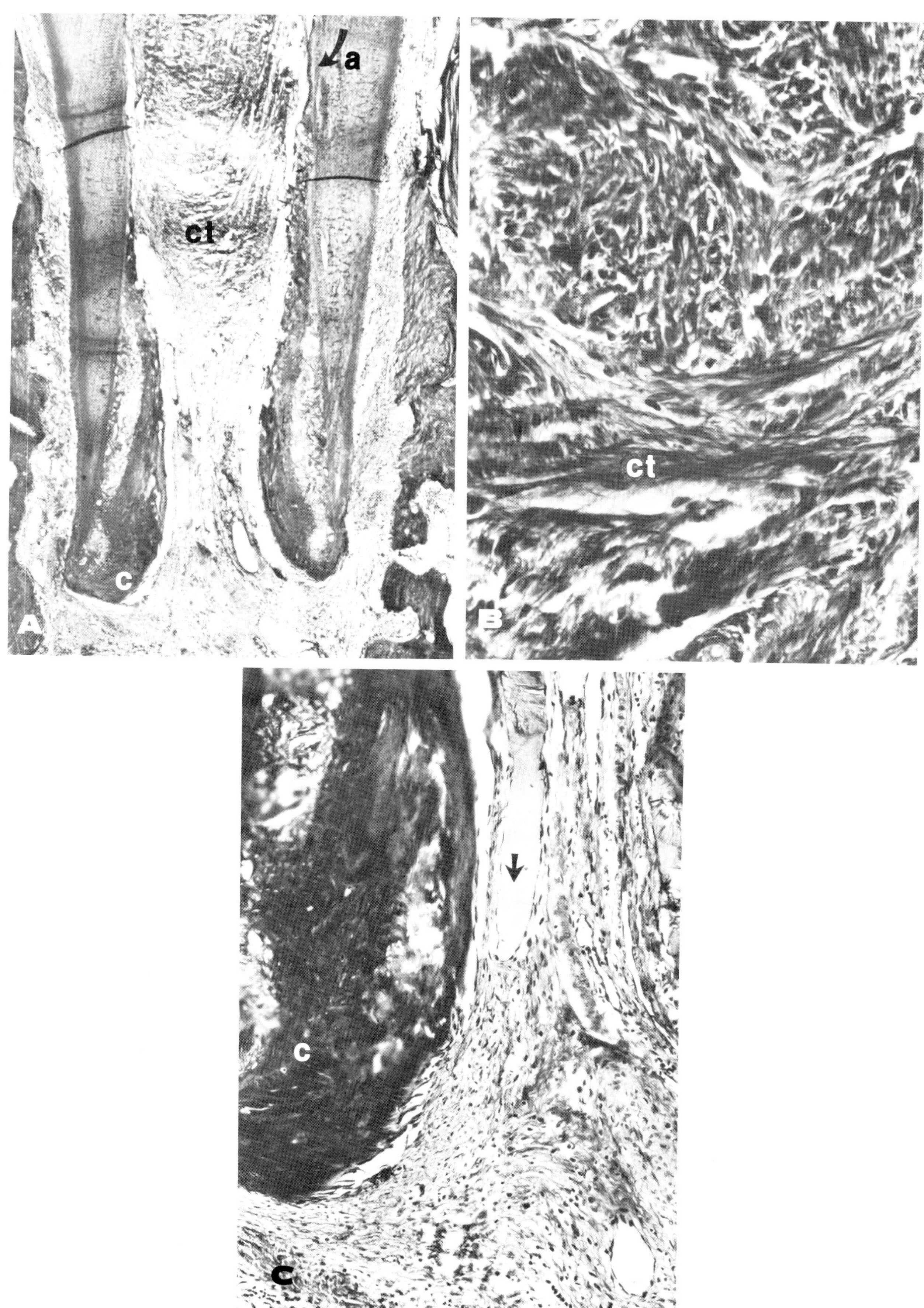

Fig. 16–8. (Legend on opposite page.)

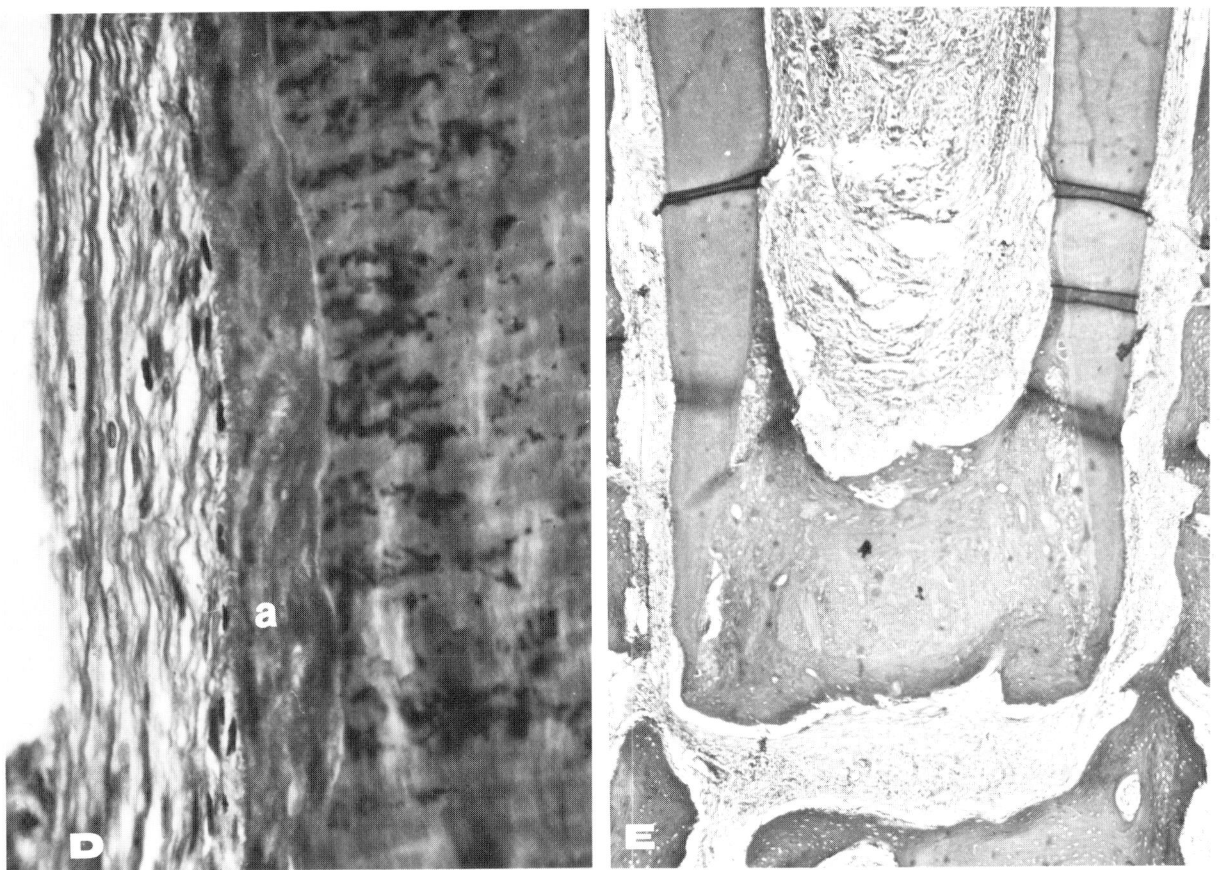

Fig. 16–8. *A,* Photomicrograph of 12-week result obtained in infected open apex incisor using collagen-calcium phosphate gel in canal. Total connective tissue ingrowth: ct, connective tissue; a, attachment; c, cementum-like tissue. *B,* Well-organized connective tissue, ct, containing sizeable blood vessels. *C,* Cementum-like tissue, c, deposited at the apex, which will lead to full closure of apexification. Remnant of gel matrix remains *(arrow). D,* Detail of ligamentous attachment, a, between connective tissue ingrowth and new cementum-like deposition within canal. *E,* Full apical closure obtained in only 12 weeks in infected mandibular incisor with open apex using collagen-calcium phosphate gel. (From Nevins, A. J., Finklestein, F., Borden, B. G., and Laporta, R.: J. Endodont., *2*:159, June, 1976.)

Initial Appointment. The initial procedure consists of the following:

1. Take an accurate radiograph for future reference.
2. Apply the rubber dam. Anesthesia is seldom necessary.
3. Prepare an optimal access cavity.
4. Irrigate the canal thoroughly with sodium hypochlorite.
5. Establish the proper length of tooth.
6. With a large blunted file, remove the necrotic canal contents and thoroughly file the entire perimeter of the canal until only clean white dentin appears. Constantly irrigate.
7. Prepare a thick, dry putty-like paste of calcium hydroxide and camphorated parachlorophenol.
8. Insert the paste into the canal and, using a long plugger, gently pack the mix to the tissue at the apex. Fill the canal completely, but avoid the pressure of overfilling (Fig. 16–9).
9. Place a dry cotton pellet over the paste, cover the ZOE temporary and place a substantial covering of oxyphosphate of zinc or polycarboxylate cement. Ask the patient to return four to six months later. The temporary filling must hold up.

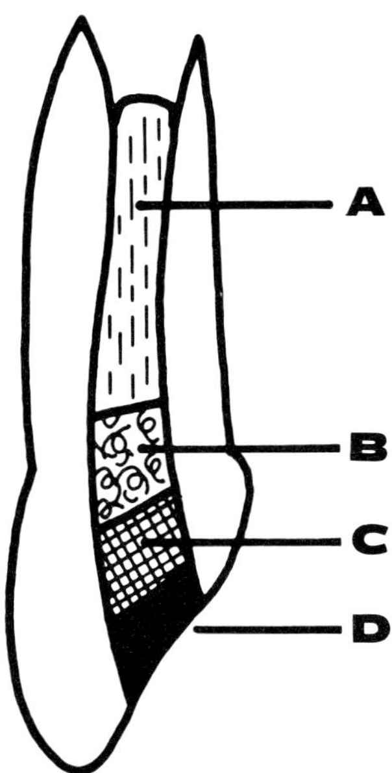

Fig. 16–9. Proper layering of filling media to stimulate apexification: *A*, calcium hydroxide-camphorated parachlorophenol up against the periapical tissue; *B*, cotton fibers, *C*, zinc oxide-eugenol first seal; *D*, zinc oxyphosphate cement top seal. (From Frank, A. L.: J.A.D.A., *74*:451, Feb., 1967.)

If symptoms of inflammation or infection occur, the patient returns, the filling and paste are removed, and the steps of the initial appointment are repeated.

Subsequent Appointments. Four to six months later, the patient returns for evaluation of the progress of the treatment.

1. A radiograph is made for a comparative evaluation of the apex. If the apex still appears to be open (and it probably will be), the procedures of the initial appointment are repeated (Fig. 16–10*A, B*).
2. It will be necessary to re-establish tooth length, for the root will probably have grown even though not closed. Record the new length and compare to the old. The patient is given another appointment.
3. In four to six months the patient again returns and an evaluation is made.

Apical closure may be verified by flushing the canal and then carefully probing with a sharp endodontic instrument against the apex. A final check may be made with a fine curved instrument (Fig. 16–10*C*). Although total closure is ideal, it is not necessary that the apex be completely calcified over. A final filling may still be condensed against this new barrier if an opening the size of the natural foramen is present. This may take anywhere from six months to two years to develop (Fig. 16–10*D, E, F*). Apexification works as well in posterior as in anterior teeth (Fig. 16–11).

There are four appearances that may be seen in the radiographs (Fig. 16–12).:

1. The apex still appears blunderbuss in shape, but is closed with a thin calcific bridge.
2. The blunderbuss appearance is the same, but a bridge has formed just below the apex.
3. The root end forms and seals, but the canal shape does not change.
4. The apex forms properly and the canal appears to fill in.

To properly fill these large tube-like canals, the reader is referred to Chapter 4, where the subject is discussed in depth.

Cementogenesis of Root Defects

Internal and external resorption are usually caused by traumatic injury to the tooth (Fig. 16–13). The ravages of tooth structure imposed by these decalcifying processes may be stopped and cemental repair instituted by applying the same biologic principles seen to work in apexification, namely, cemen-

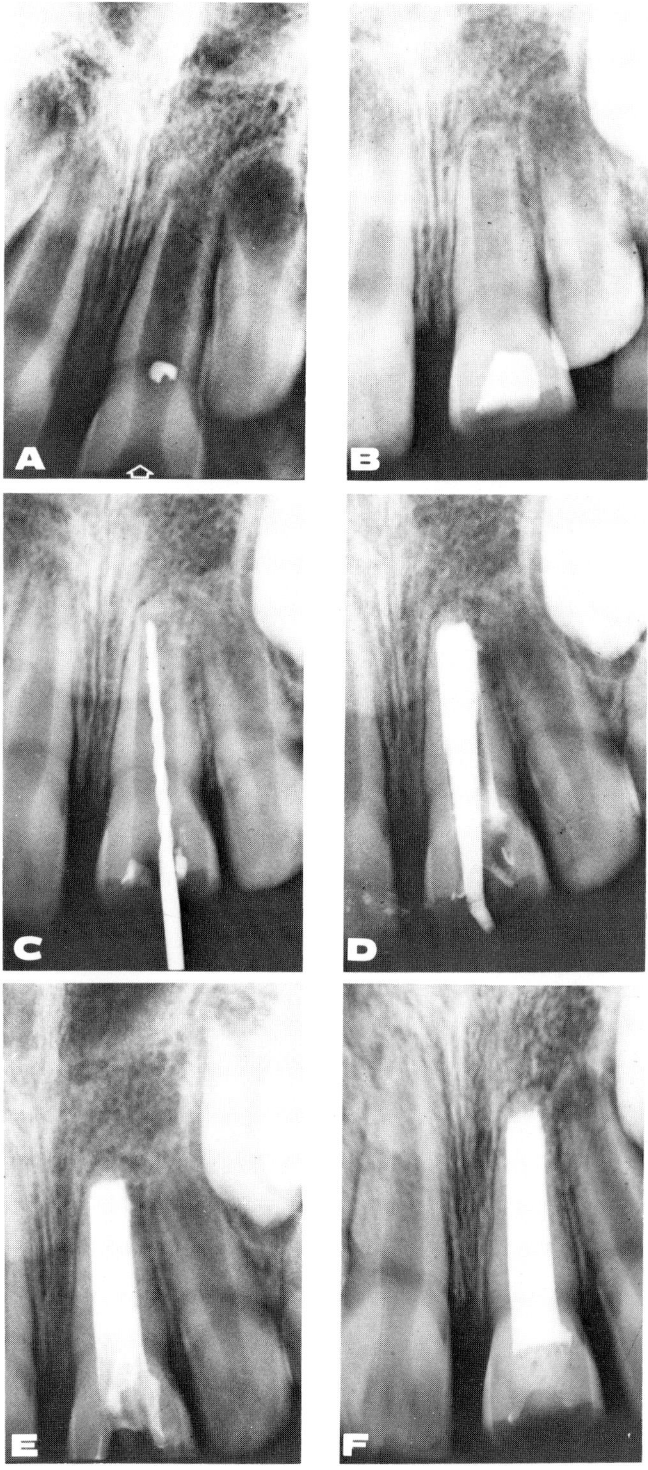

Fig. 16–10. Apexification. *A,* Pulp devitalized by trauma and root growth ceased—7-year-old male *(arrow).* Necrotic pulp is debrided and canal filed, sterilized, and filled with calcium hydroxide—CPCP mixture. *B,* Four-month recall. Cementification has elongated root and is closing apex. Calcium hydroxide mixture is replaced. *C,* Nine-month recall. Root has reached full length and apical foramen appears closed to probing. *D,* Canal is obturated with sealer and reverse gutta percha point using lateral condensation. *E,* Completed obturation indicates total closure by cementum of apex. *F,* Recall film 18 months after accident and 8 months after filling. (Courtesy Dr. Andrew E. Michanowicz.)

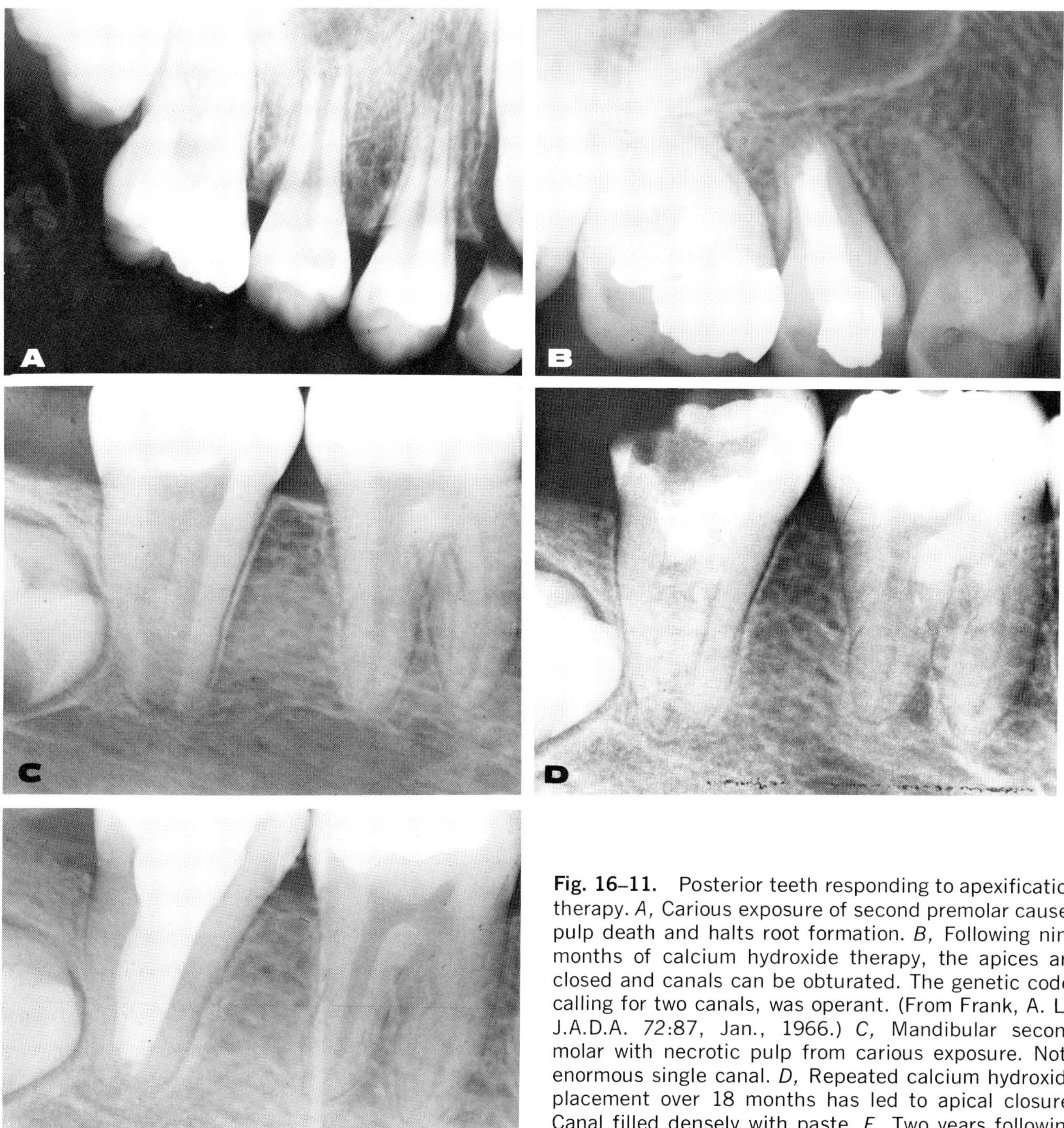

Fig. 16–11. Posterior teeth responding to apexification therapy. *A,* Carious exposure of second premolar causes pulp death and halts root formation. *B,* Following nine months of calcium hydroxide therapy, the apices are closed and canals can be obturated. The genetic code, calling for two canals, was operant. (From Frank, A. L.: J.A.D.A. *72*:87, Jan., 1966.) *C,* Mandibular second molar with necrotic pulp from carious exposure. Note enormous single canal. *D,* Repeated calcium hydroxide placement over 18 months has led to apical closure. Canal filled densely with paste. *E,* Two years following initial treatment the canal is obliterated. (Courtesy Dr. Melvin Cohen, Dr. Anthony D. Goodman, and Dr. Alfred L. Frank.)

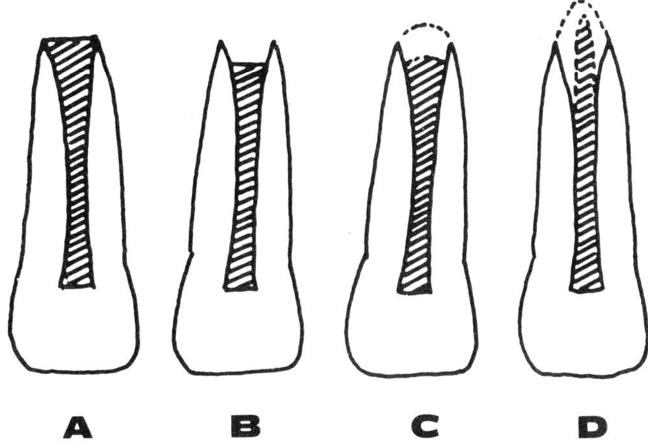

Fig. 16–12. Four basic types of apical development following calcium hydroxide therapy. (From Frank, A. L.: Dent. Clin. N. Amer., p. 675, Nov., 1967.)

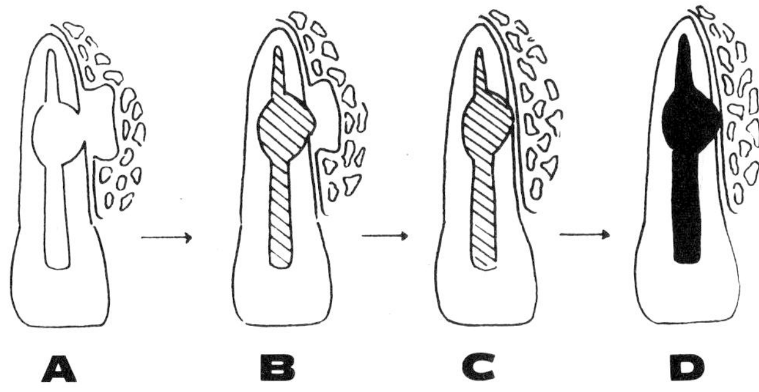

Fig. 16–13. Schematic summary of lateral cementogenesis. *A,* Periodontal destruction at the site of resorptive perforation. *B,* Placement of calcium hydroxide paste following pulpectomy and canal debridement. *C,* Healing of periodontal lesion and improvement in defect by cementogenesis. *D,* Obliteration of canal and perforation with gutta percha filling against lateral matrix of the periodontium. (From Frank, A. L. and Weine, F. S.: J.A.D.A., *87*:863, Oct., 1973.)

togenesis stimulated by biologically active chemicals. Again, Frank has succinctly written of the stimulating repair in these cases.[9,10]

Apical resorption is virtually always associated with a necrotic pulp or advanced chronic pulpitis. Obtaining closure of the apex in these cases is synonymous with the apical closure procedure in the blunderbuss canal. Apical resorption is rarely pulpal in nature, but is caused by an osteoclastic-like action from the tissue of the PDL space.

Lateral perforations, on the other hand, are usually the result of internal resorption, the pulp itself destroying an area of the tooth, breaking through to connect with the PDL space. In the latter case, internal resorption, the process can only be stopped by pulpectomy—total removal of the damaging pulp. After the pulp is removed, treating apical lesions or lateral lesions is essentially the same, introducing a biologically stimulating material and waiting for cementogenesis to occur. Calcium hydroxide is most frequently used for this process,[11] although tricalcium phosphate ceramic has been successful,[12] and a new collagen gel with stimulating chemicals has been proved effective by Nevins and his associates.[13]

Clinical Technique. If the pulp is necrotic or chronically inflamed, the degenerated tissue is removed, and the canal is thoroughly irrigated and totally cleansed and shaped. If the pulp is vital, it is removed with broaches and the canal is thoroughly cleansed and shaped. The tissue in the internal resorptive defect can be removed with a file that has had the tip severely bent to reach into the defect and "scratch" out the aberrant pulp tissue therein. Sodium hypochlorite should be left in place for some minutes to begin the proteolysis of the tissue.

Once the canal is thoroughly filed, it is dried and the thick paste of calcium hydroxide and camphorated parachlorophenol is packed into the canal, filling it to the apex. The temporary seal is then placed. Some discomfort may develop from the pressure.

The patient should be recalled about every six weeks and a radiograph made and evaluated. Gradually, the apex should be seen to close or the lesion associated with the lateral perforation begin repair (Fig. 16–13). At each recall, the calcium hydroxide paste is removed and replaced. When finally the bony lesion is filled in, it can be considered a matrix against which to fill; and a final, condensed, gutta percha root canal filling is placed (Fig. 16–14). This technique works as well with mechanical perforations as it does with pathologic ones.

Calcification

As previously stated, cases are sometimes seen in which a traumatic accident is not sufficiently severe to devitalize the pulp. In response to the injury, however, the pulp may begin to lay down reparative dentin which can eventually obliterate the entire pulp

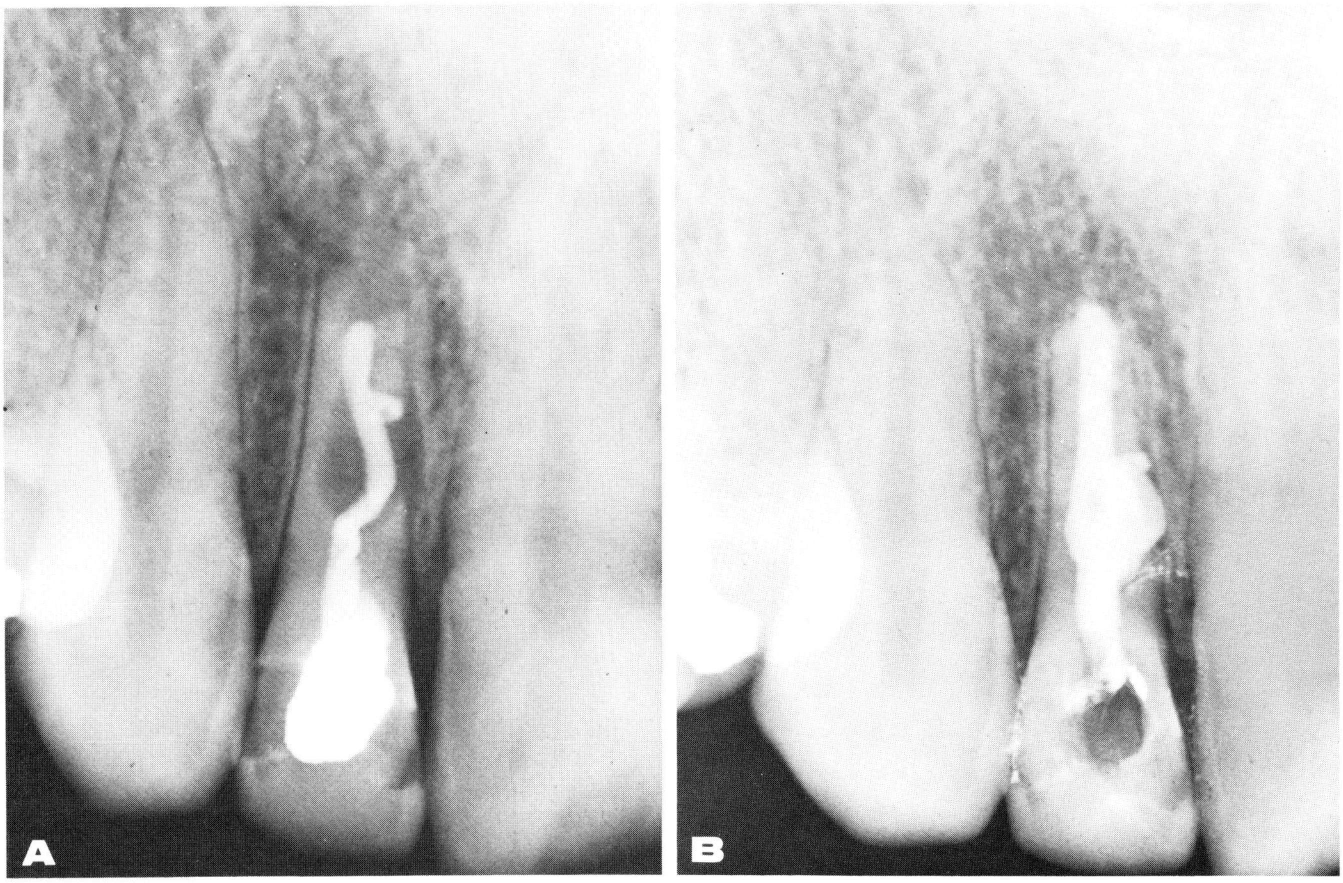

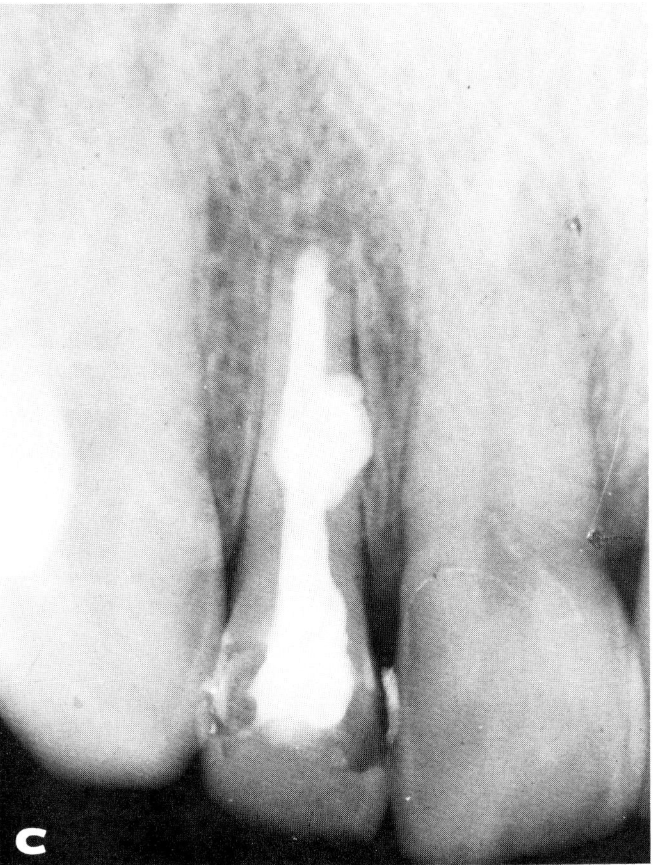

Fig. 16–14. Cementogenesis for apical and lateral perforative defects. *A,* Ineffective root canal therapy with lateral ***and*** apical resorption. Old gutta percha is removed, the canal cleansed and shaped, and calcium hydroxide paste inserted. *B,* Five weeks after calcium hydroxide therapy, obturation with gutta percha condensed with vigorous lateral and vertical pressure against new apical and lateral matrices. *C,* One-year postoperative radiograph. (From Frank, A. L. and Weine, F. S.: J.A.D.A., *87*:863, Oct., 1973.)

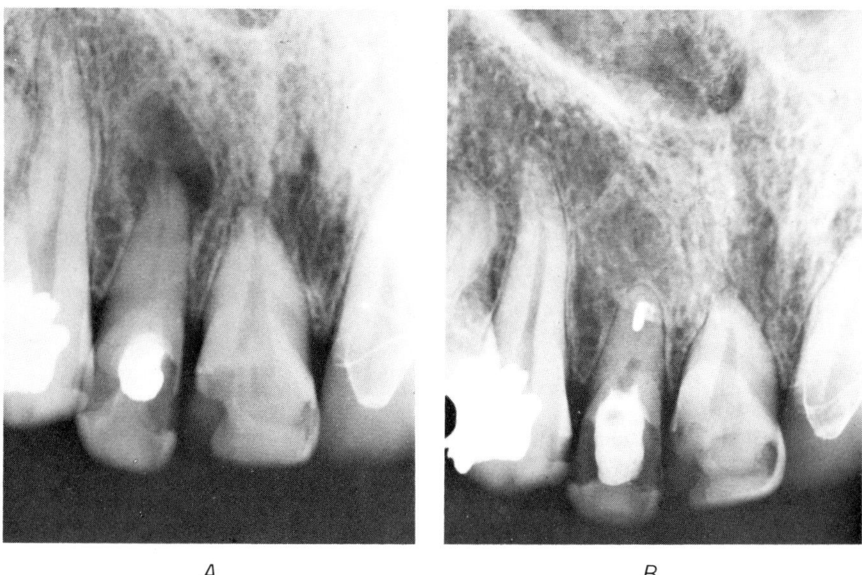

Fig. 16–15. *A*, Pulpless maxillary lateral incisor. Crown and part of root canal are calcified. *B*, Unsuccessful attempt to gain access to root canal has almost caused root perforation. Subsequent retrofilling resulted in periapical healing. Because of excessive calcification, conventional access should not have been attempted.

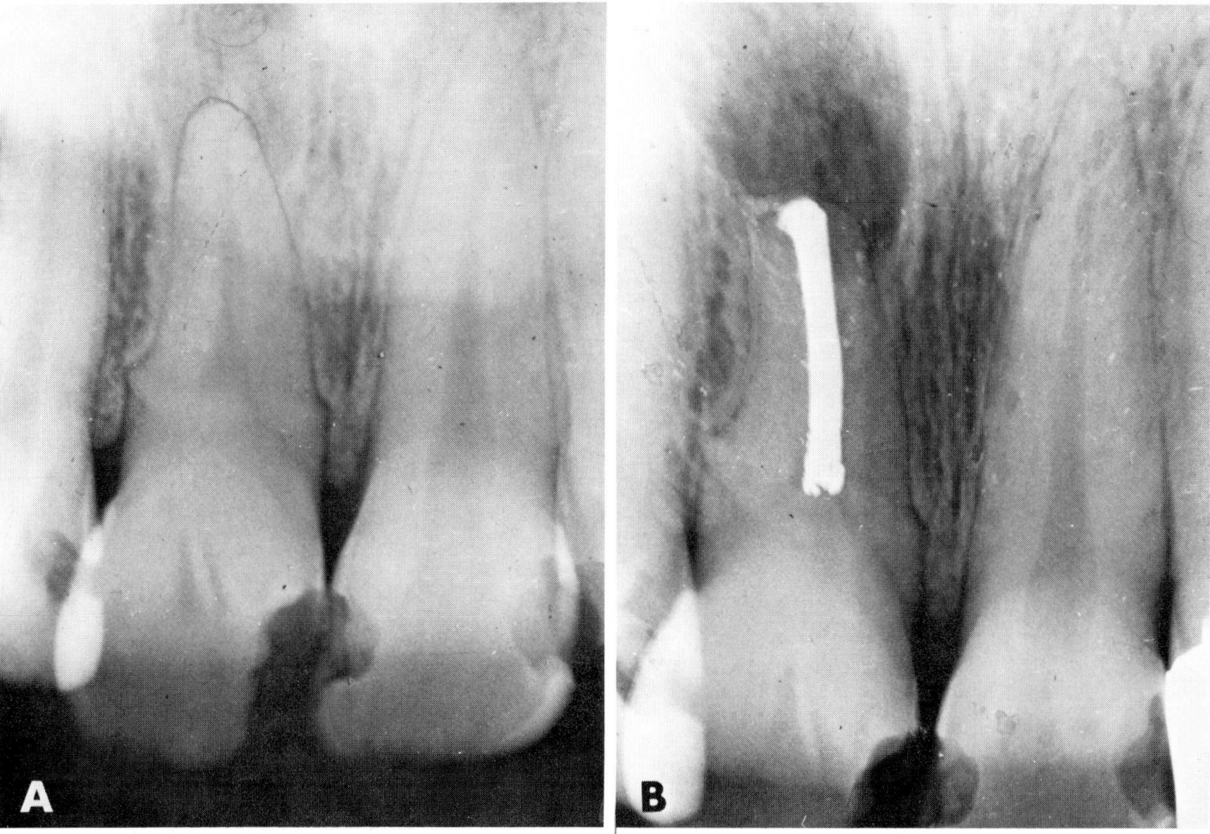

Fig. 16–16. *A*, Pulpless maxillary central incisor, years following root fracture. Callus repair of fracture is obvious. Coronal pulp remained vital and receded behind reparative dentin. Radicular pulp became necrotic. (Periapex retouched.) *B*, Access through calcified crown would be difficult and might result in crown or root perforation. Retrofilling with amalgam avoids this danger.

chamber and root canal. Teeth in which this has occurred may frequently be recognized by an opaque "lifeless" color of the crowns. These teeth often will not respond to pulp tests or will respond faintly because of the heavy pulp calcification. Roentgenographically the canal may appear totally calcified. In the absence of a periapical radiolucency or symptoms of pulpitis, one may assume that either a small portion of vital pulp is still present, or that the apical foramen has, in fact, been completely occluded by reparative dentin. In either event root canal therapy is not indicated unless painful symptoms or a periapical lesion subsequently develops. The tooth should be subjected to radiographic examination periodically to determine whether periapical changes are occurring.

In the event that the tooth responds as nonvital to pulp tests, and a periapical lesion ***is*** observed roentgenographically, root canal therapy is indicated. It is then necessary to decide whether therapy is to be carried out nonsurgically or by retrofilling. The decision should be based on the feasibility of gaining access to the patent portion of the root canal through the crown of the tooth. If calcification is considerable, and the pulp chamber and even part of the root canal are obliterated, an attempt to locate the orifice of the canal may result in excessive destruction of coronal tooth structure and possible perforation of the crown or root (Fig. 16–15). Recognition of this possibility before treatment is begun often makes it apparent that the retrosurgical approach is actually more conservative therapy than the attempt to establish coronal access. Surgical exposure of the apex and the placement of a retro-amalgam filling is the procedure of choice for the nonvital, extensively calcified pulp (Fig. 16–16).

Class II: Coronal Fracture—Pulp Not Exposed

In general, the considerations of diagnosis and treatment discussed for class I cases are also applicable to class II cases. Class II cases have added to them the problems of protection of exposed tooth structure and restoration.

If the fracture involves only enamel, or enamel and a small amount of dentin, a simple smoothing or slight contouring with stones and disks will generally provide an esthetic result. A coat of varnish should be placed over the exposed tooth structure to insulate it against thermal stimuli. Grinding and disking may also be carried out on adjacent teeth if this is necessary for esthetics. Vitality should be checked periodically throughout the area.

If the fracture involves considerable dentin, the dentin should be covered with a sedative material such as zinc oxide and eugenol, and plastic in a temporary plastic crown should be placed over the tooth (Fig. 16–17). At the end of about two months, vitality should be checked. If vitality responses are normal at this time, the tooth may be restored. The

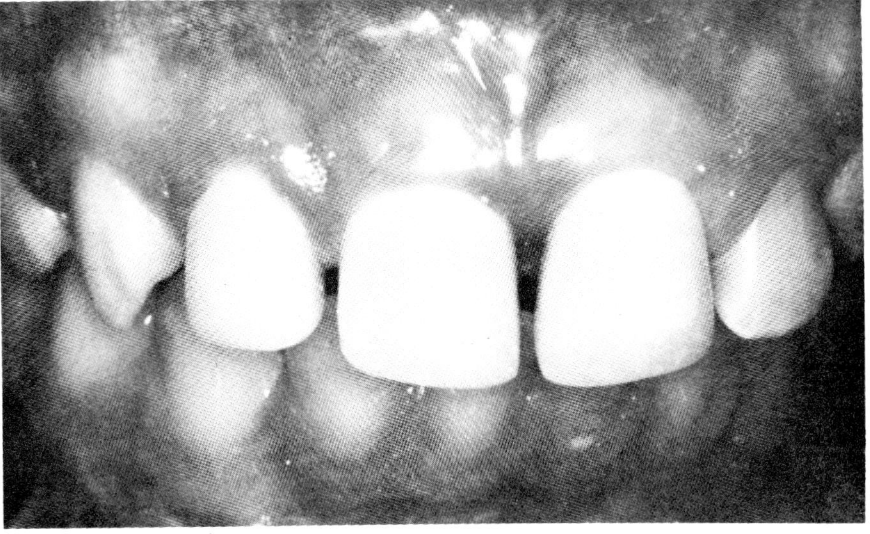

Fig. 16–17. Temporary acrylic crowns placed on maxillary central incisors and right lateral incisor after coronal fractures. Gingival margins must be carefully finished to remove acrylic "flashing" which will cause severe gingivitis.

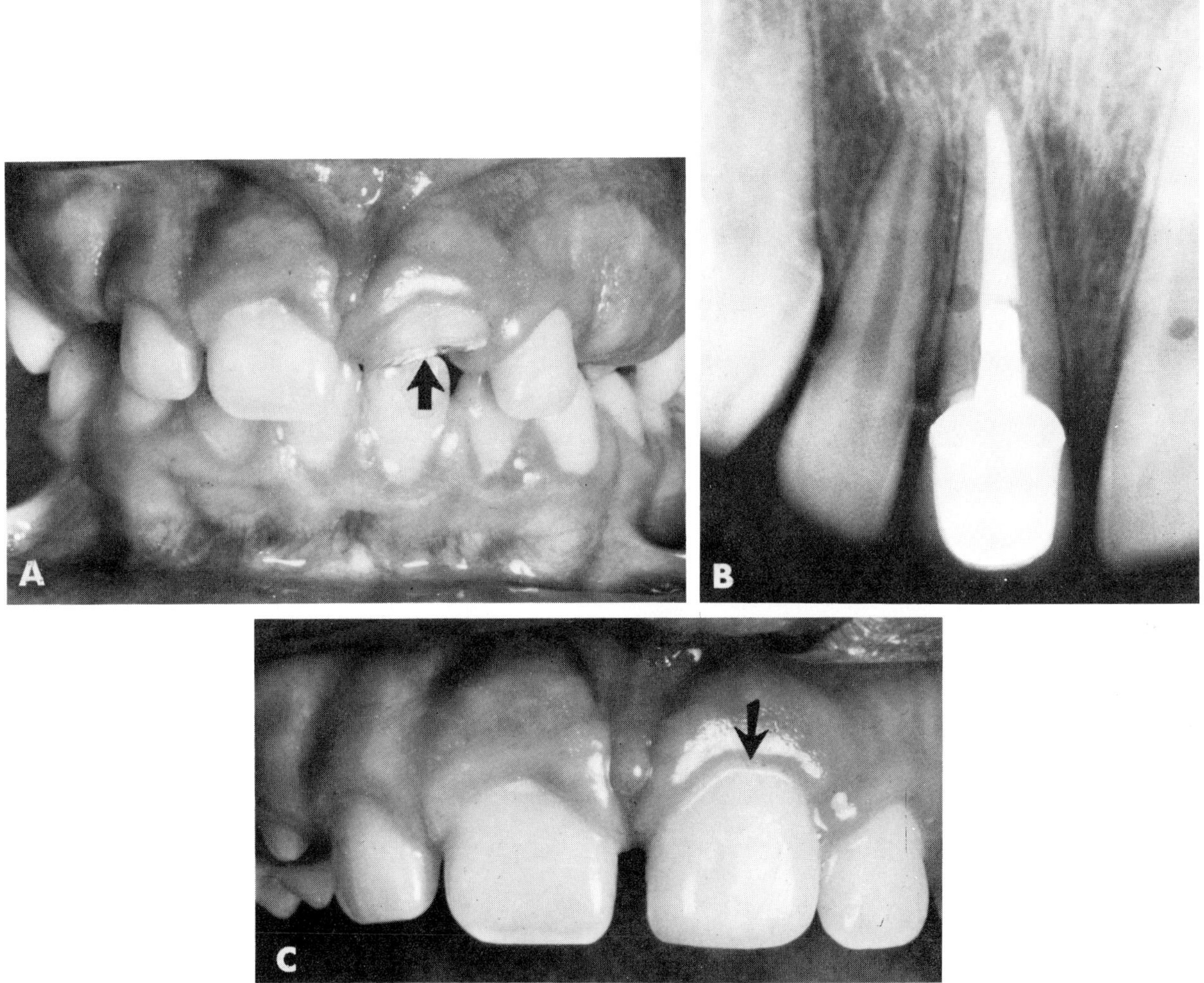

Fig. 16–18. *A*, Coronal fracture of maxillary left central incisor. *B*, Root canal therapy completed. Dowel and bonded porcelain crown placed. *C*, Bonded porcelain crown after cementation. (Courtesy Dr. Myron Warnick.)

choice of restoration will depend upon the age of the tooth and the size of the pulp chamber. If a porcelain jacket or porcelain-faced crown can be constructed without involving the pulp, one of these restorations is desirable for its superior esthetic qualities (Fig. 16–18). Several authors have reported that crowns with bonded facings may be constructed without pulp injury for most incisors, even in the younger child.[14,15]

If the pulp is liable to be exposed by a preparation for full coverage, a replacement of only the fractured portion is in order. This replacement can be made with a composite material, the fractured area being first prepared with acid etch to improve the adhesion of the composite (Fig. 16–19). The provisional restoration is quite acceptable and should well serve a youngster until the pulp recedes with age, and a shouldered or chamfered preparation may be made to receive a jacket crown. An adult with a tooth fracture not involving the pulp should have the more permanent type of crown constructed as soon as the continuing vitality of the pulp is established. Until then, a composite replacement will satisfy immediate esthetic needs.

It is commonly observed that many dentists are reluctant to recommend full coverage restorations in younger patients even when the danger of pulp exposure in preparation is negligible. This reluctance is based upon the assumption that continued rapid eruption of the crown will eventually expose the gingival margin of the restoration. The dentist

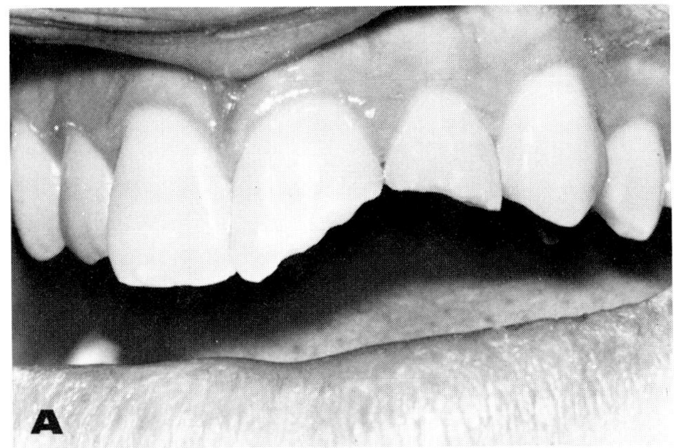

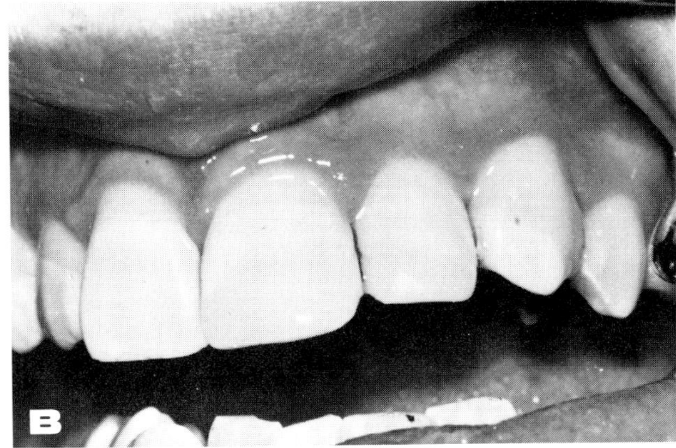

Fig. 16–19. *A*, Fractured central and lateral incisors in young patient. *B*, Restoration with composite resin restorative material. Long bevel (2 to 3 mm., if possible) of labial and lingual enamel is essential. Etching medium is applied for 90 to 120 seconds. Resin is allowed to overlap margins and is then properly finished. (From Deneky, G. E., and Fuller, J. L.: Dent. Surv., *51*:34, Nov., 1975.)

therefore will often place a less esthetic "temporary" restoration, such as a stainless steel crown, which may actually be left in place for years. Many a younger patient is thus obliged to go through difficult adolescence, self-conscious about the appearance of his teeth, until he reaches the "magic" age of twenty, and his dentist consents to restore the tooth with a jacket crown. It would seem far more desirable for the patient's psychologic well-being to place the most esthetic restoration possible at the outset. At least the parents should be made aware of the alternatives and allowed to make the choice.

Class III: Coronal Fracture—Pulp Exposed

The treatment of traumatic pulp exposures must be based on an understanding of the types of pulp therapy that can be used in such cases and the ultimate objectives of therapy. The primary objective, ***of course,*** will be the retention of the tooth. If the pulp has been devitalized, this objective can be accomplished only by complete pulp removal and root canal therapy. If the pulp remains vital after traumatic exposure, the desirability of attempting to maintain vitality must be considered. This involves the use of either of two procedures, pulp capping or pulpotomy.

Pulp capping involves the covering of a small pulp exposure with a sedative material or a material capable of stimulating repair of the exposure by reparative dentin formation.

Pulpotomy involves the removal of the coronal portion of a vital pulp, leaving the radicular portion intact. The result sought in pulpotomy is the formation of a protective layer or "bridge" of

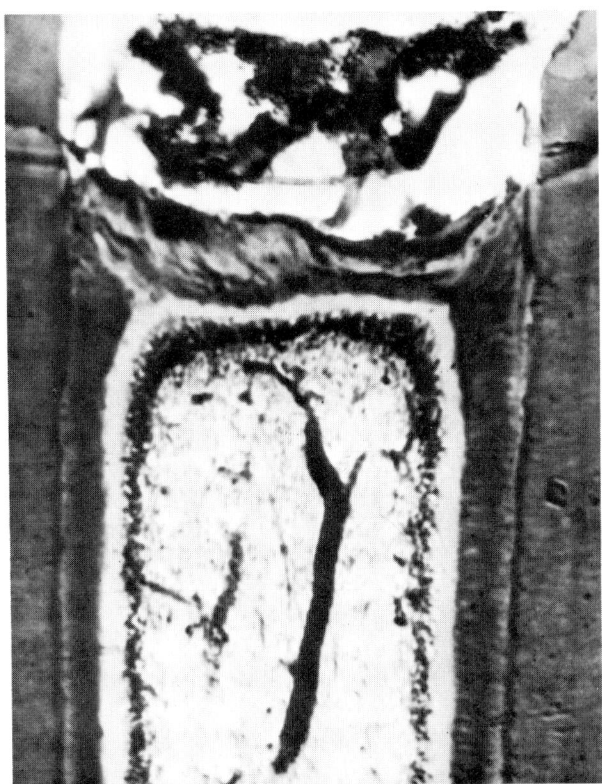

Fig. 16–20. Dentin bridge formed after calcium hydroxide pulpotomy. Note intense cellular activity below bridge. (Courtesy Dr. Seiichi Matsumiya.)

reparative dentin over the amputated surface of the pulp (Fig. 16–20).

Pulp ***capping is generally not recommended*** in cases of traumatic pulp exposure in anterior teeth. Although the capping of small fresh pulp exposures may be attempted, several factors tend to make the use of the pulpotomy more desirable:

1. Gross bacterial contamination usually occurs in traumatic pulp exposure. This contaminated surface pulp may remain if capping is carried out, but is likely to be removed by pulpotomy.
2. It is difficult to restore a pulp capped tooth without disturbing the capping. This is ***not*** true with pulpotomy.
3. It is often difficult to obtain retention in restoring a pulp capped tooth, while retention is easily obtained in the pulp chamber following pulpotomy.
4. The success of the pulpotomy procedure compares favorably with the success of pulp capping.

The relative disadvantages of pulp capping therefore make pulpotomy the indicated procedure in attempting to maintain pulp vitality after traumatic exposure.

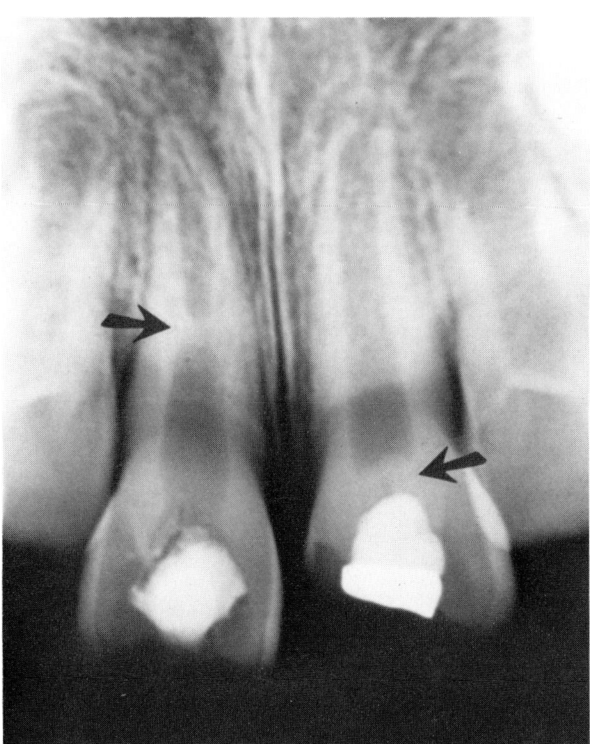

Fig. 16–21. Calcium hydroxide pulpotomy following fracture allows development of apices of central incisors. Note dentin bridge formation on both teeth.

The decision to utilize pulpotomy is based primarily on the degree of development of the root apex. If ***root formation is not complete, pulpotomy*** should be carried out whenever possible to allow continued apical development (Fig. 16–21). A successful pulpotomy will maintain the vitality of the radicular pulp, permit root-end closure, and thus eliminate the need for surgical treatment. If at a later time pulp death should occur, conservative root canal condensation can be successfully carried out against the closed root end. In the event of pulp death and a remaining open apex, apexification, stimulated by biologically active materials, is indicated. Once the root end closes, optimal obturation of the canal may be made.

Pulpotomy has also been advocated for adult teeth with closed apices, and successful cases are not unusual (Fig. 16–22). The chance of success, however, is not as great as in young teeth because of the less abundant pulp circulation and poorer ability of the adult pulp to bring about repair. In addition, since the apices of adult teeth are already closed, the primary indication for pulpotomy, which is to allow root-end development, no longer exists.

The presently favored material for covering the pulp stump after pulpotomy is calcium hydroxide used in the form of a dry powder, or as a paste with methyl cellulose (Pulpdent). Calcium hydroxide has been shown to stimulate formation of a bridge of reparative dentin over the vital pulp stump.[17,18]

However, internal resorption rather than reparative dentin formation is sometimes an unfortunate sequela to the use of calcium hydroxide (Fig. 16–23). In pulp capping experiments done by Hunter,[19] calcific bridging was observed under calcium hydroxide, magnesium hydroxide, and zince oxide-eugenol. Experiments in human teeth[18,19] failed to show bridging under zinc oxide–eugenol. Massler has shown that in rats, bridging occurs under zinc oxide–eugenol, but not as rapidly as under calcium hydroxide.[20] These differences in response to zinc oxide–eugenol may reflect differences in reaction between human and animal subjects.

The widespread use of corticosteroid drugs stimulated interest in their therapeutic value in pulp capping and pulpotomy. Fiore-Donno and Baume,[21] and Lawson and Mitchell,[22] have shown that a corticoid capping paste was capable of clinically reversing painful pulpitis. However,

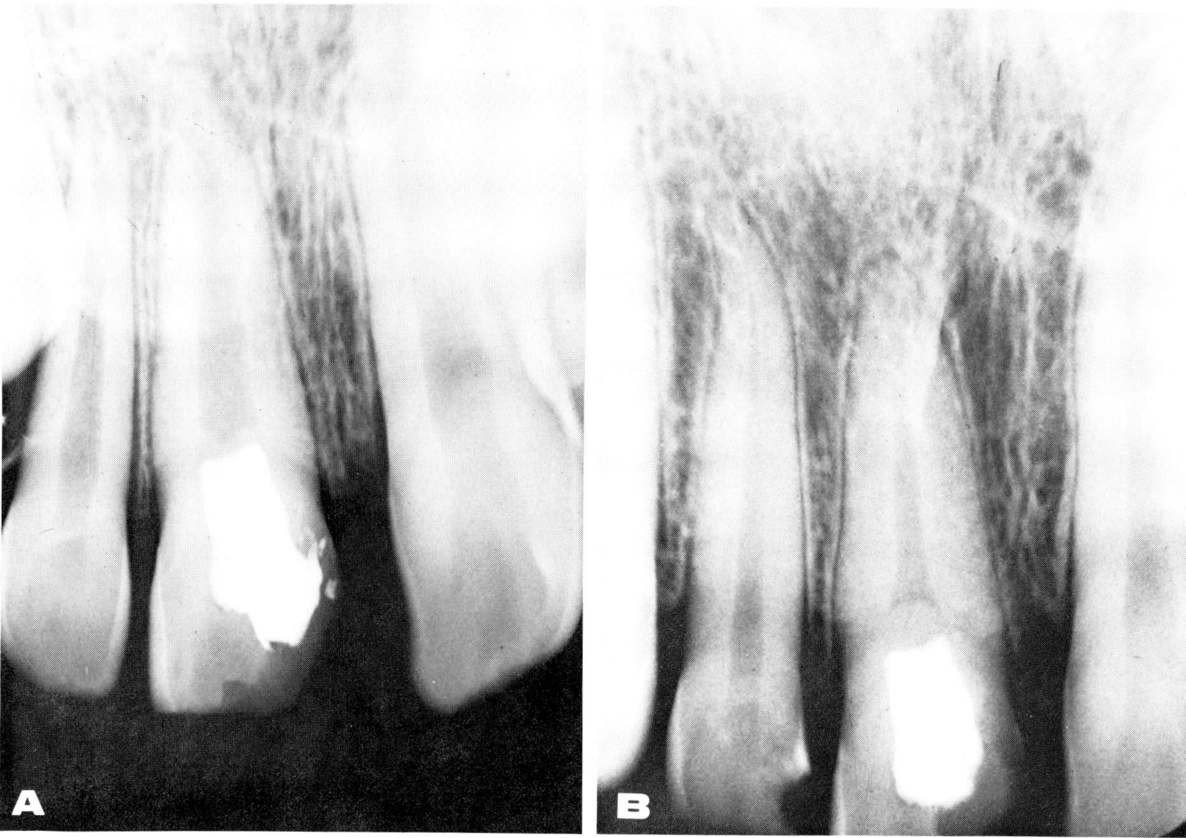

Fig. 16–22. *A,* Young adult tooth. Vital pulpotomy and calcium hydroxide placed day after accident and exposure. *B,* Pulp is still vital under visible dentin bridge 11 years later. (Courtesy Dr. Joe Merrell, Vancouver, B.C.)

calcific bridging was not observed. Experiments by Vigg indicated that bridge formation could be obtained when a corticosteroid was sealed in place by a layer of calcium hydroxide.[23]

Success Factors in Pulpotomy. Pulpotomy should not be attempted in fracture cases if there are clinical symptoms of pulpitis or if the pulp shows signs of having been devitalized. The chance of success will be improved if the exposure has occurred within the previous twenty-four hours. Exposures of longer duration will have increased the likelihood of extensive bacterial invasion of the pulp tissue. The exposed pulp should be red in color and should bleed freely when pricked with an explorer point. If these indications of vitality are present, pulpotomy may be attempted in spite of negative responses to thermal and electric pulp tests, since these tests tend to be unreliable in traumatized young teeth.

If pulpotomy is indicated, it should be carried out under the rubber dam with the use of sterile instruments.

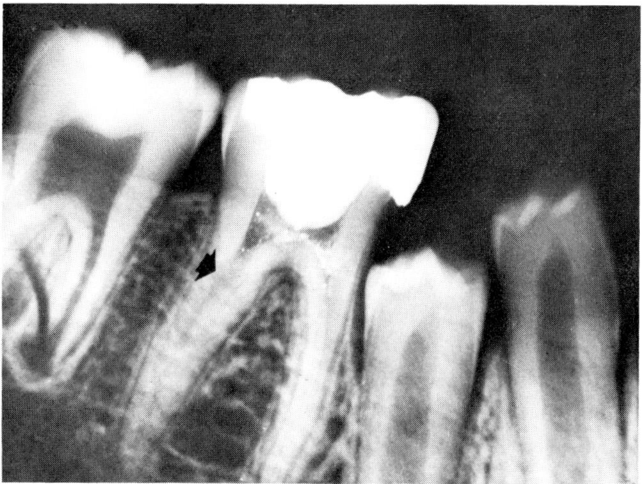

Fig. 16–23. Internal resorption *(arrow)* following calcium hydroxide pulpotomy of permanent first molar.

Pulpotomy Technique for Fractured Teeth

1. The tooth is anesthetized by block or infiltration anesthetic.
2. The rubber dam is placed and the tooth is swabbed with tincture of Zephiran.
3. Access is made through the lingual or occlusal surface of the fractured tooth and the pulp chamber is fully exposed.
4. The entire coronal pulp is amputated to the cervical level with sterile spoon excavators or curettes.
5. The pulp chamber is washed with sterile distilled water and dried with sterile cotton pellets.
6. A layer of calcium hydroxide paste (Pulpdent) is placed over the amputated pulp stump and air-dried. This is followed by placement of a creamy mix of zinc oxyphosphate cement.
7. After the zinc cement has set, a temporary (soft) silver amalgam restoration is placed for protection.

Following the pulpotomy, the patient should be recalled at one-, three-, and six-month intervals for roentgenographic examination and vitality testing. Radiographs in successful cases will show the development of calcific bridging over the pulp stump. If bridging is complete and vitality tests are normal, the tooth may be permanently restored at this time. If bridging has occurred but responses to pulp tests are negative, the patient should be re-examined at three-month intervals during the next six months to see if root development is progressing. The absence of further root development indicates failure of the pulpotomy and the necessity for employing the procedures recommended by Frank to produce apexification.[8] If and when the calcium hydroxide induced root growth is complete, final obturation of the canal and a permanent restoration may take place.

Class IV: Coronal Fracture—Extending Subgingivally

Class IV cases are similar to those in class III with respect to considerations of pulp exposure. The class IV case is further complicated by extension of the fracture beneath the gingival margin. The sight of these cases often causes the dentist to throw up his hands in despair; in many instances, however, despair is unwarranted. Most cases of subgingival fracture do not involve the root surface, and the fracture is found to extend only to the cementoenamel junction. The cementoenamel junction may be well below the gingival margin in youngsters with erupting teeth. If the lingual plate of enamel is fractured subgingivally, a simple gingivectomy generally is sufficient to expose the fractured margin. If lingual root surface is involved, an osteoectomy also may be necessary to expose the point of fracture. The resulting differences in gingival level are of little concern, since esthetic considerations are not a factor in restoration on the lingual. If, on the other hand, the fracture involves the ***labial*** plate of enamel, esthetics must be considered. It may then be necessary to extend the gingivectomy or osteoectomy to one tooth on either side of the involved tooth in order to produce a gingival level consistent with that of the fractured tooth (Fig. 16–24).

Occasionally a tooth fractures because of weakening by previous restoration, caries, or a combination of both. As a result, the crown may be completely lost, leaving intact an entirely subgingival root stump. The utilization of periodontal therapy may well be the salvation of such apparently hopeless teeth. A combination of gingivectomy and osteoectomy, extended to adjacent teeth if necessary, can accomplish the following:

1. The fractured margin and additional root structure are exposed to facilitate restoration.
2. Sufficient root structure is exposed to allow placement of a rubber dam clamp so that endodontic therapy may be carried out aseptically.
3. A suitable osseous and gingival architecture are created.

If the pulp is vital and conservative endodontic therapy is indicated, the entire endodontic procedure may be completed at the time of periodontal surgery. The amount of time involved in the combined endodontic-periodontic therapy may be no more than an hour and will spare the patient the necessity of tooth extraction and construction of a bridge or partial denture. In some cases, to avoid surgery or its unsightly result, orthodontic movement of the tooth should be considered (see Class V Fractures).

Subgingival Fracture of Posterior Teeth. Fracture in posterior teeth is rarely caused by the typical traumatic injuries affecting the anterior teeth. However, these teeth commonly suffer fracture as a result of undermining by caries, or failure to protect weakened cusps adequately. Fracture also may occur as the result of seating of tight-fitting gold inlays (Fig. 16–25).

If the fracture is subgingival but does not involve the furca area of the tooth, treatment will be the same

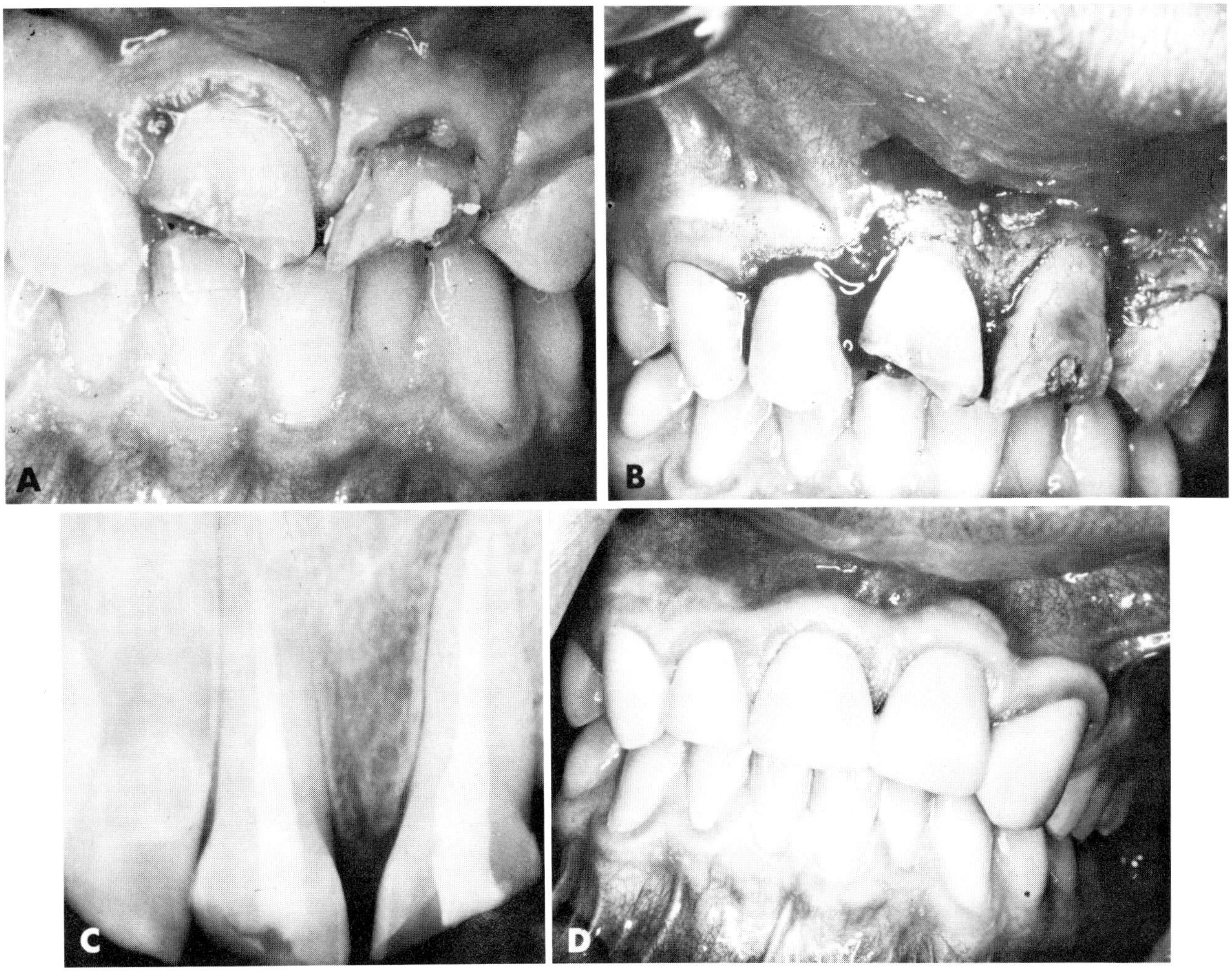

Fig. 16–24. *A*, Impact fracture of maxillary incisors. Fracture of labial enamel plate of left central and lateral incisors extends subgingivally. Temporary crown has been placed on lateral incisor. *B*, Gingivoplasty and osteoplasty expose subgingival fracture line of left central and lateral incisors. *C*, Root canal therapy completed. (Endodontic therapy by Dr. Victor Rodriguez.) *D*, Soft tissue healing complete and provisional restorations in place. (Provisional restorations by Dr. Earl Gowda.)

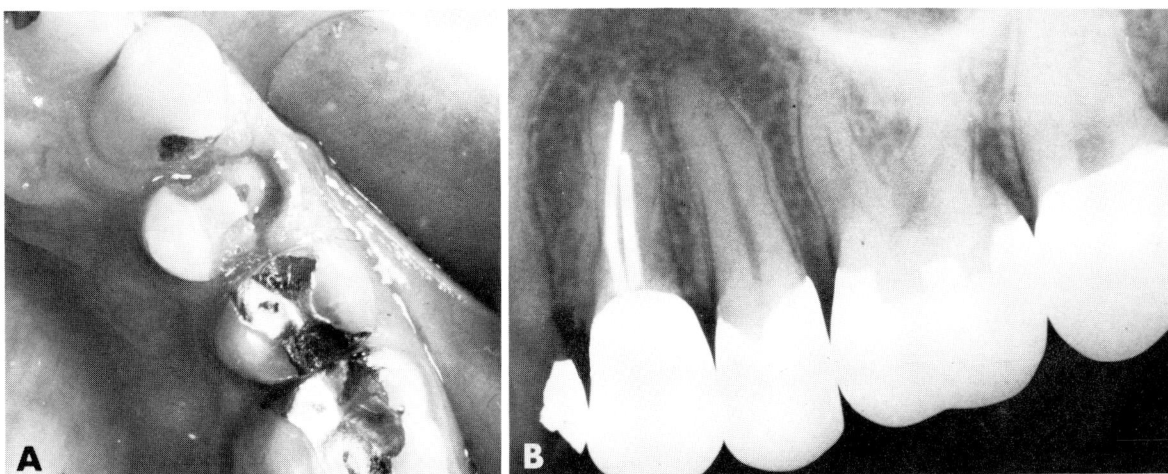

Fig. 16–25. *A*, Buccal cusp fracture and pulp exposure of first premolar following seating of gold inlay. Gingivectomy was necessary to expose subgingival fracture line. *B*, Root canal therapy completed and porcelain-faced crown placed.

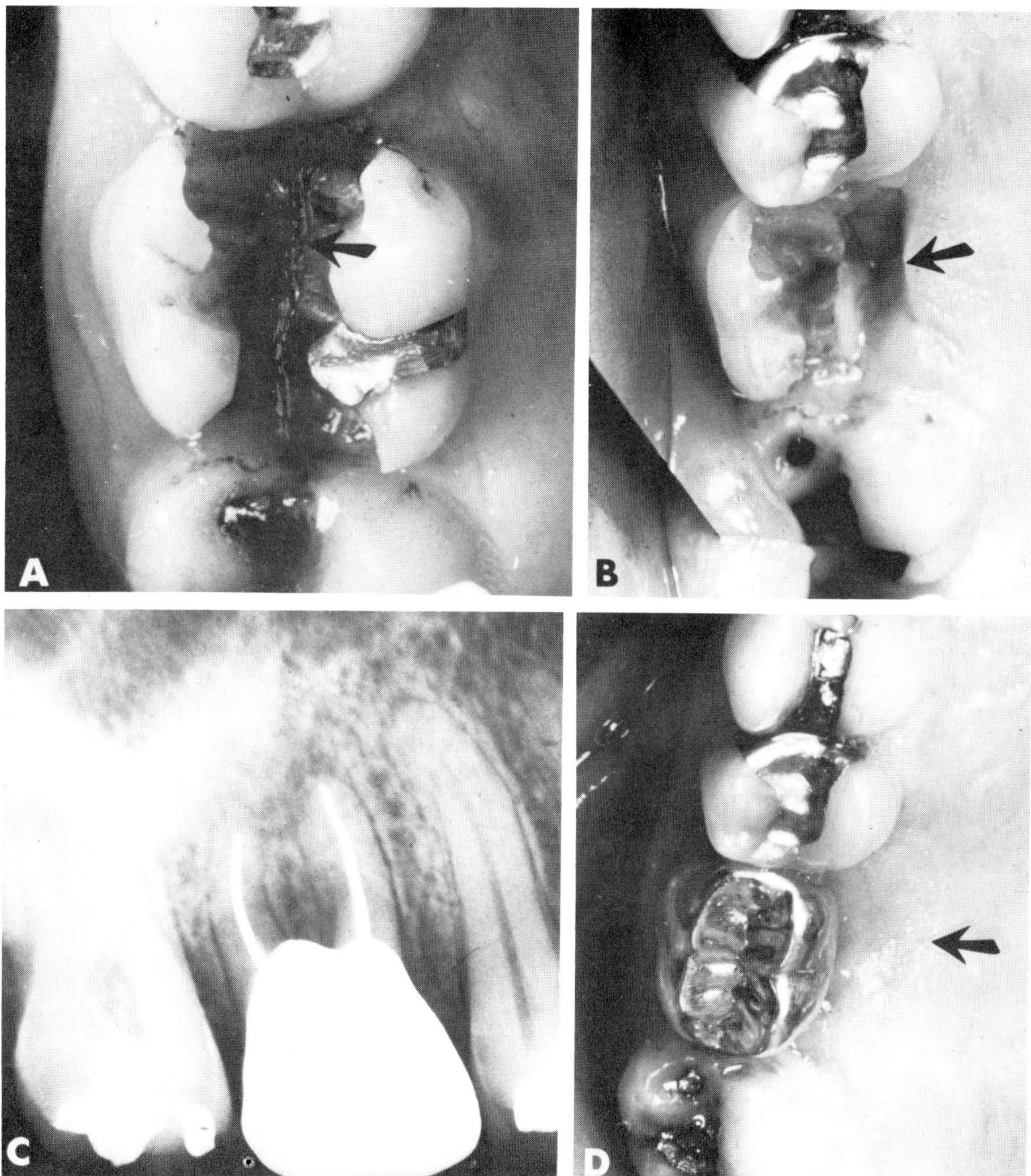

Fig. 16–26. Fracture into trifurcation of maxillary molar, treated by hemisection and endodontic therapy. *A*, Maxillary first molar. Fracture visible in floor of preparation extends into trifurcation. *B*, Lingual half of crown and palatal root extracted. Soft tissue defect must be repaired by gingivoplasty. *C*, Root canal therapy completed for remaining buccal roots and crown placed. *D*, Crown in place on first molar. Note that buccolingual diameter of occlusal table is narrower than second premolar. This reduces torquing forces on remaining buccal roots. Scar line *(arrow)* from the gingivoplasty which eliminated tissue defect is apparent. (Restoration by Dr. Leif Overby.)

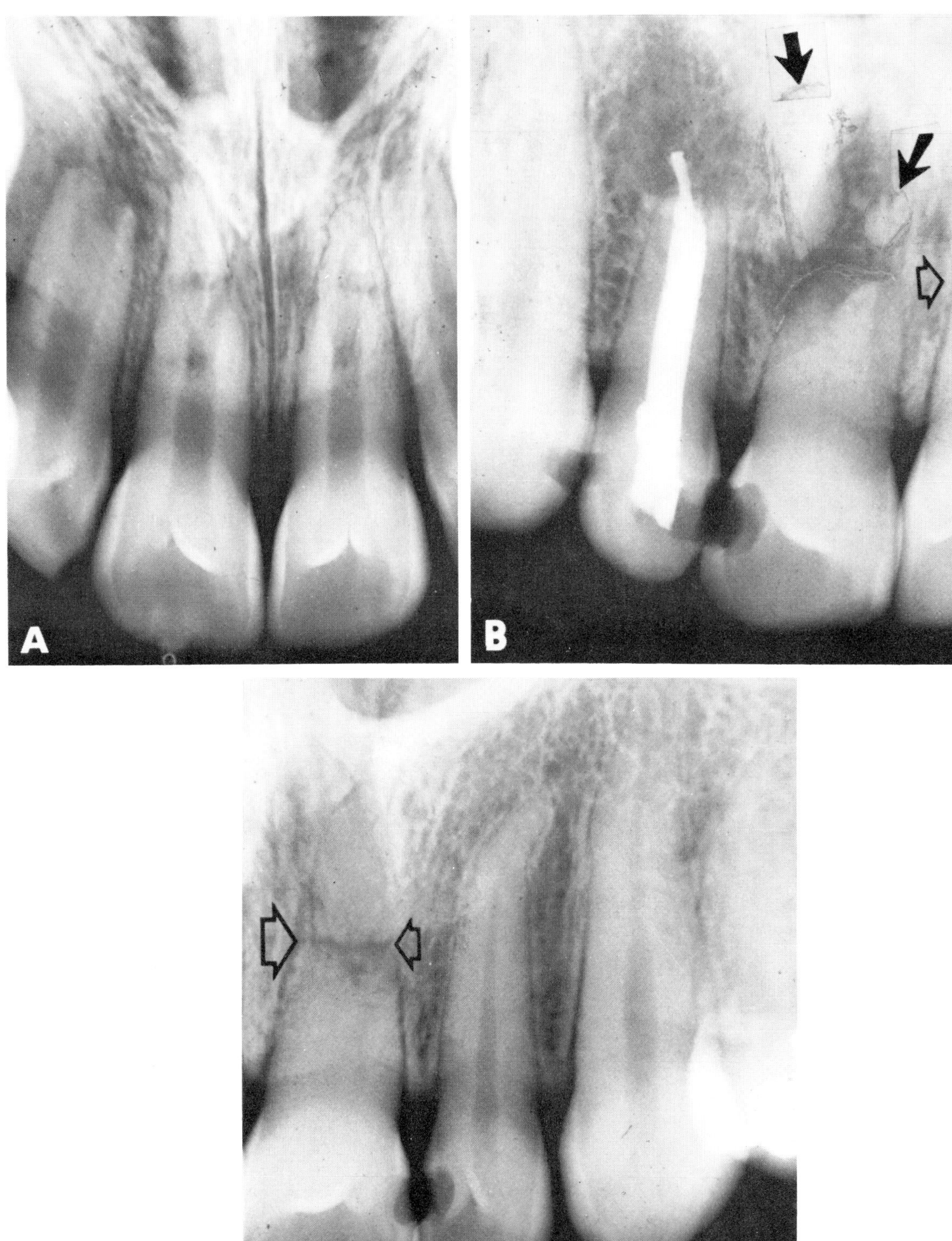

Fig. 16–27. *A,* Severe impact has fractured roots of central incisors and devitalized pulp of right lateral incisor. Pulps of central incisors have remained vital. *B,* Ten years after injury. Root tip of right central incisor has now fragmented and separated *(black arrows)* and pulp is nonvital. Root canal therapy completed for right lateral incisor ten years earlier is failing. (Retouched for clarity.) *C,* Left central incisor has remained vital and fracture has repaired *(open arrows).*

as for anterior teeth and may involve gingivectomy, osteoectomy, root canal therapy, and restoration. If the fracture extends into the furca, it may be possible to remove one of the fractured segments and its root and restore the other after root canal therapy (Fig. 16–26). The segment to be retained is the one most esthetically and functionally restorable. Gingivectomy and osteoectomy generally are required. The procedure is accomplished, in the case of the mesiodistal fracture of maxillary premolars or molars, by removal of the buccal or lingual half of the crown and its root, or, in the case of buccolingual fracture of lower molars, by removal of the mesial or distal half of the crown and its root, much like a hemisection.

Class V: Root Fracture with or without Loss Of Crown Structure

Division 1: Horizontal Fractures

Fractures of the roots of teeth may occur with or without loss of coronal tooth structure. The incidence of root fracture is negligible in the age range of seven to ten years.[24] This may well be due to the fact that at this age the roots of the permanent anterior teeth are not completely developed. They tend to be avulsed or luxated by trauma rather than fractured.[25]

With regard to fully formed adult teeth, if a horizontal fracture occurs in midroot or in the apical third, the prognosis for retention is quite favorable (Fig. 16–27). In a surprising number of these cases, both fragments remain vital. Even negative vitality readings at the time of the accident should not be taken too seriously. Vitality response frequently returns after the shock has worn off. Andreasen has discussed the problems engendered by root fracture as well as the various forms of healing.[26,27] He points out that:

1. Union of the two segments by calcified tissue may develop much as a broken bone heals (Fig. 16–28*A*).
2. A lack of union may develop in which connective tissue separates the segments and cementum grows over the fractured surfaces.

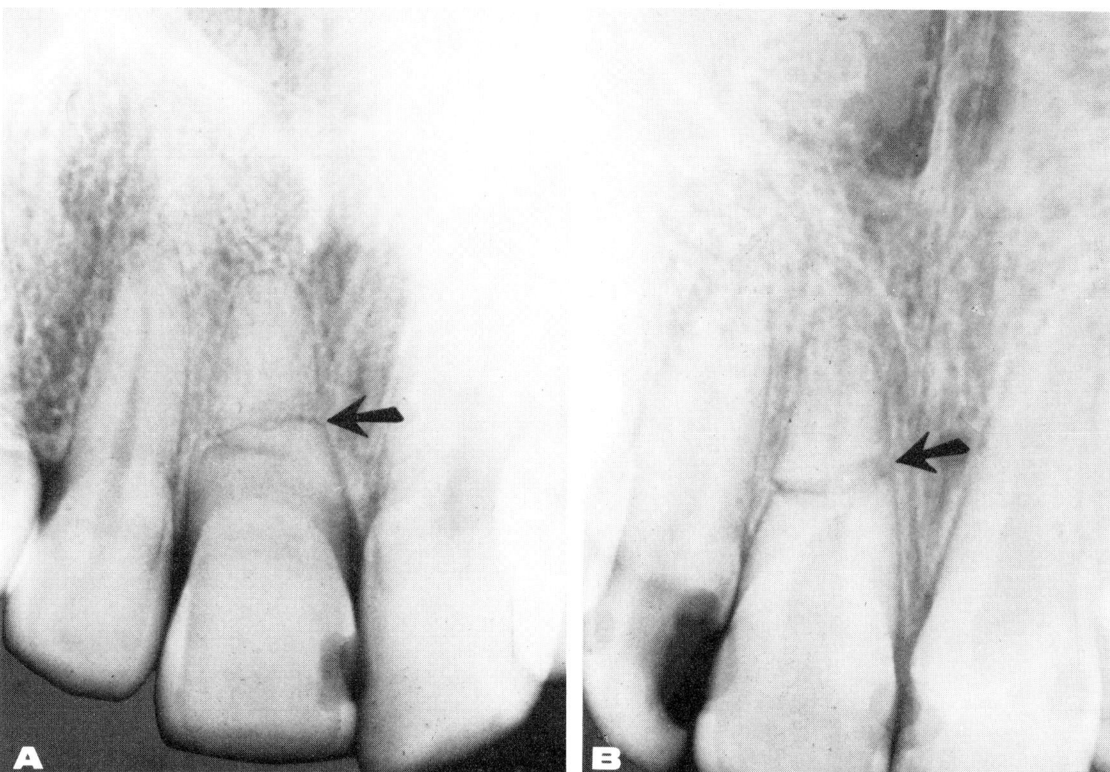

Fig. 16–28. Repair after root fracture. *A*, Repair after mid-root fracture of central incisor by callus formation. Total calcification of pulp chamber and root canal has resulted from trauma. *B*, Repair of fractured root of central incisor by deposition of connective tissue and bone in spite of displacement of apical fragment. Pulp of tooth is vital.

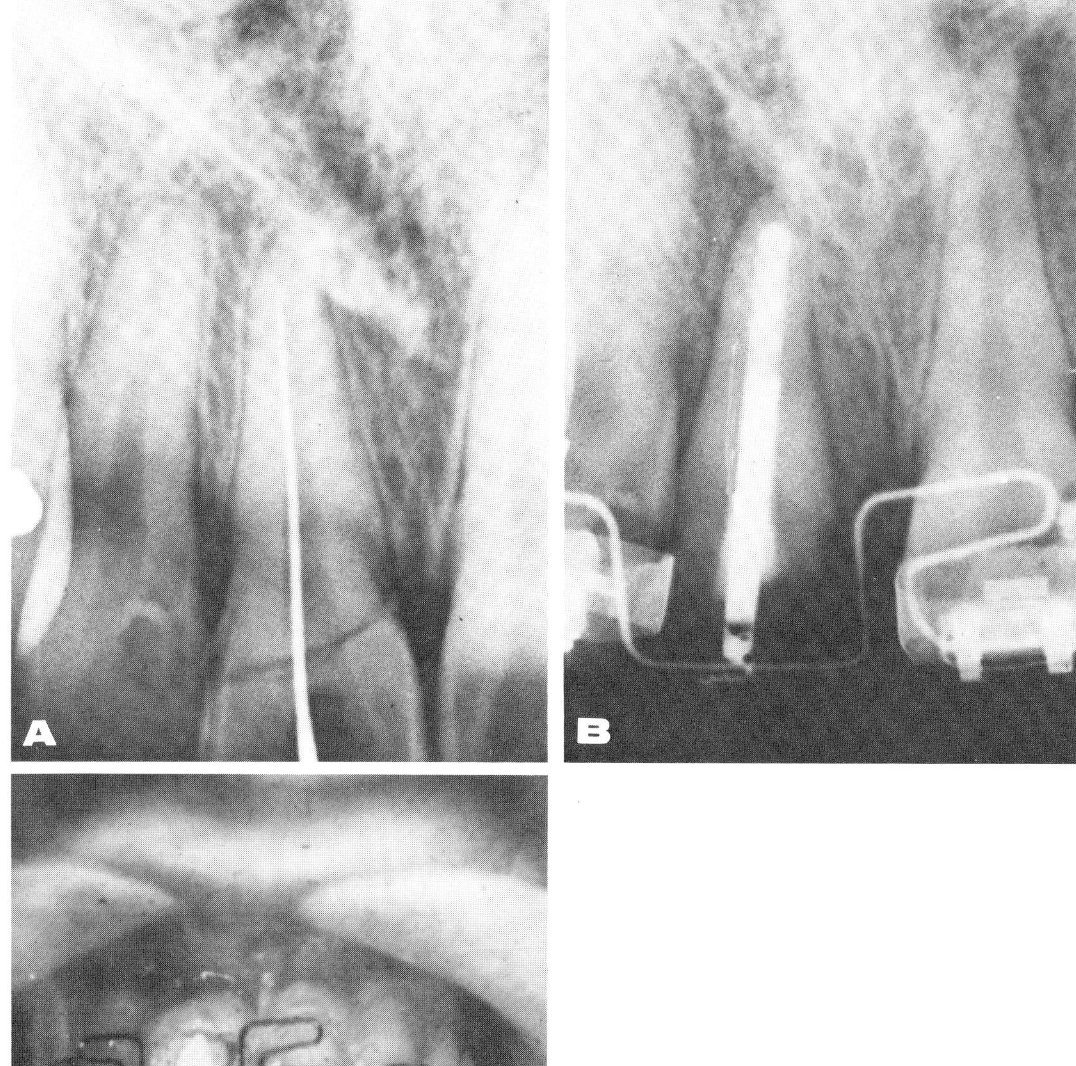

Fig. 16–29. *A*, Oblique coronal fracture below labial gingiva of central incisor. Pulp necrotic. *B*, Root canal filled and post cemented to place. Orthodontic appliance applying traction. *C*, Finger spring appliance. Continued adjustment of spring tension will "erupt" tooth to restorable position followed by two months of retention. Left canine should have also been banded. (Courtesy Dr. Andrew E. Michanowicz.)

3. A lack of union of the segments is separated by connective tissue and a bony bridge. Normal PDL is attached to the broken segments (Fig. 16–28*B*).

4. A lack of union with chronic inflammatory tissue separates the segments. The pulp of the apical fragment is most apt to remain vital, the coronal fragment becoming necrotic.

When this latter circumstance occurs (lack of union with a necrotic pulp in the coronal segment) it is suggested that cementogenesis might be stimulated early by the debridement of the short canal and the placement of calcium hydroxide. The treatment should be checked every four to six months, and if it appears to be successful, the calcium hydroxide should be replenished in the hope that the two fragments will unite or, at least, that the canal orifice will close over with cementum. A root canal filling can then be more easily placed in the coronal segment canal.

The prognosis in cases of horizontal root fracture (fracture at a right angle to the long axis of the tooth) depends primarily on the level of fracture. Teeth fractured in the ***coronal*** third of the root may have the root segment saved even though the coronal segment is lost. The terminal fragment may then be made serviceable by orthodontically moving it into position. Heithersay has detailed an orthodontic procedure to "erupt" the root segment beyond the gingiva (Fig. 16–29).[28] If the fractured crown segment is still in place, a full pulpectomy is done and both segments are filled with gutta percha. A threaded post is then placed into the root segment, and through a rectangular slot cut in the crown, an orthodontic appliance is placed to move the root into a workable position (Fig. 16–30*A*).

In the event the crown segment is missing, it is simpler to attach the same appliance (Fig. 16–30*B*). Once the root is moved into the proper position, it should be retained there for two months and then finally restored with a coping and dowel and jacket crown (Fig. 16–31).

In other cases of root fracture, wherein the coronal segment is retained but the pulp devitalized, the decision must be made whether to include the apical segment in the root canal filling or whether to remove it surgically. If the apical fragment is small or if it is considerably displaced from the coronal segment and surrounded by a lesion, it should be removed (see Fig. 16–27*B*). If the apical segment is large and in close approximation to the coronal segment, it should be retained and included in root canal instrumentation and filling. If the tooth is not mobile, root canal filling

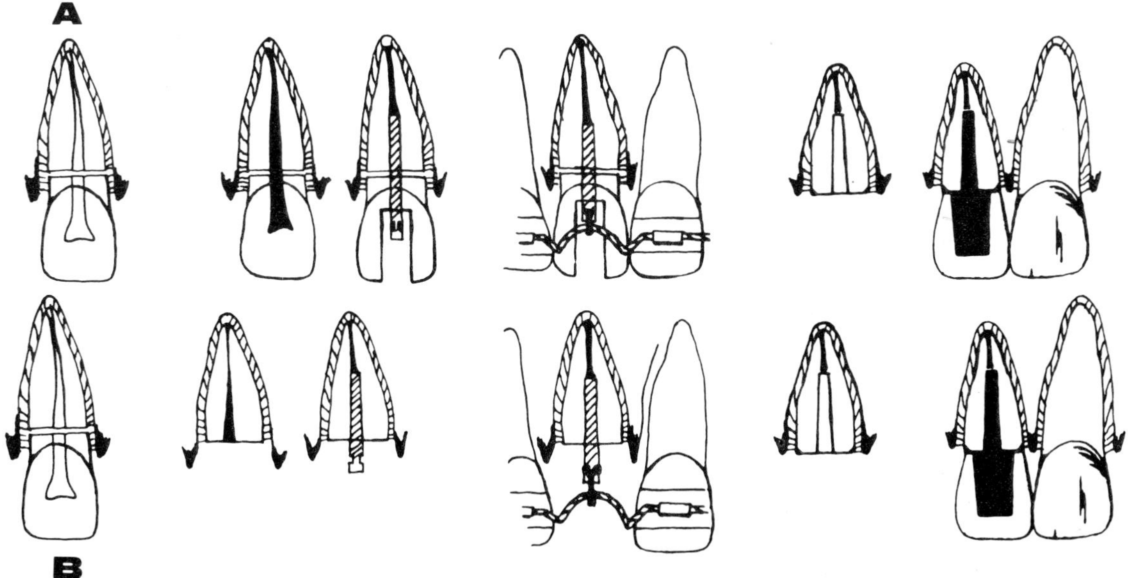

Fig. 16–30. Combined endodontic-orthodontic therapy for transverse root fracture at alveolar crest level. *A*, ***Retention of clinical crown.*** *Left to right:* transverse fracture, root canal obturated, crown incised and post placed, appliance attached, root moved to new position, post and coping crown restoration. *B*, ***Loss of clinical crown.*** *Left to right:* transverse fracture, root canal filled, post (shank of bur) placed, appliance attached, root moved to new position, post and coping crown restoration. (From Heithersay, G. S.: Oral Surg., *36*:404, Sept., 1973.)

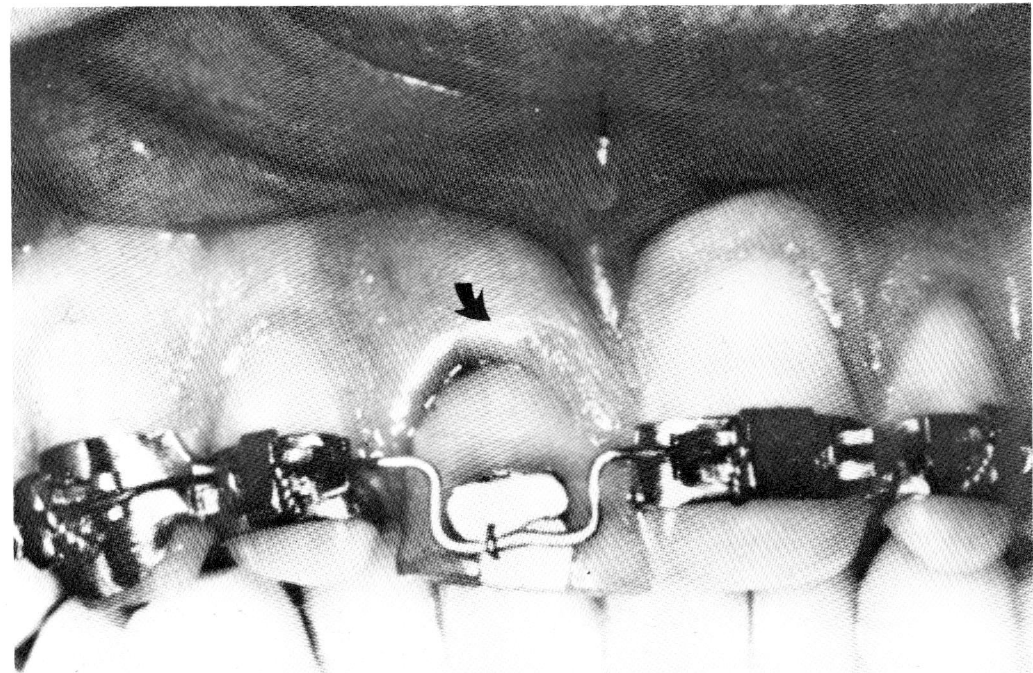

Fig. 16–31. Two months after initiation of treatment, tooth has moved downward 4 mm. and is now in retention. Notice movement of gingiva as well *(arrow).* (From Heithersay, G. S.: Oral Surg., *36*:404, Sept., 1973.)

can be carried out in a conventional manner with gutta percha (Fig. 16–32). If ***mobility*** is present, root canal filling can be carried out with a more rigid material, which will tend to splint the two segments. A chrome-cobalt endodontic implant can be used for this purpose, what Kaiser has referred to as an "orthopedic-filling," as in pinning a long bone (Fig. 16–33).[5]

If the fracture has caused mobility of the tooth, stabilization by splinting will be necessary. Plastic, band, or wire splints may be used for this purpose and should be kept in place for about six weeks. The tooth should also be ground out of occlusion to minimize trauma during the period of healing.

A novel application of the endodontic implant has been used successfully by Frank in cases of mid-root fracture in which the ***coronal*** fragment was highly mobile (Fig. 16–34).[7,10] After surgical removal of the pathologic apical fragment, conventional lingual access is obtained to the root canal of the coronal segment. The root canal is then instrumented and the largest endodontic implant is fitted in the canal to extend apically the entire length of the removed fragment. The original tooth length is thus restored by the chrome-cobalt implant. Again, it is imperative that the apical preparation be sealed by the implant passing into the bony space. Shortening the tip-end of the implant by 2-mm. segments will ensure that the point will reach the depth of the bony lesion while tightly fitting the round apical preparation. This entire procedure is thoroughly discussed in Chapter 15.

The crown should be splinted during the period of initial healing. Bone will fill in around the metal "root," and mobility will be eliminated.

It is important that the difference be pointed out between the endodontic implant that passes through the tooth into the bone, and the metal endosseous or blade implants that pass through the ***oral tissue*** into the bone. Natiella et al. have shown the disturbing incidence of failure due to inflammation around the metal blade implants.[29] Neuman, Spangberg, and Langeland found experimentally that the inflammatory response to metal implants "was significantly greater in the exposed [to the oral environment] implants than in the unexposed implants."[30]

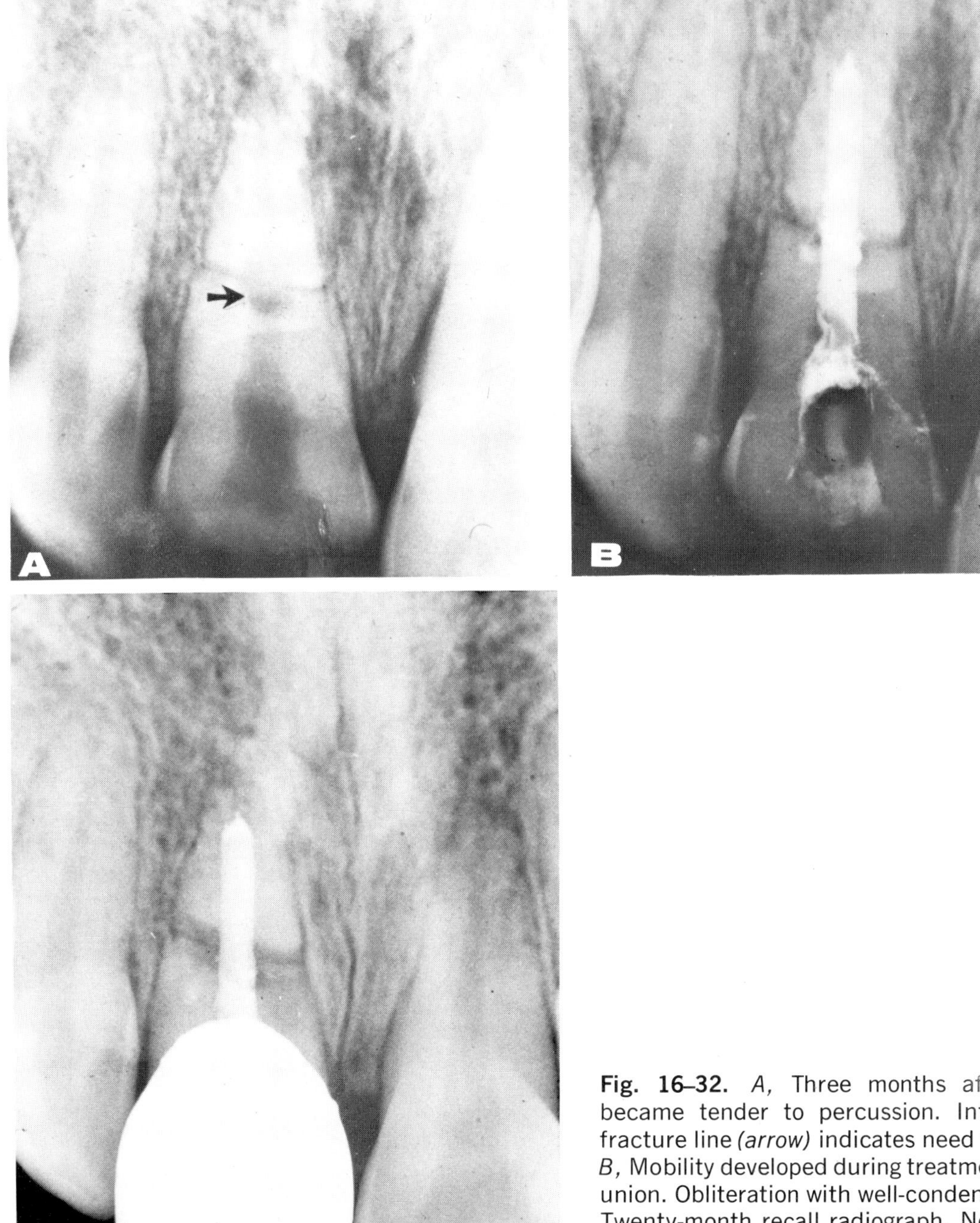

Fig. 16–32. *A,* Three months after trauma, incisor became tender to percussion. Internal resorption at fracture line *(arrow)* indicates need to remove vital pulp. *B,* Mobility developed during treatment indicating lack of union. Obliteration with well-condensed gutta percha. *C,* Twenty-month recall radiograph. No appreciable mobility. (From Frank, A. L.: Dent. Clin. N. Amer., *18*:465, Apr., 1974.)

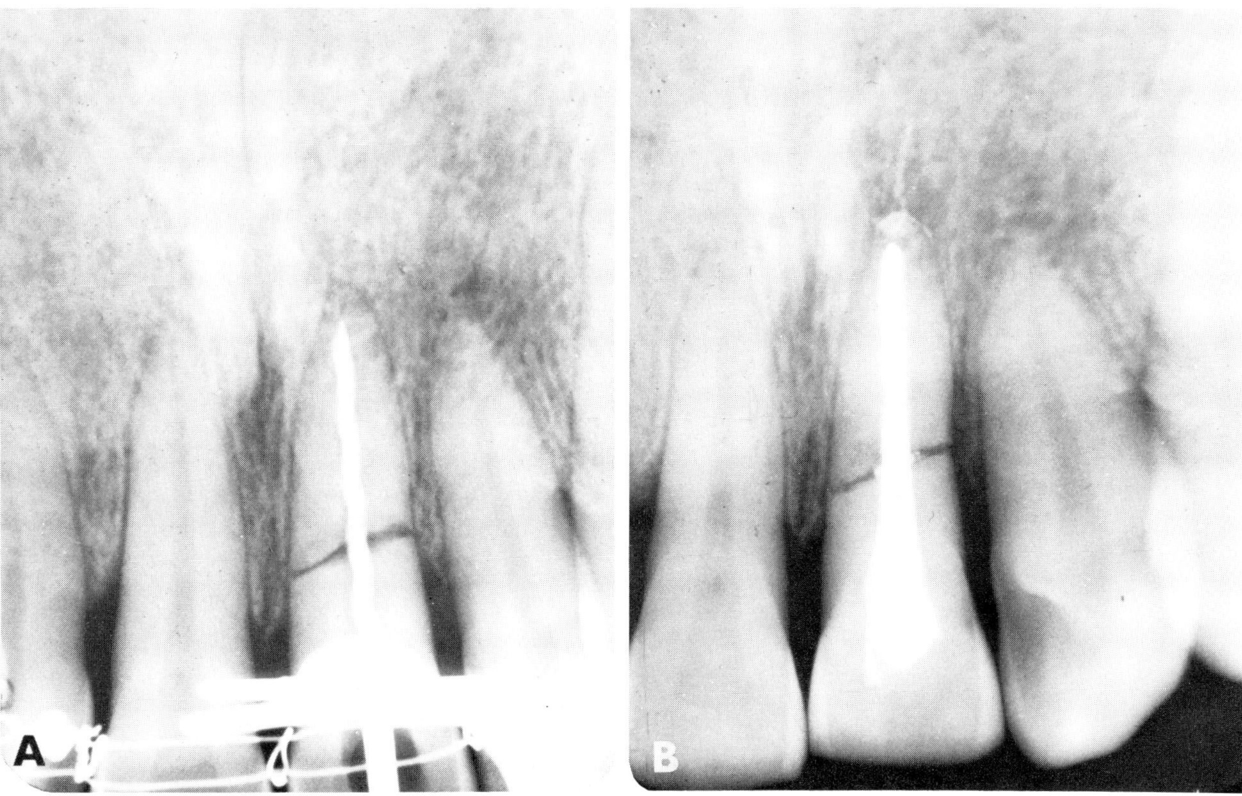

Fig. 16–33. *A*, Mid-root fracture of central incisor. Coronal fragment of tooth was highly mobile and is shown splinted to adjacent teeth during root canal therapy. *B*, Root canal therapy completed. Chrome-cobalt implant has been cemented in attempt to splint two halves of root together. Marginal periodontitis and resorption of alveolar crest complicate final result.

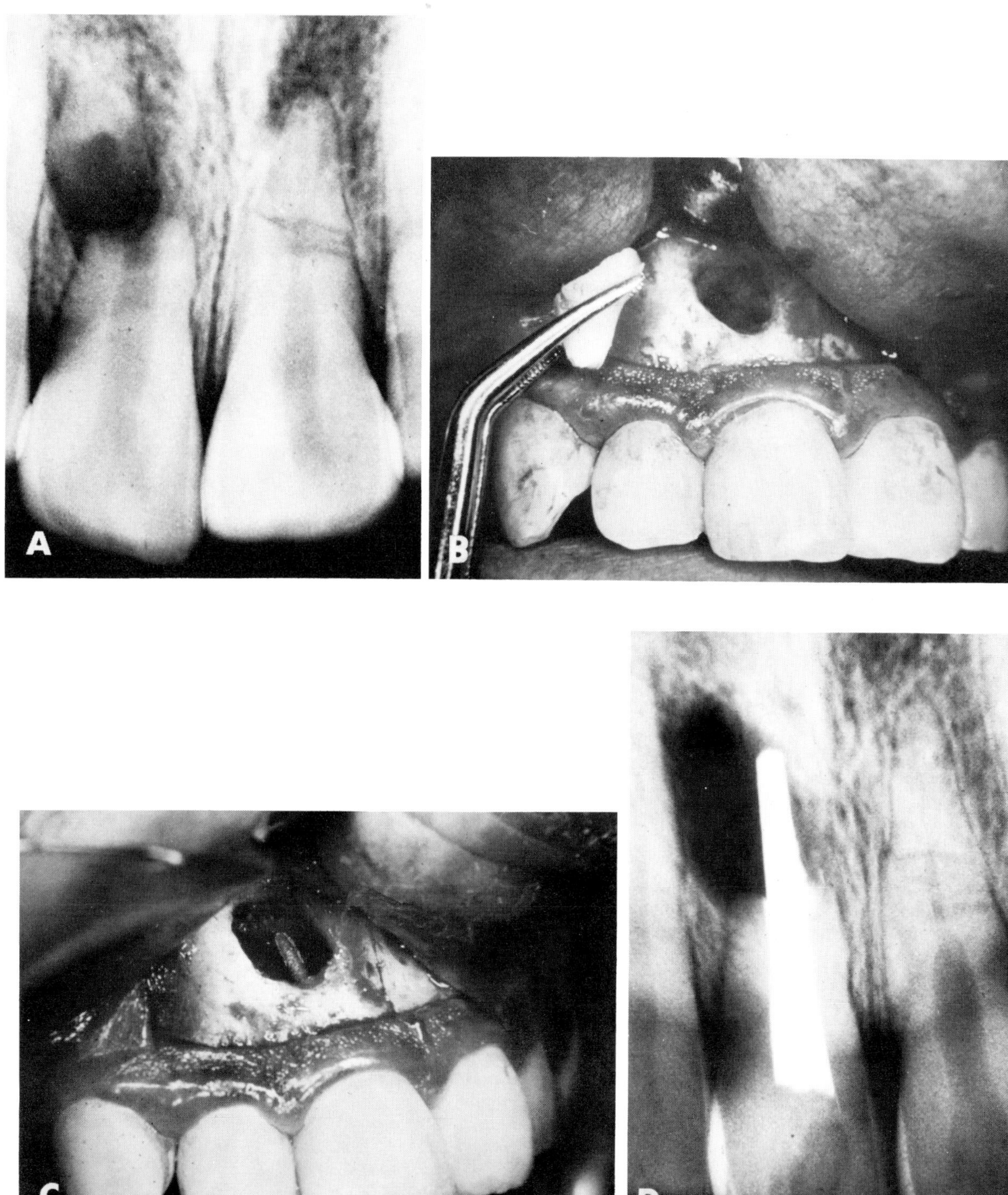

Fig. 16–34. Stabilizing fractured tooth with chrome-cobalt implant. *A*, Mid-root fracture of central incisors. Root tip of right central incisor is badly displaced and crown is highly mobile. Left incisor is vital. *B*, Surgical exposure and removal of root tip of right central incisor. *C*, After debridement and canal enlargement, extended chrome-cobalt endodontic implant has been cemented. Implant which replaces fractured root tip is seen protruding from root stump of incisor. *D*, Roentgenogram of cemented chrome-cobalt point. *(Continued)*

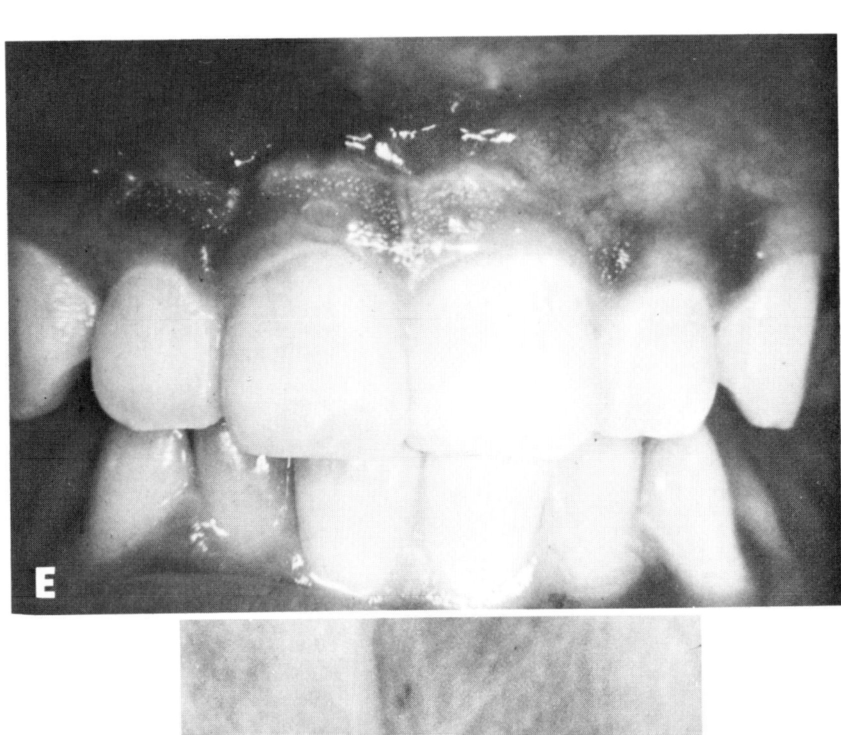

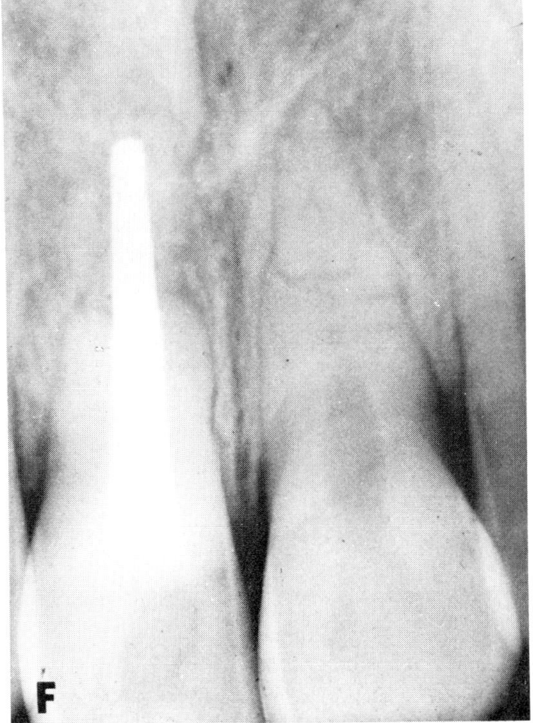

Fig. 16–34. *(Continued.) E,* Postoperative appearance of incisor teeth. *F,* One year after surgery. Bone has repaired around chrome-cobalt "root"-end and tooth is no longer mobile. Fracture of left central incisor has repaired and pulp has remained vital. (Courtesy Dr. Alfred L. Frank.)

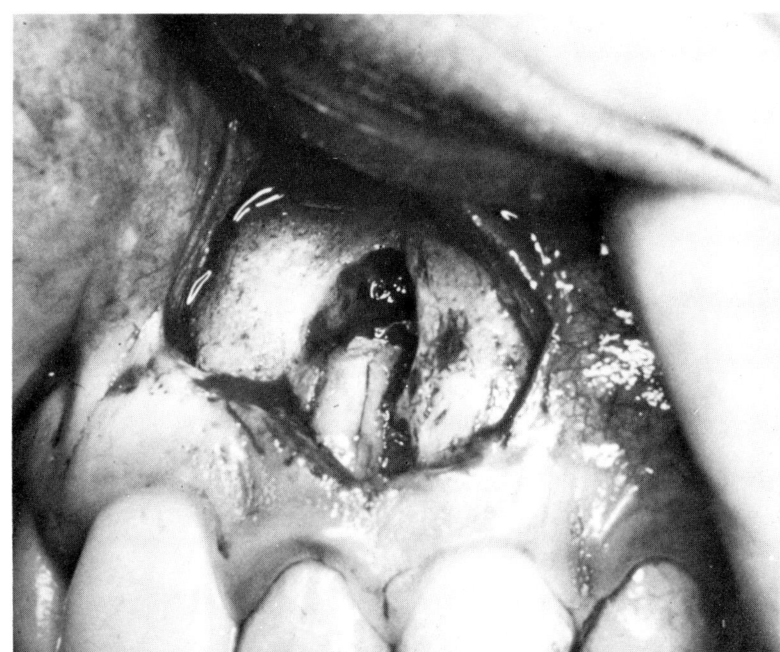

Fig. 16–35. Vertical root fracture. Surgical exposure shows that failure has resulted from vertical fracture of root. This caused both periapical and interproximal bone loss. (Courtesy Dr. Dudley H. Glick.)

Division 2: Vertical and Chisel Fractures

Vertical root fractures are those in which the fracture line is in the same direction as the long axis of the root (Fig. 16–35). Chisel fractures are those in which the labial and lingual levels of the fracture are notably different. The fractured root ends are thus evenly beveled, having a chisel-like appearance (Fig. 16–36).

The prognosis in ***vertical*** fractures is poor since the fractured segments will not generally be united by callus formation. Unfortunately, vertical fractures almost invariably involve both labial and lingual surfaces of the root, and mere repair of the labial will not provide a successful result. Extraction is therefore almost always indicated.

Vertical root fracture occasionally occurs as a result of overvigorous condensation of gutta percha (Fig. 16–37). Typically, a sharp crack is heard at the moment of fracture. The operator may then find that additional gutta percha points may be packed into the canal, seemingly without end, as the displacement of the fragments under pressure provides additional "canal" space. Roentgenogram shows displacement of the fractured segments, a large void along the gutta percha filling, or extension of gutta percha cones into the periapical region. Extraction of the tooth is the only recourse following this type of fracture.

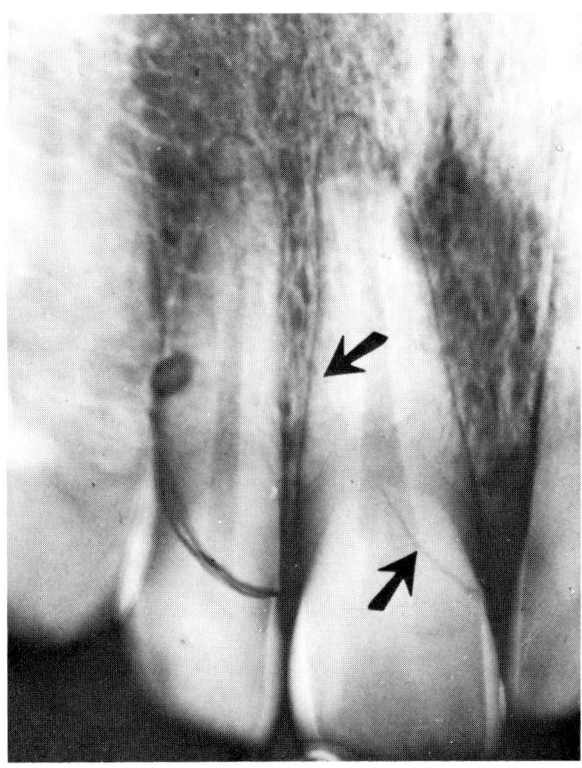

Fig. 16–36. Fractures in ***coronal*** third of roots of both central and lateral incisors. Prognosis in such cases is unfavorable because of difficulty in immobilizing coronal fragments.

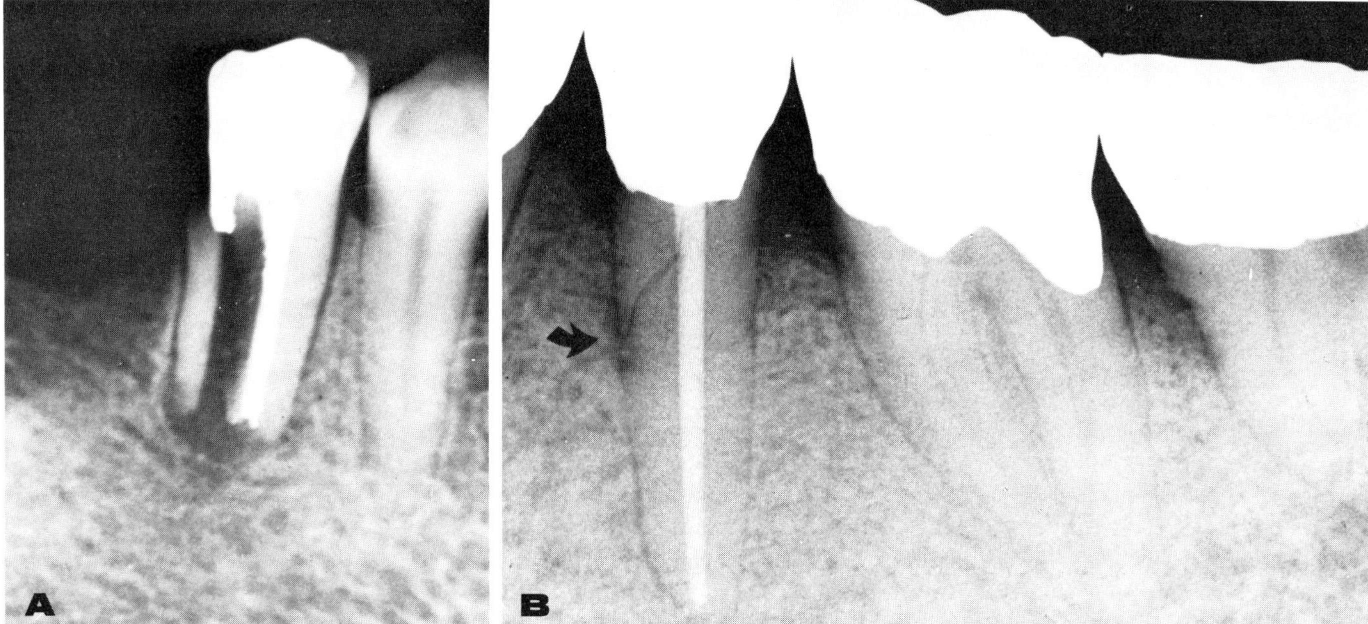

Fig. 16–37. *A,* Root of mandibular second premolar split vertically by overvigorous condensation of gutta percha. Tooth was subsequently extracted. *B,* Painful lateral lesion *(arrow)* directs attention to oblique fracture developed during obturation. Total fracture will undoubtedly develop. (Courtesy Dr. Jack Weichman.)

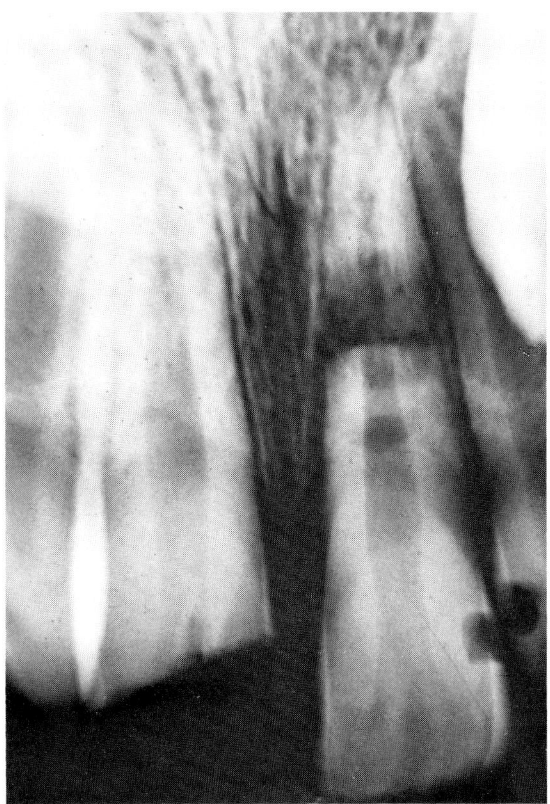

Fig. 16–38. Hopeless chisel fracture of root of left lateral incisor. Apical fragment is less radiopaque in fracture area because of its chisel-like shape. Coronal fracture of adjacent central incisor requires pulpectomy and root canal filling.

Chisel fractures have an equally poor prognosis (Fig. 16–38). The sharp beveled ends of the fractured segments tend to slide upon one another with masticatory stress, preventing union by callus formation. If the fracture occurs in the apical portion of the root, the apical fragment may be surgically removed in conjunction with root canal filling for the coronal segment. However, the coronal level of chisel fractures generally is in the coronal third of the root, and removal of the apical segment leaves only a small amount of remaining root. The solutions are, therefore, extraction or an attempt at increasing root length with the placement of an endodontic implant.

Diagnosis of Root Fracture

Diagnosis of root fracture can generally be made on the basis of roentgenographic evidence. However, in some instances displacement of the segments is so slight that the fracture line is not roentgenographically apparent. Vertical fracture may be roentgenographically undetectable for the same reason or when

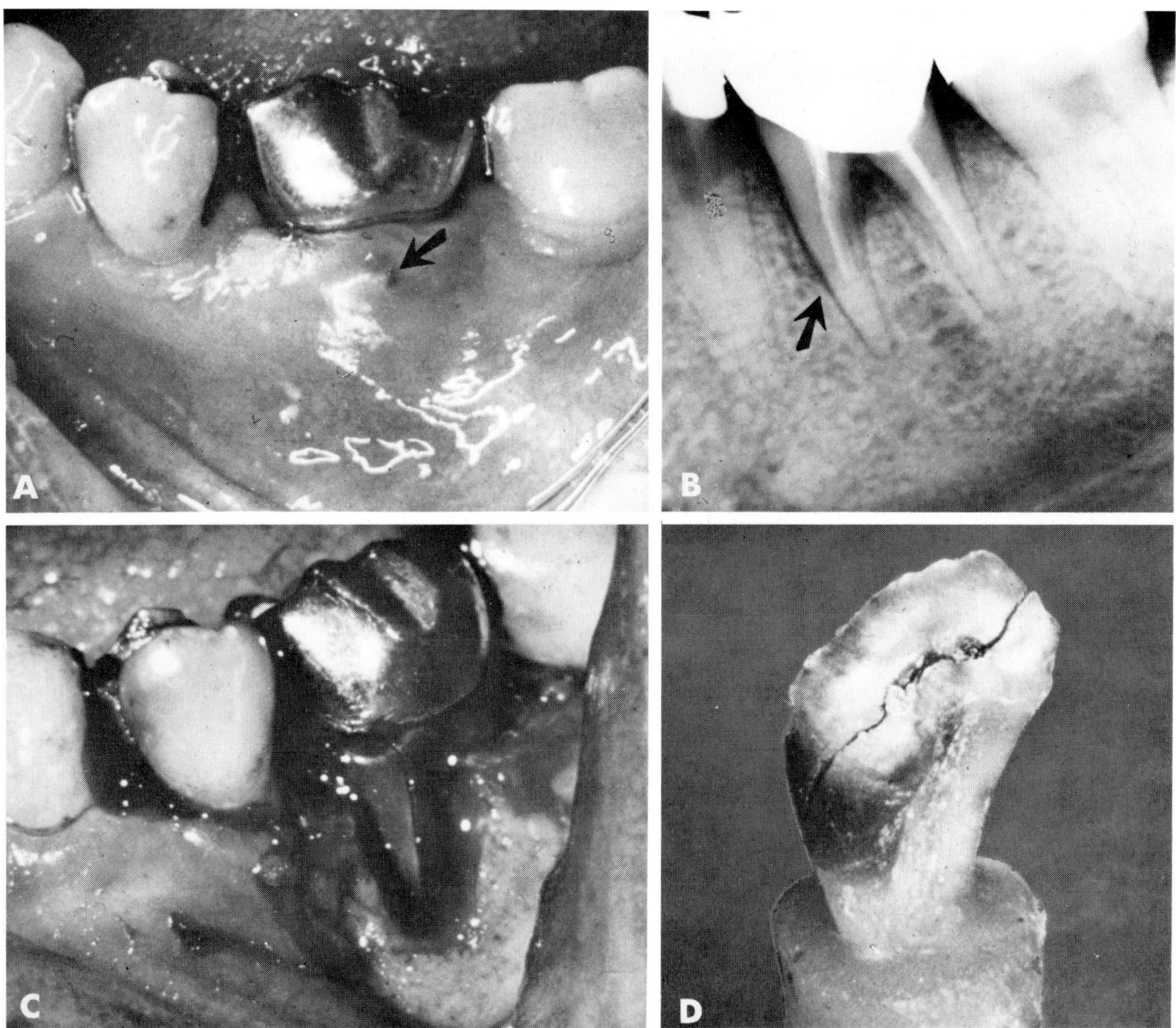

Fig. 16–39. *A,* Buccal fistula and chronic abscess *(arrow)* associated with deep periodontal pocket along mesial root of first molar. *B,* Previous root canal therapy for first molar. All canals were filled short of apex. Periapical region of both roots is normal, but vertical bone loss can be seen in furca and alongside mesial root *(arrow)*. *C,* Surgical exposure of mesial root shows extensive vertical fracture and cavernous bone loss. *D,* Amputated root clearly shows fracture. Remaining distal root and crown of tooth were retained.

the fracture is in a mesiodistal rather than a labiolingual direction. In this latter case the central x-ray beam is at right angles to the direction of fracture, and the fracture cannot be seen on the film.

Clinical symptoms of root fracture may include constant discomfort over the buccal mucosa and tenderness to percussion or palpation. A constant chronic abscess resembling a periodontal abscess is a commonly observed sign (Fig. 16–39). Occasionally a root-fractured tooth is devitalized and treated endodontically without detection of the fracture. Subsequently a radiolucent area may develop at the apex or at the side of the root at the level of fracture. In addition, a periodontal lesion may develop which extends to the level of fracture or, in the case of vertical fracture, along the entire length of the root to the apex. Linaburg and Marshall have pointed out that surgical exposure may show that the origin of the bony lesion or periodontal defect is indeed a previously undetected fracture.[31]

Class VI: Displacement of Teeth with or without Fracture

Displacement of teeth may range from a relatively slight change in tooth position on the one hand to the extreme of tooth loss (avulsion) on the other. Displacement may be complicated by crown or root fracture, although there is less tendency for displaced teeth to suffer fracture than teeth which are not displaced.

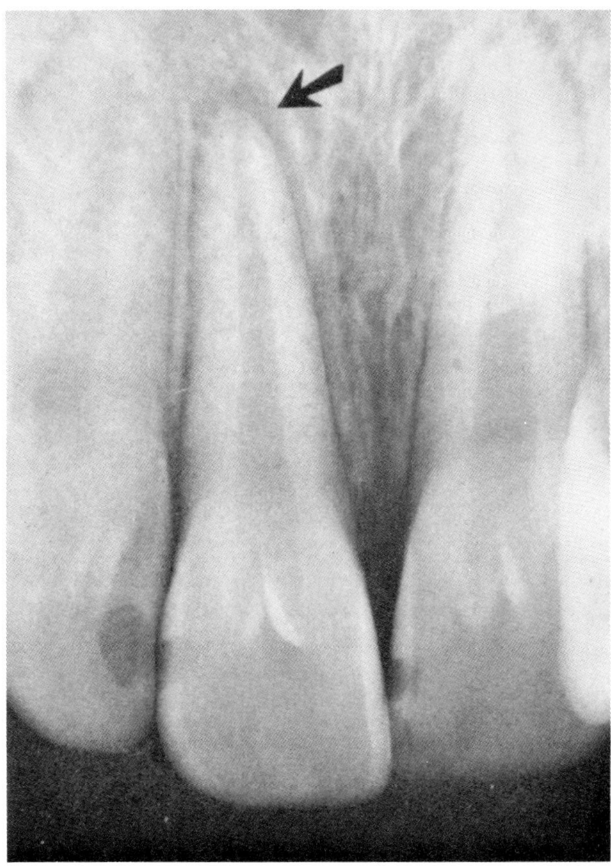

Fig. 16–40. Traumatic extrusion of right central incisor. Note outline of root socket at apex of tooth and more incisal position of crown in relation to left central incisor.

Division 1: Partial Displacement

Partial displacement may be one of the following types: (1) labial or lingual; (2) extrusion (forced out of socket); or (3) intrusion (forced into socket).

Clinical examination will determine the type of displacement and the degree of mobility. Extruded teeth and teeth displaced to the labial or lingual generally are quite mobile, whereas intruded teeth, since they have been forced into the alveolus, tend to be quite firm. Extrusion and intrusion are easily recognized because of differences in incisal level of traumatized and adjacent teeth. Roentgenograms of extruded teeth, in addition, show the outline of the tooth socket, apical to the root end (Fig. 16–40).

Although labial and lingual displacement, in most cases, are readily apparent, it is not always possible to determine the former labio-lingual position of the teeth. In patients with a large overjet or flaring maxillary anterior teeth, the mandibular arch may not serve as an accurate indicator of the position of maxillary teeth. If several of the maxillary anterior teeth are displaced, the maxillary arch itself may be of little help in determining the former position of the teeth. If this is the case, the teeth should be repositioned to provide the most reasonable esthetics and function.

Frequently, displacement of a tooth results in spreading apart of the labial and lingual alveolar plates and severing of the periodontal ligament attachment. "Traumatic pockets" thus created may extend in some instances almost to the apex along one or more surfaces of the tooth. After displaced teeth are repositioned and stabilized, the alveolar plates should be compressed against the teeth with firm digital pressure, in order to prevent the development of a permanent periodontal defect. Pocket depth should be recorded at this time. Periodontal injury

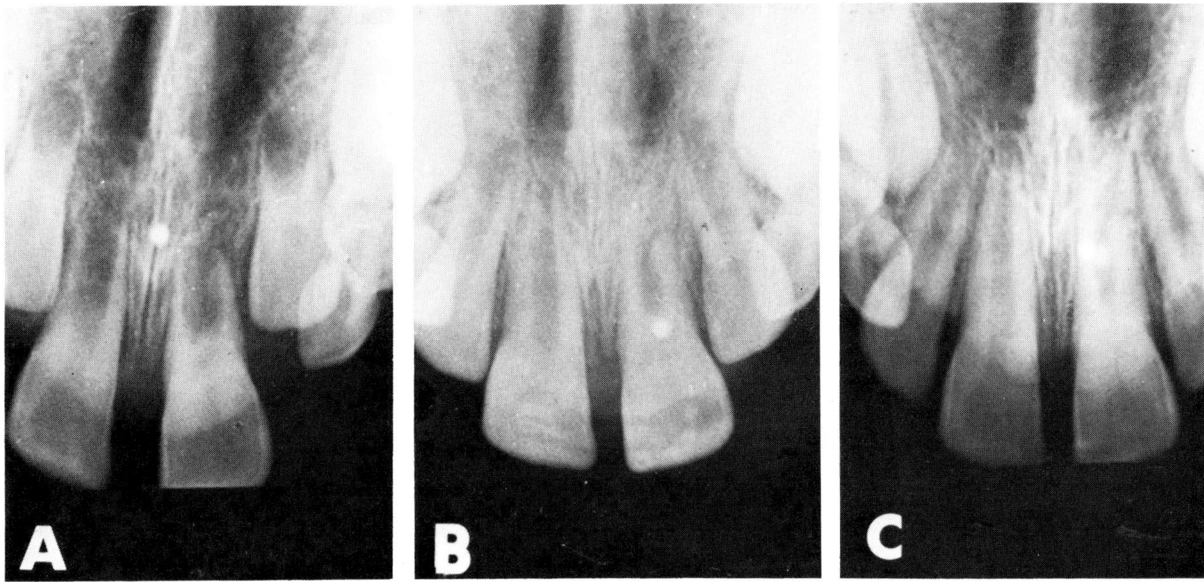

Fig. 16–41. *A,* Severe impact injury drove the central incisors lingually out of alveolus so that teeth were horizontal and faced into palate. Teeth were repositioned by finger manipulation. *B* and *C,* In spite of severe displacement, pulps of two incisors remained vital, and development of root apices continued normally. (Courtesy Dr. Max Nacht.)

created by tooth displacement generally resolves through healing of the attachment apparatus. However, if gingival inflammation develops, there is a failure of reattachment of the periodontal ligaments and a permanent defect develops. The patient therefore must keep the area scrupulously clean.

Displaced teeth should be checked for vitality and the results of tests recorded for comparison with future vitality readings. Often, in spite of severe displacement, the pulp may retain its vitality (Fig. 16–41). Root canal therapy should therefore not be instituted at the time of injury unless the pulp has been exposed by fracture.

Treatment of Extruded Teeth and Teeth Displaced Labially or Lingually. Extruded teeth or teeth displaced labially or lingually should be brought into normal position. If the teeth are mobile, this can generally be accomplished with gentle finger pressure, under a local anesthetic (Fig. 16–42). If a tooth has been displaced but is ***firm*** in its new position, the possibility of moving it into normal position with an orthodontic appliance should be considered. This slow repositioning is feasible if the displaced tooth is not interfering with normal occlusal function. Orthodontic movement is desirable since the force is applied more slowly and gently and will be less traumatic to the already traumatized pulp and periodontal structures than the force necessary in digital repositioning.

Mobile ***extruded*** teeth may resist attempts to push them back into their sockets because of the formation of blood clots in the sockets. If extrusion is slight, grinding of the incisal edge is sufficient to restore the normal incisal level. If the extrusion is great and would necessitate excessive incisal grinding, it may be necessary to create an apical "vent" to allow the release of trapped blood. This vent may be created by first making a small semilunar incision over the displaced tooth. An opening is then cut with No. 6 round bur just barely through the exposed labial plate of bone at the level of the socket apex. Blood that has collected in the socket is then released through the vent as the tooth is pushed into normal position.

Once the mobile displaced teeth have been repositioned, they must be stabilized by splinting them to the neighboring teeth. This may be done with arch bars, orthodontic arch wire, or wire ligature (Fig. 16–43). Splinting also may be done by painting on composite filling material. Careful acid etching of interproximal enamel surfaces makes for better adhesion. After reattachment of the tooth in three weeks to one month, the composite "splints" are removed and the tooth surfaces polished. Displaced teeth should be ground out of occlusion to prevent

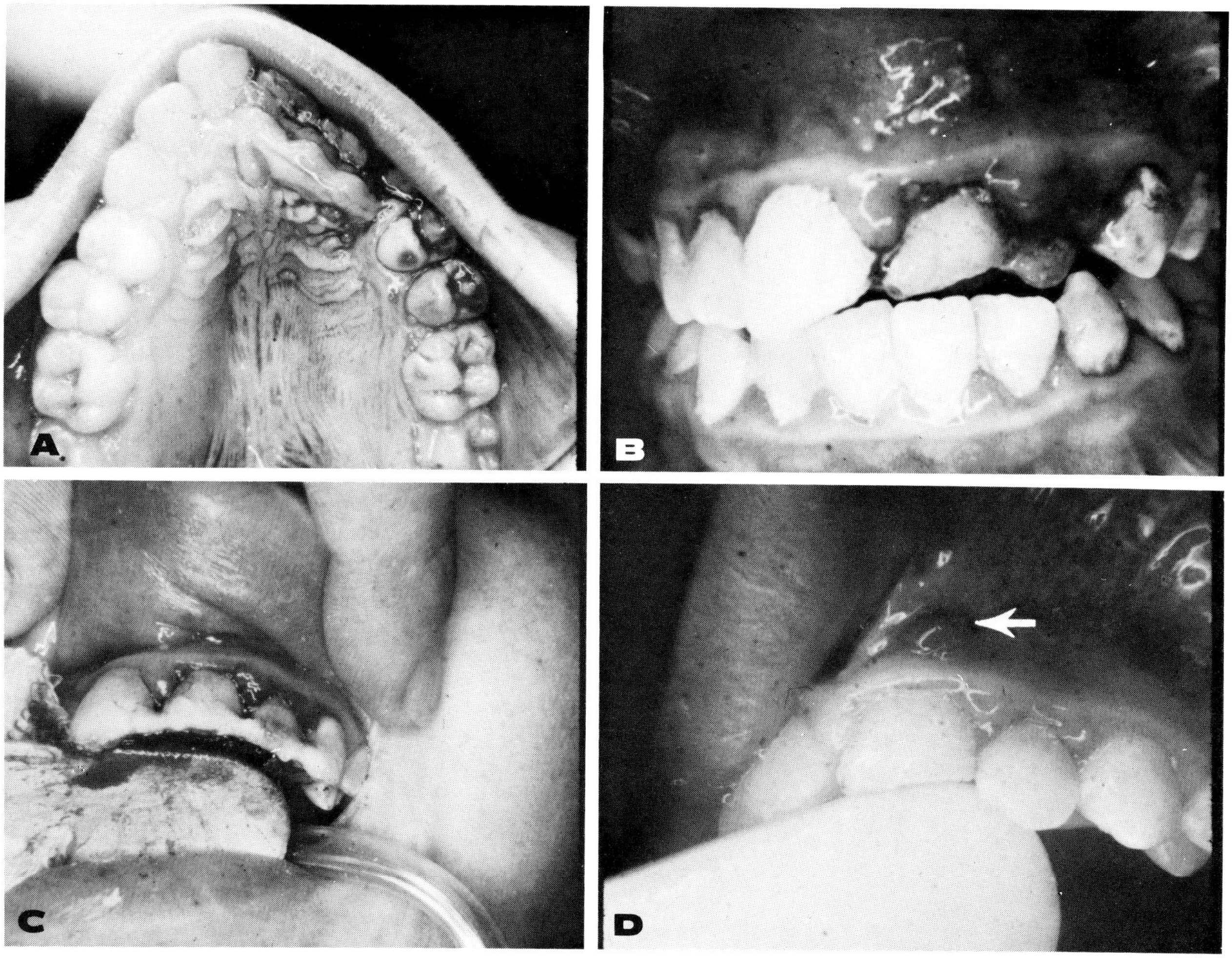

Fig. 16–42. *A*, Football accident fractures premaxilla causing misshapen arch in 14-year-old boy. *B*, Incisors fractured and devitalized and gingiva separated. *C*, Teeth repositioned and arch form restored by digital pressure. Pressure is applied from lingual by tongue blade as acrylic splint hardens. *D*, Seven days postoperative. Curvature of tongue blade shows retained rounded arch form. Fistula *(arrow)* is associated with pulpless central incisor. (Courtesy Dr. Andrew E. Michanowicz.)

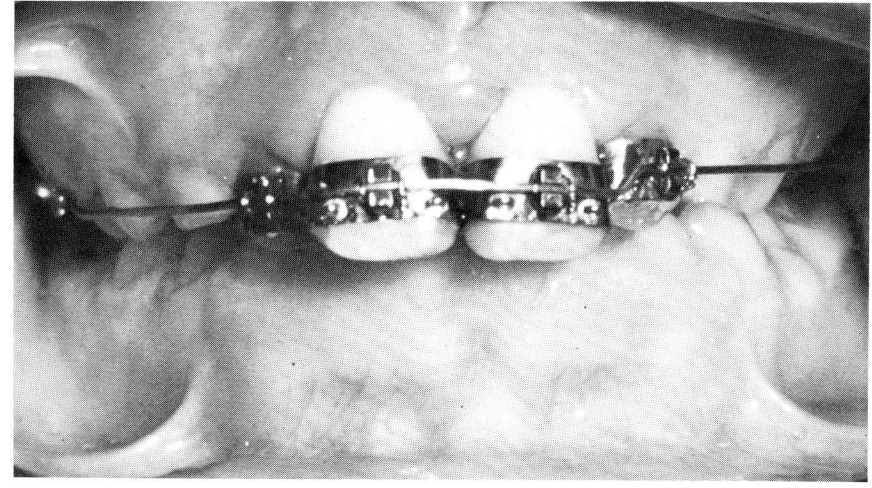

Fig. 16–43. Orthodontic band splint placed to stabilize repositioned central incisors which were partially avulsed and highly mobile.

further trauma. Splints should be kept in place from four to six weeks, after which time the traumatized teeth should be firm.

If pulpectomy or pulpotomy is required because of pulp exposure, it should be done after the placement of the splint. If pulpectomy is necessary, the pulp should be removed with broaches and a temporary seal placed. Further instrumentation and root canal filling should be deferred until the splint has been removed, unless the development of pain or swelling makes earlier treatment of the root canal necessary. If pulpotomy is required, it must, of course, be completed at the initial appointment.

Treatment of Intruded Teeth. Intruded teeth usually erupt into their original positions after a period of time, without forceful repositioning. Usually the only immediate treatment necessary is palliative treatment of the soft tissues. If eruption is slow, it may be facilitated orthodontically by means of a finger spring attached with a composite cement to the labial surface of the tooth. It has also been suggested that at the emergency appointment the intruded tooth may be brought down to position with forceps. For the tooth that has "disappeared" into the alveolar process or has been driven into the floor of the nose, this method has much to recommend it. Forcible repositioning may, however, avulse the tooth completely. Intruded teeth are invariably firmly fixed in the alveolus. Splinting therefore is not necessary unless the teeth are loosened by forcible repositioning.

In a worthwhile study, Andreasen compared results achieved by either orthodontic or spontaneous repositioning vs. "surgical" repositioning of intruded teeth.[32] As Table 16–1 shows, the gentler methods of repositioning are preferred.

Table 16–1. Results of surgical vs. orthodontic-spontaneous repositioning of intruded adult teeth

	Method of Repositioning	
Pathologic Change	*Surgical (%)*	*Orthodontic or Spontaneous (%)*
Loss of marginal bone	42	0
Ankylosis resorption	34	12
Inflammatory resorption	24	17

Division 2: Complete Avulsion

The only treatment for the completely avulsed tooth is replantation, the replacement of the tooth in its socket with the object of achieving reattachment. Replantation is most commonly attempted after accidental avulsion of a tooth; however, the intentional extraction and replantation of teeth is sometimes indicated.

Although replantation is frequently successful, the ultimate prognosis for the replanted tooth is poor because progressive root resorption almost invariably follows (Fig. 16–44). The average life span of the replanted tooth may be five to ten years; however, the period of retention may vary from a few weeks to a lifetime.

Differences of opinion exist concerning the desirability of retaining the periodontal membrane still attached to the avulsed tooth. Some authors believe that the period of retention of the replanted tooth is proportional to the amount of vital periodontal ligament on the tooth at the time of replantation.[33,34] Others,[35,36] however, claim that there is no advantage

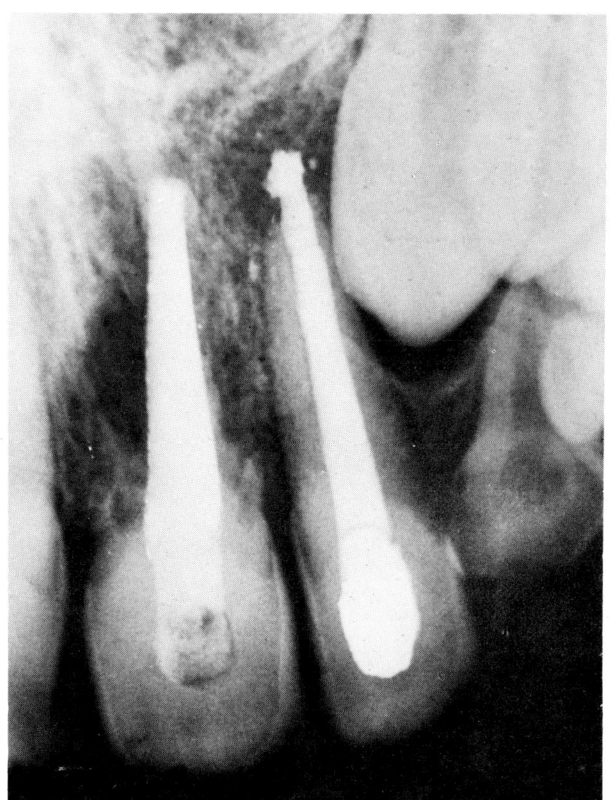

Fig. 16–44. Extensive root resorption of maxillary incisors six months following replantation.

in retaining the periodontal ligament. Experimental replantation studies of Loe and Waerhaug indicate that teeth, extracted and replanted immediately, maintain the vitality of the periodontal ligament, and ankylosis does not occur.[37] Nasjleti and his associates[37a] reported that resorption and ankylosis were not observed in replanted teeth in monkeys in 21-day to 4-month specimens, though both were apparent in the 14-day specimens. From a practical standpoint, it seems reasonable to retain the attached, vital periodontal ligament when replantation can be done soon after avulsion or extraction. If an avulsed tooth has been out of the mouth for a considerable time or has been covered with dirt or fragments of other foreign material, it is more desirable to scrub the contaminated ligament before replantation with a gauze sponge and saline solution.

The sooner that replantation can be carried out after the accident, the more favorable will be the prognosis for reattachment. Frequently the dentist is informed over the telephone by an anxious parent that her child has had a tooth "knocked out." The parent should be told to wash the tooth in cold water, and if it is not covered with debris, to replace it in the socket. If this is not possible, the tooth should be placed under the patient's tongue, and both tooth and patient brought to the dentist's office immediately.

Andreasen has presented the definitive treatise on replantation.[37b] A computer analysis of cases replanted by Danish dentists, by physicians, or by the patients themselves proved that teeth replanted by the dentists showed the poorest results. This is believed to be caused by too much intervention—the dentist's feeling that he had to "do something"; physicians and patients, on the other hand, merely replaced the tooth in the socket as soon as possible. Andreasen found histologically that healing of the PDL takes place in two weeks. In monkeys from whom incisors were extracted and replaced within 30 minutes, normal mobility was apparent at four weeks.

Andreasen describes three varieties of resorption following replantation[37b]:

1. *Surface resorption,* which is normally present and self limiting and is usually no deeper than 0.02 mm.
2. *Inflammatory resorption,* which is rapid and is related to inflammation within the space of the PDL. Inflammatory resorption may be arrested by removing a necrotic pulp, cleansing the canal, and placing $Ca(OH)_2$. Scrupulous plaque removal also prevents apical inflammatory migration from marginal gingivitis.
3. *Replacement resorption,* or ankylosis, in which alveolar bone conjoins the cementum or dentin without intervening PDL. Ankylosis is the most severe and rapid type of resorption but may be self limiting.

In a further study, Andreasen evaluated methods of storing avulsed teeth before replantation.[37b] Incisors were extracted from monkeys and stored for two hours, some to air-dry, some in saline solution, and some in the monkeys' own saliva in their buccal vestibule. The air-dried specimens all had subsequent root resorption primarily by ankylosis. After one hour in saline, no ankylosis developed, but for as long as *two hours in saliva,* there was virtually no resorption. On the basis of this experiment and clinical experience, Andreasen highly recommends that patients be instructed to place the avulsed tooth in their vestibule or under their tongue for the trip to the dentist. Parents and emergency medical service personnel (paramedics) should be so instructed or told to replace the tooth in the socket. Andreasen enjoyed 100% success if teeth were immediately replaced in the alveolus. He pointed out a rapid drop in success directly correlated with the length of time teeth are out of the socket, although saliva storage improved the chances of success. He also ***does not*** recommend removing contaminated periodontal ligament by scraping, but rather a cleansing of the root surface with a gauze sponge and saline solution.

If replantation can be done in a reasonable length of time (within minutes or hours), Andreasen found that root canal therapy should not be done first. If the tooth had been out for hours and air-dried, however, it apparently made no difference when the root canal filling was done.

Andreasen discovered in his experimental monkeys that if developing incisors with open apices were replanted within 30 minutes, root formation continued and root canal calcification developed. If the extraoral period was extended to 90 minutes, the pulp canal filled with bone with an "internal" PDL.[37b]

As far as splinting was concerned, Andreasen noted that ***rigid*** splints should be left in place only about one week, otherwise resorption increased. He recommends two to four days of penicillin therapy and a tetanus injection.

The importance of close radiographic follow-up of replanted cases has been emphasized by Andreasen. At two weeks, surface resorption should be expected—the ***self limiting*** type. If at three weeks resorption has increased, one must expect that *inflammatory resorption* has set in. This calls for immediate pulp removal, canal debridement, and $Ca(OH)_2$ placement. When inflammation appears to have ceased and a new PDL is established around the root, the canal should again be cleansed and fully obturated. Resorption at six weeks is undoubtedly ***replacement resorption*** or ankylosis, for which there is no treatment. If the alveolus has been fractured, ankylosis can be expected 80% of the time.

Andreasen has also found a direct correlation between age and the rate of replacement resorption caused by ankylosis—the older the patient, the slower the resorption. In young patients, with a fast turnover of bone, an ankylosed tooth most likely will resorb within the year. Any tooth held extraorally for an extended time, particularly if air-dried, is guaranteed of replacement resorption.

Treatment Following Replantation by the Patient. The patient must first be examined roentgenographically and clinically. If the dentist can be assured that the tooth was intact and washed free of debris before it was replaced in the alveolus, it should not be disturbed. The roentgenogram should not show any fractures, and the tooth should be relatively firm in the socket. Four or five approximating teeth, as well as the ***opposing*** teeth, should be pulp tested and the findings recorded.

Anesthesia should be administered if the area is painful and a temporary flexible acrylic splint should be placed. The splint is to be worn for about three weeks. This is the average length of time for reattachment of the periodontal ligaments to a new cemental surface. ***As soon as the tooth is firmly reattached in the alveolus, conventional root canal therapy should be completed by means of a standard technique.***

Technique for Constructing a Flexible Acrylic Splint. 1. With the tooth firmly replanted, powder and liquid of a flexible denture-reline acrylic (Audiflex Self-cure*) are mixed in accordance with the manufacturer's directions.

2. When the flexible acrylic has reached a "tacky" consistency, it is rolled in the hands to the shape of a thin frankfurter. The operator's hands should be greased with petrolatum to prevent the acrylic from sticking to them.

3. The roll is carefully centered over the incisal edges of the involved arch and should extend from premolar to premolar. The acrylic should be forcibly contoured around the involved tooth to be sure it is completely in position.

4. The patient is then asked to close in ***centric*** until the teeth are completely in occlusion.

5. The excess labial acrylic is molded against the labial surfaces of both maxillary and mandibular teeth and up onto the gingiva. The lingual excess is trimmed by the patient's tongue.

6. The patient remains closed in centric until the acrylic begins to get warm and the splint is then removed. At this stage the acrylic is still soft and can be easily trimmed with a sharp curved shears. Acrylic should not extend beyond the fornix in the vestibule. The splint should extend to the canine or first premolar on each side and excess distal to this should be removed.

7. After trimming, the splint is replaced and the patient again closes in centric until the material is fully set. If the patient complains of heat from the curing acrylic, petrolatum may be smeared under the lips.

*COE Laboratories

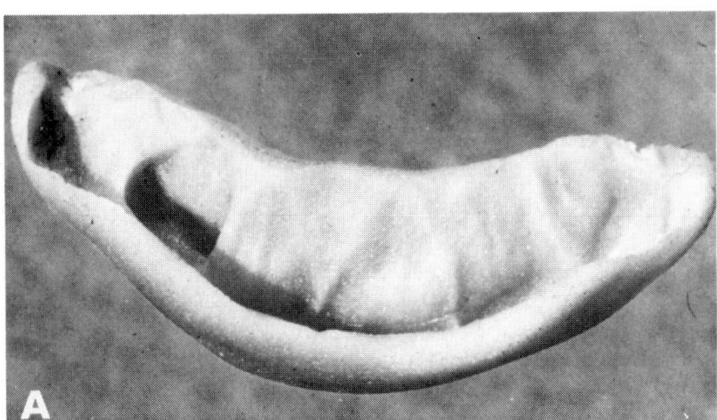

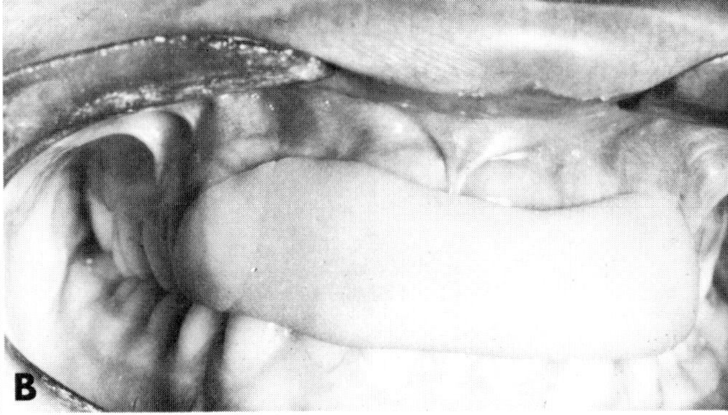

Fig. 16–45. *A*, Superior view of soft, flexible-acrylic (Audiflex) splint. Splint extends distally to include maxillary canine on each side. *B*, Splint in position with maxillary and mandibular teeth in full centric closure. It is removed only while eating and for cleaning.

8. After final set, the splint is again removed and rough edges are smoothed with disks (Fig. 16–45).

Because of its flexibility, the splint can be easily withdrawn and replaced without dislodging the replanted tooth, yet it has enough body to provide effective stabilization.

The patient is instructed to wear the splint night and day, with the teeth closed lightly together. The splint can, however, be removed at meal times. The patient should avoid eating incisive foods or hard or tough foods during the two or three weeks after replantation. The acrylic splint itself and the involved area should be kept scrupulously clean, since the development of gingivitis around the replanted tooth will prevent reattachment.

The soft acrylic splint is not indicated for adults whose occupations require extensive conversation. It is also not indicated when the tooth does not seat firmly in its socket at the time of replantation. If the tooth is quite mobile when replanted, it may be forced out of normal position during construction of the splint.

The greatest use of this emergency splint is for children. They will be conscientious about wearing the splint since they are not socially inconvenienced by its appearance or the necessity of keeping their teeth closed together. Boys are often delighted with the splint when told that it is the mouth guard used by boxers.

The advantage of the soft acrylic splint is that it is easily and rapidly constructed in an emergency situation and provides adequate stabilization in many cases. If, however, a highly rigid splint is desired, then another form of stabilization should be employed.

Preparation of the Avulsed Tooth for Endodontic Treatment. If the tooth has been out of the alveolus for a long time or is dirty and contaminated, it may be replanted with a different technique (Fig. 16–46).

1. The detached tooth is washed with a gauze sponge soaked in saline.

2. The tooth is then held in a saline-soaked 2 × 2 gauze sponge, and root canal therapy may be done in the hand before replantation. If, however, equipment for root canal treatment is not available, the tooth may first be replanted and splinted, and treated endodontically at a later time.

Endodontic Treatment. 1. Access to the pulp chamber is obtained on the lingual with 702U carbide bur and is completed with appropriate round burs.

2. The pulp is then removed with a coarse broach and the canal and pulp chambers are irrigated to remove debris and pulp remnants.

3. The canal is instrumented to the apex with reamers in accordance with "clean, white dentin" rule. The coronal portion of the canal is filed. The canal is then irrigated with sodium hypochlorite and dried with paper points and warm air.

4. A primary gutta percha point is selected and fitted.

5. A mix of root canal sealer is prepared on a sterile slab and is used to coat the root canal and the gutta percha point. The point is seated and a spreader is used to allow the introduction of additional gutta percha points.

6. When the canal has been completely packed, any excess gutta percha protruding from the apex is seared off with a hot instrument. Gutta percha and sealer are then removed from the crown of the tooth. The pulp chamber and remainder of the canal are filled with composite material.

7. If any carious lesions are present, they are excavated and can be restored with composite cement along with the lingual access cavity.

8. The tooth is replaced in saline solution while the socket is prepared for replantation.

Replantation. The replantation procedure is comprised of the following steps:

1. The region should be anesthetized. The socket should then be gently curetted and irrigated with a saline solution to remove clotted blood and any foreign material that may have entered at the time of the accident.

2. The tooth is now removed from the saline solution and gently pushed into its socket. Frequently it will be found that the tooth will not seat to its full length in the socket or, after seating, will slowly "ooze" out of the socket. This is because of resistance offered by blood, trapped apically, as the tooth is seated. In this case it will be necessary to create a surgical "vent" that will allow the release of blood, forced to the apex of the socket (Fig. 16–47). The "vent" is made in the following manner:

- *a.* A small circular incision is made at the apical level of the tooth socket.
- *b.* The flap is retracted and the labial alveolar plate is exposed.
- *c.* Using the root length as a guide a No. 6

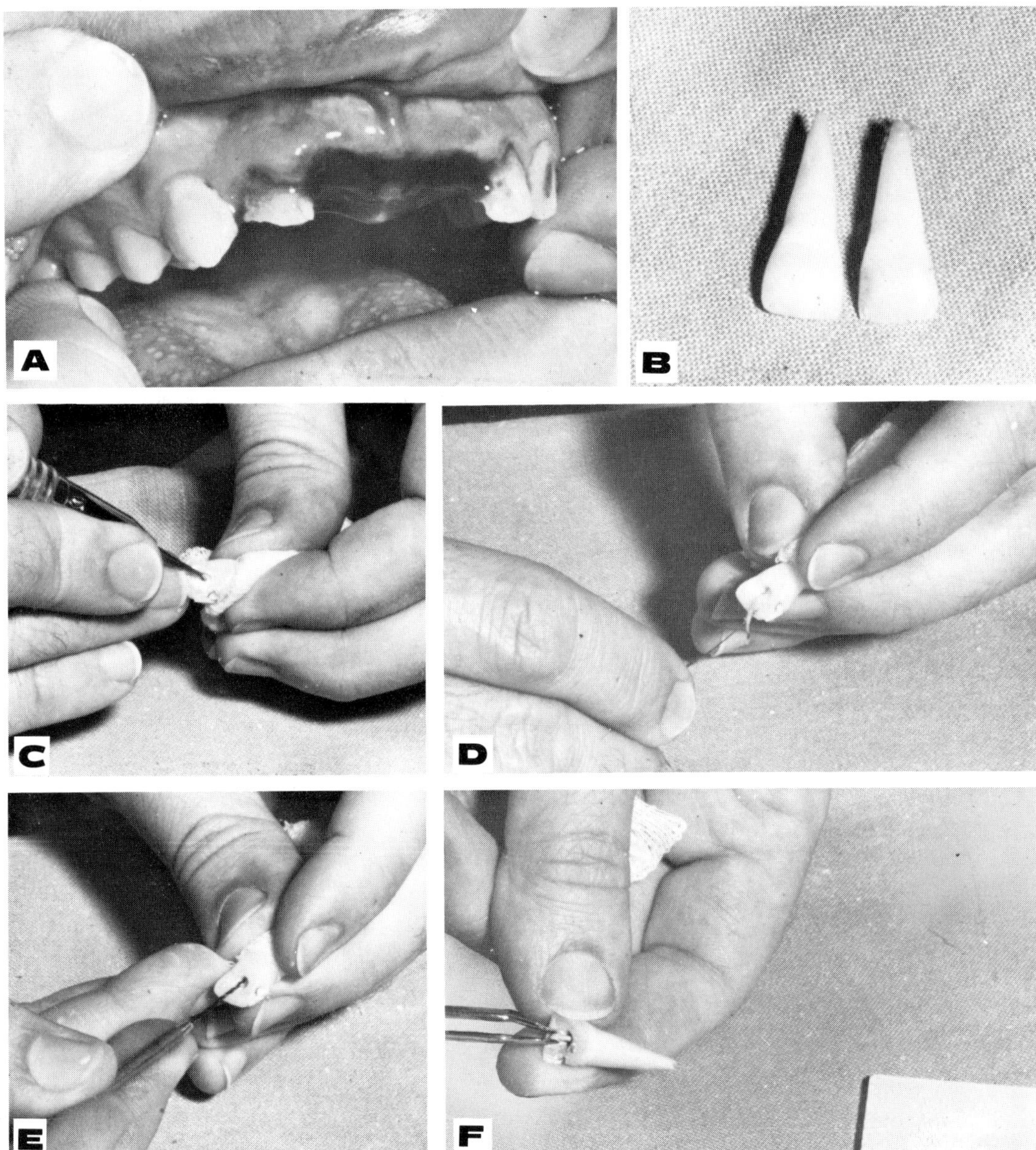

Fig. 16–46. Technique for preparation and filling prior to replantation of tooth that has been extraoral and air-dried for several hours. *A,* Photograph taken five hours after total avulsion of permanent central incisors. Crown of right lateral incisor was fractured, but pulp was not exposed. There was no fracture of alveolar cortical plate. *B,* Totally avulsed central incisors presented by patient. Contaminated periodontal ligament should be scrubbed with a gauze sponge soaked in saline solution. *C,* Access to pulp chamber is established with appropriate burs. Tooth is held in sponge soaked in aqueous Zephiran. Carious defects are to be restored prior to replantation. *D,* Coarse broach is used to extirpate pulp. *E,* Complete preparation of canals is carried out with style "D" reamers and file. *F,* After canal is irrigated and dried with paper points, primary gutta percha point is selected and fitted. After cementation of primary point, No. 3 spreader is used to displace point laterally, and additional fine points are added. Excess coronal gutta percha is removed and lingual opening is restored with silicate. (Ingle, J. I., and Dow, P. R.: Dental Digest, 59:386, Sept., 1953.)

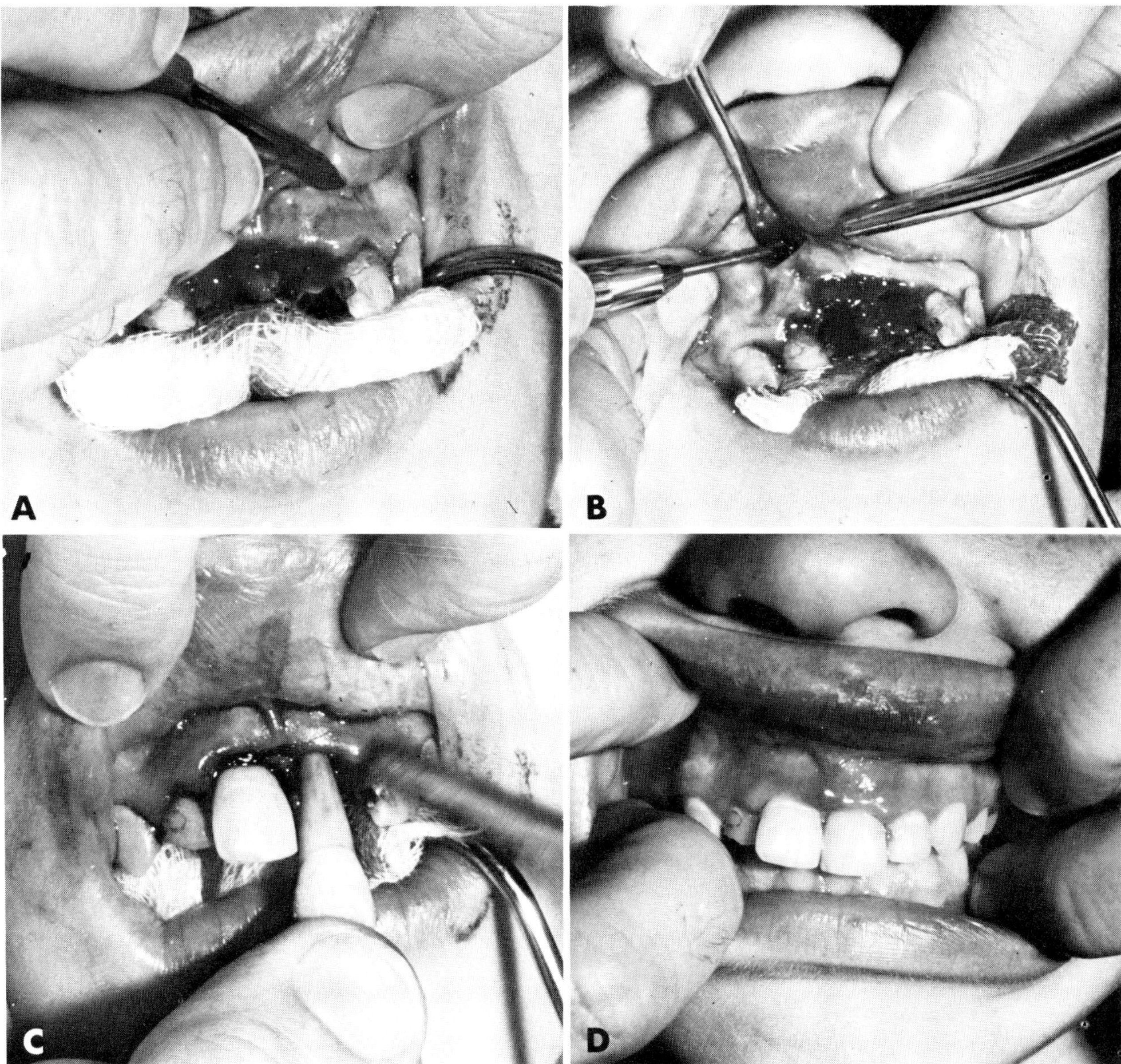

Fig. 16–47. Technique of replantation with use of apical "vent." *A,* Beginning surgical-venting procedure employed in replantation. Small incision is made at each apex. *B,* Buccal plate is perforated at apex with surgical bur to create vent for release of hydraulic pressure within alveolus. Blood clots are gently removed. *C,* Actual replantation of endodontically prepared central incisors is followed by suturing of "vent" incisions with number 000 silk thread. Pressure and fluid are released through apical "vents." Splinting (see Fig. 16–45) follows. *D,* Appearance six days after treatment. Entire area is now asymptomatic. There is firm reattachment of gingiva. (Ingle, J. I., and Dow, P. R.: Dental Digest, *59*:386, Sept., 1953.)

round bur is used to perforate the cortical plate at the apex of the socket. The aperture thus created acts as a vent for the escape of blood, which has been preventing the complete insertion of the tooth in the alveolus.

d. The tooth is now pushed into the socket until it seats firmly.

e. The venting incision is closed with a suture.

Surgical venting is not advised if the labial plate has been fractured.

3. After replantation the alveolar plates of bone should be squeezed firmly against the tooth with digital pressure as they may have been spread apart during avulsion. This will tend to prevent the development of a periodontal defect.

Splinting. The replanted tooth must be stabilized by splinting to ensure the best chance of reattachment. Splints may be constructed either of the flexible acrylic, as described, or of wire, orthodontic bands,

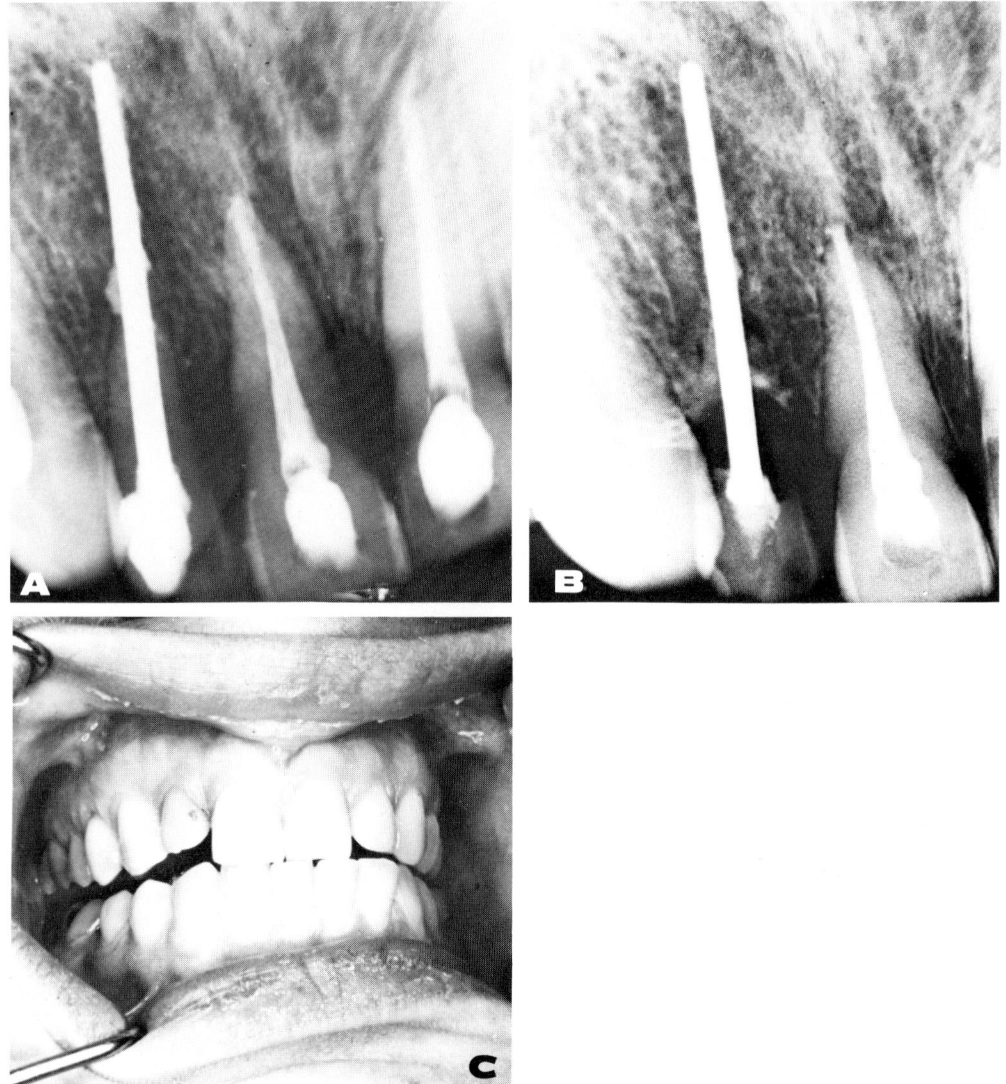

Fig. 16–48. Replantation with endodontic implant. *A,* Lateral incisor avulsed in auto accident, placed in patient's purse, and presented two days later. Tooth cleaned, replanted, and splinted. Two weeks later endodontic implant inserted. *B,* Postoperative radiograph 7 ***years*** later. Root completely resorbed and implant retaining tooth in position. *C,* Lateral incisor functioning if slightly discolored seven years later. Three months later patient bit on candy and crown fell out. Metal implant was extracted without necessity of anesthesia. (Courtesy Dr. E. H. Ehrmann, Melbourne, Australia.)

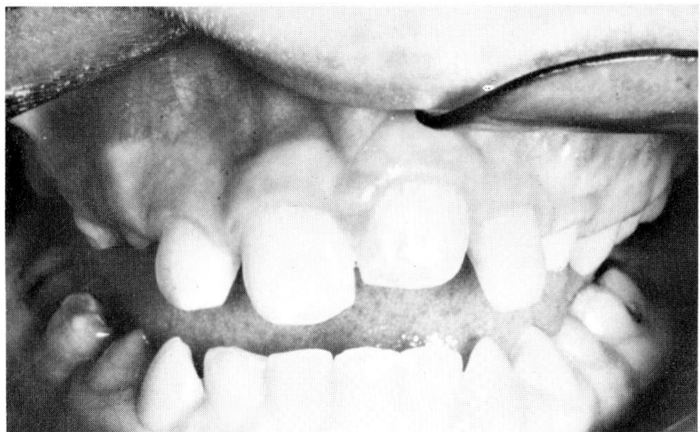

Fig. 16–49. Ankylosis of maxillary left central incisor after replantation. Adjacent teeth continued to erupt leaving replanted incisor and gingiva at former level.

quick-setting acrylic, or acid etch and composite. After splinting, the replanted tooth should be relieved from occlusion by grinding the opposing teeth. Fixed splints should be left in place for one week. At the end of this time the tooth should be firm in its socket.

Ehrmann has suggested replanting teeth avulsed for some time with an endodontic implant. As the root resorbs, the implant will retain the crown in place (Fig. 16–48).

Ankylosis Following Replantation. After replantation, ankylosis often occurs. The adjacent teeth continue to erupt leaving the replanted tooth at the former incisal level (Fig. 16–49). The replanted tooth may be restored to the new incisal level with a jacket crown. However, if the difference in level is great,

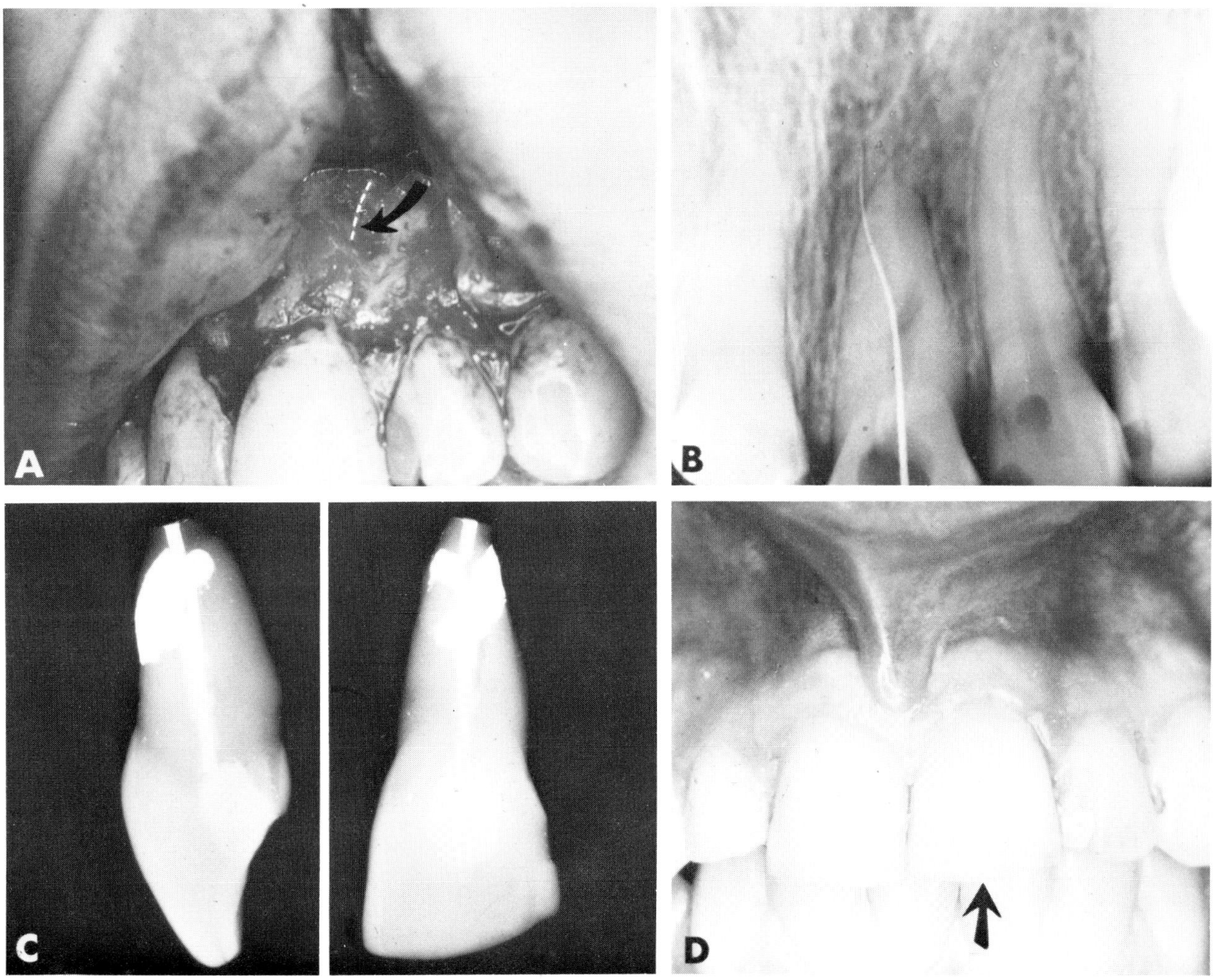

Fig. 16–50. *(Continued on opposite page)*

extraction and prosthetic replacement of the replanted tooth are indicated.

Intentional Replantation. The primary reason for intentional replantation is the inability to perform adequate root canal therapy conservatively and the inadvisability of performing endodontic surgery. ***Periapical surgery,*** for example, is ***contraindicated*** if the apices of the mandibular posterior teeth are in close ***proximity to the mandibular canal.*** In any case where periapical surgery is necessary and can be safely and successfully performed, it is preferred to intentional replantation because of the poor long-term prognosis for the replanted tooth. ***Intentional replantation should be considered when it is the only alternative to extraction.***

The patient must be forewarned that the tooth could split when it is extracted for intentional replanting.

One oral surgeon has suggested that routine root canal therapy be done by extraction, chairside root canal therapy, and replantation.[38] This ridiculous approach was condemned by Glick.[39]

In cases of intentional replantation, it is feasible to replant the tooth quickly after extraction and every effort should be made to do so in order to maintain viability of the periodontal ligament. A splint should be prepared beforehand. This will avoid unnecessary manipulation of the tooth after replantation. An appliance such as the soft acrylic removable splint can be constructed. However, since the replantation is elective and a splint can be constructed at leisure prior to extraction, a more rigid appliance such as an orthodontic band splint is preferable. The tooth to be extracted should be ground out of occlusion before extraction.

Steps in Intentional Replantation. 1. The tooth should be extracted as atraumatically as possible and

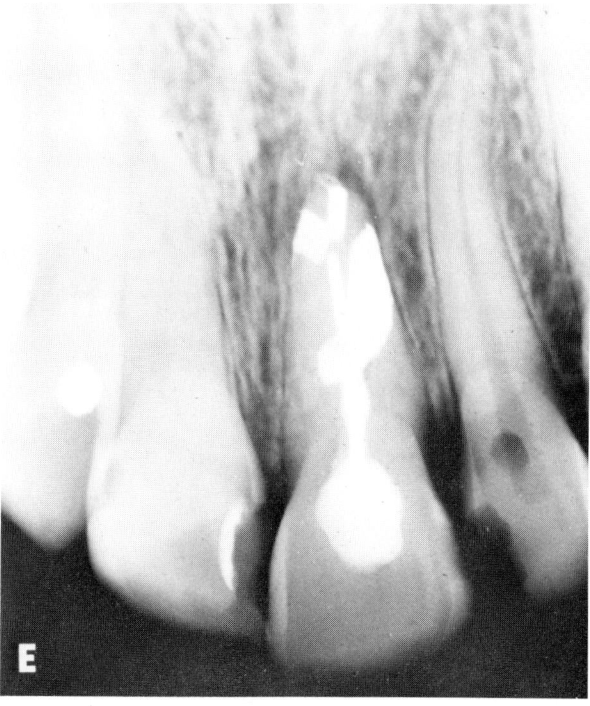

Fig. 16–50. ***Intentional*** replantation. Patient has apparent distal perforation of root of maxillary left central incisor resulting from prior root canal therapy. *A,* Root is shown surgically exposed. Note reamer extending from distal "perforation." *B,* In preparing root canal for filling, aberrant mesial canal was also discovered which was not accessible for surgical repair. To adequately repair root, it was decided to intentionally extract and replant tooth. *C,* Labial and proximal roentgenograms of extracted incisor. Mesial and distal groove-like areas have been repaired with amalgam. Root canal has been filled with silver point and apical foramen sealed with amalgam. *D,* Replanted incisor three days after replantation. At this time tooth was already quite firm in socket. *E,* Roentgenogram of replanted incisor six months after replantation. No root resorption is evident.

should be held in a sponge saturated with sterile normal saline solution during filling of the root canals.

2. If a ***posterior*** tooth is to be replanted, the root apices should be cut off since the risk of the surgical venting procedure in posterior teeth is not warranted.

3. Accessible portions of the root canals should be instrumented and filled in a conventional manner.

The root canals should then be entered apically with a small round bur and prepared for the reception of zinc-free alloy. After the preparations have been irrigated and dried, they are packed with alloy, and excess is carved away (Fig. 16–50*C*).

4. Preparations in teeth with perforations or resorption defects are similarly done. Root canal filling in these cases should be completed before repair of defects.

5. The tooth socket is lightly curetted and irrigated with saline solution and the tooth is seated to place (Fig. 16–50*D,E*).

6. The splint is now applied and should be kept in place for three weeks.

Class VII: Injuries to Deciduous Teeth

Many procedures used in the treatment of traumatic injuries of permanent teeth are equally applicable to the deciduous dentition. The desirability of attempting to retain a devitalized or avulsed deciduous tooth depends largely on how long the tooth would be retained before normal exfoliation. For example, there would be little point in attempting replantation of a deciduous central incisor for a 5½-year-old whose permanent incisors would soon be erupting.

Pulp Testing. Differences of opinion exist as to the reliability of pulp-testing procedures in the primary dentition. A study by O'Toole indicates that the electric pulp tester may be reliably used to determine vitality of the ***primary*** anterior teeth except when teeth are near exfoliation and extremely mobile.[40] McDonald, however, on the basis of clinical and histologic examination, was of the opinion that the electric pulp tester was not reliable in assessing the vitality of primary teeth.[41] Difficulties in obtaining adequate cooperation or accurate responses from the child-patient may further detract from the usefulness of pulp testing as a diagnostic procedure in the very young child.

As a general rule, one can rely on clinical signs and symptoms to determine loss of pulp vitality of a deciduous tooth. Progressive discoloration after trauma is indicative of pulp necrosis; however, immediate hemorrhagic discoloration resulting from trauma may begin to resolve within several weeks, and a waiting period should be allowed before root canal therapy is considered. Further indications of pulp death, such as fistula formation, development of a periapical lesion, percussion sensitivity, swelling and pain, should be watched for.

Complete Root Canal Therapy. Successful cases of root canal therapy in primary teeth have been reported,[42,43] and the degree of success warrants the use of the procedure.

Complete root canal therapy is indicated for a devitalized primary anterior tooth if normal root resorption is not yet extensive. Procedures of access, instrumentation, and medication of root canals are similar to those for permanent teeth. The root canals of the primary anterior teeth are usually straight and can be readily instrumented. Filling of the root canals should be done with a material that will tend to resorb at the same rate as the roots. Gutta percha and silver points are therefore not recommended.

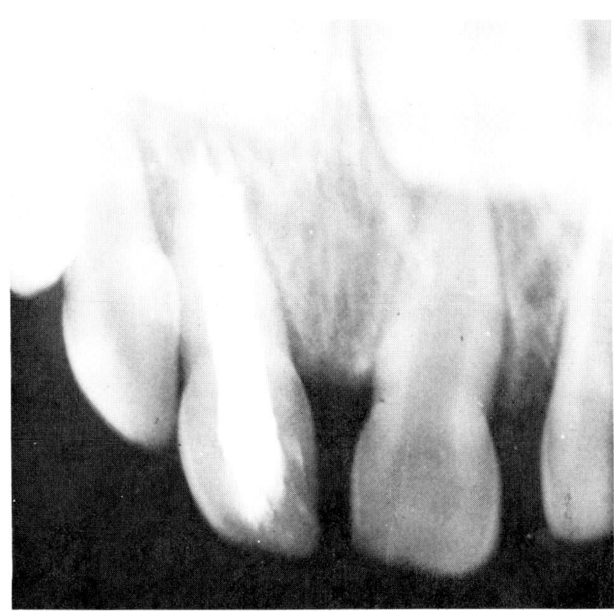

Fig. 16–51. Pulpless primary right central incisor in 2½-year-old patient. Filling material is zinc oxide-eugenol cement. Rectal chloral hydrate sedation was used to manage this young patient.

Resorbable cements such as zinc oxide and eugenol[44] (Fig. 16–51) or resorbable pastes consisting primarily of iodoform[45] also may be used. These materials do not provide as effective an apical seal as gutta percha or silver points, however, they often are adequate for the relatively short period of time needed to reach normal exfoliation. The cement or paste may be inserted into the canal with a motor-driven spiral. Pressure, then applied to the excess filling material in the pulp chamber with warm temporary stopping, will force the material to the apex.

Pulp Capping. Pulp capping is usually not indicated for traumatic exposure of the pulp for the reasons discussed for permanent teeth.

Pulpotomy. Pulpotomy may be attempted for vital traumatic pulp exposures of primary teeth. Pulpotomy for primary teeth is used simply to maintain vitality of the radicular pulp and not with the object of gaining apical closure. In choosing between pulpectomy and pulpotomy, one should remember that it is difficult to seal the root canal adequately with the paste or cement that must be used in primary teeth. Successful pulpotomy will obviate the need for root canal therapy and the possibility of failure due to inadequate apical seal. If pulpotomy fails, complete root canal therapy can be subsequently attempted. When pulpotomy is done with calcium hydroxide, a significant number of failures due to internal resorption occur.[46] It is therefore recommended that a pulpotomy technique employing formocresol[47,48] be used instead. In the technique employed by Sweet,[47] formocresol is applied to the amputated pulp stump with a cotton pledget for five minutes. The pulp stump is then protected with a layer of ZO-E cement and restored with amalgam or a stainless steel crown.

Root Fracture. Treatment of root fractures of primary teeth is similar to that employed for permanent teeth. There is often displacement of the crown associated with the root fracture and adequate stabilization may not be possible. In some instances, however, splinting may be successfully attempted.

Partial Displacement. The treatment of partial displacement is generally the same as that advised for the permanent dentition.

Intrusion is the commonest form of displacement seen in the primary dentition. The intruded primary tooth often erupts rapidly into normal position. Pulp death frequently occurs, however, and root canal therapy is necessary to retain the tooth.

Complete Displacement. Complete displacement may be treated by replantation, as in the permanent dentition. The technique of replantation is identical, except that the root canals must be filled with a resorbable paste or cement. Removal of a portion of the root apex is indicated if the replanted tooth does not remain in its socket or fails to seat to full length. Surgical venting should be avoided because of the possibility of damaging the permanent successor.

A flexible acrylic splint may be used for stabilization if the patient is old enough to cooperate in wearing it. If not, one of the fixed splints should be tried.

Intentional replantation may also be carried out for primary teeth.[50] The major indication is the inability to perform successful root canal therapy on a nonvital primary molar. Replantation of a primary molar may be difficult if the roots are widely divergent and in this event the roots may be tapered by grinding to facilitate insertion. Splinting may not be necessary if the replanted molar seems to be firm in its socket; however, some form of stabilization should be used if any mobility is present.

BLEACHING OF DISCOLORED PULPLESS TEETH

One of the most widespread misconceptions concerning the pulpless tooth is that darkening or discoloration of such a tooth is inevitable. Equally common is the general ignorance of the fact that when discoloration does occur it can often be remedied by bleaching.

Causes of Discoloration of Pulpless Teeth. A major cause of discoloration is hemorrhage into the pulp chamber, which occurs as a consequence of trauma. The hemolysis of red blood cells and penetration of the breakdown products into the dentinal tubules results in rapid darkening of the tooth. Discoloration frequently results from the decomposition of necrotic pulp tissue, even though frank hemorrhage has not occurred.

Unnecessary discoloration of pulpless teeth is often a consequence of faulty endodontic technique or the use of dentin-staining drugs or materials in root-canal therapy. Pulp material left in the pulp horns, because of failure to extend access sufficiently, is an invitation to discoloration. Failure to stop bleeding after pulpectomy may allow blood to enter the pulp chamber and may also result in discoloration. Discoloration that is almost impossible to eliminate may be caused through the use of tetracyclines, silver nitrate, or iodine solutions for root canal disinfection. Amalgam fillings or root canal sealers containing precipitated silver cause similarly intractable staining when in contact with dentin in the pulp chamber.

Careful endodontic technique and the proper choice of drugs and materials will do much to prevent discoloration from occurring after root canal therapy. However, if discoloration subsequently occurs, or is already present at the time of root canal treatment, it can often be eliminated by bleaching.

Prior to an attempt at bleaching, the dentist should inform the patient that bleaching is not always permanently successful. Some teeth may slowly discolor again and may require rebleaching. In certain instances bleaching may not be effective at all. This is especially true when staining has been caused by metals such as silver amalgam.

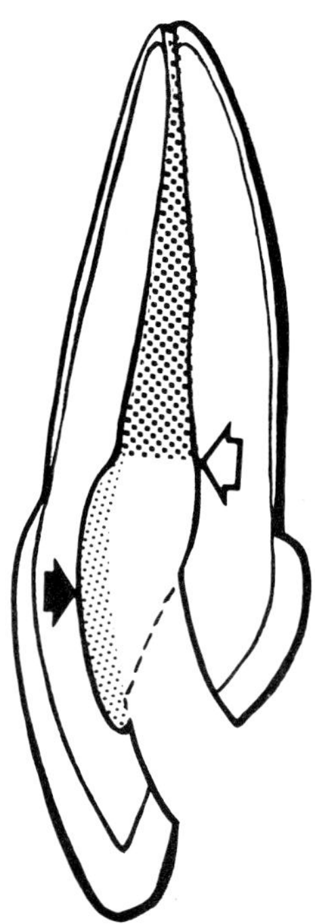

Fig. 16–52. Gutta percha and dentin removal prior to bleaching. Heavy dotted area represents gutta percha filling, which is removed to below level of labial gingiva *(open arrow)*. Light dotted area represents removal of dentin to eliminate heavy stain concentration and pulp horn material *(black arrow)*.

Bleaching Agents. The most commonly used bleaching agent is Superoxol (Merck and Co.). This is a potent oxidizing agent whose bleaching effect results from direct oxidation of stain-producing substances.

Superoxol is a 30% solution by weight of hydrogen peroxide in distilled water. It is available in amber-colored bottles, as it tends to be decomposed by light. It should be kept refrigerated and covered to prevent the possibility of explosion. A refrigerated bottle of Superoxol will retain potency for some time. Effective bleaching results have been obtained with solutions one to two years old.

Since Superoxol causes whitening of the skin upon contact, facial surfaces exposed to this agent should be washed thoroughly. The white patch on the skin disappears within an hour. Prolonged contact of Superoxol with oral tissues, however, will cause a painful burn.

Preparation for Bleaching. 1. Bleaching should not be attempted if the root canal filling does not seal the canal tightly because of the danger that bleaching agents leak into the periapical tissue. Inadequate root canal fillings should routinely be replaced ***before*** bleaching.

2. Stained or leaking silicate or plastic fillings should be removed.

3. Be certain to remove the entire roof of the pulp chamber and all material in the pulp horns.

4. Remove as much stained dentin as possible, especially in the areas of heavy stain concentration (Fig. 16–53).

5. Root canal filling material in the pulp chamber should be removed to well below the level of the labial gingiva (Fig. 16–52).

Bleaching should be done with a rubber dam in place. Only the tooth to be bleached needs to be exposed through the dam. The rubber dam must fit tightly at the cervical margin of the tooth to prevent possible leakage of the bleaching liquid onto the gingival tissue. A plastic apron should be placed over the patient's clothing to prevent damage in the event bleach is spilled.

A simplified method of bleaching has been reported by Spasser,[50] and further refined and made popular by Nutting and Poe as "The Walking Bleach."[51] In this they refer to the fact that the bleaching agents are sealed into place and the patient released; he is not held in the office for a protracted period while the Superoxol is activated by heat.

Steps in Bleaching

1. Thoroughly swab the pulp chamber with 95% alcohol and dry with an extended blast of hot air. This will dehydrate the dentin and remove fatty substances from the entrance to the tubules. Penetration of the bleach into the dentin is thus facilitated.

2. Record the shade of the discolored tooth from a shade guide. From this the progress of the bleach can be followed. Memory of both the patient and dentist is often unreliable.

3. Apply the rubber dam and petrolatum protection at the gingival. Be sure that there are no leaking restorations in the tooth and that the root canal filling is perfectly sealed at the orifice of the canal. If necessary seal off the root filling, for pressure will build up in the chamber that could leak to the periapex, leading to a painful reaction.

4. Again, wipe the inside of the cavity with a solvent—ether, alcohol, acetone, xylene, or chloroform—and place the bleaching agent. This is made by adding 2 or 3 drops of Superoxol to a sufficient quantity of powdered sodium perborate to form a thick paste. The paste should be carried into the pulp chamber with stainless instruments. Sodium peroxyborate monohydrate (Amosan) may be substituted for powdered sodium perborate. The granular form, however, should be powdered by trituration in a mechanical amalgamator using a fresh mortar and pestle.

5. Seal the bleaching agents in place by a cotton pellet and Cavit. A double seal may be necessary to prevent leakage.

6. The patient should return in 5 days and the progress checked with the shade guide. Quite possibly a second or third application may be necessary. The patient should be reappointed one month later to evaluate if the new color is stable. If the color of the treated tooth holds during this time, the prognosis for long-term color stability is good and the tooth may be restored with composite (Fig. 16–53).

Pearson has suggested that secondary discoloration after successful bleaching is due to permeability of enamel.[52] For this reason he advocates sealing of the enamel with self-curing acrylic resin monomer. The use of silicone fluid has been suggested by Grossman for restoration of translucency.[53] He claims that the silicone fluid remains permanently effective because it does not evaporate.

Nutting and Poe have shown that the walking bleach is even effective against the staining of silver nitrate, although they admit their success to be quite unusual (Fig. 16–54).[54] They have also shown the technique to be effective in discolored roots, exposed by periodontal surgery (Fig. 16–55). In this case, the root canal filling must be removed well down into the canal and the remaining filling sealed to prevent leakage toward the apex.

Freedland has shown that external enamel stains in vital teeth, such as those caused by fluorosis, may be removed by the application of a fresh solution of 30% hydrogen peroxide (Superoxol) to which has been added one part of hydrochloric acid—35%.[55] The dam and protective petroleum jelly are applied without metal clamps (Fig. 16–56), and metal instru-

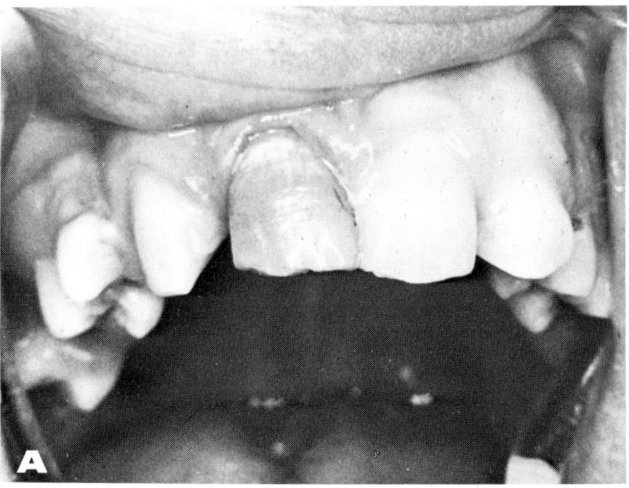

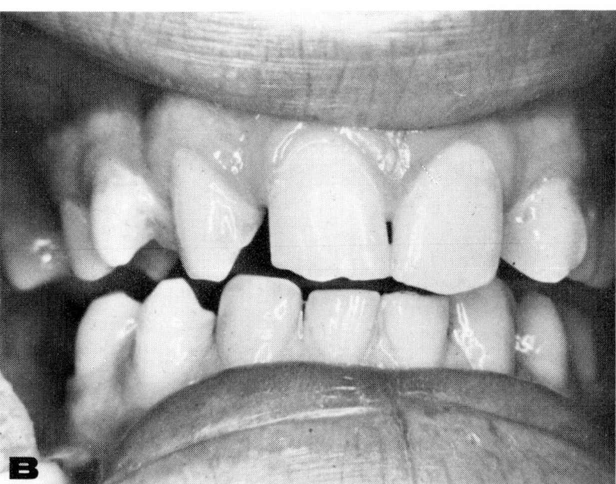

Fig. 16–53. *A,* Traumatic pulp death and dentin discoloration. *B,* "Walking bleach" following one treatment. (From Nutting, E. B., and Poe, G. S.: Dent. Clin. N. Amer., p. 655, Nov., 1967.)

ments should not be used. The solution is applied to the labial-proximal surfaces with a cotton swab. Bleaching is done in the office in five minutes, during which time the assistant constantly moistens the enamel. Heat may be applied from a light source or a bleaching instrument. The treatment may have to be repeated to be successful (Fig. 16–57).

Cooper and Kopel have suggested a similar technique to remove the enamel stains from ingested tetracycline that permeate the teeth of children who have been maintained on the drug during tooth development (Fig. 16–58).[56] The rubber dam is placed with petrolatum or Orobase and ligated around each tooth. The labial-proximal surfaces are

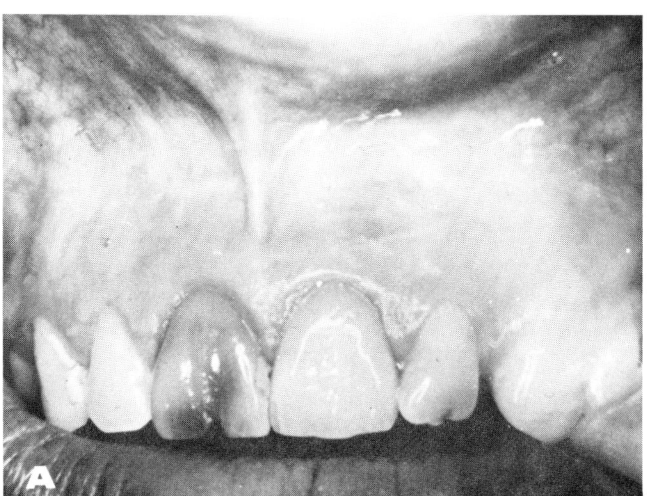

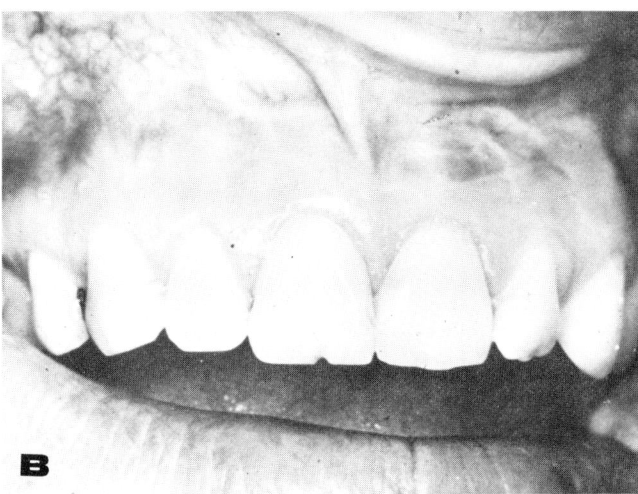

Fig. 16–54. Unusual result of bleaching a tooth stained with silver nitrate. *A,* Before treatment. *B,* After two treatments with "walking bleach." (From Nutting, E. B., and Poe, G. S.: Dent. Clin. N. Amer., p. 655, Nov., 1967.)

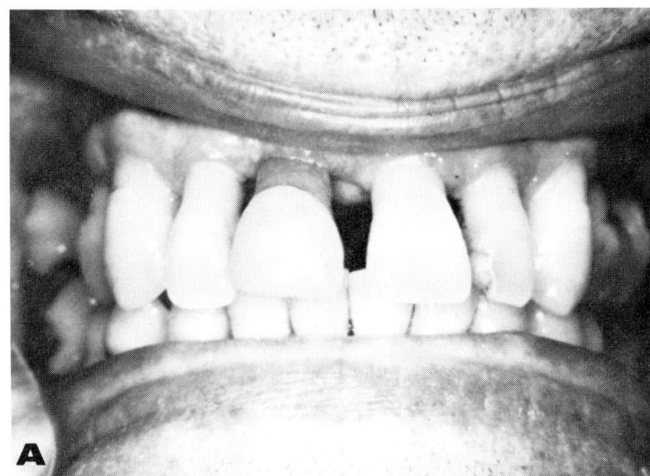

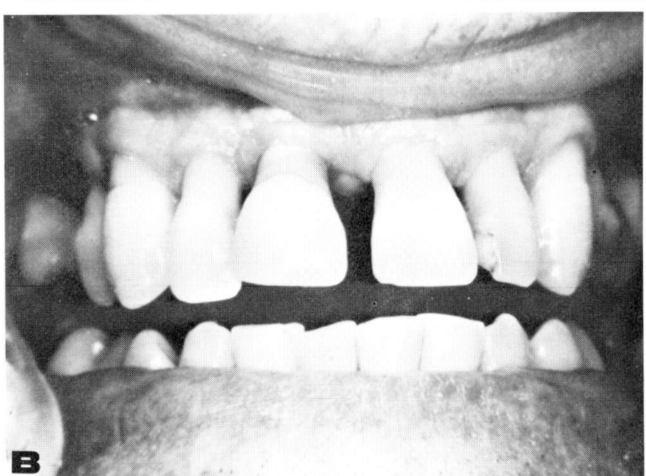

Fig. 16–55. Bleaching of discolored root surface after periodontal surgery. *A,* Before treatment. *B,* After treatment, done through porcelain jacket crown. (From Nutting, E. B., and Poe, G. S.: Dent. Clin. N. Amer., p. 655, Nov., 1967.)

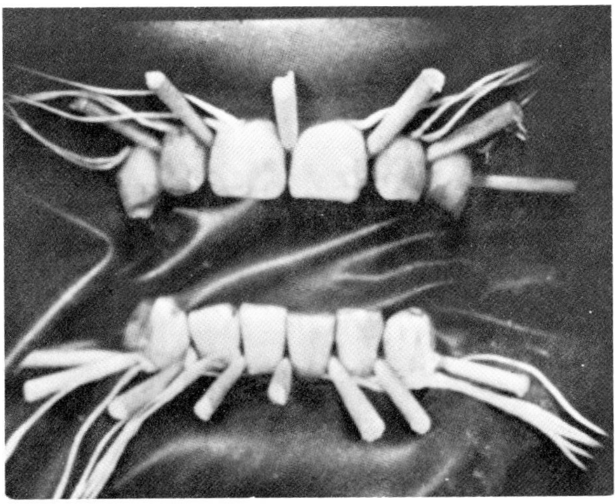

Fig. 16–56. Rubber dam placement with no metal clamps, for external bleach of enamel fluorosis. (Courtesy Dr. Jacob B. Freedland.)

then cleaned with a mixture of chloroform–alcohol and are etched with 50% phosphoric acid. A cotton mat is applied to each tooth, which is then saturated with Superoxol and ether, a 5 to 1 mixture. The bleaching process is accelerated by heating the solution with a bleaching instrument,* which operates at about 125° F. Each tooth is heated about 30 seconds and then the heat is moved on to the next tooth. The cotton is kept wet with the Superoxol solution.

*Fluroted Bleaching Instrument, Fluroted Co., Davis, California

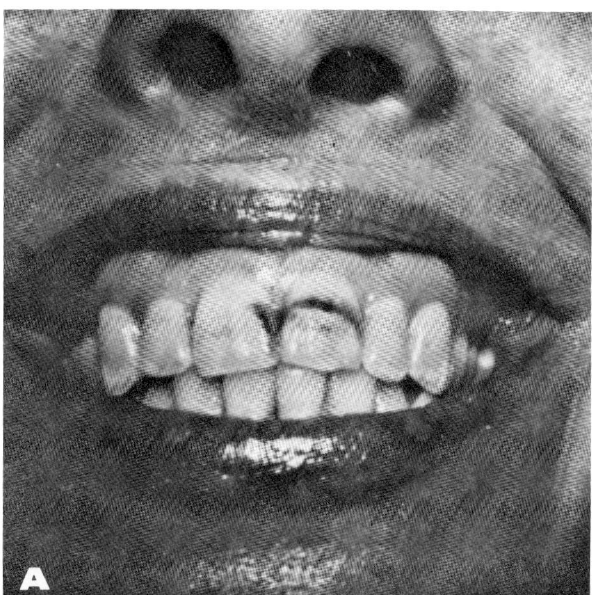

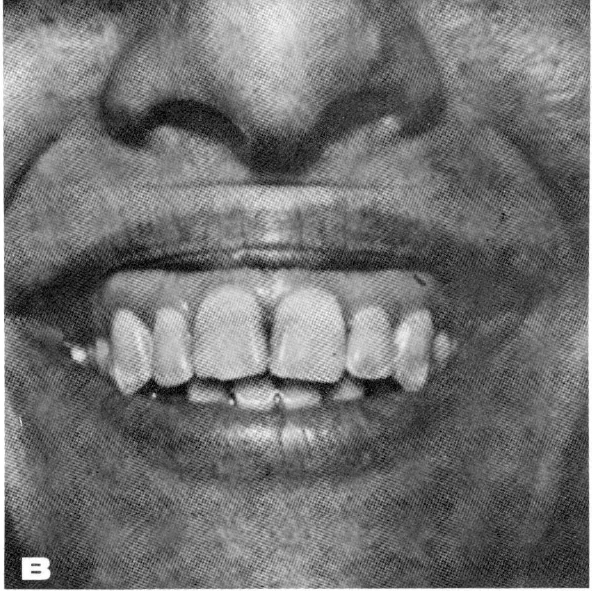

Fig. 16–57. *A,* Severe fluorosis stains of central incisors. *B,* Stain removal using Superoxol and hydrochloric acid. (Courtesy Dr. Jacob B. Freedland.)

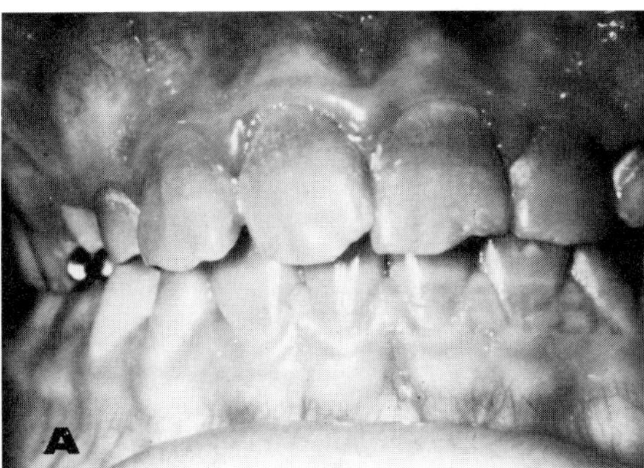

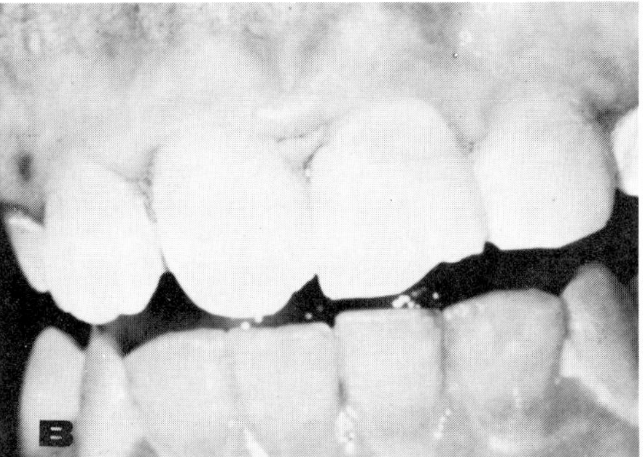

Fig. 16–58. *A,* Tetracycline stained teeth before external bleaching. *B,* After treatment with phosphoric acid (50%) etching and Superoxol. (Courtesy Dr. Hugh S. Kopel.)

The bleaching solution is washed from the teeth with water and aspiration, followed by sodium hypochlorite and again by a water rinse. Care is taken not to burn the tissue or overheat the teeth. Two to four 30-minute visits may be necessary to achieve an acceptable result. The teeth stained yellow or light brown respond better than those that are dark brown or grey.

REFERENCES

1. Andreasen, J. O.: Traumatic Injuries of the Teeth. (Copenhagen, Munksgaard) St. Louis, C. V. Mosby, 1972, 334 pp.

1a. Epstein, L. I.: Traumatic injuries to anterior teeth in children. Oral Surg., *15*:334, Mar., 1962.

2. Ellis, R. G.: *The Classification and Treatment of Injuries to the Teeth of Children.* Chicago, The Year Book Publishers, 4th Ed., 1960.

2a. International Classification of Diseases—Application to Dentistry and Stomatology. ICD–DA, Copenhagen, 1969.

3. Barker, B. C. W., and Mayne, J. R.: Some unusual cases of apexification subsequent to trauma. Oral Surg., *39*:144, Jan., 1975.

4. Nygaard-Ostby, B.: The role of the blood clot in endodontic therapy. Acta Odont. Scand., *19*:323, 1961.

5. Kaiser, J. H.: Personal communication, June, 1975.

6. Kaiser, J. H.: Presentation to the American Association of Endodontists. Washington, D.C., April, 1964.

7. Frank, A. L.: Clinical Presentation, American Association of Endodontists, Washington, D.C., April 1964.

7a. Frank, A. L.: Endodontic endosseous implants and treatment of the wide open apex. Dent. Clin. N. Amer., p. 675, Nov., 1967.

8. Frank, A. L.: Therapy for the divergent pulpless tooth by continued apical formation. J.A.D.A., *72*:87, 1966.

8a. Nevins, A. J., Finklestein, B. G., and Moodnik, R. M.: Apexification through a collagen-calcium phosphate gel. Paper presented at meeting of Am. Assoc. Endodontics, April, 1975.

9. Frank, A. L., and Weine, F. S.: Nonsurgical therapy for the perforative defect of internal resorption. J.A.D.A., *87*:863, Oct., 1973.

10. Frank, A. L.: Resorptions, perforations and fractures. Dent. Clin. N. Amer., *18*:465, Apr., 1974.

11. Torneck, C. D., Smith, J. S., and Grindall, P.: Biologic effects of endodontic procedures on developing incisor teeth. IV. Oral Surg., *35*:541, Apr., 1973.

12. Koenigs, J. F., Heller, A. L., Brilliant, D. J., Melfi, R. C., and Driskell, T. D.: Induced apical closure of permanent teeth in adult primates using a resorbable form of tricalcium phosphate ceramic. J. Endodont., *1*:102, Mar., 1975.

13. Nevins, A. J., Finklestein, F., Borden, B. G., and Moodnik, R.: Physiologic closure of the pulpless open apex tooth. Paper presented at Amer. Assoc. of Endodont., Apr. 24, 1975.

14. Law, D. B.: Prevention and treatment of traumatized permanent anterior teeth. Dent. Clin. N. Amer., p. 615, Nov., 1961.

15. Warnick, M. E.: The use of porcelain-fused-to-gold in the restoration of fractured young permanent anterior teeth. J. Dent. Children. First Quarter, 1962, p. 3–8.

16. Whynman, E.: Drugless pulpotomy in adults. Ann. Dent., *6*:125, June, 1947.

17. Glass, R. L., and Zander, H. A.: Pulp healing. J. Dent. Res., *26*:97, Apr., 1949.

18. Zander, H. A., and Glass, R. L.: The healing of phenolized pulp exposures. Oral Surg., *2*:803, June, 1949.

19. Hunter, H. A.: A study of mechanisms concerned in the deposition of lime salts in bridging over a pulp exposure. J. Dent. Res., *34*:697, Oct., 1955.

20. Massler, M.: Pulpotomy: a re-appraisal. Trans. of the Third International Conference on Endodontics. 1963, pp. 1–23.

21. Fiore-Donno, G., and Baume, L. J.: Effects of capping compounds containing corticosteroids in the human dental pulp. Helv. Odont. Acta, *6*:23, Oct., 1962.

22. Lawson, B. F., and Mitchell, D. F.: Pharmacologic treatment of painful pulpitis. A preliminary, controlled, double-blind study. Oral Surg., *17*:47, Jan., 1964.

23. Vigg, J.: Hydrocortisone in pulp therapy. Dent. Prog., *2*:53, July, 1962.

24. Ellis, R. G.: Op. cit., p. 177.

25. Sibley, L. C.: Management of root fracture. Oral Surg., *13*:1475, Dec., 1960.

26. Andreasen, J. O.: *Traumatic Injuries of the Teeth.* St. Louis, C. V. Mosby Co., 1972.

27. Andreasen, J. O., and Hjorting-Hansen, E.: Intraalveolar root fractures: radiographic and histologic study of 50 cases. Oral Surg., *25*:414, 1967.

28. Heithersay, G. S.: Combined endodontic-orthodontic treatment of transverse root fractures in the region of the alveolar crest. Oral Surg., *36*:404, Sept., 1973.

29. Natiella, J. R., Armitage, J. E., and Meenaghan, M. A.: The failing blade-vent implant. Oral Surg., *36*:336, Sept., 1973.

30. Neuman, G., Spangberg, L., and Langeland, K.: Methodology and criteria in the evaluation of dental implants. J. Endodont., *1*:193, June, 1975.

31. Linaburg, R. G., and Marshall, F. J.: The diagnosis and treatment of vertical root fractures: report of a case. J.A.D.A., *86*:679, Mar., 1973.

32. Andreasen, J. O.: Luxation of primary and permanent teeth. Presentation, American Association of Endodontists, May 1976.

33. Kromer, H.: An auxiliary device for the performance of replantation. Brit. Dent., J., *84*:210, May, 1948.

34. Hammer, H.: Replantation and implantation of teeth. Int. Dent. J., *5*:439, Mar., 1955.

35. Neuwirt, F.: Experimentelle Studie Über Zahnpflanzung', Zulni Lék, Parka, S. 145.

36. Heiss, J.: Klinische Und Histologische Unter-Suchungen Am Replantierten Zahn' Zschr. Stomat., 42, 4.

37. Löe, H., and Waerhaug, J.: Experimental replantation of teeth in dogs and monkeys. Arch. Oral Biol., *3*:176, Apr., 1961.

37a. Nasjleti, C. E., Caffesse, R. G., Castelli, W. A., and Hoke, J. A.: Healing after tooth reimplantation in monkeys. Oral Surg., *39*:361, Mar., 1975.

37b. Andreasen J. O.: Replantation of avulsed teeth. Presentation, American Association of Endodontists, May, 1976.

38. Kingsbury, B. C., Jr., and Weisenbaugh, J. M., Jr.: Intentional replantation of mandibular premolars and molars. J.A.D.A., *83*:1053, Nov., 1971.

39. Glick, D. H.: Letter to the Editor. J.A.D.A., *84*:475, Mar., 1972.

40. O'Toole, T. J.: A study of electrical stimulation of primary anterior teeth. Master's Thesis. University of Washington, 1962.

41. McDonald, R. E.: Diagnostic aids and vital pulp therapy for deciduous teeth. J.A.D.A., *53*:14, July, 1956.

42. Andrew, P.: The treatment of infected pulps in deciduous teeth. Brit. Dent. J., *98*:122, Feb., 1955.
43. Rabinowitch, B. Z.: Pulp management in primary teeth. Oral Surg., *6*:542, April; 671, May, 1953.
44. Nicholis, E.: Root canal treatment of primary teeth. Trans. of Third International Conference on Endodontics, 1964, pp. 52–66.
45. Maisto, O. A.: Personal communication (Through Dr. Ingle) 1962.
46. Via, W. F., Jr.: Evaluation of deciduous molars treated by pulpotomy and calcium-hydroxide. J.A.D.A., *50*:34, Jan., 1955.
47. Sweet, C. A.: Formocresol technique. Trans. of the Third International Conference on Endodontics, 1964, pp. 32–46.
48. Doyle, W., McDonald, R. E., and Mitchell, D. F.: Formocresol versus calcium hydroxide in pulpotomy. J. Dent. Children, *29*:86, Second Quarter, 1962.
49. Sakellariou, P. L.: Replantation of infected deciduous teeth: a contribution to the problem of their preservation until normal shedding. Oral Surg., *16*:645, June, 1963.
50. Spasser, H. F.: A simple bleaching technique using sodium perborate. N.Y. Dent. J., *27*:332, 1961.
51. Nutting, E. B., and Poe, G. S.: Chemical bleaching of discolored endodontically treated teeth. Dent. Clin. N. Amer., p. 655, Nov., 1967.
52. Pearson H. H.: Bleaching of the discolored pulpless tooth. J.A.D.A., *56*:64, Jan., 1958.
53. Grossman, L. I.: Endodontic Practice. Philadelphia, Lea & Febiger, 5th Ed., 1960, p. 393.
54. Nutting, E. B., and Poe, G. S.: A new combination for bleaching teeth. J. South. Calif. Dent. Assn., *41*:289, Sept., 1963.
55. Freedland, J. B.: Steps in bleaching vital fluorosed teeth. Personal communication, 1972.
56 Cooper, H. and Kopel, H.: Bleaching tetracycline stained teeth. Personal communication, July, 1975.

Chapter 17

Pediatric Endodontics

HUGH M. KOPEL*

Why a separate chapter on pediatric endodontics? Won't these pages be a small-scale repetition of all that has been said previously? Granted, children are smaller, their primary teeth are smaller, and child management is different from adult patient management. But there are other obvious differences—anatomic and histologic differences of primary pulps and a whole different philosophy about what constitutes success and the length of tooth survival following therapy.

That there is a need for saving children's teeth is attested to by the discouraging statistics regarding tooth loss, particularly the early loss of young permanent teeth. In spite of fluoridation and other preventive methods, the preservation of primary and young permanent teeth whose pulps have been exposed or endangered by caries, trauma, or toxic restorative materials must still be a primary objective in pediatric endodontics. Lewis and Law succinctly stated this objective as, "the successful treatment of the pulpally involved tooth to retain that tooth in a healthy condition so it may fulfill its role as a useful component of the primary and young permanent dentition."[1]

Little disagreement exists over the importance of primary and young permanent teeth in the maintenance of normal function and arch form. Premature loss of primary molars and canines may result in shortened arch length, insufficient space for the permanent teeth, impaction of premolars, mesial tipping and extrusion of permanent molars, shift of the midline with a possibility of crossbite occlusion, and the development of certain aberrant tongue positions. These sequelae of premature loss can only be prevented by either initial pulp therapy or subsequent orthodontic or prosthetic intervention. Pulp therapy is the treatment of choice. The question, however, has always been what to do about primary or young permanent molars with deep carious lesions suspected of involving the pulp.

DiMaggio et al. found that 75% of deeply carious primary and young permanent molars would have been pulpally exposed had all carious dentin been removed.[2] Eichenbaum reported that of 511 children, 213 were found to have carious exposures of primary teeth. The greatest involvement was noted between the ages of four and six. In this study, 16 children had a total of 24 ***permanent*** molars beyond repair or previously extracted[3] (Graph 17–1).

Young pulp tissue is known to be capable of healing following injury or irritation.[4–6] Our discussion concerns a sensible treatment designed to promote such healing.

In order to understand this rationale of pulp therapy, however, it is essential to know primary pulp morphology and cellular anatomy, and to understand how it responds to irritation. Furthermore, one must know that the general principles of adult pulp treatment are not often applied to the primary teeth. Special problems in dealing with primary dentition are due to differences in pulp anatomy as well to the changes caused by the normal root resorptive process.

*The author acknowledges with appreciation the assistance of Dr. Craig Coy, Dr. Geoffrey Groat, Dr. David Good, Dr. Carl Hirtzel, and Dr. Steven Mascagno.

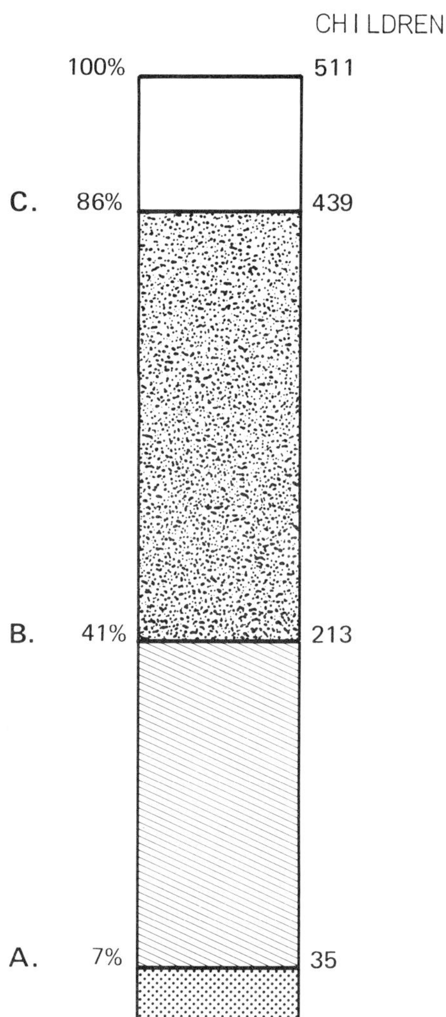

Graph 17–1. Prevalence of pulp exposures of 511 children. *A,* Only 35 (7%) were free of dental defects; *B,* 213 (41%) had necrotic pulps or carious exposures; *C,* 439 children (86%) needed dental care. (From Eichenbaum, I., and Dunn, N. A.: J. Dent. Child., *18*:8, 4th Quart., 1951.)

PULP MORPHOLOGY

In general terms, the pulp chambers of primary and young permanent teeth are similar in shape to the outer surfaces of the teeth. The mesial pulp horns of the primary molars, however, are closer to the outer surface than are the distal horns, and therefore are more readily exposed to caries or trauma.

Anatomic differences between the pulp chambers and root canals of primary teeth and those of young permanent teeth have also been demonstrated. It is conceivable that certain endodontic measures have to be modified owing to these differences.[7]

Anatomic Differences (Fig. 17–1)

When the pulp chambers of primary teeth are compared to those of young permanent teeth (1) pulp chamber anatomy in primary teeth closely approximates the surface of the crown; (2) in relation to their crowns the pulps of primary teeth are larger than those of the permanent teeth; (3) pulp horns of the primary teeth extend closer to the outer surface of the teeth than do pulp horns in permanent teeth; (4) the primary pulp horn under each cusp is longer than is suggested by the external anatomy; (5) in primary teeth, mandibular molars have proportionately larger pulp chambers than have maxillary molars; and (6) accessory canals in the primary pulp chamber floor lead directly into the intraradicular furcation.[8]

A comparison of root canals of primary teeth and those of young permanent teeth shows: (1) the roots

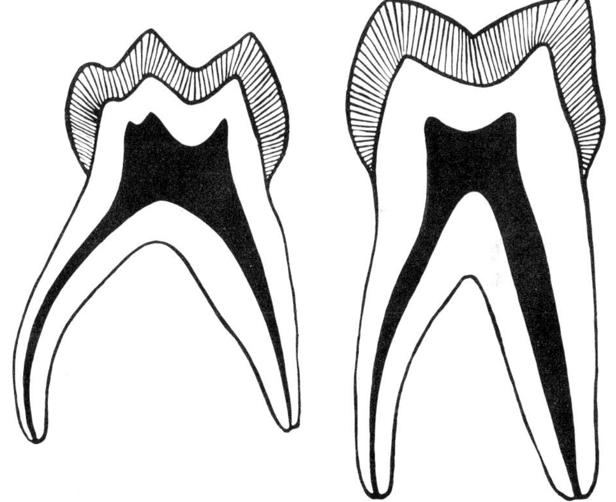

Fig. 17–1. Comparative anatomy between primary *(left)* and permanent *(right)* molars. Primary teeth are smaller in all dimensions; their enamel cap is thinner with less tooth structure protecting pulp. Primary pulp horns are higher, particularly mesial. Roots of primary molars are longer and more slender, are "pinched in" at cervical, and flare more toward apex to accommodate permanent tooth buds. All these factors tend to increase incidence of pulp involvement from caries or complicate canal preparation and obturation. (From Finn, S. B.: Clinical Pedodontics. Philadelphia, W. B. Saunders Co., 4th ed., 1973, p. 63.)

of primary teeth are longer and more slender in comparison to crown size than are those of the permanent teeth; (2) primary tooth canals are more ribbon-like than canals in the permanent teeth; (3) the roots of primary anterior teeth are narrower mesiodistally than are permanent teeth roots; (4) at the cervical region the roots of the primary molars flare outward to a greater degree than the permanent molars and continue to flare as they approach the apices.

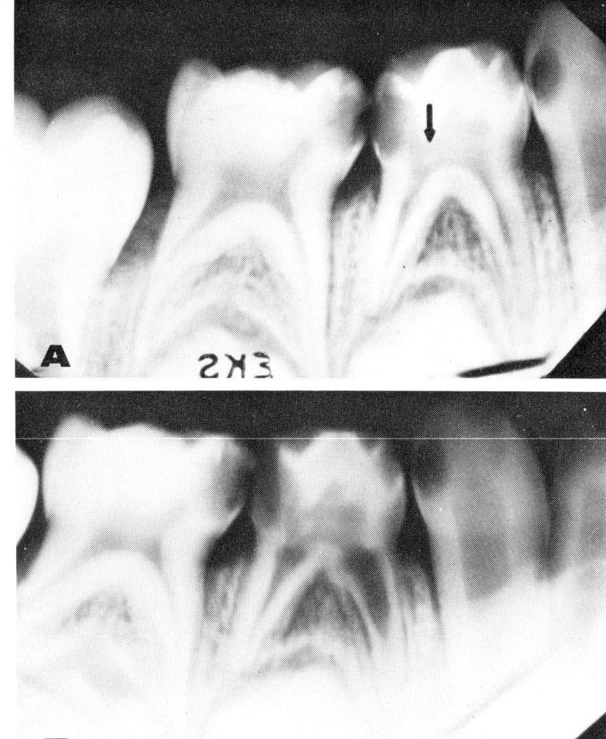

Fig. 17–2. Internal resorption triggered by inflammation. *A,* Advanced caries in 5-year-old child. Note calcification *(arrow)* in first primary molar (contraindication for pulp therapy). *B,* Same patient six months later. Marked internal resorption, forecast in earlier radiograph, indicates advanced degenerative changes. (From Law, D. B., Lewis, T. M., and Davis, J. M.: An Atlas of Pedodontics. Philadelphia, W. B. Saunders Co., 1969, p. 195.)

Histologic Differences Between Primary and Permanent Tooth Pulps

Many clinicians have noted that the pulps of primary and permanent teeth respond differently to trauma, bacterial invasion, irritation, and medication. Anatomic differences may contribute to this difference. The roots of the primary teeth have enlarged apical foramens, for example, whereas the foramens of permanent teeth are restricted. It is hypothesized, therefore, that a reduced blood supply in permanent teeth favors calcific response and healing by "calcific scarring."[9] This hypothesis is borne out in older pulps where one finds more calcified nodules and ground substance than in young pulps. Primary teeth, on the other hand, with their abundant blood supply, demonstrate a more typical inflammatory response than that seen in adult permanent teeth.

The high incidence of inflammation in primary teeth may account for the increase in both internal and external resorption to calcium hydroxide pulpotomies. The alkalinity of calcium hydroxide produces such severe pulp inflammation and subsequent metaplasia that internal resorption occurs in the roots of the primary teeth. It has been shown that the more severe the inflammation the more severe the resorption (Fig. 17–2). Although it is suspected that pulps of primary teeth have a different function from those of permanent teeth, no supporting data are available.

Some clinicians believe that primary teeth are less sensitive to pain than are permanent teeth, probably because of differences in number and/or distribution of neural elements. When comparing primary and permanent teeth, Bernick found differences in the final distribution of pulp nerve fibers. In permanent teeth these fibers terminate mainly among the odontoblasts and even in predentin. In primary teeth, pulp nerve fibers pass to the odontoblastic area, where they terminate as free nerve endings. Bernick postulated that if primary teeth were not so short-lived in the oral cavity, their nerve endings might terminate in the odontoblasts and predentin as in the permanent tooth[10] (Fig. 17–3).

Rapp has concurred with this hypothesis and has also stated that the density of the innervation of the primary tooth is not so great as that of the permanent tooth and may possibly be the reason primary teeth are less sensitive to operative procedures. He does agree, however, that as the primary teeth resorb there is a degeneration of the neural elements as with other pulp cells.[11] Neural tissue is the first to degenerate when root resorption begins, just as it is the last tissue to mature when the pulp develops.

Primary and permanent teeth also differ in their cellular responses to irritation, trauma, and medication. It has been shown, for example, that the

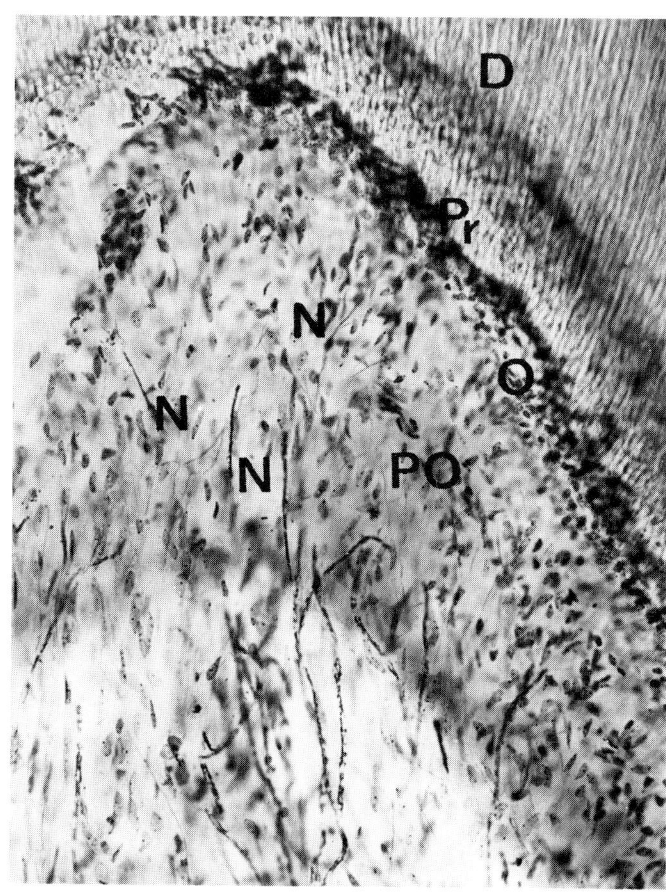

Fig. 17–3. Section of pulp from human primary molar. Note majority of nerves terminate at pulp-odontoblastic border. Only isolated nerve fiber penetrates P-O border to terminate in zone of Weil. *D,* dentin; *N,* nerve fiber; *O,* odontoblasts; *Pr,* predentin; *PO,* pulp-odontoblast border. (From Bernick, S.: Innervation of the teeth and periodontium. Dent. Clin. N. Amer., p. 503, July, 1959.)

incidence of reparative dentin formation beneath carious lesions is more extensive in primary than in permanent teeth.[12–15] McDonald also believes that the localization of infection and inflammation is poorer in the primary pulp than in pulp of permanent teeth.[16]

MANAGEMENT OF DEEP CARIOUS LESIONS AND PULP INFLAMMATION IN PRIMARY AND YOUNG PERMANENT TEETH

Pulp therapy for primary and young permanent teeth has for years been subject to change and controversy. At the same time, such pulp medicaments as zinc oxide–eugenol cement, calcium hydroxide, and formocresol have survived these controversial years. A better understanding of the reactions of the pulp and dentin to these medicaments has developed over the years, primarily through improvements in histologic techniques. Anderson et al. concluded that the pulp and dentin should be considered as one organ, and Frankl pointed out that the reaction of this pulpo-dentinal system is essentially proportionate to the intensity of, and duration of exposure to, the offending agent, whether it be caries, trauma, medicaments, or restorative materials.[17,18]

The rationale for pulp therapy has thus developed out of well-constructed clinical studies and better histologic techniques. Ongoing research, moreover, is providing modifications that will even improve upon present success.

At this time pulp therapy for primary and young permanent teeth has resolved basically into four different techniques: (1) direct pulp capping, (2) indirect pulp capping, (3) pulpotomy, and (4) pulpectomy. Three of these methods are concerned with the preservation of vital pulp tissues and dentin, and the fourth involves retaining the treated pulpless tooth.

Direct Pulp Capping

Direct pulp capping is defined as the protection of a pulp exposed by traumatic fracture or in the course of excavating deep dentinal caries. Protection is provided by placing a medicated or nonmedicated material in direct contact with the pulp tissue to promote a reparative reaction (Fig. 17–4). To initiate repair, many medicaments and materials have been

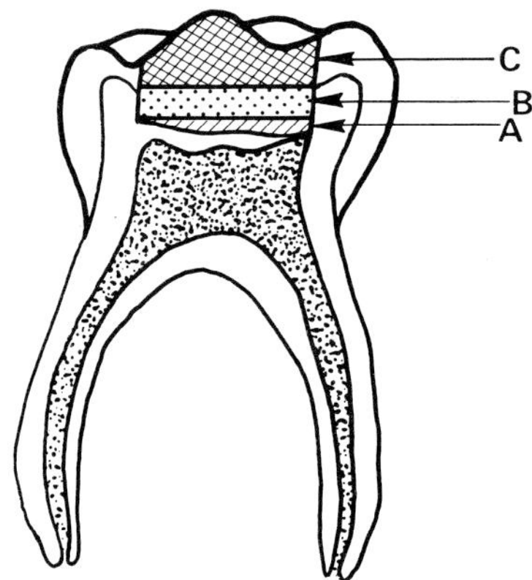

Fig. 17–4. Direct pulp-capping technique. *A*, Capping material covers pulp exposure and floor of cavity. *B*, Protective base of zinc oxide-eugenol cement. *C*, Amalgam restoration.

suggested, including Hunter's classic mixture, in 1883, of "sorgum molasses and droppum English sparrow,"[19] cappings of gold foil, thymol crystals, powdered dentin or bone, calcium hydroxide, resorbable ceramic powder, dental cements, pure or mixed with various antiseptics, antibiotics, and corticosteroids. The rationale behind these varied treatments lies in the ability of young healthy pulps to initiate a dentin bridge, walling off the exposure site[20–22] (Fig. 17–5). Controversy develops over what constitutes a young healthy pulp. McDonald has stated that the preoperative diagnosis of pulp health or disease should dictate optimal treatment for primary and young permanent teeth.[16] Starkey and Langeland et al. believe that direct capping is contraindicated if a ***carious*** exposure has occurred, because of the high probability of pulp inflammation and infection.[23,24]

Indications. It has long been emphasized that direct pulp capping must be limited to small ***mechanical*** exposures.[1,25,26] Frigoletto noted that small exposures and a good blood supply have the best healing potential.[27] A current rule of thumb limits the diameter of the exposure to less than 1.5 mm. The pulp inadvertently exposed, without previous symptoms of pulpitis, is more apt to survive if capped. The prognosis is much less favorable if an attempt is made to cap a pulp with known inflammation and/or infection due to caries or trauma.[28]

Contraindications. Contraindications to ***direct*** pulp capping include a history of: (1) severe toothache at night, (2) spontaneous pain, (3) tooth mobility, (4) thickening of the periodontal ligament, (5) radiographic evidence of pulp or periapical degeneration, (6) excessive hemorrhage at the time of exposure, and (7) purulent or serous exudate from the exposure.

Success and Failure. Even definitions of success and failure are in dispute. Glass and Zander were among the first to use the formation of a reparative dentin bridge as the criterion for success,[21] yet it has been shown by numerous investigators that a healthy vital pulp can exist beneath a direct pulp capping, even though no dentinal bridge is present.[28–30] Kakehashi et al., in a ***germ-free*** animal study, found exposures healing with bridging, even when left uncovered[31] (Fig. 17–6).

The salient features of a successful pulp capping (with or without bridging) are: (1) pulp vitality, (2) lack of undue sensitivity or pain, (3) minimum pulp inflammatory response, (4) viable odontoblastic layer, and (5) the ability of the pulp to maintain itself without progressive degeneration. The wide open apex and high vascularity of primary and young permanent teeth invite direct pulp capping.

Agents Used in Capping. The two most commonly used pulp capping materials are zinc oxide–eugenol cement and calcium hydroxide. The latter may be used alone or in combination with a variety of additives that promote new dentin in the area of exposure and the subsequent healing of the balance of the pulp. Glass and Zander and others found that zinc oxide and eugenol, in direct contact with pulp tissue, produced chronic inflammation, a lack of calcific barrier, and an end result of necrosis.[21,32,33] Weiss and Bjorvatn, on the other hand, noted negligible necrosis of the pulp in direct contact with ZO-E and stated that any calcific bridging of an exposure site was probably a layer of dentinal chips. They also found no apparent difference in the pulp reactions of primary and permanent teeth.[30]

In spite of the reported lack of success with ZO-E cement, Sveen reported that he had 87% success with the capping of primary teeth with zinc oxide–eugenol in ideal situations of pulp exposure. He offered no histologic evidence, however.[34] Tronstad, in comparing ZO-E with CaOH, found ZO-E more beneficial for inflamed, exposed pulps and felt that the production of a calcific bridge is not necessary if the pulp is free of inflammation following treatment.[35]

Since the early 1940s, calcium hydroxide has been

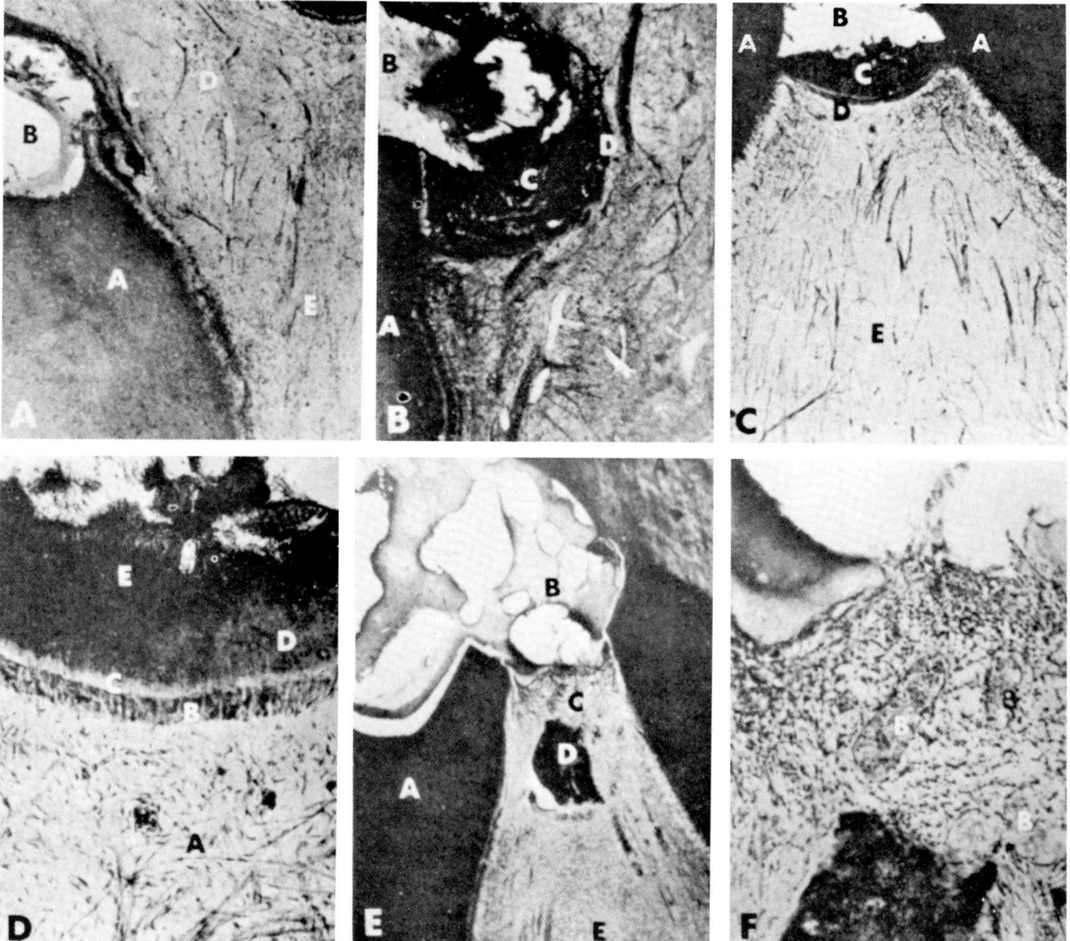

Fig. 17–5. Comparative results of capping exposed phenolized pulps with zinc oxide-eugenol or calcium hydroxide.

A, Twenty-four hours after capping with ***zinc oxide-eugenol,*** zone of necrotic tissue is seen opposite exposure site. This zone is separated from normal pulp tissue by narrow zone of inflammation. *A*, Dentin; *B*, area of pulp exposure; *C*, area of necrosis; *D*, zone of inflammation; *E*, normal pulp.

B, Twenty-four hours after capping with ***calcium hydroxide,*** zone of necrosis is similar to that in *A*, but contains precipitate of calcium proteinate. *A*, Dentin; *B*, site of exposure; *C*, area of necrosis; *D*, precipitate of calcium proteinate.

C, Ten weeks after capping with ***calcium hydroxide,*** exposure site has been walled off by bridge of new dentin. Pulp tissue below is normal and continuity of odontoblastic layer has been restored. *A*, Dentin; *B*, site of exposure; *C*, dentin bridge; *D*, new odontoblastic layer; *E*, normal pulp.

D, High magnification of dentin bridge in *C* shows calcified immature dentin adjacent to exposure site. Adjacent to immature dentin is tubular dentin containing odontoblastic processes. Predentin and odontoblasts complete structure of dentin bridge. *A*, Normal pulp tissue; *B*, odontoblastic layer; *C*, predentin; *D*, calcified dentin; *E*, calcified immature dentin.

E, Ten weeks after capping with ***zinc oxide-eugenol,*** pulp has not healed and mass of inflammatory tissue is present at site of exposure. *A*, Dentin; *B*, site of exposure; *C*, area of chronic inflammation; *D*, piece of dentin pushed into pulp tissue during exposure; *E*, normal pulp.

F, High magnification of *E* showing area of chronic inflammation. *A*, Implanted dentin fragment; *B*, new capillaries; *C*, accumulation of lymphocytes and plasma cells. (From Zander, H. A., and Glass, R. L.: Oral Surg., *2*:803, June, 1949.)

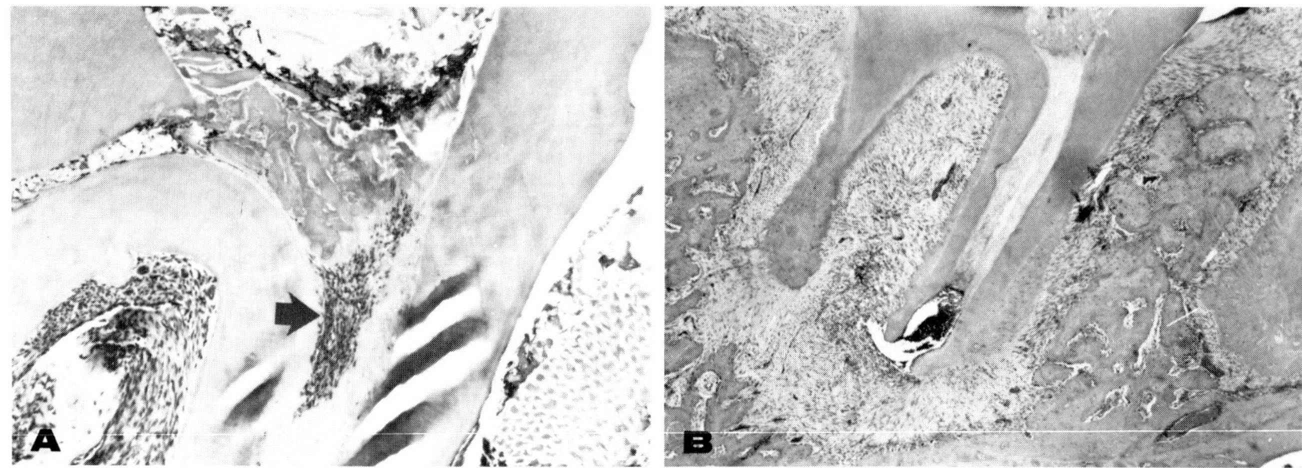

Fig. 17–6. Role of bacteria in dentin repair following pulp exposure. *A*, ***Germ-free*** specimen, obtained 14 days after surgery, with food and debris in occlusal exposure. Nuclear detail of surviving pulp tissue *(arrow)* can be observed beneath bridge consisting of dentin fragments united by new matrix. (From Kakehashi, S., Stanley, H. R., and Fitzgerald, R. J.: Oral Surg., *20*:340, Sept. 1965.) *B*, Intentional exposure of first molar in control rat (with bacteria) 28 days postoperative. Complete pulp necrosis with apical abscess. (From Clark, J. W., and Stanley, H. R.: Clinical Dentistry. Hagerstown, Md., Harper & Row, 1976.)

singled out by a myriad of authors as the medicament of choice for pulp exposures.[20–22] Jeppersen, for example, reported a long-term study on the use of a creamy mix of CaOH placed on exposed pulps of primary teeth and found 97.6% clinical success and 88.4% histologic success.[36] CaOH produces coagulation necrosis of the surface of the pulp, and directly under this, the underlying tissue differentiates into odontoblasts which then elaborate a matrix in about four weeks.

The greatest single benefit of the use of CaOH is the stimulation of a reparative dentin bridge perhaps caused by its irritating quality due to a high alkalinity of pH 11-12.[37] In this alkaline medium the enzyme phosphatase is active in releasing inorganic phosphate from the blood. Calcium phosphate then precipitates.

There is some controversy whether Ca ions are necessary for the dentinal repair of the exposure. Sciaky and Pisanti[38] and Attalla[39] stated that in their radioactive study, calcium in the capping material did not enter into the bridge formation. However, Stark et al. believed the Ca ion entered into the bridge formation in their particular pulp studies.[40] Seltzer and Bender mention the osteogenic potential of CaOH to be able to completely obliterate the pulp chamber and root canals.[41]

In some cases, the use of CaOH as a medicament has led to metaplasia of odontoblasts and a resultant internal resorption. This is not a problem with direct pulp capping when a minute pulp surface is exposed, nor is it a problem when calcium hydroxide is used in modified forms such as Dycal (Caulk), Pulpdent (Pulpdent Co.), and MPC (Kerr). With a lowered pH the action of CaOH is probably less caustic with a better chance for long-term success. The so-called necrobiotic zone is absent when these modified calcium hydroxide mixtures are used, and the dentin bridge forms directly under the commercial capping material.

Other agents suggested for direct pulp capping include a compound of calcium phosphate, neomycin, and hydrocortisone.[42] With this mixture primary tooth pulps exhibited a better ability to wall off exposed areas than did permanent tooth pulps. Dentin bridging was not a necessary prerequisite for pulp healing. Shovelton used a corticosteroid-antibiotic mixture, Ledermix, and enjoyed a high degree of success, but not significantly better than CaOH, in teeth with and without a previous history of pain.[43] Bhaskar also used cortisone with CaOH, to reduce inflammation, and concluded it would improve patient comfort and enhance the success of a CaOH pulp cap procedure.[44] A combination of the antibiotic Cleocin with the CaOH product Dycal has been reported to have a significant success rate.[45]

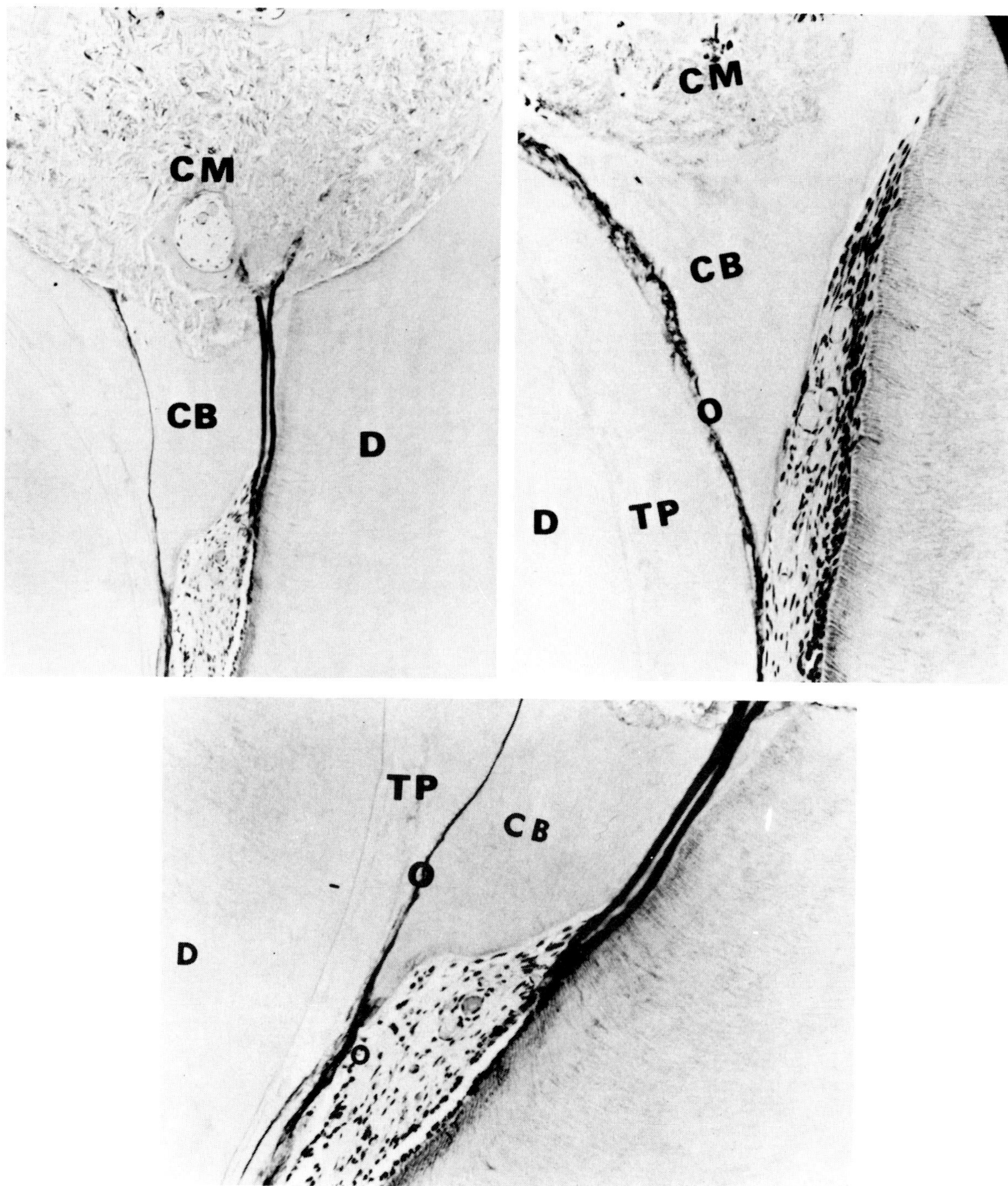

Fig. 17–7. Results of direct pulp capping with tricalcium phosphate-ceramic—24-week results. Material has been replaced by calcified matrix containing blood vessels *(upper left).* Below matrix lies forming dentin bridge mixed with blood vessels *(upper right).* Apically is wall-to-wall bridge below which lies thickened predentin and normal pulp *(bottom). CM,* calcified matrix; *CB,* calcified bridge; *D,* dentin; *O,* odontoblasts; *TP,* thickened predentin. (From Heller, A. L., Koenigs, J. F., Brilliant, J. D., Melfi, R. C., and Driskell, T. D.: J.O.E., *1*:95, Mar., 1975.)

Isobutyl cyanoacrylate has also been used as a capping agent and proved a reparative dentin bridge stimulator without causing necrosis.[46,47] It has not been used, however, in a human primary or young permanent tooth study and is not yet available on the dental market for general use.

There has also been interest in the use of formocresol mixed with ZO-E for exposed vital permanent tooth pulps. Ibrahim, Mitchell, and Healy reported, from an animal study, the absence of inflammation along with dentin bridging in 15 experimental teeth.[48] Heller et al. recently reported the use of a resorbable form of tricalcium phosphate ceramic for direct pulp capping in monkeys. Formation of a direct appositional dentinal bridge developed (Fig. 17–7). Longer term studies of human teeth were suggested.[49]

In reviewing direct pulp capping procedures for primary teeth, a rigid criteria of case selection appear to ensure a modicum of success. Direct pulp capping is less successful in primary teeth than is indirect pulp therapy or coronal amputation (pulpotomy), with healing induced with CaOH. It must be remembered, moreover, that pulp exposures are more often caused by carious excavations than by mechanical exposures. This creates a less than ideal situation in which it is difficult to apply ideal criteria.

Indirect Pulp Capping

Indirect pulp capping has been defined as a procedure wherein a small amount of carious dentin is retained in the deep areas of cavity preparation to avoid exposure of the pulp. A medicament is then sealed over the carious dentin to stimulate and encourage pulp recovery. It is understood that at a subsequent time the cavity will be re-entered, the carious material removed, and the tooth restored (Fig. 17–8).

Historical Review. Indirect pulp capping is not a new concept. Pierre Fauchard, the "father of modern dentistry," advised in the mid-18th century that all caries should not be removed in deep sensitive cavities "for fear of exposing the nerve and making the cure worse than the disease." John Tomes, in his textbook written in the mid-19th century, stated, "It is better that a layer of discolored dentin should be allowed to remain for the protection of the pulp rather than run the risk of sacrificing the tooth." Although it is true that neither of these early dental teachers referred to any specific medication of the softened dentin, they did recognize that the pulp has healing powers.

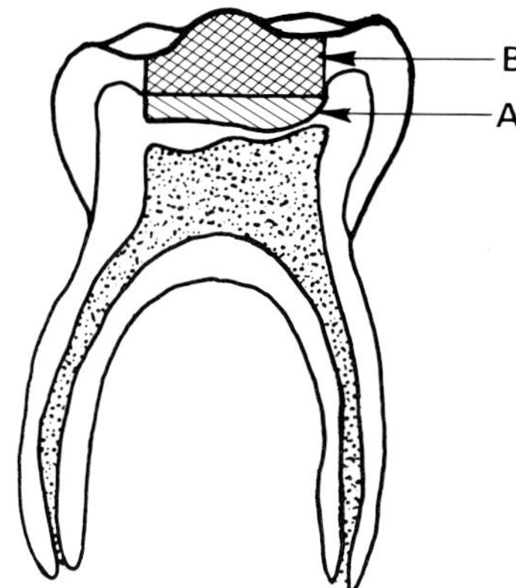

Fig. 17–8. Indirect pulp-capping technique. *A,* Medicament, either ZO-E cement or CaOH or both against remaining caries. *B,* Lasting temporary restoration. Following repair, both materials are removed along with softened caries, and final restorations placed.

One of the first to recognize the advantage of a medicament was Atkinson, who in 1866 spoke of the advantages of not exposing the pulp and reported leaving softened dentin over a vital pulp and sealing it with creosote. In 1891, Miller discussed various "antiseptics" that should be used for sterilizing dentin.[32]

This approach was reversed in the early 20th century by G. V. Black, who said, "In the interest of scientific and meticulous dental practice, in no case should any decayed or softened material be left. It is better," he stated, "to proceed by radical excavation without due regard to whether the pulp is exposed or not."[50] For years this became the standard of practice.

Since Black's time, many histologic and bacteriologic studies have shown the true nature of the carious process and the response of the dentin and pulp to infection. It is now known that the pulp is not so diseased by the initial carious attack that it cannot heal itself or withdraw from the irritation of the carious processes by laying down a calcified barrier. Indirect pulp capping is based upon the knowledge that decalcification of the dentin precedes bacterial invasion within the dentin.[51–54] Fusayama et al. demonstrated in acute caries that dentin discoloration was far in advance of the organisms, and that as much as 2 mm. of softened or discolored dentin was not infected.[55] Excavating a little deeper, Whitehead et al. compared primary and permanent teeth and demonstrated that after all softened dentin had been removed from the cavity floor, 51.5% of the permanent teeth were free from all signs of organisms and a further 34% had only one to twenty infected dentinal tubules in any one section. Primary teeth showed a much higher percentage of bacteria in the cavity floor after all soften dentin was removed.[56] Shovelton demonstrated, in a study of dentinal caries, results similar to Whitehead's: although the deepest demineralized layers of dentin are generally free from infection, the possibility of a few dentinal tubules containing organisms does exist, especially in primary teeth.[57] This also agrees with the work of Seltzer and Bender.[41] Thus, complete clinical removal of carious dentin does not necessarily ensure that all infected tubules have been removed, nor does the presence of softened dentin necessarily indicate infection.

Most investigators believe that the pulp can readily cope with minute contamination. In fact it has been shown by Reeves and Stanley,[58] as well as Shovelton,[57] that until the carious lesion was less than 1.1 mm. from the pulp (including reparative dentin when present), there was no significant disturbance within the pulp. To Massler it appeared more likely that pulp reactions under deep carious lesions are reactions to the bacterial toxins rather than to the bacteria themselves.[9] Canby and Bernier concluded that the deeper layers of carious dentin tend to impede the bacterial invasion of the pulp because of the acid nature of the affected dentin.[51]

From the results of these many studies, it is possible to identify three dentinal layers encountered in active caries: (1) necrotic, soft, brown dentin, teeming with bacteria and not painful to remove; (2) firm, but still softened, discolored dentin with fewer bacteria, but painful to remove, suggesting the presence of viable odontoblastic extensions from the pulp; and (3) hard sound dentin, a discolored area presumably with a minimal amount of bacterial invasion and painful to instrumentation.

DiMaggio and Hawes found, in histologic evaluation of teeth selected for indirect treatment, that 75% would have been pulp exposures if all the caries had initially been removed. Using clinical criteria, this same study showed a failure rate of only 1% for ***indirect*** pulp cappings compared to 25% failure for ***direct*** cappings. Histologic examination, however, raised these failure rates to 12% and 33% respectively.[2] Trowbridge and Berger stated that complete removal of softened dentin, with ensuing pulp exposure, may contribute nothing of diagnostic value in estimating the extent of existing pulp disease.[59] In fact, other studies have shown that the true picture of pulp disease cannot be assessed on the basis of such diagnostic criteria as history of pain, response to temperature change, percussion, and electric pulp testing.[60,61]

Dentin caries has been shown to be a relatively slow and intermittent process, a period of acute activity followed by a period of rest. In fact, the two stages of the carious process have been labeled as the "active lesion" and the "arrested lesion." The detailed characteristics of each period were studied by Kuwabara and Massler.[62] Diagnosis of the type of caries influences treatment planning for indirect pulp capping. In the ***active*** lesion, most of the caries-related organisms are found in the outer layers of decay, whereas the deeper decalcified layers are fairly free of bacteria. In the ***arrested*** lesions, the surface layers are not always contaminated, especially where the surface is hard and leathery. The deepest layers are quite sclerotic and free of microorganisms.

This work supports the theory that a highly mineralized sclerotic zone can block the bacterial irritants from reaching the pulp. Others have shown that deep carious dentin is even more resistant to decomposition by acids and proteolysis than is normal dentin. This was especially true in arrested caries.[63,64] Pulp reactions under arrested lesions are mild, and the pulp is capable of producing reparative dentin. Indirect pulp capping technique might not be indicated in this situation, as complete caries removal could be accomplished without fear of pulp exposure.

Two-Appointment Procedure

The number of clinical, radiographic, and histologic studies is impressive, reporting a significant reduction in the incidence of pulp exposures by using a two-appointment indirect pulp capping procedure. Only those teeth diagnosed free of irreversible symptoms should be considered for this type of treatment. Case selection is the most important factor in the success of this type of pulp therapy.

Indications. The decision to undertake the indirect pulp capping procedure is based on the following findings.

1. History
   a. Tolerable dull, mild pain associated with eating
   b. Negative history of spontaneous extreme pain
2. Clinical Examination
   a. Large carious lesion

   b. Normal mobility
   c. Normal appearance of adjacent gingiva
   d. Normal color of tooth
3. Radiographic Examination
   a. Large carious lesion with a possibility of a carious pulp exposure
   b. Normal lamina dura
   c. Normal periodontal ligament space
   d. No radiolucency in the bone about the apices of the roots or in the furcation.

Contraindications. Findings that contraindicate this procedure are listed below.

1. History
   a. Sharp, penetrating pulpalgia indicating acute pulp inflammation and/or necrosis
   b. Prolonged night pain
2. Clinical Examination
   a. Mobility of the tooth
   b. Parulis in the gingiva approximating the roots of the tooth
   c. Discoloration of the tooth
   d. Negative results to electric pulp testing
3. Radiographic Examination
   a. Large carious lesion producing definite pulp exposure
   b. Interrupted or broken lamina dura
   c. Widened periodontal ligament space
   d. Radiolucency about the apices of the roots or in the furcation

Justifications for Therapy. Indirect pulp capping therapy can be justified by the following desirable results: (1) sterilization of residual carious dentin is more readily accomplished; (2) it eliminates the need for more difficult pulp therapy by arresting the carious process and allowing the pulp reparative process to occur; (3) patient comfort is immediate; (4) rampant dental decay is halted when ***all*** carious teeth are treated; and (5) extensive endodontic and subsequent restorative procedures may not be required.

Evaluation of Therapy (Table 17–1). King and associates,[65] as well as Aponte,[66] and Parikh,[53] determined that the residual layer of carious dentin, left in the indirect technique, can be sterilized with either ZO-E cement or CaOH. On the other hand, it cannot be presumed that all the reduced infected or affected dentin becomes remineralized. It is known, however, that ***vital*** dentin will become hyper-calcified from contact with calcium hydroxide. When the cavity is re-entered after a period of time following indirect pulp capping, residual carious dentin is observed to be dry, somewhat harder, and a powdery brownish yellow. If this layer is carefully removed, under it will be found a sound layer of dentin covering the pulp itself. Sclerosis of the primary dentin, rather than a remineralization of carious dentin, has probably developed.

Histologic evaluation of pulp reactions to this technique has been reported in a varying number of samples. Law and Lewis report secondary dentin formation, an active odontoblastic layer, an intact zone of Weil, and a slightly hyperactive pulp with the presence of some inflammatory cells.[69] Held-Wydler demonstrated reparative dentin in 40 of 41 young molars in which the carious dentin was covered with ZO-E cement. The pulp tissue was either completely normal or mildly inflamed over a period of 34 to 630 days. In the histologic sections, four layers could be demonstrated (Fig. 17–9): (1) carious decalcified dentin, (2) rhythmic layers of irregular reparative dentin, (3) regular tubular dentin, and (4) normal pulp with a slight increase in fibrous elements.[70]

Sayegh, in an extensive study of the many facets of the indirect technique, found that three distinct types of new dentin had been formed: (1) cellular fibrillar dentin formed within the first two months of the

Table 17-1. Studies on Indirect Pulp Capping—Primary and Young Permanent Teeth

Author	*Agent*	*Cases*	*Observation Period*	*% Success*
Sowden, 1956	CaOH	4000	Up to 7 yr.	"very high"
Law and Lewis, 1961	CaOH	38	Up to 2 yr.	73.6
Hawes and DiMaggio, 1964	CaOH	475	Up to 4 yr.	97
Kerkhove et al., 1964	CaOH	41	12 mo.	95
	ZO-E	35	12 mo.	95
Held-Wydler, 1964	CaOH	41	35–630 days	88
King et al., 1965	CaOH	21	25–206 days	62
	ZO-E	22		88
Aponte, 1966	CaOH	30	6–46 mo.	93
Jordan and Suzuki, 1971	CaOH	243	10–12 weeks	98
Nordstrom et al., 1974	CaOH	64	94 days	84
	SnFl			90

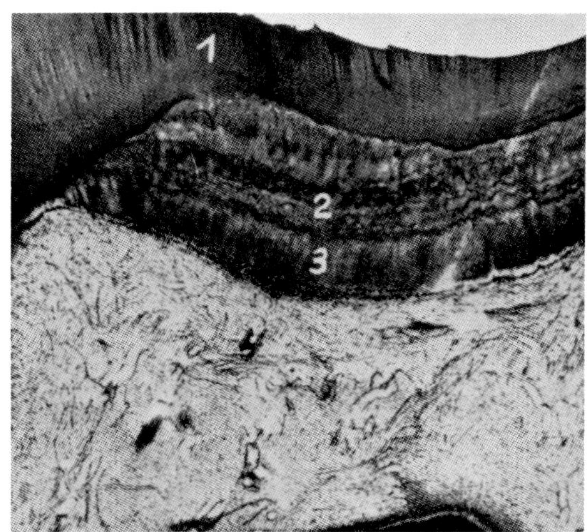

Fig. 17–9. Photomicrograph of four layers of healing under indirect pulp capping of permanent molar of 14½-year-old child. Zinc oxide-eugenol cement capping after excavation of necrotic dentin layer only. No pain 480 days later when extracted. *1,* Carious decalcified dentin. *2,* Rhythmic layers of irregular reparative dentin. *3,* Regular tubular dentin. *4,* Normal pulp with slight increase in fibrous elements. (From Held-Wydler, E.: J. Dent. Child., *31*:107, 1st Quar., 1964.)

treatment period, (2) globular dentin observed during the first three months, and (3) a more uniformly mineralized dentin, labeled tubular dentin.

In this study of 30 primary and permanent teeth, Sayegh concluded that new dentin forms fastest in teeth with the thinnest dentin remaining after cavity preparation. He also found that the longer the pulp is exposed to treatment the more new dentin is formed and that primary teeth showed considerably more dentin formation than did permanent teeth. Interestingly, males were better able than females to form new dentin.[15]

Clinical studies have shown no particular differences in the ultimate success of this technique regardless of whether CaOH or ZO-E cement is used over residual carious dentin.[67,71,72] Nordstrom et al. reported that remineralized dentin, which was wiped with a 10% solution of stannous fluoride for 5 minutes and then covered with ZO-E, was harder when compared to dentin covered with CaOH used alone. The authors further stated that no significant difference was found in failure rates of teeth treated with CaOH and those treated with stannous fluoride.[73] As so many others have also concluded, results for primary and young permanent teeth do not differ significantly.

Choice of a medicament is better based on the clinical history of any particular carious tooth. Some investigators recommend ZO-E because its obtundant properties make the pulp more comfortable. Others recommend CaOH agents because of their ability to stimulate a more rapid formation of reparative dentin. Stanley believes it makes no difference which is used since both encourage reparative dentin formation, but just in case an undetected microscopic opening into the pulp has been created during caries excavation, CaOH will better stimulate a dentinal bridge.[72] For the comfort of the patient, if the tooth has been hypersensitive, a brief application of a steroid could be placed before the ZO-E or CaOH. This might reduce the acute inflammatory process.[74]

It has been established that a minimal eight to twelve weeks should transpire to produce adequate remineralization of the cavity floor.[15, 75–77] An important consideration for success, therefore, is a good, long-lasting seal of the temporary restoration to prevent salivary and bacterial leakage[78] (Fig. 17–10).

There may be a question of the need for reentering the cavity to remove the residual carious dentin. If, at the initial visit, a proper cavity preparation was developed and all the caries was removed except the portion that would expose the pulp, re-entry might be an unnecessary step.[24] On the other hand, if the clinician had to leave considerably more caries owing to patient discomfort or management, it would be best to re-enter and check for a remineralized dentinal layer, the lack of a pulp exposure, and a sound dentinal base for a strong restoration. Should a pulp exposure occur during this second procedure, the tissue should react more favorably to a CaOH capping than it would have during the initial treatment of the carious lesion.

Pulpotomy

The pulpotomy technique has become the most accepted procedure for treating primary and young permanent teeth with carious or traumatic pulp exposures. A pulpotomy is defined as the surgical removal (amputation) of the entire coronal pulp, leaving intact the vital tissue in the canals. A suitable medicament or dressing is then placed over the remaining tissue in an attempt to promote healing and retention of this vital tissue. Dentin bridging may cover the amputated pulp (Fig. 17–11).

The major purpose of the pulpotomy technique is to remove the inflamed and infected pulp tissue at the

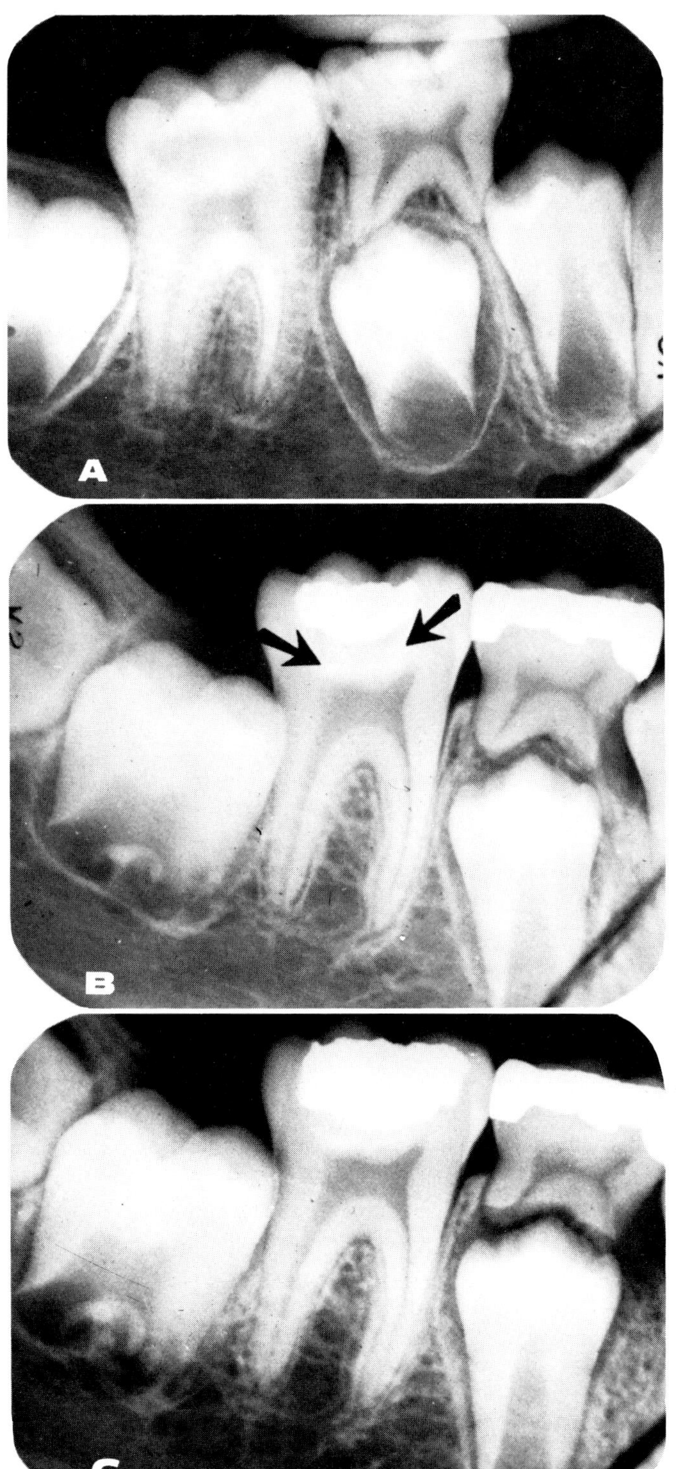

Fig. 17–10. Indirect pulp capping. *A,* First permanent molar with class I deep carious lesion. Gross caries removed without exposure. Calcium hydroxide placed over remaining caries. Tooth restored with amalgam for healing period. *B,* At three months, sclerotic dentin is seen beneath remaining caries and layer of CaOH *(arrows)*. *C,* Tooth is re-entered and remaining caries removed. Sound dentin barrier observed at base of cavity. Following complete caries removal, permanent amalgam restoration is placed. (From McDonald, R. E.: Dentistry for the Child and Adolescent. 2nd ed., St. Louis, C. V. Mosby Co., 1974, p. 149.)

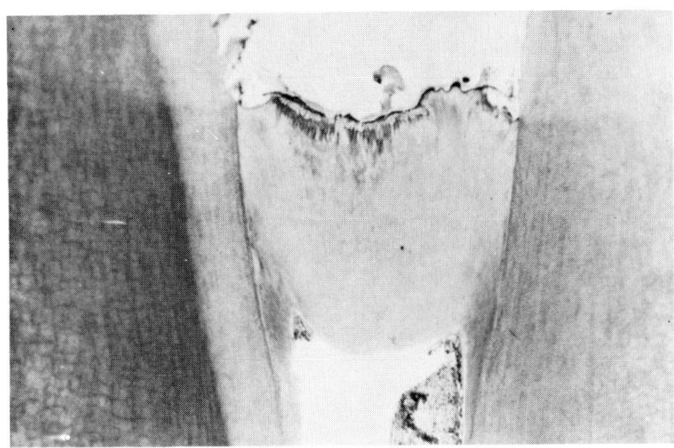

Fig. 17–11. Dentin bridge sealing canal following pulpotomy.

site of exposure, allowing the vital pulp in the root canals to heal. Whether this tissue remains vital may depend on the medicament used and the length of time it remains in contact.

Indications. Dannenberg stated that pulpotomies are performed on pulpally exposed ***primary*** teeth when their retention is more advantageous than extraction and replacement with a space maintainer.[25] The tooth, of course, should be restorable and expected to function for a reasonable period of time. At least two-thirds of root length must remain to ensure a reasonable functional life. Stainless steel crowns should be used for restoration. Pulpotomy is routinely recommended for young permanent teeth with vital exposed pulps and incompletely formed apices.

Contraindications. Pulpotomies in primary teeth are generally contraindicated if the permanent successor tooth has reached the stage of alveolar emergence (that is, no bone overlying the occlusal of the crown) or if the roots of the primary tooth are more than half resorbed regardless of the development of the permanent successor. Pulpotomies are also ***not*** indicated in teeth with significant mobility, periapical or furcal involvement, persistent toothaches, coronal pus, or no pulp hemorrhage.

Therapeutic Approaches. Currently there are two therapeutic approaches to pulpotomy. One technique uses calcium hydroxide over the amputated pulp, and the other uses formocresol. Dannenberg stated that the CaOH pulpotomy is predicated on the healing of pulp stumps under a dentin bridge, whereas the formocresol pulpotomy is predicated on sterilization of the remaining pulp and "fixation" of the subjacent tissue. Dannenberg further asserts that the so-called mummified pulp is inert, fixed, and incapable of bacterial or autolytic breakdown.[25] The extent of pulp mummification, however, depends upon the concentration of the medicament and the length of time it is in contact with the pulp.

Formocresol Pulpotomy

Formalin-containing compounds have been used in pulp therapy since the early days of the 20th century. The present-day use of formocresol for pulpotomies in primary (and permanent) teeth evolved from the use of these formalin compounds. Formocresol was introduced in 1904 by Buckley who contended that equal parts of formalin and tricresol would react chemically with the intermediate and end-products of pulp inflammation to form a "new, colorless and non-infective compound of a harmless nature."[79] This formula of Buckley, still the most frequently used, consists of tricresol, aqueous formaldehyde, glycerin, and water.

The formocresol pulpotomy technique used today is a modification of the original method reported by Sweet in 1930.[80–82] By 1953, Sweet claimed 97% clinical success in 16,651 cases.[83] It is to be noted, however, that in this report about one-half of the primary teeth exfoliated early.

Although this technique was popular on the west coast, it did not receive wide acceptance because it was regarded as a nonvital or mummification method. Histologic studies were also lacking early in its inception. Furthermore it was overshadowed by the so-called vital pulpotomy for primary teeth with calcium hydroxide used as a pulp capping material, studies that were supported with clinical and histologic evidence. As a result, interest waned in formocresol as a pulpotomy medicament. Interest in formocresol was renewed, however, with the increase of clinical failures reported with CaOH, even in the presence of dentinal bridging. At the same time an improved rate of clinical success was reported with formocresol. Subsequent clinical and histologic studies even raised doubt in labeling the formocresol method as "nonvital."

Although histologic studies showed that formalin, creosol, and paraformaldehyde are irritants to healthy connective tissue, it was recognized early on that formocresol is an efficient bactericide. It was also found to have the ability to prevent autolysis of tissue by the complex chemical binding of formaldehyde with protein. This binding reaction may be reversible as the protein molecule does not change in its basic overall structure.[84]

By 1959, Massler and Mansukhani had conducted a detailed histologic investigation of the effect of formocresol on the pulps of 43 human primary and permanent teeth in treatment intervals of one to 36 minutes and from one to three years. Fixation of the tissue directly under the medicament was apparent. Shortly after the application (7 to 14 days), the pulps developed three distinctive zones: (1) a broad eosinophilic zone of fixation, (2) a broad pale-staining zone with poor cellular definition, and (3) a zone of inflammation diffusing apically into normal pulp tissue. After sixty days, in a limited number of observed samples, the remaining tissue was believed to be completely fixed, remaining as a strand of eosinophilic fibrous tissue.[85]

In the same year, Emmerson, Myamoto, Sweet, and Bhatia also described the action of formocresol on human pulp tissue. They reported that the effect on the pulp varied with the length of time formocresol was in contact with the tissue. A five-minute application resulted in surface fixation of normal tissue, whereas an application sealed in for three days produced calcific degeneration. They concluded that formocresol pulpotomy in primary pulp therapy may be classified as either vital or nonvital, depending on the duration of the formocresol application.[83]

Spedding, in a study of 20 primary teeth in Rhesus monkeys, compared results of a one-appointment formocresol pulpotomy technique with those of the one-appointment technique with CaOH. After a period of 17 to 286 days, in most instances, the formocresol teeth exhibited normal vital tissue in the apical third of the canal. In some specimens, leucocytic infiltration and osteodentin developed in the apical areas.[86] Law and Lewis evaluated the clinical effectiveness of the formocresol technique over a four-year period, and reported a 93 to 98% success rate. Their failure rate was greatest between the first and second years.[87]

Berger compared the effects of pulpotomy and one-appointment formocresol medication with those of zinc oxide–eugenol paste on the amputated pulps of cariously exposed human primary molars. Periods of evaluation ranged from three weeks to 38 weeks postoperatively. Clinically and radiographically, the formocresol-treated teeth were judged 97% successful, whereas the zinc oxide–eugenol group was evaluated as 58% successful. Histologically, 82% of the formocresol group was judged successful compared to ***total failure*** with zinc oxide–eugenol.[88]

The intriguing part of this study was the revelation that formocresol coagulation necrosis of the pulp occurred at three weeks with total absence of cellular detail in the apical third, but by seven weeks connective tissue of a granular type had ingrown through the apical foramen. In specimens obtained after longer postoperative periods, granulation tissue progressively replaced the necrotic pulp tissue up to the coronal area. Small areas of resorption of the dentinal walls were also being replaced by osteodentin. Actually this observation was mentioned in an earlier work of Nygaard-Ostby, who found an apical ingrowth of granulation tissue being transformed into fibrous connective tissue.[89] Spamer also conducted a histologic study of caries-free human primary canines following a one-appointment formocresol pulpotomy, in which the final pulp covering was zinc oxide–eugenol. Again, the three typical zones were distinguishable including the apical one-third tissue which was normal and free of inflammatory reaction. Initially, Spamer observed an acute inflammatory reaction, succeeded by a chronic inflammation response, proliferation of odontoblasts, and an increase in collagen fibers. By six months, deposition of mature dentin and vital tissue was seen throughout.[90]

Beaver, Kopel, and Sabes investigated the differences in pulp reactions between a five-minute application of formocresol using sub-bases of either zinc oxide–eugenol cement alone or with the addition of formocresol. There was no appreciable difference in a histologic reaction of the remaining radicular pulp tissue under either of these two types of sub-bases.[91] Recently, Ranley has shown *in vitro* that formocresol can leach out from a ZO-E sub-base. He has suggested that the initial application on the pulp of a formocresol saturated cotton pellet might be an unnecessary step.[92] Venham has shown favorable histologic results based on this hypothesis and has suggested that the formocresol might be reduced to one-quarter strength.[93]

Redig has shown clinically and radiographically no significant difference in the ultimate success (85 to 90%) between formocresol application for five minutes, or application for three to five days.[94] The combined investigations of Straffon, Han, Loos, and Morawa on the clinical, histologic, and biochemical effects of formocresol has led the way for new thinking in this type of pulp therapy. Straffon and Han concluded from a study of connective tissue in hamster pulps exposed to formocresol that the medicament does not interfere with a prolonged recovery of connective tissue and may even suppress the initial inflammatory reaction.[95] In a following report, they concluded that formocresol at 1:5 strength might be equally effective and possibly a less damaging pulpotomy agent.[96] Loos concurred with the previous work in a further study of diluted formocresol.[97] Morawa et al., in a five-year clinical study of 70 cases, concluded that formocresol pulpotomy, using 1:5 concentration, is as effective as full concentration and yet has the advantage of reduced postoperative complications in the periradicular region. In only five teeth was there limited radicular internal resorption.[98]

Rolling and Thylstrup reported a clinical three-year follow-up study of pulpotomized primary molars using formocresol. Their results showed a progressively decreasing survival rate of 99% at 3 months, 83% at 12 months, 78% at 24 months, and 78% at 36 months after treatment. While failures consisted of periapical or interradicular bone lesions, no internal root resorption was observed. These investigators concluded that although their rate of success was less than previous studies had shown, the formocresol method must be considered an acceptable clinical procedure compared with other methods.[99]

The majority of pedodontic departments in North American dental schools advocate the formocresol pulpotomy as the treatment of choice for primary teeth.[100] At present, both the one-appointment and the two-appointment procedures are being used. Miyamoto suggests the two-appointment technique for uncooperative children to minimize chair time, especially on the initial operative visit.[26] The two-appointment method is also advised if hemostasis becomes a problem following coronal pulp amputation. He has also noted that in the event of failure, one of the great clinical advantages of the formocresol pulpotomy is the development of a chronic abscess rather than an acute infection requiring prompt emergency treatment. The chronic abscess may be seen clinically as internal resorption and/or a draining mucosal fistula.

Clinical experience has shown that following the pulpotomy procedure in primary molars, the restoration of choice is a well-fitted stainless steel crown. This type of restoration is required to protect the tooth from cusp fracture and to eliminate recurrent decay or filling fracture in a susceptible and changing dentition.

Formocresol Pulpotomy in Primary Teeth

Clinical and radiographic examinations are necessary to diagnose the need for pulpotomy in primary teeth. It is judicious to take bite-wing and periapical

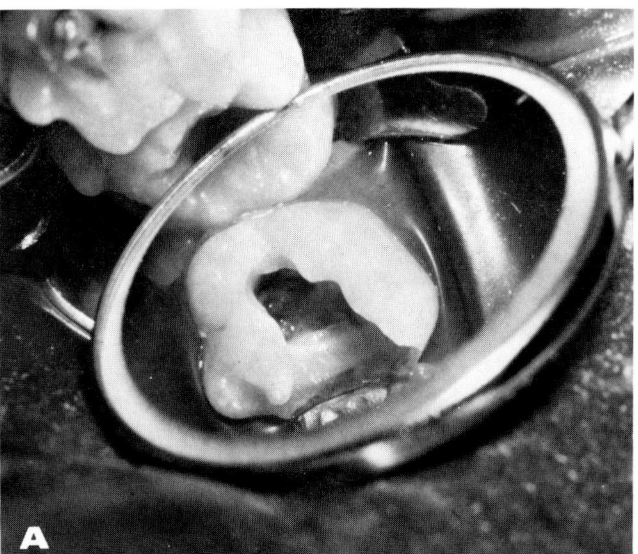

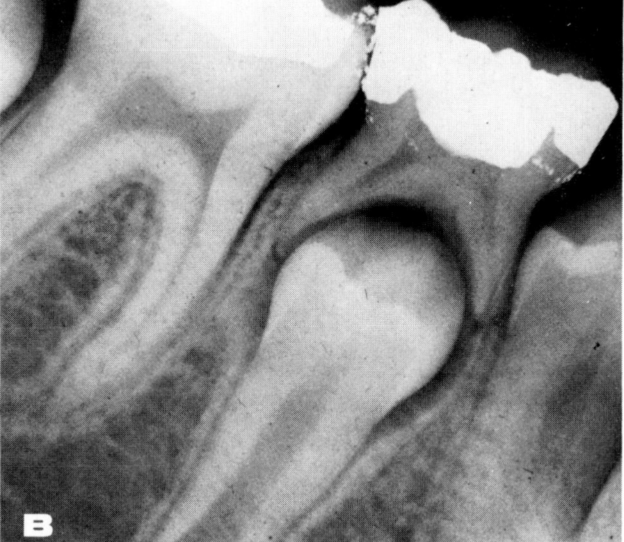

Fig. 17–12. One appointment formocresol pulpotomy. *A*, Roof of pulp chamber and coronal pulp removed. Cotton pellet with formocresol in place for 5 minutes. (Courtesy Dr. Constance B. Greeley.) *B*, Successful formocresol pulpotomy one year following treatment. (Courtesy Dr. Mark Wagner.)

radiographs so that the depth of caries may be observed and the condition of the periapical tissues determined. Correct diagnosis is essential.[101]

For successful formocresol pulpotomy in primary teeth, one must be aware of the indications and contraindications as well as reasons for employing one or two appointment treatment (Fig. 17–12).

One-Appointment Pulpotomy. ***Indications.*** This method of treatment should be carried out only on those restorable teeth in which it has been determined that inflammation is confined to the coronal portion of the pulp. When the coronal pulp is amputated, only vital, healthy pulp tissue remains in the root canals (Fig. 17–13).

Contraindications. Pulps with a history of spontaneous pain usually hemorrhage. If profuse hemorrhage occurs upon entering the pulp chamber, the one-step pulpotomy is contraindicated. Other contraindications are early or abnormal root resorption with roots two-thirds resorbed or internal root resorption, interradicular bone loss, presence of a fistula or presence of pus in the chamber (Fig. 17–14).

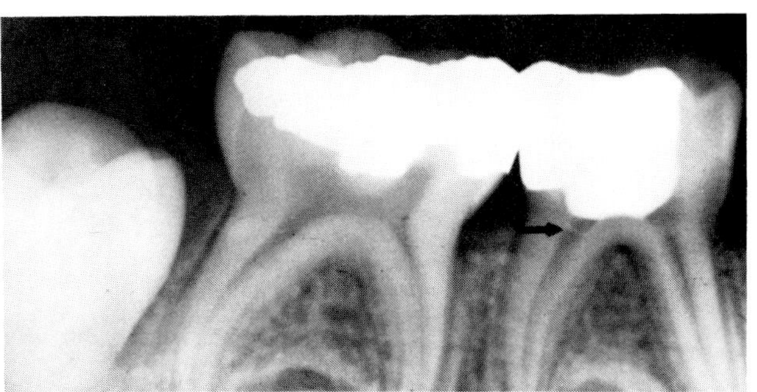

Fig. 17–13. Successful formocresol pulpotomy in first primary molar related to case selection of vital healthy pulp in canals. Dentin bridge *(arrow)* is unusual in FC pulpotomy. (From Law, D. B., Lewis, T. M., and Davis, J. M.: An Atlas of Pedodontics. Philadelphia, W. B. Saunders Co., 1969, p. 199.)

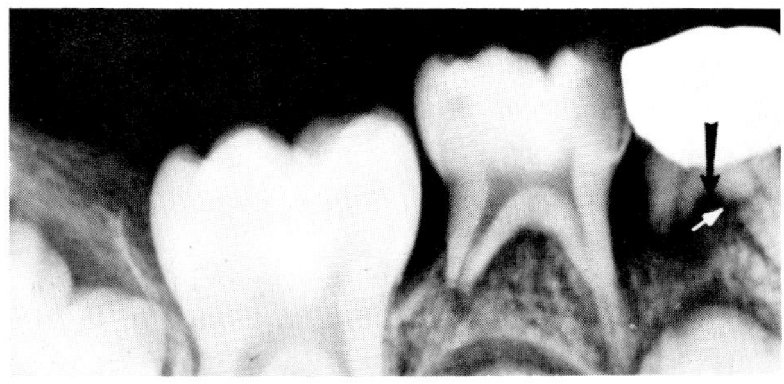

Fig. 17–14. Final failure of formocresol pulpotomy, mandibular first primary molar. Root resorption and interradicular bone loss *(arrows)* prior to treatment forecast eventual failure. Tooth was extracted. (From Law, D. B., Lewis, T. M., and Davis, J. M.: An Atlas of Pedodontics. Philadelphia, W. B. Saunders Co., 1969, p. 199.)

Procedure

1. Anesthetize the tooth and tissue.
2. Isolate the tooth to be treated with a rubber dam.
3. Remove the caries without entering the pulp chamber.
4. Remove the dentinal roof with a high-speed No. 556 or No. 700 bur (Fig. 17–15*A*).
5. Remove the coronal pulp with a sharp spoon excavator or a No. 6 or No. 8 round bur (Fig. 17–15*B*).
6. Achieve hemostasis.
7. Apply formocresol* to the pulp on a cotton pellet for 5 minutes (Fig. 17–15*C*).
8. Place a ZO-E cement base (Fig. 17–15*D*).
9. Restore the tooth with a stainless steel crown (Fig. 17–15*D*).

Two-Appointment Pulpotomy. ***Indications.*** Two appointments are indicated if there is evidence of sluggish bleeding at the amputation site or profuse difficult-to-control bleeding, if there is pus in the chamber but ***none*** at the amputation site, or if there are early bone changes in the interradicular area, thickening of the periodontal ligament, or history of pain without other contraindications.

Contraindications. For a nonrestorable tooth or one soon to be shed, or a tooth with a necrotic pulp, a pulpotomy is contraindicated.

Procedure

1. The steps are the same as for the one-appointment procedure through step 6.
2. A cotton pellet moistened with formocresol is sealed into the chamber for five to seven days. A good temporary filling is placed.
3. At the second visit the temporary filling and cotton pellet are removed.
4. A ZO-E cement base is placed.
5. The tooth is restored with a stainless steel crown.

As previously stated, the two-step pulpotomy is used when shorter appointments are necessary, as with patient management problem.

*The formocresol used in this technique may be obtained under the trade name: Buckley's Formocresol (Crosby Laboratories). Composition: 35% cresol, 19% formalin in a vehicle of glycerine and water at the pH of approximately 5.1.

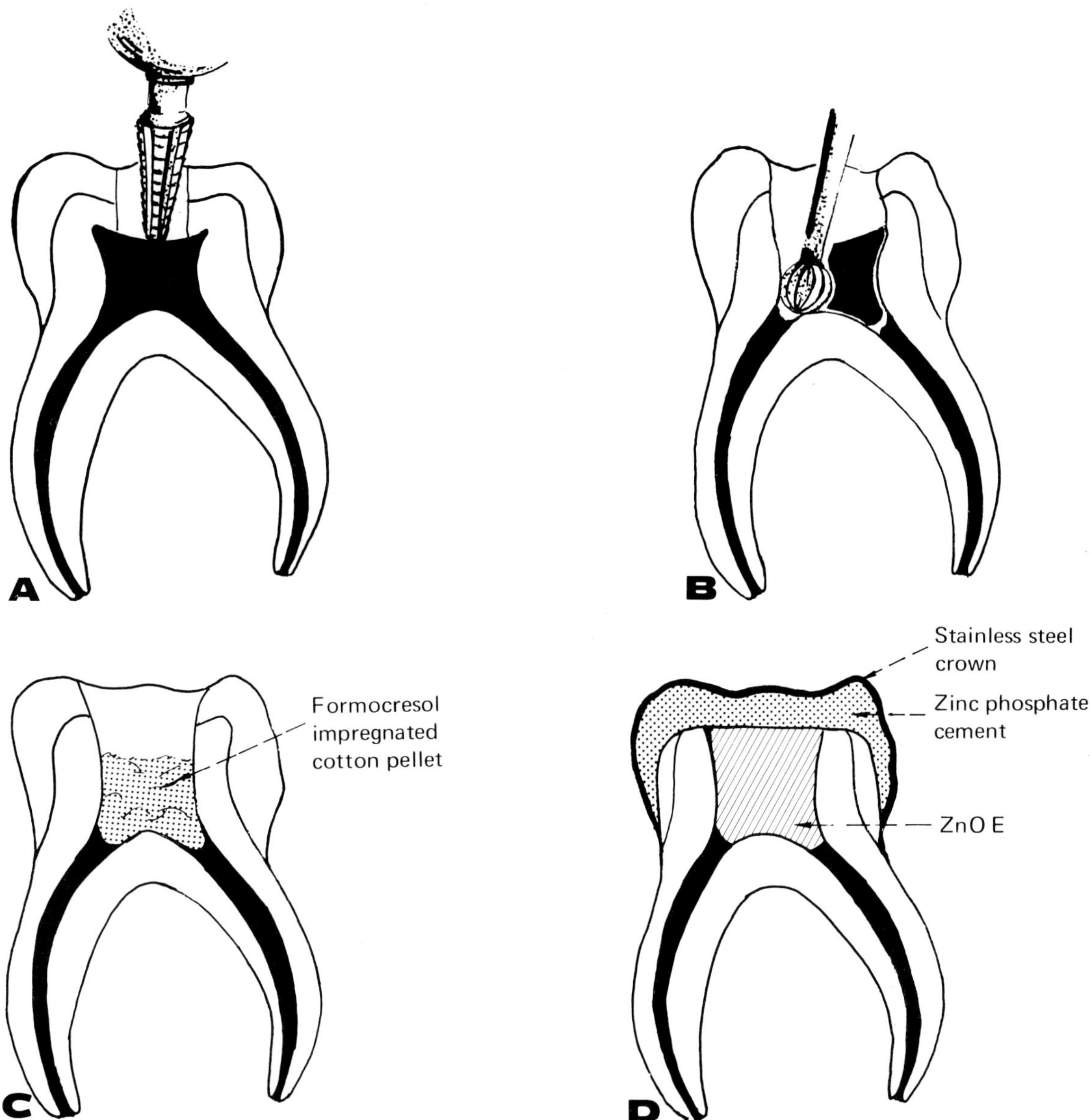

Fig. 17–15. Step-by-step technique in one-appointment formocresol pulpotomy. *A*, Exposure of pulp by roof removal. *B*, Coronal pulp amputation with round bur. Hemostasis with dry cotton or epinephrine. *C*, Application of formocresol for 5 minutes. Excess medicament is expressed from cotton before placement. *D*, Following formocresol removal, ZO-E base and stainless steel crown are placed.

Calcium Hydroxide Pulpotomy (See also pp. 704–707).

Calcium hydroxide (CaOH) pulpotomy was most favored in the 1940s and mid 1950s because it was felt to be a more biologically acceptable material, maintaining pulp vitality and promoting a bridge of reparative dentin. This rationale was introduced by Teuscher and Zander in 1938 and termed a "vital" technique. Their histologic studies showed that the pulp tissue nearest the calcium hydroxide was first necrotized by the high pH (11–12) of the calcium hydroxide; this necrosis was accompanied by acute inflammatory changes in the underlying tissue. After four weeks, a new odontoblastic layer and, eventually, a bridge of dentin developed[102] (Fig. 17–16). Later investigations showed three identifiable histologic zones under the calcium hydroxide in four to nine days: (1) coagulation necrosis; (2) deep-staining basophilic areas with varied osteodentin; and (3) relatively normal pulp tissue, slightly hyperemic, underlying an odontoblastic layer.

It should be pointed out that the presence of a dentinal bridge is not necessarily the sole criterion of success. The bridge may be incomplete and appears histologically as doughnut-shaped, dome-shaped, funnel-shaped, or filled with tissue inclusions.[26,103,104] It is also possible for the remaining pulp to be walled off by fibrous tissue with no dentin bridge evident radiographically.

Initial reports by Brown, Berk, and Shoemaker indicated a success rate with calcium hydroxide for primary and young permanent teeth in the wide range of 30% to 90%.[20,105,106] Via, in a two-year study of calcium hydroxide pulpotomies in primary teeth, had only a 31% success.[107] Law later reported only a 49% success in a one-year study.[108] In all investigations, failures were the result of chronic pulp inflammation and internal resorption. More recently, Magnusson and Schroder and Granath experienced these same high failure rates in pulpotomized primary molars. Internal resorption may be due to overstimulation of the primary pulp by the highly alkaline CaOH, causing metaplasia in the pulp tissue leading to the formation of odontoclasts[109,110] (Fig. 17–17).

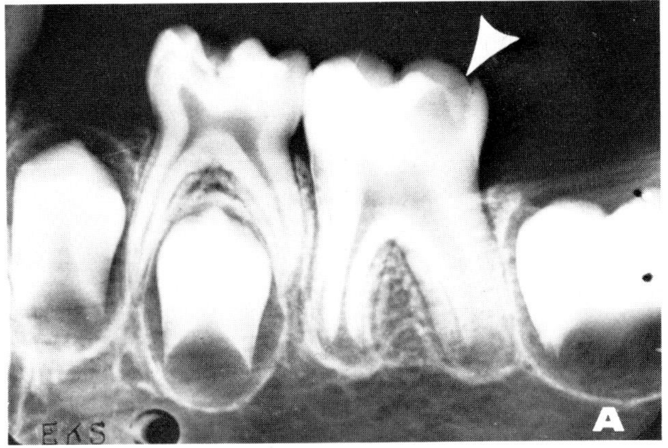

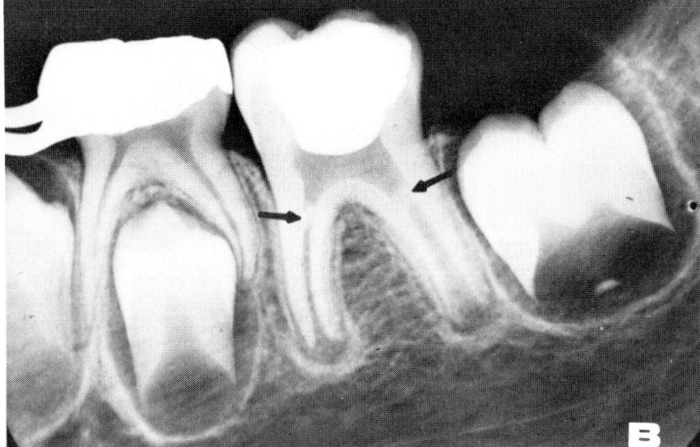

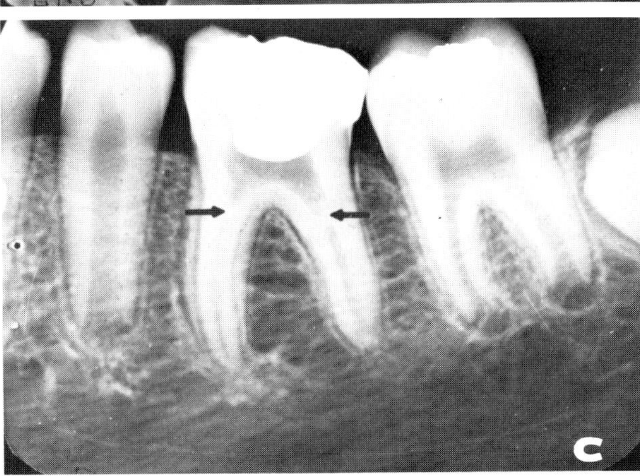

Fig. 17–16. Calcium hydroxide pulpotomy, young permanent molar. *A,* Pulp of first permanent molar exposed by caries *(white arrow)*. *B,* Calcified dentin bridges *(arrows)* over vital pulp in canals. Note open apices. *C,* Pulp recession *(arrows)* and continued root development indicative of continuing pulp vitality. (From McDonald, R. E.: Dentistry for the Child and Adolescent. 2nd ed. St. Louis, C. V. Mosby, 1974, p. 155.)

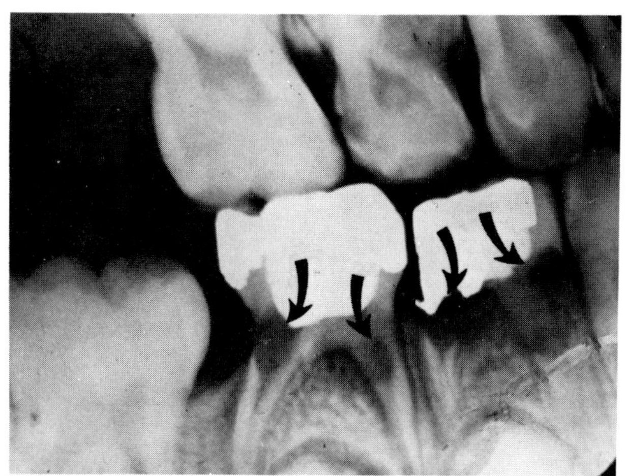

Fig. 17–17. Massive internal resorption *(arrows)* of primary mandibular molars after calcium hydroxide pulpotomy.

In spite of these earlier discouraging reports, Phaneuf, Frankl, and Ruben demonstrated significant success in calcium hydroxide pulpotomies in primary teeth using various commercial preparations of calcium hydroxide, i.e., Pulpdent, Dycal, and Hydrex. The difference in pulp response to these commercial preparations might be attributed to a lower pH. Calcium hydroxide incorporated in a methyl cellulose base, such as Pulpdent, showed earlier and more consistent bridging than did other types of calcium hydroxide preparations.[111]

Indications and Contraindications. At present, the calcium hydroxide pulpotomy technique cannot be generally recommended for ***primary*** teeth owing to its low success rate.[107–109,112] Because of the difference in cellular anatomy in ***permanent*** teeth, however, CaOH is recommended for the mechanical, carious, and traumatic exposures in ***young permanent*** teeth, particularly with incomplete apical closure (Fig. 17–18). Following the closure of the apex, it is further recommended by some that complete pulpectomy be done in order to forestall total root canal calcification.[113–115]

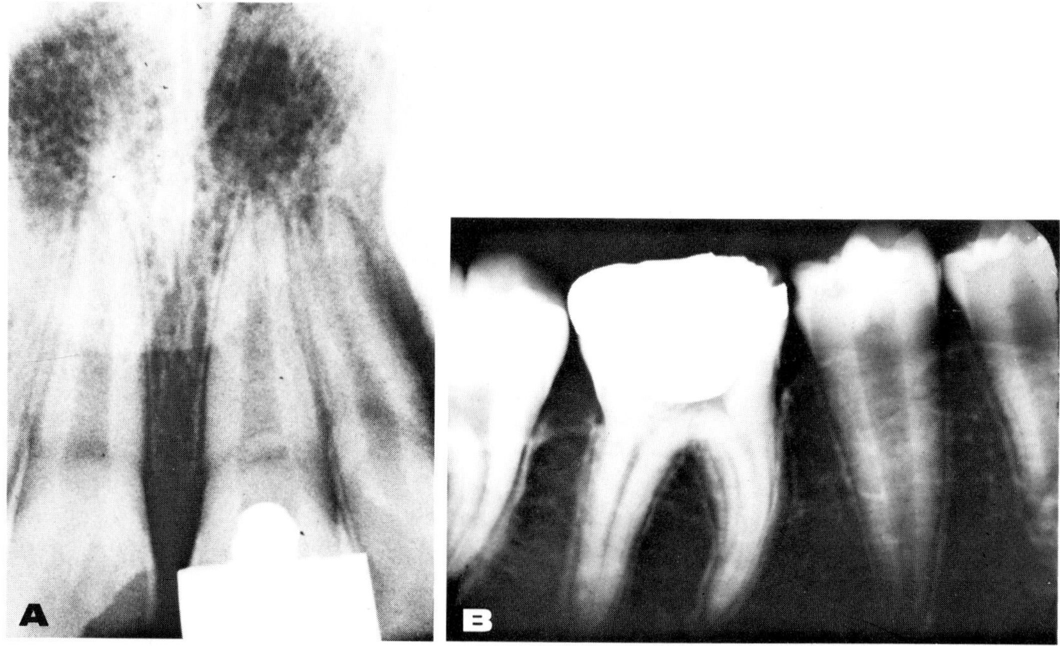

Fig. 17–18. Calcium hydroxide pulpotomies in young permanent teeth. *A,* Crown fracture exposure of central incisor. Apex was open at time of CaOH pulpotomy. Note root growth, apical closure, and dentin bridge. *B,* Partial root canal calcification following pulpotomy in young first permanent molar.

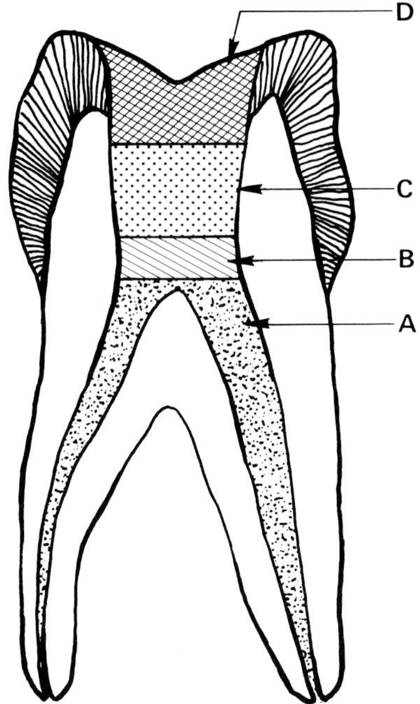

Fig. 17–19. Calcium hydroxide pulpotomy in young permanent molar. Cavity is prepared, caries and chamber roof removed, and pulp amputated to canal orifices. Following hemostasis, commercial CaOH is placed and protected with ZO-E and amalgam filling or stainless crown. *A*, Vital pulp. *B*, Calcium hydroxide. *C*, Zinc oxide-eugenol quick-set cement. *D*, Amalgam.

Procedure (Fig. 17–19)

1. A rubber dam is applied to a previously anesthetized tooth or quadrant.
2. All caries are removed without a pulp exposure if possible, and a cavity outline established.
3. The cavity is washed out with water and lightly dried with cotton pellets.
4. The roof of the pulp chamber is removed by high-speed fissure bur moving from pulp horn to pulp horn. The roof is then lifted off.
5. The coronal pulp can be amputated by a low-speed round bur running in reverse, a sharp spoon excavator or a high speed bur carefully utilized.[116]
6. Hemorrhage is stopped by wiping with a damp pellet of hydrogen peroxide and drying with cotton.
7. One of the commercial calcium hydroxide mixtures is lightly tapped into place over the root canal orifices and dried with a cotton pellet.
8. Quick setting zinc oxide–eugenol cement is then placed over the calcium hydroxide to fill up the chamber.
9. In the event the crown is severely weakened by decay, a stainless steel crown rather than an amalgam filling may be fitted and cemented in order to prevent cusp fractures.

Formocresol Pulpotomy for Young Permanent Teeth

The improved clinical and histologic success of the formocresol pulpotomy in primary teeth has aroused great interest in its use for cariously exposed young permanent teeth. Treatment of severely decayed and pulpally involved ***permanent*** teeth in the child or adolescent creates a dilemma. The ideal treatment is complete endodontic therapy and a cast full-crown restoration. However, this is time-consuming and costly in the growing dentition. Full treatment also presents problems in endodontic therapy owing to the incompletely formed roots and open apices.

As previously stated, calcium hydroxide pulpotomy has been the recommended treatment of choice in the pulpally involved vital ***permanent*** tooth. Also, as previously mentioned, the presence of a dentinal bridge below the amputation site does not always indicate a successful outcome.

Extrapolating the success with formocresol in primary teeth has led a number of pedodontists to use this medication in ***permanent*** teeth, whether the tooth tests vital or nonvital at the start of operative treatment. Using formocresol, Trask reported some success treating 43 permanent teeth with necrotic pulps in an age range of 7 to 23 years. Eight of these children were below 10 years of age when root apices are presumed to be still open. Trask sealed a small formocresol cotton pellet in the pulp chamber by amalgam restoration or stainless steel crown. The observed period of the study was 14 to 33 months. He reported asymptomatic results except in one tooth that had to be retreated in the same manner. He considered this an alternative to extraction and believed it to be a ***temporizing*** treatment only. Complete root canal therapy was advocated at a later date.[117]

Myers also conducted a clinical study of formocresol treatment in pulpless permanent molars. Sixty-six cases were evaluated clinically for periods of time ranging from 3 to 22 months. Fifty-six of the treated teeth (85%) demonstrated an elimination or marked reduction of initial periapical rarefaction. Three of the teeth (4.5%) showed no change in radiographic appearance, and seven teeth (10.6%) exhibited an increase in periapical rarefaction. An important finding showed that all the teeth treated with formocresol exhibited a continuation of apexification and an increase in root length.[118]

Fiskio undertook a five-year clinical study of 148 permanent teeth, using either a one-step or two-step formocresol treatment. Ninety-one percent required no further treatment. It was also felt that in the 9% that required further treatment, use of formocresol first did not prevent endodontic therapy from being performed at a later date. In this study, the age of the patients at the start of treatment had no significant effect on whether a tooth required further treatment.[119]

Spedding, in discussing the use of formocresol for permanent molars, stated that treatment with formocresol appears to form in root canals a "plug" of fixed tissues that can easily be removed with endodontic instruments. This is contrasted with teeth treated with calcium hydroxide. He concluded, however, that although few failures with formocresol have been reported in permanent teeth, more definite information about the failures is needed. Although this treatment rationale, according to Spedding, is empirical, its use is gaining in popularity.[86]

The philosophy behind the use of formocresol for treatment of permanent teeth has been well stated by Nishino. There is a fallacy, he believes, in extrapolating success in permanent teeth with this technique. Because they soon exfoliate, primary teeth rarely have acute or even chronic infections develop following formocresol treatment. Permanent teeth, on the other hand, provide a potential for future periapical infections or inflammation merely because of the lifetime they will be in place and exposed to developing pathologic conditions. It is conceivable though, according to Nishino, that the technique can be effective in young permanent teeth with incomplete development of an apical foramen.[120] The open apices of immature teeth would be much more conducive to ingrowth of proliferating fibroblasts.[88,121]

Other Pulpotomy Medicaments

Formocresol, calcium hydroxide, and zinc oxide–eugenol are not the only medicaments used as a pulp covering following coronal amputation. Sandler, Frankl, and Ruben sealed in Cresatin as the medicament in pulpotomy and protected it with a covering of Cavit. Clinically, there was but one failure in their test group. Histologically, tissue fixation appeared at the amputation site, while the apical-third pulp demonstrated vital tissue in 84% of the 21 cases examined[122] (Fig. 17–20).

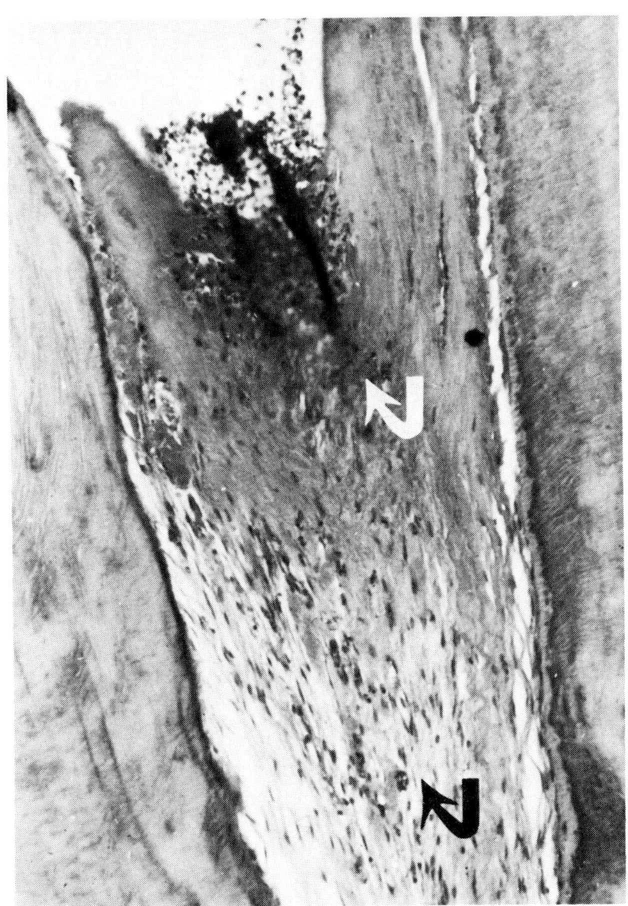

Fig. 17–20. Cellular condition of pulp 41 days after pulpotomy and ***Cresatin*** application. In homogeneous tissue adjacent to amputation site *(white arrow)*, there is paucity of cellular elements indicating nonvitality. Moving apically, tissue takes greater cellularity indicating increasing vitality *(black arrow)*. (From Sandler, E. S., Frankl, S. N., and Ruben, M. P.: J. Dent. Children, *38*:49, Jan.-Feb., 1971.)

Although it has been shown that zinc oxide–eugenol produces poor reactions in the root pulp tissue following coronal pulp amputation, the possibility of reducing these untoward reactions of ZO-E cement by the addition of a glucocorticoid has been investigated. Hansen et al., using Ledermix cement, had a clinical and radiographic success rate of 79% with this cement. Although total pulp inflammation was reduced in the glucocorticoid group, internal resorption was still a significant finding.[123]

Debridement and Filling of Pulpless Canals

The removal of necrotic pulp tissue and subsequent filling of the root canals of primary teeth have long been controversial procedures. Most negative attitudes toward primary tooth root filling have been based on the bizarre and tortuous canal anatomy of these teeth.[124] It was believed that primary canals could not be properly cleaned, shaped, and filled, particularly primary molars with their resorbing and open apices.[125,126] In addition to the problems engendered by pulp anatomy, it was believed possible to damage underlying permanent tooth buds.[37,127,128]

In spite of these fears and objections, successful root canal filling of primary teeth is not only highly recommended, but is being successfully accomplished by thousands of dentists. Pediatric endodontics, however, has had to be modified from adult endodontics because of the aforementioned anatomic differences between primary and permanent tooth pulps. For example, in primary teeth, chemical rather than mechanical canal debridement is more often used. Resorbable cements are also used for root fillings rather than solid core materials, such as gutta percha or silver points, that will not resorb along with the shedding primary roots (Fig. 17–21).

A less exacting standard of long-term success also holds in pediatric endodontics because of the limited

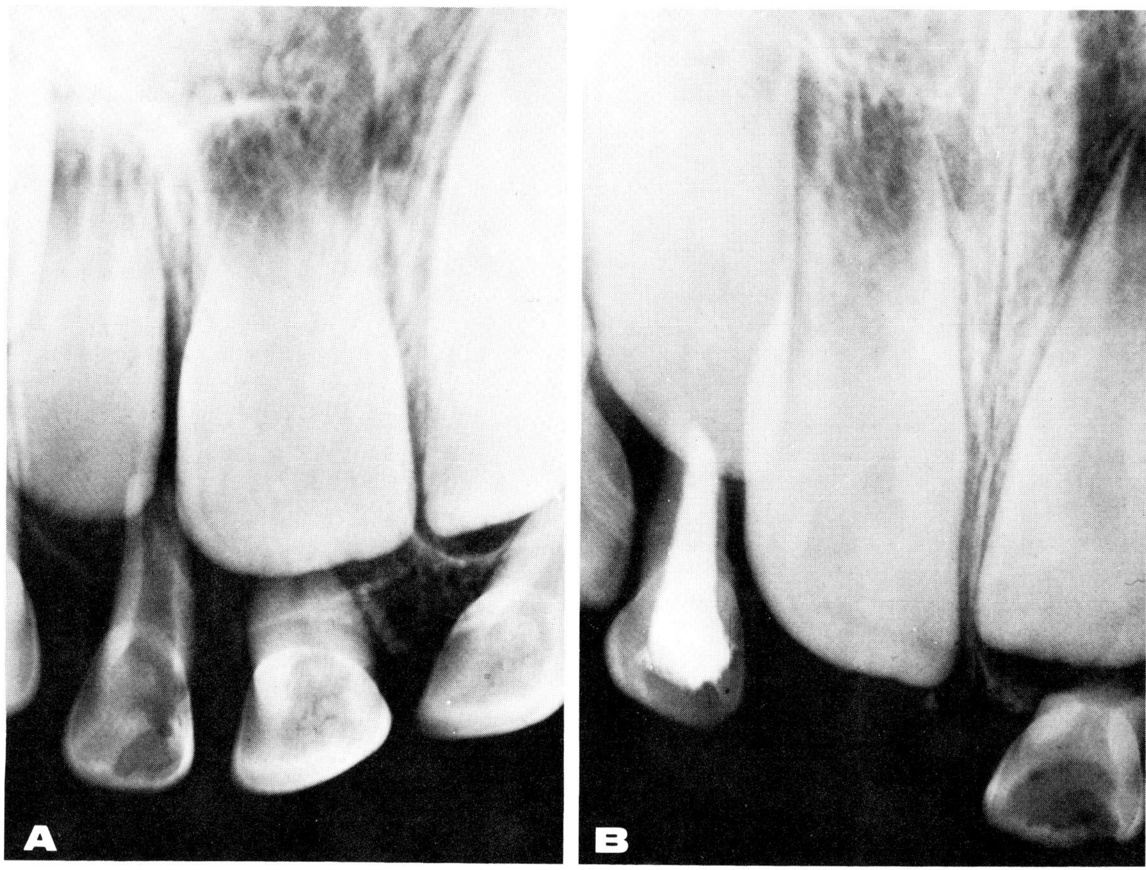

Fig. 17–21. Root canal filling of pulpless, maxillary primary lateral incisor. *A,* Carious exposure and pulp death—candidate for endodontic therapy. *B,* Six months following successful root canal filling with resorbable zinc oxide-eugenol cement. Care must be taken not to perforate the apex or overfill and injure the developing permanent tooth bud. (From Law, D. B., Lewis, T. M., and Davis, J. M.: An Atlas of Pedodontics. Philadelphia, W. B. Saunders Co., 1969, p. 206.)

time the tooth remains in function. Primary root canal therapy is judged successful if the root is firmly attached and remains in function without pain or infection until the permanent successor is ready to erupt. Fistulous tracts must also resolve. Radiographically, success is judged by the reduction of furcation or periapical lesions with re-establishment of a normal periodontal ligament.

Historical Review. Sweet described a four- or five-step technique utilizing formocresol for the treatment of pulpless teeth with and without fistulas.[80] Gerlach described the use of creosote and gutta percha for filling primary teeth, and Kelsten has recommended a ZO-E paste with Terramycin.[129,130] A study of pediatric endodontic procedures was reported by Rabinowitz in which 1,363 nonvital primary molars were treated with a two- to three-day application of formocresol followed by precipitation of silver nitrate and a sealer of ZO-E cement into the canals. While his reported success was phenomenal (only 7 failures), his procedure badly stained the teeth and involved a range of four to seventeen visits, with an average of 5.5 visits for teeth without periapical involvement and 7.7 visits for those with periapical involvement.[131] Andrew reported a study of 143 primary molars with necrotic pulps. No attempt was made to debride the canals, and beechwood creosote was sealed in for seven days. A paste containing thymol, cresol, iodoform and a zinc-oxide and glycerine was then used to fill the canals. One hundred teeth were reviewed after 12 months and 47 teeth after 18 months. Andrew's treatment proved equally successful for teeth with necrotic pulps or with vital, infected pulps.[132]

In treating primary molars, Bennett and Law and Lewis have advocated using basic adult endodontic techniques. Canals were instrumented short of the radiographic root apex, irrigated with sodium hypochlorite, dried with paper points, and medicated for three to seven days with either eugenol, camphorated parachlorophenol, or formocresol. On the second visit, the canals were mechanically prepared with files and filled with one of various resorbable mixtures, such as ZO-E cement or ZO-E mixed with iodoform crystals.[1,133]

Gould reported a clinical study of primary teeth of 27 children, age 3½ years to 8½ years, using a one-appointment technique. In 35 "frankly infected" primary molars a cotton pellet of camphorated parachlorophenol was placed in the chamber for five minutes after the canals had been debrided with files over two-thirds of their length. ZO-E cement was then pressed into the prepared canals. Over 26 months of clinical and radiographic observation, 29 of the 35 infected teeth (83%) were judged to be therapeutically successful because no lesion could be detected.[134] In asymptomatic necrotic primary teeth, Frigoletto suggested that canals be debrided with a barbed broach and washed with sodium hypochlorite, dried, and filled with root canal paste forced from a specially designed pressure syringe. If the tooth had been symptomatic, Cresatin was mixed with the paste.[27]

Today, there is no question that endodontic procedures for primary teeth are feasible and can be done with ease. The reason lies in the continued success of formocresol medication of primary teeth as advocated initially by Sweet.[80] Extension of the formocresol pulpotomy technique into treating nonvital primary teeth was a logical sequence. Vander Wall, Dowson and Shipman have shown formocresol to be more effective than either camphorated parachlorophenol or Cresatin as a root canal medicament for inhibiting bacterial growth.[135]

Starkey has described a one-appointment and a multiple-appointment method of treating the pulps of primary teeth. The one-appointment method is used in cases with vital primary pulp tissue, but with inflammation extending beyond the coronal pulp. No radiographic evidence of periapical involvement is present. In these cases Starkey recommends a partial pulpectomy, control of bleeding, and a filling of the canals and crown with a creamy mix of ZO-E cement.[23]

Starkey's multiple-appointment method is used for cases with necrotic pulps and periapical involvement. At the first appointment, coronal pulp debris is removed, but the canals are not instrumented. A medicament is then placed for two or three days. At the second visit, the canals are mechanically cleansed, and beechwood creosote or other suitable medicament is sealed in the chamber for two or three days. If the tooth is asymptomatic, the canals are filled at the final appointment with ZO-E cement to which a drop of medicament has been added (Fig. 17–22). Starkey points out that it is important to restore these treated primary teeth with full coverage— stainless steel or polycarbonate crowns.[23] Minor modifications of these procedures have been described by Kopel, Ritchey, Spedding, and Bogg.[136–139]

Because the ribbon-shaped and tortuous root

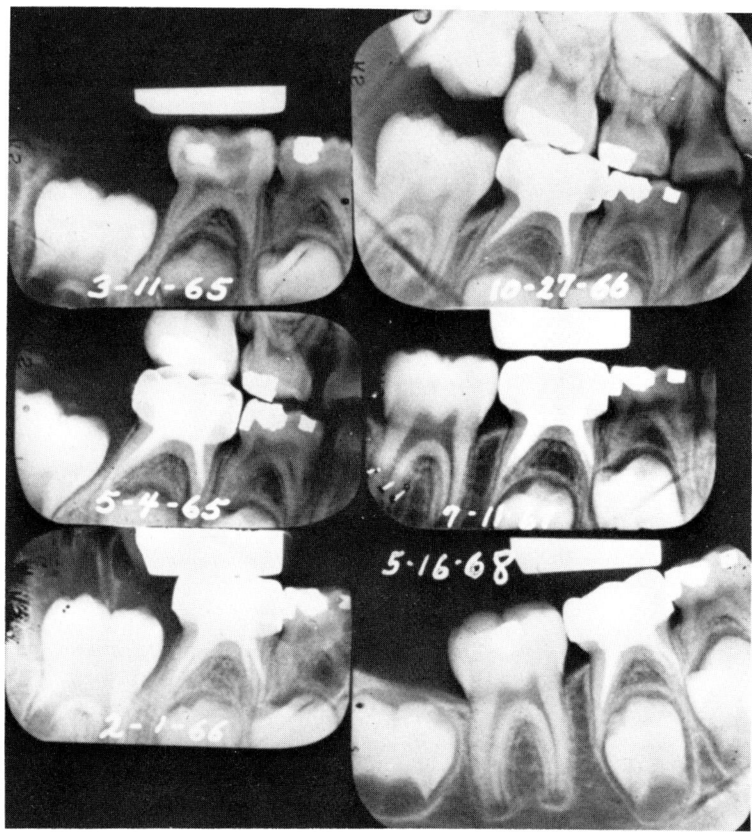

Fig. 17–22. Three-year successful root canal filling of mandibular second primary molar. (Courtesy Dr. Paul E. Starkey.) Canals have been thoroughly filed and irrigated at first appointment and medicated with formocresol or camphorated parachlorophenol. At second appointment canals were filled with resorbable zinc oxide-eugenol cement. (From Law, D. B., Lewis, T. M., and Davis, J. M.: An Atlas of Pedodontics. Philadelphia, W. B. Saunders Co., 1969, p. 208.)

canals of the primary teeth present a time-consuming problem in obtaining adequate obturation, a pressure syringe was developed by Greenberg and Katz for filling primary canals.[140] This technique has been described in detail by Krakow and Berk, Frigoletto, and Spedding.[27,138,141]

Clinical Considerations. The preceding review demonstrates the varied and confusing techniques for mastering endodontic therapy for primary teeth. Out of it all a rather standardized method has emerged. Before outlining a method, however, special considerations, indications, and contraindications should be considered.[136]

Dental Considerations

1. Clinical crowns are required that can be properly sealed and restored.
2. Chronologic and dental age must be evaluated to decide whether teeth may be saved or sacrificed.
3. Psychologic or cosmetic factors (anterior primary teeth) are important, ofttimes for the parent more than the child.
4. The number of teeth to be treated and their location may well influence treatment planning.
5. Primary molars are difficult to instrument to the apex. The walls of the curved, flattened canals are easily perforated. The floor of the pulp chamber is thin and frequently penetrated by natural accessory canals or by instruments.

General Considerations

1. The patient must be healthy and cooperative.
2. The parents must understand the procedure.
3. Informed consent must be obtained and signed.

Salvageable Primary Teeth and Indications

1. Primary teeth with pulp inflammation extending beyond the coronal pulp, but with roots and alveolar bone free of pathologic resorption.
2. Primary teeth with necrotic pulps and a minimum of root resorption and/or some bony destruction in the bifurcation.
3. Pulpless primary teeth with fistulas.
4. Pulpless primary teeth without permanent successors.
5. Pulpless primary second molars before the eruption of the permanent first molar.

6. Pulpless primary teeth in hemophiliacs.
7. Pulpless primary anterior teeth where speech, crowded arches, or esthetics are a factor.
8. Pulpless primary teeth next to the line of a palatal cleft.
9. Pulpless primary molars holding orthodontic appliances.
10. Pulpless primary molars where arch length is deficient.
11. Pulpless primary teeth when space maintainers or continued supervision are not feasible (handicapped or isolated children).*

Contraindications

1. A nonrestorable crown.
2. Periapical involvement extending to the permanent tooth bud.
3. Pathologic resorption of at least one-third of the root with a fistulous tract.
4. Excessive internal resorption.
5. Extensive pulp floor opening into the bifurcation.
6. Young patients with systemic illness such as rheumatic heart disease and leukemia, or children on long-term corticosteroid therapy.
7. Primary teeth with underlying dentigerous or follicular cysts.

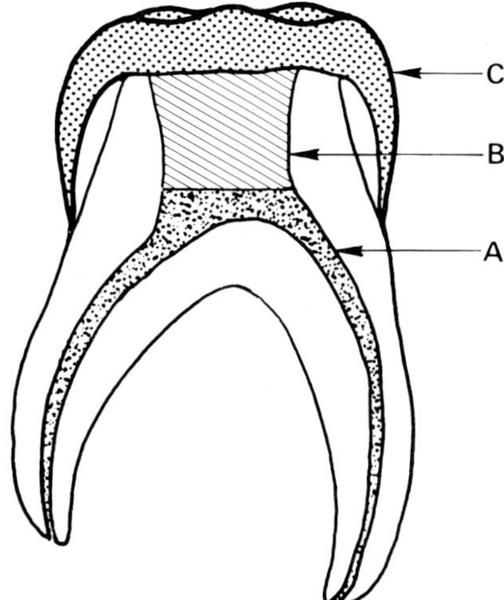

Fig. 17–23. Root canal obturation and crown restoration for pulpless primary molar. At first appointment, following mechanical and chemical canal debridement, medicament is sealed in place for one week. Canal is obturated at second appointment with resorbable zinc oxide-eugenol cement. *A,* ZO-E cement root canal filling. *B,* Oxyphosphate of zinc cement. *C,* Stainless steel crown.

Partial Pulpectomy

Generally partial pulpectomy is carried out as an extension of the pulpotomy procedure, probably as an on-the-spot decision once the chamber is entered and it becomes apparent hemorrhage is difficult to control. This situation generally presents itself in a tooth with spontaneous toothache but with negative fistula or radiographic findings.

Following anesthesia, rubber dam placement, and coronal preparation, the pulp is amputated with a high-speed round bur.[116] A Hedstrom file is then used to remove the pulp tissue about halfway down the canals or until hemorrhage is controlled. The canals and chamber are then irrigated with hydrogen peroxide followed by sodium hypochlorite and then dried with blunted paper points and cotton pellets. If hemorrhage is impossible to control, all the pulp tissue must be removed from the bleeding canal.

*Due to isolation of the children involved in its Indian Bureau of Health Affairs, the United States Public Health Service has recommended root canal filling of primary teeth, whenever feasible, rather than space maintainers requiring lengthy supervision.[142]

A cotton pellet, squeezed dry of formocresol, is then placed in the chamber and the cavity sealed over with Cavit, or a stainless steel crown is placed with zince oxide–eugenol mixed with petroleum jelly for easy removal at the next appointment.

One week later, if all adverse symptoms are absent, the medicament is removed and the canals and chamber may be filled with a mix of zinc oxide–eugenol cement. The cement is teased down the canals with a lentulo spiral or wiped and pumped there with a sterile instrument and paper point. A plastic "jiffy" tube or cement syringe may also be used.

To fill the chamber and improve the density of the canal fillings, fast-setting ZO-E cement is placed under pressure in the chamber with a damp cotton pellet and amalgam pluggers. A drop of 10% zinc acetate will hasten the set. A radiograph is then taken, and if the canals appear to be adequately filled, a stainless steel crown is placed as a permanent restoration. The week of pulp canal medication recommended here prevents post-treatment infection. Starkey has suggested that this same technique be used in one appointment[143] (Fig. 17–23).

Necrotic Canal Treatment

The child who is presented with pulp necrosis is an entirely different challenge to treatment. In some situations the tooth may be acutely or chronically abscessed—loose, painful, and with swollen periodontal tissues. At this appointment, the child may be apprehensive and irritable, so that relief of pain and swelling is a first-order priority.

Under gently secured anesthesia, the pulp chamber is carefully opened to relieve the pressure. A high-speed round bur and spoon excavator clean out the pulp chamber, which is then irrigated. At this point, the chamber of the acute case may be left open with a cotton pellet in place, or the chronic case may be closed with a formocresol dressing sealed in the pulp chamber. In neither case should canal instrumentation be undertaken. The child with acute symptoms should be placed on antibiotic therapy and pain relieved with analgesics.

At the end of one week, or when acute symptoms subside, the chamber may be reopened under a rubber dam and the canals debrided with copious irrigation and careful cleaning with broaches and Hedstrom files. Tooth length should be carefully estimated and not exceeded. Once again, a "dry" dressing of formocresol is sealed in the chamber. If a fistula is present it should be punctured to improve drainage—a painless procedure.

Again, at the end of one week, if all symptoms including a fistula have resolved, final canal preparation is completed with hydrogen peroxide-sodium hypochlorite irrigation and debridement and canal enlargement with Hedstrom files.

The canals may now be filled with a paste of ZO-E cement. Again, obturation is sought with a lentulo spiral or syringe application of paste filling. By radiograph the canal fillings are evaluated for voids and corrected by additional pressure on the ZO-E cement in the chamber.

Final restoration with a stainless steel crown is indicated.

Less demanding techniques than the one described here, usually centering around one appointment treatment, have been reported as successful by Ripa, Velling, Droter, Ritchey and Bly, the latter author even cautioning not to force the filling paste into the canals.[137,144–148]

Concern has been expressed whether primary teeth treated endodontically are subject to early resorption and exfoliation. Nacht found that vital primary molars treated by pulpotomy and Oxpara (containing paraformaldehyde) did resorb early.[149] Lauterstein noted a faster eruption rate of permanent teeth beneath primary molars subjected to calcium hydroxide pulpotomy. He stated though that prior extensive caries, pulp inflammation, and abscess formation may also have contributed to the accelerated rate.[150] Starkey, on the other hand, believes delayed eruption of the permanent premolars follows formocresol treatment of primary molars.[143]

There appears to be a tendency for delayed eruption of permanent successor teeth under root canal treated primary molars, with some minor deflection in the eruption path. The most important factor, however, is not whether the tooth erupts early or late, but rather that the infection was eliminated, the primary tooth remained healthy in the dental arch, and the space became available for the eventual eruption of the permanent tooth. In spite of the many inherent endodontic problems presented by primary teeth, there are overwhelming indications for such procedures. Satisfactory results apparently may be obtained through several methods. By adherence to sound endodontic principles in case selection and technique, the feasibility and practicality of this therapy become obvious.

One should bear in mind that a successful pediatric endodontic outcome is based upon the re-establishment of normal periodontal tissues and nonpathologic root resorption rather than concern about the complete obturation of all the root and accessory canals. (See also pp. 734–735.)

REFERENCES

1. Lewis, T. M., and Law, D. C.: Pulpal treatment of primary teeth. Chapt. 10. In *Clinical Pedodontics*. 4th ed. Edited by S. B. Finn. Philadelphia, W. B. Saunders Co., 1973.
2. DiMaggio, J. J., Hawes, R. R., and Kiryati, A.: Histological evaluation of direct and indirect pulp capping. IADR Abst. 22 & 23, Mar., 1963.
3. Eichenbaum, I., and Dunn, N. A.: Prevalence of pulpally involved primary teeth. J. Dent. Child., *18*:8, 4th Quar., 1951.
4. Langeland K.: Response of the adult tooth to injury. In *Biology of the Dental Pulp Organ: A Symposium*. Edited by S. B. Finn. Univ. Alabama Press, 1968.
5. Masterson, J. B.: The healing of wounds of the dental pulp of man. Brit. Dent. J., *120*:213, March 1, 1966.
6. Stanley, H. R., White, C. L., and McCray, L.: The rate of tertiary (reparative dentin) formation in the human tooth. Oral Surg., *21*:180, Feb., 1966.
7. Finn, S. B.: Morphology of the primary teeth. Chapt. 4. In *Clinical Pedodontics*. 4th Ed. Edited by S. B. Finn. Philadelphia, W. B. Saunders Co., 1973.

8. Moss, S. J., and Addleston, H.: Histologic study of the pulpal floor of deciduous molars. J.A.D.A., *70*:372, Feb., 1965.
9. Massler, M.: Preventive endodontics: vital pulp therap. Dent. Clin. N. Amer., p. 663, Nov., 1967.
10. Bernick, S.: Innervation of the teeth and periodontium. Dent. Clin. N. Amer. p. 503, July, 1959.
11. Rapp, R., Avery, J. K., and Strachan, D. C.: The distribution of nerves in human primary teeth. Anat. Rec., *159*:89, Sept., 1967.
12. Benzer, G., and Bevelander, S.: Morphology and incidence of secondary dentin in human teeth. J.A.D.A., *30*:1075, July, 1943.
13. Ireland, R. I.: Secondary dentin formation in deciduous teeth. J.A.D.A., *28*:1626, Oct., 1941.
14. Corbett, M. D.: The incidence of secondary dentin in carious teeth. Brit. Dent. J., *114*:142, Feb. 19, 1963.
15. Sayegh, F. S.: Qualitative and quantitative evaluation of new dentin in pulp capped teeth. J. Dent. Child., *35*:7, Jan., 1968.
16. McDonald, R. E.: Diagnostic aids and vital pulp therapy for deciduous teeth. J.A.D.A., *53*:14, July, 1956.
17. Anderson, A. W., Sharav, Y., and Massler, M.: Reparative dentin formation and pulp morphology. Oral Surg., *26*:837, Dec., 1948.
18. Frankl, S. H.: Pulp therapy in pedodontics. Oral Surg., *34*:192, Aug., 1972.
19. Hunter, W.: Saving pulps, a queer process. Dental Items of Interest, *5*:352, Sept., 1883.
20. Berk, H.: Effect of calcium hydroxide methylcellulose paste on the dental pulp. J. Dent. Child., *17*:65, 4th Quar., 1950.
21. Glass, R. L., and Zander, H. A.: Pulp healing. J. Dent. Res., *28*:97, Apr., 1949.
22. Nyborg, H.: Healing processes in the pulp on capping. Acta. Odont. Scand., *13*:9–130, Suppl. 16, 1955.
23. Starkey, P. E.: Methods of preserving primary teeth which have exposed pulps. J. Dent. Child., *30*:219, 4th Quar., 1963.
24. Langeland, K.: Capping exposed pulpal tissue. Clin. Dent., *2*:1, Jan.-Feb., 1974.
25. Dannenberg, J. L.: Pedodontic endodontics. Dent. Clin. N. Amer., *18*:367, Apr., 1974.
26. Miyamato, O.: Current status of pulpal therapy on primary and young permanent teeth. J. Acad. Dent. Hand., *1*:27, Nov., 1974.
27. Frigoletto, R. T.: Pulp therapy in pedodontics. J.A.D.A., *86*:1344, June, 1973.
28. Mitchell, D. F.: Pulp reaction to commonly used pulp capping materials. J. Dent. Child., *28*:150, 2nd Quar., 1961.
29. Tannenbaum, H. I.: Pulp capping with zinc oxide-eugenol and CaOH. J. Dent. Child., *18*:16, 3rd Quar., 1951.
30. Weiss, M. D., and Bjorvatn, K.: Pulp capping in deciduous and newly erupted permanent teeth of monkeys. Oral Surg., *29*:769, May, 1970.
31. Kakehashi, S., Stanley, H. R., and Fitzgerald, R. J.: The effects of surgical exposures of the dental pulp in germ free and conventional laboratory rats. Oral Surg., *20*:340, Sept., 1965.
32. Miller, W. D.: What antiseptics should be used for sterilizing cavities before filling. Dent. Cosmos, *33*:337, 1891.
33. Mohammed, Y. R., et al.: Filling base materials and the unexposed and exposed tooth pulps. J. Prosth. Dent., *11*:503, May-June, 1961.
34. Sveen, O. B.: Pulp capping of primary teeth with zinc oxide–eugenol. Odont. Tidskr., *77*:427, Dec., 1969.
35. Tronstad, L., and Mjor, I.: Capping of the inflamed pulp. Oral Surg., *34*:477, Sept., 1972.
36. Jeppersen, K.: Direct pulp capping on primary teeth—a long-term investigation. J. Internat. A. Dent. Child., *2*:10, June, 1971.
37. Shiere, F. R., and Frankl, S. N.: The effect of deciduous tooth infection on permanent teeth. Dent. Prog., *2*:59, Oct., 1961.
38. Sciaky, I., and Pisanti, S.: Localization of calcium placed over amputated pulps in dogs teeth. J. Dent. Res., *39*:1128, Nov.-Dec., 1960.
39. Attalla, M. N. and Noujaim, A. A.: Role of calcium hydroxide in the formation of reparative dentin. Canad. Dent. Assoc. J., *35*:267, May 1969.
40. Stark, M. M., et al.: The localization of radioactive CaOH (Ca 45) overexposed pulps in Rhesus monkey teeth: a preliminary report. J. Oral Therap. and Pharm., *3*:290, Nov., 1964.
41. Seltzer, S., and Bender, J. B.: The Dental Pulp. Philadelphia, J. B. Lippincott, 1965, pp. 108, 192.
42. Brosch, J. W.: Capping pulps with a compound of calcium phosphate, neomycin and hydrocortisone. J. Dent. Child., *33*:42–8, Jan., 1966.
43. Shovelton, D. S.: Studies of dentin and pulp in deep caries. Internat. Dent. J., *20*:283, June, 1970.
44. Bhaskar, S., Cutright, D. E., and Van Osdel, V.: Tissue response to cortisone-containing and cortisone-free calcium hydroxide. J. Dent. Child., *36*:1, May-June, 1969.
45. Soldali, G. D.: Pulp capping with antibiotics. Fla. Dent. J., *46*:18, Spring, 1975.
46. Bhaskar, S., et al.: Pulp capping with isobutyl cyanoacrylate. J.A.D.A., *79*:640, Sept., 1969.
47. Berkman, M. D., et al.: Pulpal response to isobutyl cyanoacrylate in human teeth. J.A.D.A., *83*:140, July, 1971.
48. Ibrahim, S. M., Mitchell, D. F., and Healy, H. G.: A histopathologic study of the effects of formocresol in pulp capping of permanent teeth. Egypt Dent. J., *16*:219, July, 1970.
49. Heller, A. J., et al.: Direct pulp capping of permanent teeth in primates using a resorbable form of tricalcium phosphate ceramic. J.O.E., *1*:102, March, 1975.
50. Black, G. V.: A work on operative dentistry. Vol. 2, Chicago, Medico-Dental Publ. Co., 1908.
51. Canby, C. P., and Bernier, J. L.: Bacteriologic studies of various dentin. J.A.D.A., *23*:2083, Nov., 1936.
52. Dorfman, A., Stephan, R. M., and Muntz, J. A.: In vitro studies of carious dentin. II Extent of infection in carious lesions. J.A.D.A., *30*:1901, Dec., 1943.

53. Parikh, S. R., Massler, M., and Bahn, A.: Microorganisms in active and arrested carious lesions of dentin. New York State Dent. J., *29*:347, Oct., 1963.
54. Shovelton, D. S.: Studies of dentin and pulp in deep caries. Internat. Dent. J., *20*:283, June, 1970.
55. Fusayama, T., Okuse, K., and Hosoda H.: Relationship between hardness, discoloration and microbial invasion in carious dentin. J. Dent. Res., *45*:1033, July-Aug., 1966.
56. Whitehead, F. I., MacGregor, A. B., and Marsland, E. A.: The relationship of bacterial invasion of softening of the dentin in permanent and deciduous teeth. Brit. Dent. J., *108*:261, April 5, 1960.
57. Shovelton, D. S.: A study of deep carious dentin. Internat. Dent. J., *18*:392, June, 1968.
58. Reeves, R., and Stanley, H. R.: The relationship of bacterial penetration and pulpal pathosis in carious teeth. Oral Surg., *22*:59, July, 1966.
59. Trowbridge, H., and Berger, J.: The clinical management of deep carious lesions. Calif. Dent. J., *47*:26, Fall, 1971.
60. Ishibaski, M.: A comparison between results of clinical and histo-pathological diagnosis of disease of deciduous tooth pulp. Dent. Abstr., *3*:547, Sept., 1958.
61. Reynolds, R. L.: The determination of pulp vitality by means of thermal and electrical stimuli. Oral Surg., *22*:231, Aug., 1966.
62. Kuwabara, R. K., and Massler, M.: Pulpal reactions to active and arrested carious lesions. J. Dent. Child., *33*:190, May, 1966.
63. Bradford, E. W.: The dentin, a barrier to caries. Brit. Dent. J., *109*:387, Nov. 15, 1960.
64. Young, M. A., and Massler, M.: Some physical and chemical characteristics of carious dentin. Brit. Dent. J., *115*:406, Nov. 19, 1963.
65. King, J., Crawford, J., and Tindahl, R.: Indirect pulp capping: a bacteriologic study of deep carious dentin in human teeth. Oral Surg., *20*:663, Nov., 1965.
66. Aponte, A. J., Hartsook, J. T., and Crowley M. C.: Indirect pulp capping verified. J. Dent. Child., *33*:164, May, 1966.
67. Kerkhove, B. C., et al.: A clinical and television densitometric evaluation of the indirect pulp capping technique. J. Dent. Child., *34*:192, May, 1967.
68. Mjor, I. A., Finn, S. B., and Quigley, M. B.: The effects of calcium hydroxide and amalgam on noncarious vital dentin. Arch. Oral Biol., *3*:283, June, 1961.
69. Law, D. B., and Lewis, T. M.: The effects of calcium hydroxide on deep carious lesions. Oral Surg., *14*:1130, Sept., 1961.
70. Held-Wydler, E.: "Natural" (indirect) pulp capping. J. Dent. Child., *31*:107, 2nd Quar., 1964.
71. Ehrenreich, D. W.: A comparison of the effects of zinc oxide-eugenol and calcium hydroxide in carious dentin in human primary molars. J. Dent. Child., *35*:451, Nov., 1968.
72. Stanley, H. R.: Pulpal response to dental techniques and materials. Dent. Clin. N. Amer., *15*:115, Jan., 1971.
73. Nordstrom, D. O., Wei, S. H., and Johnson, R.: Use of stannous fluoride for indirect pulp capping. J.A.D.A., *88*:997, May, 1974.
74. Schroder, A.: Indirect capping and the treatment of deep carious lesions. Internat. Dent. J., *18*:381, June, 1968.
75. Eidelman, E., Finn, S. B., and Koulorides T.: Remineralization of carious dentin treated with calcium hydroxide. J. Dent. Child., *38*:218 4th Quar., 1965.
76. Jordan, R. E., and Suzuki, M.: Conservative treatment of deep carious lesions. Canad. Dent. Assoc. J., *37*:337, Sept., 1971.
77. Pittman, J. L.: Clinical evaluation of an indirect technic for capping dental pulps. Univ. Mich. School of Dentistry, M. S. Thesis, 1963.
78. Hutchins, D. W., and Parker, W. A.: Indirect pulp capping: a clinical evaluation using polymethyl methacrylate reinforced zinc oxide-eugenol cement. J. Dent. Child., *39*:55, Jan., 1972.
79. Buckley, J. P.: The chemistry of pulp decomposition with a rational treatment for this condition and its sequelae. J.A.D.A., *3*:764, Nov., 1904.
80. Sweet, C. A.: Procedure for treatment of exposed and pulpless deciduous teeth. J.A.D.A., *17*:1150, June, 1930.
81. Hobson, P.: Pulp treatment for deciduous teeth. I. Factors affecting diagnosis and treatment. Brit. Dent. J., *128*:232, March 3, 1970. II. Clinical investigation. *128*:275, March 17, 1970.
82. Sweet C. A.: Treatment of vital primary teeth with pulpal involvement—therapeutic pulpotomy. Colorado State Dent. Assoc. J., *33*:10, June, 1955.
83. Emmerson, C. C., Miyamoto, O., Sweet, C. A., Sr., and Bhatia, H. D.: Pulpal changes following formocresol applications on rat molars and human primary teeth. South. Calif. Dent. Assoc. J., *27*:309, Sept., 1959.
84. Berger J. E.: A review of the erroneously labeled "mummification" techniques of pulp therapy. Oral Surg., *34*:131, July, 1972.
85. Massler, M., and Mansukhani, H.: Effects of formocresol on the dental pulp. J. Dent. Child., *26*:277, 4th Quar., 1959.
86. Spedding, R. H., Mitchell, D. F., and McDonald, R. E.: Formocresol and calcium hydroxide therapy. J. Dent. Res., *44*:1023, Sept.-Oct., 1965.
87. Law, D. B., and Lewis, T. M.: Formocresol pulpotomy in deciduous teeth. J.A.D.A., *69*:601, Nov., 1964.
88. Berger, J.: Pulp tissue reaction for formocresol and zinc oxide and eugenol. J. Dent. Child., *32*:13, 1st Quar., 1965.
89. Nygaard-Ostby, B.: The role of the blood clot in endodontic therapy. Acta Odonto. Scand., *19*:323, Dec., 1961.
90. Spamer, R. G.: The formocresol pulpotomy: a histological study of a single application of formocresol on the dental pulp of human primary teeth. Univ. Wash. School of Dent., Seattle, M. S. Thesis, 1965.

91. Beaver, H. A., Kopel, H. M., and Sabes, W. R.: The effect of zinc oxide-eugenol cement on a formocresolized pulp. J. Dent. Child., *33*:381, Nov., 1966.
92. Ranley, D. M., Montgomery, E. H., and Pope, H. O.: The loss of 3H-formaldehyde from zinc oxide–eugenol element—an *in vitro* study. J. Dent. Child., *43*:48, Mar.-Apr., 1975.
93. Venham, L. J.: Pulpal responses to variations on the formocresol pulpotomy technique. Ohio State Univ. College of Dentistry, M. S. Thesis, 1967.
94. Redig, D.: A comparison and evaluation of two formocresol pulpotomy techniques utilizing Buckley's formocresol. J. Dent. Child., *35*:22, Jan., 1968.
95. Straffon, L. H., and Han, S. S.: The effect of formocresol on hamster connective tissue cells: a histologic and quantitative radioautographic study with proline H3. Arch. Oral. Biol., *13*:271, Mar., 1968.
96. Straffon, L. H., and Han, S. S.: Effects of varying concentrations of formocresol on RNA synthesis of connective tissue in sponge implants. Oral Surg., *29*:915, June, 1971.
97. Loos, P. J., Straffon, L. H., and Han, S. S.: Biological effects of formocresol. J. Dent. Child., *40*:193, May-June, 1973.
98. Morawa, A. P., et al.: Clinical studies of human primary teeth following dilute formocresol pulpotomies. IADR Abstr. No. 859, 1974.
99. Rolling, I., and Thylstrup, A.: A three-year clinical follow up study of pulpotomized primary molars treated with the formocresol technique. Scand. J. Dent. Res., *83*:47, Mar., 1975.
100. Spedding R. H.: Pulp therapy for primary teeth—a survey of North American dental schools. J. Dent. Child., *35*:360, Sept., 1968.
101. Koch, G., and Nyborg, H.: Correlation between clinical and histological indications for pulpotomy of deciduous teeth. J. Internat. A. Dent. Child., *1*:3, Sept., 1970.
102. Teuscher, G. W., and Zander, H. A.: A preliminary report on pulpotomy. Northwest. Univ. Grad. Bull., *39*:4, 1938.
103. Dowden, W. E., et al.: A histologic evaluation of formocresol and calcium hydroxide. IADR Abstr. No. 835, 1971.
104. Ulmansky, M., Sela, J., and Sela, M.: Scanning electromicroscopy of calcium hydroxide induced bridges. J. Oral Path., *1*:244, 1972. (Annual)
105. Brown, W. E., Jr.: The vital pulpotomy technique for the management of vital exposed pulps in primary and young permanent teeth. Univ. Mich. Alumni Bull., *48*:14–16, Aug., 1947.
106. Shoemaker, C. P.: Results of 28 pulpotomies. J.A.D.A., *50*:71, Jan., 1955.
107. Via, W. R., Jr.: Evaluation of deciduous molars treated by pulpotomy and calcium hydroxide. J.A.D.A., *50*:34, Jan., 1955.
108. Law, D. B.: An evaluation of the vital pulpotomy technique. J. Dent. Child., *23*:40, 1st Quar., 1956.
109. Magnusson, B.: Therapeutic pulpotomy in primary molars—clinical and histological follow-up. Odonto. Revy., *21*:415, Dec., 1970.
110. Schröder, U., and Granath, L. E.: On internal dentin resorption in deciduous molars treated by pulpotomy and capped with calcium hydroxide. Odonto. Revy., *22*:179, No. 2, 1971.
111. Phaneuf, R., Frankl, S. H., and Ruben, M. P.: A comparative histological evaluation of calcium hydroxide preparations on the human primary dental pulp. J. Dent. Child., *35*:61, Jan., 1968.
112. Doyle, W. A., McDonald, R. E., and Mitchell, D. E.: Formocresol versus calcium hydroxide in pulpotomy. J. Dent. Child., *29*:86, 2nd Quar., 1962.
113. Hallett G. E., and Porteus, J. R.: Fractured incisors treated by vital pulpotomy. Brit. Dent. J., *115*:279, Oct. 1, 1963.
114. Luks, S.: Pulpotomy—a critical evaluation. J. Dent. Child., *21*:249, 4th Quar., 1954.
115. Patterson, S. S.: Pulp calcification due to operative procedures—pulpotomy. Internat. Dent. J., *17*:490, June, 1967.
116. Harris, S.: A preliminary histologic investigation of three amputation techniques with formocresol pulpotomies in normal primary teeth. Univ. So. Calif. School of Dentistry, M. A. Thesis, 1969.
117. Trask, P. A.: Formocresol pulpotomy in young permanent teeth. J.A.D.A., *85*:1316, Dec., 1972.
118. Myers, D. A.: Effects of formocresol on pulps of cariously exposed permanent molars. Univ. Tennessee School of Dentistry, M. S. Thesis, 1972.
119. Fiskio, H. M.: Pulpotomies in vital and non-vital permanent teeth. J. Acad. Gen. Dent., *22*:27, Jan.-Feb., 1974.
120. Nishino, P. K.: Apical histologic response to formocresol pulpotomy. Chron. Omaha Dent. Soc., *22*:242, Dec., 1974.
121. Granath, L. E., et al.: First permanent molars subjected to mortal amputation before maturation of roots. Odonto. Revy., *21*:319, No. 3, 1970.
122. Sandler, E. S., Frankl, S. N., and Ruben, M. P.: The histological response of the dental pulp to Cresatin. J. Dent. Child., *38*:49, Jan.-Feb., 1971.
123. Hansen, H. P., et al.: Vital pulpotomy in primary molars. Scand. J. Dent., *79*:13 1971.
124. Hibbard, E. D., and Ireland, R. L.: Morphology of the root canals of the primary molar teeth. J. Dent. Child., *24*:250, 4th Quar., 1957.
125. Hartsook, J. T.: Pulpal therapy in primary and young permanent teeth. Dent. Clin. N. Amer., p. 385, July, 1966.
126. Nicholls, E.: Root canal treatment of primary teeth. In Transactions of the Third International Conference on Endodontics. Edited by L. I. Grossman. University of Pennsylvania School of Dentistry, Philadelphia, 1963.
127. Binns, W. H.: Primary tooth infections can affect permanent tooth buds. Penn. Dent. J., *33*:44, Feb., 1966.

128. McCormack, J., and Filostrat, D. J.: Injury to the teeth of succession by abscess of the temporary teeth. J. Dent. Child., *34*:501, Nov., 1967.
129. Gerlach, E.: Root canal therapeutics. Dent. Survey, *8*:68, May, 1932.
130. Kelsten, L. B.: Pedodontics for the general practitioner. Brooklyn Dent. Items of Interest, p. 396, 1956.
131. Rabinowitz, B. Z.: Pulp management of primary teeth. Oral Surg., *6*:542, Apr., 1953; *6*:671, May, 1953.
132. Andrew, P.: Treatment of infected pulps in deciduous teeth. Brit. Dent. J., *98*:126, Feb. 15, 1955.
133. Bennett, C. G.: Pulpal management of deciduous teeth. Pract. Dent. Monogr., May-June, 1965.
134. Gould, J. M.: Root canal therapy for infected primary molar teeth—preliminary report. J. Dent. Child., *34*:23, July-Aug. No. 3, 1970.
135. Vander Wall, G. L., Dowson, J., and Shipman C.: Endodontic medicaments. Oral Surg., *25*:238, Feb., 1972.
136. Kopel, H. M.: Root canal therapy for primary teeth. Mich. Dent. A. J., *52*:28, Feb., 1970.
137. Ritchey, W. H.: A very simple technic for abscessed deciduous teeth. Tex. Dent. J., *82*:5, Aug., 1964.
138. Spedding, R. H.: Root canal treatment for primary teeth. Dent. Clin. N. Amer., *17*:105, Jan., 1973.
139. Bogg, D. S.: Simple technique for treating non-vital deciduous teeth—a study. Northwest Dent., *48*:102, Mar.-Apr., 1969.
140. Greenberg, M.: Filling root canals of deciduous teeth by an injection technique. Dent. Digest, *67*:574, Dec., 1961.
141. Krakow, A. A., and Berk, H.: Efficient endodontic procedures with the use of the pressure syringe. Dent. Clin. N. Amer., p. 387, July, 1965.
142. Glauser, R. O.: Preventive orthodontics and limited treatment procedures. U. S. Public Health Service, Div. of Indian Health, 1967.
143. Starkey, P. E.: Management of deep caries of pulpally involved teeth in children. In *Current Therapy in Dentistry*. Edited by H. M. Goldman et al. Vol. III, St. Louis, C. V. Mosby Co., 1968.
144. Ripa, L. W.: Pulp therapy for the primary dentition. II. The treatment of teeth with non-vital or degenerating pulps. Connecticut State Dent. Assoc. J., *44*:210, Oct., 1970.
145. Velling, R. J.: A study of the treatment of infected and necrotic primary teeth. J. Dent. Child., *28*:213, 3rd Quar., 1961.
146. Droter, J. A.: Formocresol in vital and non-vital teeth—a clinical study. J. Dent. Child., *30*:239, 4th Quar., 1963.
147. Droter, J. A.: Pulp therapy in primary teeth. J. Dent. Child., *34*:507, Nov., 1967.
148. Bly, P. E.: One setting treatment for pulpless teeth. Dent. Surv., *46*:27, Jan., 1970.
149. Nacht, M.: A devitalizing technique for pulpotomy in primary molars. J. Dent. Child., *23*:45, 1st Quar., 1956.
150. Lauterstein, A. M., Pruzansky, S., and Barber, T. K.: Effect of deciduous molar pulpotomy on the eruption of succedaneous premolars. J. Dent. Res., *41*:1367, Nov.-Dec., 1962.

Chapter 18

Restoration of the Pulpless Tooth. Preparation for the Overdenture

ALFRED L. FRANK, STEPHEN TEEL, and DAVID H. WANDS

The restoration of function to the pulpless tooth has received increased interest and attention. No longer is the pulpless tooth treated as a temporary measure and, as such, worthy only of an inadequate temporary restoration. With improved endodontic techniques, the well-treated pulpless tooth will remain an integral part of the dental apparatus as long as it is adequately restored.

In spite of the continuous trend toward more specialized areas in dentistry, the interdependence among the many disciplines is obvious. This is particularly true in the field of endodontics, which cannot be disassociated from restorative dentistry.

The procedures presented in this chapter are time-tested. The approach will reiterate and re-emphasize principles and procedures known to every

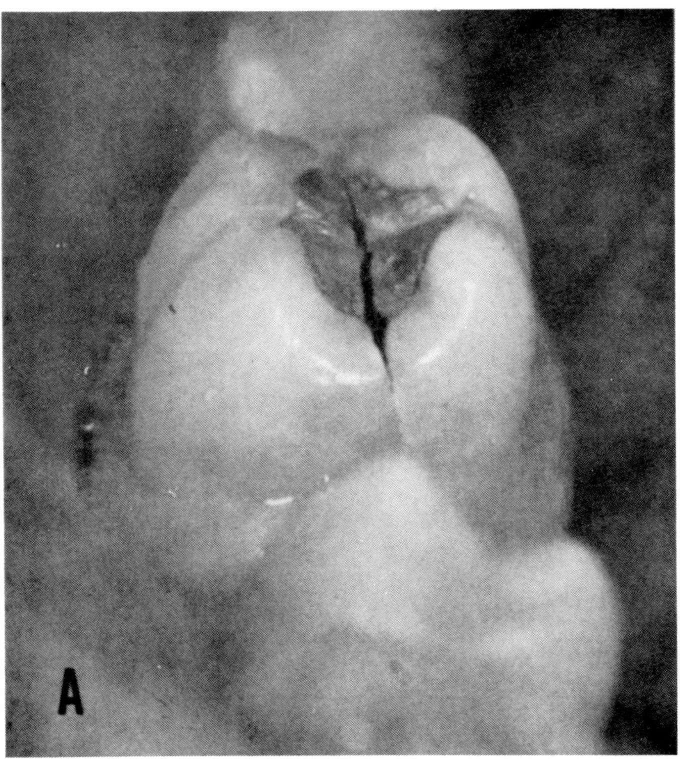

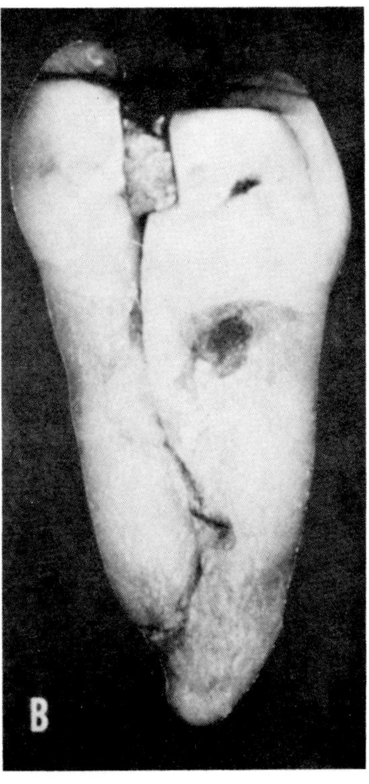

Fig. 18–1. Fractures of endodontically treated teeth that could have been prevented by adequate restoration. *A,* Mesiodistal fracture of mandibular molar. *B,* MOD onlay should have been restoration of choice.

dental practitioner. Although they are elementary, these procedures represent the most neglected phase of endodontic therapy. How frustrating to see a well-treated pulpless tooth end in the beaks of the exodontist's forceps because the restorative procedure was withheld or not executed properly (Fig. 18–1). The proper restoration of the pulpless tooth is no less important a step than the proper initial access cavity.

It has never been adequately shown that the pulpless tooth is a more brittle tooth. Some dentists, however, have seen fragmentation during the extraction of such a tooth, and have noted a glass-like brittleness. Whether this represents actual brittleness of the tooth or whether this brittle nature is due to the extensive loss of tooth structure is relatively unimportant in this discussion. Whatever the reason, the conclusion may be drawn that pulpless teeth are vulnerable to fracture.

In light of this conclusion, it is imperative that the utmost care and preoperative planning be utilized in the selection of the final restoration. Only by such

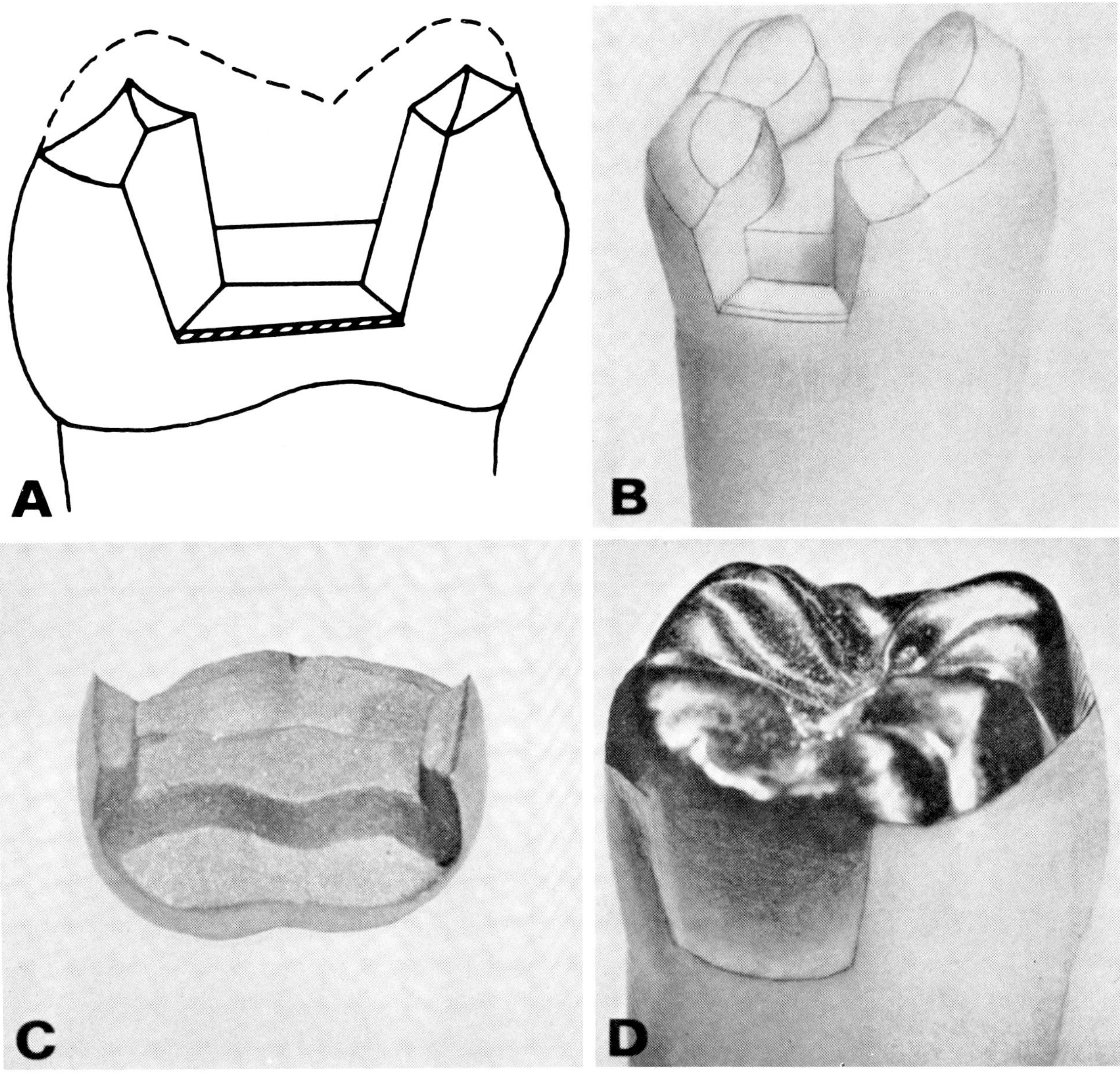

Fig. 18–2. MOD onlay restoring pulpless mandibular first molar. *A*, Schematic drawing of cavity preparation. *B*, Preparation which emphasizes cuspal protection. *C*, Internal surface of casting. *D*, Restoration in place.

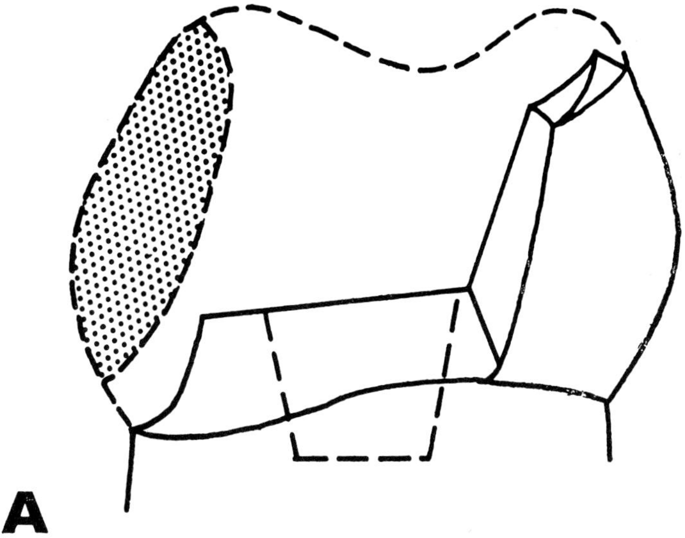

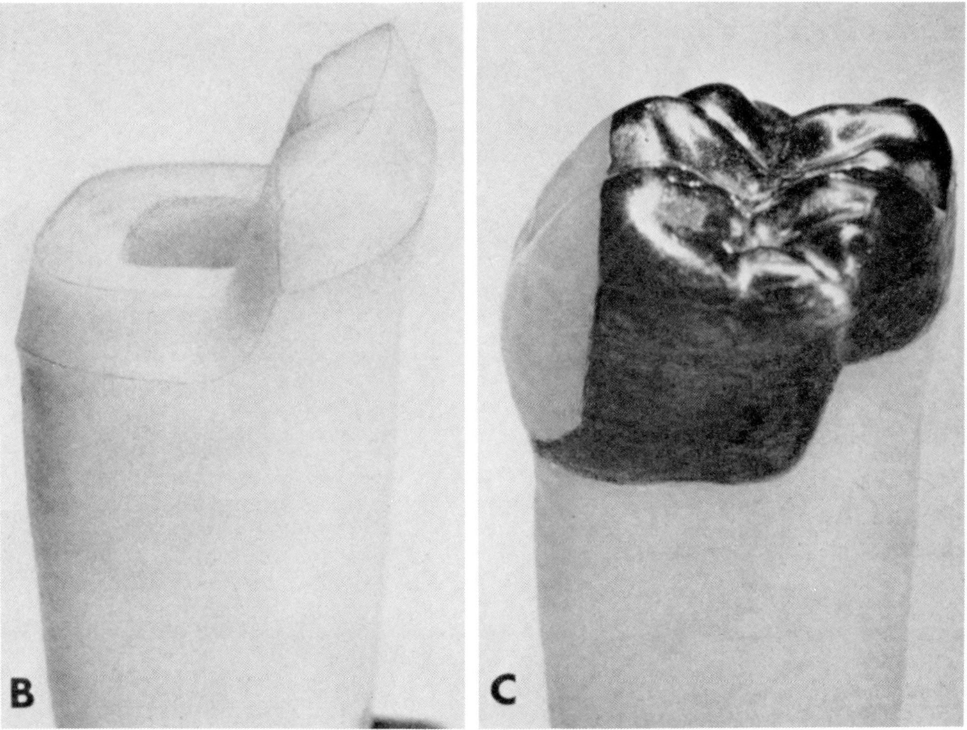

Fig. 18–3. Restoration of fractured buccal cusp with reverse three-quarter crown and dowel. Total preparation of remaining lingual cusp for full crown would have sacrificed retentive features of remaining wall. *A*, Schematic drawing of crown and dowel preparation. *B*, Completed preparation carried over lingual surface of lingual cusp. *C*, Restoration with porcelain facing cemented to place.

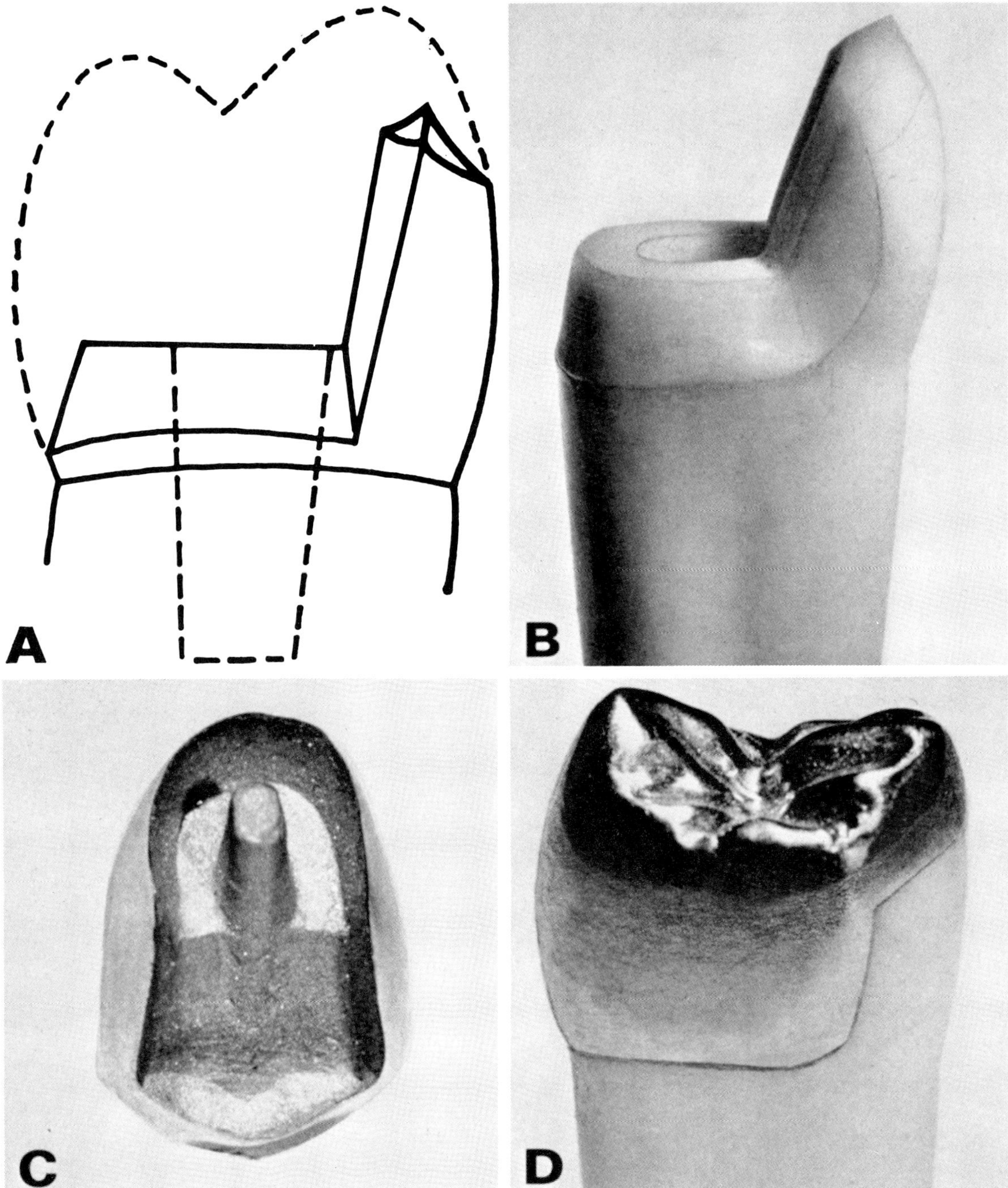

Fig. 18–4. Three-quarter crown used to restore fractured lingual cusp utilizing dowel retention. *A,* Schematic drawing emphasizing buccal cusp protection. *B,* Preparation emphasizing gingival chamfer. *C,* Internal surface of casting. Note length and bulk of dowel. *D,* Casting cemented in place. Protective features are apparent.

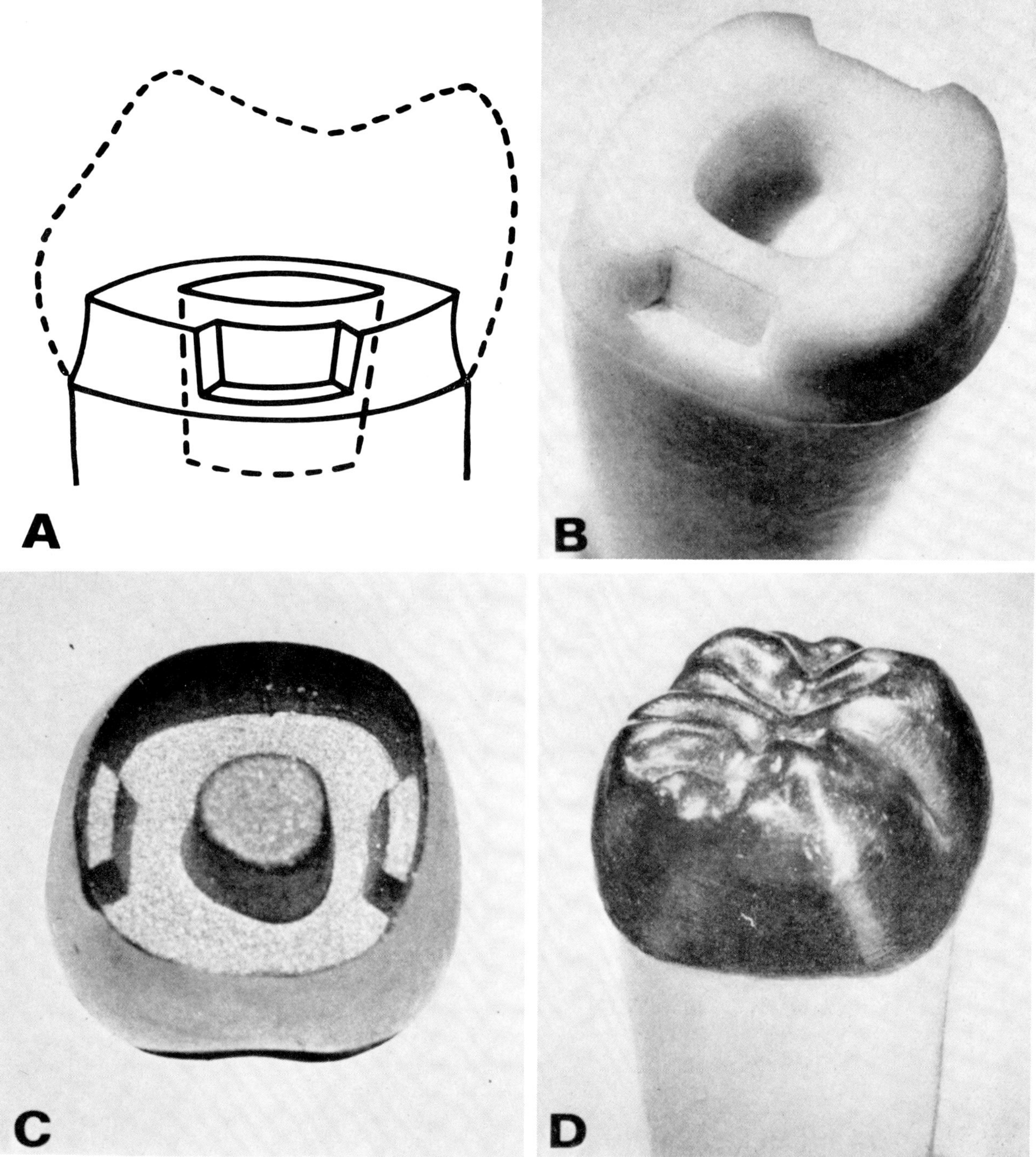

Fig. 18–5. Full crown preparation with dowel and retentive steps. *A,* Schematic drawing of preparation showing long chamfer, retentive step, and dowel preparation. *B,* Preparation showing depth and bulk of dowel preparation and steps. *C,* Internal surface of casting. *D,* Full crown casting cemented in place.

consideration can the maximum strength and retention be realized from what little usable tooth structure remains.

PRINCIPLES OF PREPARATION

Whenever the marginal ridge of a pulpless tooth is no longer intact, the buccal and lingual cusps should be capped or tied together to give the coronal portion of the tooth a ***chain of continuous strength.*** The MOD onlay is probably the most widely utilized technique employing the continuous chain principle (Fig. 18–2). Failure to cap or shoe these cusps has been the major shortcoming in restoring the tooth in which a root canal filling has been placed. The onlay preparation should be the ***minimum*** preparation for a posterior tooth with any appreciable amount of dentin destruction. The condition of the proximal walls should determine the number of surfaces to be included.

Full and Partial Coverage

The badly broken-down tooth should have full coverage whenever necessary. Many times, however, preparation for a full crown would sacrifice additional sources of retention, such as parallel walls, and would leave in its stead a frail unsupported spur of tooth (Fig. 18–3). It is obvious in such a situation that little advantage is derived from full crown preparation. Utilization of a remaining cusp adds retentive features otherwise lost. With the dowel and collar preparation, additional strength and power of retention are imparted to the tooth. This preparation is indicated after a fracture of the buccal or lingual cusp on teeth that initially were not properly protected (Fig. 18–4).

In the event full coverage is needed in a badly broken down posterior tooth additional retention may be gained by the use of retentive proximal box forms (Fig. 18–5). The more internal surface developed in the preparation, the more retention is gained. Composite resins or polycarboxylate cements should be used to extensively build up these teeth prior to cavity preparation. Zinc phosphate cements lack the crushing strength needed to withstand the forces of displacement. Self-threading pins may be placed for better retention of the resin base.

THE DOWEL PREPARATION

Whenever feasible, for additional strength and retention, the mechanical advantage of the dowel should be utilized. In preparation for the dowel, every effort should be made to obtain as much retention as possible: first, by making the dowel as long as practical, and second, by increasing the width of the walls to extend the area of lateral contact. ***There is a direct correlation between the lateral area of the dowel and the retention that it affords.***

Caution in Dowel Preparation. The basic precautionary measures in dowel preparation are as follows:

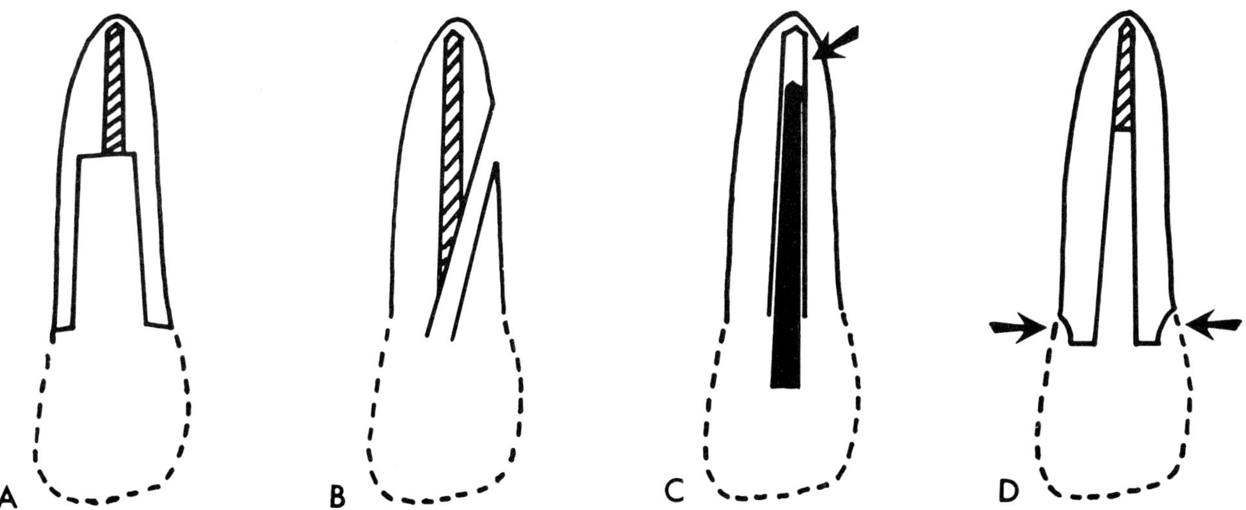

Fig. 18–6. Precautions to be observed in dowel preparation. *A,* Avoid overpreparation. *B,* Avoid lateral perforation. *C,* Avoid dislodging root canal filling material *(arrow). D,* Preparation must include retentive collar of gold *(arrows)* to encircle tooth.

1. Avoid overpreparation, which only leaves a thin shell of dentin surrounding the dowel (Fig. 18–6*A*).

2. Avoid lateral perforation by exactly planning the direction of the dowel (Fig. 18–6*B*).

3. Avoid dislodging the root canal filling material, especially when silver points have been used (Fig. 18–6*C*).

4. Improve retention and assure exact position by utilizing a collar of gold, encircling more than half the circumference of the tooth. It is necessary to tie the root portion of the dowel and the coronal aspect together (Fig. 18–6*D*).

It behooves the operator to plan ahead for restoration. Every effort is made to employ gutta percha in filling. Silver points are not recommended for obturation if a dowel is to be used.

With careful dowel preparation, an impression may be taken employing standard impression techniques, whether it be hydrocolloid, rubber base, or silicone. The dowel impression may be strengthened by inserting paper clips, tooth picks, or nylon fibers into the preparation. These measures will prevent breakage of the impression during removal of the tray.

Gerstein and Burnell have described a technique of dowel preparation in which standardized root canal reamers are used along with corresponding sizes of prefabricated precious metal precision dowels (Endopost) (Fig. 18–7).[1] This dowel is positioned in the

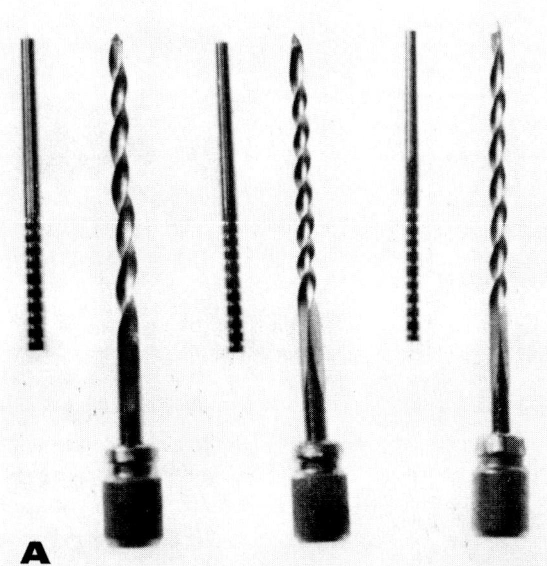

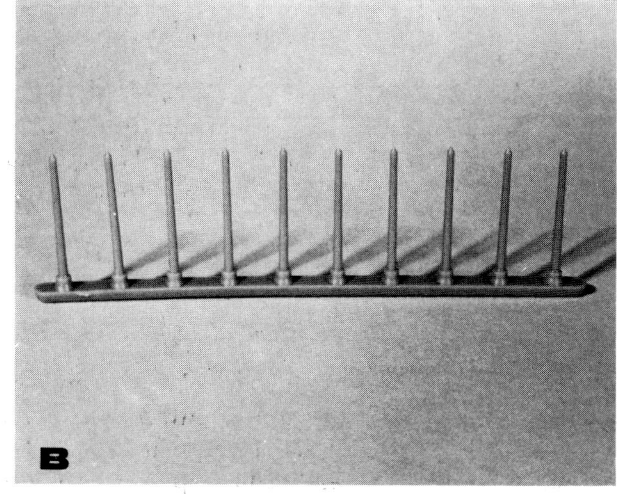

Fig. 18–7. *A,* Precious metal dowels (Endopost) manufactured to size and shape of standardized endodontic instruments. Smooth end of post perfectly fits into canal preparation, which is done with hand instruments. Safety in preparation by hand instruments over power-driven instruments is apparent. *B,* "Endowel" posts made of plastic to burn out completely at casting temperature. Available in five color-coded sizes, 80 to 140, matching standardized reamers. (Courtesy Star Dental Manufacturing Co.)

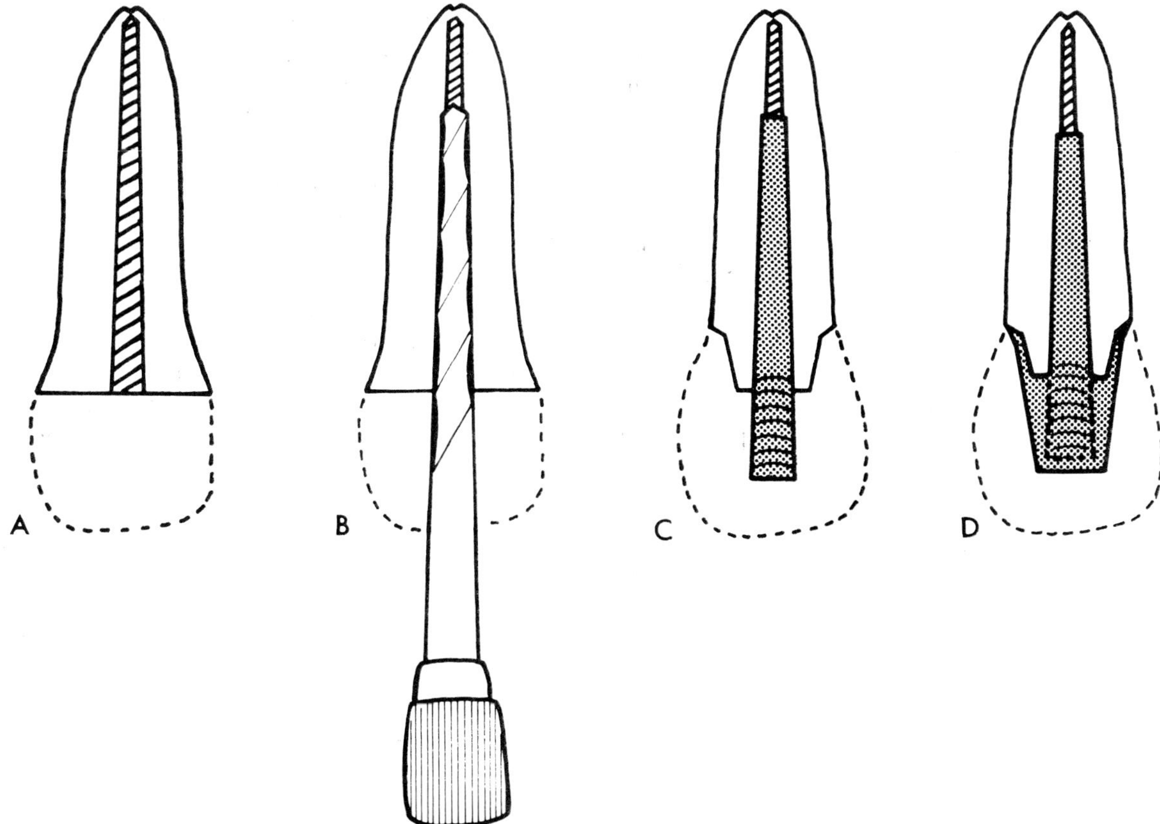

Fig. 18–8. Technique of using Endopost as suggested by Gerstein and Burnell.[1] *A,* Root canal therapy is completed and canal is totally obliterated with gutta percha. *B,* Large standardized endodontic instrument (size 70–120) is used to reprepare cavity to receive dowel. *C,* Corresponding Endopost is positioned and knurled, coronal end is shortened to proper length. Preparation of stump is completed to include a gingival retentive collar. Post is removed in impression and coronal extension is waxed and cast from laboratory model. Posts are also supplied in plastic, which burns out prior to casting. *D,* Dowel extension crown with coping is cemented to place to be restored by porcelain jacket or porcelain-faced crown.

prepared canal, it is removed in the impression, and models are poured. A laboratory technique follows in which the coronal preparation is waxed and cast to the dowel, allowing for an accurately fitting doweled restoration. This preparation is then covered by a porcelain jacket or a porcelain-faced crown (Fig. 18–8).

Restoring the Anterior Tooth

In restoring anterior teeth that have been destroyed or fractured near the gingival level, it is important that a full coping with collar and dowel be used (Fig. 18–9). The crown built up in metal can then be esthetically restored with a jacket crown. In this manner the tooth may serve in the future as a base for restorations of any type (Fig. 18–9), thus eliminating risk if the crown has to be remade, a decided advantage in full mouth rehabilitation (Fig. 18–10).

The dowel and cast extension should be used instead of the full coping when tooth structure is adequate to make a full coping unnecessary, but not sufficient for an adequate length of preparation. The dowel and cast extension also permits the tooth to be a strong restorable member as does the full coping (Fig. 18–11). Esthetic restoration, along with the freedom for future change, makes this an important technique (Fig. 18–12).

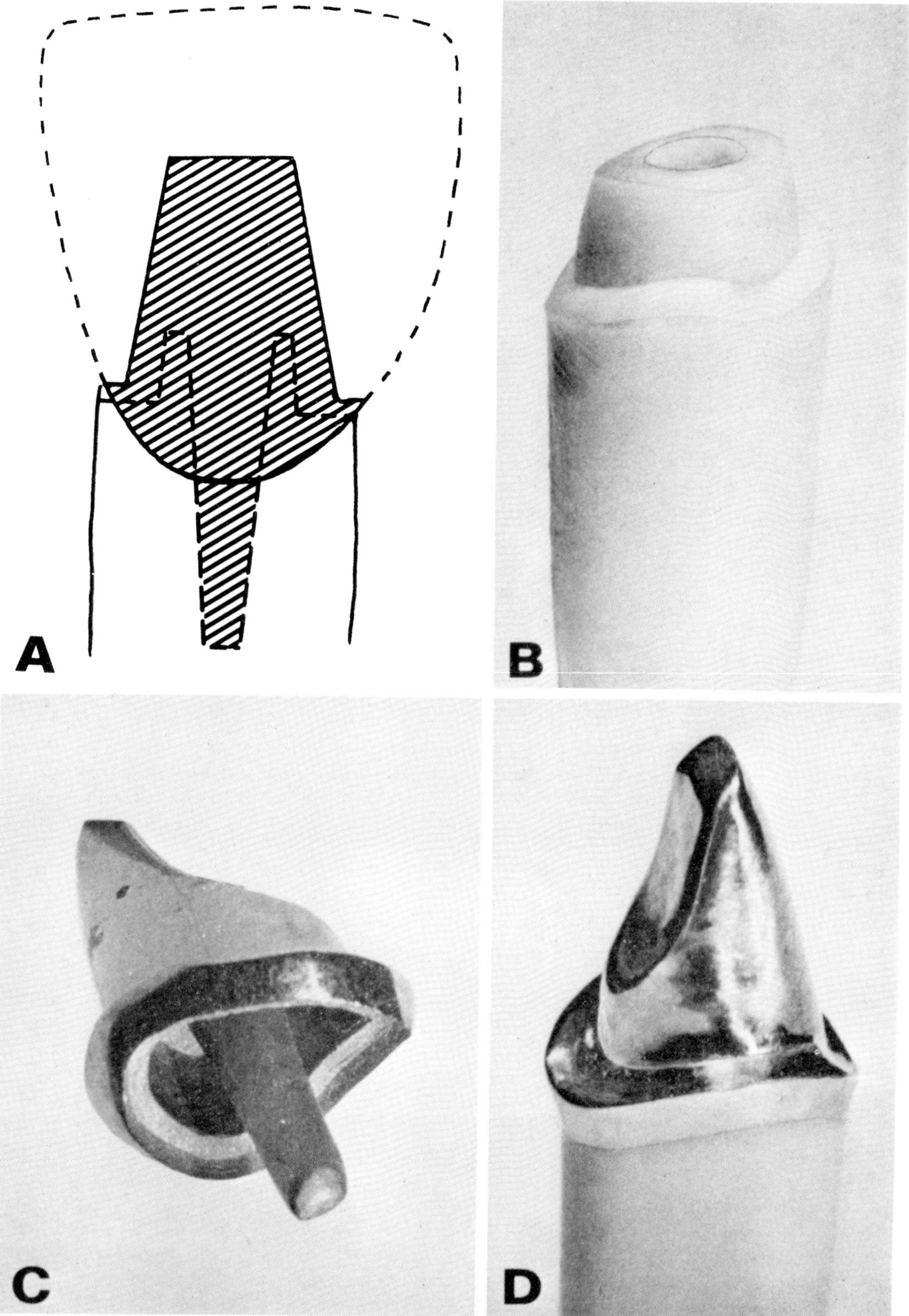

Fig. 18–9. Full coping with collar and dowel. Preparation for restoration with jacket crown. *A,* Schematic drawing of preparation and casting. *B,* Preparation which emphasizes subgingival shoulder. *C,* Internal surface of casting. Note shoulder, collar, and bulk and length of dowel. *D,* Casting cemented in place. Restoration with jacket crown will complete case.

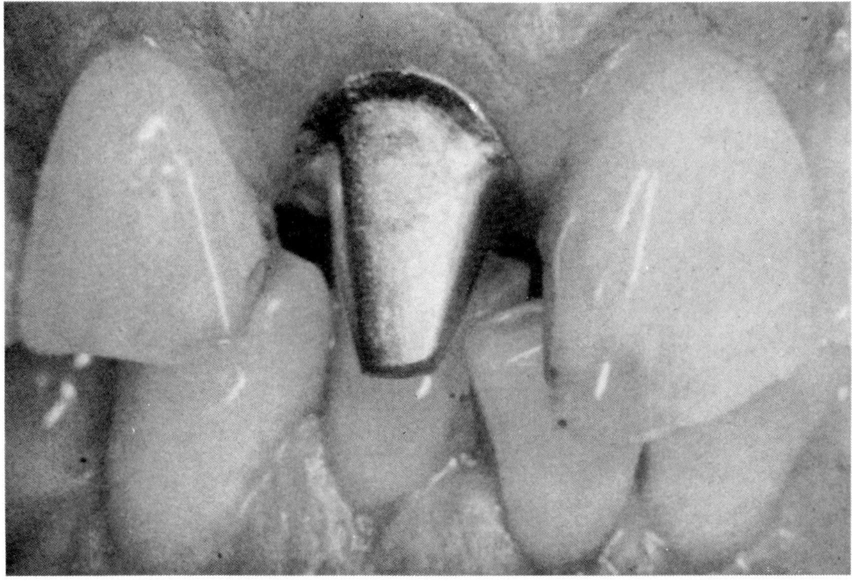

Fig. 18–10. Coping and built-up crown remains intact following second accident which fractured away previous jacket crown. Gold preparation may serve again as base for restoration with new jacket. Note excellent tissue tolerance to subgingival collar of gold.

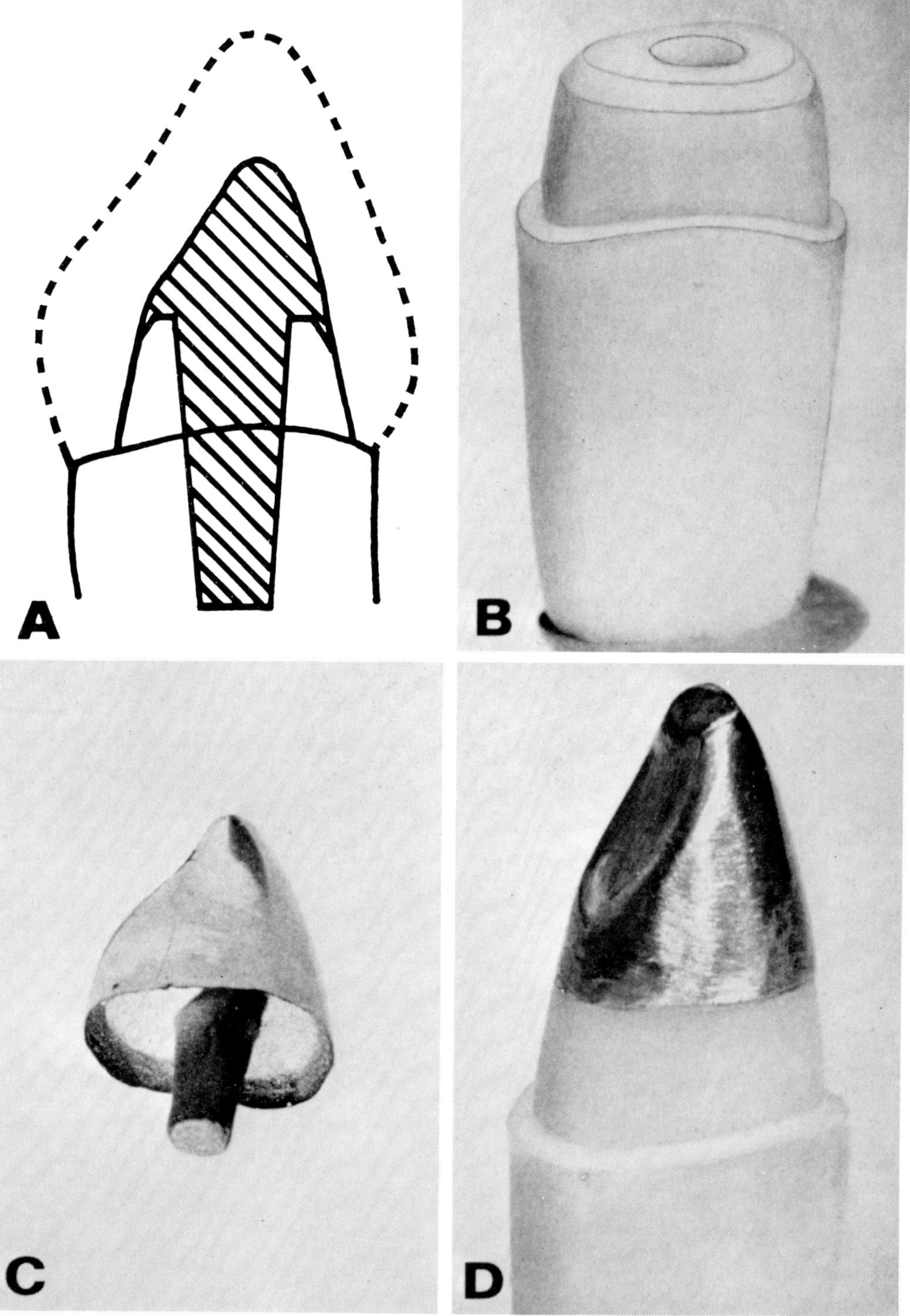

Fig. 18–11. Dowel and extension for increasing length of preparation of fractured crown. *A,* Schematic drawing. *B,* Preparation for coping to extend length of remaining tooth. *C,* Internal surface of casting. Note collar and bulk and length of dowel. *D,* Casting cemented in place ready for impression for jacket coverage.

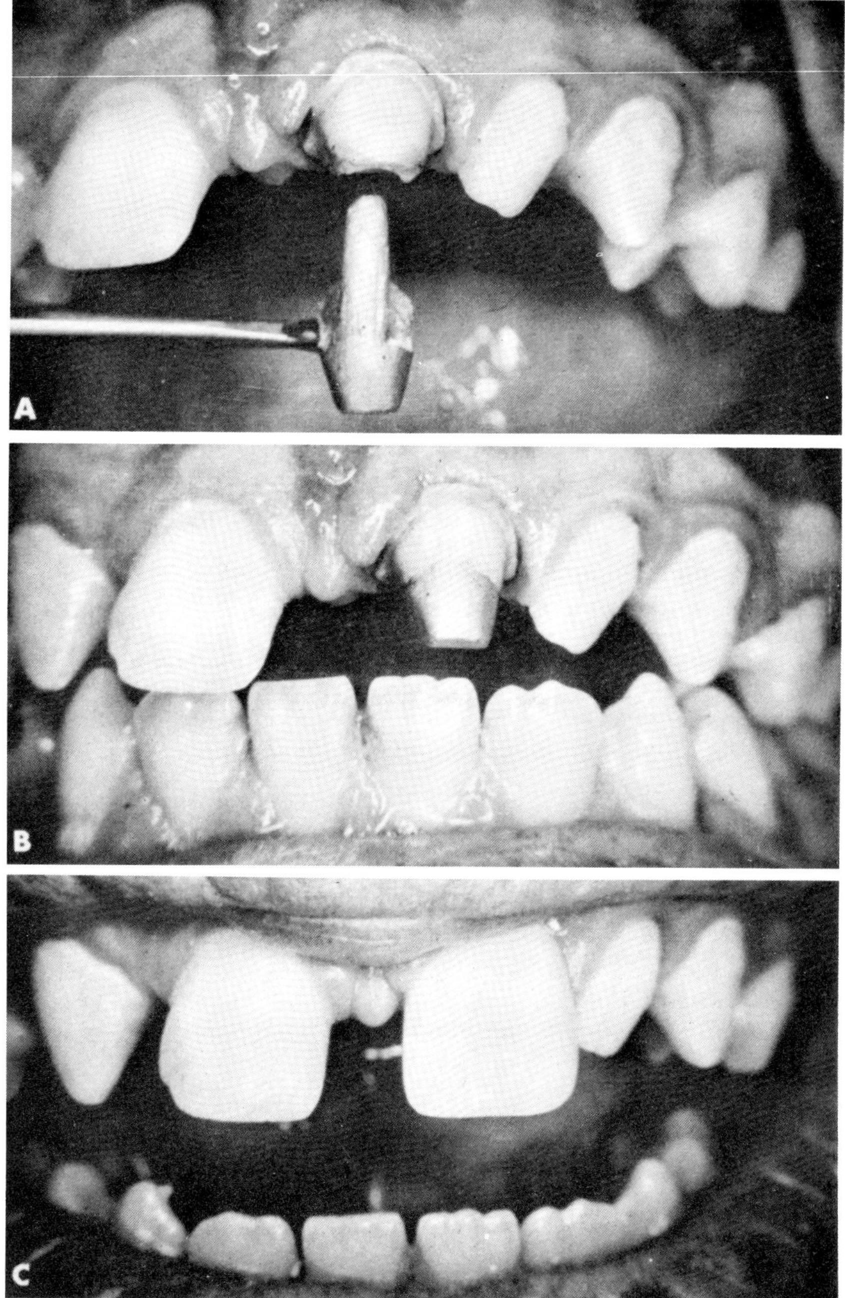

Fig. 18–12. Restoration of fractured central incisor in 12-year-old boy just prior to orthodontic therapy. Richmond crown is contraindicated because of possibility that later changes will be necessary. *A,* Dowel and crown extension is being carried to place into preparation. *B,* Cast extension of preparation allows flexibility for necessary future changes. *C,* Jacket crown restoring fractured incisor. Orthodontic treatment may now be undertaken.

Double Abutments

Many a condemned pulpless tooth could have served as an abutment for a fixed or removable partial denture. By judicious double-abutting, the strength of the adjacent tooth is imparted to its weaker neighbor (Fig. 18–13). The advantage of the multiple-abutting should be considered if any doubt exists as to the dependability of the restored broken-down pulpless tooth. This method is also recommended for the support of periodontally involved teeth strengthened through the use of the endodontic implant.

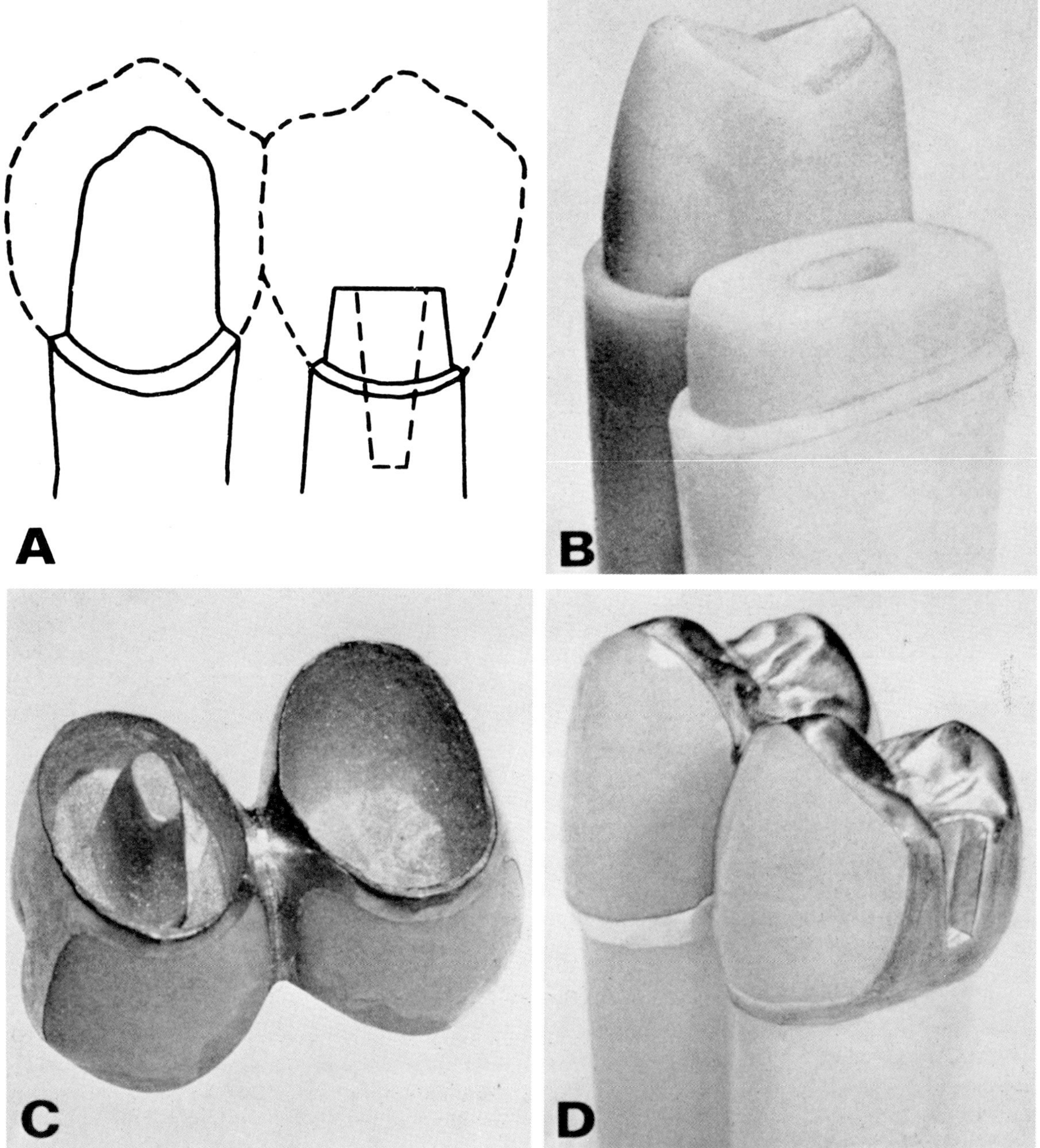

Fig. 18–13. Double abutment to impart additional strength to pulpless tooth. *A*, Schematic drawing showing full crown preparation, and dowel crown preparation on pulpless tooth. *B*, Preparation with subgingival retentive collar. *C*, Internal surface of soldered castings with porcelain facings. *D*, Porcelain-faced crowns cemented in place. Partial denture retentive rest in pulpless distal abutment.

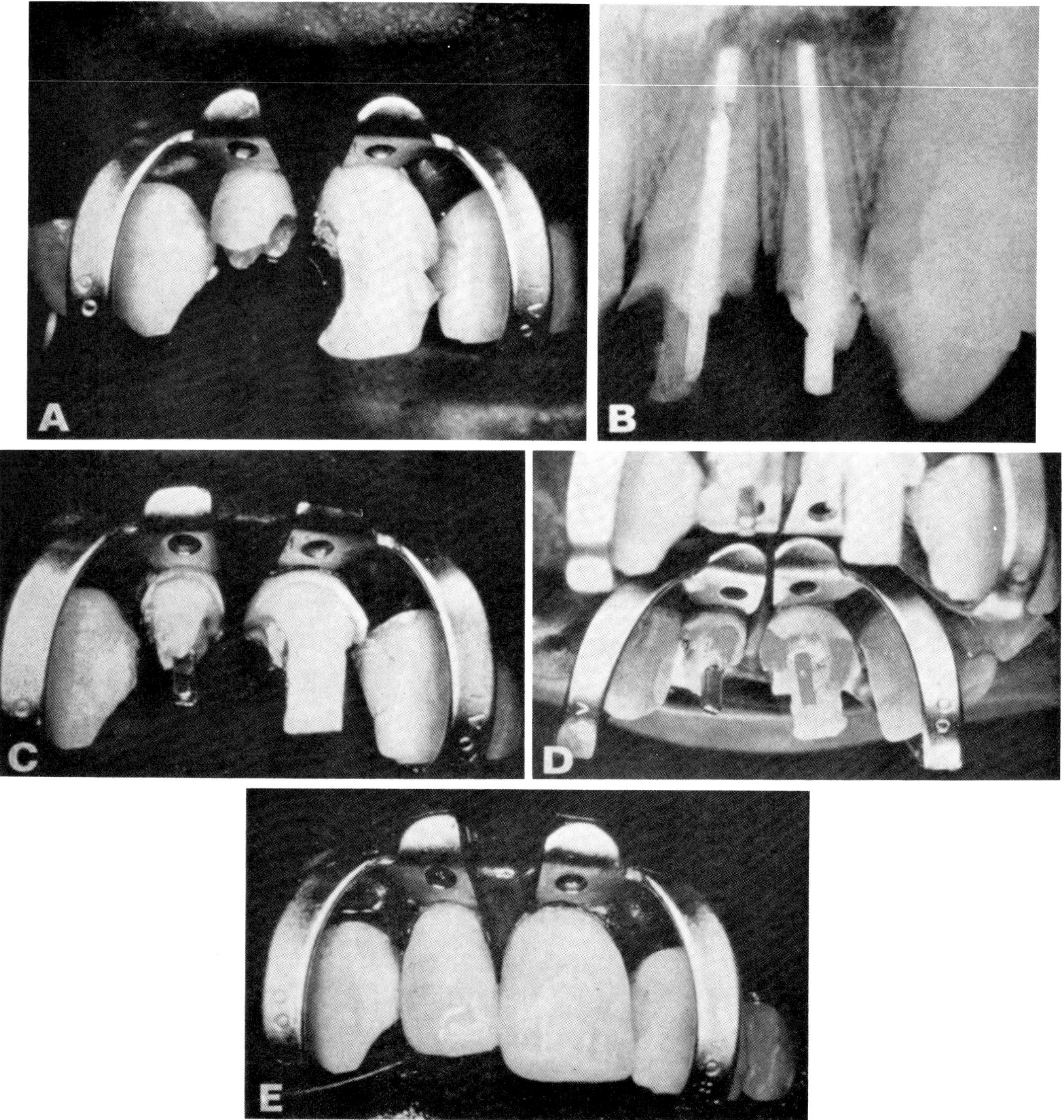

Fig. 18–14. Provisional restoration for esthetics in adolescent girl. *A*, Pulpless maxillary incisors decimated by dental caries. *B*, Root canal therapy completed and retentive posts cemented to place. *C*, Crown preparation with finishing shoulder apparent. *D*, Lingual mirror view of completed preparation which shows importance of rubber dam clamp placement. *E*, Esthetic, plastic, provisional restorations. Care must be exercised in finishing to leave no flashings past gingival should which would act as tissue irritants. (Courtesy Dr. F. Lloyd Jacobson.)

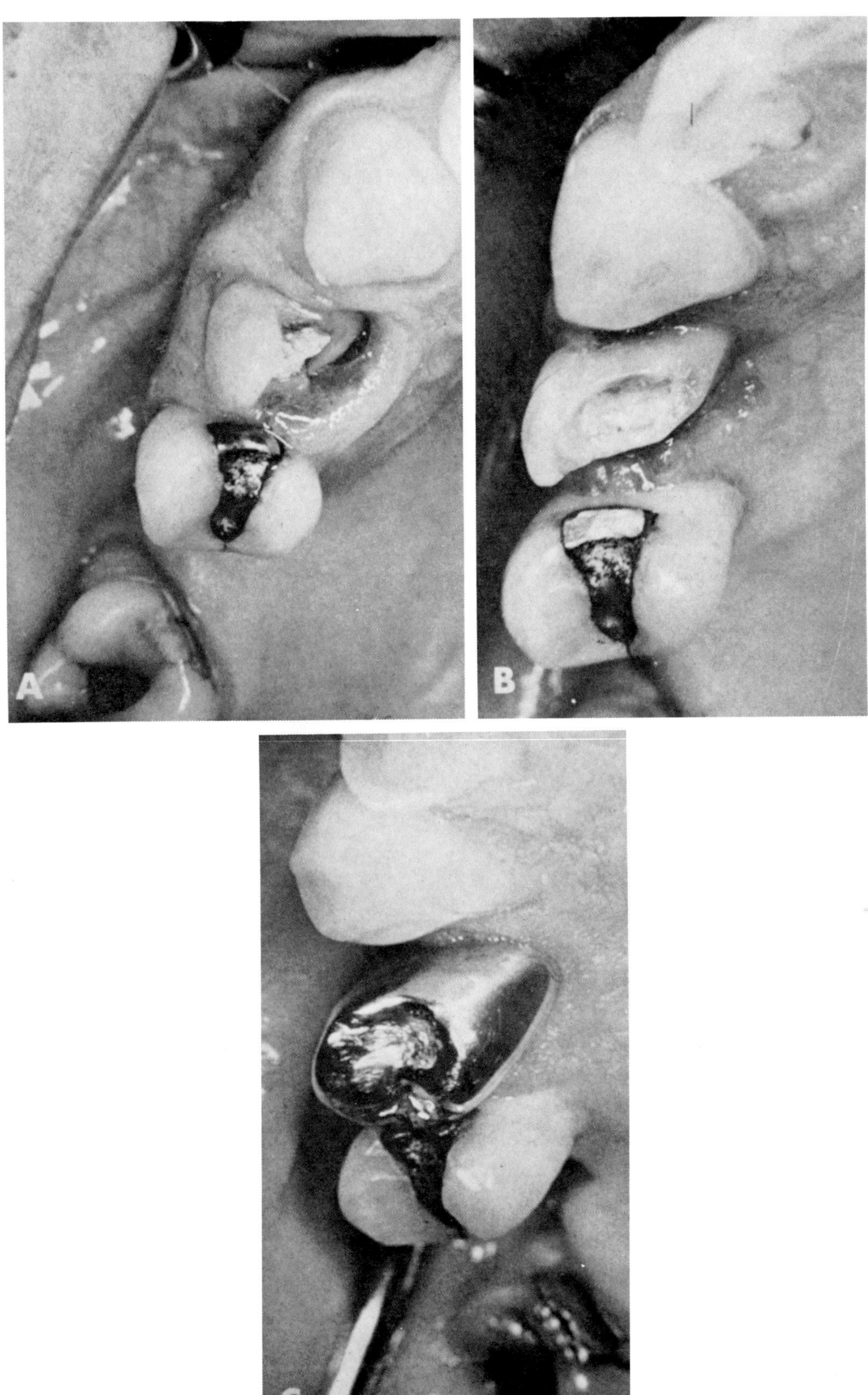

Fig. 18–15. Periodontal preparation for restoration of fractured pulpless premolar. *A*, Subgingival fracture could have been prevented by protective restoration. *B*, Palatal gingivoplasty exposes depth of fracture, allowing operator to establish lingual finish line for preparation. *C*, Three-quarter crown restoration with healthy gingival adaptation.

Provisional Restoration

Frequently the dentist sees a dentition that is decimated by rampant dental caries. Teeth are fractured away, pulps exposed and carious lesions involve over half the tooth (Fig. 18–14*A*). The adolescent, often in the lower income group, is the most pathetic victim of this destruction. In the past, full-mouth extractions and dentures were the only future available to these youngsters. Today, these cases can be treated by root canal therapy (Fig. 18–14*B*) and restored provisionally with quick-setting plastics in crown forms. Dowels should be used to strengthen the crowns, and care taken to establish a definite finish line, so that a flashing of plastic will not extend as a gingival irritant (Fig. 18–14*C,D*). Following this esthetic restoration, the improvement in personality exhibited by these young people is heartwarming (Fig. 18–14*E*).

Periodontal Consideration

Periodontal therapy is needed to preserve the tooth that has been fractured below the gingiva or the alveolar crest. Invariably, the cusp fracture extends subgingivally. By performing a gingivectomy (and osteoplasty, if necessary for preparation access), it is possible to retain an otherwise condemned tooth (Fig. 18–15). If necessary, the tooth may also be "elongated" by orthodontic movement (see Chap. 16).

Summary

It is important to remember that root canal filling alone is not the final effort in the preservation of a pulpless tooth. Consideration must be given various restorative and periodontal techniques to protect the pulpless tooth or to restore the fractured tooth which previously was not properly restored.

Failure to consider the coronal restoration of the pulpless tooth at the time of the endodontic therapy is a disservice to the patient. Moreover, the patient should be advised of the necessity of this coronal protection during the original diagnosis. Every available technique should be considered to restore the tooth properly with the permanence that is its due. All too often we are so blinded by success at the apical level that we allow coronal destruction to occur.

PREPARATION FOR THE OVERDENTURE

"The overdenture is a complete denture supported by retained teeth and the residual alveolar ridge."[2]

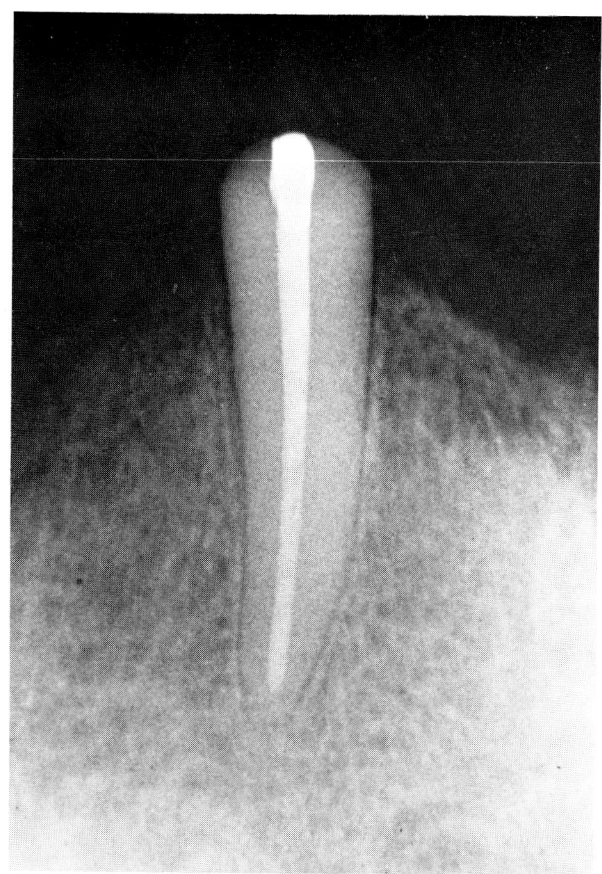

Fig. 18–16. Overdenture abutment, well obturated and restored with amalgam. Notice excellent bony support. (Courtesy Dr. David H. Wands.)

Because the "retained teeth" are shortened, contoured, and altered to be covered, root canal therapy is imperative to their retention (Fig. 18–16).

In 1969, Lord and Teel coined the term "overdenture" and described the combined endodontic-periodontic-prosthodontic technique applied thereto.[3] As early as 1916, however, Prothero had referred to the use of root support, stating, ". . . Oftentimes two or three widely separated roots or teeth can be utilized for supporting a denture."[4] It should also be noted that much earlier, in 1789, George Washington's first lower denture, constructed of ivory by John Greenwood, retained a left mandibular premolar.[5]

Retaining roots in the alveolar process is based on the proved observation that as long as the root remains, the bone surrounding it remains (Fig. 18–17). This overcomes the age-old prosthetic prob-

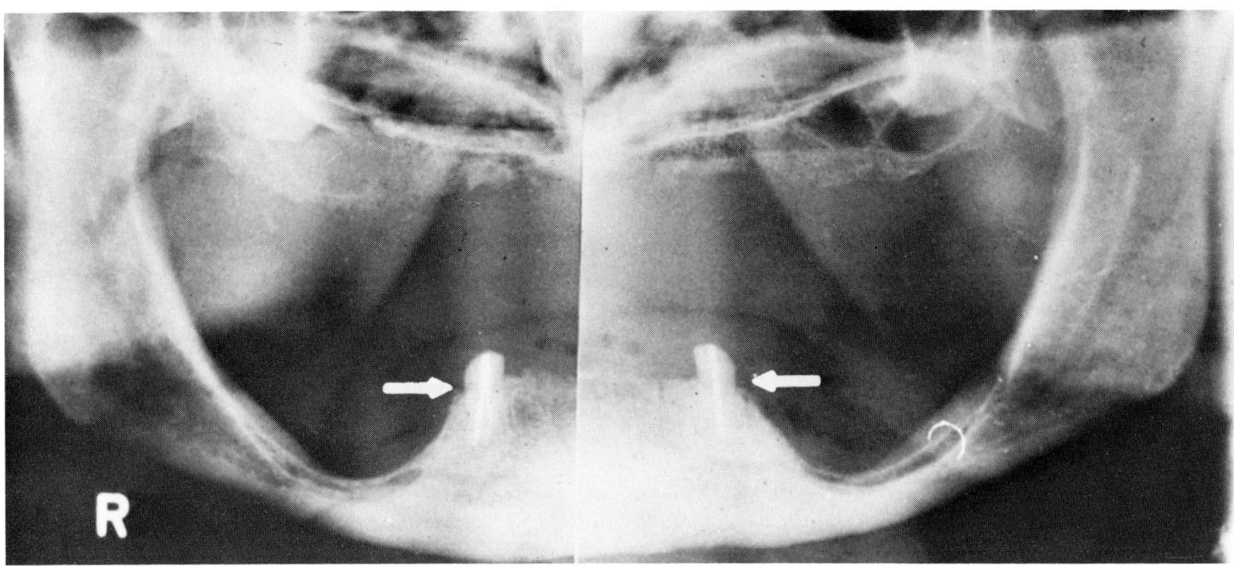

Fig. 18–17. Dramatic demonstration of alveolar bone remaining around retained canines and badly resorbed under full upper and posterior lower partial dentures. (From Lord, J. L., and Teel, S.: J. Prosth. Dent., *32*: 41–51, July, 1974.)

lem of ridge resorption. Ideally, then, retaining four teeth, two molars and two canines—one each at the four divergent points of an arch—should guarantee perfect balance and long "life" to a full overdenture. Unfortunately, patients requiring prostheses seldom present just these ideal conditions, and the dentist must make-do with the best he can devise from the dentition that remains. One situation to be warned against, however, is the diagonal cross-arch arrangement—a molar abutment on one side, for example, and a canine on the opposite side. The rocking and torquing action set up by this arrangement leads to problems and loss of one or both abutments. The molar abutment alone is preferable to the diagonal cross-arch situation.

If the selected abutment teeth are reduced to a short rounded or bullet shape—literally "tucking" the abutments inside the denture base— the crown-root ratio of the tooth is vastly improved, especially when periodontally involved teeth have lost some alveolar support. Bone loss dangerously lengthens the crown lever arm of the crown-root ratio. These loosened teeth are often too weak to serve as abutments for removable partial dentures. As shortened teeth, however, they will serve admirably as abutments for full overdentures.

Indications and Advantages. The indications for overdenture include the psychic support some patients receive from ***not*** being totally edentulous. Even more important is the preservation of the alveolar ridge and the shielding of the ridge from stress provided by firm abutment teeth. One should also be aware that vertical dimension is better preserved if ridge height is maintained. A bonus to all these advantages is the support, the stability and retention derived from firm abutments. All these advantages are heightened in the young patient doomed to dentures for years to come.

Complete overdentures should be considered for virtually every patient for whom full-mouth extractions are indicated. Some of these "hopeless" teeth can be treated and retained as abutments to support an overdenture, especially when opposed by natural teeth or a removable partial denture. The overdenture better resists the occlusal forces that can be exerted by the natural teeth than does the full denture completely tissue-borne. Some attribute this resistance to the proprioceptive sensory mechanism derived from the retained roots under the overdenture. Application of the overdenture to partial denture support is also indicated, even if only one abutment is available.

Contraindications. The overdenture technique is contraindicated when remaining alveolar support is so lacking that no tooth can be retained very long. Conversely, overdentures are contraindicated if the remaining natural teeth are adequate to restore the mouth with fixed or removable partial dentures. It should be no pathway to expediency.

Abutment Tooth Selection. "A healthy abutment tooth for an overdenture must have minimal mobility, a manageable sulcus depth, and an adequate band of attached gingiva."[2]

If these prerequisites are lacking, pocket depth can be reduced and attached gingiva developed by proper periodontal procedures.

Abutment Tooth Location. The ideal teeth to retain are those whose occlusal forces wreak greatest destruction upon the ridges. Opposite a natural dentition, the canine teeth are ideal to retain. In edentulous patients, the anterior portion of the arches are particularly susceptible to resorption, so canines and premolars are again first choice to be saved, with incisors second choice. It is especially important to save mandibular teeth because of difficulties encountered in retaining lower dentures. Even saving a single tooth, a molar in particular, may contribute greatly to long-term denture success.

Technique. After the selection of the proper abutment teeth, the key to successful overdenture

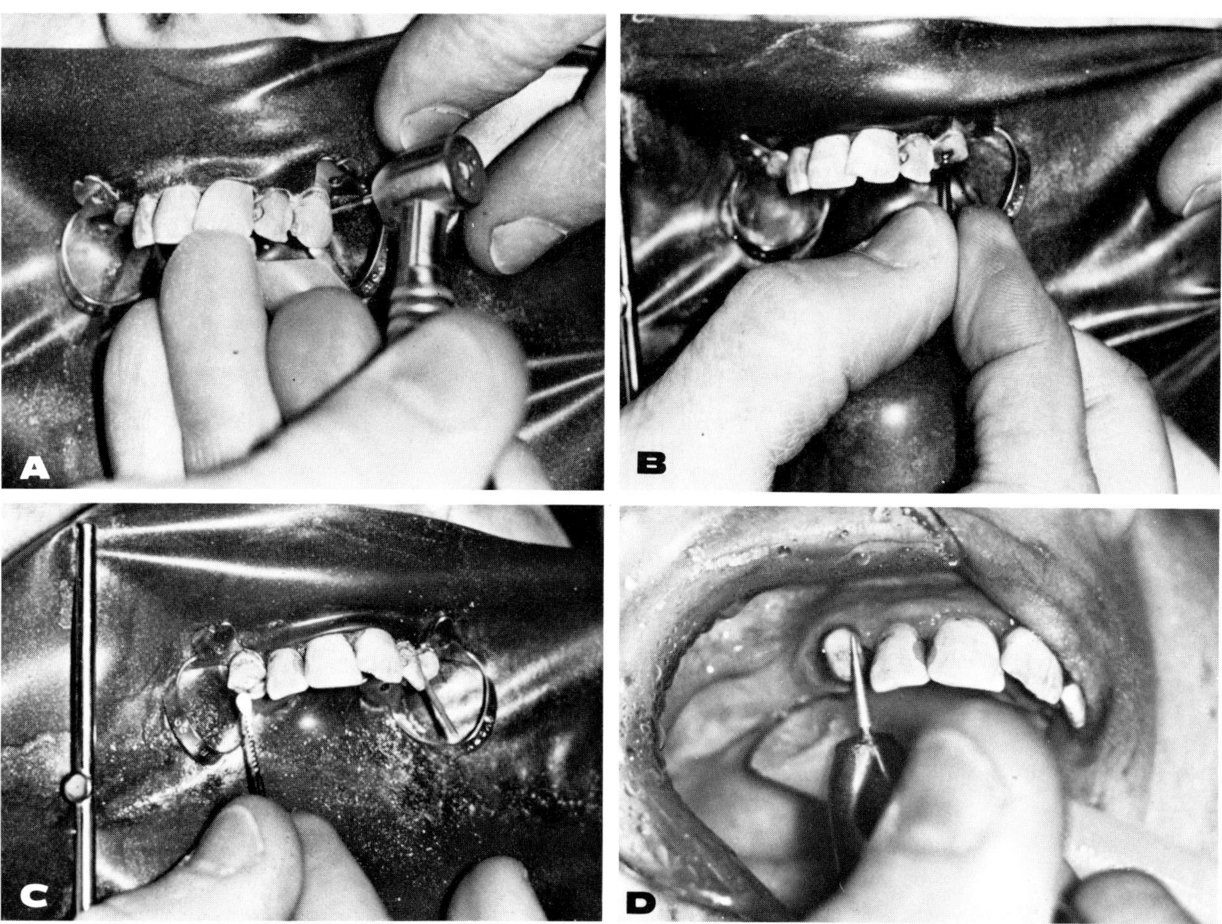

Fig. 18–18. *A,* Under anesthesia and rubber dam, vital abutment teeth are sectioned 3 to 4 mm. from cervical. *B,* Unconventional access to canal greatly simplifies pulpectomy, cleaning and shaping canal. Establishing length of tooth is imperative. *C,* Canals are obturated with sealer and gutta percha laterally condensed. *D,* Following placement of amalgam restoration, stump is properly shaped. Top of preparation should be about 3 mm. above sulcus depth. If gingival surgery is necessary, tissue will shrink. (From Lord, J. L. and Teel, S.: J. Prosth. Dent., *32*:41–51, July, 1974.)

construction is simplicity of technique. If an immediate denture is to be placed, the endodontic therapy, extractions, and periodontal treatment may all be done at the insertion appointment. The teeth to receive root canal fillings are anesthetized and a rubber dam placed. The crowns of these teeth are then amputated 3 to 4 mm. above the gingival level. With an endodontic instrument, the length of the remaining tooth is established radiographically, and the pulps are removed. The canals are then properly cleaned, shaped, and obturated with gutta percha, by means of the filling technique appropriate to the canal anatomy (Fig. 18–18*A, B, C*). The coronal 5 to 6 mm. of the gutta percha filling is then removed, the preparation is undercut, and a well-condensed amalgam filling is placed to cap the canal obturation. At this time as well, the abutments should be properly shaped to rise 2 to 3 mm. above the tissue (Fig. 18–18*D*), and to be rounded or bullet-shaped with a slope back from the labial to accommodate the denture tooth to be set above it. They should then be highly polished (Fig. 18–19). The abutments must not be too short or the tissue will grow over them as a

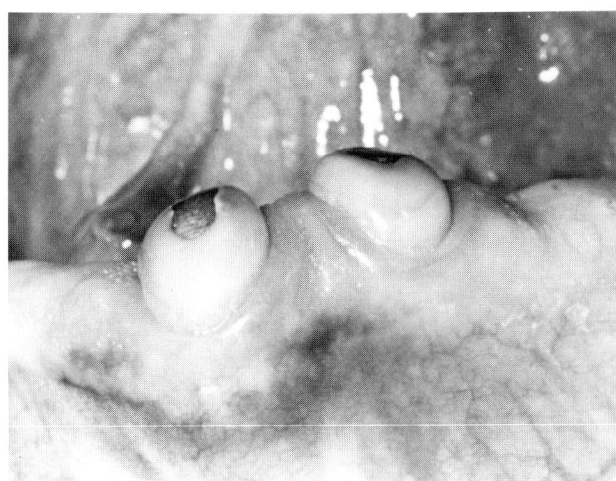

Fig. 18–19. Overdenture abutment teeth at two-year recall. Note glassy smooth surface, bullet shape, well condensed amalgam filling, and healthy attached gingiva. (Courtesy Dr. David H. Wands.)

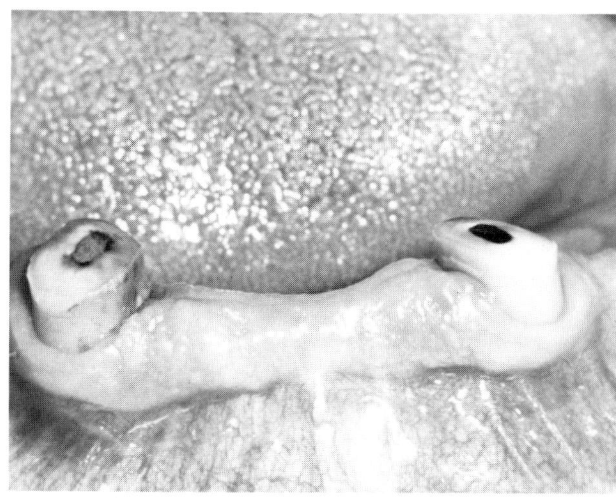

Fig. 18–20. Improperly contoured overdenture abutments. Square edge invites grip by overdenture and torquing action. Prominent buccal contour and extra height compromised contour of overdenture. (Courtesy Dr. David H. Wands.)

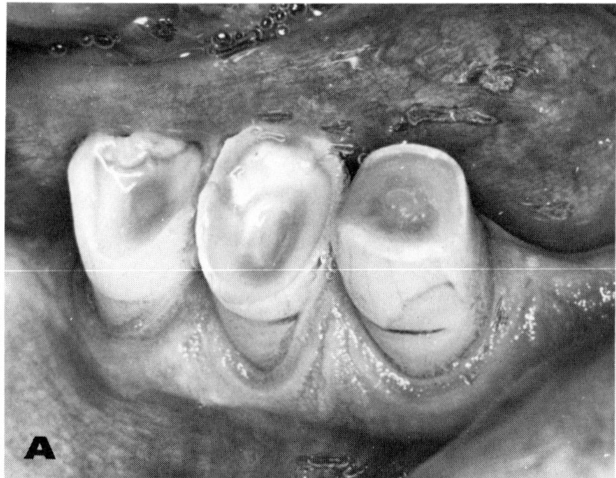

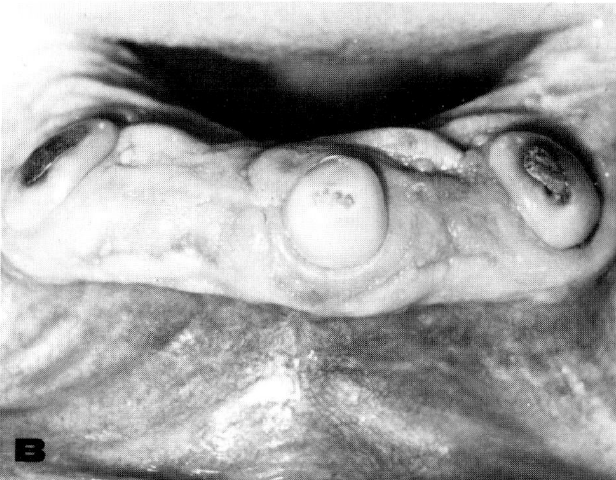

Fig. 18–21. *A,* Vital teeth with severe abrasion and receded pulps—ideal overdenture abutments. *B,* Incisor overdenture abutment which did not require root canal therapy due to pulp recession. Calcified pulp area should be carefully explored for pulp horn. (Courtesy Dr. David H. Wands.)

"lawn grows over a sidewalk";[2] nor should they be too long, compromising the denture contour and placing greater stress on the supporting teeth (Fig. 18–20).

The denture is relieved over the abutment teeth until it fits securely on the tissue without touching the abutment teeth. It is then related to the abutment teeth with a small amount of self-curing acrylic. This proper relationship of denture to tissue and tooth is important for denture stability and to keep the stresses on the teeth within physiologic limits.

This entire operation is neither complex nor time consuming. Removing the crown from the tooth greatly simplifies and speeds the endodontic therapy and should materially reduce the fee as well. Some candidates for overdenture abutment teeth may not need root canal therapy. The pulpless teeth may already have been successfully treated. Other teeth may be so abraded that the pulp has receded to a level where the tooth only needs shortening, proper contouring, and polishing (Fig. 18–21). This, too, reduces the cost to the patient.

In the event the abutment teeth are involved periodontally or are not surrounded by a good collar of attached gingiva, periodontal therapy will be needed to correct these aberrations (Fig. 18–22).

Problems. A number of problems have arisen with overdentures, most of them related to poor case selection and lack of patient cooperation.

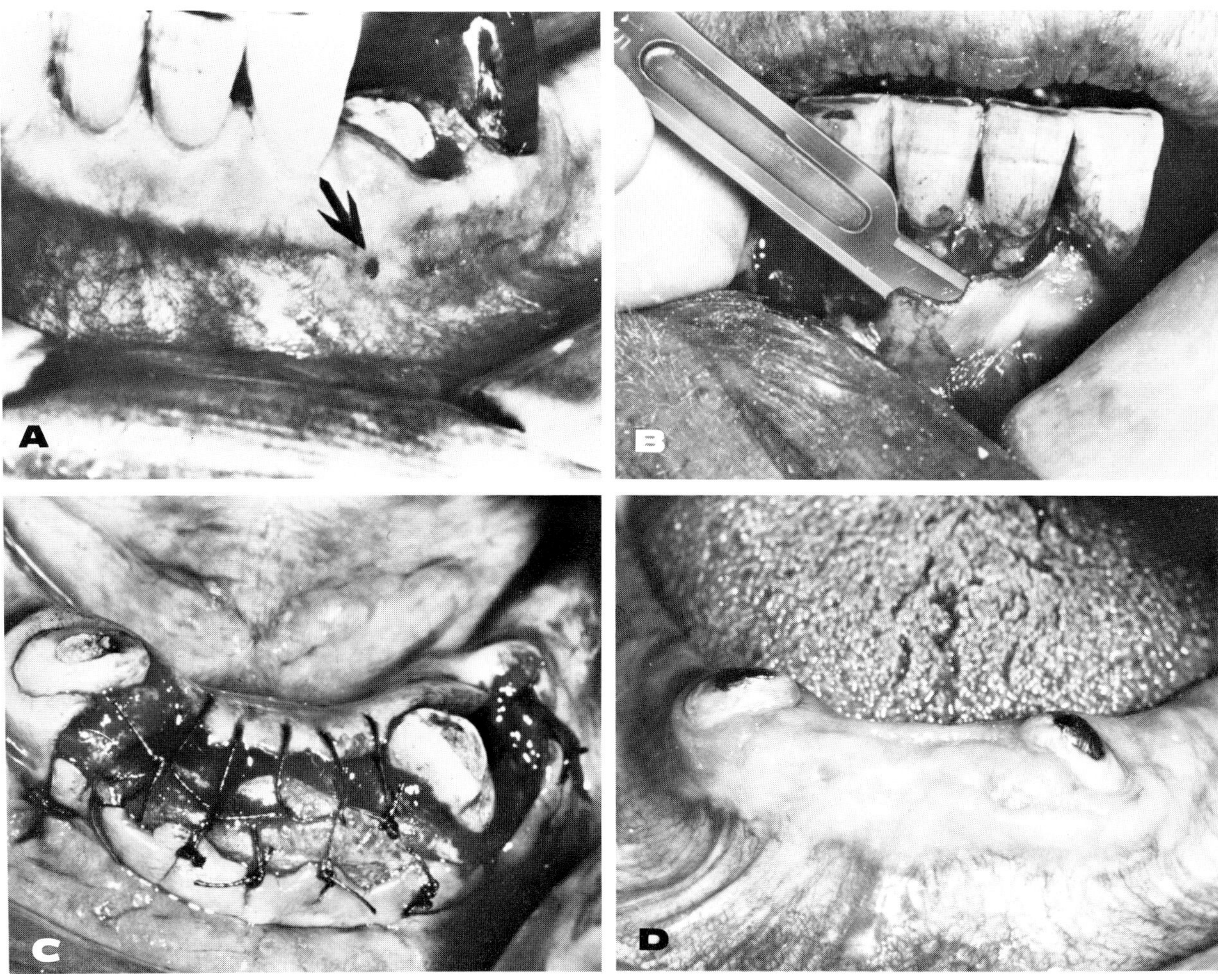

Fig. 18–22. *A,* Pocket depth marked *(arrow)* on labial gingiva of prepared overdenture abutment tooth transverses mucogingival junction. Periodontal preparation is necessary. *B,* Sharp dissection is used to retract flap, leaving periosteum intact. *C,* Incisors are extracted, and labial flap is apically repositioned and sutured to periosteum. Labial periodontal pockets are eliminated and wider band of attached gingiva established. *D,* Three-year follow-up reveals wide band of gingiva attached labially to overdenture abutments and covering anterior residual ridge. (From Lord, J. L., and Teel, S.: J. Prosth. Dent., *32*:41–51, July, 1974.)

In the first instance, it has been found that teeth close together (Fig. 18–23) make poor abutments, that tissue and bone between the teeth break down from the stress applied. Another problem is the matter of torquing rotation that centers around one abutment, usually a mandibular anterior tooth.

The most serious problems, however, are concerned with dental caries and periodontal disease. One must remember that, throughout their lives, candidates for full dentures have usually been neglectful of their teeth and supporting structures and have a history of extensive dental disease. That is why they have reached this sad point (Fig. 18–24*A*,*B*). In recommending overdentures, the dentist takes an obvious chance that the patient's habits will change, and that he will become motivated and adept at oral hygiene to retain the vestiges of his dentition. That some do not should come as no surprise (Fig. 18–25). The importance of good home care must be emphasized to the overdenture patient—scrubbing the abutments and surrounding tissue at least once a day as well as scrubbing the inside of the denture.

This does not seem to be asking too much, but apparently it is. The Department of Prosthodontics at the University of Southern California recently recalled their original 50 overdenture cases for long-term evaluation.[6] The average case had been in place

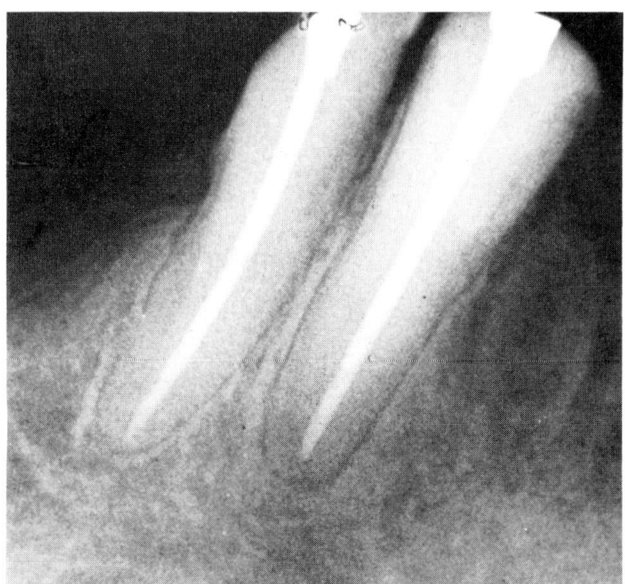

Fig. 18–23. Two mandibular overdenture abutment teeth too close together. Interproximal tissue and bone tend to break down from overdenture stresses. (Courtesy Dr. David H. Wands.)

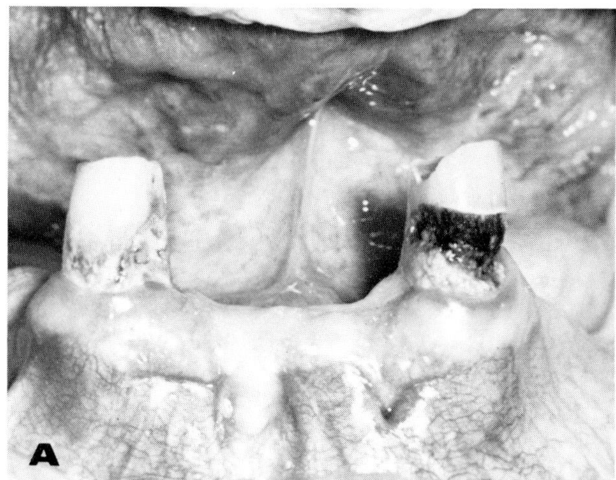

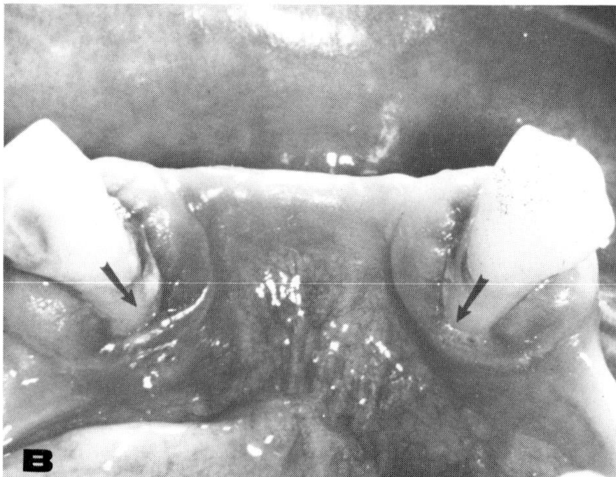

Fig. 18–24. *A*, Rather typical neglect by many denture patients. Caries and periodontal disease forecast probable lack of future patient cooperation. *B*, Mirror view of lingual gingiva of two possible overdenture abutments. Because it is virtually impossible to develop attached gingiva in area, use of these teeth as abutments is ***contraindicated.*** (Courtesy Dr. David H. Wands.)

19 months and some of the cases as long as four years. Although only two teeth were lost among the 50 patients with 131 support teeth, the prosthodontists were not pleased with the periodontal condition around the abutments. Attached gingiva was lost in over 40% of the patients. It is interesting that the cases judged "failing" by the prosthodontists were "functioning satisfactorily" as far as the patients were concerned. Caries was also a problem, but of a lesser nature.

Possible Solution to the Problems. Quite naturally the prime solution to the caries-periodontal problem is better patient cooperation in home care. Recently a special fluoride gel has been introduced to be placed in the "well" in the base plate to remineralize the dentin. This, of course, will do nothing for periodontal disease, which can only be controlled by plaque removal and by proper and equal force placed on the abutments. More frequent denture relines may also be required.

Another solution to the caries problem is to construct cast copings to cover and properly contour the abutment teeth (Fig. 18–26). However, this seems to be an expensive solution to a problem that might have been solved with a toothbrush.

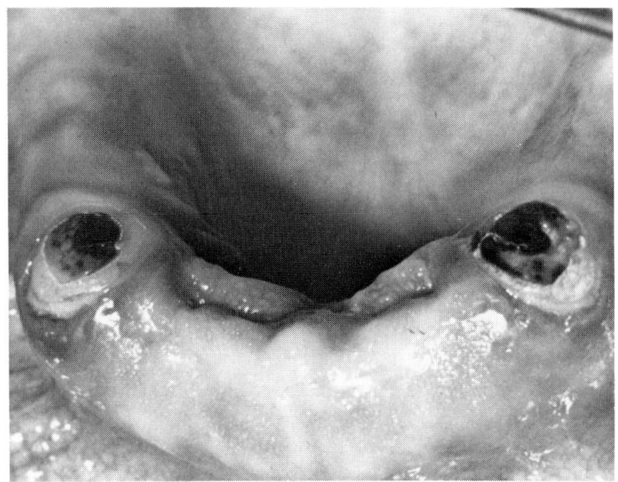

Fig. 18–25. Two-year recall reveals advanced caries and periodontal disease of abutments. Patient did not remove denture for days at a time. (Courtesy Dr. David H. Wands.)

A possible solution to inadequate denture retention or to the rotational problem centering around the single anterior abutment tooth may be with denture attachments. There are a number on the market usually named for their designer. One of the problems with attachments, of course, is increased cost for the attachments themselves and the cost, time, and effort required for placement.

Two of the attachments, the Gerber and Rotherman types, require placing the male portion of the attachment in the tooth. The female portion is processed in the denture (Fig. 18–27). In the Zest attachment, this is reversed, with the female portion in the tooth (Fig. 18–28). These attachments all have an added disadvantage, which is the extensive tooth preparation needed. This may be too much for a narrow mandibular anterior tooth. Perforations may also be a problem with the overzealous. There is no question that some patients may feel more secure having their overdentures attached, although in the majority of cases, it should be quite unnecessary.

One final problem and solution should also be considered—the apparently hopeless periodontally involved abutment tooth. Frank has recommended that endodontic implants be used to extend the length, and thus the life, of these seriously involved teeth (Fig. 18–29).

In any event, one comes to appreciate even more the importance of retaining the natural dentition rather than making such a heroic stand to retain a poor substitute.

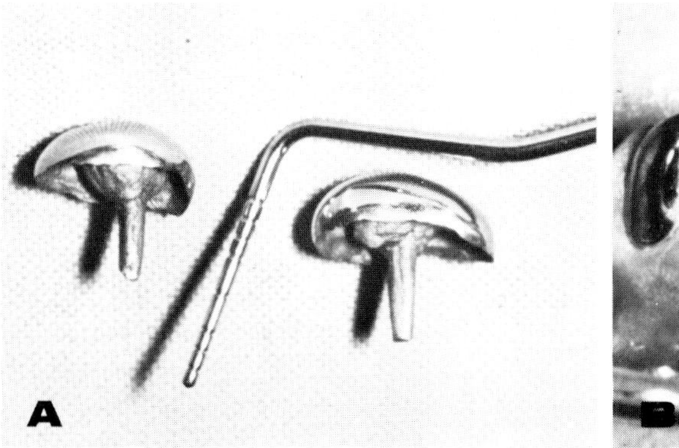

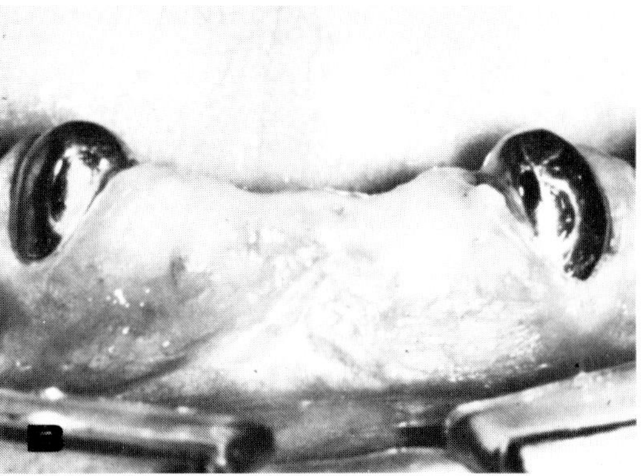

Fig. 18–26. *A,* Cast post and copings, properly contoured and polished to restore abutment teeth. *B,* Two-year recall shows healthy response to this ideal, albeit expensive, restorative method. (From Lord, J. L., and Teel, S.: Dent. Clin. N. Amer., *13*:871–881, 1969.)

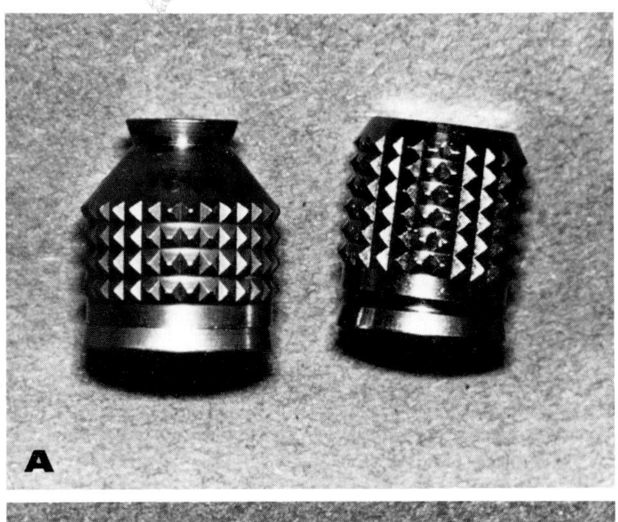

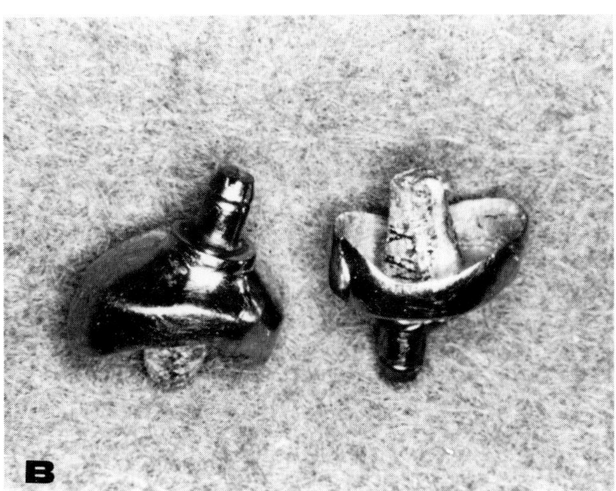

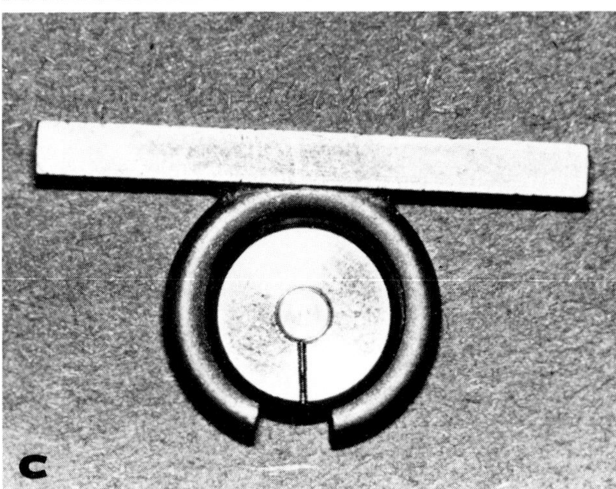

Fig. 18–27. *A,* Female portion of Gerber attachment to be embedded in denture. Denture contour and tooth placement may be compromised to provide room for attachment. *B,* Male portion of Gerber attachment positioned by cast post and coping. Obvious expense of construction figures highly in decisions of utilization. *C,* Rotherman attachment similar to clothing "gripper." Circle and bar embed in denture and spring-load male portion *(center)* attaches to abutment tooth by post. (Courtesy Dr. David H. Wands.)

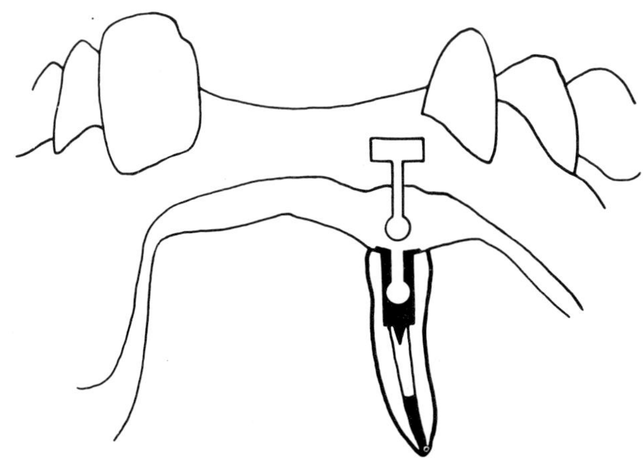

Fig. 18–28. Zest anchor attachment derives its retention from within root. Precise root preparation to receive female portion could lead to thinning of root or perforation. Male portion is in denture. (From Zamikoff, I. I.: J.A.D.A., *86*:853, April, 1973.)

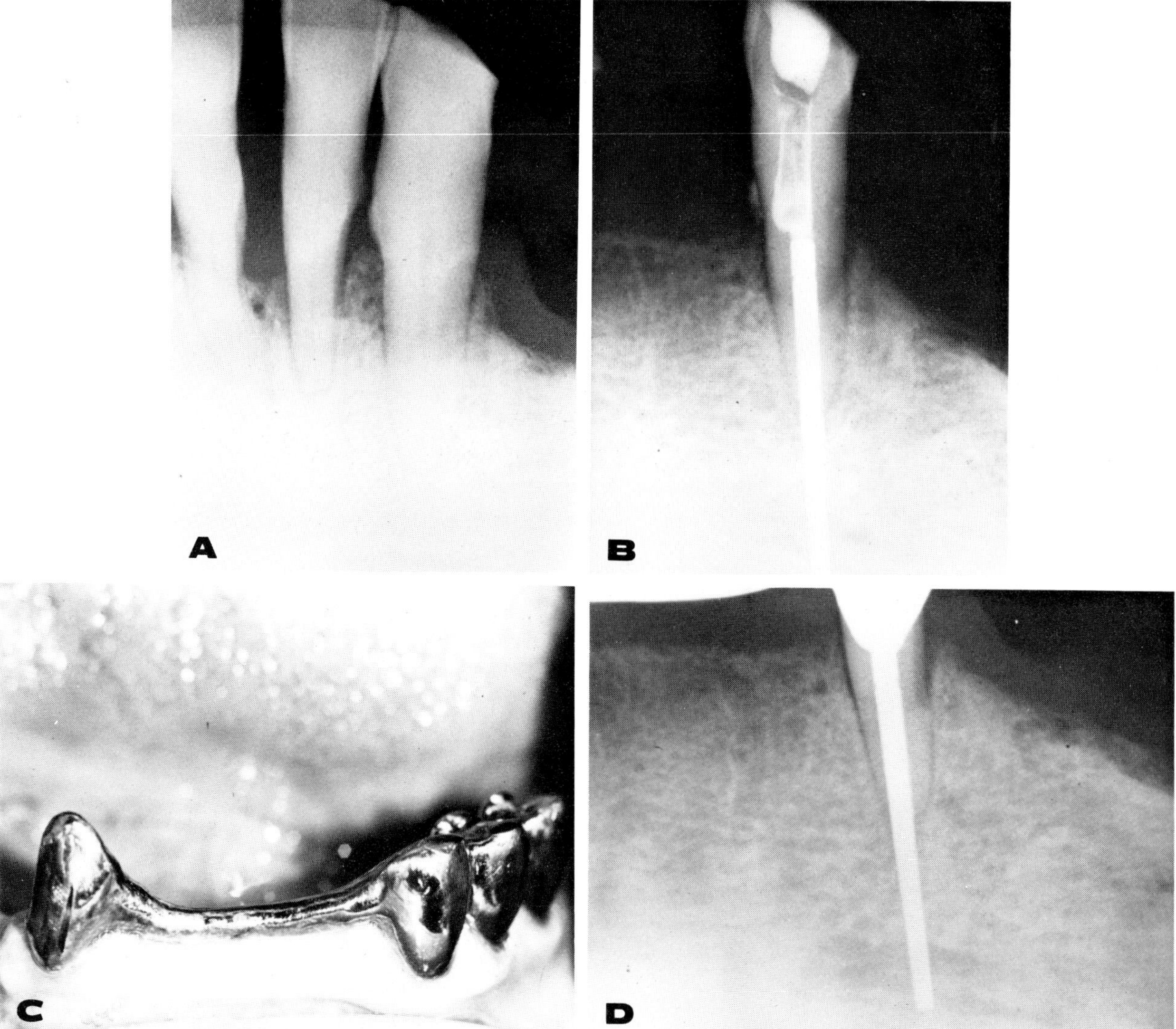

Fig. 18–29. Stabilizing tooth to be used as abutment for fixed prothesis and overdenture. *A,* Preoperative radiograph. Canine to be retained—incisors to be sacrificed. *B,* Postoperative film following implant and incisor extraction. *C,* Stabilized fixed prosthesis as base for overdenture. Gingival tissue health is apparent. *D,* Eight-month recall. Improved periodontal condition and great stability. (Courtesy Dr. Calvin Lau and Dr. Alfred L. Frank.)

REFERENCES

1. Gerstein, H., and Burnell, S. C.: Prefabricated precision dowels. J.A.D.A., *68*:787–791, June, 1964.
2. Lord, J. L., and Teel, S.: The overdenture: patient selection, use of copings, and follow-up evaluation. J. Prosthet. Dent., *32*:41–51, July, 1974.
3. Lord J. L., and Teel, S.: The overdenture. Dent. Clin. N. Amer., *13*:871–881, 1969.
4. Prothero, J. H.: *Prosthetic Dentistry,* 2nd Ed. Chicago, Medico-Dental Publishing Co., 1916, pp. 476 and 519.
5. Sognnaes, R. F.: America's most famous teeth. Smithsonian, *3*:47–51, Feb., 1973.
6. Reitz, P. V., Weiner, M. G., and Levin, B.: An overdenture survey: a preliminary report. To be published. Prosth. Dent., 1976.

Author Index

Subject Index